AF813544

Pediatric Surgery

Subhasis Roy Choudhury
Editor

Pediatric Surgery

A Guide to Clinicians

Second Edition

Springer

Editor
Subhasis Roy Choudhury
Director Professor, Pediatric Surgery
Lady Hardinge Medical College
and Associated Kalawati Saran
Children's Hospital
New Delhi, Delhi, India

ISBN 978-981-96-1256-7 ISBN 978-981-96-1257-4 (eBook)
https://doi.org/10.1007/978-981-96-1257-4

© The Editor(s) (if applicable) and The Author(s), under exclusive license to Springer Nature Singapore Pte Ltd. 2018, 2025

This work is subject to copyright. All rights are solely and exclusively licensed by the Publisher, whether the whole or part of the material is concerned, specifically the rights of translation, reprinting, reuse of illustrations, recitation, broadcasting, reproduction on microfilms or in any other physical way, and transmission or information storage and retrieval, electronic adaptation, computer software, or by similar or dissimilar methodology now known or hereafter developed.
The use of general descriptive names, registered names, trademarks, service marks, etc. in this publication does not imply, even in the absence of a specific statement, that such names are exempt from the relevant protective laws and regulations and therefore free for general use.
The publisher, the authors and the editors are safe to assume that the advice and information in this book are believed to be true and accurate at the date of publication. Neither the publisher nor the authors or the editors give a warranty, expressed or implied, with respect to the material contained herein or for any errors or omissions that may have been made. The publisher remains neutral with regard to jurisdictional claims in published maps and institutional affiliations.

This Springer imprint is published by the registered company Springer Nature Singapore Pte Ltd.
The registered company address is: 152 Beach Road, #21-01/04 Gateway East, Singapore 189721, Singapore

If disposing of this product, please recycle the paper.

Dedicated to my parents, family, patients and students

Foreword

It is a privilege to write the foreword for this outstanding contribution to the field of pediatric surgery in the second edition of the book titled *Pediatric Surgery: A Guide to Clinicians*, edited by Dr. Subhasis Roy Choudhury—an eminent surgeon, educator, and thought leader whose work has influenced generations of clinicians and students alike.

Pediatric surgery is a demanding discipline that balances intricate technical precision with a profound sense of compassion. In the second edition of this book, Dr. Roy Choudhury brings together decades of surgical experience, academic rigor, and clinical wisdom to create a resource that is as instructive as it is inspiring. With clarity of thought and a deep understanding of the unique physiological and emotional needs of children, he presents a comprehensive guide revised and written by several eminent authors in their respective field of practice and teaching in pediatric surgery, which will benefit not only residents and young surgeons but also experienced practitioners seeking to refine their knowledge.

Throughout his distinguished career extending from India, the United Kingdom, and the United States, Dr. Roy Choudhury has been known for his unwavering commitment to patient care and medical education. His contributions in the operating room are matched by his excellence as a mentor and his dedication to advancing pediatric surgical standards across institutions. This book reflects those very qualities—carefully constructed, deeply insightful, and always anchored in the realities of clinical practice.

This book, a culmination of several eminent authors' vast clinical experience and academic insight, is a current and authoritative resource focusing on some of the most significant and transformative areas in the field: *fetal and neonatal surgery*, *minimally invasive techniques*, *organ transplantation*, and *recent technological advances*. These domains not only represent the cutting edge of surgical care but also the future of pediatric surgery as a whole.

More than just a technical manual, this work encourages critical thinking, ethical practice, and a holistic approach to pediatric healthcare. Whether it is the management of complex congenital anomalies or the nuances of perioperative care, the authors approach each topic with both scientific acumen and humanistic sensitivity sharing contemporary clinical practice across the globe.

As we look toward the future of pediatric surgery, resources like this will be essential in shaping a new generation of surgeons committed to the care of children. I am confident that this book will serve as a cornerstone reference in pediatric surgical education for years to come.

Former Professor and Head,
Pediatric Surgery
PGIMER, Chandigarh, India
10th September 2025

Soumen Kumar Mitra, FRCS

Preface

The second edition of this book has been inspired by the overwhelming response and appreciation of the first edition from the readers particularly the trainees in pediatric surgery.

In the rapid pace of scientific development, the advancement of knowledge in pediatric surgery has been very fast. Current medical knowledge is getting obsolete even faster, and our need to upgrade frequently has become a necessity. We shall briefly delve into all the issues relevant to Pediatric Surgeons after the last edition of this book was published.

In this book, the common surgical diseases affecting children are presented in a concise format with up-to-date information. The text is presented in an easy-to-read language supported with clinical photographs and illustrations for rapid reference and assimilation. An attempt has been made to provide the information in a systematic pattern like embryology, incidence, approach to diagnosis, and management with the help of flowcharts and algorithms wherever appropriate. The aim is to make the reader familiar with pediatric surgical conditions and plan a simple approach to the management. This book covers the subject of pediatric surgery and its allied subspecialties of pediatric urology, thoracic surgery, gastrointestinal surgery, oncology, tropical diseases, organ transplantation and trauma in a concise and reader-friendly manner with the latest and up-to-date information. The recent advances in pediatric surgery including antenatal diagnosis, fetal interventions, and minimally invasive surgery have been covered. I acknowledge the help of several eminent authors for contributing to the revisions/new chapters. I extend my gratitude to my colleagues for their inspiration in the pursuit of excellence. The support and suggestions of my wife Dr. Ruma and daughter Dr. Shayeri were invaluable. In compilation of the material in this book, several textbooks and original published articles of several authors and websites have been consulted, which are gratefully acknowledged. I thank the staff of Springer India for their constant encouragement and support, without which it would not have been possible to publish this book. My heart goes out to all the patients who have taught me and many others through their suffering. I hope that the medical students, pediatricians, resident doctors in pediatrics and surgery, and general and nursing practitioners treating children will find the information in this book very useful.

New Delhi, Delhi, India — Subhasis Roy Choudhury

Contents

Part III Trauma

Part IV Head, Neck and Spine

Part V Thorax

About the Editor

Subhasis Roy Choudhury M.S., D.N.B., M.Ch., M.D., is currently holding the position of Director Professor (Professor of Excellence), Department of Pediatric Surgery at the Lady Hardinge Medical College and affiliated Kalawati Saran Children's Hospital, New Delhi, India. After graduating from the NRS Medical College, Kolkata, in 1984, he completed his postgraduate studies in surgery and pediatric surgery (M.Ch.) at the PGIMER, Chandigarh, India. Subsequently, he received further training in pediatric surgery at Birmingham Children's Hospital, United Kingdom, and at Children's Mercy Hospital, Kansas City, United States. He has over 30 years of teaching experience in pediatric surgery, 120 publications to his credit and has presented papers, orations and CME lectures at numerous national and international conferences. He has guided over 40 theses and dissertations for postgraduate students. He is an active reviewer of several national and international journals and a board member of several institute bodies, e.g., AIIMS, PGIMER, BHU, SGPGI, NBE, NMC, CSIR. In addition to patient care, he has a keen interest in teaching and research and is a recognized postgraduate teacher for M.Ch. course in pediatric surgery affiliated with the University of Delhi, India.

Part I

General

1 Fluid and Electrolyte Balance in Children

Partap Singh Yadav and Subhasis Roy Choudhury

1.1 Introduction

Managing fluids is a critical aspect of care for seriously ill children. The physiology of water and electrolytes in neonates and children is markedly distinct from adults due to ongoing developmental processes. Healthcare providers must understand the mechanisms behind water and electrolyte disturbances to effectively restore equilibrium.

In fetal development, water accounts for 90% of body weight, with about 60% located in the extracellular fluid (ECF). As gestation progresses, total body water (TBW) and ECF decrease gradually. In newborns, TBW comprises 70–80% of their body weight compared to 60% in adults. In adults, TBW is divided into approximately one-third extracellular fluid (ECF) and two-thirds intracellular fluid (ICF). However, in neonates, ECF forms around 45% of body weight, while ICF accounts for 55%. Since ECF is more susceptible to loss and infants have a proportionally larger body surface area, they are at an increased risk of dehydration compared to adults.

At birth, neonates have an excess of TBW, primarily within the ECF compartment. During the first week, they lose 5–10% of their body weight as part of a normal diuresis process. In preterm infants, this loss can be as high as 15–20%. On their first day, neonates typically produce minimal urine (oliguria), followed by physiological diuresis over subsequent days. With growth, the proportion of TBW and ECF decreases, while the ICF compartment increases. Insensible water loss (IWL), which occurs mainly through the skin and respiratory tract, is significant in neonates because of their relatively large surface area. Preterm infants are particularly prone to higher IWL, which ranges between 20 and 50 mL/kg/day, depending on factors such as gestational age. Conditions like fever, the use of radiant warmers, and phototherapy further increase IWL. Covering preterm neonates with transparent plastic films can help minimize these losses.

Neonatal kidneys have a lower filtration capacity and reduced ability to concentrate urine, which makes them more vulnerable to both dehydration and fluid overload. Initially, neonatal kidneys can concentrate urine to only about 400 mOsm/L (500–600 mOsm/L in term infants), compared to 1200 mOsm/L in adults. As a result, neonates require a higher urine output of 2–4 mL/kg/h to eliminate their renal solute load, while older children and adults need only 1–2 mL/kg/h and 0.5–1 mL/kg/h, respectively. Urine output less than 1 mL/kg/h is classified as oliguria.

P. S. Yadav (✉)
Department of Pediatric Surgery, LHMC, New Delhi, Delhi, India

S. Roy Choudhury
Pediatric Surgery, Lady Hardinge Medical College and Associated Kalawati Saran Children's Hospital, New Delhi, Delhi, India

© The Author(s), under exclusive license to Springer Nature Singapore Pte Ltd. 2025
S. Roy Choudhury (ed.), *Pediatric Surgery*, https://doi.org/10.1007/978-981-96-1257-4_1

When planning fluid therapy for neonates undergoing surgery, it is important to consider all potential sources of fluid and electrolyte loss. These include stool output (as seen in conditions like short gut syndrome or ostomy), nasogastric tube drainage, losses from chest or abdominal drains, burns, and cerebrospinal fluid drainage.

1.2 Accessing Fluid and Electrolyte Status

1.2.1 History

Maternal factors such as the administration of hypotonic fluids and medications like oxytocin, angiotensin-converting enzyme (ACE) inhibitors, indomethacin, and furosemide can negatively impact a neonate's renal function.

1.2.2 Clinical Evaluation

Regular weight checks are vital for pediatric care. Monitoring weight, urine production, and electrolytes is key to detecting hydration and electrolyte abnormalities, allowing adjustments to intravenous (IV) fluid rates and composition. In certain conditions, such as prolonged paralytic use, sepsis, or peritonitis, an infant's weight may increase due to fluid accumulation in the interstitial compartment, even without an increase in blood volume.

Signs of dehydration, including sunken anterior fontanelles, sunken eyes, dry mucous membranes, and altered skin elasticity, can provide clues but are not always reliable for identifying electrolyte imbalances.

1.2.3 Cardiovascular Signs

Cardiovascular instability may appear as tachycardia, prolonged capillary refill, or hepatomegaly, which could indicate congestive heart failure.

1.2.4 Laboratory Evaluation

Evaluating serum electrolytes, blood urea nitrogen, creatinine, urine electrolytes, specific gravity, and plasma osmolality provides insight into fluid and electrolyte status. Metabolic acidosis observed in blood gas analysis may signal inadequate tissue perfusion.

1.2.5 Fluid and Electrolyte Balance

During the first 12–24 h, neonates typically do not require sodium, potassium, or chloride supplementation. During this period, 10% dextrose at 60–80 mL/kg/day ensures a glucose infusion rate of 6–7 mg/kg/min. After the initial days, N/5 in D10 is administered for neonates, while older children are generally provided with N/2 or N/3 in D5 (N = normal saline, D = dextrose).

Electrolyte requirements for full-term neonates include:

- Sodium: 2–3 mEq/kg/day (with increased requirements of 6–8 mEq/kg/day in small preterm neonates)
- Potassium: 1–2 mEq/kg/day
- Chloride: 3–5 mEq/kg/day

1.3 Maintenance Fluid Requirements

Maintenance therapy accounts for urine production and insensible water loss, as fecal fluid loss in healthy children is minimal. Preterm infants have a reduced ability to excrete sodium and are vulnerable to both sodium loss and fluid overload. Excessive intravenous fluids can lead to complications such as patent ductus arteriosus, bronchopulmonary dysplasia, enterocolitis, and intraventricular hemorrhage. Daily fluid needs should consider:

1. Urinary water losses
2. Gastrointestinal losses
3. Insensible water losses
4. Surgical losses

Initial Fluid Therapy for Neonates (mL/kg/day)

Birth weight (kg)	<24 h	24–48 h	>48 h
<1	100–150	120–150	140–190
1–1.5	80–100	100–120	120–160
>1.5	60–80	80–120	120–160

Maintenance Fluid Requirements for Older Children (Holliday–Segar Method):

- For the first 10 kg: 100 mL/kg.
- For 11–20 kg: 1000 mL + 50 mL/kg for each additional kg for 11–20.
- For >20 kg: 1500 mL + 20 mL/kg for each additional kg more than 20.
- Maximum daily fluid intake is usually capped at 2400 mL.

Hourly fluid calculations (rule of 4-2-1):

- 4 mL/kg/h for 0–10 kg
- 40 mL/h + 2 mL/kg/h for 10–20 kg
- 60 mL/h + 1 mL/kg/h for >20 kg

1.4 Replacement Fluids

The typical composition of gastric fluid includes:

- Sodium (Na): 60 mEq/L
- Potassium (K): 10 mEq/L
- Chloride (Cl): 90 mEq/L

Nasogastric losses are replenished using N/2 saline in D5W with 10 mEq/L potassium chloride (KCl) every 1–6 h. Biliary losses, which have higher sodium content (Na: 130 mEq/L, K: 5–15 mEq/L, Cl: 80–120 mEq/L), should be replaced volume-for-volume with normal saline (NS) containing 10 mEq/L KCl or Ringer's lactate (RL).

1.5 Deficit Therapy

1.5.1 Calculating Fluid Deficit

The most accurate way to assess fluid deficit is by determining weight loss. Fluid deficit equals the difference between the pre-illness weight and the current weight. When the preillness weight is unknown, clinical signs of dehydration should guide calculations, with 1% dehydration corresponding to 10 mL/kg of fluid loss.

Percentage dehydration can be calculated using the formula:

Percentage dehydration = Preillness weight – Current weightPre-illness weight × 100\text{Percentage dehydration} = \frac{\text{Pre-illness weight – Current weight}}{\text{Pre-illness weight}}\times 100Percentage dehydration = Pre-illness weightPre-illness weight – Current weight × 100

1.5.2 Phases of Fluid Therapy

1. *Initial resuscitation*

   Dehydrated infants require urgent treatment to improve tissue perfusion. Isotonic solutions, such as normal saline or Ringer's lactate, are administered in boluses of 20 mL/kg to rapidly restore intravascular volume in older children. For neonates, smaller boluses of 10 mL/kg are used due to immature renal function. Resuscitation is considered complete once adequate circulation and perfusion are restored. In cases of metabolic alkalosis, such as hypertrophic pyloric stenosis, lactated Ringer's should be avoided as it can exacerbate alkalosis.
2. *Deficit and ongoing losses correction*

   This phase addresses both maintenance needs and the replacement of fluid deficits. Potassium should only be added after confirming normal renal function. Calculate the 24-h fluid requirement (maintenance + deficit), subtract any fluids already given as boluses, and administer the remainder over 24 h.

1.6 Signs of Dehydration

Dehydration is classified as mild, moderate, or severe, based on clinical observations and weight loss.

1. *Mild dehydration*
   - *Weight loss*: ~3% in older children (~30 mL/kg) or ~5% in infants (~50 mL/kg).
   - *Clinical signs*: skin appears normal, mucous membranes are dry, and eyes are normal. The anterior fontanelle is flat, heart rate is normal, and urine output is only slightly reduced.
2. *Moderate dehydration*
   - *Weight loss*: ~6% in older children (~60 mL/kg) or ~10% in infants (~100 mL/kg).
   - *Clinical signs*: skin tents when pinched, oral mucosa is dry, and eyes are deep-set. The fontanelle is slightly depressed, heart rate shows mild tachycardia, pulse volume becomes weak, and capillary refill time is delayed. Urine output decreases, showing mild oliguria.
3. *Severe dehydration*
   - *Weight loss*: ~9% in older children (~90 mL/kg) or ~15% in infants (~150 mL/kg).
   - *Clinical signs*: skin tents significantly when pinched, mucosa is parched, and eyes are sunken. The fontanelle is significantly sunken, heart rate shows marked tachycardia, and pulse volume is feeble or nonpalpable. Capillary refill time exceeds 3 s, and urine output is severely reduced or absent (anuria).

1.6.1 Distribution of Fluid Losses

Fluid loss distribution depends on the duration of illness. For illnesses lasting less than 3 days, 80% of the fluid deficit is from the extracellular fluid (ECF) compartment, and 20% is from the intracellular fluid (ICF) compartment. In illnesses exceeding 3 days, the deficit shifts to 60% from ECF and 40% from ICF. Sodium and chloride are the predominant ions in the ECF, while potassium and phosphate dominate in the ICF.

1.6.2 Fluid Therapy Examples

1. *Isonatremic dehydration*

   A child weighing 10 kg preillness with 10% dehydration (current weight 9.3 kg) and a duration of illness of 5 days requires fluid therapy.

   Maintenance fluid is calculated as 1000 mL with 30 mEq of sodium and 20 mEq of potassium.

   The fluid deficit is 700 mL (preillness weight - current weight).

   Sodium deficit is calculated as 61 mEq, while potassium deficit is 42 mEq.

   The total 24-h requirement is 1700 mL of fluid with 91 mEq of sodium and 62 mEq of potassium.

   Half the deficit is given in the first 8 h (683 mL with 35 mEq sodium and 24 mEq potassium), and the remaining is given over the next 16 h (1016 mL with 56 mEq sodium and 38 mEq potassium).
2. *Hyponatremic dehydration*

   An infant weighing 7 kg preillness with 10% dehydration (current weight 6.3 kg) and serum sodium of 115 mEq/L requires fluid therapy.

   Maintenance fluid is 700 mL with 21 mEq sodium and 14 mEq potassium.

   The fluid deficit is 700 mL.

   Sodium deficit is calculated as 61 mEq, and excess sodium deficit (based on 135 mEq/L desired sodium) is 84 mEq.

   Potassium deficit is 42 mEq.

   The total 24-h requirement is 1400 mL of fluid with 166 mEq sodium and 56 mEq potassium.

   Half of the deficit is given in the first 8 h (583 mL with 80 mEq sodium and 26 mEq potassium), and the rest over the next 16 h (817 mL with 86 mEq sodium and 30 mEq potassium).
3. *Hypernatremic dehydration*

   For a 1-year-old child weighing 7 kg preillness with 10% dehydration, a serum sodium of 155 mEq/L, and a duration of illness exceeding 3 days, sodium reduction must proceed slowly to prevent cerebral edema. Sodium should decrease by no more than 10 mEq/L per day.

Free water deficit (FWD) is calculated as 280 mL using the formula:

FWD = 4 mL/kg × preillness weight × (serum sodium − desired sodium)

The solute fluid deficit (SFD) is the difference between total fluid deficit and FWD, amounting to 420 mL.

Maintenance fluid is 700 mL with 21 mEq sodium and 14 mEq potassium.

Fluid deficit is also 700 mL with similar electrolyte composition.

So, the total 24-h requirement is 1400 mL of fluid with 58 mEq sodium and 39 mEq potassium.

For the first 24 h, the child receives 1260 mL (700 mL maintenance +420 mL SFD + 140 mL FWD).

1.6.3 Pediatric Shock

Shock is a clinical condition characterized by inadequate tissue perfusion and oxygen delivery, leading to organ dysfunction and cellular derangements. It is important to note that while hypotension is a feature of shock, shock itself is not defined solely by hypotension.

1.6.4 Types of Shock

Shock is classified into the following categories:

1. *Hypotensive shock*
2. *Distributive shock*
3. *Obstructive shock*

Combinations of these types can occur, such as in septic shock.

1.6.5 Assessment of Shock

To monitor and evaluate shock, both clinical and laboratory parameters are essential:

- *Clinical assessment*: vital signs, such as heart rate, blood pressure, and pulse pressure, are critical. Additional clinical signs include capillary refill time, central venous pressure (CVP), temperature, level of consciousness, and reduced urine output (oliguria or anuria).
- *Laboratory parameters*: key markers include arterial-venous oxygen gradients (A-V O_2), mixed venous oxygen saturations (SvO_2), acid–base status, and lactate levels. Arterial blood gas analysis provides a straightforward way to assess oxygenation and acid–base balance. Elevated serum lactate indicates poor tissue perfusion and impaired oxygen delivery.

1.6.6 Management of Shock

1.6.6.1 Monitoring and Environment

Children with shock require intensive care unit monitoring for active clinical surveillance.

1.6.6.2 Fluid Resuscitation

Fluid resuscitation is the first-line treatment. Most children can tolerate intravenous fluid administration up to 60 mL/kg, but children with heart disease may require adjustments to avoid pulmonary edema. Improvement in blood pressure, peripheral perfusion, and urine output signals successful resuscitation.

Central venous pressure (CVP) and arterial monitoring are useful in guiding fluid and resuscitation efforts. The goal of therapy should be rapid and goal directed.

1.6.6.3 Laboratory Workup and Antibiotics

Basic investigations include a complete blood count, electrolytes, blood glucose, coagulation profile, blood cultures, and blood gas analysis. In cases of septic shock, broad-spectrum antibiotics should be started immediately after collecting blood cultures.

1.6.6.4 Repeat Fluid Boluses

Boluses of intravenous fluids can be repeated up to 60 mL/kg over an hour, with close monitoring for signs of pulmonary edema.

1.6.6.5 Advanced Interventions

If the patient does not respond to fluid resuscitation, intubation and invasive monitoring are recommended, and inotropic support should be initiated. The resuscitation goals include:

- CVP >10 mm Hg
- Mean arterial pressure within age-appropriate ranges

  Blood transfusion is reserved for patients with significant hypovolemia or anemia, typically when hemoglobin (Hb) is less than 7 g/dL.

1.6.7 Inotropic Therapy

- *Warm shock*: persistent low systolic blood pressure with peripheral vasodilation and SvO_2 > 70%. Recommended treatments include norepinephrine (0.1–3 μg/kg/min) and/or vasopressin.
- *Cardiogenic shock*: normal blood pressure with poor perfusion and SvO_2 < 70%. Treatments include milrinone (0.3–0.7 μg/kg/min), nitroprusside, or dobutamine (4–20 μg/kg/min).
- *Cold shock*: low blood pressure, poor perfusion, and SvO_2 < 70%. Management includes optimizing Hb >10 g/dL and administering epinephrine (0.02–0.3 μg/kg/min).

  If shock persists despite fluids and inotropic therapy, consider adrenal insufficiency as a cause and treat with hydrocortisone (2 mg/kg). Dopamine (2–20 μg/kg/min) is another frequently used inotropic agent.

1.6.8 Extracorporeal Membrane Oxygenation (ECMO)

Extracorporeal membrane oxygenation (ECMO) is an option for patients who fail all other resuscitative efforts but have a potential for recovery. It is often utilized in postoperative cardiac surgery patients, those with congenital diaphragmatic hernia, or cases of refractory septic shock.

1.6.9 Blood Volume and Replacement

The approximate blood volume for different pediatric age groups is:

- *Premature infants*: 85–100 cc/kg
- *Term newborns*: 85 cc/kg
- *Infants*: 70–80 cc/kg

  If blood loss exceeds 10% of total blood volume, replacement with blood products is necessary.

1.7 Electrolyte Disturbances

Electrolyte imbalances are a critical component of pediatric care, as they significantly impact cellular and organ functions. Below are details of common electrolyte disturbances, their causes, effects, and management.

1.8 Sodium Disturbances

1.8.1 Hyponatremia

Defined as a serum sodium concentration below 135 mEq/L, hyponatremia causes water to shift from the extracellular fluid (ECF) into intracellular fluid (ICF) to maintain osmotic equilibrium. This results in cellular swelling, which is particularly dangerous in the brain, where space is limited, leading to increased intracranial pressure. Neurological symptoms include anorexia, vomiting, lethargy, confusion, agitation, seizures, and coma.

1.8.1.1 Causes of Hyponatremia

1. *Pseudohyponatremia*: due to hyperosmolality caused by hyperlipidemia, mannitol, or sucrose.
2. *Extrarenal losses*: seen in conditions like short gut syndrome, diarrhea, stoma losses, vomiting, or nasogastric suction.
3. *Renal losses*: conditions include renal tubular acidosis, cerebral salt wasting, postobstructive diuresis, thiazide or loop diuretic use, and certain genetic kidney diseases.
4. *Euvolemic hyponatremia*: caused by syndrome of inappropriate antidiuretic hormone secretion (SIADH), hypothyroidism, or water intoxication (e.g., from faulty feeding practices or psychogenic polydipsia).
5. *Hypervolemic hyponatremia*: common in congestive heart failure, cirrhosis, nephrotic syndrome, renal failure, or protein-losing enteropathy.

1.8.1.2 Management of Hyponatremia

Treatment depends on the underlying cause. Correcting hyponatremia too quickly risks central pontine myelinolysis. In symptomatic patients (seizures or coma), hypertonic saline is used to slightly increase serum sodium, avoiding normalization within 24 h.

- Sodium deficit can be calculated as:
- Sodium Deficit = (Desired Na − Current Na) × 0.6 × Weight (kg).
- Each mL of 3% NaCl increases serum sodium by 1 mEq/L.
- Avoid correcting by more than 12 mEq/L per 24 h or 18 mEq/L over 48 h.

1.8.2 Hypernatremia

Hypernatremia is defined as serum sodium levels exceeding 145 mEq/L and often results in dehydration. Fluid shifts from ICF to ECF maintain intravascular volume, but neurological complications like irritability, high-pitched crying, lethargy, and even seizures or coma can occur. Severe cases may lead to brain hemorrhage due to tearing of intracerebral vessels.

1.8.2.1 Causes of Hypernatremia

1. *Excess sodium*: hypertonic saline, sodium bicarbonate excess, or hyperaldosteronism.
2. *Water deficit*: seen in nephrogenic diabetes insipidus, central diabetes insipidus, phototherapy, radiant warmers, or prematurity.
3. *Combined water and sodium deficit*: conditions include burns, diarrhea, chronic kidney disease, and osmotic diuresis.

1.8.2.2 Management of Hypernatremia

- Correct serum sodium gradually at a rate of <12 mEq/L per 24 h or 0.5 mEq/L per h to prevent cerebral edema.
- Water deficit can be calculated as:
- Water Deficit = Body Weight × 0.6 × (Current Na/140–1)
- Fluid choices depend on clinical conditions:
  – Hypotensive patients: normal saline.
  – Hypernatremic dehydration: half-normal (N/2) or quarter-normal (N/4) saline.
  – Sodium overload: use D5 water (sodium-free fluid).

1.9 Potassium Disturbances

1.9.1 Hyperkalemia

Hyperkalemia is defined as serum potassium exceeding 5.5 mEq/L and results in significant cardiac effects due to its role in membrane polarization. electro cadio graphy (ECG) changes include peaked T waves, ST depression, widened QRS complexes, and flattened P waves. Neurological signs include paresthesias, fasciculations, and weakness, with ventricular fibrillation or asystole being life-threatening complications.

1.9.1.1 Causes of Hyperkalemia

1. *Spurious causes*: hemolysis, thrombocytosis, or tissue ischemia.
2. *Increased intake*: potassium supplementation or blood transfusions.
3. *Transcellular shifts*: seen in acidosis, rhabdomyolysis, or tumor lysis syndrome.
4. *Reduced excretion*: common in renal failure, obstructive uropathy, or ACE inhibitor use.

1.9.1.2 Management of Hyperkalemia

- Stop all potassium intake.
- Stabilize the heart with calcium gluconate to prevent arrhythmias.
- Shift potassium intracellularly using insulin with glucose, bicarbonate, or nebulized beta-agonists.
- Remove potassium via sodium polystyrene sulfonate (orally) or dialysis in severe cases.

1.9.2 Hypokalemia

Hypokalemia is defined as serum potassium less than 3.5 mEq/L and can lead to muscle weakness, cramps, ileus, and ECG changes like flattened T waves, ST depression, and U waves.

1.9.2.1 Causes of Hypokalemia

1. *Transcellular shifts*: alkalosis, adrenergic agonists, or refeeding syndrome.
2. *Reduced intake*: anorexia nervosa or malnutrition.
3. *Extrarenal losses*: diarrhea, laxative use, or excessive sweating.
4. *Renal losses*: postobstructive diuresis, renal tubular acidosis, or loop diuretics.

1.9.2.2 Management of Hypokalemia

- Assess renal function and urine output before supplementation.
- Oral potassium is preferred, with doses of 2–4 mEq/kg/day. For severe cases, IV potassium may be administered at a rate of 0.5–1 mEq/kg/h, with a maximum concentration of 40 mEq/L in IV fluids.
- Address underlying causes, such as restoring intravascular volume in cases of metabolic alkalosis and volume depletion.

1.9.3 Hypocalcemia

1.9.3.1 Definition and Causes

Hypocalcemia occurs when total serum calcium falls below 7 mg/dL or ionized calcium is less than 4 mg/dL. Common causes include prematurity, hypoparathyroidism, vitamin D deficiency, pancreatitis, tumor lysis syndrome, or hypomagnesemia.

1.9.3.2 Clinical Features

Hypocalcemia increases neuromuscular excitability, leading to symptoms such as weakness, laryngospasm, seizures, and cardiac arrhythmias. Signs include *Trousseau's sign* (carpal spasm) and *Chvostek's sign* (facial twitching).

1.9.3.3 Management

Calcium supplementation should be done cautiously under cardiovascular monitoring. For symptomatic cases, 10% calcium gluconate (100–200 mg/kg) is infused slowly over 10 min. Maintenance calcium is added to IV fluids if symptoms persist.

Suggested Reading

Arcara K, Tschudy M. The Harriet Lane handbook. 20th ed. Philadelphia, PA: Mosby Elsevier; 2014.

Kliegman R, Stanton B, Geme JS, Nelson SN. Textbook of pediatrics. 20th ed. Philadelphia, PA: Saunders, Elsevier; 2015.

Simmons CF Jr. Fluid and electrolyte management. In: Cloherty JP, Stark AR, editors. Manual of neonatal care. 4th ed. New York: Lippincott Raven; 1997. p. 100.

2 Fetal Circulation and Neonatal Physiology

Vishnu Mohan Murukesan
and Subhasis Roy Choudhury

2.1 Introduction

Understanding the basics of foetal circulation and its transition at birth and the neonatal period (first 28 days of life) is essential in managing neonates, particularly preterm infants of varying gestational age. The neonatal period is the most exciting part of human life as abrupt physiological changes in the cardiovascular and respiratory systems occur during it. The maturation of the central nervous system, renal, gastrointestinal, hepatic and endocrine systems with the post-conceptual age is worth knowing in managing various medical and surgical conditions in the neonatal period and their further follow-up.

2.2 Foetal Circulation

Normally, the umbilical cord contains three vessels: *two umbilical arteries (UAs)* and *a single umbilical vein (UV)*. The *UA* carries the deoxygenated blood from the foetus to the placenta, where it is oxygenated. From there, the oxygenated blood is then carried back to the foetus via the *UV*.

The three important foetal shunts which come into play in foetal circulation are

Ductus venosus (DV)—a shunt between the umbilical vein and inferior vena cava
Foramen ovale (FO)—opening between left and right atrium
Ductus arteriosus (DA)—connects the pulmonary artery to the descending aorta

Blood from the UV enters the foetal heart en route to the liver or *DV* and is preferentially passed across the *FO* into the left atrium by the Eustachian valve. Oxygenated blood passes from the left atrium into the left ventricle and is pumped into the aorta to supply the head and the upper trunk.

The right atrium receives deoxygenated blood from the head and the upper trunk via the superior vena cava and myocardial blood via the coronary sinus. This right atrial blood is passed into the right ventricle and then into the pulmonary artery; only 8–10% of this blood passes through the high-resistance pulmonary circulation, and the remaining majority of blood from the pulmonary artery is shunted via the *DA* into the descending aorta. Blood in the descending aorta either goes to the placenta via the *UA* for oxygenation or continues to supply the lower limbs.

Intra and extra-cardiac shunts achieve preferential blood splitting into parallel circulations (the left ventricle provides 35%, and the right ventricle provides 65% of cardiac output) (Fig. 2.1).

V. M. Murukesan (✉)
Lady Hardinge Medical College, New Delhi, Delhi, India

S. Roy Choudhury
Pediatric Surgery, Lady Hardinge Medical College and Associated Kalawati Saran Children's Hospital, New Delhi, Delhi, India

© The Author(s), under exclusive license to Springer Nature Singapore Pte Ltd. 2025
S. Roy Choudhury (ed.), *Pediatric Surgery*, https://doi.org/10.1007/978-981-96-1257-4_2

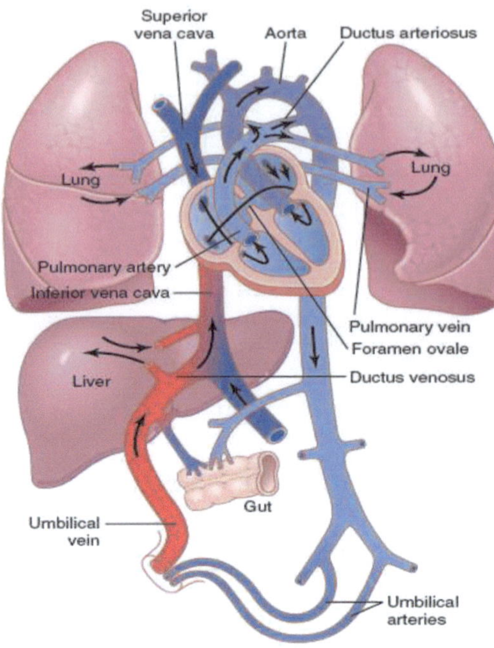

Fig. 2.1 The foetal circulation

2.3 The Transition from Foetal to Postnatal Circulation

As a result of the clamping of the umbilical cord (which results in umbilical vessel constriction, leading to higher systemic vascular resistance, as well as the initiation of breathing which helps in reducing the pulmonary vascular resistance), there would be a drastic improvement in the pulmonary circulation, reduced blood flow through the inferior vena cava (IVC), and closure of shunts.

Clamping of the umbilical cord results in poor blood flow from the placenta to *DV*, leading to its functional closure within several minutes and reducing IVC blood flow. Reduced IVC flow decreases the right atrial pressure due to poor filling and as the systemic vascular resistance rises, the left atrial pressure increases. With these changes in right and left atrial pressures after birth, the *FO* closes as the anatomical properties of the atrial septum do not favour left-to-right flow through it.

Moreover, the high systemic resistance and low pulmonary resistance bring about a reversal in *DA* flow, becoming left-to-right flow as compared to right-to-left flow in *DA*. These culminate in higher PaO_2 exposure to DA, stimulating closure. Any stimuli like low PaO_2 or low pH and raised prostaglandin levels worsen the scenario by increasing the pulmonary vascular resistance, resulting in non-closure of *FO* and *DA*, which allows a right-to-left shunt, reaggravating hypoxia.

Table 2.1 Closure of shunts after birth

Shunt	Closure—functional	Closure—anatomical	Remnant
Ductus venosus	Within minutes	3–7 days	Ligamentum venosum
Foramen ovale	Within minutes	Around 1 year	Fossa ovalis
Ductus arteriosus	10–96 h	14–21 days	Ligamentum arteriosus

2.4 Remnants of Foetal Structures

The right umbilical vein disappears. Remnants of the left umbilical vein, the two umbilical arteries, the ductus arteriosus, and the ductus venosus become the ligamentum teres of the liver, the medial umbilical ligaments, the ligamentum arteriosum, and the ligamentum venosum, respectively (see Table 2.1).

Closure of patent ductus arteriosus (PDA): Inhibitors of prostaglandin synthesis like indomethacin and ibuprofen are used in clinical practice to close those patent ductus arteriosus causing haemodynamically significant disturbances to the infant. PDA closure by a percutaneous transcatheter occlusion device (minimally invasive method) and transthoracic open PDA ligation are methods to close a large-sized significant PDA.

2.5 Systemic Changes After Birth

2.5.1 Respiratory System

Newborn with their first gasp at birth generates inspiratory pressures of up to −70- to −100 cm H_2O, which assist in the clearance of airway fluids and lung expansion. During the initial expirations at birth, pressures of 18–115 cm H_2O are generated, and thus, amniotic fluid is squeezed out from the respiratory tract (see Fig. 2.2).

With the cutting of the umbilical cord, due to a sudden drop in PaO_2 and an increase in $PaCO_2$, a transient fall in blood pH occurs, stimulating the respiratory centre located in the brainstem and carotid artery chemoreceptors to aid breathing. Furthermore, a decrease in environmental temperature, and stimuli such as tactile, auditory and visual promote breathing at birth. Alveolar distension, epinephrine, and cortisol stimulate the type II pneumocytes to produce lung surfactant. Surfactant prevents the lung from collapsing by lowering the surface tension in the alveolar air/fluid interface.

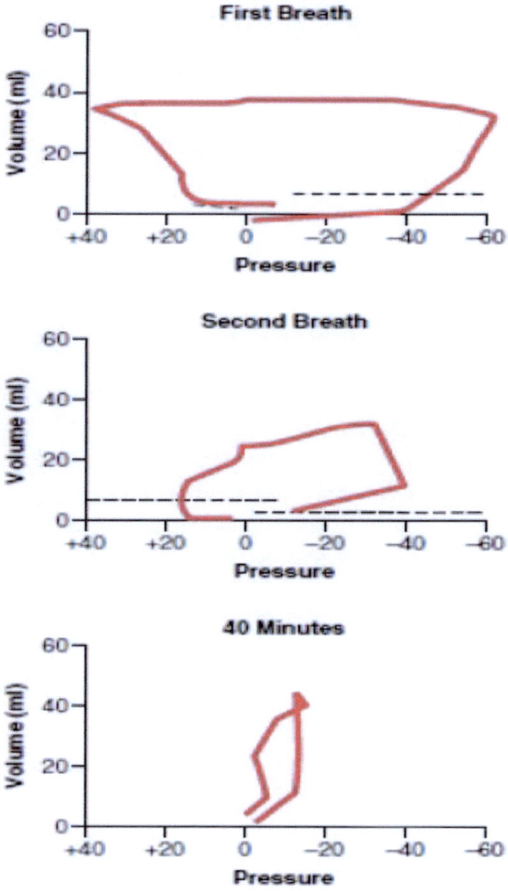

Fig. 2.2 Pressure–volume loop in neonates during the first hour of life

There are a few structural differences in the neonatal period when compared to older children. The main muscle of inspiration in the newborn period is the diaphragm, which is predominantly composed of type 2 muscle fibres (with fast contractility and high fatigability). Whereas the type 1 muscle fibres (with slow, sustained contractility and low fatigability) are present in very low proportion at 25%, there is a risk of diaphragmatic fatigue during hyperventilation. In preterm infants, the proportion is even lower at 10%. With the increase in age, the proportion alters; by the age of 2 years, only 55% of muscle fibres are type 2.

In addition, the more horizontally placed ribs in the newborn favour thoracic expansion in an inferior direction. Abdominal distention from intestinal obstruction, necrotising enterocolitis (NEC), or ascites inhibits diaphragmatic movements and reduces lung expansion. The temporary cessation of breathing (apnoea), mostly seen in preterm infants, improves with maturity but may persist up to 50 weeks post-conceptual age.

Moreover, the anatomical and physiological differences between infants and adults are depicted in Tables 2.2 and 2.3 and in Fig. 2.3.

2.5.2 Cardiovascular System

The chief determinant of neonatal cardiac output is the heart rate (chronotropic property); other important factors, although limited, influencing the cardiac output are preload, cardiac contractility (ionotropic effect) and afterload. When compared to adults, the neonatal cardiac ventricles are less compliant; they are more fibrous and restrictive, and hence, preload/afterload changes have less effect on cardiac output and are more

Table 2.2 Comparison of normal respiratory values in infants and adults

Parameter	Infant	Adult
Respiratory frequency	30–50	12–16
Tidal volume (mL/kg)	7	7
Dead space (mL/kg)	2–2.5	2.2
Alveolar ventilation (mL/kg/min)	100–150	60
Functional residual capacity (mL/kg)	27–30	30
Oxygen consumption (mL/kg/min)	7–9	3

Table 2.3 Differences between paediatric and adult airway

Anatomy	Pediatric	Adult
Tongue	Large	Normal
Eiglottis shape	Floppy, omega shaped	Firm, flatter
Epiglottis level	Level of C3–C4	Level of C5–C6
Trachea	Smaller, shorter	Wider, longer
Larynx shape	Funnel shaped	Column
Larynx position	Angles posteriorly away from glottis	Straight up and down
Narrowest point	Sub-glottic region	At level of vocal cords
Lung volume	250 ml at birth	6000 ml as adult

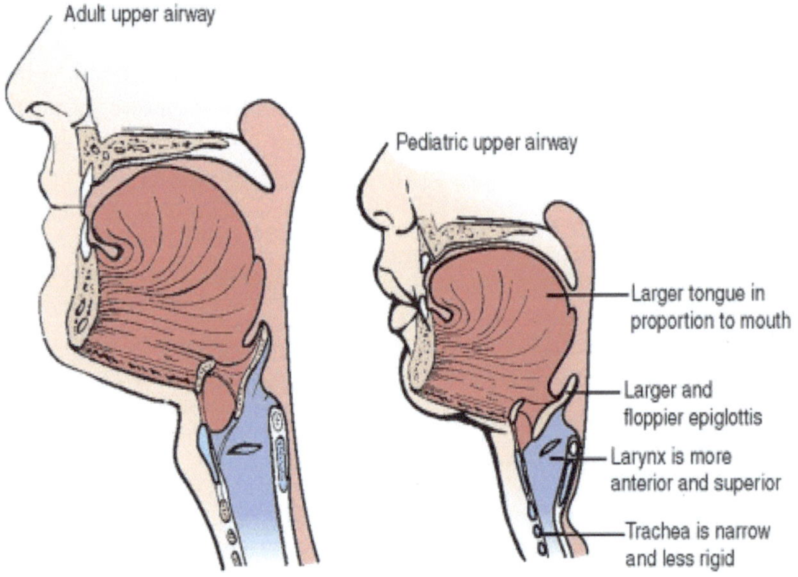

Fig. 2.3 Comparison of paediatric upper airway with adult upper airway

dependent on heart rate. Bradycardia due to stress, apnoea, raised intracranial pressures, or drugs should be dealt with immediately as the newborn circulation would be compromised.

A relatively stable neonate can tolerate left ventricular cardiac output as low as 120 mL/kg/min. The right ventricle cardiac output in term newborns ranges from 150 to 300 mL/kg/min, almost double the left ventricle output. With the increase in age, the right ventricular predominance decreases as the pulmonary pressure drops.

2.5.3 Central Nervous System

Neonates, especially preterm babies, lack cerebral autoregulation, and hence, there is an increased risk for intraventricular hemorrhage (IVH) If blood pressure fluctuates. The immature blood–brain barrier in newborns is more permeate to drugs, especially lipid-soluble drugs and hence exhibits higher sensitivity to them. The neonatal spinal cord and dural sac terminate at L3 and S4, respectively, whereas in adults, they end at L1 and S2. The increased amount of cerebrospinal fluid (CSF) and the immature myelination in neonates shorten and decrease the potency of local anaesthetics.

2.5.4 GI/Hepatic System

The feeding route in neonates depends on the maturation of feeding skills (sucking, swallowing and coordination between swallowing and breathing). Stable babies born at >34 weeks of gestation can be put on direct breastfeeds. Paladai/cup or gavage feeding is needed for babies born at

<34 weeks, depending on their feeding skills. Neonates are more prone to gastro-oesophageal reflux as the lower oesophageal sphincter tone is low. Moreover, the type of feed also influences the gastric transit time, and the emptying time is more with formula feeds than breast milk. Hypertonic feeds could cause bowel ischaemia and necrotising enterocolitis (NEC), particularly in premature infants due to intestinal immaturity and increased intestinal trophic demands.

Immaturity of neonatal hepatic function impairs glucose levels, and reduced hepatic blood flow results in delayed drug metabolism. The cytochrome p450 enzymes essential for the metabolism of various drugs are very low in newborn infants, at only one-third of the adult levels. Glycogen reserves in the liver and muscles are very minimal in preterm infants. Therefore, fasting is detrimental to the blood glucose levels and requires high glucose infusion rates at 6–8 mg/kg/min to avoid hypoglycaemia. On top of that, there is a transient hyperinsulinaemia state in preterm infants and low birth weight (LBW) babies, especially intra-uterine growth-retarded infants.

Neonatal jaundice is another entity common in newborn infants. Most commonly seen is physiological jaundice (presents with unconjugated hyperbilirubinaemia) as a result of decreased entero-hepatic circulation and immature liver, attributed to poor biliary conjugation. In any neonates presenting with conjugated hyperbilirubinaemia (if >20% fraction of total bilirubin is conjugated type) or prolonged jaundice after 2 weeks of life, diagnostic workup for cholestasis is to be commenced, and always raise the suspicion of surgical causes like biliary atresia, if pale or clay-coloured stools are found.

2.5.5 Renal System

The neonatal renal system is considerably immature, and the glomerular filtration rate (GFR) is low (the GFR at term corrected age is only 20–40 mL/min/1.73 m^2, compared to adult values of 120 mL/min/1.73 m^2). Since the renal osmotic gradient is diminished in newborns, the renal tubules lack the ability to concentrate urine. Furthermore, in contrast to the adult system, the medullary tubules are lesser in newborn infants, and the scenario in preterm infants is even worse. The urine osmolality is 600 mOsm/kg in preterm infants and 800 mOsm/kg in term infants. These properties make neonates more prone to fluid imbalances, dyselectrolytaemia, such as hyponatraemia, and metabolic acidosis due to renal bicarbonate wasting.

Additionally, precautions are to be made while reading the serum creatinine levels in the first week of life, as they reflect elevated maternal values. Any serial increase in creatinine levels should be a concern rather than relying on a single high value. Oliguria is defined as urine output less than 1 mL/kg/h after the first day for both term and preterm neonates.

2.5.6 Thermoregulation

The normal temperature of neonatal infants is 36.5–37.5 °C. The higher body surface area to weight ratio (approximately double the adult ratio), reduced subcutaneous fat percentage, and the different mechanisms to produce body heat (non-shivering thermogenesis) altogether make the neonates prone to hypothermia (<36.0 °C). Various modes of heat loss in newborns are by radiation and convection (the two most common causes) followed by evaporation and conduction. Nursing the babies in a thermoneutral environment (during the first week of life—30–33 °C in infants with birth weight >2.5 kg and 34–35 °C for very low birth weight babies (<1.5 kg)) will help in reducing heat loss, basic metabolic requirements, and dehydration.

2.6 Methods to Reduce Heat Loss

Setting the room temperature of delivery and operating room to 26 °C, routine care for babies over the mother's abdomen immediately after delivery, nursing sick babies in servo-controlled radiant warmers or incubators, adequate dressings (hat, covering blankets), and providing kangaroo mother care for stable babies are to be practised to prevent hypothermia.

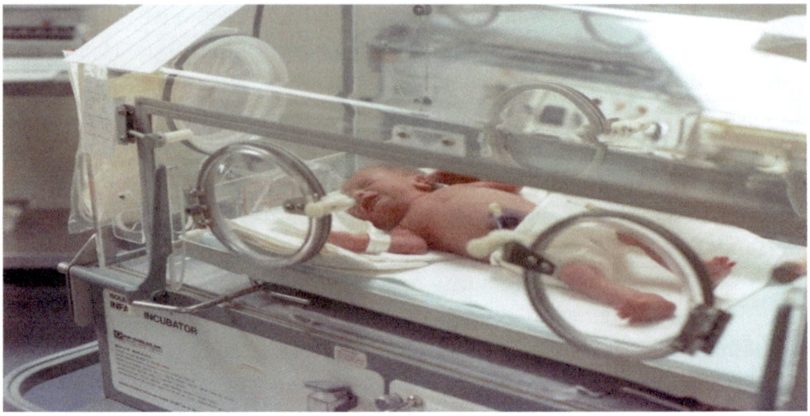

Fig. 2.4 A neonate placed inside a double-walled neonatal incubator

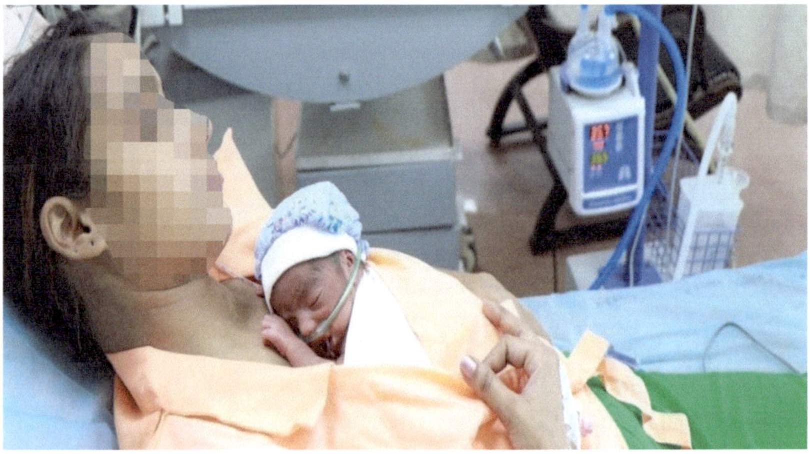

Fig. 2.5 Kangaroo mother care: easy, safe and effective way of neonatal nursing compared to costly incubators

Sufficient humidification maintenance is another entity which helps prevent weight loss, dehydration, loss of skin integrity, and temperature instabilities. Nursing babies in incubators during the first 2 weeks of life provides an adequate humidified environment for low birth weight babies (see Fig. 2.4).

1. Kangaroo mother care (placing baby in skin-to-skin contact with mother or other caregiver as shown in Fig. 2.5) is the standard of care to prevent hypothermia in stable preterm or LBW (<2500 g) babies.

Suggested Readings

Chakkarapani AA, Roehr CC, Hooper SB, Te Pas AB, Gupta S, ESPR Neonatal Resuscitation Section Writing Group. Transitional circulation and hemodynamic monitoring in newborn infants. Pediatr Res. 2023;

Gleason CA, Taylor sawyer. Avery's diseases of the newborn. 11th ed. Elsevier; 2023.

Elshazzly M, Anekar AA, Shumway KR, et al. Physiology, Newborn. [Updated 2023 Sep 4]. In: StatPearls [Internet]. Treasure Island, FL: StatPearls Publishing. p. 2024.

Kooi EMW, Richter AE. Cerebral autoregulation in sick infants: current insights. Clin Perinatol. 2020;47(3):449–67.

Martin RJ, Fanaroff AA, Walsh MC. Fanaroff and Martin's neonatal-perinatal medicine: diseases of the fetus and infant. 11th ed. Elsevier; 2020.

Van Vonderen JJ, Roest AA, Siew ML, Walther FJ, Hooper SB, te Pas AB. Measuring physiological changes during the transition to life after birth. Neonatology. 2014;105(3):230–42.

Zhu L-B, Xu Y-H, Li J-F, Hu X, Lu C-Y, Li R-L, Shi C-P, Yuan M. The effect of kangaroo mother care after duodenal obstruction in neonates. Front Surg. 2022;9:813052.

Hypoglycemia, Hypothermia, Neonatal Hyperbilirubinemia

3

Partap Singh Yadav and Subhasis Roy Choudhury

3.1 Hypoglycemia

Neonatal hypoglycemia is a frequent metabolic condition, defined as a blood glucose level below 30 mg/dL in the first 24 h of life and less than 45 mg/dL thereafter. Although the exact threshold for abnormality is debated, a practical value of <40 mg/dL is often used to guide treatment decisions.

3.2 Symptoms

The clinical manifestations include hypotonia, lethargy, apathy, poor feeding, jitteriness, seizures, cyanosis, apnea, and hypothermia.

3.3 Management

- Asymptomatic hypoglycemia: in neonates with blood glucose levels above 25 mg/dL, oral feeding can be attempted.
- *Symptomatic hypoglycemia*: treat with an intravenous (IV) bolus of 10% dextrose at 2 mL/kg. Following the bolus, continue an IV glucose infusion at a rate of 5–8 mg/kg/min in neonates and 3–5 mg/kg/min in older children to maintain adequate glucose levels.

If hypoglycemia persists for more than 5–7 days or if a glucose infusion rate exceeding 12 mg/kg/min is required for longer than 24 h, further diagnostic evaluation is necessary.

3.4 Persistent Hyperinsulinemic Hypoglycemia of Infancy (PHHI)

PHHI is a rare but significant cause of severe neonatal hypoglycemia. Early diagnosis is critical to prevent irreversible neurological damage or life-threatening episodes.

3.5 Management of PHHI

- *Medical therapy*: includes glucose infusion rates exceeding 10 mg/kg/min to maintain glucose levels above 54 mg/dL, continuous glucose feeding, and administration of diazoxide, octreotide, or glucagon infusions.
- *Surgical intervention*: if medical therapy fails, near-total pancreatectomy (removal of 95% or more of the pancreas) is performed, except in cases of focal lesions.

P. S. Yadav (✉)
Department of Pediatric Surgery, LHMC, New Delhi, Delhi, India

S. Roy Choudhury
Pediatric Surgery, Lady Hardinge Medical College and Associated Kalawati Saran Children's Hospital, New Delhi, Delhi, India

© The Author(s), under exclusive license to Springer Nature Singapore Pte Ltd. 2025
S. Roy Choudhury (ed.), *Pediatric Surgery*, https://doi.org/10.1007/978-981-96-1257-4_3

3.6 Hypothermia

Newborns are at high risk of hypothermia due to heat loss through evaporation, conduction, convection, and radiation. Surgical neonates are particularly vulnerable during procedures.

3.7 Mechanism of Heat Regulation

Neonates generate heat by increasing their metabolic activity and utilizing brown adipose tissue stored in the neck, axillae, and interscapular regions.

3.8 Severe Hypothermia

When the body temperature falls below 35 °C, symptoms such as lassitude, apnea, bradycardia, hypoglycemia, hyperkalemia, metabolic acidosis, shock, elevated blood urea nitrogen (BUN), and oliguria may develop. This condition, known as neonatal cold injury syndrome, is particularly significant in preterm infants, those undergoing prolonged surgery, and cases with exposed bowel (e.g., gastroschisis).

3.9 Prevention and Management

Effective temperature management is crucial, particularly during surgery and transport:

1. *Pre-warming*: ensure operating theatres and recovery rooms are preheated to around 25 °C.
2. *Transport incubators*: use incubators with ambient air temperatures of 34–38 °C and warm, humidified air set to 40–80%.
3. *Intraoperative techniques*:
   - Use humidified and warmed inhalant gases during anesthesia.
   - Employ warm saline solutions for peritoneal washing.
   - Utilize servo-controlled heating mattresses and continuously monitor the core body temperature.
4. *Radiant heaters*: during procedures or extended examinations, use servo-controlled radiant warmers to maintain an optimal body temperature

3.10 Neonatal Hyperbilirubinemia

Hyperbilirubinemia affects approximately *85% of term infants* and nearly all premature infants. It results from an imbalance between *bilirubin production and elimination***.** Clinical jaundice becomes visible when bilirubin levels exceed *7 mg/dL*.

3.10.1 Physiologic Jaundice

1. *Onset and progression*:
   - Clinical jaundice appears on day 2–3 of life.
   - Total bilirubin levels rise by less than 5 mg/dL per day.
   - Peak bilirubin levels occur at 3–5 days of life and are:
     - <12 mg/dL in term infants.
     - <15 mg/dL in preterm infants.
   - Jaundice resolves by 2 weeks in term infants and 3–4 weeks in preterm infants.

3.10.2 Pathological Jaundice

1. *Onset and progression*:
   - Jaundice appears before 24 h of age.
   - Bilirubin rises by more than 0.2 mg/dL/h.
   - Peak bilirubin concentrations exceed 12 mg/dL in term infants and 15 mg/dL in preterm infants.
   - Clinical jaundice:
     - Persists beyond 8 days in term infants and 14 days in preterm infants.
     - Recurs after initially resolving.
     - Involves direct bilirubin levels exceeding 1.5 mg/dL.

3.10.3 Causes of Neonatal Hyperbilirubinemia

1. *Overproduction*: excessive hemolysis due to blood group incompatibility.
2. *Undersecretion*: associated with metabolic and endocrine disorders or obstructive conditions.
3. *Mixed causes*: seen in sepsis or infections.
4. *Uncertain mechanisms*: examples include breast milk jaundice.

3.10.4 Kernicterus

Kernicterus occurs due to bilirubin deposition in the brain, particularly in regions like the hippocampus, thalamus, striatum, and auditory nuclei.

3.10.5 Management

Two primary treatment approaches include:

1. *Phototherapy*
2. *Exchange transfusion*

3.10.6 Indications for Phototherapy and Exchange Transfusion

1. *Infants >35 weeks of gestation*: treatment depends on bilirubin levels, age in days, gestational age, and risk factors. Clinical charts guide decisions on therapy.
2. *Infants <35 weeks of gestation*: thresholds are based on body weight:
   - *<1000 g*: phototherapy at *10–12 mg/dL*, exchange transfusion at bilirubin levels of *10–12 mg/dL*.
   - *1000–1500 g*: phototherapy at *7–9 mg/dL*, exchange transfusion at *12–15 mg/dL*.
   - *1500–2000 g*: phototherapy at *10–12 mg/dL*, exchange transfusion at *15–18 mg/dL*.
   - *2000–2500 g*: phototherapy at *13–15 mg/dL*, exchange transfusion at *18–20 mg/dL*.

3.10.7 Mechanism of Phototherapy

Phototherapy reduces bilirubin through three mechanisms:

1. *Photooxidation*: converts bilirubin into water-soluble molecules.
2. *Configurational isomerization*: changes bilirubin to a more soluble form for easier excretion.
3. *Structural isomerization*: produces forms that can bypass hepatic conjugation.

3.10.8 Conjugated Hyperbilirubinemia

Management depends on the underlying cause. See Chap. 34 on infantile obstructive cholangiopathy for more details.

Suggested Reading

Arcara K, Tschudy M. The Harriet Lane handbook. 20th ed. Philadelphia, PA: Mosby Elsevier; 2014.

Kliegman R, Stanton B, Geme JS, Nelson SN. Textbook of pediatrics. 20th ed. Philadelphia, PA: Saunders, Elsevier; 2015.

Simmons CF Jr. Fluid and electrolyte management. In: Cloherty JP, Stark AR, editors. Manual of neonatal care. 4th ed. New York: Lippincott Raven; 1997. p. 100.

4 Vascular Access in Children

Partap Singh Yadav and Subhasis Roy Choudhury

4.1 Challenges in Pediatric Vascular Access

- *Small vessel size*: pediatric patients have narrower vessels, making access technically demanding.
- *Uncooperative behavior*: fear and anxiety in children can hinder the process.
- *Congenital anomalies*: structural abnormalities may complicate vascular access.
- *Parental anxiety*: anxious caregivers can further complicate the process.

4.2 Classification of Vascular Access

Vascular access in children can be categorized into three broad types (Fig. 4.1):

1. *Arterial or venous access*
   - Arterial access is typically used for invasive blood pressure monitoring and arterial blood gas sampling.
   - Venous access is more common and used for the administration of medications, fluids, and nutrition.
2. *Peripheral or central venous access*
   - *Peripheral venous catheters*:
     - Indicated for short-term use such as administering IV fluids, antibiotics, and other medications.
     - Easily inserted but unsuitable for long-term or high-concentration therapies.
   - *Central venous catheters (CVCs)*:
     - Essential for long-term treatments like chemotherapy, total parenteral nutrition (TPN), and monitoring central venous pressure.
3. *Intraosseous access*
   - Used in emergency situations when venous access is not feasible.
   - Provides a rapid and reliable route for the administration of fluids and medications during resuscitation.

P. S. Yadav (✉)
Department of Pediatric Surgery, LHMC, New Delhi, Delhi, India

S. Roy Choudhury
Pediatric Surgery, Lady Hardinge Medical College and Associated Kalawati Saran Children's Hospital, New Delhi, Delhi, India

© The Author(s), under exclusive license to Springer Nature Singapore Pte Ltd. 2025
S. Roy Choudhury (ed.), *Pediatric Surgery*, https://doi.org/10.1007/978-981-96-1257-4_4

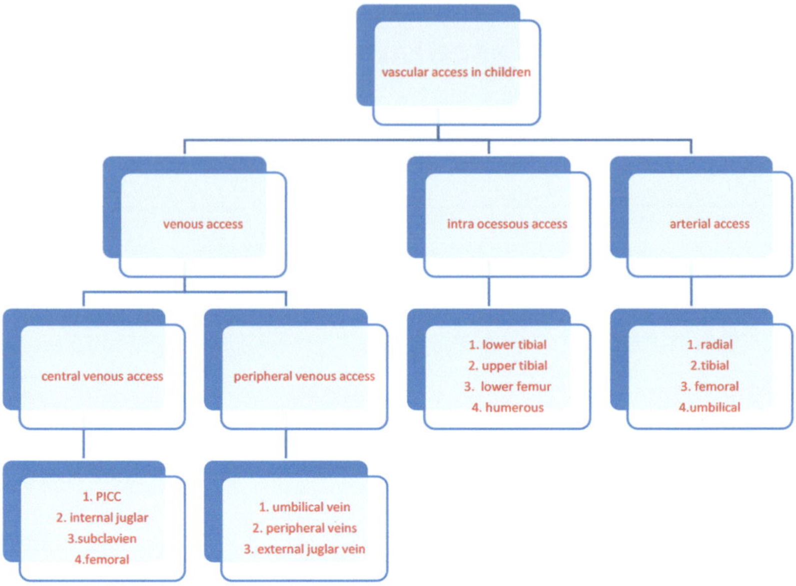

Fig. 4.1 Classification and sites of vascular access

4.3 Types of Catheters

4.3.1 Peripheral Venous Catheters

Peripheral venous catheters are the most widely used option due to their safety and ease of insertion. However, complications such as dislodgement and occlusion are common concerns.

4.3.2 Preferred Insertion Sites

- Dorsum of the hand and feet
- Scalp veins (especially in neonates)
- Saphenous vein

4.3.3 Additional Sites

- Cephalic, basilic, and femoral veins may also be utilized but are often reserved for peripherally inserted central catheters (PICC).
- The external jugular vein can be used but is harder to maintain in children due to their shorter neck anatomy.

4.4 Venous Cut-Down Catheters

Venous cutdown is a method used when vascular access is difficult, particularly in emergency situations. It provides reliable catheter placement but requires surgical expertise and a thorough understanding of vascular anatomy.

4.4.1 Preferred Site

- *Saphenous vein*: this is the first-choice site due to its consistent anatomy and ease of access.
  - A linear incision is made just anterior and above the medial malleolus**.** Blunt dissection using artery forceps exposes the vein for venotomy and catheter insertion (Fig. 4.2a).

4.4.2 Alternative Sites

- Veins of the arm (antecubital vein, cephalic vein) (Fig. 4.2b)
- Femoral vein (Fig. 4.2c)

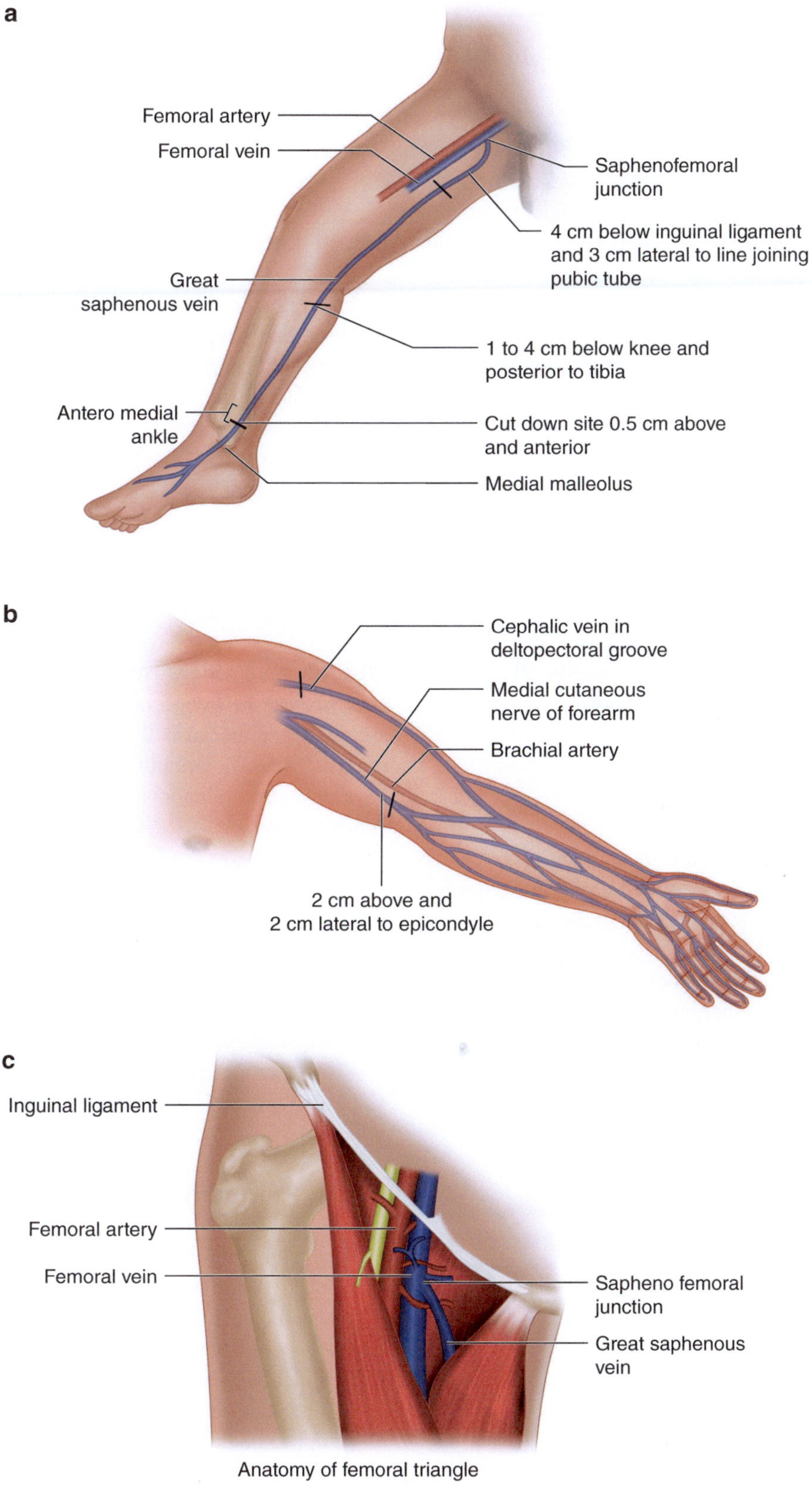

Fig. 4.2 (**a**) Saphenous vein cut down landmarks. (**b**) Basilic and cephalic vein cut down landmarks. (**c**) Femoral and great saphenous vein in femoral triangle

4.5 Complications of Peripheral Catheters

Proper securing of the catheter is critical to maintain functionality and prevent complications. The most frequent complication associated with peripheral catheters is dislodgement or occlusion, which may lead to extravasation of fluids into the surrounding tissues. If extravasation occurs, the catheter should be promptly removed. Potential consequences of extravasation include:

- *Tissue necrosis*
- *Compartment syndrome*

4.5.1 Intraosseous Catheters

The intraosseous route is reserved for life-threatening situations in critically ill children when vascular access is difficult.

4.5.2 Procedure

- A large-bore needle or cannula (16–18G) is inserted into the proximal tibia, approximately 1–2 cm below and medial to the tibial tuberosity (Fig. 4.3).
- This route uses the noncollapsible veins in the medullary sinuses of the bone marrow, which drain into the central circulation via emissary veins.

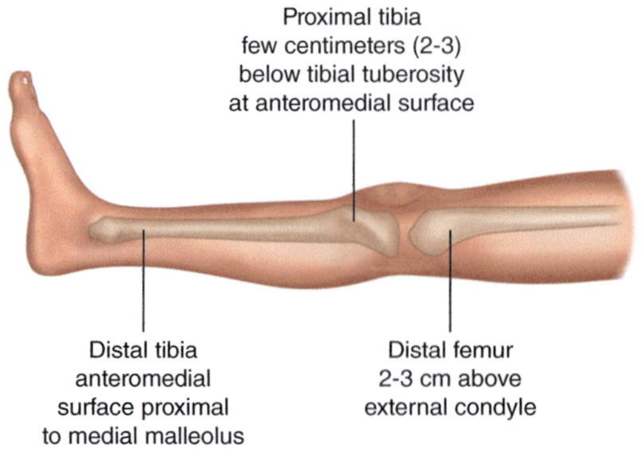

Fig. 4.3 Landmarks for intraosseous access

4.5.3 Applications

- Delivery of resuscitation drugs, fluid boluses, and blood products.

4.5.4 Limitations and Complications

- The catheter should not remain in place for more than 12–24 hours.
- Potential complications include:
  - Leakage
  - Osteomyelitis
  - Fractures
  - Occlusion

4.6 Peripherally Inserted Central Catheters

PICC lines are widely used for patients requiring *intermediate to long-term venous access*. They are preferred because they can be placed and removed *bedside* without general anesthesia and have fewer complications than traditional central venous catheters.

4.6.1 Preferred Insertion Sites

- Veins of the cubital fossa:
  - Basilic vein.
  - Cephalic vein.
  - Antecubital vein.
- Great saphenous vein (Fig. 4.4a and b).

4.6.2 Procedure

- A vein appropriate for the size of the PICC line is selected (ultrasound guidance can assist).
- The catheter is inserted through *an introducer needle* and advanced to a larger central vein.
- The ideal tip position is at:
  - The superior vena cava-atrial junction (for upper-body PICC lines).
  - *The inferior vena cava* at the level of the diaphragm (for lower-body PICC lines).

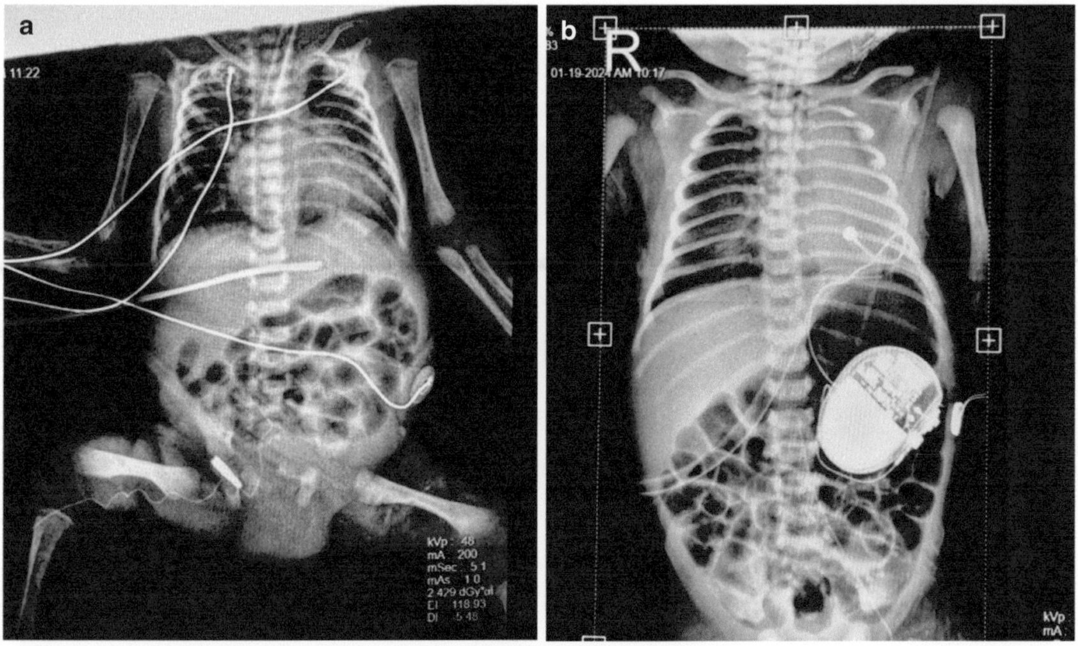

Fig. 4.4 (**a**) Percutaneously inserted central catheter (PICC) through saphenous vein, X-ray showing tip in inferior vena cava (IVC). (**b**) Proximal saphenous PICC X-ray showing catheter position

- Tip placement is confirmed with a chest or abdominal radiograph.

4.6.3 Uses

PICC lines are versatile and can be used for:

- Total parenteral nutrition (TPN)
- Chemotherapy
- Administration of inotropes
- Blood sampling

4.6.4 Types of PICC Lines

1. *Open PICC*:
   - Requires regular flushing with heparinized saline to prevent clot formation.
2. *Groshong PICC*:
   - Features a two-way pressure-sensitive valve that prevents blood backflow.
   - Does not require locks, clamps, or regular heparinized flushing.

4.7 Central Venous Catheters (Tunneled/ Nontunneled and Implantable Devices)

4.8 Central Venous Catheters (CVCs)

Central venous catheters are inserted into the femoral, subclavian, or internal jugular veins (Fig. 4.5a and b) and are primarily used in chronically ill patients. They are suitable for long-term use and can deliver:

- Large-volume infusions
- Blood products
- Total parenteral nutrition (TPN)
- Chemotherapy

Additionally, CVCs are useful for blood sampling and critical care monitoring.

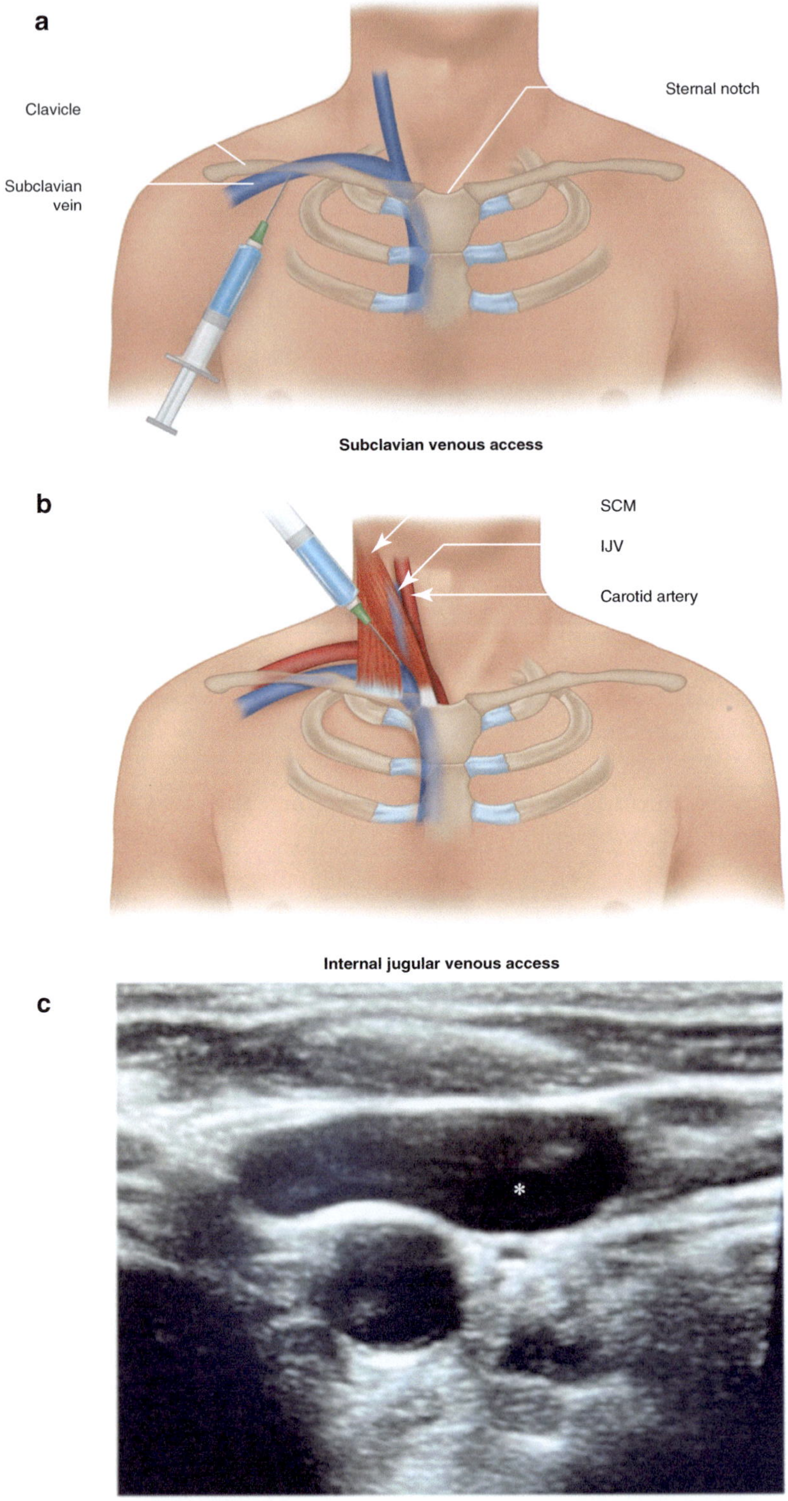

Fig. 4.5 (**a**) Percutaneous internal jugular venous access. (**b**) Percutaneous subclavian vascular access. The needle is guided toward the sternal notch from just below the mid-clavicular point. (**c**) Ultrasound-guided internal jugular venous access * internal jugular vein

4.9 Types of Central Venous Catheters

1. Percutaneous polyethylene catheters
   - Material: made of polyethylene, suitable for short- to medium-term use.
   - Procedure:
     - Inserted under local anesthesia with mild sedation and strict asepsis using the Seldinger technique.
     - Preferred site:
       - Right internal jugular vein: chosen for its straight course into the right atrium, located between the two heads of the sternocleidomastoid muscle and directed toward the ipsilateral nipple while avoiding the carotid artery (medial to the vein) (Fig. 4.5a).
       - Subclavian vein: accessed laterally and inferior to the midclavicular bend, directed toward the suprasternal notch at a 30° angle to the chest wall (Fig. 4.5b). Pneumothorax is a common complication with this site.
   - Uses: ideal for short- to medium-term therapies.

4.9.1 Ultrasound-Guided CVC Insertion

Ultrasound-guided techniques are increasingly favored as they improve precision, reduce complications, and ensure a high success rate during catheter placement (Fig. 4.5c).

Position of the catheter tip can be checked with an x-ray (Fig. 4.6a and b).

1. Silicone CVCs (e.g., Hickman, Broviac Catheters)
   - Material: made of silicone, which is more pliable and less irritant to the veins, making it suitable for long-term use.
   - Procedure:
     - Inserted using an open surgical technique.
     - Features:
       - Proximal cuff: provides fixation and reduces the risk of dislodgement.
       - Tunneling: the catheter is tunneled under the skin and exits from a separate site away from the venous insertion point, enhancing durability and reducing infection risk.
     - Sites: internal jugular, femoral, and subclavian veins can be used.

4.10 Implantable Vascular-Access Devices (Ports)

An implantable port system comprises a reservoir placed in a subcutaneous pocket, connected to a tunneled central line that drains into a central vein. These devices allow multiple drug administrations through the reservoir using specialized needles, with the capacity for up to 1000 punctures.

4.10.1 Key Features

1. Maintenance:
   - Requires minimal upkeep as the skin acts as a natural barrier against infection.
   - Patients can engage in regular activities without the need for special handling or dressing.
2. Applications:
   - Primarily used for long-term central venous access, particularly in patients requiring:
     - Cancer chemotherapy.
     - Long-term antibiotic therapy.
3. Commercially available devices:
   - Examples include Port-A-Cath and Vascuport.
4. Advantages:
   - Excellent durability.
   - Lower infection risk compared to external devices.
5. Limitations:
   - Higher cost.
   - Requires surgical insertion and removal.
   - Special needles are needed for repeated access, limiting ease of use.

This system is particularly beneficial for patients requiring long-term treatment with minimal interference in daily life.

4.11 Other Vascular-Access Sites

4.11.1 Umbilical Vein

- The umbilical vein is the largest and thin-walled vessel in the umbilical cord, located at the 12 o'clock position in the umbilical stump.
- The procedure involves an open technique with freshening the umbilical stump, identifying the vein, and inserting the catheter into its lumen to the desired length, with the tip ideally located in the inferior vena cava (Fig. 4.7a).
- Position confirmation: can be done with an abdominal radiograph (Fig. 4.7b).
- *Contraindications*:
  - Newborns with abdominal defects, necrotizing enterocolitis, or peritonitis.
- *Uses*: fluid administration, drug delivery, and blood sampling.

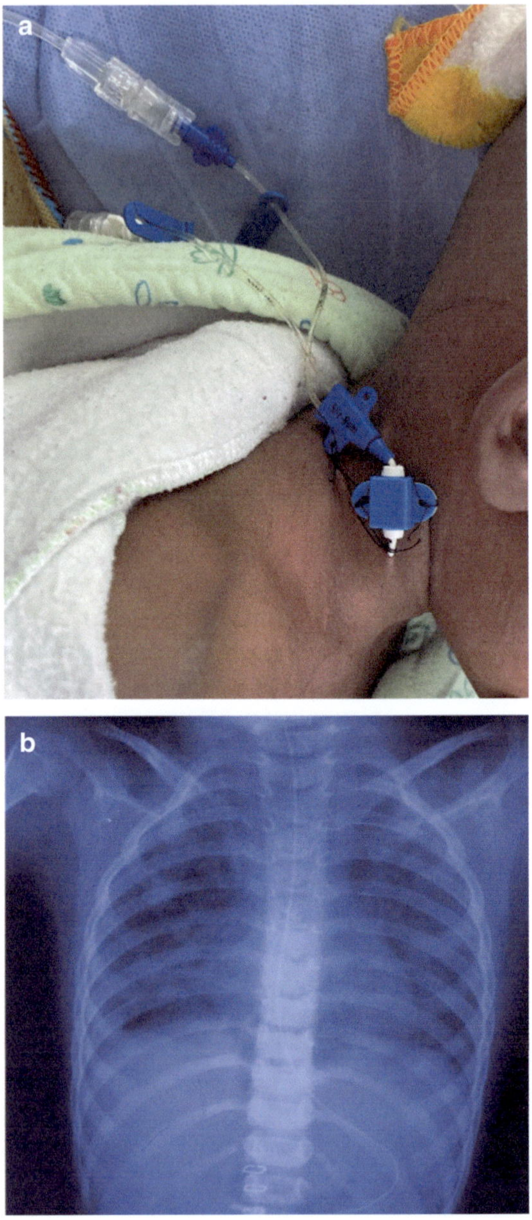

Fig. 4.6 (**a**) Internal jugular central venous catheter (double lumen). (**b**) Radiograph confirming correct positioning of tip of catheter

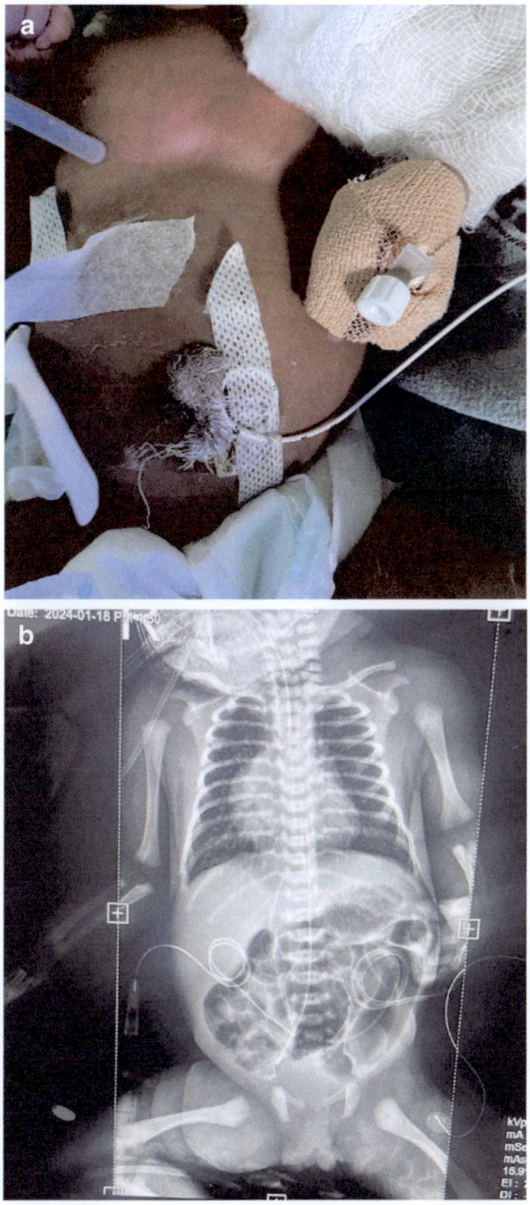

Fig. 4.7 (**a**) Umbilical venous access. (**b**) X-ray showing catheter tip in IVC

4.12 Miscellaneous Venous Access Sites

Other veins that may be utilized include:

- Azygous, hemiazygous, intercostal, hepatic veins, inferior vena cava, and unusual collateral vessels.
- Inferior epigastric and lumbar veins can also be accessed using a surgical cutdown technique.

4.13 Arterial Vascular Access

4.13.1 Indications

Arterial access is essential for:

- Repeated blood gas analysis.
- Invasive blood pressure monitoring in critically ill patients.

4.13.2 Common Sites

- Radial artery (preferred due to accessibility and safety).
- Posterior tibial and dorsalis pedis arteries.
- Femoral artery: generally avoided in small children due to higher risk of complications.

  Procedure for radial artery cannulation

- Perform the Allen test to assess collateral blood flow.
- Use two fingers to locate the radial artery and mentally visualize its course. Cannulation is performed carefully under sterile conditions.

4.14 Principles of General Care for Vascular Access

1. Aseptic technique:
   - Clean the site with 2% chlorhexidine in 70% alcohol or 10% povidone–iodine.
   - For central venous access, wear a sterile gown and gloves and create a sterile field.
2. Child comfort:
   - Parental presence, distraction techniques, and sedation can help calm the child.
   - For neonates:
     – Non-nutritive suckling, holding the baby in the mother's lap, or gentle rocking can reduce anxiety.

   - Topical anesthetics (e.g., prilocaine) and oral sucrose solution can alleviate post-procedure pain.
3. Adjuncts for difficult vascular access:
   - Tourniquet, vein tapping, or local warming for vasodilation.
   - Transillumination, infrared vein finders, ultrasound, or fluoroscopy to visualize veins.

4.14.1 Fluid Choices for Venous Infusion

Characteristic	Central venous access	Peripheral venous access
Type of fluid	Hyper-/ hypo-osmolar	Isotonic
Dextrose concentration	>12.5%	<12.5%
Osmolality	>600 mOsm/L	<600 mOsm/L
Irritant fluids	Yes	No

4.15 Complications of Vascular Access

4.15.1 Acute Complications

- Pneumothorax (most serious with subclavian or jugular access)
- Air embolism
- Arrhythmias
- Arterial puncture
- Brachial plexus injury
- Cardiac tamponade
- Guidewire knotting or fracturing
- Hematoma, hemorrhage, or hemothorax
- Thoracic duct injury
- Vascular perforation or dissection

Note: obtain a chest radiograph to rule out pneumothorax following central venous access placement.

Long-term complications

- Catheter-related bloodstream infections and sepsis.
- Thrombosis (e.g., deep vein thrombosis or pulmonary embolism).
- Catheter migration, displacement, or occlusion.
- Line fracture or embolization.
- Phlebitis of the cannulated vessel.

Specific complications

1. Catheter dislodgement and migration:
   - Common long-term issue causing malfunction or, in severe cases, perforation of the vessel wall.
2. Infection:
   - Most frequent complication of long-term vascular access.
   - Signs: fever, positive blood cultures, or catheter tip cultures.
   - Management: administer broad-spectrum antibiotics via the catheter. If the infection persists or the patient is septic, remove the catheter and place a new one at a different site.
3. Thrombosis:
   - Regular flushing with heparinized saline minimizes thrombotic occlusion.
   - Agents such as streptokinase, tissue plasminogen activator, or heparin can be used for partial thrombosis.

4.16 Summary

- Pediatric vascular access is a highly specialized procedure, requiring skill and proper care.
- Imaging technologies and adherence to care protocols help reduce complications and improve success rates.
- Meticulous aseptic techniques and regular maintenance are critical to preventing complications like infection and thrombosis.

Suggested Reading

Biasucci DG, Disma NM, Pittiruti M, editors. Vascular access in neonates and children. 1st ed. Springer.

Holcomb GW III, Murphy PJ, St Peter SD, editors. Holocomb and Ashcraft's pediatric surgery. 7th ed. Philadelphia: Elsevier; 2020.

5 Parenteral Nutrition in Children

Partap Singh Yadav and Subhasis Roy Choudhury

5.1 Parenteral Nutrition

Parenteral nutrition is the administration of balanced nutrition intravenously to meet daily energy requirements and help anabolism and support weight gain.

5.2 Normal Paediatric Growth

A term newborn grows at a rate of 25–30 g/day leading to doubling of birth weight by 5 months of age. The birth weight triples by 12 months in an average infant. Acute nutritional deprivation affects the body weight, thus altering the weight for height ratio, whereas length is a good indicator for long-term body growth. Chronic malnutrition results in a lag in both weight and height.

5.3 Indications

Infants who remain in a fasting state for more than 5 days should be considered for nutritional supplementation. Enteral route of feeding should always be considered and tried first and even if full feedings are not tolerated, small volumes of "trophic" feedings are useful to maintain intestinal function.

Certain indications for parenteral nutrition are:

(a) Congenital anomalies: gastroschisis, bowel atresia's, volvulus, meconium ileus.
(b) Gastrointestinal disorders: short bowel syndrome, malabsorption, intractable diarrhoea, inflammatory bowel disease, high output enterocutaneous fistula.
(c) Others: radiation enteritis, chemotherapy resulting in intolerance to oral feeds, severe respiratory distress syndrome in preterm babies and sever acute pancreatitis.
(d) All babies born <31 weeks of gestation.
(e) All babies born >31 weeks of gestation, with failure to establish enteral feeding 72 h after birth.
(f) If enteral feeds have been stopped and it is unlikely to be resumed in 48 h.

5.4 Administration of Total Parenteral Nutrition (TPN)

Total parenteral nutrition (TPN) for less than 15 days duration can be given by peripheral access (<12.5% dextrose); for longer duration of parenteral nutrition, central access is ideal. Percutaneously inserted central venous catheters are now the most commonly used venous access

P. S. Yadav (✉)
Department of Pediatric Surgery, LHMC, New Delhi, Delhi, India

S. Roy Choudhury
Pediatric Surgery, Lady Hardinge Medical College and Associated Kalawati Saran Children's Hospital, New Delhi, Delhi, India

© The Author(s), under exclusive license to Springer Nature Singapore Pte Ltd. 2025
S. Roy Choudhury (ed.), *Pediatric Surgery*, https://doi.org/10.1007/978-981-96-1257-4_5

for TPN. Ideal position of the tip of the central venous catheter is at the junction of the superior vena cava and right atrium. Peripheral TPN solution should have osmolality less than 600–900 mOsm/L and a maximum dextrose concentration of 12.5% to prevent thrombophlebitis.

5.5 Composition of Parenteral Formulas

Parenteral nutrition can be partial or total (TPN). Parenteral nutrition provides both macro- and micro-nutrients.

5.6 Amino Acids

Amino acids are provided in crystalline form and provide both essential and non-essential amino acids. They provide 4 kcal/g, and approximately 10–15% of total calories are provided by amino acids. Amino acids are started at the rate of 1.5–2 /kg/day and advanced to the goal of 3.5 g/kg/day by 4 days onwards. One should ensure adequate nonprotein calories to prevent catabolism of proteins for calorie, and maintain nonprotein nitrogen to nitrogen ratio 150–250:1. Patients with liver failure and encephalopathy require lower amounts of amino acids.

5.7 Dextrose

Dextrose provides the major chunk of calories (50–60%) and acts as a protein-sparing substrate. Hydrous dextrose provides 3.4 kcal/g. Dextrose is started at glucose infusion rate (GIR) of 6 mg/kg/min and increase up to a maximum GIR of 9–16 mg/kg/min by day 4 of TPN. The target blood sugar range is 100–120 mg/dL and the GIR can be titrated based on blood sugar monitoring. Blood sugar should be monitored 1–2 h after the change of GIR. It should be frequently monitored in babies with hypoglycaemia and sepsis. Symptomatic hypoglycaemia (or < 40 mg/dL) should be treated with a bolus of D10W at 2 cc/kg followed by readjustment of GIR.

5.8 Lipid Emulsions

Lipids are a condensed source of energy and essential fatty acids (EFAs) providing 9 kcal/g. Lipids are available in 10%, 20%, and 30% concentrations. Lipids are iso osmolar and hence can be given through a peripheral line. Most of the current available lipids are derived from soyabean, and other source is fish oil which is rich in omega 3 fatty acids. Lipids provide 20–30% of total calories. They are initiated at the rate of 1 g/kg/day and advanced by 0.5–1 g/kg/day to a maximum of 3–4 g/kg/day. There are two essential fatty acids: alpha-linolenic acid (omega 3 fatty acid, anti-inflammatory) and linoleic acid (omega 6 fatty acid pro inflammatory). Soy-based lipids have an omega 6 to omega 3 ratio of 7:1; a ratio of 1:4 is present in fish-based lipids which is desirable. Deficiency of essential fatty acid (EFA) is associated with poor wound healing capacity and dryness of skin. Patients who develop parenteral nutrition-associated cholestasis benefit from a reduction of lipid content and switching over to fish oil-based lipids. Hypertriglyceridemia (>250 mg/dL) and thrombocytopenia warrant a reduction in lipid infusion.

5.9 Multivitamins

Parenteral nutrition solutions should contain both water and fat-soluble vitamins. Paediatric formulations are currently unavailable; however, adult multivitamin infusion at the rate of 1.5 mL/kg/day can be used.

5.10 Trace Elements

TPN solutions should provide zinc, copper, manganese, chromium and selenium. Trace element solution is usually given at the rate of 0.15 mL/kg/day.

5.11 Electrolytes

Sodium, potassium, chloride, acetate, calcium and phosphate are added in the TPN solutions depending on the patient's daily requirement. Premature babies are deficient in both calcium and phosphorus and need them for skeletal development. They have significant requirements and are usually provided in 1:1 ratio. Precipitation of calcium with other anions can occur.

5.12 Heparin

0.5–1 IU/mL heparin is added to TPN solution to maintain the patency of venous catheter.

5.12.1 Administration of Parenteral Nutrition

Pre-formulated paediatric and neonatal TPN is generally not available. They need to be formulated based on individual needs under a laminar flow with strict asepsis. The TPN in neonates is usually given by peripherally inserted central catheters (PICC) and in children central intravenous access through internal jugular veins is preferrred.

5.12.2 Calculation of TPN

1. Maintenance fluid requirement.
2. Calculation of caloric needs.
3. Caloric distribution into components: 30–40% from fat, 50–60% from carbohydrates, and 8–12% from protein.
4. Calculate electrolyte and trace elements.
5. Calculate GIR: %glucose × mL/kg/day/144.

Example—for a 3 kg weight child at day 3 of life, if we have to calculate day 1 TPN:

Total fluid requirement—300 mL/day.
Total calorie requirement approx. 300 kcal/day.
Total protein requirement = 1 g/kg/day = 3 g/day = 30 mL 10% solution.
Total lipid requirement = 1 g/kg/day = 3 g/day = 15 mL 20% solution.
Total dextrose requirement @ 6 mg/kg/min = 6× 3× 60× 24 = 26 g/day.
Total sodium requirement = 3 mEq/kg/day = 9 mEq/day =18 mL 3% NaCl.
Total potassium required = 2 mEq/kg/day = 6 mEq/day = 3 mL KCl.
Total calcium = 1 mEq/kg/day = 3 mEq/day = 3 mL/day.

So, the composition of TPN for this 3-kg child will be as follows:

210 mL 10% dextrose (21 g) + 20 mL 25% dextrose (5 g)+
30 mL Aminoacid solution (10%) + 15 mL (20%) lipid solution +
18 mL 3% NaCl +3 mL KCl + 3 mL Ca gluconate+ $MgSO_4$ 0.5 mL + trace elements solution 0.5 mL.

5.12.3 Stopping TPN

Once adequate enteral nutrition is established at 120–140 mL/kg/day, TPN can be withdrawn. If there are concerns of sepsis or cholestasis, it can be stopped early at 100 mL/kg/day of enteral feeds.

5.13 Monitoring Patients on TPN

Monitoring patients on TPN is essential; complete blood count, blood glucose, blood urea nitrogen, creatinine, serum electrolytes and liver function tests need to be monitored. Patients on long-term TPN require special monitoring of trace elements to prevent toxicity and deficiencies.

5.14 Complications

(a) Metabolic complications: hyperglycaemia, hypoglycaemia, hypertriglyceridaemia, metabolic acidosis and electrolyte disturbances.

(b) Hepatobiliary complications: cholestasis, steatosis, and cholelithiasis.
(c) Infectious complications: sepsis is the most frequent and serious complication of central TPN administration. Catheter-related infections are the most frequent cause of sepsis.
(d) Complications from venous catheters: pneumothorax, cardiac arrhythmias, vessel thrombosis and catheter dislodgment.
(e) Complications from overfeeding: osmotic diuresis, immunologic suppression.
(f) Parenteral nutrition-associated liver disease (PNALD): it is a heterogenous clinical syndrome characterised by cholestasis, fibrosis and in late stages even cirrhosis. Persistent direct hyperbilirubinemia develops. Other causes of liver damage should be ruled out. PNALD is the cause of long-term morbidity and mortality in patients receiving TPN. Preterm, patients with necrotizing enterocolitis (NEC), gastro intestinal (GI) surgeries, sepsis, type of lipid and presence of antioxidants are some of the factors affecting the development of PNALD. Initiating enteral feeds (minimal enteral nutrition), cycling PN, and substituting soy lipid with fish-based products reduces the incidence.

Suggested Reading

Arcara K, Tschudy M. The Harriet Lane handbook. 20th ed. Philadelphia, USA: Mosby Elsevier; 2014.
Kliegman R, Stanton B, Geme JS, Schor N. Nelson textbook of pediatrics. 20th ed. Philadelphia: Saunders, Elsevier; 2015.

Anesthetic Management of Pediatric Surgical Patients

6

Raksha Kundal

6.1 Introduction

Neonates, Infants, and young children have morphological, physiological, pharmacological, emotional, and social characteristics entirely distinct from those of adults.

Children who get anesthesia have specific needs, and all children have a right to the best possible care in the appropriate setting. It is prudent for surgeons to know about their patient's anesthesia plan, including preparation, optimization, and the analgesia options available for a particular surgery. Knowledge of operating surgeons regarding pediatric anesthesia practices may improve patient outcomes.

6.2 Preanesthetic Evaluation and Preparation

Preanesthesia checkup in a preanesthetic clinic is essential for the preoperative preparation of children undergoing surgery. During this checkup, the management of any comorbid condition is optimized before surgery. Parents are made to understand fasting instructions, and children are categorized as per the American Society of Anaesthesia Physical status (ASA-PS) classification.

Anxiety issues of children related to surgery are dealt with during this visit.

Proper preoperative evaluation of children before surgery needs close coordination of the pediatric surgeon, pediatrician, and anesthesiologist. During preanesthesia consultation, history of the present illness is sought, and any derangement of hemodynamics or fluid status is assessed. Thorough medical history of the patient is taken; birth asphyxia and other events in the neonatal period are recorded. The immunization status of a child is also noted.

Investigations are planned per the patient's medical status and the type of surgery the patient is undergoing.

6.3 Preoperative Consideration in Children with Systematic Respiratory Disorders

A significant cause of morbidity and mortality is respiratory events among children in the perioperative period. Few conditions are upper respiratory tract infection (URTI), lower respiratory tract infection (LRTI), asthma, bronchial hyperreactivity, and passive smoking. Chances of laryngospasm and apnea are more in infants because of the high vagal tone in infants.

All respiratory conditions should be optimized before surgery. There is still a debate about the

R. Kundal (✉)
Department of Anaesthesia and Critical Care, All India Institute of Medical Science, Vijaypur, J&K, India

© The Author(s), under exclusive license to Springer Nature Singapore Pte Ltd. 2025
S. Roy Choudhury (ed.), *Pediatric Surgery*, https://doi.org/10.1007/978-981-96-1257-4_6

period of postponing surgery in a patient with an active URTI. Due to a hyperreactive airway, children with URTI are at risk for adverse respiratory outcomes. As the airway remains hyperactive for 4–6 weeks, it is prudent to defer elective surgery for 4 weeks. It is suggested that if children have a running nose, a dry cough, or minor surgery scheduled that does not require tracheal intubation, an evaluation of the risk–benefit ratio can be used to decide whether to proceed with the procedure. However, surgery should be deferred in infants or children with a profuse running nose, productive cough, wheezes in the chest, or fever.

6.4 Preoperative Consideration in Children with Cardiovascular Ailments

All children with the symptomatic cardiac disease need proper preoperative cardiac evaluation by a pediatric cardiologist. Symptoms of cardiac disease include (1) failure to thrive, (2) cyanosis, (3) spells of loss of consciousness, (4) recurrent chest infections, (5) tachypnea, (6) sweating in an infant during feeding, etc.

All children with corrected cardiac anomalies like the patent ductus arteriosus and ventricular septal defects can be safely anesthetized after cardiac clearance. For infective endocarditis prophylaxis of various cardiac conditions, National Institute for health and care excellence (NICE) guidelines are followed (Box 6.1).

Box 6.1 NICE Guideline (Infective Endocarditis Prophylaxis)

High risk of infective endocarditis prophylaxis
Acquired valvular heart disease with stenosis or regurgitation. Valve replacement surgery. Structural congenital heart diseases, including surgically corrected or palliated structural conditions, but excluding isolated atrial septal defect, fully repaired ventricular septal defect, or fully repaired patent ductus arteriosus, and closure devices that are judged to be endothelialized. Previous infective endocarditis. Hypertrophic cardiomyopathy.
Antibiotic prophylaxis against IE is not recommended
For patients undergoing dental procedures. For patients undergoing non-dental procedures like lower gastro-intestinal tract, genitourinary tract, Ent procedures, bronchoscopy, upper and lower respiratory tract procedures.

Source:www.nice.org.uk

Risk to patients undergoing surgery is stratified by The American Society of Anaesthesiologists Physical Status risk stratification system (Box 6.2).

Box 6.2 The American Society of Anaesthesiologists Physical Status (ASA-PS) risk stratification system

ASA PS classification	Definition	Examples
ASA I	Healthy patient	Healthy (no acute or chronic disease), normal BMI percentile for age
ASA II	Mild systemic disease	Asymptomatic congenital cardiac disease, well-controlled dysrhythmias, asthma without exacerbation, well-controlled epilepsy, non-insulin-dependent diabetes mellitus, abnormal BMI percentile for age, mild/moderate obstructive sleep apnea (OSA), oncologic state in remission, autism with mild limitations
ASA III	Severe systemic disease	Uncorrected stable congenital cardiac abnormality, asthma with exacerbation, poorly controlled epilepsy, insulin-dependent diabetes mellitus, morbid obesity, malnutrition, severe OSA, oncologic state, renal failure, muscular dystrophy, cystic fibrosis, history of organ transplantation, brain/spinal cord malformation, symptomatic hydrocephalus, premature infant, post conceptional age (PCA) <60 weeks, autism with severe limitations, metabolic disease, difficult airway, long term parenteral nutrition. Full-term infants <6 weeks of age.
ASA IV	Systemic disease which is a constant threat to life	Symptomatic congenital cardiac abnormality, congestive heart failure, active sequelae of prematurity, acute hypoxic-ischemic encephalopathy, shock, sepsis, disseminated intravascular coagulation, automatic implantable cardioverter-defibrillator, ventilator dependence, endocrinopathy, severe trauma, severe respiratory distress, advanced oncologic state.
ASA V	Moribund patient not expected to survive without operation	Massive trauma, intracranial hemorrhage with mass effect, patient requiring ECMO, respiratory failure or arrest, malignant hypertension, decompensated congestive heart failure, hepatic encephalopathy, ischemic bowel or multiple organ/system dysfunction.
ASA VI	Brain dead patient for organ removal	

Source:asahq.org

[a]Addition of E stands for emergency surgery

Box 6.3 Preoperative fasting guidelines for children

Nature of fluid or food	Hours of fasting recommended
Water and clear liquids	2
Breast milk	4
Formula milk or cow milk	6
Solid food, sweets (including lollipops, swallowed chewing gums)	6

6.5 Preanesthetic Medications and Calming an Anxious Child

The preoperative period is stressful for children due to thoughts of parental separation and limited knowledge of operation theater (OT) and its proceedings. Anxiolysis is very much needed to allay the fears of these children.

Nonpharmacological means to reduce anxiety

(a) Preoperative counseling of children in front of parents: this psychological intervention gives parents and children a chance to ask questions regarding OT, surgical, and anesthesia proceedings and thus reduce their anxiety.
(b) Music therapy: it is proved by certain studies that music therapy helps in reducing anxiety in children.

6.6 Pharmacological Premedication

Premedication helps reduce children's anxiety, provides anterograde amnesia, eases parental separation, and reduces physiological stress, postoperative behavioral changes, and adverse outcomes.

Various drugs and routes of giving them have been described as a part of premedication regimens. Premedication drugs can be provided through intravenous (IV), oral, Intramuscular (IM), nasal, sublingual, or rectal routes.

Different drugs used as a premedication are:

1. *Benzodiazepines*
   (a) Midazolam: commonly used premedication produces anterograde amnesia, and memory is usually impaired 10 minutes after oral administration.
   (b) Diazepam: has prolonged half-life, is not a chosen premedicant, and is known to be neurotoxic in neonates. Oral dose –0.1-0.3 mg/kg.
   (c) Lorazepam: slow onset and slow offset, metabolized in the liver to inactive metabolites recommended only in inpatients. IV formulation is known to be toxic in neonates.

   Oral or IV dose 0.025–0.05 mg/kg.
2. *Ketamine*

   Ketamine acts by antagonizing N-methyl-D-aspartate receptors in the brain, causing dissociation of the cortex from the limbic system. It is associated with excessive secretion, so concurrent use of antisialogogues like Inj glycopyrrolate is recommended. Also, it is related to side effects like hallucination and emergence delirium; to counteract these, coadministration of benzodiazepines is advised.
3. *Opioids*

   Opioids are used as premedication in children having painful conditions; caution should be exercised as they are associated with respiratory depression, nausea, vomiting, and pruritus. They are not advised in neonates.
4. *Chloral Hydrate*

   It has a bitter taste and no analgesic property, should not be given to children with liver disease and neonates. Oral or rectal dose 20–75 mg/kg acts within 30–45 minutes.
5. *$\propto$ 2 Agonists*

   Dexmedetomidine is commonly used these days; it provides sedation, analgesia, and anxiolysis without respiratory depression.

Box 6.4 Showing commonly used premedication, route, and doses

Drug	Oral	IV	IM	Transmucosal	Rectal
Midazolam	0.25–0.75 mg/kg	0.025–0.1 mg/kg	0.1–0.2 mg/kg	0.2 mg/kg	1 mg/kg
Ketamine	4–6 mg/kg	0.25–0.5 mg/kg; onset 1–2 min	IM-1-2 mg/kg; onset 3–4 min	Nasal –3-5 mg/kg, onset 10–15 min	Rectal-5 mg/kg
Fentanyl	10–15 μgm/kg	1–2 μgm/kg		Nasal 1–2 μgm/kg	
Dexmedetomidine	2.5–4 μgm/kg			1–2 μgm/kg: Onset is 30–70 minutes	

6.7 Topical Local Anesthesia for IV Cannulations

Use of an eutectic mixture of local anesthetics (2.5% lidocaine and 2.5% prilocaine), known as EMLA cream, is recommended 1 hour before cannulation on the intact skin of the child where cannulation is planned. There is a risk of methemoglobinemia in infants younger than 3 months.

Other agents available include 4% tetracaine.

6.8 Anesthetic Management in Operation Theater

Before entering OT, consent for anesthesia and surgery should be checked, and the fasting status of the child should be reconfirmed.

Children's preferences should be kept in mind, and induction of anesthesia should be smooth and pleasant for kids. Sedative premedications generally improve anesthesia face mask acceptance. Inhalational induction is the preferred method in those without IV cannula; however, in the absence of a cannula, an inhalational agent is used to aid the insertion of an IV cannula. The inhalational drugs used to induce anesthesia in kids are sevoflurane and halothane. Desflurane and isoflurane are inappropriate since they are strong and create irritated airways. Sevoflurane is chosen over halothane because it induces less cardiovascular depression and faster induction.

Anaesthesiologists use sevoflurane in increments up to 8% for quick inhalational induction. After the child falls asleep, the IV line is secured, and other drugs are given as per the plan of anesthesia.

6.8.1 Intraoperative Monitoring

Monitoring equipment is used to support clinical findings and helps in minimizing unfavorable outcomes. Essential and desirable monitoring required for anesthesia to be administered safely in children is illustrated in (Box 6.5).

Box 6.5 Intraoperative monitoring

Essential monitoring	Desirable monitoring	Monitoring in special situations
Heart rate (HR) monitoring with electrocardiogram (ECG). Noninvasive blood pressure (NIBP). A pulse oximeter (SpO_2). Monitoring of end-tidal carbon dioxide ($EtCO_2$). Temperature monitoring. Precordial stethoscope.	Anesthesia gas monitoring (oxygen, carbon dioxide, and anesthetic gases) monitoring. Mean airway pressure, pressure–volume loops, and plateau pressure monitoring. Peripheral nerve stimulator or ultrasound monitoring for placing regional nerve block.	Invasive blood pressure monitoring. Central venous pressure monitoring. Cardiac output monitoring. Intracranial pressure monitoring.

Desirable monitoring (necessary for the best results, but the absence of which will not jeopardize the child's safety).

6.8.2 Inhalational Agents

Several inhalation agents are available for the induction and upkeep of anesthesia. The choice of agent is based on the child's age and the nature of the procedure. Each agent has both general and unique benefits and drawbacks. None of the inhalational agents guarantees stable hemodynamics. Inhalation agents are typically avoided in kids with substantial cardiac depression or hemodynamic instability or should be administered at significantly lower doses. Regardless of age, most inhalation agents can be used safely and effectively on healthy children. Often inhalational agents are used to aid the insertion of an IV cannula. Still, there is a risk of bradycardia, hypotension, and even cardiac arrest at higher concentrations of inhalational agents. The introduction of newer inhalation agents like sevoflurane has added safety to inhalational induction compared to earlier used halothane. Age-related differences in absorption, the need for anesthesia, and the sensitivity of the cardiovascular system are all thought to contribute to the prevalence of unwanted effects from powerful inhalation medications in preterm or critically ill newborns. Various factors like variations in blood-gas solubility coefficients, blood-tissue solubility coefficients, body composition, the ratio of alveolar ventilation to functional residual capacity, and the distribution of cardiac output are responsible for the pace of induction of anesthesia with an inhalational agent. The minimum alveolar concentration can be used to titrate the volatile anesthetic amount to obtain and maintain a safe level of anesthesia. The minimum alveolar concentration (MAC) is the lowest concentration of an inhalation anesthetic at 1 atm of pressure required to prevent 50% of patients from moving their skeletal muscles in reaction to a surgical incision.

Halothane is a nonirritant, nonpungent inhalational agent that can be used for inhalational induction in children. Still, it is not a good induction agent as it is associated with bradycardia, hypotension, and arrhythmias.

Sevoflurane has a sweet odor and a low blood-gas partition coefficient, thus suitable for hastened induction in children. It is associated with less cardiovascular depression as compared to halothane. It is the induction agent of choice in pediatric patients. However, no inhalational agent is idle.

Prolonged use of sevoflurane is associated with emergence delirium (ED). Children with ED exhibit inconsolable, irritable, uncompromising, or uncooperative behaviors or a mix of these behaviors.

Isoflurane has a pungent odor, irritable to the airway; thus not appropriate for inhalational induction. It maintains heart rate and is less arrhythmogenic but sometimes is associated with bradycardia in neonates.

Desflurane has a very low blood-gas partition coefficient, so induction is fast. However, it has a very pungent odor and is irritant to the airway, associated with high chances of laryngospasm, so poor choice as the induction agent.

It is also associated with emergence delirium and is expensive too.

6.8.3 Nitrous Oxide

It is a nonpotent inhalational agent, most commonly used in adjunct to other potent inhalational agents; it has a high MAC (105%), so it facilitates early induction by carrying other gases along and thus reducing their side effects.

Advantages—it is inexpensive, odorless, and reduces vasodilatation or cardiac depression caused by other inhalational agents.

Disadvantages—incapable of providing general anesthesia alone, precautions to be taken as it expands the air in closed spaces like the middle ear, intestine, etc. There is a risk of expansion of pneumothorax or pneumocephalus with its use. Its exposure in the operating room is related to the cause of neuropathies. Nitrous oxide is a potent greenhouse gas and is associated with ozone depletion.

6.9 Intravenous Agents

Propofol is the most commonly used drug in day-care surgeries. It has a quick onset and quick off-set; it is also used for procedural sedation and monitored anesthesia care. It has the advantage of reducing postoperative nausea and vomiting; however, it is a respiratory depressant and causes vasodilation. Propofol injection alone is painful, so it should be mixed with inj Lignocaine (0.5–1 mg/kg), and a large vein should be chosen for injection. Its use should be avoided in children allergic to eggs as it causes allergic reactions.

Thiopentone—among barbiturates, thiopentone is ultra short-acting and the most commonly used induction agent; its dose varies with the child's age, and the requirement is usually higher in children than adults. It has a quick onset (30–45 sec) but a very long half-life inside the body, so it is inappropriate for daycare anesthesia or enhanced recovery after anesthesia. Thiopentone decreases intracranial pressure, depresses the myocardium, and is a respiratory depressant. It comes in yellow amorphous powder, which must be reconstituted with sterile water to make a 2.5% solution for children and a 1% solution for neonates and infants. This is the only available induction agent for rapid sequence induction.

Ketamine—it produces a trans-like state (dissociative anesthesia). Ketamine has analgesic properties, is an effective bronchodilator, and preserves airway reflexes, so it is used for procedural sedation. It is associated with side effects like excessive secretions and agitation post-anesthesia, so concurrent use of benzodiazepines and anticholinergics is recommended.

Its use as an induction agent is beneficial in patients with congenital heart diseases with the right-to-left shunts, e.g., tetralogy of Fallot.

Etomidate—it is the most cardiostable induction agent, so it is a chosen drug for anticipated hemodynamic instability. But it is associated with a risk of adrenal depression even with a single dose in some patients.

Box 6.6 Showing IV induction agents and their doses

	Propofol	Thiopentone	Ketamine	Etomidate
Neonate	3–4 mg/kg bw IV	2.5–3 mg/kg IV		
Infant	2.6–3.4 mg/kg bw IV	6–7 mg/kg IV	2 mg/kg bw IV	0.3 mg/kgbw IV
Children	2.5–3 mg/kg bw IV	5–6 mg/kg IV	2 mg/kg bw IV	0.3 mg/kgbw IV

6.10 Airway Devices and Ventilation Strategies in the Operating Room

Airway devices are the connection between anesthetized patients and ventilation equipment.

Various equipment can be used as the interface to aid ventilation, e.g., anesthesia face mask, nasopharyngeal airway, supraglottic airway devices, and endotracheal tubes.

6.10.1 Anesthesia Face Mask

Pediatric anesthesia masks are available in various sizes to fit children of all ages, from newborns to teenagers. Selecting the correct size mask is crucial to achieving a good fit and a strong seal. Rendell-Baker Soucek masks with low dead space are used for neonates and infants. Scented transparent masks are available for pleasant induction of anesthesia and easy visualization of

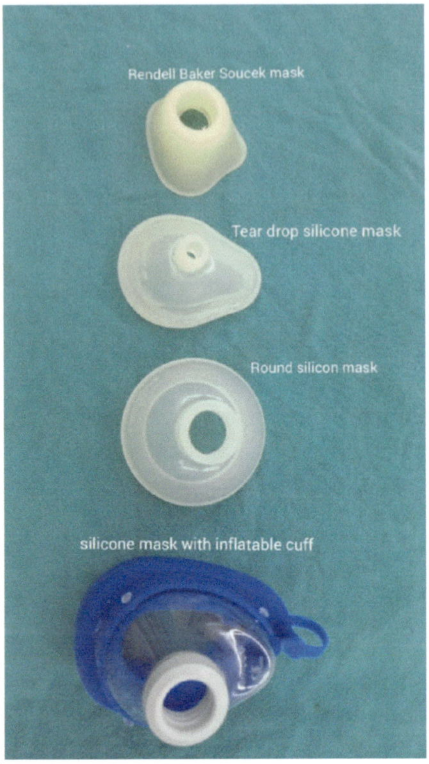

Fig. 6.1 Showing different types of anesthesia face mask (pediatric)

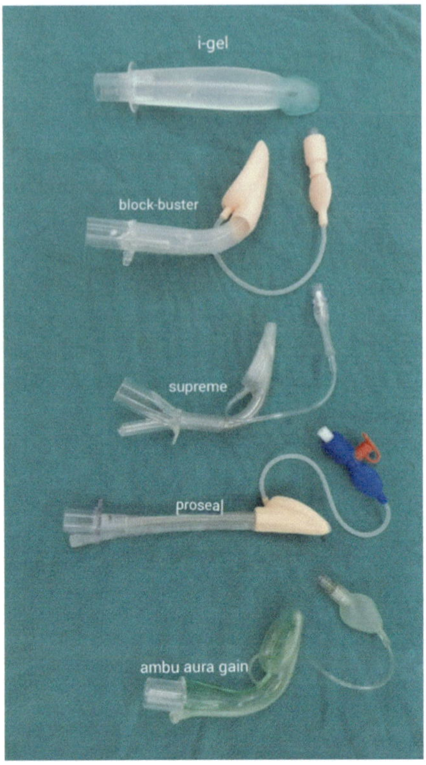

Fig. 6.2 Showing the different varieties of laryngeal mask airway devices

any secretion or vomitus. Different types of face masks are available as shown in Fig. 6.1.

Proper positioning of the mask is ensured by holding the apex of the mask on the nasal bridge and base between the lip and chin and pressing it down with the index finger and thumb in a C shape, simultaneously elevating the jaw up with the last three fingers in the form of E.

6.10.2 Supraglottic Airway Devices

They are used as rescue airway devices in case of failed endotracheal intubation. They are used in all surgeries except those involving body cavities and are broadly classified into first generation (without gastric channel) and second generation devices (with gastric channel for stomach decompression). Different varieties of devices are shown in Fig. 6.2 and their available sizes are shown in Box 6.7.

Box 6.7 Different types of LMA, sizes, and special features

Name of device	Sizes available	Special features
LMA Proseal	1, 1.5, 2, 2.5, 3, 4, 5	Reusable LMA with inflatable cuff and gastric drain tube
LMA supreme	1, 1.5, 2, 2.5, 3, 4, 5	Disposable preformed LMA, gastric tube
I-gel	1, 1.5, 2, 2.5, 3, 4	Noninflatable cuff, gastric tube integrated bite block
LMA ambu aura gain	1,1.5,2,2.5,3,4,5,6	Gastric channel, preformed airway tube (can be used as a conduit for endotracheal intubation)
Blockbuster LMA	1, 1.5, 2, 2.5, 3, 4, 5	Intubating LMA, comes with flexo metallic endotracheal tube

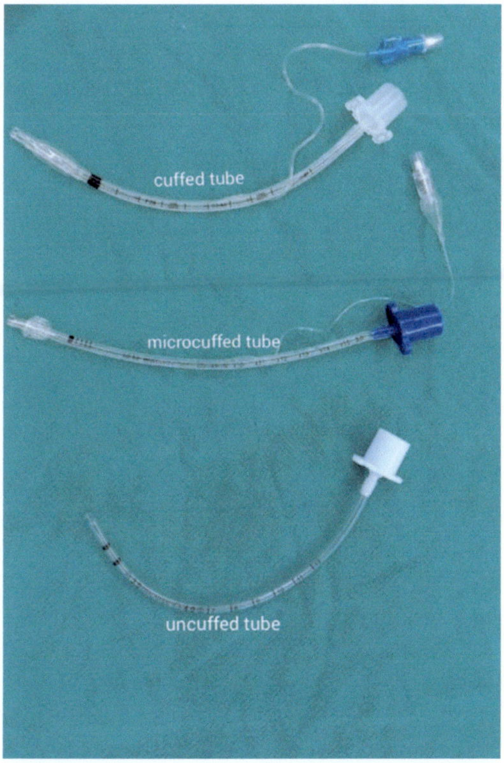

Fig. 6.3 Showing different types of endotracheal tubes

6.10.3 Endotracheal Tubes (ETT)

A few years back, only uncuffed tubes were preferred in children below 6 years of age, considering cricoid cartilage as the narrowest part, but now it is clear that the narrowest part is subglottis which is elliptical and has a long anteroposterior diameter. So, the availability of microcuffed tubes (thin, distally placed polyurethane cuff) is a boon. Such ETTs can be used in small children with minimized leaks and better ventilation, thus improving oxygenation. So, cuffed, uncuffed, and microcuffed endotracheal tubes are available in pediatric patients. Maintaining intracuff pressure between 20 and 30 cmH_2O for cuffed endotracheal tubes is recommended. Various sizes of endotracheal tubes are shown in Fig. 6.3, and Box 6.8 shows the calculation of tube size and determination of the fixation length of the tube depending on the age of the patient.

Tracheal intubation technique: a slight roll beneath the shoulders is helpful in neonates and newborns because of their large heads. A head ring can stabilize the head, but care must be taken to avoid hyperflexion, making laryngoscopy and intubation challenging. In older children, head extension is needed for intubation; a pillow is not necessary, but stabilizing the head is essential. Initial settings of the ventilator in the Intensive care unit (ICU)/ward according to age are shown in Box 6.9.

Box 6.8 Endotracheal tube size calculation

Age	Endotracheal tube size	Depth of fixation
Preterm neonate	2.5 mmID	Usually at 7–8 cm
Term neonate	3.0 mmID	Usually at 9–10 cm
1–10 years (uncuffed)	(age/4) + 4	12 + age/2 = length of tube in cm
1–10 years (cuffed)	(age/4) + 3	Same as above

Box 6.9 Initial setting for mechanical ventilation in ICU/ward

Pressure control mode ventilator settings	<1 Year	1–12 Years
FiO_2	Start with 100%, wean rapidly to 60%	Start with 100%, wean rapidly to 60%
Respiratory rate in breaths per min	20–30	15–25
Pressure support in cm H_2O	6–10	6–10
PEEP in cm H_2O	3–7	3–7
PIP in cm H_2O	16–25	16–25
Flow trigger in L/min	0.25–0.5	0.8–2

FIO_2 fraction of inspired oxygen, *PEEP* peak end-expiratory pressure, *PIP* peak inspiratory pressure (note that settings have to be adjusted as per clinical status of the patients)

6.11 Postoperative Pain Assessment and Pain Management

Scales used to assess pain include behavior observational scale (validated in<3 years), F-Face, L-Legs, A-Activity, C-Cry, C-Consolability (FLACC) scale (validated in 2–7 years), Cheops (validated in 1–7 years), Wong-Baker Faces scale, C-Crying, R-Requires oxygen, E-Expression, S-Sleeplessness (CRIES), and N-Non crying facial expression, I-Infant cry, P-Posture of arm/leg, State of arousal (NIPS) (validated in <1 year).

Postoperative pain management varies with the type of surgery, but multimodal analgesia techniques are usually used to manage pain in the post-anesthesia care unit.

Analgesia plan may include paracetamol, nonsteroidal medications, opioids, local anesthesia, nerve blocks, regional anesthesia, patient-controlled IV analgesia, or patient-controlled epidural analgesia.

Analgesia options to manage postoperative pain are shown in Box 6.10.

Box 6.10 Analgesia option to manage postoperative pain

Drug	Dose
Oral paracetamol	15 mg/kg bw
Oral ibuprofen	10 mg/kg bw
IV Ketrolac	0.2–0.5 mg/kg
IV fentanyl	0.5–2 μgm/kg

6.11.1 Local Anesthetics

Local anesthetics act by interrupting the propagation of nerves by blocking sodium channels. They are broadly categorized into aminoesters (metabolism by plasma pseudocholinesterase and other nonspecific esterases) and aminoamides (undergoing hepatic metabolism). Their examples and maximum dose limit are shown in Box 6.11.

Box 6.11 Types of local anesthetic agents and their doses

Aminoesters	Maximum dose in mg/kg	Maximum dose with epinephrine (mg/kg)	Aminoamides	Maximum dose in mg/kg	Maximum dose with epinephrine (mg/kg)
Cocaine			Bupivacaine	3 mg/kg	3 mg/kg
Procaine	7 mg/kg	10 mg/kg	Levobupivacaine	3 mg/kg	3 mg/kg
Tetracaine			Lidocaine	5 mg/kg	10 mg/kg
Benzocaine			Prilocaine	7 mg/kg	10 mg/kg
Chloroprocaine	7 mg/kg	10 mg/kg	Ropivacaine	4 mg/kg	Epinephrine not needed

Overdose of the local anesthetic agent or accidental injection in the intravascular compartment may result in local anesthesia systemic toxicity (LAST). It comprises cardiovascular and neurological symptoms.

CVS symptoms include tachycardia, hypotension, myocardial depression, arrhythmia conduction blocks, and cardiac arrest in severe cases.

CNS premonitory symptoms include confusion, agitation, dizziness, perioral tingling, slurred speech, tinnitus, visual disturbances, and auditory disturbances. Tremors and muscle twitching in the face and extremities follow. This excitatory stage ends in tonic and clonic generalized convulsions, eventually progressing into the depressing stage of respiratory arrest and coma. Children's early excitatory phase is concealed because they frequently receive sedation or general anesthesia before receiving regional or peripheral blocks.

6.11.1.1 Management of LAST

Early treatment of LAST is recommended; on noticing initial symptoms, immediately stop local anesthetic injection, start oxygen, and manage symptomatically. As per guideline, intralipid treatment should be considered as soon as LAST is detected, especially if there are notable neurological (like seizures) or cardiovascular symptoms (like hypotension, arrhythmias, or cardiac arrest). The disease can be stopped from developing into a serious cardiovascular collapse by using it early.

(a) Seizure management:
  (i) 100% oxygen and airway management (mask ventilation or tracheal intubation).
  (ii) Inj midazolam 0.05 mg/kg IV or Inj diazepam 0.1–0.2 mg/kg IV.
  (iii) Inj phenytoin 5 mg/kg slow IV over minutes.

(b) CVS symptom management:
  (i) 100% oxygenation with mask ventilation or tracheal intubation as per the situation.
  (ii) Administer sodium bicarbonate at 2 mg/kg bw IV to prevent metabolic acidosis.
  (iii) In case of persistent bradycardia Inj atropine 0.02 mg is recommended.
  (iv) For persistent hypotension, IV inotropic medications, such as epinephrine (0.1 mL/kg of a 1/10,000 solution), dopamine or dobutamine (2–10 g/kg/minute) or isoprenaline 0.1 μg/kg (rarely necessary) can be used.
  (v) For cardiac arrest, administration of intralipid emulsion (ILE) to be used alongside Advanced Cardiac Life Support (ACLS) to reverse LA- induced cardiac\arrest.
  (vi) Administration of intralipid emulsion (ILE) can be used to reverse LA-induced cardiac\arrest

Dose of intralipid bolus of 20% ILE at 1.5 mL/kg; infusion 10–15 mL/kg/hr. (maximum dose 12 mg/kg).

Treatment for newborns with methemoglobinemia caused by prilocaine poisoning involves an IV injection of 1–5 mg/kg of methylene blue. It instantly transforms methemoglobin into hemoglobin.

6.11.1.2 Central Neuraxial Blocks

All central neuraxial blocks given in adults can be placed in the pediatric population, including spinal anesthesia, epidural anesthesia, and caudal block. But they slightly differ as sedation or general anesthesia is often required before placing these blocks.

Spinal anesthesia-spinal block can be placed in all pediatric patients, including neonates. It is easy and quick in onset and requires only a small amount of local anesthetic agent. The drug is injected into the lumbar cerebrospinal fluid, resulting in excellent analgesia, anesthesia, and motor blockade. Spinal block in children is often given under sedation.

Indications are given in Box 6.12.

Box 6.12 Indications for spinal anesthesia

Indications of spinal anesthesia in pediatric patients
Lower body surgery, including lower abdominal, inguinal, urologic, and lower limb operations. Surgical procedures performed on high-risk, premature newborns (inguinal hernia). Children with recent upper respiratory tract infection where general anesthesia and airway instrumentation have to be avoided. Emergency surgery feasible in a spinal block in full-stomach patient. Difficult airway Comorbidities like lung diseases, neuromuscular disease, malignant hyperthermia susceptibility, as well as cardiac surgery, suppressing the stress response, and resource-poor settings, are associated comorbidities.

Box 6.13 Local anesthetic dose for spinal block

Weight of the patient	Inj bupivacaine/Inj levobupivacaine Dose	Inj ropivacaine Dose
<5 kg	0.5–0.6 mg/kg (0.1–0.12 mL/kg)	0.5–1 mg/kg (0.1–0.2 mL/kg)
5–15 kg	0.4 mg/kg (0.08 mL/kg)	0.5 mg/kg (0.1 mL/kg)
>15 kg	0.3 mg/kg (0.06 mL/kg)	0.3–0.4 mg/kg

Equipment, drug, and dosing—special small sizes varying from 2 to 5 cm and thicknesses of 25–27 gauze pediatric spinal needles are available for performing lumber punctures. Drugs and doses are shown in Box 6.13. Duration of the spinal block is usually shorter (80–90 minutes).

6.11.1.3 Epidural Block

Local anesthetic agent is deposited in the epidural space. An epidural block is usually given as an adjunct to general anesthesia in children to manage intraoperative and postoperative pain. Depending on the surgery level and the analgesia requirement, it can be placed in a lumbar epidural or thoracic epidural space. Single-shot drug injection and continuous drug infusion through the epidural catheter are manageable.

Equipment, drug, and dosages.

Three different sizes—Tuohy needles with or without catheters are available in the market 18, 19, and 20 Gauze. Tiny 5 cm needles are used in <10 kg patients. Drugs and dosages are shown in Box 14.

Box 6.14 Local anesthetic doses for epidural analgesia

Local anesthetic agent	Initial loading dose	Maintenance bolus dose	Infusion dose
Bupivacaine or Levobupivacaine preservative free	0.25%concentration up to 20 kg: 0.75 mL/kg From 20 to 40 kg: 8–10 mL >40 kg: Adult doses	0.125–0.2% concentration 0.1–0.3 mL/kg every 6–12 hr	Age < 4 months: 0.0625% of drug @ of 0.3 mL/kg Age 4–18 months: 0.0625% of drug@ of 0.4 mL/kg Age > 18 months 0.0625% of drug@ of 0.6 mL/kg
Ropivacaine	0.2% concentration @ same dose as bupivacaine	0.1–0.2%concentration @ 0.1–0.3 mL/kg every 6–12 hr	0.1–0.2%concentration@ same dose as bupivacaine

6.11.2 Caudal Block

Caudal block is most commonly performed regional procedure in pediatric patients for below umbilicus surgeries. It is straightforward and relatively easy to learn.

Indications include lower abdomen surgery, inguinal hernia repair, orchidopexy, circumcision, lower limb, and pelvic orthopedic surgery. A sole block without General Anaesthesia (GA) can be placed in premature neonates for inguinal hernia repair—contraindications: local infection, local anesthetic toxicity, sacral defects, etc.

Needles used: special caudal needles varying in size (20G, 22G, 25G) are available in the market. For small neonates, hypodermic needles can be used to place caudal blocks.

Dose and volume of drug: recommended dose is 0.5 mL/kg for the sacral block,1 mL/kg for the thoracolumbar block, and 1.25 mL/kg for the mid thoracic block.

6.12 Common Anesthesia-Related Complications

1. *Airway obstruction and arterial oxygen desaturation*: switch to 100% oxygen. Correct the underlying cause (equipment failure, airway device displacement, obstruction, bronchospasm, laryngospasm, etc.).
2. *Laryngospasm*: reflex closure of vocal cords resulting from hyperstimulation of the airway, hypersensitive airway, recent URTI/LRTI, etc. Manage with 100% oxygen along 5–10 cm of continuous airway pressure, deepening plane of anesthesia with propofol, inj lidocaine 1.0–1.5 mg/kg or inj succinylcholine 0.5–1.0 mg/kg is recommended.
3. *Bronchospasm*: treatment options include salbutamol via metered dose inhaler through the endotracheal tube. In persistent bronchospasm, IV adrenaline at 1–2 μgm/kg is recommended.
4. *Bradycardia*: common causes of bradycardia in children are hypoxia and vagal stimulation. Treatment is to address the underlying cause and 20 μgm/kg of IV atropine.

6.13 Conventional Ventilation in Neonates

Mechanical ventilation is commonly required in case of ventilatory failure in neonates and is potentially life-saving.

Mechanical ventilation ensures adequate gas exchange. With the advancement in medical science and technology, delivering small tidal volumes and flow through sophisticated ventilation modes is possible, even for premature neonates.

The goal of mechanical ventilation in neonates:

1. To oxygenate the neonate.
2. Ensure the removal of carbon dioxide.
3. To avoid damage to the lung.

Modes of ventilation used for neonates: conventionally, positive pressure ventilation is used for ventilating neonates, but with advanced ventilators, minimal flow, and tidal volume can be delivered. So, volume-targeted ventilation is emerging as a choice mode of ventilation.

Components of neonatal mechanical ventilation.

1. Tidal volume (V_T): the amount of gas inspired during a single spontaneous breath or by breath delivered through mechanical inflation. It is normally 4–6 ml/kg in neonates.
2. Minute ventilation (V_E): normal 0.2–0.3 L/min/kg in neonates.
   (V_E) = (V_T) in ml x RR/F Per min.
   V_T—tidal volume.
   RR—respiratory rate.
   F—respiratory frequency.
3. Inspiratory time (i time)

Inspiration is spontaneously breathing neonates in an active process of 0.35–0.40 sec in full-term infants, whereas it is near about 0.30–0.30 sec in a preterm neonate.

So inspiratory time is to be set around 0.30–0.40 sec.

In the case of stiff lungs, inspiratory time may be required to increase to improve oxygenation.

Increasing inspiration time on the ventilator increases air flow into the lung and generates enough pressure to open up the alveoli. Thus, helping in the diffusion of air/oxygen in the lungs.

Volume targeted ventilation: aim tidal volume of 4–6 mL/kg body weight and set alarm limits for minute ventilation should be set 10–20% above. The limit of minute ventilation is 0.20–0.30 L/min/kg.

Expiration—elastic recoil of the lung is mainly responsible for expiration which is a passive process.

Elastic recoil of the lung depends on lung tissue elasticity, surface tension due to our liquid interface, and the structure of the rib cage.

The airway may collapse at the end of the expiration resulting in atelectasis; this can be prevented by positive end-expiratory pressure.

Positive end-expiratory pressure (PEEP): PEEP is recommended ranging from 4 to 6 cm of H_2O.

Concept of wasted ventilation in neonates.

Anatomic dead space: the part of respiratory gases that fail to arrive at the level of the respiratory bronchioles and alveoli but remain in the conducting airway is known as anatomic dead space.

The volume of anatomic dead space is 1.5 mL/kg; adding to this is usually fixed (Tube connector, flow sensor, Y-Piece). The total dead space is generally significant in extremely low birth weight neonates.

Alveolar dead space: tidal volume delivered to unperfused or less perfused alveoli is alveolar dead space.

A combination of anatomic dead space and alveolar dead space is physiologic dead space (V_{DS}).

Wasted ventilation = V_{DS}/V_{T}.

So, wasted ventilation is the amount of tidal volume not taking part in actual gas exchange.

There is more wasted ventilation in a 500 g preterm than in a term baby.

Thus, the tidal volume required by preterm neonates is more, i.e., 5 ml/kg, whereas it will be around 4 mL/kg in a term baby.

6.14 High-Frequency Oscillation (HFO) Ventilation

High-frequency oscillatory ventilation (HFOV) is a mode of mechanical ventilation that decreases ventilator-induced lung damage and enhances clinical outcomes. It delivers breaths at a very high rate with the tidal volume either less than or equal to anatomical dead space where mean airway pressure is kept constant. HFO ventilation is often utilized in conditions of diffuse alveolar damage. Since the lung volume is the primary determinant of oxygenation during HFO ventilation, the strategy is to keep alveoli open by repeated recruitment maneuvers. The indications for HFOV are imprecise and mainly depend on the attending physician's preferences. HFOV is often only used as an option if traditional mechanical ventilation fails.

6.14.1 Extracorporeal Membrane Oxygenation (ECMO)

Extracorporeal membrane oxygenation refers to bypassing patients' failed cardiopulmonary or only pulmonary system. The components of the ECMO machine are (1) a mechanical pump, (2) a membrane oxygenator, and a heat exchanger.

Two primary ECMO types are (a) venovenous (VV) and (b) venoarterial (VA).

Venovenous ECMO can be utilized in conditions where cardiac functions are preserved, and isolated lung failure exists. Cannulas are placed in a large venous line; blood is drawn and circulated through a membrane oxygenator, warmed, and recirculated in the venous system. Thus, bypassing lungs and improving oxygenation.

Venoarterial ECMO has a role in conditions where there is a total cardiopulmonary failure. A cannula for drainage of deoxygenated blood is inserted in the internal jugular vein; blood is passed through the membrane oxygenator, warmed, and infused into a large artery like the internal carotid artery. Venoarterial ECMO thus provides mechanical hemodynamic support along with improved oxygenation.

Referring patient for ECMO.

Parameter for impaired gas exchange is oxygenation index (OI).

OI = Mean airway pressure × FiO_2 × 100/PaO_2.

Consider transfer if OI >25 in conditions like respiratory distress syndrome, pulmonary hypertension, congenital diaphragmatic hernia, pneumonia, meconium aspiration syndrome, etc.

Summary box

1. Neonates, infants, and young children have morphological, physiological, pharmacological, emotional, and social characteristics entirely distinct from adults.
2. Any acute or chronic condition should be optimized before elective surgery in children.
3. Children with URTI are at risk of adverse respiratory events; it is prudent to defer elective surgery for 4 weeks.
4. The presence of procedure-appropriate consent is to be ensured.
5. Electrocardiography, pulse oximetry, noninvasive blood pressure monitoring, temperature, and end-tidal carbon dioxide monitoring are components of minimal mandatory monitoring.
6. Anesthetic agents like sevoflurane and propofol are used in daycare surgeries.
7. Age and weight-appropriate airway devices are needed to be selected for safe airway management.
8. All neuraxial and regional blocks are equally possible and effective in pediatric patients as in adults.
9. Multimodal analgesia is recommended for postoperative pain management.
10. Prompt detection and early supportive treatment of local anesthesia toxicity are recommended.
11. High-frequency oscillatory ventilation is an alternative ventilation strategy.
12. Extracorporeal membrane oxygenation can be utilized in lung or cardiopulmonary failure situations.

Suggested Reading

Boric K, Dosenovic S, Jelicic Kadic A, et al. Interventions for postoperative pain in children: an overview of systematic reviews. Paediatr Anaesth. 2017;27:893.

Cravero JP, Havidich JE. Pediatric sedation—evolution, and revolution. Paediatr Anaesth. 2011;21:800.

Mitchell MC, Farid I. Anesthesia for common pediatric emergency surgeries. Surg Clin North Am. 2017;97:223.

Suresh S, Ecoffey C, Bosenberg A, Lonnqvist P-A, de Oliveira GS Jr, de Leon Casasola O, de Andrés J, Ivani G. The European Society of Regional Anaesthesia and Pain Therapy/American Society of Regional Anesthesia and PainMedicine Recommendations on Local Anesthetics and Adjuvants Dosage in Pediatric Regional Anesthesia. Reg Anesth Pain Med. 2018;43:211.

Vargas A, Sawardekar A, Suresh S. Updates on pediatric regional anesthesia safety data. Curr Opin Anaesthesiol. 2019;32:649.

7 Antenatal Diagnosis and Management of Fetal Anomalies

Manisha Kumar and Subhasis Roy Choudhury

7.1 Introduction

Major congenital anomalies are seen in 3% of live births, 15% of cases with perinatal death. Antenatal screening tests are universally recommended for all pregnant women for the early detection of fetal anomalies. After detection of the anomaly, counseling the family regarding its prognosis and outcome becomes necessary. This is currently best done by the team of experts from obstetrics, fetal medicine, pediatric surgery, neonatology, and radiology.

7.2 Antenatal Diagnosis and Counseling

The role of antenatal counseling is to provide information to prospective parents regarding the cause, prognosis, possible interventions, timing, and the route of delivery, apart from information regarding the expected postnatal outcome and follow-up. The benefit includes antenatal transfer to the appropriate center where the newborn would receive appropriate treatment and preparedness of the facility and the parents to cope with the adverse circumstances due to the anomaly. The care of such patients should begin early and counseling should include follow-up and information regarding the risk of recurrence.

7.3 Procedures Currently Available for Fetal Diagnosis Are

- Ultrasonography, fetal echocardiography
- Procedures—amniocentesis, chorionic villous sampling, cordocentesis
- Genetic tests—karyotyping, fluorescent in situ hybridization, chromosomal microarray (CMA), enzymatic assays, and whole-exome sequencing.
- Fetal MRI

Ultrasonography is the ideal screening test. A detailed structural sonography done at 18–20 weeks detects major structural abnormalities (Table 7.1).

M. Kumar (✉)
Lady Hardinge Medical College, New Delhi, India

S. Roy Choudhury
Pediatric Surgery, Lady Hardinge Medical College and Associated Kalawati Saran Children's Hospital, New Delhi, Delhi, India

© The Author(s), under exclusive license to Springer Nature Singapore Pte Ltd. 2025

S. Roy Choudhury (ed.), *Pediatric Surgery*, https://doi.org/10.1007/978-981-96-1257-4_7

Table. 7.1 1st and 2nd trimester marker for aneuploidy

Soft markers	Major malformation
First trimester Nuchal translucency Absent nasal bone *Second trimester* Echogenic intracardiac focus Pylectasis Short humerus and femur Echogenic bowel Nuchal fold thickness (>6 mm) Mild ventriculomegaly Hypoplastic nasal bone	Cardiac defect Duodenal atresia Cystic hygroma Non-immune hydrops Omphalocele CDH/EA Limb anomalies Orofacial anomalies Renal anomalies

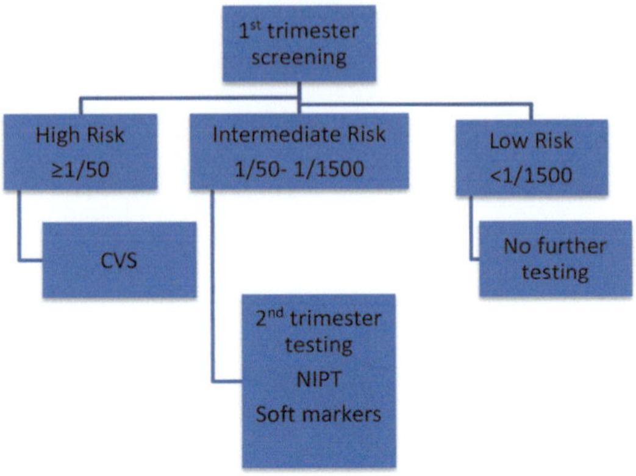

Fig. 7.1 Contingent screening test

7.3.1 Fetal Malformations Which Can Be Detected by Antenatal Ultrasonography

- Spina bifida and hydrocephalus
- Craniofacial/limb anomalies
- Twins/conjoint twins
- Abdominal wall defects (gastroschisis, exomphalos)
- Intestinal atresias (esophageal, duodenal, bowel)
- Congenital lung lesions
- Renal tract disease
- Congenital diaphragmatic hernia (CDH)
- Bladder/cloacal exstrophy
- Cardiac defects
- Tumors: teratomas, lymphangiomas

7.3.2 Screening Tests

In the first trimester, the combined test which involves maternal age, nuchal translucency, and biomarkers pregnancy associated plasma protein A (PAPP-A) and free beta human chorionic gonadotrophin (hCG) estimation gives the aneuploidy detection rate of 85% at 5% false-positive rate. In the second trimester (15–20 weeks), quadruple test can be performed which includes maternal age along with biomarkers alpha fetoprotein, human chorionic gonadotrophin (hCG), unconjugated estriol (uE3), and inhibin A. The test requires pre- and post-test counseling, usually 1:250 is taken as cut-off to be considered for recommending further definitive testing. To reduce the false-negative report and to increase the detection, contingent screening is advised (Fig. 7.1).

Currently, cell-free fetal DNA testing in the maternal blood offers an effective screening test for aneuploidy in high-risk women. However, because of its limitation of detecting fetal abnormalities and questionable cost effectiveness, combined first-trimester screening is still the choice in low-risk women.

7.4 Antenatal Diagnosis and Treatment

Antenatal diagnosis helps in planning further management.

The following modes of management may be adopted for antenatally detected anomalies

- *Managed by termination*: medical termination of pregnancy can be opted by the couple and is allowed as per medical termination of pregnancy (MTP) act of different countries for malformations that are considered incompatible with life or having major degree of handicap. Anencephaly, hydranencephaly, holoprosencephaly, severe chromosomal anomalies like trisomy 13, bilateral renal agenesis, infantile polycystic renal disease, metabolic diseases like Tay-Sachs disease, and lethal bone dysplasia are some examples.

- *Correction after term delivery*: most of the malformations are managed by this mode. A pediatric surgical team should be available to manage the newborn. Some examples include esophageal and gastrointestinal atresias, cysts, duplications, meconium ileus, small omphalocele or gastroschisis, unilateral hydronephrosis, craniofacial, limb or chest wall deformities, small cystic hygromas, teratomas, mesoblastic nephromas, neuroblastoma, cysts like choledochal, ovarian, mesenteric, duplication, cystic lung malformations without hydrops and diaphragmatic hernia without much lung hypoplasia.
- *Cesarean delivery*: for large lesions that may interfere with normal delivery. It may be needed in conjoint twins, large hydrocephalus or meningomyelocele, giant omphalocele, large sacrococcygeal or cervical teratoma.
- *Induced preterm delivery*: where continuing with pregnancy is considered harmful. Intrauterine growth retardation, progressively enlarging hydrocephalus, hydrothorax, abdominal wall defects with damaged bowel, intestinal ischemia, and necrosis secondary to volvulus or meconium ileus.
- Ex utero intrapartum procedure (EXIT): the fetus is maintained on uteroplacental circulation till the airway is secured. This is done for fetuses with compromised airway, e.g., congenital high airway obstruction syndrome, large cervical teratoma, mass (like cystic hygroma) obstructing airway, congenital chest masses preventing lung expansion, and lung immaturity requiring ECMO.
- *Fetal interventions.*

7.4.1 Fetal Surgery

7.4.1.1 Defects Treated by Open Fetal Surgery

- Congenital cystic adenomatoid malformation, pulmonary sequestration
- Congenital heart disease
- Myelomeningocele
- Sacrococcygeal teratoma

7.4.1.2 MIS (Minimally Invasive) Fetal Surgery

The current indications for minimally invasive fetoscopic surgery (Fetendo) are

- Twin–twin transfusion syndrome—laser ablation of vessels supplying the parasitic twin
- Fetal bladder obstructions—vesicoamniotic shunt, fetoscopic valve ablation
- Aortic or pulmonary valvuloplasty, atrial septostomy
- Congenital diaphragmatic hernia—balloon tracheal occlusion (plug lung until it grows (PLUG))
- Spina bifida—fetoscopic closure of the malformation

7.5 Indications for In-Utero Fetal Intervention

7.5.1 Antenatal Diagnosis of Lower Urinary Tract Obstruction (LUTO)

Fetuses with abnormal ultrasound findings before 24 weeks fare worse than those who develop features of obstruction after 24 weeks of gestation. Ultrasonographic features of bilateral hydroureteronephrosis (Fig. 7.2a), enlarged bladder (Fig. 7.2b), dilated posterior urethra, and oligohydramnios in a male baby with normal karyotype and no other life-threatening malformation are considered for intervention. Urinary electrolytes such as sodium if less than 100 mEq/L, chloride less than 90 mEq/L, osmolality less than 210 mEq/L, or β_2-microglobulin levels less than 6 mg/L are considered to be associated with favorable outcome.

Ruano et al. proposed a classification of LUTO according to the severity from mild to severe with or without potential for prevention of renal impairment and pulmonary hypoplasia (Table 7.2).

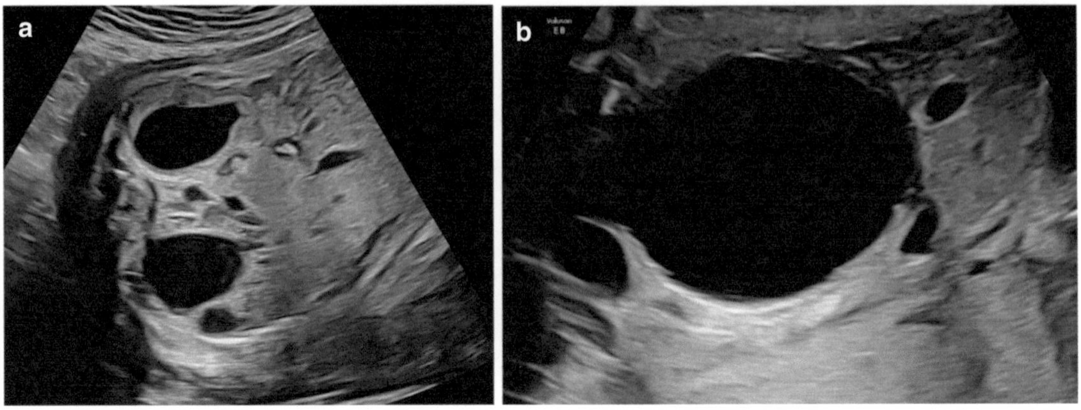

Fig. 7.2 (**a**) Bilateral hydroureteronephrosis with (**b**) distended bladder sign of LUTO

Table 7.2 Proposed classification of fetal lower urinary tract obstruction (LUTO) according to severity

	Stage I (mild LUTO)	Stage II (severe LUTO, with prenatal findings suggestive of preserved fetal renal function)	Stage III (severe LUTO, with prenatal findings suggestive of fetal abnormal renal function)
Amount of amniotic fluid	Normal	Oligohydramnios or anhydramnios	Oligohydramnios, but usually anhydramnios
Echogenicity of fetal kidneys	Normal	Hyperechogenic	Hyperechogenic
Renal cortical cysts	Absent	Absent	Can be present
Renal dysplasia	Absent	Absent	Can be present
Fetal urinary biochemistry	Favorable	Favorable within three consecutive evaluations	Not favorable after three consecutive evaluations
Fetal intervention	Not indicated	Indicated to prevent pulmonary hypoplasia and severe renal impairment	May be indicated to prevent pulmonary hypoplasia but not postnatal renal impairment; further studies are necessary

Adopted from Ruano R et al., Ultrasound in Obetetrics & Gynaecology 2016;48: 476–482
The disease can progress from Stage I to Stage II and then to Stage III during pregnancy

7.5.2 Management of Fetal LUTO (Fig. 7.3)

7.5.2.1 Fetal Interventions

(a) Vesicoamniotic shunt. A double pigtail stent is inserted with one end in the bladder and the other in the amniotic cavity.

(b) Fetal cystoscopy. A 1–1.3 mm cystoscope is inserted in the fetal bladder and guided in the posterior urethra for valve ablation.

The definite advantage of percutaneous vesico-amniotic shunting for fetal LUTO (PLUTO trial) is unclear. Despite improved survival rates with fetal intervention, there has been no difference in the long-term renal outcome.

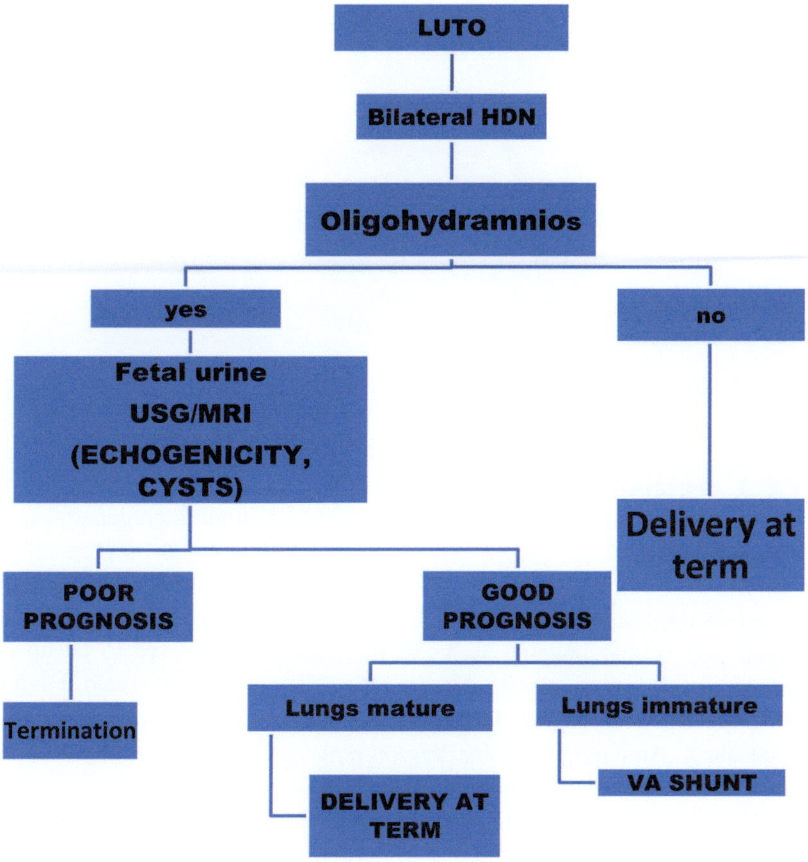

Fig. 7.3 Management algorithm for fetal LUTO

7.6 Fetal Management for Ventriculomegaly

Ventriculomegaly is defined as fetal lateral ventricular measurement (at atria) >10 mm.

Detailed workup for associated abnormalities includes family history, maternal toxoplasma, rubella, cytomegalovirus, Herpes Simplex (TORCH) serology, blood sugar status, neurosonogram, fetal MRI, invasive procedure for chromosomal and genetic tests, DNA extraction, and storage. Routine follow-up ultrasound needs to be done.

7.6.1 Management

With associated intracranial and other systemic abnormalities, termination of pregnancy should be considered. Fetuses with isolated hydrocephalus with stable mild ventricular dilatation may be observed till term. For those with progressive ventricular dilatation and gestational age > 32 weeks, delivery and shunting may be considered. Fetal therapy and in utero shunting procedures are not recommended for clinical practice.

7.6.2 Fetal Procedures Are

(a) Serial cephalocentesis
(b) Ventriculo-amniotic shunt

Fetal treatment has no obvious documented benefit at present.

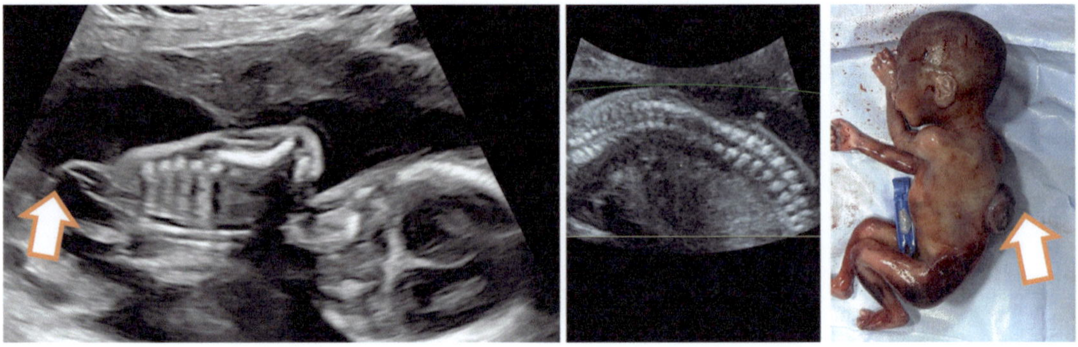

Fig. 7.4 Spina bifida with meningomyelocele

7.6.3 Fetal Diagnosis of Spina bifida and Meningomyelocele (MMC)

A second-trimester ultrasonography with detailed spinal and cranial imaging is a recommended screening test for neural tube defects (Fig. 7.4). Antenatal MRI can be useful to assess and aid in counseling. Amniotic fluid for karyotyping or chromosomal microarray may be offered. Spina bifida is often associated with Arnold-Chiari malformation type II. This occurs due to herniation of the medulla, fourth ventricle, and vermis of the cerebellum through the foramen magnum into the spinal canal causing obstructive hydrocephalus as seen in 70–80% cases of spina bifida.

The *lemon sign* is the scalloping of the frontal bone, resulting in the cranium appearing as lemon and is known as lemon sign. The *banana sign* is due to the obliteration of cisterna magna giving rise to an elongated shape of the cerebellum associated with type II Chiari malformation. The prognosis depends on the level of the defect; it is poor with higher defects, the presence of hydrocephalus, and the severity of the Chiari malformation.

The family should be counseled and explained the prognosis with the following options: (a) fetal surgery, for selected fetuses which is currently available in a limited number of centers, (b) continuing pregnancy and post-natal surgery, (c) termination of pregnancy. There is no documented benefit of cesarean delivery over normal vaginal delivery. The recurrence risk in next pregnancy is considered to be up to 4%. Hence, preconceptional folic acid at 4–5 mg daily starting 3 months before conception and continuing 12 weeks post gestation along with appropriate screening tests is advised.

7.7 Fetal Therapy for Meningomyelocele

7.7.1 The Rationale for Fetal Treatment

The fetuses with 19–25 weeks of gestation, with lesions below T1, and having associated Chiari II malformation qualify for fetal surgery, generally offered around 26 weeks. The reasons for benefit of intrauterine surgery are that the neural tissue is primarily normal in this defect and gets damaged due to exposure to amniotic fluid and covering of defects in utero may improve neurological outcome. Current fetal surgical treatment is open repair of meningomyelocele indicated in fetus with an open defect having herniation of hindbrain.

A prospective randomized controlled trial of prenatal versus postnatal repair of meningomyelocele has been completed in the USA (myelomeningocele study (MOMS) trial).

Fetal repair of spina bifida was found to be superior to postnatal repair in terms of the following:

- Incidence of Chiari malformation was found less in the fetal repair group.
- The need for a ventricular shunt was found less in the fetal repair group.
- Motor skills were better in the fetal repair group.

However, there remains a significant risk of prematurity and serious maternal complications with fetal surgery.

7.8 Fetal Therapy for Congenital Cystic Adenomatoid Malformation/Congenial Pulmonary Airway Malformation (CPAM)

7.8.1 Diagnosis by Imaging (Fig. 7.5a, b)

Macrocystic lesions are cysts >5 mm in diameter. Microcystic lesions are solid echogenic masses. Sequestrations are solid echogenic lesions with an anomalous systemic blood supply.

7.8.2 Monitoring

The parameters are

$$\text{CCAM Volume ratio}(\text{CVR}):(\text{Height}\times\text{width}\times\text{depth}\times 0.523)\div\text{head circumference}(\text{in cm})$$

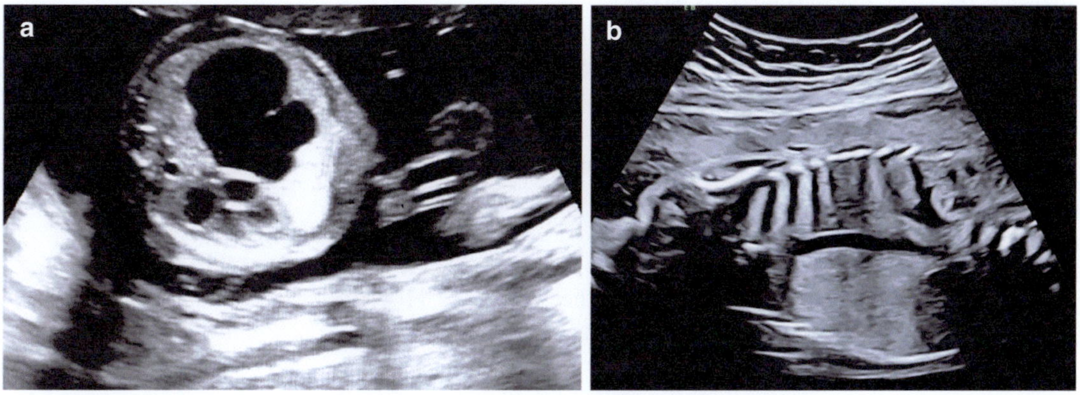

Fig. 7.5 Antenatal scan showing a. Macrocystic CPAM b. Microcystic CPAM (solid lesion)

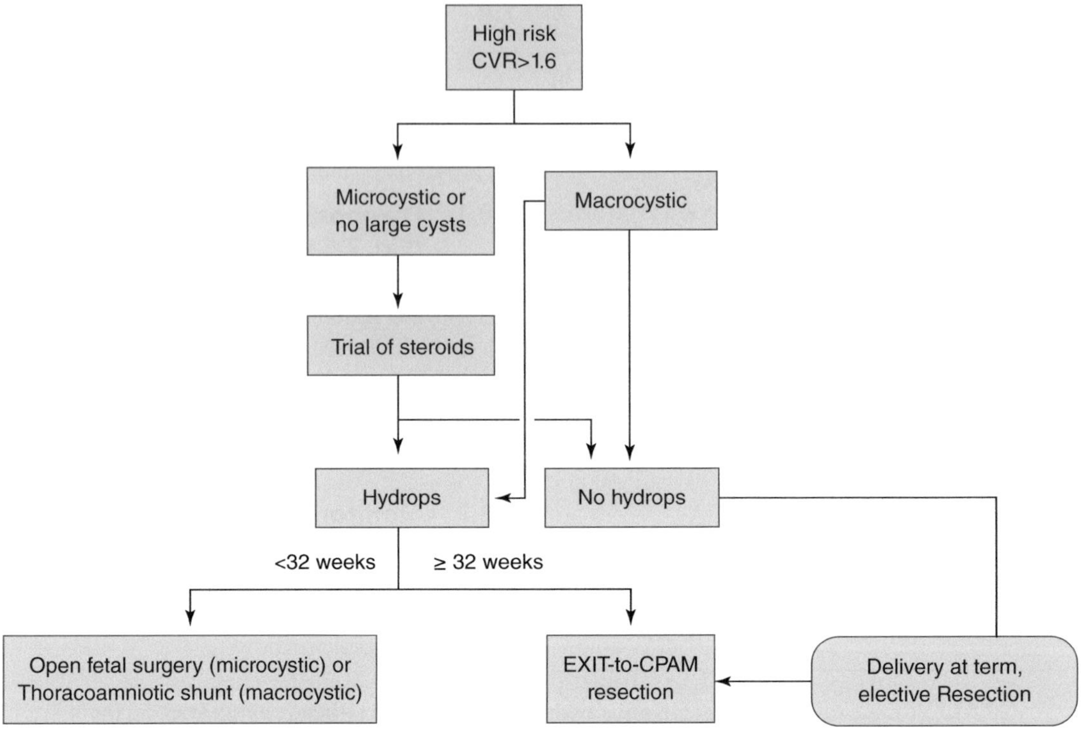

Fig. 7.6 Fetal management of CPAM

CVR > 1.6 is predictive of increased risk of hydrops; the value plateaus after 28 weeks

Indications for in-utero intervention (Fig. 7.6) (thoracic-amniotic shunt or fetal lobectomy) are

(a) Evidence of early hydrops
(b) High risk of pulmonary hypoplasia (large lesion with mediastinal shift before 24 weeks of gestation)

Role of steroid therapy: administration of systemic steroid (dexamethasone) to the mother between 24 and 28 weeks has been associated with better lung maturity and favorable outcome. It appears to be more effective for microcystic CPAM.

7.8.3 Outcome

In fetuses with hydrops without intervention, the mortality rate can be as high as 100%. Postintervention survival rates as high as 74% have been reported.

7.9 Fetal Management of Congenital Diaphragmatic Hernia

The diagnostic accuracy of ultrasound is very high for CDH although it is often detected late after 20 weeks (Fig. 7.7a, b).

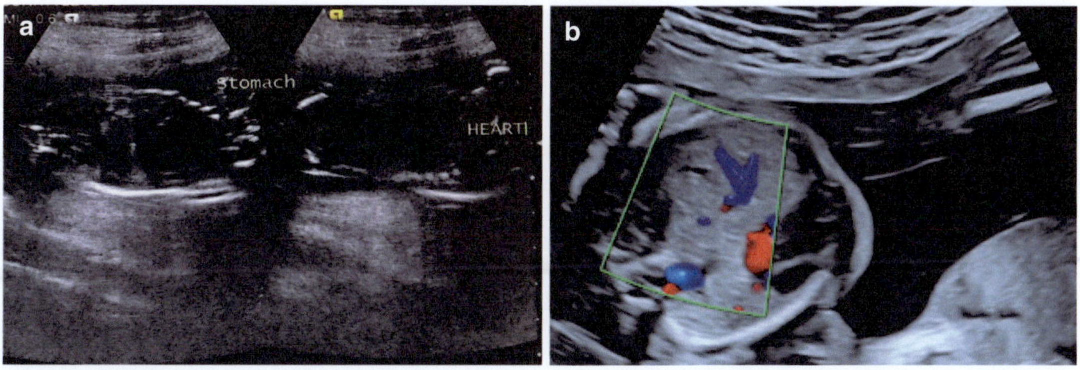

Fig. 7.7 (**a**) Antenatal scan at 16 weeks showing stomach in the chest; (**b**) heart shifted to the right, the liver in thorax suggestive of congenital diaphragmatic hernia

Performing procedure such as plug lung until it grows (PLUG) is currently introduced to reverse pulmonary hypoplasia in CDH. Fetal tracheal occlusion is done to promote lung growth by preventing egress of fluid from the lung, facilitating its expansion.

Indication for fetal interventions in CDH is high-risk fetuses with lung to head ratio (LHR) < 1 or equivalent. LHR less than one carries a poor prognosis and more than 1 has better survival rate.

There is disproportionate growth of the chest in the later part of gestation resulting in spontaneous improvement in LHR. To account for this observed/expected LHR is used. O/E LHR <25% has 12–30% survival whereas value <35% has 65–88% survival. The presence of liver in the chest is associated with poor outcome.

Fetal endoscopic tracheal occlusion. A 1.3 mm scope can be used to place a balloon in the trachea. Balloon is placed at 26–29 weeks, and deflated by ultrasound (USG)-guided puncture/tracheoscopy at 34–36 weeks or by EXIT (ex utero intrapartum treatment).

7.10 Antenatal Diagnosis and Management of Abdominal Wall Defects

Accurate prenatal diagnosis of the type of defect is important (gastroschisis, omphalocele, exstrophy/cloacal exstrophy) for planning the management (Fig. 7.8a–c).

It has been seen that an isolated defect has good prognosis whereas the presence of chromosomal and genetic syndromes affects patient management and prognosis (Fig. 7.9a, b). The clinical outcome of antenatally diagnosed abdominal wall defects is favorable with adequate postnatal treatment (see Chap. 32).

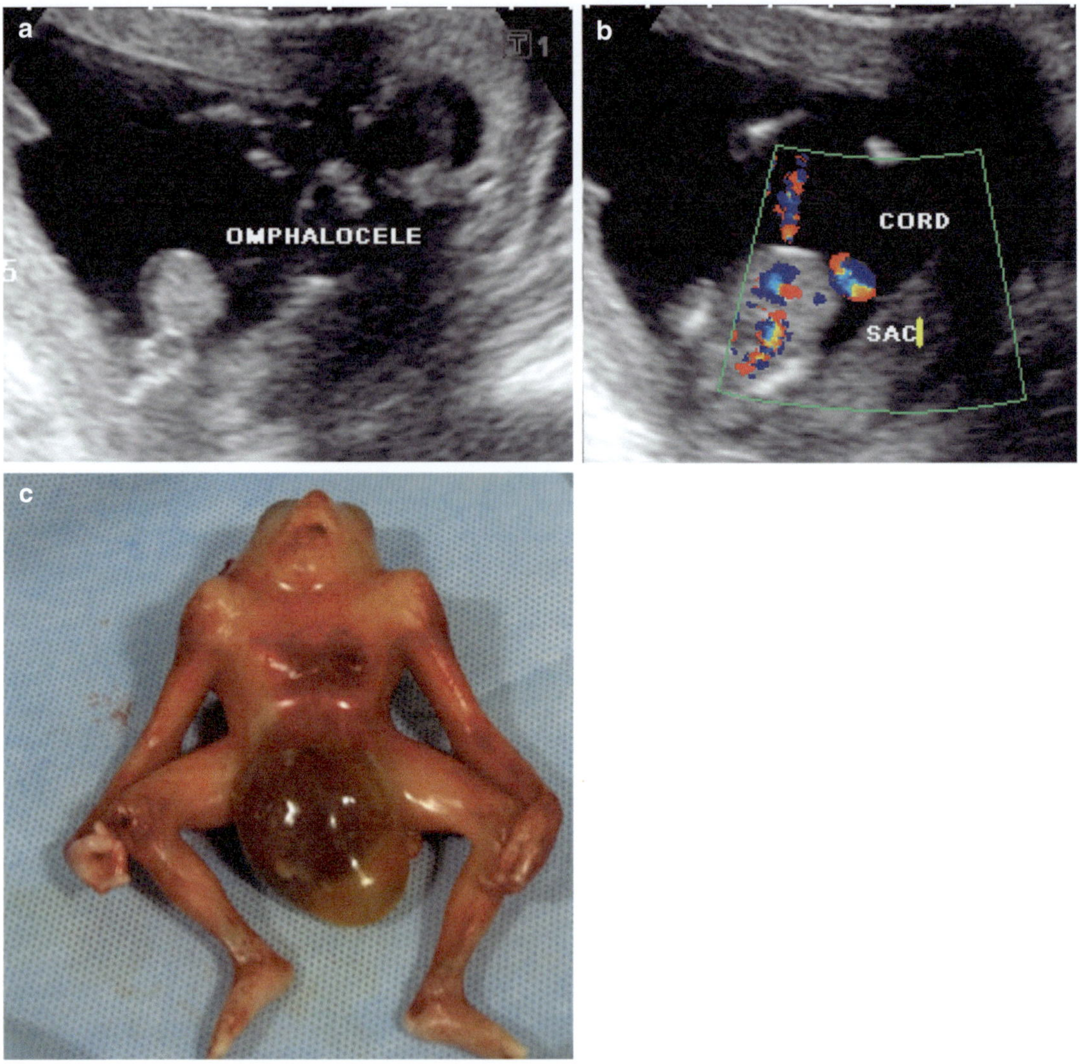

Fig. 7.8 (**a**, **b**) Antenatal scan showing omphalocele, (**c**) Large omphalocele with sac and multiple anomalies

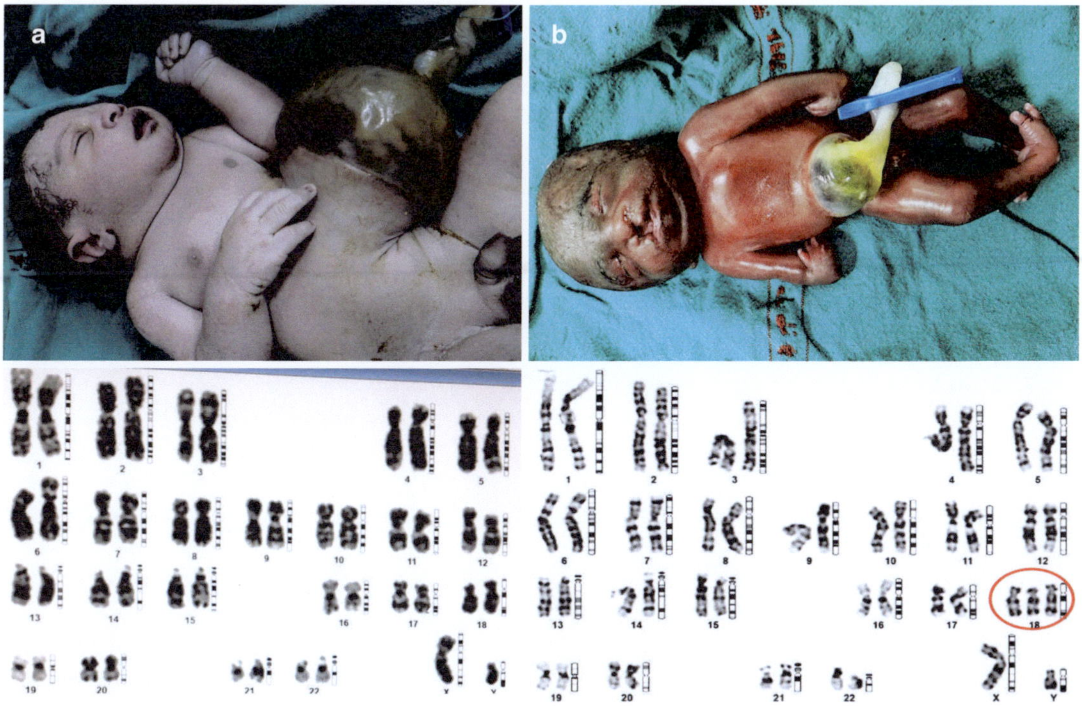

Fig. 7.9 (**a**) Huge omphalocele with normal fetal karyotype, (**b**) omphalocele with multiple anomalies, such as limb defects and median cleft having trisomy 18

7.11 Antenatal Diagnosis and Management of Intra-abdominal Anomalies

The examples of intra-abdominal anomalies are duodenal atresia (Fig. 7.10a, b), intra-abdominal calcification (Fig. 7.11), meconium pseudocyst (Fig. 7.12) and other cystic conditions like choledochal cyst, ovarian cyst, mesenteric cyst. Fetal intra-abdominal calcifications can be due to intrauterine infections (cytomegalovirus), meconium peritonitis, or teratoma. Fetuses with isolated calcifications generally have a good prognosis. Those with multiple lesions should be offered amniocentesis and fetal karyotype and cystic fibrosis mutation analysis.

For antenatal diagnosis and management of fetal sacrococcygeal teratoma (Fig. 7.13), see chapter on SCT (Chap. 61).

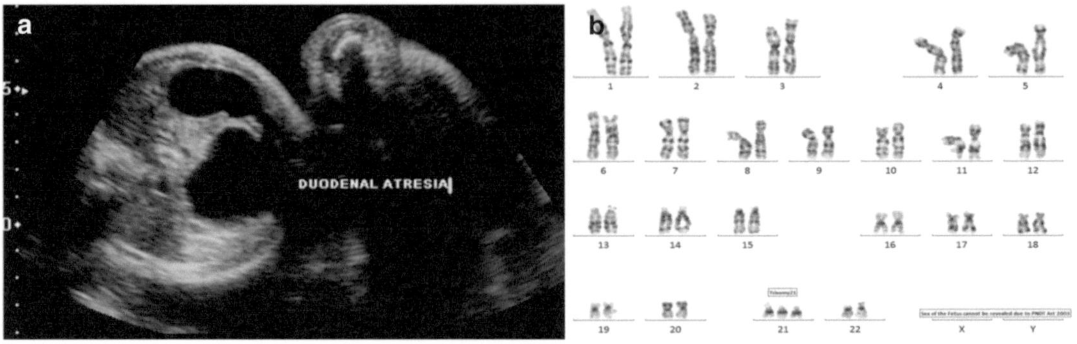

Fig. 7.10 (**a**) Antenatal scan showing duodenal atresia with (**b**) trisomy 21

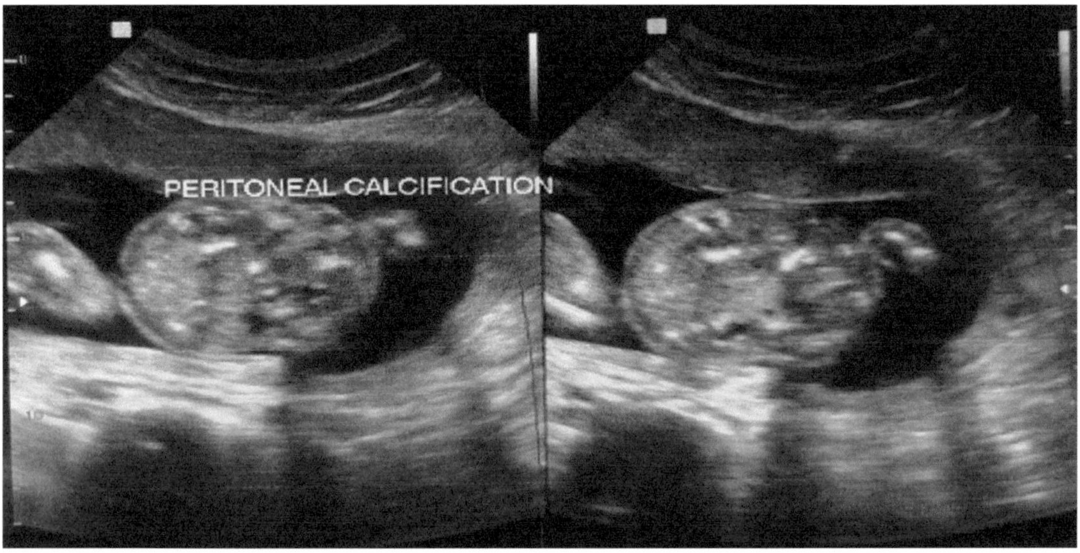

Fig. 7.11 Antenatal scan showing intraperitoneal calcification (meconium peritonitis)

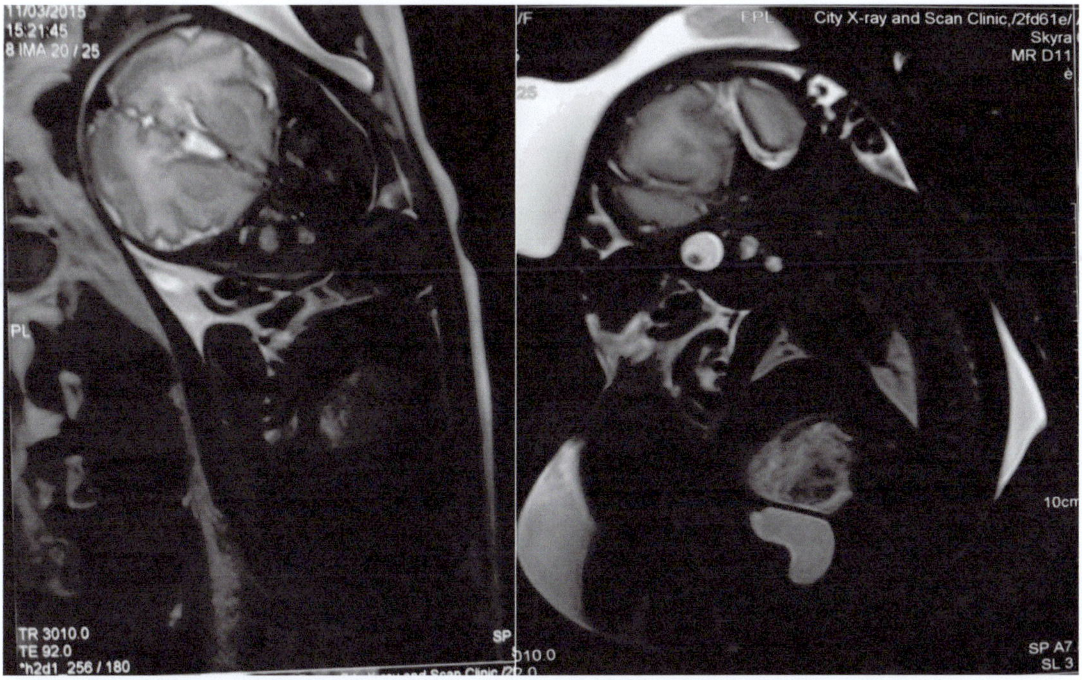

Fig. 7.12 Fetal MRI showing a large cystic lesion in the abdomen, meconium pseudocyst

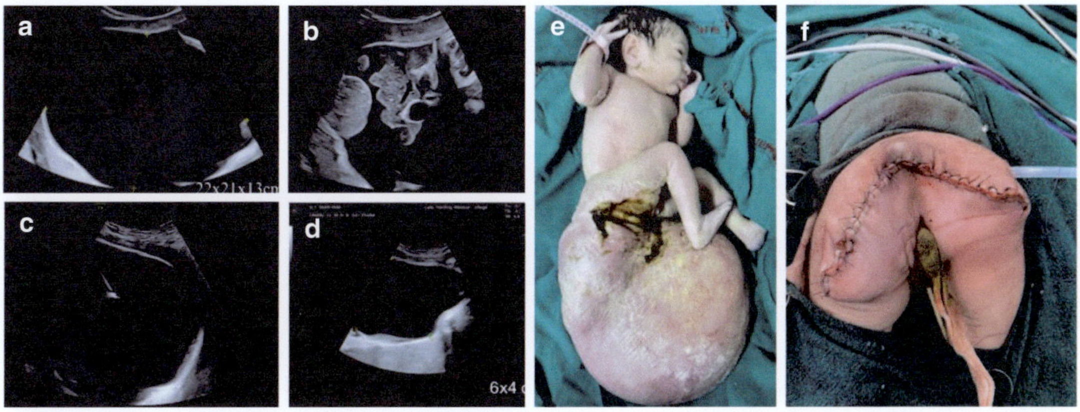

Fig. 7.13 Antenatal scan showing the cystic (**a**) and solid component (**b**) of the teratoma; drainage of cyst (**c**) compression after drainage (**d**); picture of the baby post delivery (**e**) and post surgery (**f**)

7.12 Summary

Early diagnosis of fetal anomalies remains the mainstay for planning subsequent management. Proper evaluation and prognostication are essential for counseling the family. With the advancement of fetal diagnosis and therapy, a multidisciplinary team of specialists is required to provide appropriate care leading to a satisfactory outcome. Majority of the structural anomalies can be managed postnatally; however, fetal intervention currently has some role in specific situations.

Suggested Reading

Joglekar A, Choudhury SR, Vibhash C, Kumar M, Gupta A. Risk factors and outcome of antenatally diagnosed congenital diaphragmatic hernia. Monaldi Arch Chest Dis. 2025;95(2). https://doi.org/10.4081/monaldi.2024.2880.

Holocomb GW III, Murphy JP, St Peter SD, editors. Holocomb and Ashcraft's pediatric surgery. Philadelphia: Elsevier; 2020.

Bianchi MD, Crombleholme TM, Malone FD. Fetology: diagnosis and management of the fetal patient. 2nd ed. Mc Graw Hill Education, United States; 2010.

Ruano R, Sananes N, Wilson C, et al. Fetal lower urinary tract obstruction: proposal for standardized multidisciplinary prenatal management based on disease severity. Ultrasound Obetetr Gynaecol. 2016;48:476–82.

8 Vascular Anomalies

Subhasis Roy Choudhury and Vishesh Jain

There are several confusing nomenclatures for vascular malformations like nevus, angiomas, hemangiomas, etc. However, the classification needs to be based on the growth of blood vessels (angiogenesis), biological and clinical behavior which has implication for diagnosis and treatment.

8.1 Classification

Currently, the classification suggested by International Society for the Study of Vascular Anomalies is being followed (Fig. 8.1).

Hemangiomas are distinctly different from vascular malformations as shown below.

Hemangiomas	Vascular malformations
Infantile Hemangiomas: true *neoplasm*, arise from endothelial hyperplasia 30% are *visible at birth* *Common in females* *Proliferative & involuting phase* *Responds* to *pharmacologic* therapy *GLUT-1 positive*	*They occur due to Dysmorphogenesis.* Normal endothelial cell turnover *Always present at birth* M/F *equal ratio* Grow and expand throughout life, *Do not involute* *Do not respond* to pharmacologic therapy *GLUT-1 Negative*

S. Roy Choudhury
Pediatric Surgery, Lady Hardinge Medical College and Associated Kalawati Saran Children's Hospital, New Delhi, Delhi, India

V. Jain (✉)
Department of Pediatric Surgery, AIIMS, New Delhi, India

© The Author(s), under exclusive license to Springer Nature Singapore Pte Ltd. 2025
S. Roy Choudhury (ed.), *Pediatric Surgery*, https://doi.org/10.1007/978-981-96-1257-4_8

Fig. 8.1 Classification of vascular anomalies

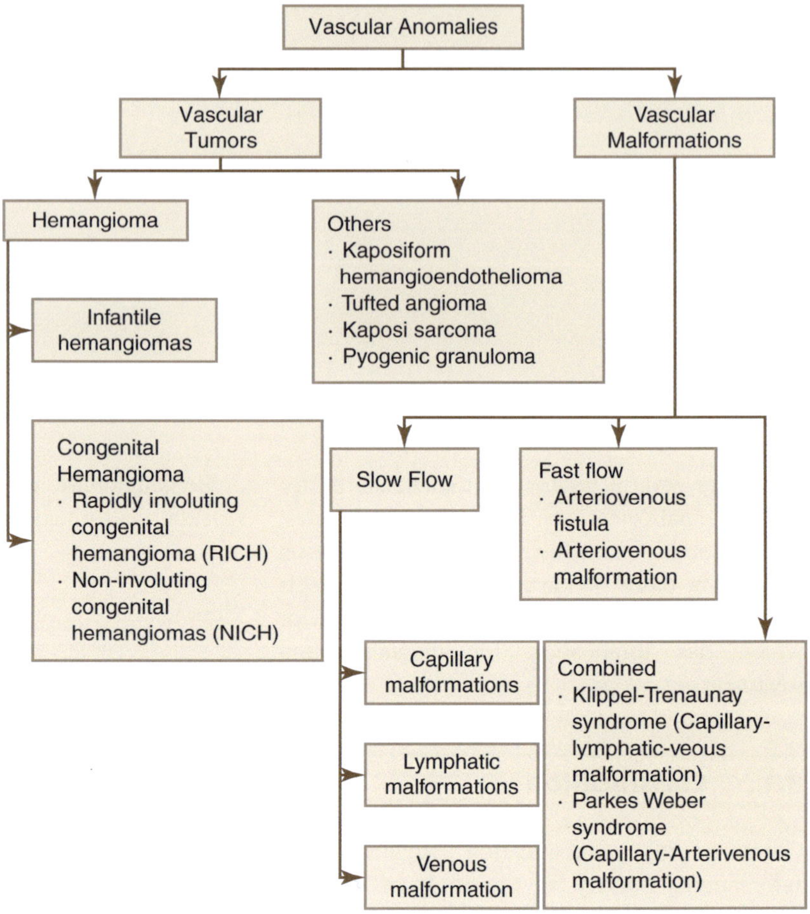

8.2 Infantile Hemangioma (IHs; Figs. 8.2a,b, 8.3, and 8.4)

Infantile hemangiomas are the most prevalent benign vascular tumors in infants, affecting approximately 4–10% of children. These lesions typically emerge within the first few weeks after birth, undergo rapid growth during a proliferative phase, and gradually regress over several years. Growth usually peaks by 5 months of age, with most involution completed by 3–5 years. Although the precise cause remains unclear, current hypotheses suggest that localized hypoxia triggers abnormal vascular growth through angiogenesis and vasculogenesis mechanisms. IHs can occur in various anatomical locations, including the skin, internal organs, and mucosal surfaces. They are classified based on depth (superficial, deep, or mixed) and distribution (localized, segmental, or multifocal). Glucose transporter 1 (GLUT-1) immunohistochemical staining is a reliable diagnostic marker that differentiates IHs from other vascular anomalies (Figs. 8.5 and 8.6).

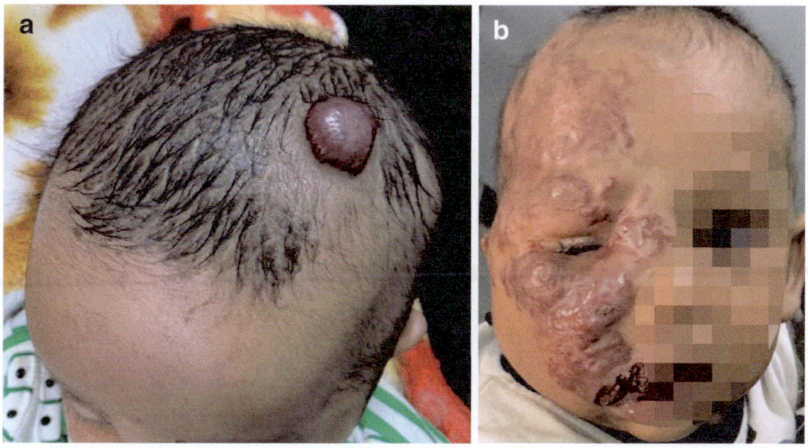

Fig. 8.2 Infantile hemangioma (**a**) scalp and (**b**) face

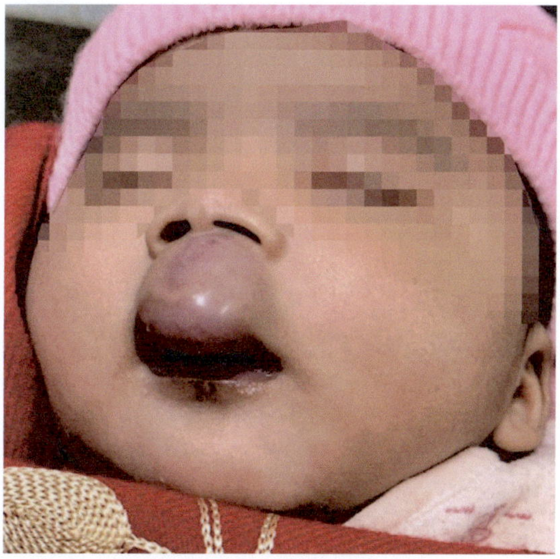

Fig. 8.3 Infantile hemangioma lip

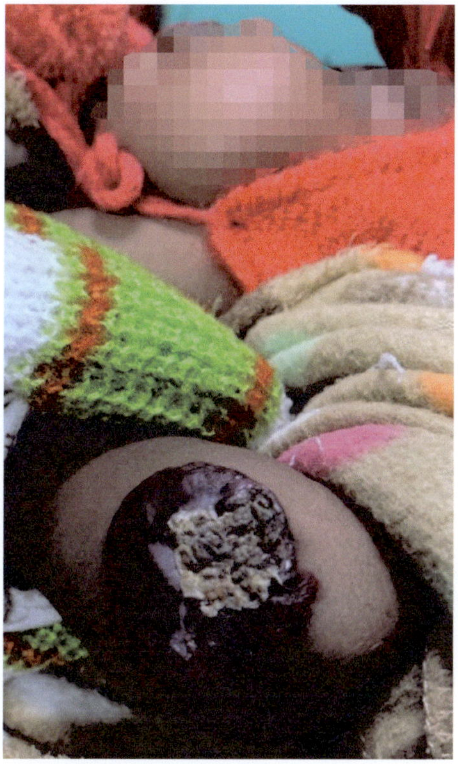

Fig. 8.4 Deep hemangioma, arm

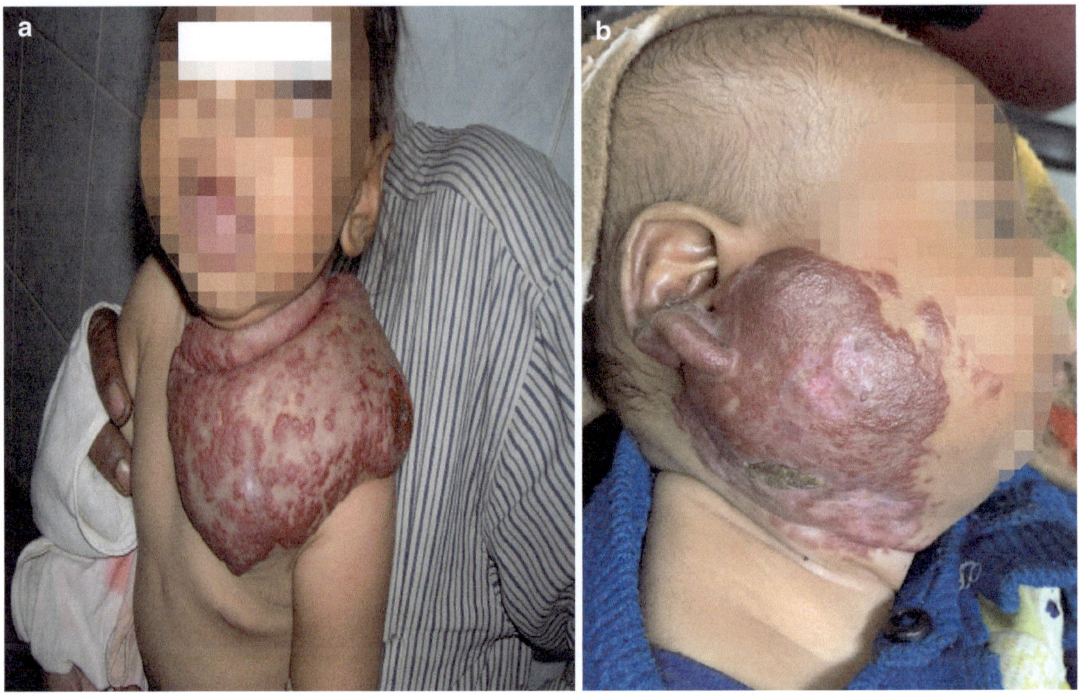

Fig. 8.5 (**a**) Large infantile hemangioma neck and chest, (**b**) parotid region

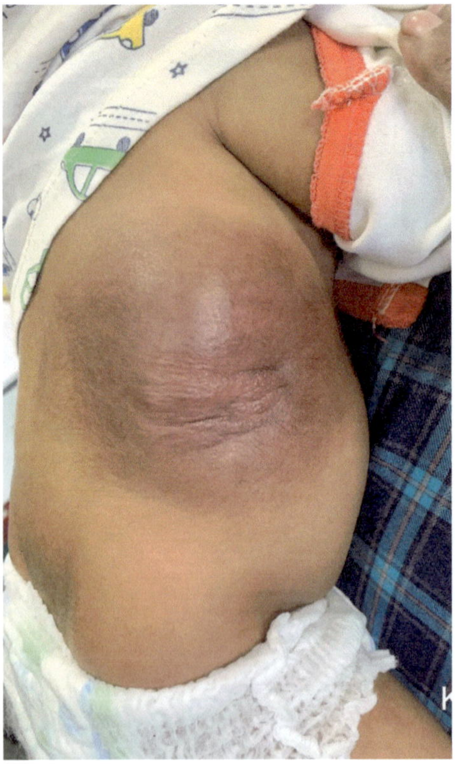

Fig. 8.6 Large hemangioma with platelet trapping (Kasabach–Merritt phenomenon)

8.3 Congenital Hemangiomas (CHs)

Congenital hemangiomas, unlike IHs, are fully developed at birth and exhibit variable growth patterns. They are classified into rapidly involuting (RICH), non-involuting (NICH), and partially involuting (PICH) subtypes. Unlike IHs, CHs do not exhibit a postnatal proliferative phase. Genetic mutations in GNAQ and GNA11 have been implicated in their development, highlighting a distinct pathophysiological origin.

CHs are typically large, firm, and well-defined lesions, often appearing on the head, neck, or extremities. They may show features such as telangiectasias, pallor, and ulceration. While RICH lesions regress completely within the first year, NICH lesions persist with no significant regression, and PICH lesions exhibit partial regression followed by stabilization.

Large hemangiomas, particularly those with extensive vascularity, may lead to platelet sequestration and consumption, resulting in thrombocytopenia, a condition termed *Kasabach-Merritt phenomenon (KMP)*. This phenomenon is more commonly associated with congenital hemangiomas and other vascular tumors such as Kaposiform hemangioendotheliomas (KHE). Additionally, high-flow vascular shunting within these lesions can result in *high-output cardiac failure*, necessitating careful monitoring and timely intervention.

Facial hemangiomas, especially those located in the *"beard" distribution*, carry a higher likelihood of concurrent *subglottic hemangiomas*, which can compromise the airway and necessitate urgent evaluation and treatment. In infants presenting with *five or more cutaneous hemangiomas*, abdominal ultrasonography (USG) is recommended to screen for *visceral hemangiomas*, which may otherwise remain asymptomatic.

8.3.1 Investigations

- Ultrasound is only needed when the diagnosis is uncertain or to rule out visceral lesions.
- USG with Doppler—seen as high flow lesions especially during the proliferative phase.
- Magnetic resonance imaging (MRI): solid lesion with vascularity and flow voids.

If the number is more than 5, then exclude visceral lesions.

8.3.2 Treatment

(a) Observation with reassurance and regular photography to monitor the progress. Observation over a period gives the best cosmetic result with spontaneous involution.

(b) Pharmacotherapy: intervention is needed for large ulcerated hemangiomas, hemangiomas interfering with limb function or encroachment to vital structures like eye, nose, airway, etc. The decision for pharmacotherapy should be made early if possible before the period of rapid growth.

- Beta blockers: propranolol has recently been discovered to be useful in the management of IH and has now become the first line in pharmacotherapy for IH due to good efficacy and minimal side effects. Propranolol is gradually increased to a dose of 2 mg/kg body weight orally for 3–6 weeks or even longer till 9–12 months of age so as to suppress the proliferative phase. They act initially by causing vasoconstriction, later by inhibiting angiogenesis and in the long term promote apoptosis in the lesion. It is important to rule out family history of asthma and heart block in the family.
- Steroids (high dose, systemic/intralesional), prednisolone—2 mg/kg body weight orally for 2 weeks and then are gradually tapered, response rate is 80–90%. Gastritis is frequent complication so antacids are also prescribed. All live vaccines are withheld till the child is on steroids. Steroids act by inhibiting angiogenesis.
- Vincristine.
- Interferon 2 alpha a, b (out of favor).
- Local application of 0.5% timolol maleate gel twice a day for 6 months has been associated with early resolution during the proliferative phase of the infantile hemangioma.

Laser treatment is not ideal.

Surgery is indicated for ulceration, hemorrhage, interference with vital structures and functions and where pharmacotherapy has failed or for primary treatment of small pedunculated lesions.

8.4 Kaposiform Hemangioendothelioma (KHE)

Kaposiform hemangioendothelioma (KHE) is a rare, locally aggressive vascular tumor commonly diagnosed in infancy, with half of cases present at birth. It frequently involves the extremities, but deeper lesions may affect retroperitoneal or thoracic regions. KHE is characterized by

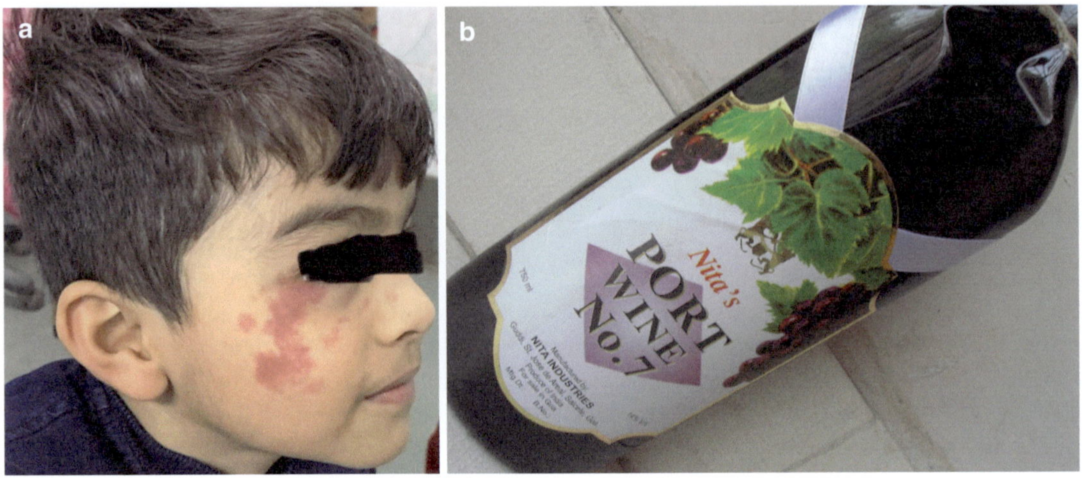

Fig. 8.7 (**a**, **b**) Port wine capillary malformation

firm, purpuric, or ecchymotic skin lesions, often associated with pain and swelling. KHE is strongly associated with Kasabach-Merritt phenomenon (KMP).

8.4.1 Port Wine Stain (Capillary Malformation)

They are flat, pink, purple lesions with geographical distribution (Fig. 8.7a, b).

Associations are Sturge-Weber syndrome (trigeminal distribution), spina bifida, and encephalocele.

If untreated, they persist in the adulthood, the color darkens, and the skin thickens.

8.4.2 Treatment

Indication for treatment is mainly cosmetic.

Flash lamp pulse-dye laser can be applied.

Result of therapy: lightening of color occurs in 70% of cases and complete disappearance in 15–20% cases.

Disadvantages: need for anesthesia, multiple sitting, cost of treatment.

Complications: thinning, hypo/hyperpigmentation, scarring, and pain.

8.4.3 Venous Malformations

8.4.3.1 Clinical Features

These lesions are dark colored, diffuse, spongy, compressible, and involve deeper tissue (Fig. 8.8a, b). There is slow flow in these lesions and due to stasis in these lesions, thrombus may form. This may cause local swelling along with low fibrinogen along with raised d-dimers.

8.4.4 Diagnosis

Imaging with USG Doppler, MRI and MR venography aids in the diagnosis. The presence of slow flow lesion along with calcifications (phleboliths) helps in making the diagnosis.

8.4.5 Treatment

- Graduated compression stocking may be helpful.
- Intralesional sclerotherapy with agents like alcohol, sodium tetradecyl sulfate (setrol), ethanolamine oleate, doxycycline, or policodanol is used with variable success rate. Multiple sittings may be required. Compression the lesion to decreased blood in

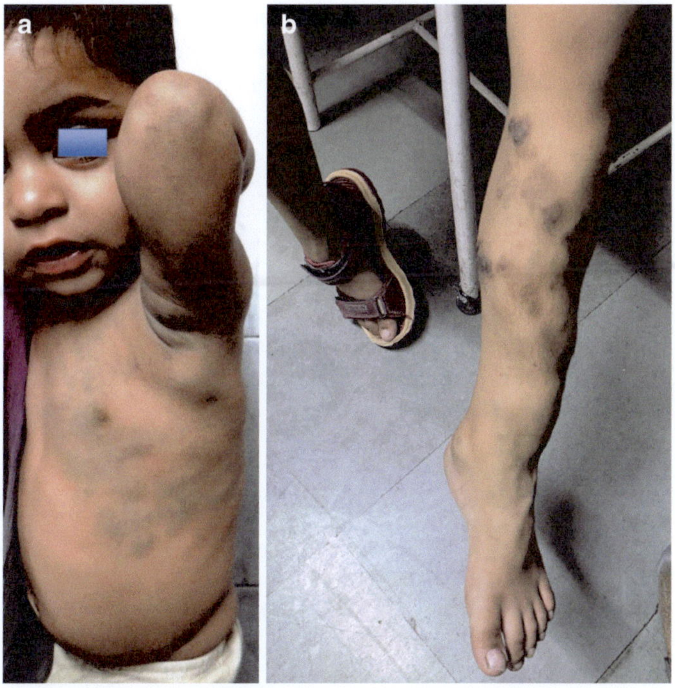

Fig. 8.8 (**a**) Venous malformation chest wall and upper limb, (**b**) lower limb

the lesion and injecting multiple sites with post-injection compression improves the success rate. The injections are administered every 6 weeks to 3 months. In an extensive lesion involving the limb, the injections are started from proximal to distal. These injections have an inherent risk of pain, swelling, infection, and embolization of the sclerosant.

- *Sirolimus* has recently been used with favorable outcomes in complex and extensive low-flow malformation (venous and lymphatic malformation). It is an mTOR inhibitor, targets the *PIK3CA/AKT/mTOR* pathway involved in endothelial proliferation, making it effective for treating complex or refractory lymphatic and venous malformations. It reduces lesion size, alleviates symptoms like pain and swelling, and improves quality of life.
- Surgical resection for well-localized lesion can be done.
- Argon/ Nd Yag lasers are indicated for only superficial lesions, and are associated with a high recurrence rate.

8.4.6 Lymphatic Malformation (See Chap. 9)

8.4.6.1 Diagnosis

Lymphatic malformations (LMs) are low-flow vascular anomalies arising from developmental errors in the lymphatic system. They are benign, commonly detected at birth or within the first few years of life, with an incidence ranging from 1 in 2000 to 1 in 16,000 and no gender or racial predisposition.

LMs present as cystic masses, classified into microcystic, macrocystic, or mixed forms. These lesions often grow proportionally with the child but may enlarge rapidly following infection or trauma. Histologically, they consist of endothelial-lined cystic spaces filled with proteinaceous fluid.

Diagnosis is based on clinical examination and imaging studies. Ultrasonography is the first-line imaging modality, showing anechoic or hypoechoic cystic spaces with septations. Magnetic resonance imaging (MRI) provides detailed anatomic relationships and is particularly useful for assessing extent and depth. Absence of vascularity in contrast-enhanced MRI is useful for differentiating from venous malformation.

8.4.6.2 Treatment

- Treatment of infection if present.
- Sclerotherapy for macrocystic lesion (bleomycin, doxycycline, picibanil).
- Sirolimus for extensive malformation.
- Surgery for microcystic lesions, residual lesion after sclerotherapy.
- Radiofrequency ablation (for low-flow lesions).

8.5 Arterio-Venous Malformation (AVM)/Arterio-Venous Fistula.

Diagnosis: high-flow lesion that could be pulsatile. Limb and tissue overgrowth often occurs (Figs. 8.9a, b and 8.10).

MR angiography is diagnostic.

8.5.1 Treatment

- Angio embolization.
- Surgical excision.
- Embolization followed by surgical excision.

Vascular malformations involving lip (Fig. 8.11), breast (Fig. 8.12), parotid region (Fig. 8.13), and involuting hemangioma with central scarring (Fig. 8.14).

8.5.2 Combined Vascular Malformation (Fig. 8.15)

(a) Klippel–Trenaunay syndrome, slow-flow, capillary-lymphatico-venous malformation.
(b) Parkes-Weber syndrome, fast-flow, capillary arteriovenous malformation.

Diagnosis: MRI.

Treatment: combination of different therapy.

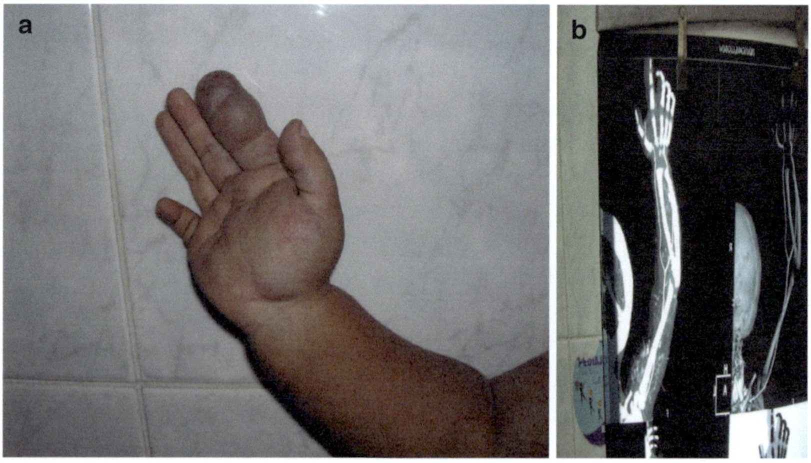

Fig. 8.9 (**a**) Overgrowth of limb due to arteriovenous malformation, (**b**) MRA angiography showing AVM

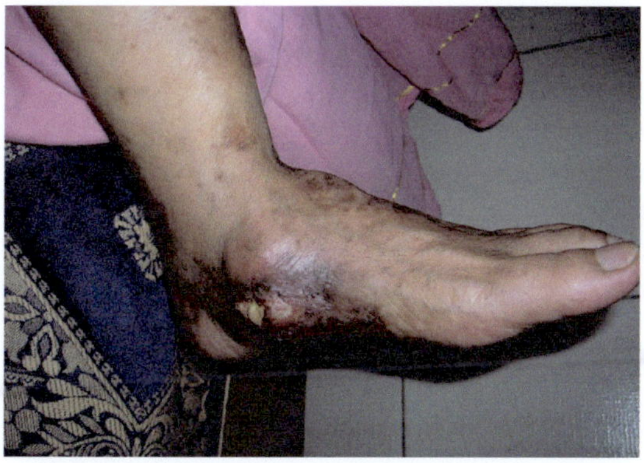

Fig. 8.10 Arteriovenous malformation foot, pulsatile lesion, note dilated vessels around the lesion

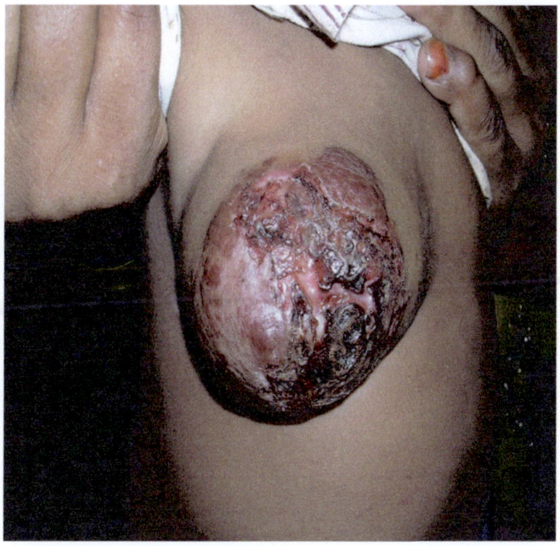

Fig. 8.12 Vascular malformation involving breast

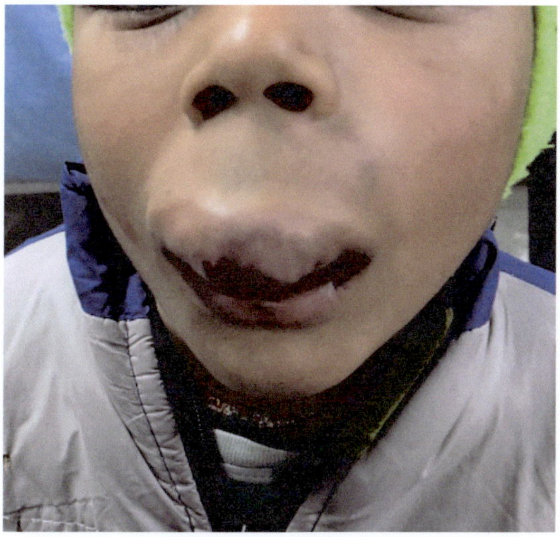

Fig. 8.11 Vascular malformation of lip

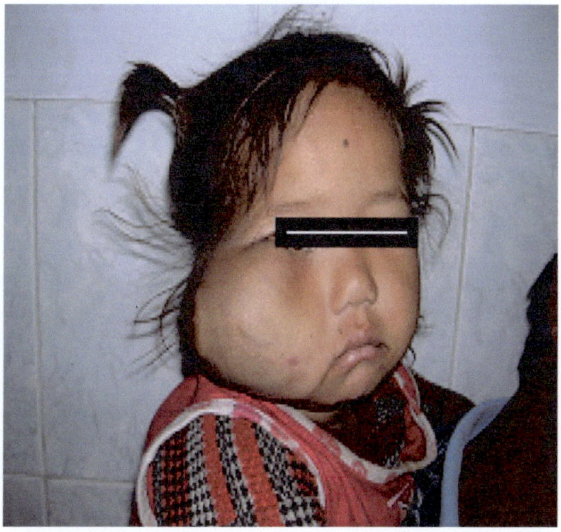

Fig. 8.13 Vascular malformation parotid region

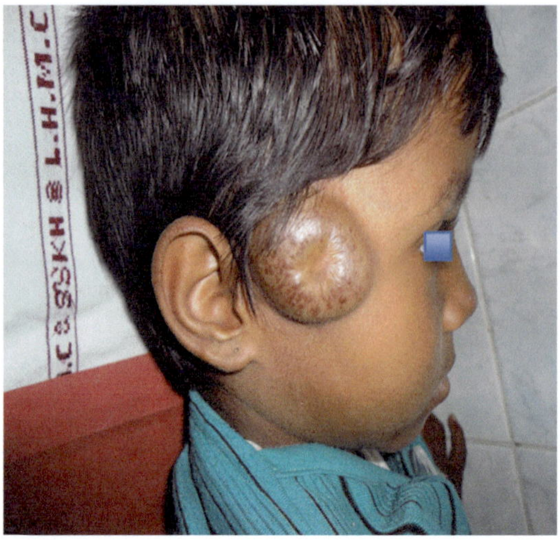

Fig. 8.14 Involuting hemangioma

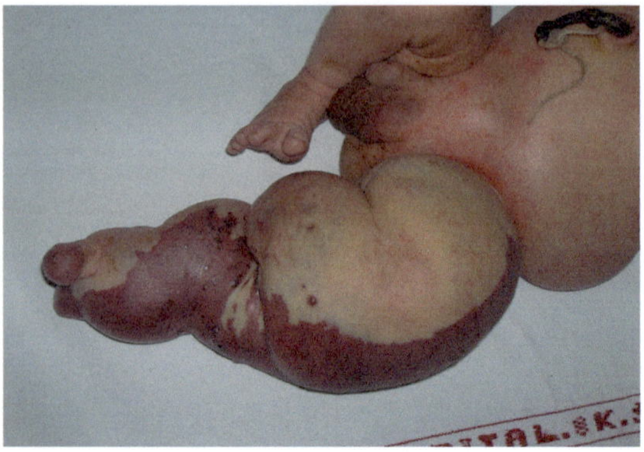

Fig. 8.15 Combined malformation, limb gigantism, consumptive coagulopathy

8.5.3 Summary of Treatment

Type of lesion	Treatment
Infantile hemangioma	Observation/pharmacotherapy/surgery
Capillary malformations	Laser therapy
Venous malformations	Sclerotherapy, compression therapy, surgery
Lymphatic malformations	Sclerotherapy, surgery
Arterial malformations	Embolization, surgery
Combined malformation	Combination therapy

Suggested Reading

Coran AG, Caldamone A, Scott Adzich N, Krummel TM, Laberge JM, editors. Pediatric surgery. 7th ed. Oxford: Elsevier Limited; 2012.

Gupta DK, Sharma S, Azizkhan RG, editors. Pediatric surgery—diagnosis and management. 1st ed. New Delhi: Jaypee Brothers; 2009.

9 Lymphatic Malformations

Subhasis Roy Choudhury and Vishesh Jain

9.1 Introduction

Lymphatic malformations (LMs) are a variety of congenital hamartomatous malformations of the lymphatic system. The lesions can be superficial or deep and may have mixed venous elements. The term lymphatic malformations should not be used interchangeably with old misnomers like lymphangioma and cystic hygroma. Lymphangioma would literally mean a tumor of the lymphatic system, which is not the case. The term cystic hygroma is reserved for antenatally diagnosed bilateral cystic swelling in the occipito-cervical areas of the fetus. It is important to differentiate this entity from lymphatic malformation as cystic hygroma is associated with chromosomal abnormalities in 50% and is prone to develop hydrops.

Embryology In the sixth week of intrauterine life, the primitive lymph sacs (principal pair) develop between the jugular and subclavian veins. Sequestration of a portion of the jugular lymph sac from the lymphatic system accounts for this malformation.

Pathology It consists of multiple cysts giving the appearance of a mass of soap bubbles—a larger cyst on the surface and smaller ones infiltrating into muscle and tissue planes. This makes surgical excision challenging. There are *macrocystic* (>1 cm) *or microcystic* (<1 cm) varieties depending on the predominant size of the cysts. It contains clear lymphatic fluid and is lined with endothelium. The fluid is lymphocyte rich which can aid in pathological diagnosis. In comparison with cystic hygroma, lymphatic malformations are generally larger lesions, situated more anteriorly in the head and neck and not associated with other malformations, hence have a better prognosis.

9.2 Sites

They can occur anywhere. Lower third of the posterior triangle of the neck is a common site, other sites being the check, axilla, groin, mediastinum, intrathoracic, intra-abdominal, and tongue (Figs. 9.1 and 9.2).

Clinical features The lesion may present at birth or appear early in infancy. Large swelling may obstruct labor. The characteristics of the swelling are soft, cystic, and partially compressible due to the intercommunication of cysts. It may increase in size with cough or cry, and usually brilliantly trans illuminant (Fig. 9.3). Clinical behavior is uncertain, as it may increase in size due to infection (Fig. 9.4) or hemorrhage, and

S. Roy Choudhury
Pediatric Surgery, Lady Hardinge Medical College and Associated Kalawati Saran Children's Hospital, New Delhi, Delhi, India

V. Jain (✉)
Department of Pediatric Surgery, AIIMS, New Delhi, India

© The Author(s), under exclusive license to Springer Nature Singapore Pte Ltd. 2025

S. Roy Choudhury (ed.), *Pediatric Surgery*, https://doi.org/10.1007/978-981-96-1257-4_9

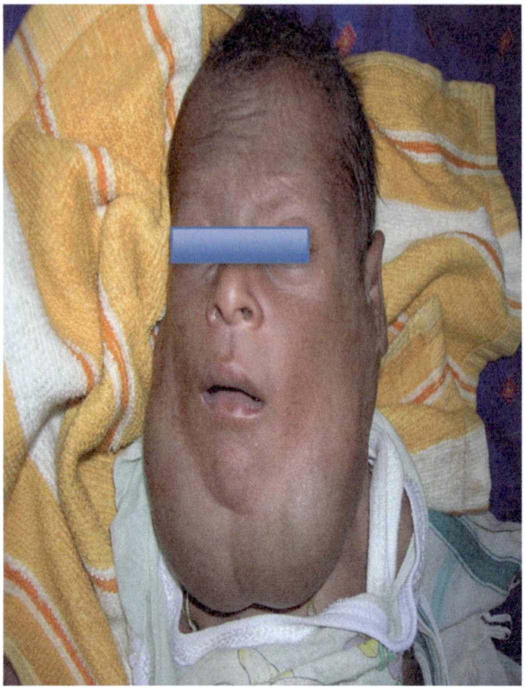

Fig. 9.1 Extensive lymphatic malformation of the neck

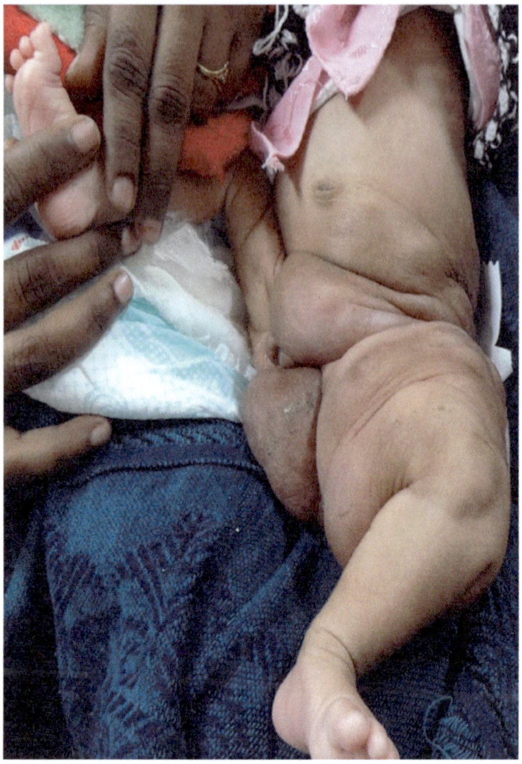

Fig. 9.2 Extensive lymphatic malformation involving groin and extremities

Fig. 9.3 (**a**) Lymphatic malformation of the chest wall, (**b**) brilliantly trans illuminant

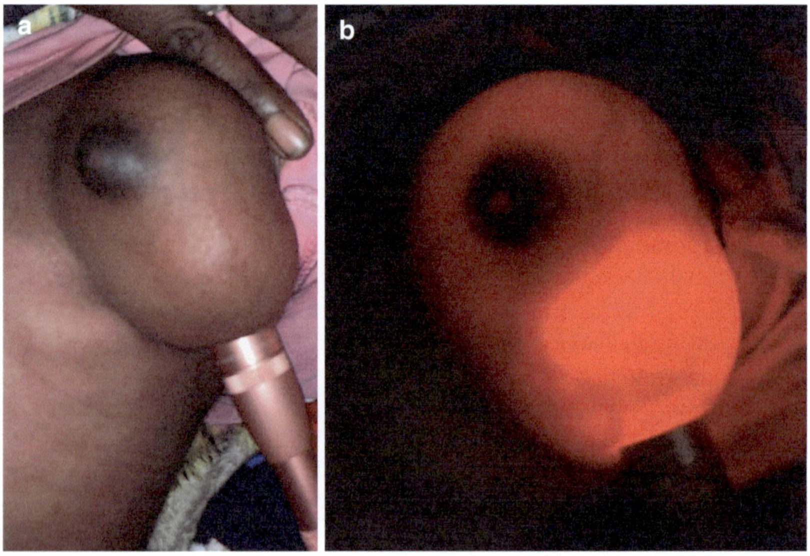

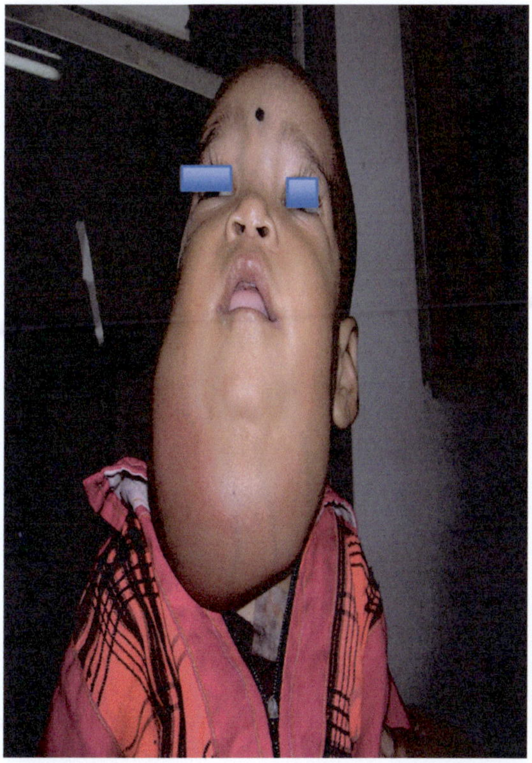

Fig. 9.4 Lymphatic malformation of neck with infection

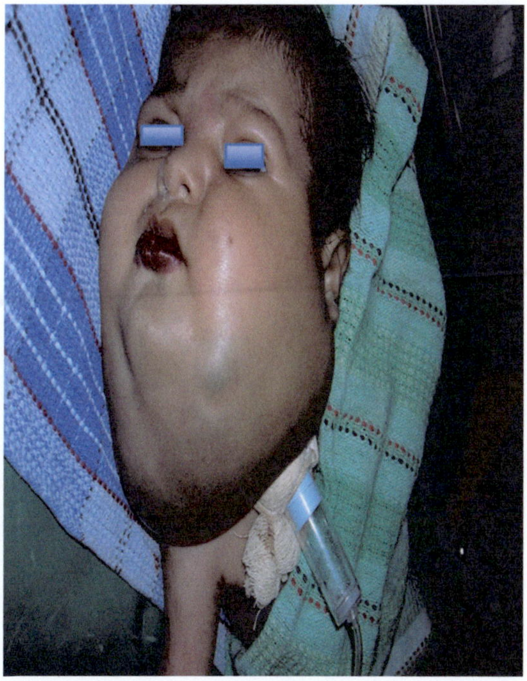

Fig. 9.5 Airway obstruction due to lymphatic malformation

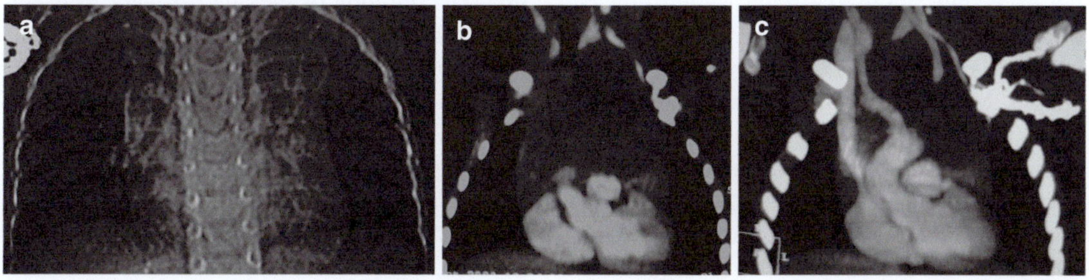

Fig. 9.6 Chest X-ray (**a**) and CT scan (**b**, **c**) showing lymphatic malformation involving neck with mediastinal extension, note insinuation between the vessels

may cause airway obstruction (Fig. 9.5). It may even decrease in size and disappear. Neck lesions may have intrathoracic extension (Fig. 9.6).

9.3 Investigation

Ultrasonography is useful for diagnosis as it shows the cystic nature of the swelling. Imaging may show a fluid level in case of bleeding into the cyst. However, the detailed anatomical extent can be better defined with magnetic resonance tomography (MRI). MRI with contrast may also be helpful in ruling out an associated slow-flow venous malformation.

Complications Infection, hemorrhage, and airway obstruction (Fig. 9.5) are common complications.

Treatment In antenatally diagnosed large lesions involving the neck, assessment should be made regarding the possibility of airway compromise after birth. In such cases, ex utero intrapartum procedure can be performed in which the airway of the neonate is intubated while the baby is still attached to the mother through the placenta.

Lesions involving small babies and asymptomatic small lesions may be observed. For large and symptomatic lesions, injection sclerosant therapy is effective.

Sclerosant injection after aspiration of the cyst fluid is usually successful in the macrocystic variety. However, results are unsatisfactory when it is used for the microcystic (solid) type. The different agents used are hypertonic saline, bleomycin, sodium tetradecyl sulphate, doxytetracycline, and OK 432 therapy (lyophilized mixture of group A *Streptococcus pyogenes* and benzylpenicillin).

Intralesional bleomycin is injected under ultrasound guidance under sedation. The dose of injection bleomycin is 0.2 IU/kg body weight, not exceeding 0.5 mg/kg body weight repeated at intervals of 2–3 weeks with a maximum cumulative dose not exceeding 5 mg/kg body weight. Majority responds between 1 and 4 sittings of sclerotherapy (Fig. 9.7). Very often due to an inflammatory response, there is an increase in the size of the swelling in the first few days after sclerotherapy. This is usually self-limiting but caution should be exercised in large infiltrative cervical lesions as they may compromise the airway. Application of gentle compression after sclerosant injection improves the effectiveness and avoids hematoma formation. Complications of bleomycin include mild flu-like symptoms, erythema, edema, and pigmentation. Febrile response following bleomycin sclerotherapy is common and usually managed with antipyretics like paracetamol. Sclerotherapy results in obliteration of lymphatic channels with minimal fibrosis. The mechanism of action is probably cytokine-mediated damage to endothelial cells.

The presence of infection requires treatment with antibiotics with or without aspiration of the contents. The macrocystic lesion often responds favorably to injection sclerotherapy but the microcystic variety often has a poor response (Fig. 9.8a, b).

Novel drugs like sirolimus synonymous with rapamycin, due to their antilymphangiogenetic properties by inhibition of mammalian target of rapamycin (mTOR) and vascular endothelial growth factor have been tried successfully in the management of microcystic or difficult infiltrative lesion. The dose is 0.8 mg/m^2 per dose twice daily to achieve a target blood level of 10–15 ng/mL. The duration of therapy can vary from few months to years, and the potential side effects are hyperlipidemia, leucopenia, and infections.

Surgical excision is usually done for the residual lesion after sclerotherapy or for easily removable lesions. Primary surgical excision for extensive lesions infiltrating into nerves, vessels, or vital structures is challenging and better avoided.

Airway obstruction may require tracheostomy or urgent cyst aspiration.

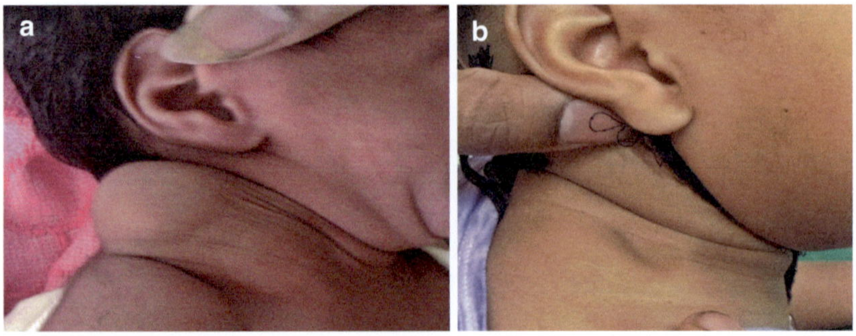

Fig. 9.7 (**a**) Cervical lymphatic malformation, (**b**) resolution after one course of bleomycin sclerotherapy

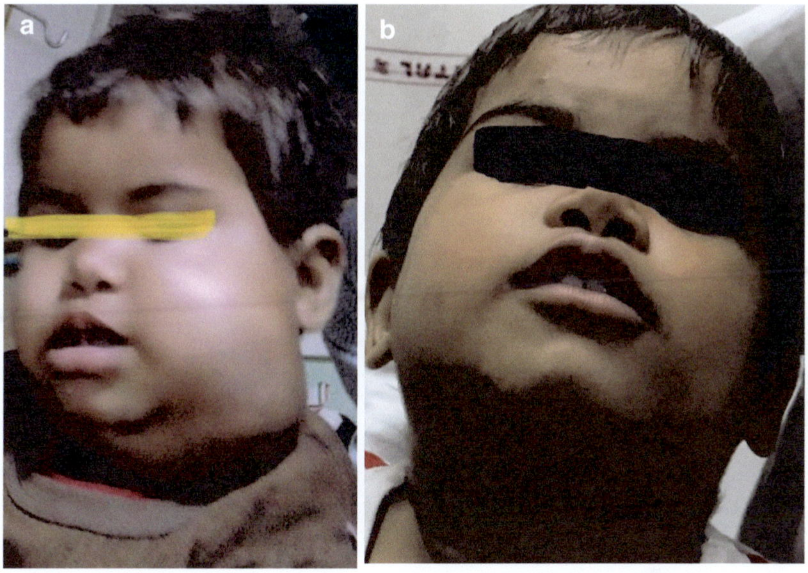

Fig. 9.8 (**a**) Large lymphatic malformation, left cheek, (**b**) response after bleomycin sclerotherapy

Summary: Lymphatic Malformations

1. Congenital hamartomatous lesion involving the lymphatic system, often with mixed venous or other tissue elements.
2. Presents usually in infancy, and common sites are the neck, axilla, groin, mediastinum, abdomen, and tongue.
3. Grossly, the lesions may be macrocystic (>1 cm), microcystic (<1 cm), and mixed, large lesions may obstruct vital structures like airway. Complications like infection and hemorrhage are common.
4. Imaging with ultrasound and MRI usually shows infiltration of the malformed tissues into anatomical tissue planes, rendering complete surgical excision difficult.
5. Management varies from observation to sclerotherapy to surgical excision.
6. Macrocystic variety responds well to injection sclerotherapy. For complicated and extensive lesions, sirolimus can be tried.

Suggested Reading

Coran AG, Scott Adzich N, Krummel TM, Shamberger RC, Caldamone A, Laberge JM, editors. 2012 Pediatric surgery. 7th ed. Oxford: Elsevier; 2012.

Gupta DK, Sharma S, Azizkhan RG, editors. Pediatric surgery—diagnosis and management. 1st ed. New Delhi: Jaypee Brothers; 2009.

Holcomb GW III, Murphy PJ, St Peter SD, editors. Holocomb and Ashcraft's pediatric surgery. 7th ed. Philadelphia: Elsevier; 2020.

Kumar V, Choudhury SR, Yadav PS, Khanna V, Gupta A, Chadha R, Anand R. Results of injection sclerotherapy with bleomycin in pediatric lymphatic malformations. J Indian Assoc Pediatr Surg. 2021;26:223–7.

Wiegand F, Dietz A, Wichmann G. Efficacy of sirolimus in children with lymphatic malformations of the head and neck. Eur Arch Otolaryngol. 2022;279:3801–10.

Part II

Organ Transplantation in Children

10 Liver and Kidney Transplantation in Children

Sanjay Rao

10.1 Certain Basic Facts About Organ Transplantation

Organ transplantation (Tx) is one of the most dramatic and successful developments in modern medicine. A collaborative effort among different specialties—surgeons, physicians, immunologists, radiologists, intensive care specialists and basic scientists has ensured that advances in the laboratories have been rapidly brought to the bedside, thereby improving outcomes. Presently, Tx remains the sole life-saving option for patients with end-stage liver disease and the preferred option for those with end-stage renal disease (ESRD).

Kidneys and livers remain the most common organs transplanted. Heart, lungs, pancreas, and intestines are the other solid organs transplanted as part of routine clinical care.

Composite grafts such as hand and limb transplants, facial transplants, and uterine transplants are still in stages of development and refinement.

Over the years, early outcomes of transplantation have improved exponentially. However, many transplanted organs deteriorate over the years and fibrose—this is thought to be due to poorly understood immune responses. Hence, transplant immunology is an extremely important aspect of solid organ transplantation.

10.2 The Concept of Self and Non-self: A Brief Look into Transplant Immunology

Our innate immunity has the ability to recognise 'self' from 'non-self'. This fundamental, but complex, ability is responsible for our ability to survive in this highly antigenic world. Our immune system has the ability to recognise multiple different antigens and retains the ability to recognise newer ones that are presented to it over a lifetime. Also retained is a memory of antigens that it has interacted with previously, and the ability to mount rapid immune responses to similar antigens. Even though understanding has improved, much of this extraordinarily complex system remains unexplained.

The main players in this complex orchestra of antigen recognition are:

(i) *The Major Histocompatibility Complex (MHC)*
In humans, this is called the human leucocyte antigen (HLA) system. These are a group of antigens that are both *species (allo-)* and *individual (auto-)* specific. It is able to recognise self-proteins, proteins from other humans and non-human proteins. This system is encoded on a set of genes on the short

S. Rao (✉)
Department of Pediatric Surgery, Division of Solid Organ Transplantation, Narayana Health Hospitals, Bangalore, India

© The Author(s), under exclusive license to Springer Nature Singapore Pte Ltd. 2025
S. Roy Choudhury (ed.), *Pediatric Surgery*, https://doi.org/10.1007/978-981-96-1257-4_10

arm of Chromosome 6, at loci 6p21–31. These encode a series of proteins called HLA proteins, which are of three types:

A. Class I: they are expressed on all nucleated cells and are recognised by CD8+ (cytotoxic-T) lymphocytes. There are HLA-A, HLA-B, and HLA-C antigens.
B. Class II: these are expressed only on antigen-presenting cells—macrophages, dendritic cells and B cells. These are recognised by CD4+ (Helper T) lymphocytes. These are HLA-DP, DR and DQ. Of these, HLA-DR is thought to be important in the genesis of rejection.
C. Class III: their role is not clearly understood. These include C4B, Bf, C2, TNF A and B.

The MHC genes are inherited, one allele from each parent, and are co-dominant. This inheritance pattern results in great heterogeneity and provides each individual with a specific immunological signature.

(ii) *Effector cells*: T lymphocyte, B lymphocytes, NK cells, and macrophages.
(iii) *Soluble elements*: such as antibodies, complement factors, cytokines, and interleukins.

All these elements process every antigen that is presented to the host—this includes the antigens coming with the graft organ. An immune reaction is mounted by the recipient and this is called rejection. Left uncontrolled, this inflammation will destroy the graft organ and cause serious harm to the recipient. The science and art of controlling this process is called *post-transplant immune suppression*.

Rejection can happen at different stages after transplant, and these are summarised in Table 10.1.

Various immunological tests are used to ensure compatibility between the donor organ and the recipient. The tests look to identify the presence, in the recipient serum, of preformed antibodies against the donor HLA antigens. Presence of such antibodies increases the risk of hyperacute/acute rejection. (At this time, there is no test that predicts chronic rejection.)

Table 10.1 Types of rejection seen after organ transplantation

Hyperacute rejection	Acute rejection	Chronic rejection
Occurs soon after reperfusion Immediate graft destruction	Usually in the first 6 months post Tx	Usually, after 6 months of transplantation
From preformed antibodies from previous transplants or blood transfusion	Either T cell-mediated or antibody-mediated or both	Antibody mediated
Characterised by intravenous thrombosis and interstitial haemorrhage	Characterised by cellular infiltration of graft with inflammatory cells	Myointimal proliferation in graft arteries, leading to ischaemia and graft fibrosis
Kidney is particularly vulnerable	Can lead to early graft injury	Most common cause of long-term graft loss

1. *Blood group compatibility*: the first test is a blood group. The donor blood group must be identical or compatible with the recipients. Though across the blood group transplantation is feasible and performed regularly, the immune suppression requirements, in the early post-operative period, are higher.
2. Complement-dependent cytotoxicity *cross match*: this is the oldest and traditional method. Donor lymphocytes are mixed with recipient serum and complement. If preformed antibodies exist, the test is termed positive.
3. *Flow cytometry-based crossmatched*: here too, donor lymphocytes are mixed with recipient serum and fluorescent labelled anti-HLA antibodies. Cells are then run through a flow cytometry to identify anti-HLA antibodies.
4. *Virtual cross match*: here, there is donor lymphocytes used. Instead, the recipient serum is mixed with beads coated with a standard panel of human antigens. Each bead can be coated with a single or multiple antigens. The test has high sensitivity and specificity. The advantage is that logistically, there is no need

to get donor samples to the testing laboratory.

10.3 Post-transplant Immunosuppression

The goal is to modify the immune response in such a way that organ rejection is prevented. At the same time, the immune system must retain its ability to battle infections and neoplasia.

Eventually, it is hoped that the host will achieve a level of 'tolerance', characterised by the acceptance of specific 'non-self' antigens without medication; however, this goal has not been reached in solid organ transplantation.

The various techniques used to control rejection are described in Table 10.2.

Majority of long-term complications after solid organ transplantation are related to the consequences of prolonged immune suppression, especially true in children, who after transplant, are looking at decades of immune suppression. Complications include renal dysfunction, dyslipidaemia and metabolic syndrome and post-transplant lymphoproliferative disease (PTLD).

Current immunosuppression regimens successfully limit hyperacute and acute rejection.

Table 10.2 Commonly used drugs and techniques to control rejection after organ transplantation

Drugs	Monoclonals	Physical techniques
Calcineurin inhibitors: Tacrolimus, cyclosporine *Anti-metabolites*: Azathioprine, mycophenolate *Corticosteroids* *m-TOR inhibitors*: Rapamycin	ATG, anti-thymocyte globulin Basiliximab (IL-2 receptor blocker, anti-CD25, T-reg cells, regular T cells) OKT-3 (muromonab, first monoclonal used in Tx of rejection, blocks CD3, which is a T cell that activates CD4, CD8)	Plasmapheresis Immune adsorption Splenectomy

However, they have not been very successful in limiting damage to the graft from chronic immunological effects–which results in chronic graft fibrosis and dysfunction. This is a major problem in paediatric transplantation as children are expected to have many decades of survival after their transplantation.

10.3.1 Source of Grafts

The original source of grafts was from compatible cadaveric brain-dead donors. A single donor could provide organs to up to 6–7 individuals. The laws governing brain death are well defined. India was one of the countries to adopt the concept of brain death quite early. The Transplantation of Human Organs Act (THOA) is a central law that regulates all transplant-related activity in the country. Each state has created state-specific rules under the umbrella of the THOA.

In India, the system is governed by the National Organ and Tissue Transplantation Organisation, set up under the Director of Health Services, Ministry of Health and Family Welfare, Government of India. Each state has SOTTO, under the corresponding state ministry. There are Regional OTTO (ROTTO) proposed (these will coordinate donor and organ sharing between adjacent states—there are five ROTTOS proposed).

However, as transplantation became more successful, the waitlist for organs grew longer. The challenge is even more acute in Asia, as the social acceptance of cadaveric donation is low. There was high wait-list mortality—especially in the case of liver. (Kidney failure patients could be maintained on dialysis). This problem was even more acute for children, for whom finding size-matched cadaveric donors was difficult. This led to the development of several strategies to reduce pre-transplant waitlist mortality. These include:

(i) *Marginal donor organs*: these included utilising organs from elderly donors, donors with comorbidities, donors with prolonged hypoxia/hemodynamic instability, infections, etc.

(ii) *Reduced liver grafts*: here, 2–4 segments of a donor liver are used for the child and the rest is discarded. While this provided more organs to children, it also led to wastage.
(iii) *Split liver grafts*: here, the left lateral segments from an adult cadaveric donor are transplanted to a small child, while the remaining right lobe is provided to a suitable-sized adult; in this way, two patients are transplanted from one donor liver. However, this process is technically challenging and requires specific expertise.
(iv) *Donation of cardiac death*: in many cases, a dying person does not fit the criteria of brain death. In such instances, the organs can be harvested after cessation of cardiac activity. Naturally, this leads to a longer warm ischaemia time and this can affect graft function and the success of the transplant.
(v) *Living donor transplants*: organs are procured from health voluntary donors. A healthy person could donate one kidney or a part of their liver to a person in need. In this instance, donor safety is paramount. The downside of this technique was the problems related to organ trade. Despite its challenges, living donor organ donation remains the mainstay of liver and kidney transplantation in India and most of Asia. It is an optimal technique for infants and small children, needing a liver transplant.

10.3.2 Ischaemia Time

During the transplantation process, the graft is ischaemic. There are two phases:

(i) *Warm ischaemia*: this occurs from the time of clamping of arterial inflow in the donor, up to the time that the organ is completely perfused with cold perfusion fluid. In the case of live donor and donation after brain death, this period is relatively short lasting 15–30 minutes. However, in donation of cardiac death, the warm ischaemia time can run up to an hour or more. Maximum injury to tissues occurs during warm ischaemia time and this needs to be kept to the minimum.
(ii) *Cold ischemia*: this starts from the time the organ is fully perfused with cold perfusion fluid and cooled with ice. It ends when the organ is reperfused after completion of vascular anastomosis in the recipient. This time includes time taken for bench work, packing, transportation, and implantation. Cooling of the organ decreases the metabolic rate of tissues and reduces oxygen consumption. The perfusion fluid has chelating agents that chelate toxic products of anaerobic metabolism. This has allowed the transport of organs over long distances to ensure optimal usage of this precious resource. The two common perfusion fluids are histidine–tryptophan–ketoglutarate (HTK) and University of Wisconsin solutions.

The ischaemia time should be kept as short as possible. However, a kidney can survive ischaemia times of up to 8–12 hours if properly prepared, while a liver can be used even after 6–8 hours of ischaemia time.

Organ	Optimal (Hr)	Maximum (Hr)
Heart, lungs	<3	8
Pancreas	<10	24
Liver	<12	24
Kidney	<24	48

On unclamping the vessels in the recipient, the organ is reperfused with warm blood. This ischaemia reperfusion is known to cause varying degrees of organ injury and can result in delayed graft function.

10.3.3 Normothermic Machine Perfusion

This is a recent technique where the organ is placed in a bath and perfused with processed blood at body temperature. As there is no ischaemia-reperfusion injury, organs are better preserved, and can be kept viable for long periods of time—even up to 24 hours. The other benefit is that biochemistry of venous blood from the organ allows accurate assessment of graft function before transplant—this is especially useful when marginal grafts are used.

Table 10.3 Varioius factors that determine outcomes in organ transplants

Patient-related factors	Graft-related factors	Immunological factors
Surgical factors and technical issues	Degree of ischaemic injury to organ—Both before and after harvest	Degree of compatibility between donor and recipient
Pre-existing morbidities-especially those that will not correct with the transplant	Age and comorbidities in donor	Pre-existing sensitisation of recipient (previous transplant, blood transfusion)
Extremes of age	Haemodynamic and metabolic instability	Compliance with immune suppression regimen
	Ischaemia times	
	Technical issues during harvest	

10.4 Factors Determining Outcome of Transplantation

These are enumerated in Table 10.3.

10.5 Liver Transplantation

The first successful liver transplantation was performed in 1967, by Thomas Starzl, in a child with biliary cirrhosis secondary to biliary atresia. However, challenges related to organ availability and immune suppression continued to hinder its rapid adoption. With the advent of efficient drugs such as cyclosporine and adoption of brain death criteria, transplantation became more commonplace during the 1980s and 1990s, in adults. Since the late 1990s, paediatric liver transplantation has also grown rapidly. Over the next 2 decades, refinements in techniques, intensive care and immunosuppression have made paediatric liver transplantation a routine procedure, even in small infants.

10.5.1 Indications of Liver Transplantation in Children

LTx remains the only, and life-saving, option in children with end-stage liver disease, whatever the cause. Biliary atresia accounts for about 50% of all liver transplants performed in children. The common indications are illustrated in Fig. 10.1.

LTx may have to be performed as an emergency in some situations. Fulminant hepatic failure occurs due to acute viral hepatitis, paracetamol toxicity, and some toxins such as yellow phosphorus. Also emergency retransplant is required in patients who develop acute hepatic artery (HAT) or portal vein thrombosis (PVT) or primary nonfunction.

10.5.2 When Does One Refer a Patient to a Transplant Centre?

A patient should be referred to a transplant centre early, once a transplant is considered a therapeutic option. In cases of biliary atresia, if at the end of 2–3 months post Kasai Portoenterostomy, referral to a transplant centre is recommended. Similarly, in patients with cirrhosis of the liver (from any cause, even if they are reasonably well compensated), pretext III or IV hepatoblastoma are potentially patients who may require a liver transplant, and an early contact with the transplant centre helps.

On referral, the transplant team—paediatric hepatology, surgeons, anaesthetists, social work, and coordinators—will review the child and the family. The child will be optimised with special focus on nutritional rehabilitation, infection treatment and prevention (cholangitis, spontaneous bacterial peritonitis, bacterial colonisation, cytomegalovirus (CMV)), immunisation, identification, and optimisation of comorbidities. The family will be educated about transplantation and its sequelae. If there is a voluntary donor is available from the family, donor evaluation will also

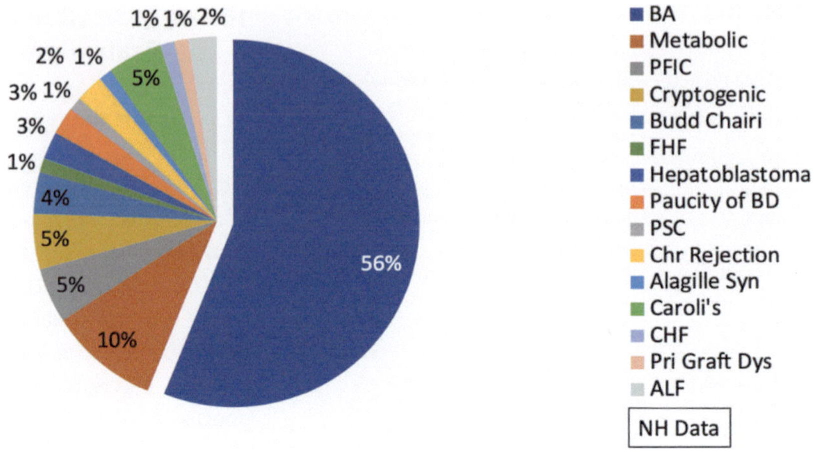

Fig. 10.1 Indications for liver transplantation in children

be commenced. Help and advice to raise finances will be often provided. An assessment will be made about the need for and the potential timing of a liver transplant.

This early referral allows time for the transplant team to work with the child and the family. Also, the child and family become familiar with the transplant process and teams. This goes a long way in ensuring transparency, trust and optimal therapy—all of which are essential for a high stakes interventions like transplantation.

10.5.3 Donor Evaluation and Estimation of Graft Size

Children requiring transplantation vary in age from infancy to teenage, with weights from a few kilograms to 50–60 kg. The optimum size of the graft required is calculated using the *Graft Recipient Weight Ratio* (GRWR). An ideal GRWR is between 1% and 3%. For example, for a 10-kg child, a graft weight between 100 and 300 g is ideal. A graft that is less than 0.8% or more than 4% in GRWR is associated with a higher risk of complications and poorer outcomes. Current imaging technologies allow accurate assessment of segmental volume/weight in the donor liver. Based on these findings, resections for graft procurement can be planned—a left lateral segment graft is often adequate for most children in the first decade. Larger grafts—either a full left lobe or even a right lobe—would be required for bigger children.

In case of cadaveric donation, it is not possible to perform detailed imaging and clinical assessment during at the time of organ retrieval relied upon. This calls for some experience and expertise.

The potential living donor is thoroughly evaluated to ensure they do not have comorbidities that could increase surgical risks. The liver is carefully assessed for vascular and biliary anatomy and fat content. A triphasic CT scan, MRI scan, and fibro scans are all used in varying combinations. Vascular and biliary anatomy needs to be closely looked at. This is to ensure that safe retrieval is feasible, the residual liver in the donor is not jeopardised and the graft anatomy allows for a safe implantation in the recipient.

10.5.4 The Transplant Operation

10.5.4.1 Anaesthetic Considerations

The anaesthetic preparation for a liver transplant includes robust vascular and central venous access, invasive monitoring of cardiorespiratory and renal physiology, temperature maintenance and close monitoring of hemodynamic, biochemistry, coagulation, fluid and electrolytes. Close and continuous communication between the anaesthetic team and the surgical team is essential for a successful outcome. Point-of-care monitoring greatly facilitates timely management.

Surgery commences with a generous upper abdominal incision. In case the patient has had previous abdominal surgery, incorporation of the previous scars in the incision is preferred. The surgery progresses in 3 phases.

10.5.5 Phase One: Explanation of Native Liver

After gaining entry into the peritoneal cavity, the liver is completely mobilised by dividing all its moorings the left and right triangular and falciform ligaments. In children who have had a previous Kasai portoenterostomy or any previous laparotomy, the abdomen is usually full of inflammatory adhesions which are all vascular. This occurs due to portal hypertension that is a part of biliary cirrhosis. The transverse colon and hepatic flexure, duodenum, stomach and small bowel are usually densely adherent to the liver capsule. Careful and meticulous dissection is essential to allow for safe separation of the bowel from the liver and minimise blood loss. Once colon and duodenum are taken down, the lesser sac and the porta hepatitis are exposed. Major vascular structures—inferior vena cava above and below the liver, portal vein, hepatic arteries—are identified, dissected and looped. In case the child has had a kasai portoenterostomy (KPE) previously, the roux loop is carefully taken down from the liver and preserved for later use. This phase of surgery is often tedious and is associated with significant blood and fluid loss. Careful monitoring and interventions from the anaesthetics to replenish fluid and blood products are essential. The liver is completely mobilised, and the retrohepatic inferior vena cava (IVC) is separated from the posterior abdominal wall by dividing several small tributaries that might exist.

10.5.6 Phase 2: Explanation and the Anhepatic Phase

Once it is confirmed that the donor graft is ready and being prepared, explanation of the recipient liver commences (Fig. 10.2). Clamps are applied across the IVC, an inferior clamp just cranial to renal veins and a superior clamp above the insertion of the hepatic veins, close to the diaphragm. The portal vein and hepatic arteries are controlled with a vascular clamp and divided close to the liver. The liver is then separated from the IVC by dividing the three hepatic veins. The cirrhotic liver is removed. The child is now anhepatic (Fig. 10.3). Haemostasis is confirmed and then anaesthetic team optimises haemodynamics, acid base and coagulation.

10.5.7 Phase 3: Implantation and Neo Hepatic Phase

The graft liver is now brought into the field and implantation starts (Fig. 10.4). The first anastomosis to be performed is an end-to-side anastomosis between the hepatic veins and the IVC. This anastomosis is usually made at the site of the

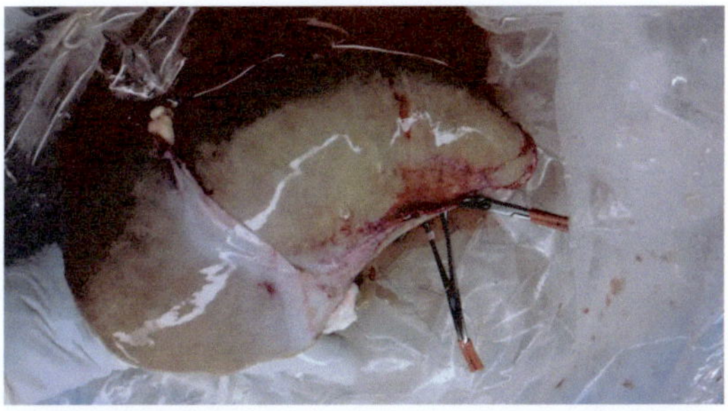

Fig. 10.2 Cadaveric full liver graft, for implantation in size-matched donor

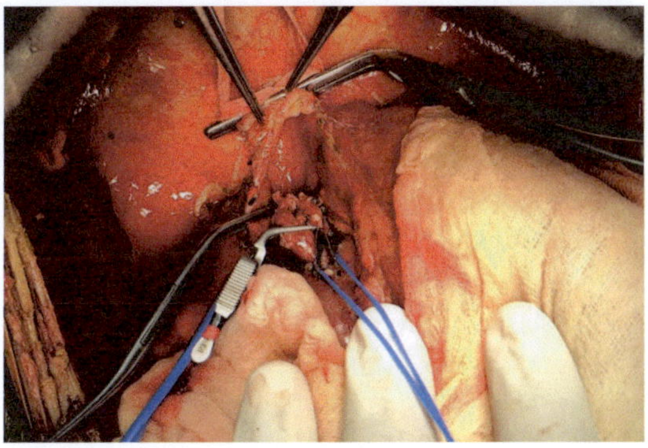

Fig. 10.3 A hepatic phase. Clamps on suprahepatic and subhepatic IVC, bulldogs on portal vein and hepatic artery

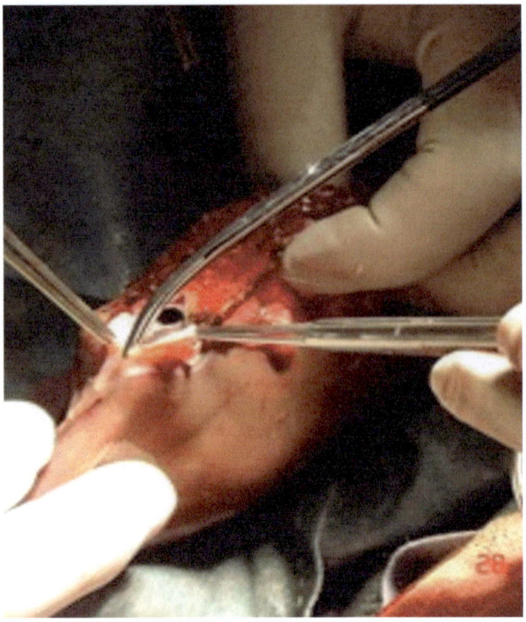

Fig. 10.4 Bench work in progress, hepatic veins being prepared in live donor left lateral segment liver graft

original left and middle hepatic veins with a generous extension caudally. A triangular configuration is achieved to ensure an absence of kinking and adequate flow. Next, an end-to-end anastomosis between the patient and graft portal vein is carried out. Often, in children with biliary atresia, the native portal vein is of poor quality, very narrow and with poor flow. Techniques to enhance hepatopetal portal flow are often required. Once a secure anastomosis of the portal vein is completed, IVC and portal vein clamps are removed and the new liver is perfused with portal blood. This is the neo hepatic phase (Fig. 10.5).

Neo hepatic phase is often associated with haemodynamic instability as backed up acidotic, blood from below the diaphragm suddenly rushes into the heart. The anaesthetist has to be especially vigilant to rapidly correct these abnormalities. Meanwhile, the surgical team ensures a proper flow across the anastomosis and secure haemostasis. Once the child is haemodynamically stable and haemostasis has been insured, the hepatic artery anastomosis is done. Use of microvascular techniques has resulted in a significant reduction in hepatic artery thrombosis rates.

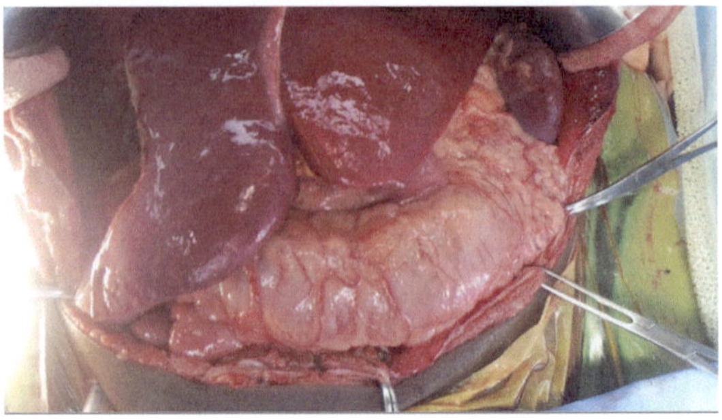

Fig. 10.5 Left lobe liver graft, after reperfusion–neohepatic phase

Biliary drainage is usually achieved by use of a roux y jejunal loop, either a fresh one or the pre-existing one done during the KPE. Bile duct to duct anastomosis is feasible in older children where the transplantation is being performed for metabolic indications.

A thorough lavage is done, haemostasis rechecked and the abdomen closed after placing drains. In small recipients, often anatomical closure of the abdominal wall risks abdominal compartment syndrome and in such instances just skin and fascial closure is performed, leaving a ventral hernia. This is repaired some weeks down the line.

The child is shifted to the intensive care unit (ICU) on the ventilator. Over the next few hours, haemodynamic and biochemistry are stabilised. Early graft function is assessed by falling lactate levels, euglycaemia, stable haemodynamics and improving coagulation. Early next morning, an ultrasound Doppler is performed to ensure graft health and satisfactory flows through all the vascular anastomosis. The child is extubated and monitored for steady recovery over the next few days. Generally, graph function stabilisers over the next 48–72 hours as reflected by falling transaminases and passage of normal coloured stools. Early feeding is commenced and the child is shifted to the wards.

10.5.8 Immunosuppression

Immunosuppression is commenced with the administration of 5 mg/kg of methyl prednisolone before reperfusion of the graft. In specific instances, induction using biologicals such as basiliximab (an IL6 receptor blocker) is administered. Tacrolimus is commenced on return to the ICU and is administered enterally, in a dose of 0.15 mg /kg/day in two divided doses. Our practice is to wean steroids rapidly and have the child on a single drug by the end of 2 months. Tacrolimus dosage is titrated based on trough levels.

The child is generally discharged 3–4 weeks after the transplantation.

10.5.9 Early Post-operative Complications

Early vascular thrombosis (hepatic artery—HAT and portal vein—PVT) and the most serious surgical complications. If recanalisation cannot be achieved, the graft undergoes irreversible damage and survival is low in the absence of an emergency re-transplantation. The incidence of vascular thrombosis varies between 5% and 15%. It is higher in technical variant grafts, living donor grafts and in children with biliary atresia. Other surgical complications include early bleeding, biliary leaks, and intestinal complications such as perforations and obstruction. Close surveillance and early response to these are essential to limit morbidity and enhance recovery.

Sepsis remains one of the most common complications in the post-operative period. Many of these children are chronically hospitalised, are heavily colonised with resistant bacteria, malnourished and immunosuppressed—all these add to the risk of sepsis. Delayed graft function, hepatorenal syndrome, and hepatopulmonary syndrome are other well-known complications.

10.5.10 Long-Term Complications Could Be Surgical or Medical

Surgical complications are related to biliary stricture, vascular stenosis and adhesive intestinal obstruction. Medical complications are almost all related to the adverse effects of immunosuppression. These include infections (CMV, ebstein barr virus (EBV), fungal), renal dysfunction, metabolic syndrome, cytomegalovirus (CNS) effects and PTLD. Careful monitoring of immunosuppression is essential to limit these side effects.

10.5.11 Outcomes

After a successful transplant, children catch up in growth and milestones and have a good quality of life. However, lifelong care and medication are essential.

Thirty-day mortality is about 5%. Long-term survival is about 80%. About 10–15% of children will require re-transplantation as a result of chronic rejection.

10.6 Renal Transplantation

Kidney transplantation is the second most common solid organ transplantation performed in children. Children are defined to have end stage renal disease (ESRD) when their glomerular filtration rate (GFR) is <15 mL/min/1.73 m^2. At this point, children require renal replacement—either dialysis or renal transplantation.

Peritoneal dialysis (long-term, domiciliary) and haemodialysis are both feasible options in children. However, these carry significant morbidity and long-term results are poorer as compared to transplantation. The longer a child remains on dialysis before transplant, the worse the outcomes of transplant. Hence, there is a large push for pre-emptive transplant—that is renal transplant as primary treatment of ESRD, without spending a significant time on dialysis.

The general principle of renal transplantation is like that of liver transplant. However, as the kidney does not have the capacity to regenerate (unlike the liver), outcomes are marginally less than that for liver. The kidney is also more immunogenic than the liver and more prone to acute and chronic rejections.

10.6.1 Indications for Renal Tx

The general indication for renal transplantation in children includes

(i) ESRD, unresponsive to medical therapy.
(ii) Progressive growth failure.
(iii) Severe renal osteodystrophy.
(iv) Developmental delay.
(v) Inability to maintain dialysis (peritoneal or haemodialysis).

10.6.2 Threshold for Renal Replacement

Most children will require renal replacement therapy when GFR <15 mL/min/1.73 m^2. This is grade V of chronic kidney disease (CKD), also referred to as end-stage renal disease (ESRD).

The common causes for ESRD in children are listed in Table 10.4.

10.6.3 Renal Transplant in Children with Lower Urinary Tract Anomalies

Establishment of safe, low-pressure storage and unobstructed drainage before transplantation is essential. As most of these children are not anuric, bladder assessment is possible by standard techniques. A detailed history of voiding aided by uroflowmetry and an ultrasound of the kidney, ureter, bladder (KUB) system looking at bladder wall thickness, capacity and post-void residue provides valuable information and guides the requirement of more invasive tests. A video urodynamic study is performed when necessary.

Major lower urinary tract reconstructions such as Mitrofanoff and augmentation, if required, should ideally be done before transplant. However, these procedures will lead to a worsening of the baseline renal function and should be embarked upon only when a clear path to transplant is in place. Ideally, the transplant should happen about 4–6 weeks after these reconstructions.

Unlike in liver transplant, where the liver is placed in the orthotopic position, the graft kidney is placed in a heterotopic position, usually in the right iliac fossa. This position allows for easy access to the common iliac vessels, aorta and IVC to reconstruct a robust blood supply to the graft. In addition, the bladder is close by and reimplantation of the graft ureter is without tension.

Table 10.4 Common causes of ESRD in children

Surgical causes	Medical causes
Posterior urethral valve	Glomerulonephritis
Obstructive uropathy	Diabetic nephropathy
Bilateral renal dysplasia	Hypertensive nephropathy
Neurogenic bladders	Renal vascular disease
Recurrent pyelonephritis (VUR)	Drug-induced nephropathy
Polycystic kidney disease	Metabolic diseases, primary oxalosis

10.6.4 Role of Native Kidney Nephrectomy

Native nephrectomy is required in a minority of cases. Indications for native nephrectomy are

(i) Proven focus of infection in the kidney.
(ii) Severe proteinuria.
(iii) Large kidneys, such as in those with autosomal recessive polycystic kidney disease (ARPKD), to allow space for the graft kidney.

Managing an anephric patient is extremely challenging. Hence, native kidney nephrectomies are performed as close to, or along with, the renal transplant. In a child, it is easy to perform a right native kidney nephrectomy, by slightly extending the usual renal transplant incision cranially. A laparoscopic left nephrectomy can be performed if required a few weeks before the transplant.

10.7 The Renal Transplant Procedure

In cases of living donor, usually, the left kidney is harvested from the donor. The long left renal vein allows for comfortable vascular reconstruction in the recipient. The donor nephrectomy is performed laparoscopically, and the kidney is removed via a small incision in the lower left abdomen. Donor nephrectomy is a standardised procedure and rapid recovery is the norm.

10.7.1 Recipient Operation

An incision is made in the right lower abdomen, in a hockey stick fashion. If the child has a previous Pfannenstiel incision, the same can be extended laterally and upwards. The extraperitoneal space is entered and peritoneum is reflected medially to expose the iliac artery and veins. Usually, the kidney vessels are anastomosed in an end-to-side fashion to the common iliac artery and external iliac vein in the recipient (Fig. 10.6). In younger recipients, the anastomosis is usually at a higher level, even at the aorta and IVC if required. This is essential to ensure a good pressure head for the child's circulation to perfuse the adult graft kidney. Once the vascular anastomosis is complete, the bladder is filled and identified. An extravesical Lich-Gregoir type ureterovesical anastomosis is performed, a double j stent is inserted before completion of the anterior wall. In patients who have had previous augmentation, it is preferable to implant the ureter in the native bladder if this can be identified. If not, it is anastomosed to the augment itself. Haemostasis is ensured, a perinephric drain is placed, and the abdomen closed. If the kidney is large, only the anterior sheath is closed; it is important to avoid compression of the graft. In smaller children, the kidney can be placed intraperitoneally, as there is insufficient space in the retroperitoneum.

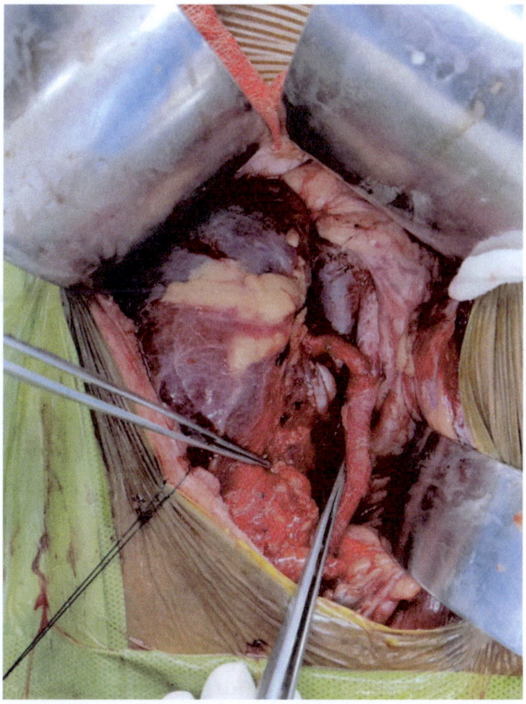

Fig. 10.6 Renal transplant completed, renal artery anastomosed end-to-side to common iliac artery, renal vein end-to-side to common iliac vein

10.7.2 Outcomes of Renal Transplantation in Children

The overall graft survival is about 75% at 10 years. Unlike in the case of liver, the kidney is more prone to chronic immunological injury and long-term graft fibrosis. The outcomes are somewhat poorer in those with lower urinary tract anomalies, possibly due to effects from recurrent urinary infections and a hostile bladder in these children. These children also carry a higher risk of mortality as compared to those with normal lower urinary tracts. A second transplant is usually required when the transplant is performed in younger children and hence limiting sensitisation is important.

10.7.3 Combined Liver–Kidney and Multi-visceral Transplant

Dual organ transplants are standard procedures now. A combined liver and kidney transplant is performed in certain conditions, a classical example being primary oxalosis. Here, there is an enzymatic defect in the liver that results in stone formation from an early age—which in turn damages the kidney. A combined liver–kidney transplant helps cure the problem. Similarly, a combined liver and intestinal transplant is performed for children with short gut who have end-stage liver disease from total parenteral nutrition (TPN) cholestasis. A liver–heart transplant is performed in children who develop 'Fontan Hepatopathy'. A kidney–pancreas transplant benefits patients with severe insulin-dependent diabetes with diabetes induced renal failure. These procedures are technically more challenging and need large multidisciplinary teams to achieve good results.

10.8 Special Considerations-Paediatric Recipients

Children who develop CKD and chornic liver disease (CLD) in early childhood carry a lifelong burden-first from their organ failure and then from the sequelae of transplant and immunosuppression. These are major challenges; the child and the family require support and care for a lifetime. Even after a successful transplant, children are susceptible to the adverse effects of lifelong immune suppression. It is imperative that their care also be taken to ensure that the medical team continuously addresses the child's continued development, education, social interactions and psychological well-being. As these children enter teenage, high-risk behaviour and non-compliance with medications become major issues and lead to a high incidence of graft loss in the mid-teens to mid-twenties. Careful support and hand-holding are essential to ensure that the young transplant recipient navigates these challenges successfully.

10.9 Conclusions

Transplantation remains the standard of care for end-stage organ failure and provides the best chance of optimal long-term survival and quality of life. However, it is not without its challenges—especially those related to long-term immune suppression. However, with the advent of multispecialty transplant teams and a better understanding of the science and art of transplantation, outcomes are steadily improving. It is hoped that, in the future, techniques will be available to ensure immune tolerance and the holy grail of one child one transplant for life.

Further Reading

Martinez OM, Rosen HR. Basic concepts in transplant immunology. Liver Transpl. 2005;11(4):370–81.

Transplantation of Human Organs and Tissues Act. 1994. https://www.indiacode.nic.in/handle/123456789/1962.

Dunn SP, Horslen S. Solid organ transplantation in infants and children. Springer; 2018. https://doi.org/10.1007/978-3-319-07284-5.

Pancreas Transplantation

11

Sukrit Singh Shah

History of human organ transplantation

- First successful renal transplant was done by Joseph Murray in 1954 in identical twins.
- Simultaneous pancreas and kidney transplantation (SPK) 1966 by William Kelly and Richard Lillehei at the University of Minnesota.
- 1974—David Sutherland—pancreatic islet transplantation.

11.1 Introduction

Unlike other solid organ transplants, whole pancreas transplantation in the pediatric population is not common and usually is done as a component of multivisceral or composite organ transplantation. It is rare to find devastating sequelae of type 1 diabetes mellitus in children; pancreatic transplantation is generally done in the setting of acute recurrent or chronic pancreatitis and not for diabetes mellitus.

More importantly, islet cell autotransplantation is essential post-total pancreatectomy wherein pancreatectomy removes the foci of chronic pain while autologous islet cell transplantation aims to preserve endocrine function.

Limited studies done to date have found satisfactory outcomes with glycemic control, freedom from chronic opioid use and consequently improved quality of life (QOL) scores in patients of chronic pancreatitis operated for total pancreatectomy and autologous islet cell transplantation.

11.2 SPK Transplantation (Simultaneous Pancreas and Kidney Transplantation)

- The simultaneous transplantation of the kidney and pancreas can render a patient free of both lifelong usage of insulin injections and the need for dialysis. It can occasionally reverse the end-stage disease.
- How is it done?
- Systemic venous drainage to the right iliac vein and bladder drainage of the pancreas exocrine secretions through a duodenocystostomy.
- Donor splenic artery, the donor superior mesenteric artery (SMA), joined by a Y-graft constructed from the donor common external/internal iliac artery complex anastomosed to the recipient common iliac artery.
- The mid-duodenum is anastomosed to the posterior dome of the bladder, and the duodenal stumps are oversewn (Fig. 11.1).

S. S. Shah (✉)
Lady Hardinge Medical College, New Delhi, Delhi, India

© The Author(s), under exclusive license to Springer Nature Singapore Pte Ltd. 2025
S. Roy Choudhury (ed.), *Pediatric Surgery*, https://doi.org/10.1007/978-981-96-1257-4_11

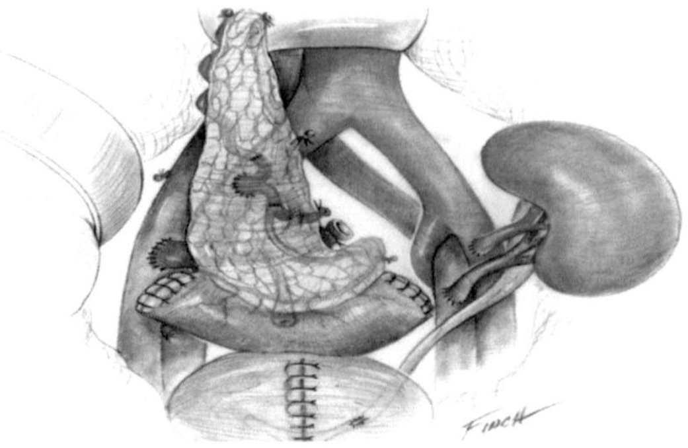

Fig. 11.1 Simultaneous pancreatic and kidney transplant showing placement of grafts and outflow and inflow communications (see text for description)

11.3 Pancreas–Duodenal Transplantation

- Pancreas–duodenal transplantation with systemic venous drainage and enteric drainage of graft exocrine secretions to a proximal loop of the recipient jejunum.
- End-to-side two-layer duodenojejunostomy, using the distal end of the graft duodenum, and the anastomosis is located 40–80 cm distal to the ligament of Treitz.
- Alternatively, a side-to-side stapled or hand-sewn duodenojejunostomy, with or without a Roux-en-Y loop, can be done.

11.4 Islet Cell Transplantation

- Islet cell transplantation into the portal vein using an embolization technique to the liver, where at least some islets will survive by nutrient diffusion until revascularization occurs.
- Done either as an autograft of islet cells isolated from the excised specimen after total or distal pancreatectomy.
- Or as an allograft of cells isolated from a donor for the treatment of a patient with type 1 diabetes,
- Islet autotransplantations have had a relatively high success rate in preventing diabetes after total pancreatectomy.
- Dr. Shapiro and colleagues (2000) at the University of Alberta in Edmonton achieved diabetes reversal in seven of seven recipients by using islets from more than one donor pancreas.

Suggested Reading

Balamurugan AN, Elder DA, Abu-El-Haija M, Nathan JD. Islet cell transplantation in children. Semin Pediatr Surg. 2020;29(3):150925.

Principles of Immunosuppression Therapy in Organ Transplants in Pediatric Age Group

12

Madhavi Redkar

12.1 Introduction

Significant advances in modern medicine characterize the achievements of healthcare industry. Rapid and newer advances of antimicrobials, widespread vaccination and transplantation have revolutionized modern medicine. Transplantation includes solid organs, blood and blood products, and more recently, stem cell transplants.

Organ transplantation is the best therapy for terminal and irreversible organ failure. However, despite many improvements, it still encounters persistent issues. Medically, the recipient's immune system poses the most significant challenge since it orchestrates several defense processes to eliminate the allogeneic transplant, which it detects as "foreign." Although immune response plays a significant part in rejecting or accepting donor organs, multiple cell, and molecular mechanisms ultimately determine whether the transplant will be successful.

Over the past few decades, a wide range of immune suppressants has been created to manage the various types of rejection. The survival duration of the transplant has significantly increased thanks to immunosuppressive treatment and improved surgical and preservation technologies. Despite this, immune suppressants have many drawbacks. Significant iatrogenic effects can result from their targets' tissue distribution and molecular state.

12.2 Immunology

Understanding the immune system's identification and reaction to foreign tissue is a pivotal aspect of transplant immunology. This has become a topic of great medical interest and research.

After transplantation, recipient T cells become activated by the donor tissue's major histocompatibility complex (MHC) antigens, commonly referred to as human leukocyte antigens (HLAs). Both antibody-mediated and cellular-mediated mechanisms are involved when the recipient immune system is activated.

M. Redkar (✉)
Department of Pharmacology, BKL Walawalakar Rural Medical College and Hospital, Kasarwadi, At Post Sawarde, Chiplun, Maharashtra, India

© The Author(s), under exclusive license to Springer Nature Singapore Pte Ltd. 2025

S. Roy Choudhury (ed.), *Pediatric Surgery*, https://doi.org/10.1007/978-981-96-1257-4_12

Antibiotic-mediated immune response takes place via B-cells, activated by CD4+ T-cells, which produce donor-specific antibodies, whereas cellular immune response involves cytotoxic T cells, natural killer cells, macrophages, and neutrophils.

This immune response triggered by host cells can potentially damage the transplanted organ. Therefore, post-transplant immunosuppression therapy aims to modify these immune responses to minimize damage to the transplanted organ caused by the recipient's immune system.

12.3 Tissue Typing

Potential transplant candidates undergo HLA tissue typing before listing to lower the chance of rejection. Class I (HLA-A, B, and C) and class II (HLA-DP, DQ, and DR) HLA antigens are used to classify patients.

An individual has the ability to express up to six Class-I and six Class-II molecules because everyone has two chromosomes and the paternal and maternal chromosomes produce different HLA molecules.

HLA matching before organ allocation has the role of identifying the best match between the donor organ and recipient, as this will ensure an optimal outcome and minimize the risk of rejection.

12.3.1 Types of Immunity

The immune system consists of mainly two subdivisions: innate (natural) and adaptive (humoral) immunity.

Innate immunity is nonspecific and has no memory. It is the first-line protection against foreign antigens.

Adaptive immunity is antigen-specific and has a memory function. Cytokines are crucial for the development and differentiation of immune cells.

Both types of immunities can activate each other and play a role in transplant rejection. To cite an example, ischemia-reperfusion injury during transplantation is an important cause of transplant rejection. Both types of immunities are in play in this process.

Innate immunity is activated by the expression of damage-associated molecular patterns. These cause further tissue damage and release of donor antigens.

This process, in turn, involves the activation of B and/or T lymphocytes, a part of adaptive immunity. This may cause subsequent allograft rejection. This, in turn, increases the chances of sepsis or infection and failure of transplants. Understanding the fundamental principles of immunology is crucial for effective transplant management.

Immunosuppressive drugs are medications that suppress or reduce the activity of the immune system. They are commonly used in various medical conditions, including organ transplantation, autoimmune disorders, and certain inflammatory conditions.

Immunosuppressive drugs can be classified into several categories based on their mechanism of action and target within the immune system. Here are the main classes of immunosuppressive drugs (Table 12.1).

Table 12.1 Immunosuppressive drugs

Class of therapeutic agents	Examples	Place in therapy
Glucocorticoids	Prednisone Budesonide Prednisolone	The first line of immunosuppression Induction and maintenance agents
Small-molecule drugs Immunophilin-binding drugs Calcineurin inhibitors Cyclophilin-binding drugs: FKB12-binding drugs. Target-of-rapamycin inhibitors	Cyclosporine Tacrolimus, modified release tacrolimus Sirolimus, everolimus	Initial postoperative immunosuppression Tacrolimus is the first line of immunosuppression in most centers Early maintenance agents of immunosuppression
Inhibitors of nucleotide synthesis Purine synthesis (IMDH) inhibitors Pyrimidine synthesis (DHODH) inhibitors Antimetabolites. Sphingosine-1-phosphate-receptor antagonists.	Mycophenolate mofetil Enteric-coated mycophenolic acid (EC-MFS) Mizoribine (MZR) Leflunomide FK778 Azathioprine (Aza) FTY720 (fingolimod)	Acute to early immunosuppression. Acute to early immunosuppression
Protein drug Depleting antibodies (against T cells, B cells, or both). Nondepleting antibodies and fusion proteins.	Polyclonal antibody: Horse or rabbit antithymocyte globulin Mouse monoclonal anti-CD3 antibody (muromonab-CD3) Humanized monoclonal anti-CD-52 antibody (alemtuzumab) B-cell-depleting monoclonal anti-CD-20 antibody (rituximab) Humanized or chimeric monoclonal anti-CD25 antibody (basiliximab) Fusion protein with natural binding properties: CTLA4-Ig (belatacept)	Immunosuppression-inducing drugs Early maintenance drug/induction Early maintenance drugs
C5 inhibitor	Eculizumab	
Janus Kinase inhibitors	*Tofacitinib*	Newer and rescue immunosuppressive drugs

12.4 Modern Immunosuppression

The primary objective of immunosuppression is to prevent graft rejection and minimize unfavorable reactions. Presently, immunosuppression regimens used are associated with rejection rates between 35% and 40%, but due to the emergence of various molecules and modern modalities, graft loss due to rejection is much less.

Immunosuppressive drugs are also classified into three categories: induction, maintenance, and anti-rejection. Presently, immunosuppressive agents are administered as combination therapies. The specific combinations depend on individual patient factors and the circumstances of the surgery, as summarized in the accompanying table. A brief mention of the pharmacology of various drugs is given below.

12.5 Induction Agents

Include various classes of drugs like the following:

12.5.1 Monoclonal Antibodies (MAB)

Basiliximab is a monoclonal antibody that blocks interleukin-2 (IL-2) receptors, inhibiting IL-2-induced T-cell activation. It is primarily used as an induction agent in kidney transplantation and is also employed in some steroid-free protocols for pancreas transplantation.

The administration of basiliximab as an induction agent facilitates early withdrawal of steroids and significantly reduces the need for other immunosuppressive medications shortly after transplantation.

Alemtuzumab is a monoclonal antibody that specifically targets CD52, which is widely expressed on the surface of immune cells, including all B and T cells, most macrophages, and natural killer cells. This makes Alemtuzumab an effective lymphocyte-depleting agent.

It is generally used for patients at high immunological risk.

While it is effective in lowering the risk of organ rejection, its use is associated with a heightened risk of postoperative opportunistic infections and post-transplant lymphoproliferative disease.

12.5.2 Interleukin Inhibitors

These drugs target specific cytokines, such as tumor necrosis factor-alpha (TNF-alpha), interleukin-1, or interleukin-6, to reduce inflammation and immune activity. Examples include drugs like adalimumab, infliximab, and tocilizumab.

12.6 Early Maintenance Agents

12.6.1 Calcineurin Inhibitors

Calcineurin inhibitors (CNIs), such as cyclosporine and tacrolimus, are potent inhibitors of the T-cell response. They work by blocking the production of interleukin-2 (IL-2).

CNIs are the primary agents used for initial postoperative immunosuppression, with tacrolimus being the first-line immunosuppressant in most transplant centers.

These medications are nephrotoxic due to their vasoconstrictive effects, so it is important to regularly monitor their levels, as they have a narrow therapeutic window.

In addition to nephrotoxicity, CNIs can cause other side effects. Common adverse reactions include hypertension, neurotoxicity, diabetes mellitus, and hyperlipidemia. Tacrolimus, more commonly associated with and presenting as tremors, headaches, and irritability, is more neurotoxic.

Cyclosporine has specific adverse effects as well, including hirsutism and gingival hyperplasia.

12.6.2 Antiproliferatives

Mycophenolate mofetil (MMF) and azathioprine are the most commonly used antiproliferative agents.

Their main mechanism of action involves inhibiting nucleotide synthesis, with the most notable side effect being severe myelosuppression.

First-pass metabolism converts MMF into the active compound mycophenolic acid (MPA). MPA inhibits lymphocyte proliferation by blocking DNA formation.

12.6.3 Mammalian Target of Rapamycin (mTOR) Inhibitors

Mammalian target of rapamycin (mTOR) inhibitors, such as sirolimus and everolimus, disrupt intracellular signaling pathways and inhibit the activation and proliferation of T-cells.

Both sirolimus and everolimus can be used in conjunction with low-dose calcineurin inhibitors (CNIs) in recipients experiencing CNI-induced nephrotoxicity; The aim is to improve renal function while maintaining the effectiveness of the immunosuppressive regimen.

These agents are seldom employed as primary immunosuppressants. The side effects reported include bone marrow suppression, hyperlipidemia, peripheral edema, and delayed wound healing.

Immunosuppressive antibiotics Some antibiotics, such as cyclophosphamide and methotrexate, have immunosuppressive properties and are used in certain autoimmune disorders and organ transplantation.

12.7 Corticosteroids

Corticosteroids, also known as glucocorticoids (GCs), have a wide range of anti-inflammatory and immunosuppressive effects. Glucocorticoids (GC) are powerful, nonspecific anti-inflammatory agents used in both the induction and maintenance of immunosuppression. They work by binding to intracellular receptors.

These effects primarily occur through genomic mechanisms, although some occur via nongenomic pathways.

The genomic effects of GCs typically have a delayed onset. They occur when GCs bind to their cytosolic receptors, enter the nucleus, and activate glucocorticoid response elements. This process induces the expression of anti-inflammatory genes (known as transactivation).

Additionally, GCs repress the activation of genes that promote inflammation, such as those regulated by nuclear factor kappa-light-chain enhancer of activated B-cells and activator protein-1, a process referred to as transrepression.

In the innate immune system, glucocorticoids (GCs) reduce the production of proinflammatory cytokines, such as tumor necrosis factor-alpha (TNF-α) and interleukin-1 beta. In dendritic cells, GCs inhibit the upregulation of costimulatory molecules, including CD40, CD80, CD83, CD86, and MHC-II.

GCs are also the first-line treatment for acute cellular rejection, typically administered as high-dose intravenous methylprednisolone.

However, prolonged use of glucocorticoids can lead to numerous side effects, including diabetes mellitus, hypertension, increased susceptibility to infections, osteoporosis, hyperlipidemia, delayed wound healing, and neuropsychiatric symptoms.

To mitigate the long-term complications associated with corticosteroids, steroid withdrawal protocols, which include mycophenolate mofetil (MPA) plus a calcineurin inhibitor (CNI), are currently employed.

12.7.1 Long-Term Maintenance Therapy

After transplantation, the prophylaxis against rejection can be gradually reduced as the patient enters the late maintenance phase. This typically involves tapering steroids and progressively lowering calcineurin inhibitor (CNI) levels. Treatment regimens can vary between centers and among patients, but they generally involve one or two main therapies.

However, long-term maintenance therapy is linked to several health risks, including an increased likelihood of cardiovascular issues and nephrotoxicity associated with CNIs. Additionally, there is a heightened risk of opportunistic infections, such as cytomegalovirus and *Pneumocystis jirovecii*, as well as an increased risk of certain malignancies, including post-transplant lymphoproliferative disorder.

The specific medical condition, individual patient factors, and the required level of immunosuppression influence the choice of immunosuppressants. Healthcare professionals must carefully monitor and manage these medications to balance the benefits of immune suppression with the risks of infections and other potential side effects.

12.7.2 Organ Rejection

Despite the employment of immunosuppressive therapies, organ rejection may still occur at times.

Recipient responses to donor organs can be classified into hyperacute rejection, acute rejection, or chronic rejection. The presentation varies depending on the transplanted organ, but a tissue biopsy is required for definitive diagnosis.

Hyperacute rejection is a rapid and destructive response triggered by preformed cytotoxic antibodies that target donor HLA or ABO antigens. If not addressed immediately, graft destruction can occur within a mere 24 hours.

The critical importance of preventing hyperacute rejection cannot be overstated; meticulous preoperative blood group and HLA matching are essential strategies to safeguard against this potentially devastating outcome.

Acute rejection The most frequent form of rejection is acute rejection, affecting up to 50% of grafts. It typically happens within the first 6 months after the transplant.

It is primarily caused by a T-cell-mediated immune response against the graft's major histocompatibility complexes (MHCs).

Acute rejection is higher in individuals with a history of HLA sensitizing episodes, such as previous transplants or blood transfusions.

Treatment for acute rejection usually involves high-dose steroids. If the response is not adequate, second-line treatment options may include plasma exchange or intravenous immunoglobulin.

Chronic rejection typically occurs after 6 months and is characterized by a gradual decline in organ function.

The causes of chronic rejection are multifactorial, including immune-mediated injury, ischemia-reperfusion injury, and toxicity from immunosuppressive agents.

Unfortunately, immunosuppressive therapies are often limited in their ability to reverse chronic rejection.

12.7.3 Newer Research Areas

Soluble mediators of immune response are being researched as potential therapeutic targets. Focus in recent times is on the increasing role of the innate immune system in solid organ transplantation and solid allograft rejection. While the adaptive immune system has been the focus of previous research studies, recent evidence suggests that the innate immune system and its soluble mediators play a more important role in these processes. The role of novel soluble mediators involved in innate immune activation during allo-immune response and solid allograft rejection is being researched worldwide. New treatments to stop allograft loss in solid organ transplantation may result from a better knowledge of these soluble mediators.

Cytokines, miRNAs, eATP, pentraxin 3 (PTX3), and soluble receptor for advanced glycation end products (sRAGE) are a few of the unique soluble mediators. These mediators activate the innate immune system during solid allograft rejection and the allo-immune response.

Potential diagnostic/prognostic indicators and therapeutic targets for allograft injury and protection are found to be PTX3 and sRAGE.

12.8 Recent Advances

Recent advances in immunosuppressive strategies are vital for organ transplantation, as they help prevent the recipient's immune system from rejecting the transplanted organ. Some key developments in this field are:

- *Targeted therapies*: researchers have been exploring targeted immunosuppressive drugs that aim to inhibit specific immune system components involved in rejection, such as certain immune cells or cytokines. These targeted therapies may offer more effective immunosuppression with fewer side effects compared to traditional broad-spectrum immunosuppressive agents.
- *Personalized medicine*: the advances in genetic testing enhance the understanding of how individual variations in drug metabolism shape personalized medicine regimes in transplant immunosuppression.
  Customizing the immunosuppressive treatment based on a patient's genetic profile may enhance the effectiveness of the therapy while reducing side effects.
- *Tolerance induction*: tolerance induction refers to strategies that are oriented at achieving donor-specific immunological tolerance. This allows the recipient's immune system to accept the transplanted organ without requiring lifelong immunosuppression.

Various approaches, such as mixed chimerism, regulatory T cell therapy, and immune tolerance biomarkers, are being studied to induce tolerance and reduce or eliminate the need for immunosuppressive drugs.

- *Immunotherapies and new drug combinations*: the introduction of innovative immunotherapies has significantly transformed the field of oncology.
  Recent advancements in checkpoint inhibition therapies, tumor-infiltrating lymphocyte therapies, chimeric antigen receptor T cell therapies, and cancer vaccines have demonstrated great potential for improving cancer treatment outcomes.
  Researchers are currently exploring new drug combinations to enhance the effectiveness of immunotherapy while minimizing side effects. Immunotherapies work by enhancing different stages of the immune response, helping the body recognize, target, and eliminate cancerous cells more effectively.
  Combining immunotherapies with other treatment modalities aims to boost the immune response, reduce immunosuppression, and address signaling and resistance pathways. This approach offers a more durable and long-lasting treatment compared to traditional therapies and immunotherapies used alone for cancer.
- *Optimal monitoring and management strategies*: further research is essential to identify the best strategies to monitor and manage pediatric patients undergoing immunosuppressive therapy. These strategies may involve the determination of the ideal frequency and methods to track drug levels, immune function, and possible complications. Establishing clear guidelines and standardized approaches can help healthcare professionals deliver consistent and evidence-based pediatric healthcare.
- *Biomarker-guided immunosuppression*: biomarkers are measurable indicators that can help predict the risk of organ rejection or other complications. By using biomarkers to guide immunosuppressive therapy, healthcare providers can achieve more precise dosing and adjustments of medications based on an individual's immune response. This approach has the potential to reduce the risk of rejection and minimize side effects.
- One biomarker that has gained prominence recently is tumor mutational burden (TMB). TMB measures the number of somatic mutations in a tumor's genome across its coding sequence. Studies have shown that a high TMB is associated with better response rates in patients undergoing treatment.

It is worth noting that these advances are an ongoing area of research and may not be readily available or widely implemented in clinical practice. Also, some promising molecules that may be in clinical trial stages involve adult patients. Their utility in the pediatric age group may require long-term studies and risk–benefit analysis.

12.9 Summary

The array of therapeutic immunosuppressive agents is rapidly increasing as newer modalities are being researched. Although many promising molecules are in the pipeline, it will take some time to use them in children.

Suggested Reading

Ali HA, Todd J, Palmer S. Rejection after lung transplantation? Am J Respir Crit Care Med. 2016;193(10):P17–8. https://doi.org/10.1164/rccm.19310P17. PMID: 27174487.

Barbari C, Fontaine T, Parajuli P, Lamichhane N, Jakubski S, Lamichhane P, Deshmukh RR. Immunotherapies and combination strategies for Immuno-oncology. Int J Mol Sci. 2020;21(14):5009.

Dashti-Khavidaki S, Saidi R, Lu H. Current status of glucocorticoid usage in solid organ transplantation. World J Transplant. 2021;11(11):443–65.

Goodman AM, Kato S, Bazhenova L, Patel SP, Frampton GM, Miller V, Stephens PJ, Daniels GA, Kurzrock R. Tumor mutational burden as an independent predictor of response to immunotherapy in diverse cancers. Mol Cancer Ther. 2017;16:2598–608.

Grinyó JM. Why is organ transplantation clinically important? Cold Spring Harb Perspect Med. 2013;3(6). PMID: 23732857; PMCID: PMC3662355.

Hussain Y, Khan H. Immunosuppressive drugs. In: Encyclopedia of infection and immunity. 2022. pp. 726–40. Epub 2022 Apr 8.

Organ Transplantation: Research perspectives. Collective Expert Report. Summary and Recommendations. Inserm [Institut National de la Santé et de la Recherche Médicale] (National Institute for Health and Medical Research). 2008.

Parlakpınar H, Günata M. Transplantation and immunosuppression: a review of novel transplant-related immunosuppressant drugs. Immunopharmacol Immunotoxicol. 2021;43:1–15.

PDQ Pediatric Treatment Editorial Board. Complications, Graft-Versus-Host Disease, and Late Effects After Pediatric Hematopoietic Stem Cell Transplantation (PDQ®): Health Professional Version. 2022. In: PDQ Cancer Information Summaries [Internet]. Bethesda (MD): National Cancer Institute (US); 2002-. Available from: https://www.ncbi.nlm.nih.gov/books/NBK577669/

Reyes J, Murase N, Starzl TE. Principles of transplantation. In: Pediatric surgery editor in chief Conran AG, vol. 1. Elsevier Saunders; 2012. p. 605–15.

Shrestha B. Immune system and kidney transplantation. JNMA J Nepal Med Assoc. 2018;56 https://doi.org/10.31729/jnma.3375.

Sykes M. Hematopoietic cell transplantation for tolerance induction: animal models to clinical trials. Transplantation. 2009;87(3):309–16. PMID: 19202432; PMCID: PMC2723946.

Usuelli V, Loretelli C, Seelam AJ, Pastore I, D'Addio F, Nasr MB, Fiorina P. Novel soluble mediators of innate immune system activation in solid allograft rejection. Transplantation. 2022;106(3):500–9.

Part III

Trauma

Head Injury in Children

13

Pinaki Ranjan Debnath, Gali Divya, and Subhasis Roy Choudhury

Head injury is the most common cause of trauma-related deaths in children. A total of 85% of the injuries sustained by children are mild and non-life-threatening and on the other hand, half of the deaths resulting from blunt trauma are because of brain injuries. Most common causes are falls and motor vehicle accidents. Use of child restraints and helmets can decrease the incidence of traumatic head injuries.

13.1 Types of Brain Injuries

Focal
Diffuse

13.1.1 Focal Injuries

Immediately apparent on initial neuroimaging, e.g., skull fractures, contusions, lacerations, and hematoma.

Skull fractures—majority of them do not require any treatment. Multiple or complex fractures are associated with high-energy impact.

Contusions—most common and majority of them are neurologically silent and only discovered on initial computed tomography (CT) scans.

Traumatic intracerebral hematomas—unusual in pediatric age, results from disruption of central arterial blood vessels. Traumatic intracerebral hematomas are distinguished from hemorrhagic contusions by their lack of contact with the surface of the brain. Surgical evacuation may be required if the intracranial pressures (ICPs) are high. Penetrating injuries are also possible but rare. Penetrating injuries with cerebrovascular injury or subarachnoid hemorrhage may require magnetic resonance imaging (MRI) with MR angiography or CT angiography.

13.1.2 Diffuse Injuries

These are due to angular or translational accelerations or decelerations and the injury is due to the direct result of energy dissipation within the substance of brain. Diffuse axonal injury, cerebral concussion, global ischemia, systemic hypoxia, and diffuse vascular injury are some of examples of diffuse injuries. Only minimal or no changes on early neuroimaging despite drastic changes in neurologic function clinically. Small but widespread intracerebral hemorrhages and intraventricular hemorrhages are a typical finding.

P. R. Debnath (✉)
Pediatric Surgery, ABVIMS and Dr. RML Hospital, New Delhi, India

G. Divya
Department of Pediatric Surgery, All India Institute of Medical Sciences, New Delhi, India

S. Roy Choudhury
Pediatric Surgery, Lady Hardinge Medical College and Associated Kalawati Saran Children's Hospital, New Delhi, Delhi, India

© The Author(s), under exclusive license to Springer Nature Singapore Pte Ltd. 2025

S. Roy Choudhury (ed.), *Pediatric Surgery*, https://doi.org/10.1007/978-981-96-1257-4_13

Subdural hematomas may occur in association with diffuse axonal injury. These patients with diffuse axonal injury (DAI) are unconscious from the time of injury and remain so for a prolonged period. Decerebrate posturing and pupillary changes may also be noted. CT scan findings include multiple petechial hemorrhages in the deep white matter even though the initial CT may appear normal. Intraventricular hemorrhage or focal subarachnoid hemorrhage in the prepontine cistern is highly suggestive of DAI.

13.2 Nonaccidental Injuries

Clinical presentation with altered consciousness, retinal hemorrhage, acute intracranial hemorrhage on CT, new or healing skeletal fractures or other solid organ injuries are pathognomonic features of inflicted injuries especially if the history is not known or reported to be minor. These children need multidisciplinary management.

13.3 Assessment of Children with Head Injury

1. The severity of injury is measured by Glasgow Coma Scale Score (GCS) (Table 13.1)
2. CT Scan

Computed tomography is indicated if there is loss of consciousness, seizure, cranial penetration, cerebrospinal fluid (CSF) leak, headache, persistent vomiting, lethargy, or irritability

3. Magnetic Resonance Imaging

The advantage of MRI over CT scan is that it poses no risk of radiation

4. Pediatric Trauma Score (Table 13.2)

Table 13.1 Pediatric glasgow coma scale

Pediatric Glasgow Coma Scale (PGCS)				
	>1 Year		**<1 Year**	**Score**
Eye opening	Spontaneously		Spontaneously	4
	To verbal command		To shunt	3
	To pain		To pain	2
	No response		No response	1
Motor response	Obeys		Spontaneous	6
	Localizes pain		Localizes pain	5
	Flexion-withdrawal		Flexion-withdrawal	4
	Flexion-abnormal (decorticate rigidity)		Flexion-abnormal (decorticate rigidity)	3
	Extension (decerebrate rigidity)		Extension (decerebrate rigidity)	2
	No response		No response	1
	>5 Years	**2–5 Years**	**0–23 months**	
Verbal Response	Oriented	Appropriate words/ phrases	Smiles/coos appropriately	5
	Disoriented/confused	Inappropriate words	Cries and is consolable	4
	Inappropriate words	Persistent cries and screams	Persistent inappropriate crying and/or screaming	3
	Incomprehensible sounds	Grunts	Grunts, agitated, and restless	2
	No response	No response	No response	1
Total Pediatric Glasgow Coma Score (3–15):				

Table 13.2 Pediatric trauma score

Assessment component	Score +2	+1	−1
Weight	>20 kg (>44 lb)	10–20 kg (22–44 lb)	<10 kg (<22 lb)
Airway	Normal	Oral or nasal airway, oxygen	Intubated, cricothyroidotomy, or tracheostomy
Systolic Blood Pressure	>90 mm Hg; good peripheral pulses and perfusion	50–90 mm Hg: carotid/ femoral pulses palpable	<50 mm Hg: weak or no pulses
Level of Consciousness	Awake	Obtunded or any loss of consciousness	Coma, unresponsive
Fracture	None seen or suspected	Single, closed	Open or multiple
Cutaneous	None visible	Contusion, abrasion, laceration <7 cm not through fascia	Tissue loss, any gunshot wound or stab wound through fascia
Totals:			

Source: Adapted with permission from Tepas JJ. Mollitt DL Talbert JL, et al. The pediatric trauma score as a predictor of injury severity in the injured child. *Journal of Pediatric Surgery* 1987; 22(1)15

13.4 Management

13.4.1 Mild Head Injuries

Children with these injuries recover without any intervention. Airway, breathing, and circulation should be assessed. Advanced trauma life support (ATLS) guidelines should be followed during the initial resuscitation phase

13.4.2 Severe Injuries

Child should be arranged for pediatric intensive care unit admission. Secure airway if GCS < 8 or worsening neurological status. The head of the bed should be elevated (without hip flexion). The child's head should be kept in the midline, neutral position (to avoid jugular venous compression and spinal cord injury). Child should be mechanically ventilated if necessary. Aggressively treat hypotension with intravenous (IV) fluid boluses and vasopressors. Provide adequate analgesia (morphine) and sedation (midazolam). Paralyze with muscle relaxants. Mannitol should be given at a dose of 0.5–1 g/kg (2.5–5 mL/kg of 20% mannitol) by intravenous infusion over 20 min. Consider hypertonic saline (3–5 mL/kg of 3% saline) intravenous bolus (if given rapidly may result in drop in blood pressure). Monitor intracranial pressure (ICP) if GCS <8 by ventriculostomy and maintain ICP <20 mm Hg by CSF drainage if necessary. Hyperthermia should be avoided (>37.5 °C). All pediatric head-injured patients who require intravenous fluid for maintenance or resuscitation must receive 0.9% NaCl ±10 mmol KCL/500 mL. Further management is dependent on CT scan findings and consultation with a pediatric neurosurgeon.

Anterior basilar skull fractures may be manifested by periorbital ecchymoses, nasal hemorrhage, and CSF rhinorrhea is a contraindication to the placement of a nasogastric tube until the integrity of the anterior cranial skull base can be determined.

13.4.3 The Warning Signs to Watch by the Parents After Discharge

After discharge, child should be under close observation. If there are any symptoms like unusual sleepiness, jerking movements of arms, legs, or face—"a fit," severe headache, that paracetamol does not relieve, vomiting, confusion or unusual behavior, any change in the way your child walks or uses their arms/legs, blurred vision or slurred speech. Such signs should be immediately reported to the hospital.

Summary Box

- Most common causes are falls and motor vehicle accidents
- They can be focal, diffuse or nonaccidental injuries
- Injuries can be assessed by GCS, CT, or MRI and pediatric trauma score.
- Surgical evacuation may be required in cases of focal intracerebral hematomas with raised intracranial pressures.
- Use of child restraints and helmets can decrease the incidence of traumatic head injuries

Suggested Reading

ATLS guidelines – 10th edition; 2018.

Coran AG, Caldamone A, Scott Adzich N, Krummel TM, Laberge JM, editors. Pediatric surgery. 7th ed. Oxford: Elsevier Limited; 2012.

Wesson DE, Cooper A, Stylianos S, editors. Pediatric trauma pathophysiology diagnosis and treatment. 1st ed. New York: Taylor & Francis; 2006.

14 Abdominal Trauma in Children

Pinaki Ranjan Debnath, Gali Divya,
Arnab Kumar Saha, and Subhasis Roy Choudhury

Abdominal trauma accounts for 10% of overall trauma and is the third most common cause of death in children after head and thoracic injuries. It can be blunt abdominal trauma, which is most common (85%) or penetrating injury (15%). Most injured organs are the spleen, liver, kidney, pancreas, and less frequently small bowel and bladder. Short and pliable thoracic cage fails to protect upper abdominal organs like liver, spleen, and kidney and pelvis fails to protect the bladder below, as it is intraperitoneal organ initially.

14.1 Epidemiological Aspects

Different modes of injury are road traffic accidents (RTA), pedestrian hit by motor vehicle, fall from height, sports injuries, direct blows to abdomen, assaults, and child abuse. The age group most involved is 6–12 years. Males are affected more commonly. Waddell's triad comprises head injury, splenic laceration, and fracture of femur. Seat belt syndrome includes transverse bruise or contusion over the abdomen, anterior compression fracture of the lumbar spine, and visceral trauma rarely abdominal aortic injury. Parental education, child health education, strict enforcement of traffic regulations, proper supervision of children at home and play area can decrease the incidence of pediatric trauma.

14.2 Assessment of a Trauma Child

Different protocols which help in proper management of a trauma child include—Advanced Trauma Life Support, Pediatric Advanced Life Support, Advanced Pediatric Life Support, and Pediatric Emergency Trauma Advanced Life Support. Arizona-Texas-Oklahoma-Memphis-Arkansas Consortium algorithm has been validated in most pediatric trauma centers currently. The structured approach to a trauma child includes:

- Primary survey
- Initial resuscitation
- Secondary survey
- Definitive management

Focused assessment with sonography for trauma (FAST) is an important screening diagnostic tool in abdominal trauma. FAST-positive unstable patient even after resuscitation

P. R. Debnath (✉)
Pediatric Surgery, ABVIMS & Dr. RML Hospital, New Delhi, India

G. Divya
Department of Pediatric Surgery, All India Institute of Medical Sciences, New Delhi, India

A. K. Saha
Department of Surgery, Rohilkhand Medical College, Bareilly, India

S. Roy Choudhury
Pediatric Surgery, Lady Hardinge Medical College and Associated Kalawati Saran Children's Hospital, New Delhi, Delhi, India

© The Author(s), under exclusive license to Springer Nature Singapore Pte Ltd. 2025

S. Roy Choudhury (ed.), *Pediatric Surgery*, https://doi.org/10.1007/978-981-96-1257-4_14

may need laparotomy, and FAST-positive stable child should undergo computed tomography (CT) with intravenous (IV) contrast.

14.2.1 Primary Survey and Initial Resuscitation

Primary survey includes assessment of airway, breathing, circulation, neurological deficit, and exposing the child completely to search for any missed injuries (ABCDE). It includes identification of immediate and potential life-threatening injuries (Table 14.1).

The 2010 American Heart Association resuscitation guidelines changed the sequence of A-B-C to C-A-B for adults and children as checking for pulse and starting cardiac compressions should be before turning attention to airway.

14.2.2 Resuscitation

14.2.2.1 Airway

In addition to securing a patent airway, there are indications for mechanical ventilation including severe brain injury that requires controlled ventilation, where airway cannot be maintained, the patient showing signs of ventilatory failure, and a child who has suffered significant hypovolemia and has a depressed sensorium or requires operative intervention.

14.2.2.2 Breathing

Breathing should be assessed rapidly. Children have smaller functional residual volume, greater oxygen consumption, and increased chest wall compliance which can predispose to airway collapse and hypoxia. Tension pneumothorax, open pneumothorax, hemothorax, and flail chest should be identified rapidly which needs urgent intervention.

Table 14.1 Life-threatening injuries after trauma

Immediate life-threatening injuries	Potential life-threatening injuries
Airway obstruction	Simple pneumothorax
Tension pneumothorax	Hemothorax
Open pneumothorax	Pulmonary contusion
Massive hemothorax	Tracheobronchial injury
Cardiac tamponade	Cardiac contusion
Aortic disruption	Flail chest
	Diaphragmatic injury

14.2.2.3 Circulation

It can be assessed by evaluating heart rate, arterial pressure, capillary refill time, color and mental status (Table 14.2). Children can tolerate >25–40% blood volume loss. Hypotension is a sign of decompensated shock; tachycardia is an early sign when compared to hypovolemia. In an injured child of age < 6 years, if no intravenous (IV) access is achieved within 90 seconds, it is better to get an intraosseous access. Initial resuscitation fluid includes warm isotonic crystalloid either Ringer lactate or normal saline (NS). Large volumes of NS can lead to hyperchloremic acidosis.

14.2.2.4 Disability

It consists of brief neurological examination to determine the conscious level which is assessed by A-Alert, V-response to Voice, P-response to Pain, U-Unresponsive score, pupil size, and reactivity.

14.2.3 Secondary Survey

It includes a detailed head-to-toe examination to identify all traumatic injuries. Abdominal examination is done in the secondary survey. Inspection of the abdomen should document all abrasions and contusions as they indicate associated intra-abdominal injury. Tenderness on palpation suggests an intraperitoneal process like hemorrhage or perforation. Examiner should also look for abdominal distension, rebound tenderness, absent bowel sounds, and upper abdominal mass (duodenal hematoma). There is continued reassessment of ABCs even during secondary survey.

14.2.3.1 Tertiary Survey

It is performed 24 hours after admission which includes follow-up head-to-toe examination to reduce the risk of missed injuries.

Table 14.2 Normal vital functions as per age

Age group	Weight range (kg)	Heart rate (beats/min)	Blood pressure (mm Hg)	Respiratory rate (breaths/min)	Urinary output (mL/kg/h)
Infant (0–12 months)	0–10	<160	>60	<60	2.0
Toddler (1–2 years)	10–14	<150	>70	<40	1.5
Pre school (3–5 years)	14–18	<140	>75	<35	1.0
School age (6–12 years)	18–36	<120	>80	<30	1.0
Adolescent (≥13 years)	36–70	<100	>90	<30	0.5

14.2.3.2 Laboratory Evaluation

Routine trauma panel includes hematological and biochemical tests including complete blood picture along with hematocrit; glucose, liver enzymes, pancreatic enzymes, serum electrolytes, serum creatinine, and urine analysis because even microscopic hematuria is also associated with significant renal trauma.

Six clinical factors that help in identifying intra-abdominal injury are hypotension as per age, abnormal abdominal examination, low hematocrit, rise in aspartate aminotransferase, elevated amylase, and hematuria.

14.2.3.3 Imaging

Plain X-ray films of the thorax can give some information like air under the diaphragm and air fluid levels. Abdomino-pelvic radiographs help in assessing pelvic skeletal integrity.

14.2.3.4 Ultrasonography (USG)

Focused assessment with sonography in trauma (FAST) is highly sensitive in detecting free fluid in the peritoneal cavity; it has a sensitivity of 80% and a specificity of 96% but does not provide information regarding the grade of injury. Focused assessment by ultrasound in trauma (FAST) is advocated as initial evaluation in trauma. A FAST exam consists of sonographic evaluation of the pericardium, right upper quadrant, including Morrison's pouch, left upper quadrant, and the pelvis. This evaluation is to identify the presence of blood.

Contrast-enhanced USG is an emerging alternative in which second-generation intravenous contrast agent is used.

14.2.3.5 Computed Tomography (CT)

It is the gold standard investigation to identify injuries in blunt abdominal trauma. It gives a reliable characterization of solid organ injury. CT should be done in hemodynamically stable patients with intravenous contrast injection and oral contrast should be reserved only for some special cases. Hollow viscus injuries are difficult to detect on CT. In order to reduce ionizing radiation to children, Pediatric Emergency Care Applied Research Network established seven clinical indicators to undergo CT, which includes: abdominal wall bruising, glasgow coma scale (GCS) score <14, abdominal pain, vomiting, thoracic trauma, decreased breath sounds, abdominal tenderness. To reduce radiation exposure, as low as reasonably achievable principle helps in reducing the radiation delivered with each imaging study.

CT angiography is indicated in cases of pulseless limbs or any evidence of vascular compromise. Routine use of pan scans (whole-body CT scans) should be avoided. Contrast extravasation on CT does not need prompt embolization or surgery in a stable child.

14.2.3.6 Diagnostic Laparoscopy

It has both diagnostic and therapeutic applications; it can be applied for the assessment of both blunt and penetrating injuries. It helps in reducing exploratory laparotomies and associated morbidity. It is useful in managing hemodynamically stable patients suspected with early intra-abdominal injuries but is less valuable in patients with delayed presentation.

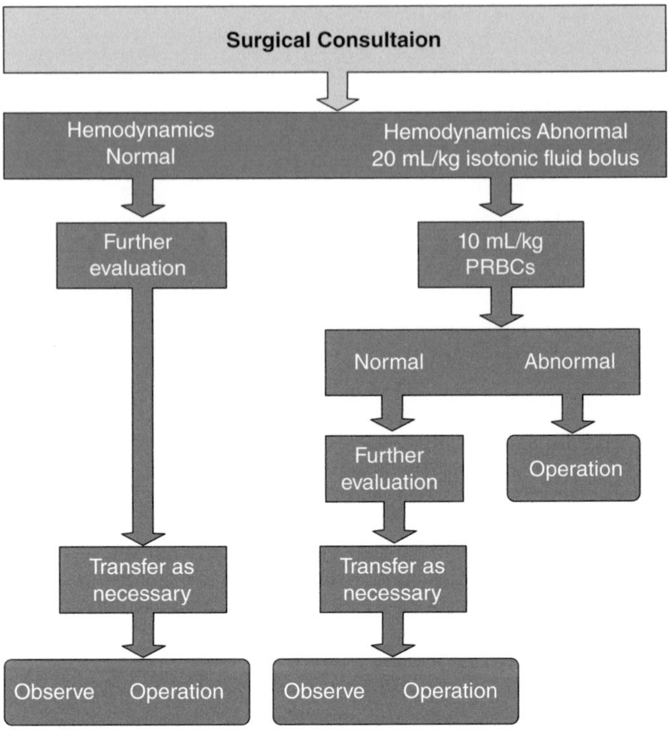

Fig. 14.1 Resuscitation flow diagram for pediatric patients with normal and abnormal hemodynamics

14.2.4 Management (Fig. 14.1)

Nonoperative management (NOM) is the standard of care for solid organ injuries and is successful in 90–95% of cases. Hemodynamic status plays an important role in decision making. If contrast extravasation is demonstrated on CT, then embolization of the bleeding vessel is also an option. Renal injuries with collecting system involvement and extravasation of urine can be treated with nonaggressive options like percutaneous nephrostomy or stents. Failure rate of NOM is approximately 3.2% and the most common indications for laparotomy being hemorrhage and persistent hypovolemic shock, hollow viscus injuries, and diaphragmatic injuries.

14.3 Solid Organ Injuries

Children are more susceptible for solid organ injuries because of their relatively large size, less subcutaneous fat, lack of sufficient protection by chest wall and abdominal musculature. Management of solid organ injuries should be based on hemodynamic status rather than grade of injury.

14.3.1 Splenic Injuries

Spleen and liver are the two most injured organs in blunt abdominal trauma, followed by kidney and pancreas. Spleen and liver account to one-third of injuries. Splenic laceration is one of the most common isolated injuries. Nonoperative management (NOM) is the standard of care and the success rate approaches 90–95% in patients with liver and splenic injuries.

A CT scan of abdomen helps in grading the trauma (Fig. 14.2). Nonoperative management (NOM) for all grades of splenic injury (Table 14.3) is currently the standard of care and the success rate approaches 90–95%. NOM includes: bed rest, monitoring of vital signs, complete blood count every 4–6 hourly, restricted activity for 4 weeks, avoidance of contact sports for 3 months. Spleen preservation remains the goal of the nonoperative care to reduce postsplenectomy infections.

14.3.1.1 Indications for Surgical Intervention

Patients who become hypotensive or tachycardiac and remain hemodynamically unstable even after adequate resuscitation are considered to have failed nonoperative management. They can be explored for splenectomy, or splenic salvage.

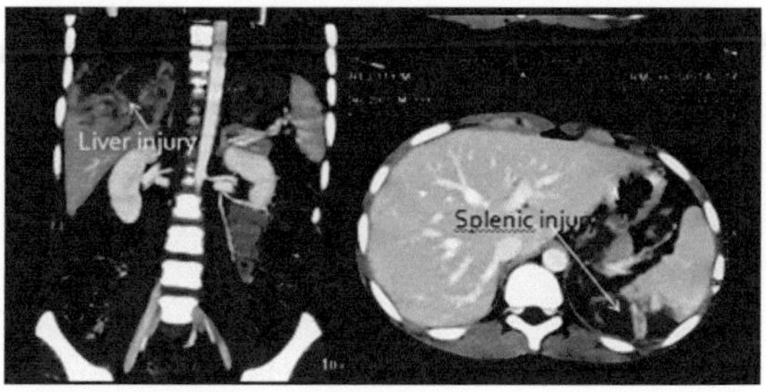

Fig. 14.2 CECT abdomen showing liver and splenic injuries

Success of conservative treatment for splenic injury in children exceeds 90%.

14.3.2 Liver Injuries

Liver and spleen are placed in the right and left upper quadrants of abdomen. These are partially protected by pliable ribs and extend below the costal margin. These are relatively more commonly injured in children than adults. CT scan is the standard imaging study in trauma for hemodynamically stable patients (Fig. 14.2). Grading for severity of injuries is also based on CT scan examination (Table 14.3). Extravasation of contrast demonstrated on CT scan suggests active bleed from the injury site and further intervention may be warranted.

Table 14.3 The American Association for the Surgery of Trauma grading of injury to different organs

Grade	Liver	Spleen	Kidney
I	Hematoma: <10% subcapsular surface area Laceration: capsular tear <1 cm	Hematoma: <10% subcapsular surface area Laceration: capsular tear <1 cm	Contusion: microscopic or gross hematuria Hematoma: subcapsular, nonexpanding, no parenchymal tear
II	Hematoma: 10–50% subcapsular area, <10 cm intraparenchymal hemorrhage Laceration: capsular tear 1–3 cm deep, <10 cm length	Hematoma: 10–50% subcapsular area, <5 cm intraparenchymal hemorrhage Laceration: capsular tear, 1–3 cm deep not involving a trabecular vessel	Hematoma: nonexpanding perirenal hematoma confined to retroperitoneum Laceration: <1 cm parenchymal depth of renal cortex without collecting system rupture or urinary extravasation
III	Hematoma: >50% expanding subcapsular surface area, ruptured subcapsular hematoma with active bleeding, or intraparenchymal hematoma ≥2 cm or expanding Laceration: >3 cm parenchymal depth	Hematoma: ruptured subcapsular or parenchymal hematoma, intraparenchymal hematoma>5 cm or expanding Laceration: >3 cm parenchymal depth involving trabecular vessels	Laceration: >1 cm parenchymal depth of renal cortex without collecting system rupture or urinary extravasation
IV	Hematoma: ruptured parenchyma with active bleeding Laceration: parenchymal disruption involving 25–75% of hepatic lobe	Hematoma: ruptured parenchyma with active bleeding Laceration: hilar vessels with major devascularization (>25% of spleen)	Laceration: parenchymal laceration extending through the renal cortex, medulla, and collecting system Vascular: main renal artery or vein injury with contained hemorrhage
V	Laceration: parenchymal disruption involving > 50% of hepatic lobe Vascular: juxtahepatic venous injuries (retrohepatic vena cava, central major hepatic veins)	Laceration: completely shattered spleen Vascular: hilar vascular injury with total devascularization	Laceration: completely shattered kidney Vascular: avulsion of renal hilum with devascularization of kidney
VI	Vascular: hepatic avulsion		

Grades I–III can be treated nonoperatively, but extensive tissue destruction or posterior lacerations involving hepatic veins need exploration.

14.3.2.1 Operative Management

A hemodynamically unstable patient despite aggressive fluid resuscitations and blood transfusions or an associated hollow viscus injury requires emergent exploratory laparotomy.

Large packs are placed posteriorly, inferiorly, and superiorly to control the bleeding and then removed slowly one by one to assess the damage. Pringle maneuver (occlusion of the porta between the thumb and forefinger or using a vascular clamp) is done in case of uncontrolled hemorrhage and limited visualization due to blood. The following interventions could be done, depending on the degree of injury to the liver: a) simple repair, b) exploration of expanding hematomas, c) debridement of devitalized tissue, d) rarely a lobectomy.

14.3.2.2 Role of Interventional Radiology in Liver Injury

Angioembolization has become the mainstay in the management of liver injuries for hemodynamically stable patients with active bleeding. CT-guided percutaneous drainage procedures can also be used to manage symptomatic biloma, liver, and intra-abdominal abscesses.

14.3.3 Kidney Injuries

Kidney is the most commonly injured organ in the genitourinary system but less frequent than the liver and spleen. Nonoperative management in a stable child with renal injury has become the standard of care. Bed rest, hydration, catheterization, antibiotics avoiding aminoglycosides, serial vital, hemoglobin and urine sample monitoring are done routinely. Risk factors for failure of NOM include urinoma >4 cm, collecting system hematomas, dissociated renal fragments, interpolar extravasation. Indications for operative management in renal trauma are life-threatening hemorrhage, renal pedicle avulsion, major urinary leak or pulsatile/expanding retroperitoneal hematoma. Control of vascular pedicle is the most essential step in renal exploration.

Renal pelvic and ureteric injuries can be picked up on imaging by contrast CT. The arterial and venous phase can identify active extravasation, whereas delayed phase images assess the renal collecting system and ureteric continuity. Angioembolization, percutaneous drainage, and internal drainage are also the options in selected cases.

14.3.4 Pancreatic Injuries

Pancreatic trauma ranges from 0.3% to 0.7% of overall trauma and 3–12% of children sustaining abdominal trauma. Because of its location in the protected retroperitoneum, pancreatic injuries are less when compared to other solid organ injuries. Handle bar injury is the most common mechanism of injury which causes compression of pancreatic neck and body against lumbar vertebra. contrast enhanced computed tomography (CECT) abdomen remains the most sensitive imaging modality to pick up injuries to pancreas (Fig. 14.3). Raised serum amylase and lipase also aid in diagnosis. Management remains mostly conservative with NPO, bed rest, pain relief, total parenteral nutrition (TPN), IV fluids, and IV antibiotics. Contusions and minor lacerations, i.e., grades I and II are best managed by NOM

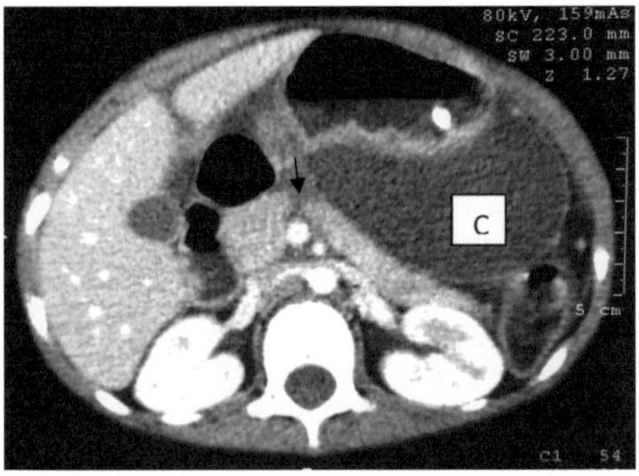

Fig. 14.3 Traumatic transaction of the pancreas between the pancreatic head and body (arrow) with large peripancreatic collection (C)

whereas early distal pancreatectomy has fewer complications in cases of pancreatic duct transaction at the body of the pancreas. Pancreatic secretions collected in the retroperitoneum can form a pseudocyst, which can be drained via cystogastrostomy few weeks later.

14.3.5 Hollow Viscus Injuries

Incidence of hollow viscus injuries in case of polytrauma ranges from 1% to 23%. Presence of free fluid in the peritoneal cavity without solid organ injury indicates either mesenteric tear or hollow viscus perforation. Rapid acceleration or deceleration of bowel near a point of fixation (like ligament of Treitz or ileocecal valve) or due to the trapping of the intestine between the seatbelt and the spine is the mechanism causing injury. Small bowel injuries are most common, followed by duodenal, colonic and stomach injuries.

14.3.5.1 Small Intestine

Jejunal perforation is most common among hollow viscus injuries (Fig. 14.4). Mesenteric injuries compromise blood supply to small intestine which can cause delayed perforation due to ischemic necrosis. In these injuries, signs and symptoms like pain and tenderness may appear 12–24 hours after injury.

14.3.5.2 Duodenum

Significant force should be applied to cause duodenal injury because of its location in the retroperitoneum. Fall and impact with a bicycle handle-bar is a common cause. Hematoma and perforation are the most common injuries. Compression against the vertebral column produces a hematoma, which can cause partial or complete obstruction. Perforations are rare and should always be managed operatively if present. Early diagnosis is important because the time gap between the injury and intervention correlates with mortality and morbidity.

14.3.5.3 Colon

Transverse colon is at risk for crush injuries from compression against the spine. Sigmoid colon is at risk for perforation in case of rapid deceleration injuries because it is tethered at its junction with the rectum. Colonic perforations should always be treated operatively.

14.3.5.4 Stomach

Distensibility, mobility, and shielding by the rib cage protect the stomach from being injured. After a meal, stomach distends and extends below the ribcage, making it more vulnerable to injury. Perforation is the most commonly reported injury, which mandates surgical repair. Rich blood supply of the stomach helps in successful healing.

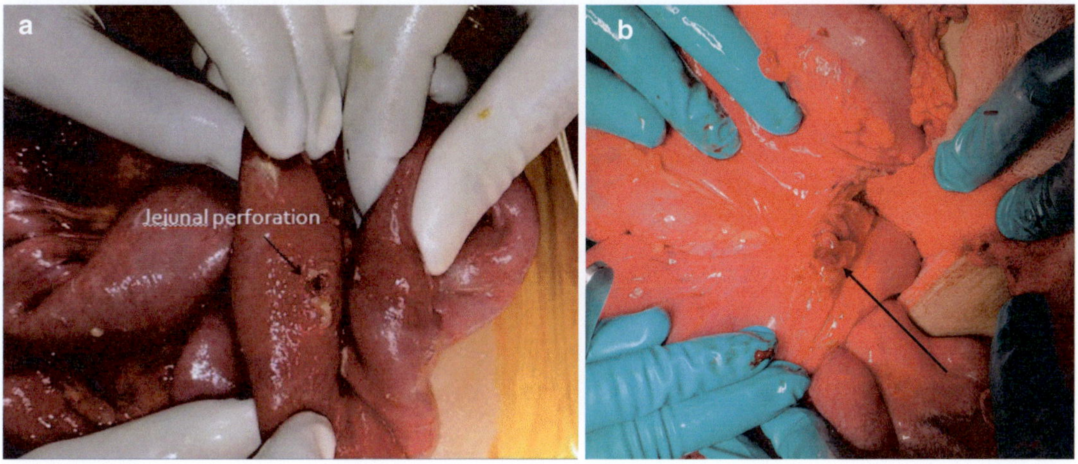

Fig. 14.4 Intraoperative picture showing. (**a**) Traumatic jejunal perforation. (**b**) Perforation at the duodeno-jejunal flexure

14.3.6 Bladder Injuries

Bladder is usually protected in the bony pelvis but in younger children it becomes more abdominal especially when it is full. Hence, dome of the bladder is more susceptible to injury. Bladder injury is more common if there is any associated pelvic fracture. Tear drop deformity of the bladder will be seen in case of large pelvic hematoma.

American Pediatric Surgical Association recommended hospital stay of "grade of injury plus one" in days (e.g., if grade of injury is III, then hospital stay will be 4 days) and return to normal activity will be after "grade of injury plus two weeks" (e.g., in grade III injury, it will be 5 weeks). In case of visceral perforations, laparotomy or laparoscopy is the gold standard. Laparoscopy plays an important role in hemodynamically stable children for both diagnosis and treatment in case of hollow viscus injury.

14.3.7 Complications and Outcome

After single organ injury, prognosis is usually good. One should be aware about the possibility of overwhelming postsplenectomy infections. Kidneys may heal with scarring in case of severe contusions but rarely cause functional deficiency and late hypertension is uncommon. Morbidity and mortality are high with pancreatic injuries. Complications after laparotomy in cases of hollow viscus perforation include wound infection, septic shock, bowel obstruction due to adhesions or strictures.

Summary

- Abdominal trauma is the third most common cause of trauma-related deaths in children.
- Multisystem involvement is common in children because of their small size.
- The structured approach includes primary survey, initial resuscitation, secondary survey and definitive management.
- FAST plays an important role in the initial evaluation and management.
- Conservative management is the gold standard in case of solid organ injuries in children with few exceptions like active bleeding.
- Treatment of children at pediatric trauma care centers has a better outcome when compared to management at adult trauma centers. Hence, early referral to pediatric trauma care centers helps in achieving better outcomes.

Suggested Reading

Coran AG, Caldamone A, Scott Adzich N, Krummel TM, Laberge JM, editors. Pediatric surgery. 7th ed. Oxford: Elsevier Limited; 2012.

Hegde S, Bawa M, Kanojia RP, Mahajan JK, Menon P, Samujh R, et al. Pediatric trauma: management and lessons learned. J Indian Assoc Pediatr Surg. 2020;25:142–6.

Kundal VK, Debnath PR, Sen A. Epidemiology of pediatric trauma and its pattern in urban India: a tertiary care hospital-based experience. J Indian Assoc Pediatr Surg. 2017;22:33–7.

Thoracic Trauma in Children

15

Pinaki Ranjan Debnath, Gali Divya,
and Subhasis Roy Choudhury

15.1 Introduction

Trauma is the leading cause of morbidity and mortality in children more than 1 year of age. Thoracic trauma accounts for 5–12% of the trauma-related admissions. Despite their low incidence, chest injuries have high mortality because the thoracic cavity contains vital structures like the heart, lungs, and major vessels. Blunt injuries are more common when compared to penetrating injuries and these penetrating injuries are more common in adolescents which can be stab wounds or gunshot wounds. Different mechanisms of injury include motor vehicle accidents, fall from height, or child abuse. Isolated chest trauma is rare in children, because of their small-size multisystem involvement is more common.

There are some anatomical and physiological differences between adult and pediatric patients which need to be kept in mind while managing the children with thoracic trauma. The muscular layer around the bony rib cage is very thin in children, ribs are not ossified, and the chest wall is very compliant and elastic. Physiological variation in children is that they can tolerate up to 40% loss of blood volume. Hypotension is a late sign. Even though they had good cardiac reserve, pulmonary reserve is low in children when compared to adults.

Pulmonary contusion is the frequently encountered injury in children with thoracic trauma, and other injuries were rib fractures, flail chest, pneumothorax, hemothorax, pulmonary laceration, tracheobronchial injuries, diaphragmatic injury, aortic rupture, and esophageal injuries. Children with chest trauma should be treated according to the principles of the Advanced Trauma Life Support Program of the American College of Surgeons, which includes

1. Primary survey
2. Resuscitation of vital functions
3. Detailed secondary survey
4. Definitive care

Primary survey is of first priority which focuses on identifying immediate life-threatening injuries. Resuscitation should also be done simultaneously during the primary survey. The conditions which need immediate attention are tension pneumothorax, open pneumothorax, cardiac tamponade, massive hemothorax, and flail chest. In the initial emergency workup airway, breathing and circulation (A-B-C) should be assessed and appropriate intervention should be done at every step. American

P. R. Debnath (✉)
Pediatric Surgery, ABVIMS and Dr. RML Hospital, New Delhi, India

G. Divya
Department of Pediatric Surgery, All India Institute of Medical Sciences, New Delhi, India

S. Roy Choudhury
Pediatric Surgery, Lady Hardinge Medical College and Associated Kalawati Saran Children's Hospital, New Delhi, Delhi, India

© The Author(s), under exclusive license to Springer Nature Singapore Pte Ltd. 2025

S. Roy Choudhury (ed.), *Pediatric Surgery*, https://doi.org/10.1007/978-981-96-1257-4_15

Heart Association resuscitation guidelines changed the sequence from A-B-C to C-A-B for both children and adults in the year 2010. If there is any airway obstruction because of secretions or blood, it should be cleared by suctioning. Stridor is a sign of partial airway obstruction. Jaw thrust maneuver can also help in maintaining a patent airway. Sometimes they may need endotracheal intubation and assisted ventilation. In cases where endotracheal intubation is difficult or impossible or if it is contraindicated, then cricothyrotomy can be considered. After stabilizing the airway, breathing pattern should be checked. Respiratory failure can be because of underlying pathology like tension or open pneumothorax or massive hemothorax; hence, they should be addressed. Circulation should be taken care after airway and breathing. Heart rate, quality of pulse, and capillary refill are better indicators than blood pressure because hypotension is a late sign in children with blood loss. Urine output is a better predictor of hydration status.

Secondary survey is the detailed examination of the child with chest trauma which should be done after initial stabilization. Care givers should keep monitoring the vital signs by pulse oximetry, electrocardiogram, and blood gas analyses. Mechanism of injury must be inquired to identify the high-impact acceleration–deceleration injuries. Abnormal respiratory rate, hypoxemia, respiratory distress, distended neck veins, ecchymoses or abrasions over the chest wall, crepitus or subcutaneous air, paradoxical chest wall movement and abnormal breath sounds signify underlying chest injuries. Then, necessary imaging and laboratory tests should be done.

15.2 Imaging

Plain X-ray of the chest in anteroposterior view can identify hemothorax, pneumothorax, and any abnormalities of mediastinum. Ultrasonography (USG) especially Extended Focused Assessment with Sonography in Trauma can identify not only fluid in the abdomen but also pleural and pericardial fluid. Computed tomography can be advised whenever necessary especially in suspected cases of vascular/aortic injuries and tracheobronchial injuries but radiation exposure should be kept in mind. Magnetic resonance imaging is recommended to identify injuries to the thoracic spine. Transthoracic echocardiography can better identify intracardiac injuries. A 12-lead electrocardiogram should be done in cases of suspected cardiac contusion to rule out arrhythmias.

Laboratory tests, which include complete blood count, arterial blood gas analysis, and coagulation profile, including prothrombin time and activated thromboplastin time, should be done. Blood grouping and cross-matching should be done and blood products should be ordered if there is any suspicion of massive blood loss requiring transfusion. Troponin I levels should be done in cardiac injuries. Definitive care differs in each condition of thoracic injury.

15.3 Pulmonary Contusion

Pulmonary contusions are seen in 34–100% of children with thoracic trauma. They cause damage at the level of alveoli with hemorrhage and edema leading to impairment of oxygen and carbon dioxide exchange. Diagnosis can be done with chest X-ray or CT chest; role of USG in diagnosing pulmonary contusion has also been described. Minor contusions can be treated with supportive care like supplemental oxygen, analgesics for pain, chest physiotherapy, and pulmonary toileting and severe contusions may require mechanical ventilation. Most of the children show spontaneous resolution and children with severe contusions may develop acute respiratory distress syndrome.

15.4 Rib Fractures and Flail Chest

They are infrequent in children because the bones are resilient and not ossified; they are more common in adolescents. It requires significant force for the child to sustain rib fracture. If rib fractures are present, it indicates severe underlying injury and multisystem injuries. Concomitant pulmonary contusions are more common. They can be treated by high-flow oxygen, pain relief by analgesics, and ventilatory support if needed. Fractures infants should raise the suspicion of child abuse. Abused children have more ribs fractured than accidentally sustained rib fractures. In nonaccidental injuries, concurrent extrathoracic injuries are common.

Flail chest is defined as a fracture of two or more ribs at two or more points. The flail segment moves paradoxically during breathing. Severe pain associated with the injury, in turn, impairs spontaneous breathing in these children. Stabilization of the flail segment should be done, if not it can cause contusion of the underlying lung parenchyma. Children with large flail segments may require positive pressure ventilation. Surgical stabilization may be required in some cases.

15.5 Pneumothorax and Hemothorax

Pneumothorax and hemothorax are the second most commonly encountered injuries in children with thoracic trauma after pulmonary contusion. Pneumothorax occurs if there is injury to any air-containing organs like the trachea, bronchi, lung parenchyma, and esophagus. Mild pneumothorax may not be symptomatic but large pneumothorax may manifest symptoms like tachypnea and respiratory distress. On clinical examination, there may be decreased movement of the chest on the affected side which will be hyper-resonant on percussion with decreased or absent breath sounds. Tension pneumothorax is more common in children when compared to adults. In emergency situation, needle thoracostomy can be done in the midclavicular line in the second intercostal space.

Hemothotrax can be a consequence of injury to blood vessels of the thoracic wall or intrathoracic vessels, lung parenchyma, or great vessels. It should be addressed promptly as hypotension is a late sign and child can tolerate up to 40% of blood volume loss. Minimal hemothorax can resolve spontaneously but large hemothorax requires drainage via tube thoracostomy. Arrangement for blood transfusion should be made because drainage of the hemothorax can aggravate bleeding by sudden decompression. Continuous bleeding of >2 mL/kg/hour requires emergency thoracotomy to control the bleeding.

15.6 Pulmonary Laceration

It is seen after penetrating injuries or displaced rib fractures. Associated pulmonary contusion or hemo-pneumothorax is common. Treatment is by supportive measures like oxygen supplementation, analgesics, and ventilator support if required. Major persistent air leaks may require surgical correction.

15.7 Other Injuries

Pneumomediastinum is seen in injury to mediastinal structures like the trachea, bronchi, and esophagus. Other rare injuries include diaphragmatic rupture, aortic injuries, traumatic asphyxia, blunt cardiac injury, and commotion cordis. Diaphragmatic rupture requires surgical repair after stabilizing the child, and esophageal injuries can usually be treated by conservative management in children with pleural drainage, intravenous antibiotics, and parenteral nutrition. Aortic injuries can be treated with a synthetic patch, endovascular stent graft. Chylothorax occurs if there is any injury to the thoracic duct. Most of the patients recover spontaneously with only nutritional support (TPN or elemental diet with medium chain triglycerides). Some patients may require thoracic duct ligation.

Summary

- Thorax in children is highly resilient
- Considerable amount of force is required to cause injuries like rib fractures and if rib fractures are present, they indicate significant underlying injuries
- Pulmonary contusions are the most common injuries seen in children with chest trauma and other common injuries are rib fractures, hemothorax, and pneumothorax
- Most of the injuries can be managed conservatively with supplemental oxygen, analgesics, and mechanical ventilation if required
- Tube thoracostomy should be done to drain hemo or pneumothorax

Suggested Reading

Haxhija EQ, Nöres H, Schober P, Höllwarth ME. Lung contusion-lacerations after blunt thoracic trauma in children. Pediatr Surg Int. 2004;20(6):412–4.

Kleinman ME, Chameides L, Schexnayder SM, Samson RA, Hazinski MF, Atkins DL, et al. Part 14: pediatric advanced life support: 2010 American heart association guidelines for cardiopulmonary resuscitation and emergency cardiovascular care. Circulation. 2010;122(18 Suppl 3):S876–908.

Moore MA, Wallace EC, Westra SJ. The imaging of paediatric thoracic trauma. Pediatr Radiol. 2009;39:485.

Moore MA, Wallace EC, Westra SJ. Chest trauma in children: current imaging guidelines and techniques. Radiol Clin North Am. 2011;49(5):949–68.

Nakayama DK, Ramenofsky ML, Rowe MI. Chest injuries in childhood. Ann Surg. 1989;210(6):770–5.

Özdülger A. Thoracic trauma in children. Turk Gogus Kalp Dama. 2024;32(Suppl 1):S21–8. https://doi.org/10.5606/tgkdc.dergisi.2024.25746.

Sartorelli KH, Vane DW. The diagnosis and management of children with blunt injury of the chest. Semin Pediatr Surg. 2004;13:98.

Sharp NE, Holcomb GW III. The role of minimally invasive surgery in pediatric trauma: a collective review. Pediatr Surg Int. 2013;29:1013–8.

Tovar JA, Vazquez JJ. Management of chest trauma in children. Paediatr Respir Rev. 2013;14(2):86–91.

Weerdenburg KD, Wales PW, Stephens D, et al. Predicting thoracic injury in children with multitrauma. Pediatr Emerg Care. 2019;35:330.

Woosley CR, Mayes TC. The pediatric patient and thoracic trauma. Semin Thorac Cardiovasc Surg. 2008;20(1):58–63.

Pediatric Burns

16

Pinaki Ranjan Debnath and Gali Divya

16.1 Introduction

One-fourth of burn injuries occur in children, and majority of them are seen in children below 5 years of age. Different types of burn injuries in children include scalds, fire/flame-induced burns, electrical, and chemical burns. Scalds are the most common type of injury in children below 5 years of age. In older children, fire injuries are more common and nonthermal burns or child abuse is common in children less than 2 years of age who are nonverbal. Majority of them involve less than 10% of the body surface area and are nonfatal, and the mortality rate in children with burn injuries is 3–4. In India, 17–25% of burn admissions are due to pediatric burns.

16.2 Classification

Classifying the burn injuries has some implications on the fluid management of these children. They are classified based on the depth of the burn wound and also the total body surface area (TBSA) involved.

1. *Superficial (first-degree) burns*:
   Only the epidermis is involved with clinical features like erythema, pain, and desquamation. Dermis is not involved. It resolves without scarring within 7–10 days. For example, sunburns.
2. *Superficial partial-thickness (second-degree):*
   Epidermis and papillary dermis are involved. Clinical features include blisters, erythema, and edema. There will be blanching with pressure and a brisk capillary refill.
3. *Deep partial-thickness (second-degree)*:
   Reticular dermis is involved in this and it exhibits a more sluggish capillary refill. Wound is moist and edematous and there will be complete loss of sensation. Generally, they require surgical therapy.
4. *Full-thickness (third-degree)*:
   Entire epidermis and dermis are involved. Injury extends till the subcutaneous tissue and can have a leathery appearance. They require surgical excision and grafting.
5. *Subdermal (fourth-degree)*:
   There are the deepest subgroup of burns in which there will be involvement of the fascia, muscles, and bone. They also require surgical intervention.

There is a difference in estimating the body surface area involved in adults and children. Lund and Browder chart is used for the estimation of the total body surface area involved in children. Involvement of head (front and back)

P. R. Debnath (✉)
Pediatric Surgery, ABVIMS and Dr. RML Hospital, New Delhi, India

G. Divya
Department of Pediatric Surgery, All India Institute of Medical Sciences, New Delhi, India

© The Author(s), under exclusive license to Springer Nature Singapore Pte Ltd. 2025
S. Roy Choudhury (ed.), *Pediatric Surgery*, https://doi.org/10.1007/978-981-96-1257-4_16

-18%, front of torso—18%, back of the trunk—18%, each upper limb—9% and each lower limb—13.5% and the perineum—1%.

16.3 Pathophysiology

After any burn injury, there will be a local response as well as a systemic response. Children are more prone to hypothermia because of a high body surface area to mass ratio. Disruption of healthy skin after thermal injury leads to increased permeability, capillary leakage, significant fluid loss, and edema. The extent of injury depends on the temperature and specific heat of the causative agent, duration of exposure, and skin thickness. Thermal injury causes coagulative necrosis of the local tissue.

16.4 Local Tissue Response

Local response is characterized by three zones, which are zone of coagulation, zone of stasis, and zone of hyperemia. Jackson described the three zones of burn in 1947.

Zone of coagulation: this is the area of maximal insult with irreversible damage to the tissue and necrosis.

Zone of stasis: there is decreased tissue perfusion in this zone. The damage caused to the tissues in this zone is reversible; hence, the resuscitation measures are mainly focused on improving the tissue perfusion to this zone. However, additional factors like hypotension and infection may further damage the tissues in this zone and lead to complete tissue loss.

Zone of hyperemia: this is the outermost zone, and there is increased perfusion in this area and it usually recovers unless there is sepsis.

16.5 Systemic Response

The systemic response in children with burns is due to the release of cytokines and other inflammatory mediators. The release of these vasoactive mediators, catecholamines and inflammatory markers, leads to systemic inflammatory response syndrome. It is seen in children with burns involving more than 30% of the total body surface area.

Cardiovascular system–increased capillary permeability leads to escape of fluid into the interstitial space, which further causes decreased venous return and stroke volume causing reduced myocardial contractility and hypotension.

Respiratory system–inhalational injury may lead to upper airway obstruction, bronchospasm, airway edema, respiratory failure, and acute respiratory distress syndrome. This can happen with inhalational burn and facial burn.

Renal–because of decreased blood flow, there is decreased glomerular filtration rate. Activation of stress-induced hormones and mediators like angiotensin, vasopressin, and aldosterone further compromises renal blood flow which can progress to acute tubular necrosis, acute kidney injury, and renal failure.

Neurological–agitation, confusion, ataxia, abnormal posturing, seizures, and transient loss of consciousness can occur. Cellular hypoxia can lead to increased intracranial pressure and cerebral edema.

Hepatic–there will be altered drug metabolism and coagulopathy.

Gastrointestinal–decreased gastric emptying, gastritis, ulcers, and bleeding. Translocation of gut bacteria and sepsis, vasoconstriction in the splanchnic circulation causes transient mesenteric ischemia, atrophy of small bowel mucosa.

Immune system–immunosuppression is seen in children with major burns which makes them more prone to infections.

16.6 Management of Children with Burns

Children with burns are managed in a phased manner

Phase 1–initial assessment and triage
Phase 2–fluid resuscitation
Phase 3–burn wound management
Phase 4–supportive and critical care
Phase 5–rehabilitation

16.6.1 Initial Assessment and Triage

Evacuation from the source of burn injury should be the priority. Burning clothing and metal jewelry must be quickly removed to prevent further injury. In the primary survey airway, breathing and circulation and any life-threatening conditions should be assessed. In the secondary survey, estimation of the depth and extent of the burns with total body surface area involved is assessed. Inhalational injury should be suspected if there is dyspnea, hoarseness of voice, stridor, singed nasal hair, decreased level of consciousness, increased work of breathing, and facial burns. Oxygen therapy should be given in all children with inhalational burns and be considered for endotracheal intubation preemptively. American Burn Life Support indications for early intubation: signs of airway obstruction (hoarseness, stridor, sternal retraction and accessory respiratory muscle use), extent of the burn (total body surface area burn) > 40–50%, burns inside the mouth, extensive and deep facial burns, significant edema or risk for edema, difficulty swallowing, decreased level of consciousness where airway protective reflexes are impaired, anticipated patient transfer of large burn with airway issue without qualified personnel to intubate en route, signs of respiratory compromise like inability to clear secretions, respiratory fatigue, poor oxygenation or ventilation.

After securing the airway, adequate ventilation must be ensured. If there are circumferential burns involving the chest and abdomen, escharotomy should be performed. After airway and breathing, circulation should be taken care of to maintain adequate intravascular volume by fluid resuscitation.

16.6.2 Fluid Resuscitation

Adequate fluid resuscitation is of paramount importance in managing a child with burns. It is recommended for all children with involvement of more than 10% total body surface area (TBSA). Inadequate resuscitation can lead to tissue ischemia, renal failure, hypotension, increase in the depth of the burn wound, and overhydration can cause pulmonary edema and heart failure.

Parkland formula—lactated Ringer solution; 4 mL/kg/%TBSA burn
50% volume in the first 8 hours, remaining in subsequent 16 hours

The disadvantage with the Parkland formula or other weight-based formulas is that they underestimate the fluid required to resuscitate. Hence, the Parkland formula is modified to add the additional fluid required for maintenance.

Modified Parkland formula:

Total requirement in first 24 hours = 4 mL/kg/%TBSA + 1500 mL/m^2 BSA

Crystalloids like Ringer's lactate are the preferred for initial resuscitation and addition of dextrose is recommended in children less than 20 kg weight, to prevent hypoglycemia. As children are more prone to hypothermia, especially in infants, administration of warmed fluids is recommended. Adequacy of fluid resuscitation can be assured by maintaining urine output of 1–2 mL/kg/hour in children <30 kg and 0.5–1 ml/kg/hour in children ≥30 kg; during the resuscitation, hemodynamic stability, mental status, base deficit, and lactate levels should be monitored.

16.6.3 Burn Wound Management

Superficial burns with intact epidermis do not require any topical antimicrobials or dressings. The burn wound management includes cleaning, debridement, topical antimicrobials, and dressing changes. Cleaning should be done with mild soap and water and debridement can be done by scraping or brushing, proteolytic enzymes also have a role. Different topical antimicrobials used in the management of burn wounds include silver sulfadiazine, mafenide acetate, sulfamylon, and 0.025% sodium hypochlorite. Petroleum-based antimicrobial ointments such as bacitracin, polymyxin B, and polysporin can be used.

Synthetic dressings have the advantage of eliminating frequent painful dressing changes and potential tissue fluid loss; they also allow rapid spontaneous re-epithelialization of the involved burn areas. Different synthetic dressings like Opsite, Biobrane, Trancyte, and Integra are available for use in burn wound management. Surgical management in these children includes excision of the necrotic tissue, grafting, and reconstruction. Early excision and grafting decrease the length of hospital stay. Skin grafts can be split thickness or full thickness. The advantage with split thickness graft is coverage of a large area with less donor skin and the advantage with full-thickness graft is good cosmesis but limited availability of donor area.

16.6.4 Supportive Care

It includes managing the nutrition, antibiotic treatment, and pain management.

16.6.4.1 Nutrition

Children with burns have increased calorie requirements because of the hypermetabolic state. And the nutritional requirement in these children can be calculated by using the Curreri formula or the Galveston revised formula:

Curreri formula – 25 kcal/kg plus 40 kcal/% TBSA burned

Galveston revised formula –

Daily calorie requirement: 1800 kcal/m^2 + 1300 kcal/m^2 TBSA burned

16.6.4.2 Antibiotic Treatment

Broad-spectrum antibiotics like third-generation cephalosporin and fluoroquinolones can be given initially. Sensitive antibiotic based on the culture report (either blood culture/culture from swab taken at the burn wound) should be started as soon as possible. Antibiotics against the gram –ve bacteria and antifungals should be given in children with chronic burns. Common pathogens which are isolated from the burn wound are *Staphylococcus aureus*, *Streptococcus pyogenes* and *Pseudomonas*; hence, drugs against these pathogens should be considered.

16.6.4.3 Pain Management

Non-steroidal anti-inflammatory drugs, opioid drugs like morphine and fentanyl, are used to manage pain in these children with burns. Benzodiazepines like lorazepam and diazepam are used to relieve anxiety; they also enhance the effect of narcotics. Ketamine (1–2 mg/kg intravenous (IV) or 5–7 mg/kg intramuscular (IM)) can be used as a sedative to manage procedure-related pain. Local or regional anesthesia may be required in some children.

16.6.5 Rehabilitation

Post burn contractures are the most common sequelae after recovery from the acute phase; hence, active limb movements and exercises should be advised. Splinting to maintain joint alignment, even in the early phase of treatment, will prevent contractures. Hypertrophic scars or keloids can also occur which can be managed either medically or by surgical excision.

16.7 Nonaccidental Injuries

Children between 1 and 3 years of age are more vulnerable to this type of injury. Chronically ill children, unwanted children, nonbiological parents, or caregivers are some of the risk factors. If there is any inconsistency between history and the examination findings, changing history and delay in seeking medical care should alert the medical professionals to suspect nonaccidental injuries. They can be immersion burns or contact burns. Typical bilateral symmetrical "stocking distribution" is seen in these children. If nonaccidental injuries are suspected, they should be reported.

16.8 Electrical Burns

These are very rare in children accounting to 5–7% of total burns. Severity of injury depends on the type of current, voltage, wetness of skin, and duration of exposure. Boys and older children are more prone. All children should undergo electrocardiogram; urine examination should also be done to look for myoglobinuria. Supportive treatment should be given. Proper maintenance of power lines and educating the parents regarding safety measures will prevent electrical burns.

Summary Box

- Scalds are the most common type of burns in children.
- Burns can be classified as first degree, second degree, third and fourth degree based on the depth of the burn wound.
- Fluid resuscitation in the first 24 hours is very crucial. Children's fluid resuscitation guidelines should be based on Body surface area (BSA) rather than weight based, because weight-based formulas can overhydrate or underhydrate the child.
- Inhalational injuries need proper evaluation and treatment; endotracheal intubation may need to be done preemptively.
- Burns that are bilaterally symmetrical or stocking-glove distribution in conjunction with a delay in seeking medical care should raise the suspicion of child abuse.

Suggested Reading

Hettiaratchy S, Dziewulski P. ABC of burns: pathophysiology and types of burns. BMJ. 2004;328(7453):1427–9.
Lee J, Herndon D. The pediatric burned patient. In: Total burn care. 3rd ed. Elsevier; 2007. p. 485−495.
Palmieri TL. Problems in general surgery, vol. 20. In: Pediatric burn management. Philadelphia: Lippincott Williams and Wilkins; 2003. p. 27–36.
Palmieri TL. Pediatric burn resuscitation. Crit Care Clin. 2016;32(4):547–59.
Srivastava S, Patil AN, Bedi M, Tawar RS. Paediatric electrical burn injuries: experience from a tertiary care burns unit in North India. Ann Burns Fire Disasters. 2017;30(3):185–8.
Warden GD. Fluid resuscitation and early management. In: Herndon D, editor. Total burn care. Philadelphia: WB Saunders Co; 1996. p. 53–60.

Part IV

Head, Neck and Spine

Hydrocephalus

17

Monika Bawa and Subhasis Roy Choudhury

17.1 Introduction

Hydrocephalus is a common entity encountered in pediatric patients. In this chapter, we shall primarily focus on the pathophysiology, classification, and causes of hydrocephalus in children. The natural history of the disease, along with the clinical manifestations and the management options, will also be discussed.

Hydrocephalus is defined as a disproportionate increase in the amount of cerebrospinal fluid (CSF) in the cranium resulting from an imbalance between the CSF production, absorption, and obstruction to its flow.

Physiology of CSF flow: total amount of CSF is 150mL; daily production is 500 mL; circulation of CSF is 3–4 times/day. About 80% of CSF produced from the choroid plexus, the rest from ventricular ependyma and brain parenchyma.

Normal CSF: clear odorless, white blood cell (WBC) count—0–5, proteins—15–45, glucose 50–80 with a pressure of 50–180 cm of H_2O.

Production is an active transport process regulated by the homeostatic environment, and alteration in CSF pressure (hydrostatic gradient between CSF and venous sinuses).

CSF drainage: after being produced in the lateral ventricles, CSF flows in a caudal direction, first into the third ventricle through the foramen of Monroe (two on each side) then to the fourth ventricle through the aqueduct of Sylvius, and then exits from the ventricles into the cortical and spinal subarachnoid space via the foramen of Luschka (lateral, two) and Magendie (medial) (Fig. 17.1a, b). CSF then travels through the tentorial incisura, passes over the hemispheric convexity, and is absorbed in the venous system at the level of the arachnoid villi. CSF absorption is pressure dependent: hydrostatic gradient existing between the CSF in subarachnoid space and the arachnoid villi in the venous system. Small amounts are reabsorbed via the sleeves of nerve roots.

Incidence: 2–4 in 1000 population

Etiology

Imbalance in the CSF circulation due to

- Overproduction: choroid plexus papilloma
- Decreased absorption: (communicating) at the level of arachnoid villi
- Obstruction in the CSF flow pathway (obstructive/noncommunicating)

M. Bawa (✉)
Pediatric Surgery, PGIMER, Chandigarh, India

S. Roy Choudhury
Pediatric Surgery, Lady Hardinge Medical College and Associated Kalawati Saran Children's Hospital, New Delhi, Delhi, India

© The Author(s), under exclusive license to Springer Nature Singapore Pte Ltd. 2025
S. Roy Choudhury (ed.), *Pediatric Surgery*, https://doi.org/10.1007/978-981-96-1257-4_17

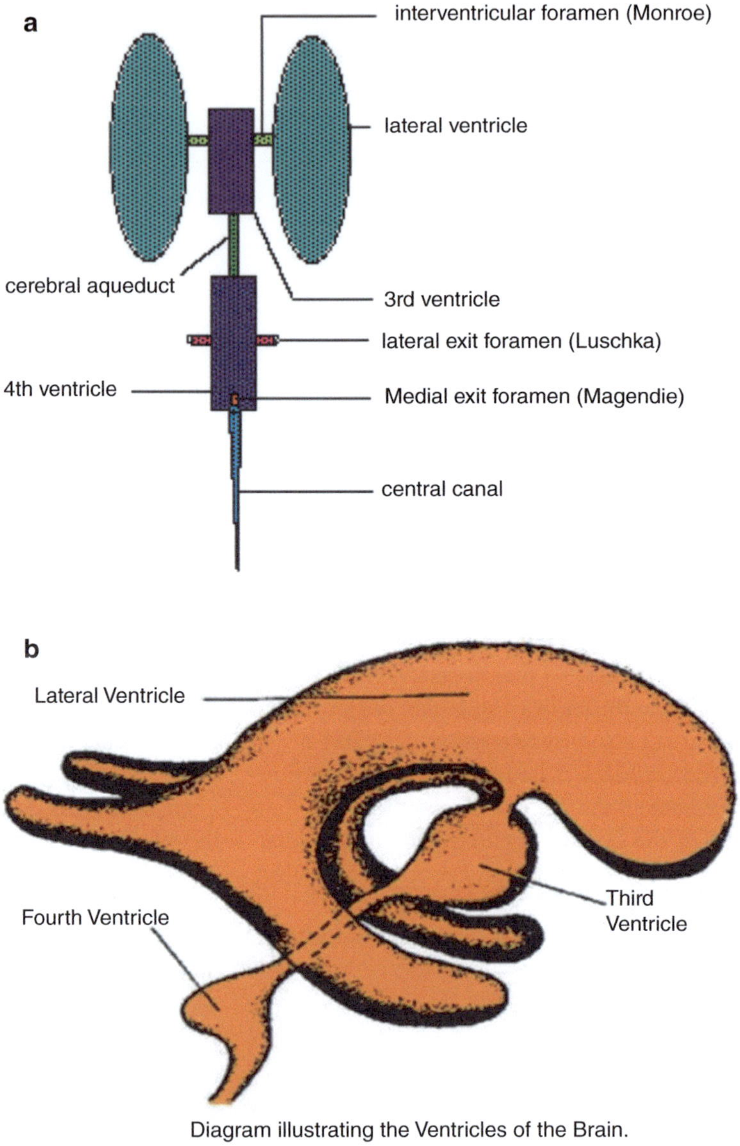

Fig. 17.1 (**a**, **b**) Diagram of ventricles of the brain. (**a**) Coronal. (**b**) Lateral view

17.2 Types

17.2.1 Congenital

- Arnold-Chiari malformation with spina bifida (Fig. 17.2)
- Dandy Walker cyst—large fourth ventricle due to obstruction of the foramen of Luschka or Magendie

17.2.2 Acquired

- Brain tumors
- Premature babies—intracerebral and intraventricular hemorrhage, infections
- Postinfective: pyogenic meningitis, tuberculosis

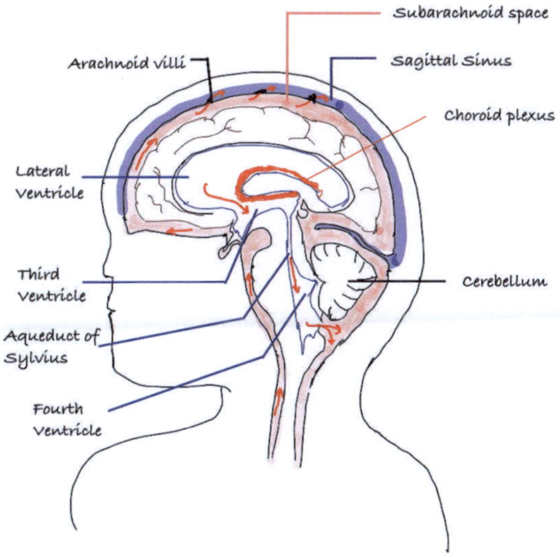

Fig. 17.2 Arnold-Chiari malformation

17.2.3 Noncommunicating (Obstructive)

- Aqueductal stenosis (the commonest cause of congenital hydrocephalus)
- Colloid cyst of the third ventricle
- Ependymal cyst of the fourth ventricle
- Craniopharyngioma
- Pineal, cerebellar tumor

17.2.4 Communicating (Nonobstructive)

- Meningitis
- Subarachnoid hemorrhage

17.3 Types of Arnold-Chiari Malformation

Type	Presentation
1	Herniation of cerebellar tonsils
2	Associated with meningomyelocele due to herniation of vermis of cerebellum
3	Associated with occipital encephalocele
4	Lack of cerebellar development

17.3.1 Clinical Features

- Neonates and infants—increased head circumference, tense fontanelle, sutural diastasis, dilated scalp veins, Sun-set sign, difficulty in feeding, excessive sleepiness, brief, shrill high pitched cry, slow growth, Crack-pot sign on percussion (Fig. 17.3)
- Children and adults: headache, nausea, vomiting, somnolence, drowsiness, sixth nerve palsy, papilledema on fundoscopy, urinary incontinence, gait disturbance, secondary endocrine features like diabetes insipidus, visual impairment, developmental delay

17.3.2 Clinical Diagnosis

Normal head circumference—35–37 cm at birth

Increase in the occipito-frontal head circumference > 1.5 cm/week is suggestive of hydrocephalus

17.3.2.1 Neurological Examination

- Spasticity—stretching of the fibers from the motor cortex around the dilated ventricles may result in spasticity of the extremities, especially the legs.
- Compression of the third or sixth cranial nerve—diplopia.
- Pressure on the midbrain may result in impairment of upward gaze—"setting-sun" sign
- Fundus—papilledema
- Spine—stigmata of an acquired Chiari II malformation associated with spinal dysraphism
- Growth and pubertal development—accelerated pubertal development and disturbed growth may result from the pressure of the dilated third ventricle on the hypothalamus
- Syndromic features—infants and children with suspected hydrocephalus should also be examined for associated congenital anomalies

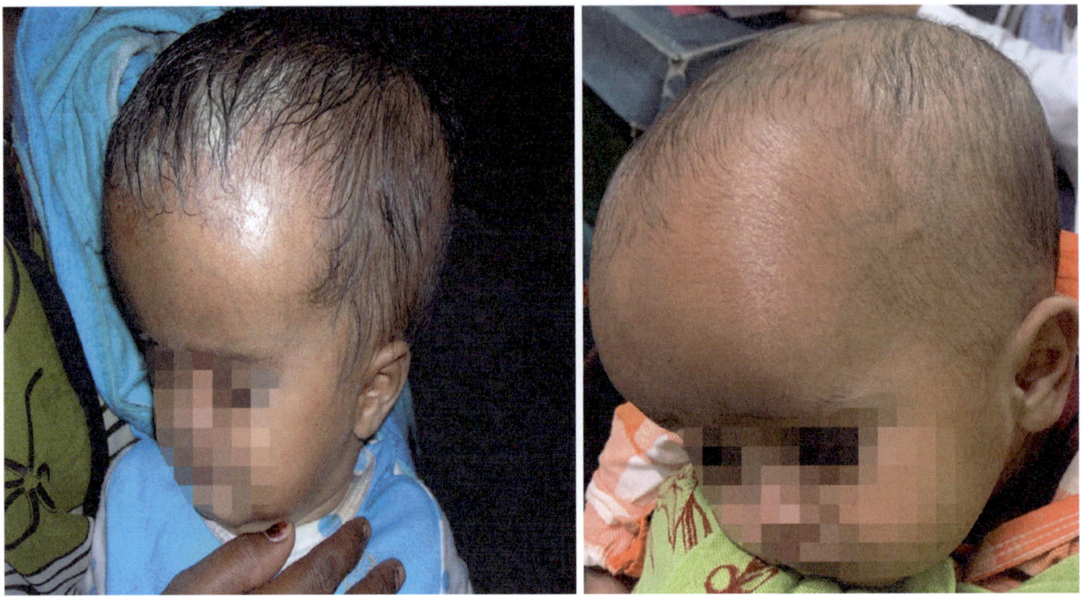

Fig. 17.3 Large head due to hydrocephalus

17.3.3 Antenatal Diagnosis and Follow-Up

- Fetal cerebral lateral ventricles
  - Normal (< 10 mm)
  - Mild/borderline Ventriculomegaly (VM) (10–12 mm)
  - Moderate VM (13–15 mm)
  - Severe VM (> 15 mm)
- Ventricle–hemisphere ratio (VHR)
- No role for fetal surgery
- Antenatal hydrocephalus
  - Mortality—70%
  - Normal intellectual development—50%

17.3.4 Investigations

- *Trans Cranial Ultrasonography (USG)*
  It is done through an open fontanelle and measures the ventricular dilatation. Ventriculo-parenchymal ratio of more than 33% indicates hydrocephalus. Single lateral ventricular dilatation indicates obstruction of foramen of Monro. Also useful for evaluating subependymal and intraventricular hemorrhage.

$$\text{Doppler Resistive Index} - \frac{\text{Peak systolic velocity} - \text{lowest diastolic velocity}}{\text{Peak systolic velocity}}$$

- *X-Ray*—"Copper beating" of skull, erosion of pituitary fossa
- *CT-Scan*—greater anatomic details, to distinguish between communicating and noncommunicating hydrocephalus, to look for any tumors, abscess or any bleeding (Fig. 17.4).
- Findings suggestive of hydrocephalus on CT
  - Size of both temporal horns greater than 2 mm
  - Evan's ratio—ratio of the largest width of the frontal horns to maximal biparietal diameter >30%
  - Transependymal exudates
  - Mickey Mouse ventricles—ballooning of frontal horns of lateral ventricles and third ventricle
- *Contrast MRI* for visualization of brain stem and posterior fossa
  - Upper bowing of the corpus callosum on sagittal section

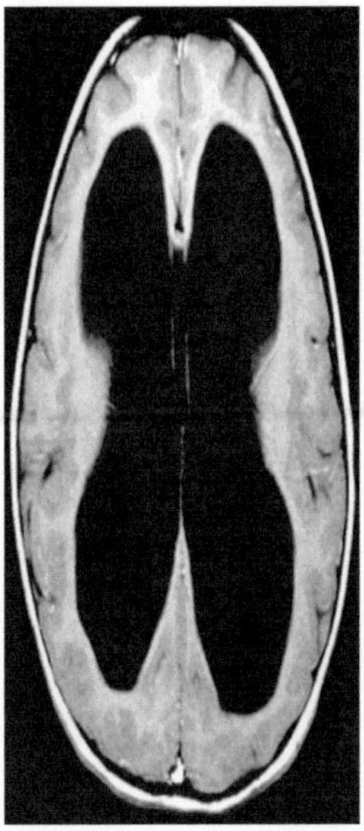

Fig. 17.4 MRI head showing hydrocephalus

17.3.5 Medical Management

17.3.5.1 Indications

- Patients temporarily not suitable for shunt placement, e.g., coagulopathy
- Patients with oligosymptomatic secondary hydrocephalus waiting for treatment for the underlying cause
- Patients in whom the shunt alone is not able to control the hydrocephalus

17.3.5.2 Pharmacotherapy

- Acetazolamide/Diamox—is a carbonic anhydrase inhibitor which causes preferential vasoconstriction of the choroidal arteries. Recommended dose is 50–100 mg/kg/day and the major side effect noted with it is metabolic acidosis.
- Osmotic diuretics—like isosorbide (2–3 g/kg), mannitol, urea, glycerol (2 mg/kg qid) have also been tried, though they have a very limited role.
- Post—pyogenic meningitis hydrocephalus—needs appropriate antibiotics.
- Posttubercular meningitis hydrocephalus—should be treated with antitubercular drugs along with steroids when indicated.
- Posthemorrhagic hydrocephalus in premature infants
  - Gr 1,2 observe.
  - Gr 3,4—acetazolamide, frusemide, ventriculoscopy and irrigation, shunt.

Ventricular tap: is usually done through the lateral angle of the anterior fontanelle in case of raised intracranial tension.

In case of acute rise in intracranial pressure (headache, vomiting, drowsiness), urgent drainage (tap) followed by shunt operation should be done; otherwise, there could be loss of vision, loss of brain parenchyma, and loss of intellectual function.

17.3.6 Surgical Management

17.3.6.1 Indications

- Rapidly progressive Hydrocephalus (HCP) uncontrolled with 3–6 m medical management
- Adverse effect on medical management
- Symptomatic, raised ICP
- Head size>2 SD, Occipito-frontal circumference (OFC) >2 cm/week, >97th centile
- Falling IQ during follow-up
- Papilledema of fundoscopy, periventricular ooze on CT
- Postinfectious HCP after infection control
- Thinning of the cortical mantle on follow-up or thickness <1 cm on initial investigations

17.3.6.2 Contraindications

- Ventriculitis, meningitis—high CSF protein
- Acute Intra-ventricular hemorrhage (IVH)
- Irrecoverable optic atrophy with gross hydrocephalus
- Extreme brain pathology

17.3.7 Surgical Treatment

1. Removal of obstructing lesion, e.g., tumor
2. Decrease CSF production—ablation of choroid plexus
3. Bypassing a block to normal CSF flow by Cannulation of Aqueduct of Sylvius, *3rd ventriculostomy*, ventriculo-cisternostomy
4. External drainage in case of infection
5. *Internal drainage—shunt, most commonly performed operation for hydrocephalus*

17.4 Shunt Operations (Figs. 17.5 and 17.6)

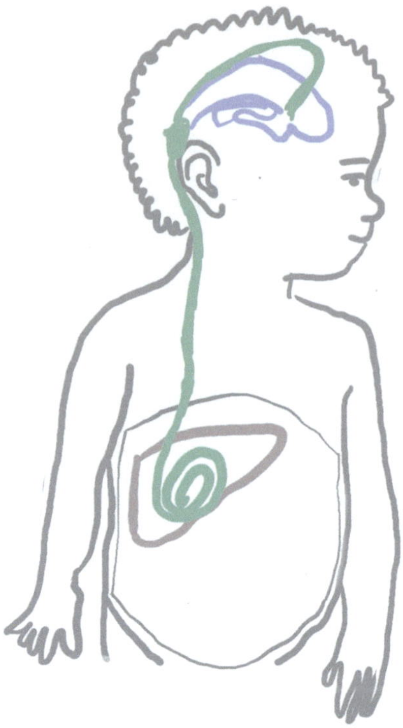

Fig. 17.5 Ventriculo-Peritoneal shunt

Protocol to be Followed for Any Shunt Procedure—to Reduce the Infection Rates
The protocol needs to be strictly followed while doing the shunt surgeries so as to reduce the shunt-related complications specially the infection rates. Intravenous antibiotics should be given before incision. Paint the surgical field properly and wait for 3 minutes. Handscrub by the entire surgical team (antiseptic cream not allowed) and double gloves should be worn by the entire team. Ioban is applied to the surgical field after painting and draping. A single dose of antibiotic dose is enough postoperatively if the surgical team abides by the above guidelines.

Preoperative planning The surgeon selects the side for the shunt depending on the patient's intracranial anatomy and other cranial or extracranial factors (other recent surgical procedures, skin abrasions or infections).

The choice of anterior (coronal) or posterior (occipital or parieto-occipital) entry site may be based on factors such as intracranial anatomy, recent surgical procedures, skull shape, or surgeon experience.

Ventriculo Peritoneal (VP) Shunt (Most Commonly Done)
Chhabra VP Shunt—most commonly used shunt in the Indian scenario

- Proximal catheter tantalum tip
- Barium coated for x-ray visibility
- Differential pressure >opening pressure
  - Low 5 cm H_2O
  - Medium 10 cm H_2O
  - High 15 cm H_2O
- Anti-siphon mechanism
- Proximal slit valve in the shunt chamber is girdled by a stainless steel spring, which helps in maintaining the opening pressure

Procedure for insertion—normally inserted through a burr hole in the right parieto-occipital region (keen's point) and the valve will usually sit

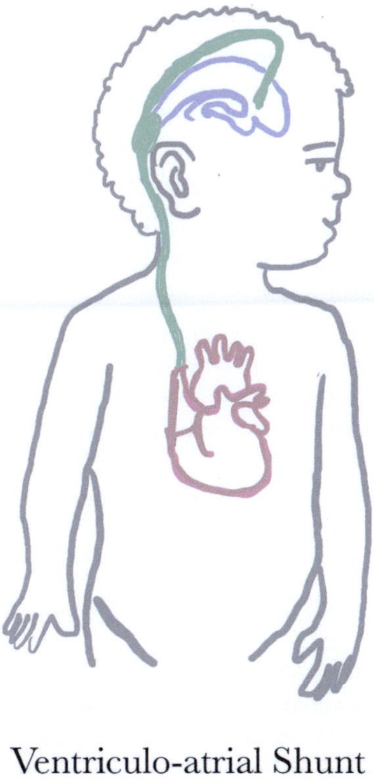

Fig. 17.6 VA shunt

behind the right ear. The distal catheter is tunneled subcutaneously down to another incision in the abdomen, where it is then placed into the peritoneal cavity, preferably in the suprahepatic region.

Ventriculo-atrial Shunt
This involves placing the distal tip in the right atrium just above the tricuspid valve. Externally, the point of insertion is between T4 and T7. The procedure is usually through open venotomy or percutaneous technique (fluoroscopic, sonographic or electrocardiographic guidance). The entrance is usually through common facial vein into the jugular vein and then to superior vena cava. Few serious complications like pulmonary embolism, Cor pulmonale, septicemia, shunt nephritis (immune complex), cardiac mural thrombi, and cardiac tamponade have been reported.

Lumboperitoneal Shunt
It is done only in communicating type of hydrocephalus. The procedure is similar to lumbar puncture with the Seldinger technique, tunneled subcutaneously to enter peritoneum near umbilicus.

Ventriculo-Pleural Shunt
It is viable alternative if the peritoneum is not available. It is usually avoided in infants and children <8 yrs due to the risk of persistent pleural effusion and pneumothorax. Usual location is the 4th–6th intercostal space along anterior axillary line. It is recommended only for >7 yrs of age.

Torkildsen Shunt
This shunts ventricles to the cisternal space and is effective only in acquired obstructive hydrocephalus, as children with congenital hydrocephalus frequently do not develop normal subarachnoid CSF pathways.

Miscellaneous: when the distal end is placed in either the gall bladder, ureter or bladder—rarely done when all the above-mentioned shunt procedures are not feasible.

17.4.1 Postoperative Care

A sterile dressing should be done for 48 hours. Intravenous anitibiotics are recommended to prevent shunt infection. Shunt series (skull, chest, abdomen) baseline X-ray and 1 month postoperative neuroimaging should be done. Keep a watch for complications.

17.4.2 Shunt Complications (Figs. 17.7 and 17.8)

- Malfunction:
  - Obstruction
  - Disconnection or fracture
  - Shunt migration
- Shunt infection
- Overdrainage
  - Slit ventricle syndrome
  - Subdural/extracerebral CSF collections
  - Craniosynostosis
- Seizures
- Pneumocephalus
- Isolated ventricle syndromes

17.4.3 Complications of Shunt Assembly

- Obstruction
  - Upper end block—abnormal position, blockage by choroid plexus
  - Lower end block—peritonitis, pseudocyst formation
- Disconnection and migration
- Fracture especially at connectors
- Overdrainage—low pressure symptoms, slit ventricle on CT scan
- Loculation
- Infection

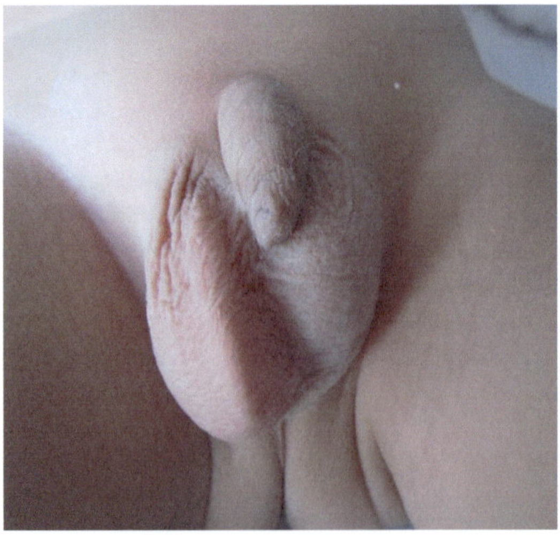

Fig. 17.7 Shunt migration into the scrotum

17.4.4 Other Complications Related to a Particular Procedure

- Cardiac complications:
  - Mural thrombosis
  - Endocarditis
  - Cardiac arrhythmias, tamponade
  - Distal shunt migration
  - Superior vena cava obstruction
- Pulmonary complications:
  - Pulmonary thromboembolism
  - Pulmonary hypertension and cor pulmonale
  - Pleural effusion, pneumothorax, parenchymal injury
- Peritoneal complications:
  - Inguinal hernia and hydrocele
  - Ascites
  - Cyst formation
  - Intestinal volvulus and obstruction
  - Bowel perforation, bladder perforation
  - Intraperitoneal spread of infection
  - Malignancy
- Shunt nephritis

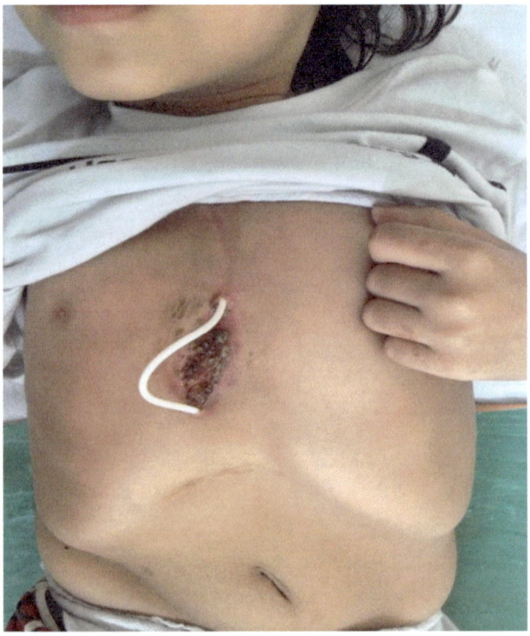

Fig. 17.8 Image shows an exposed shunt tubing through the overlying eroded chest wall

17.4.5 Causes of Shunt Malfunction (Fig. 17.9)

- Mechanical causes
  - Kinking
  - Discontinuity/disconnection
  - Break/fracture
  - Functional failure of the valve/shunt apparatus
  - Migration
- Overdrainage
  - Epidural, subdural or intracranial hematoma
  - Slit ventricle syndrome
- Infection

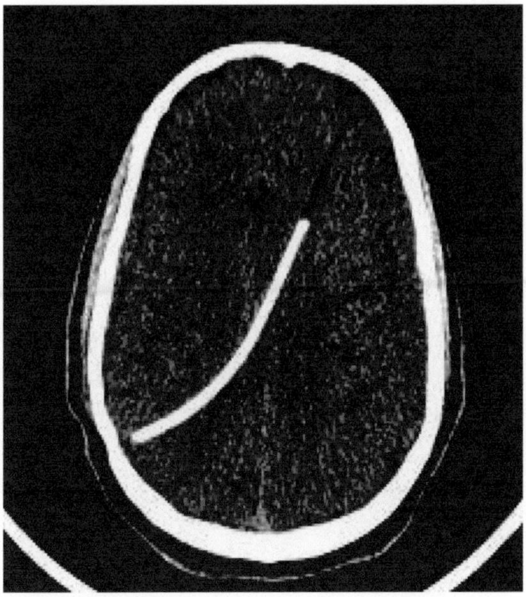

Fig. 17.9 CT image of a patient with slit ventricle syndrome

17.4.6 Shunt Infections

Incidence of shunt infections has been reported as 6% with a mortality of about 60%.

Majority of the infections occur within 2 months with 90% in 6 months. Shunt infection can lead to ventriculitis, scarring, and loculation. The common organisms implicated are *Staphylococcus aureus*, epidermidis, Gram-negative bacilli. The risk factors for infections include young age, premature, postoperative CSF leak, glove holes, previous infections, intraventricular hemorrhage, shunt revision, and long duration of surgery.

Treatment includes externalization or removal of shunt along with IV antibiotics and shunt reimplantation after resolution of infection on contralateral side.

17.4.7 Slit Ventricle Syndrome

Usually develops in patients who have been shunted for many years. The slit ventricle triad of symptoms consists of chronic, intermittent headaches with slowly refilling shunt reservoir on physical examination and "slit" ventricles on radiographic evaluation

Treatment is initially medical management with acetazolamide or mannitol. If it fails, revision of the shunt with higher pressure/flow control with anti-siphon mechanism should be done. Few patients might require subtemporal decompression.

17.5 Endoscopic Third Ventriculostomy (ETV)

Endoscopic Third Ventriculostomy is becoming popular because it is done by a minimally invasive endoscopic technique and no foreign material is inserted (Fig. 17.10). The floor of third ventricle is opened to basal cisterns for CSF drainage bypassing the obstruction.

- Indications:
  - Obstructive hydrocephalus—highest success rates >75%
  - Shunt infection (removal of hardware), previously failed shunts, shunt complications

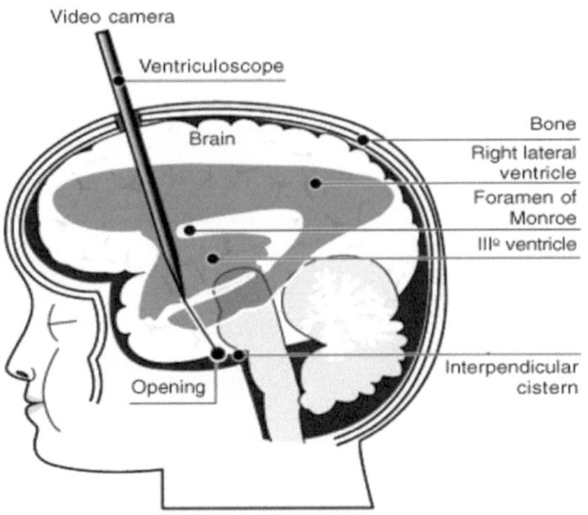

Fig. 17.10 Neuroendoscopic third ventriculostomy

  - Patients with subdural hematomas (shunt removed before ETV is performed)
  - Slit ventricle syndrome
  - Older patients >2 years
- Contraindications:
  - Communicating hydrocephalus
  - Previous radiation leading to subarachnoid scarring
  - Infants with Meningomyelocele (MMC), hemorrhage, infection—poor response
  - Small ventricles, crowded basilar cisterns
  - Smaller children <6 months—restoration of cortical thickness faster with shunting

17.6 Choroid Plexus Cauterization

In early 2000s, choroid plexus cauterization (CPC) was added to ETV to improve the efficacy of ETV alone in very young patients especially those less than 1 year of age. It involves cauterization of the entire choroid plexus throughout both lateral ventricles. The efficacy of the procedure is proportional to the amount of choroid plexus cauterized.

- Indications
  - Communicating slowly progressing HCP in infants
  - Choroid plexus papilloma/hyperplasia
  - Abdominal complications-precluding shunts, e.g., necrotizing enterocolitis
  - Intractable shunt failure
- Contraindication
  - Obstructive hydrocephalus

Other Causes of Large Head

- Achondroplasia
- Metabolic disease
- Vitamin A toxicity

17.7 Other Types of Hydrocephalus

17.7.1 Posthemorrhagic Hydrocephalus

It is usually due to neonatal intraventricular hemorrhage (Respiratory distress syndrome (RDS)/atelectasis/hypertension) or subarachnoid hemorrhage or traumatic brain injury in adults. It is seen in 15–20% of premature babies (due to germinal matrix hemorrhage). The treatment is shunt surgery, or alternatively ETV + CPC (not routinely practiced).

17.7.2 Hydrocephalus in MMC

There is fourth ventricle outflow obstruction with a high tentorial angle and isolation of cranial and spinal compartments which leads to anatomical obstruction. Also, there is venous congestion which leads to impaired absorption. >80% of the patients of MMC have associated hydrocephalus (the higher the level, the greater the incidence). Chiari II malformation and aqueductal stenosis are usually associated, if not treated it is usually progressive.

Treatment—Timing of Shunt in MMC—Opposing Views

MMC first followed by Shunt surgery—closing the MMC first allows for a period of observation to demonstrate the absence of infection related to the initial open defect.

It also allows observation to determine which patients will actually need CSF diversion.

Simultaneous management—simultaneous repair of the MMC defect and insertion of a ventriculoperitoneal shunt is recommended by a few. Similar infection rates have been reported when compared to the staged approach, reduced anesthesia and reduced CSF fistula formation from MMC repair leakage

Open myelomeningocele with delayed repair may already have CSF infection documented by CSF microbiologic testing—external ventricular drainage should be performed for 7–10 days in conjunction with antibiotic treatment, until the CSF infection is controlled and a shunt can be inserted.

17.8 Outcome and Prognosis

Prenatal hydrocephalus is usually associated with a poor prognosis with only one-third of the patients having an IQ > 80. Hydrocephalus associated with other congenital anomalies has a mortality of about 80% in first 5 years. About 50% of the untreated patients usually die. Postsurgery survival is about 50–90%. Patients with a cortical mantle thickness (CMT) <2 cm are uneducable; those with CMT of 2–3 cm have an IQ < 100. Ones with CMT >3 cm have a normal IQ. Average life of the shunt is 6 years.

Other causes of hydrocephalus

- Normal pressure hydrocephalus due to dementia/Alzheimer's disease
- Arrested hydrocephalus
- Hydrocephalus-ex-vacuo—due to cerebral agenesis or decrease brain substance
- Porencephalic cyst

17.9 Recent Advances

- Stereotactic shunt placement—infrared optical tracking systems or electromagnetic technology
- Reduced rate of poor shunt placement compared with standard blind shunt placement
- Antibiotic-impregnated shunt systems reduced infection rates by 1.5–4%
- Development of intracranial pressure transducers that are remotely readable and can be programmed to drain according to a patient's needs and symptoms
- Implantation of the ventricular catheter using an endoscopic technique
- Magnetically adjustable pressure valves—allow individually tailored CSF drainage
- Future "Smart Shunt" systems—electronic flow, posture detection sensors and instant adjustment circuits will provide better performance

17.10 Summary

Congenital hydrocephalus should be treated at the earliest to have good neurological outcomes. Surgical management is the treatment of choice and a shunt procedure should be done under strict aseptic precautions. Ventriculoperitoneal shunts continue to be the preferred choice although associated with multiple complications. In the recent times, endoscopic third ventriculoctomy has gained popularity mainly for obstructive hydrocephalus due to aqueductal stenosis.

Suggested Reading

Bajpai M. Congenital hydrocephalus occurs in approximately 1 case for every 2,000 live or stillborn births. Indian J Pediatr. 1997;64(6 Suppl):1–3.

Coran AG, Caldamone A, Scott Adzich N, Krummel TM, Laberge JM, editors. Pediatric surgery. 7th ed. Oxford: Elsevier Limited; 2012.

Flannery AM, Mitchell L. Pediatric hydrocephalus: systematic literature review and evidence-based guidelines. Part 1: introduction and methodology. J Neurosurg Pediatr. 2014;14(Suppl 1):3–7. https://doi.org/10.3171/2014.7.PEDS14321.

Hochstetler A, Raskin J, Blazer-Yost BL. Hydrocephalus: historical analysis and considerations for treatment. Eur J Med Res. 2022;27(1):168. https://doi.org/10.1186/s40001-022-00798-6. PMID: 36050779; PMCID: PMC9434947

Konar SK, Maiti TK, Bir SC, Kalakoti P, Nanda A, Robert H. Pudenz: (1911-1998) and ventriculoatrial shunt: historical perspective. World Neurosurg. 2015; https://doi.org/10.1016/j.wneu.2015.05.080.

Youmans and Winn Neurological Surgery, 7th ed.

18 Neural Tube Defects

Monika Bawa and Subhasis Roy Choudhury

Neural tube defects (NTD) occur due to failure of the normal neural tube development. They are broadly classified into two types based on the coverings of the defect:

1. *Open*: the neural tube and its membranous coverings are abnormal, the neural tube is exposed, and the overlying skin is lacking. Examples—anencephaly (without a brain), myeloschisis/rachischisis [the most severe form with exposed spinal cord and cerebrospinal fluid (CSF) leak], and myelomeningoceles.
2. *Closed*: the defect is as above, but the overlying skin is intact, and the neural tissue is not exposed. Examples—spina bifida occulta, lipomeningomyelocele, encephalocele, etc.

The spinal defects can be further classified as below (Table 18.1).

Spina bifida aperta (open neural tube defect, Fig. 18.1): there is a defect in the posterior vertebral arch with no skin cover, CSF leak, and a chance of meningitis. Example: syringocele (open spinal canal) and rachischisis (open bony defect).

Spina bifida cystica (Fig. 18.2): this is a variant of spina bifida aperta with cystic swelling. It is usually of two types: meningocele-CSF contained sac without neural tissue and meningomyelocele (MMC)—when there is neural tissue within the sac.

Spina bifida occulta (Fig. 18.3): this is due to a defect of the posterior vertebral arch, but there is no herniation of the neural tube. Various changes may be seen on the skin cover—like hairy patch (Fig. 18.4a, b), pigmentation, fatty lump, and dermal sinus. There may be associated intradural lesions like—lipoma, dermoid, epidermoid tumor, tethering of the cord with thickening of filum terminale, and diastematomyelia (bony spur). Bony spina bifida is found in 10% of the normal population.

M. Bawa (✉)
Pediatric Surgery, PGIMER, Chandigarh, India

S. Roy Choudhury
Pediatric Surgery, Lady Hardinge Medical College and Associated Kalawati Saran Children's Hospital, New Delhi, Delhi, India

© The Author(s), under exclusive license to Springer Nature Singapore Pte Ltd. 2025

S. Roy Choudhury (ed.), *Pediatric Surgery*, https://doi.org/10.1007/978-981-96-1257-4_18

Table 18.1 Classification of spinal dysraphism

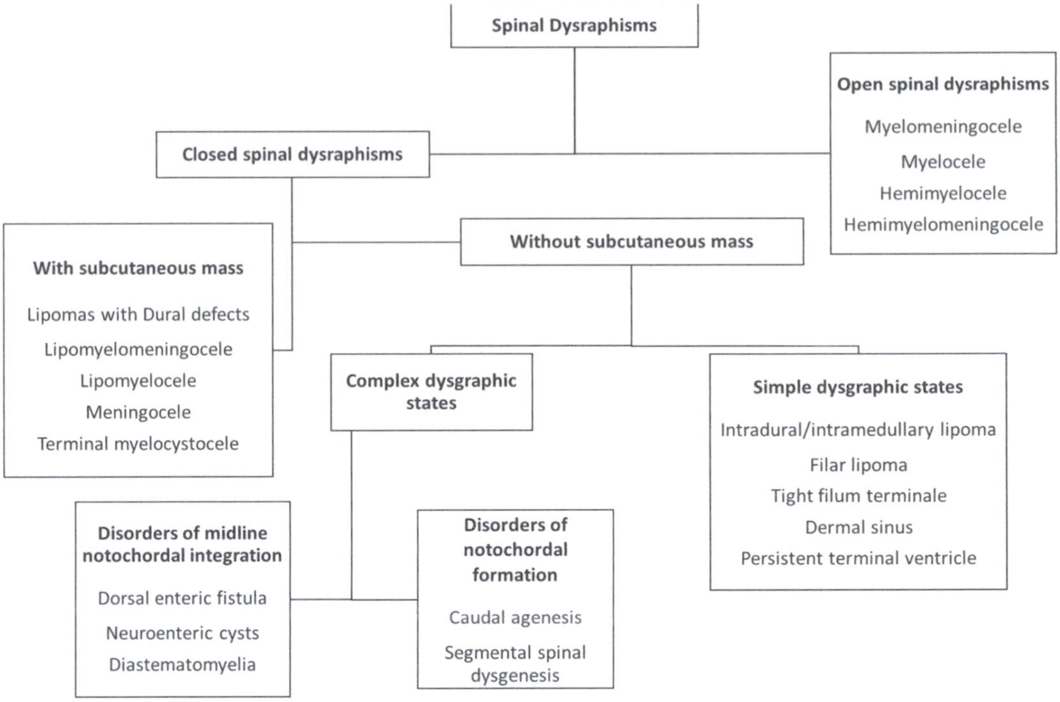

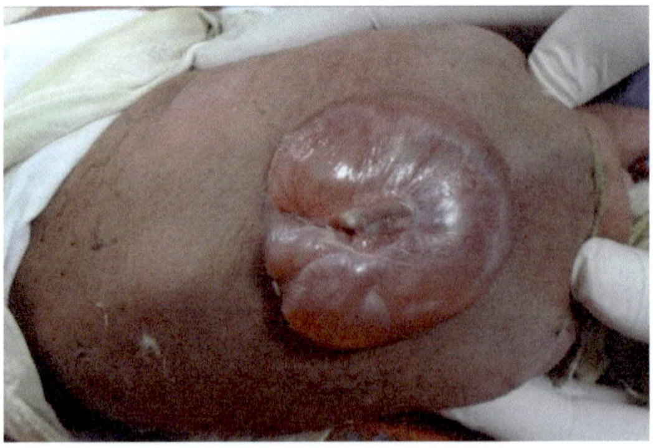

Fig. 18.1 Open neural tube defect over lumbosacral area

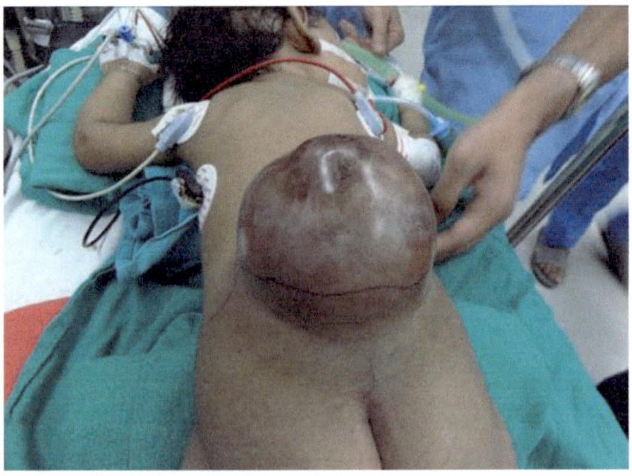

Fig. 18.2 Lumbosacral meningomyelocele

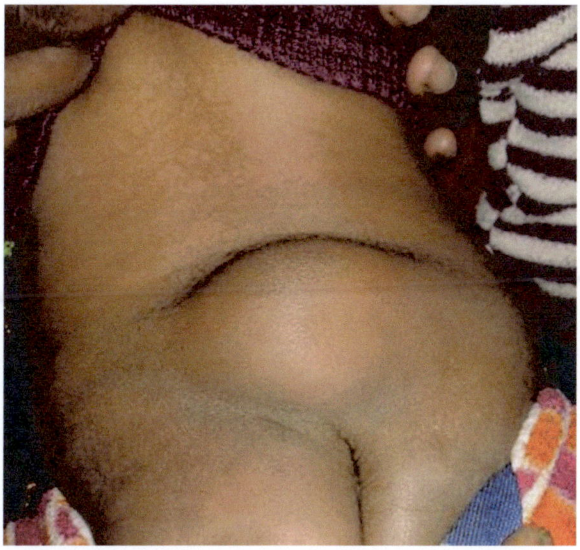

Fig. 18.3 Lipomeningocele

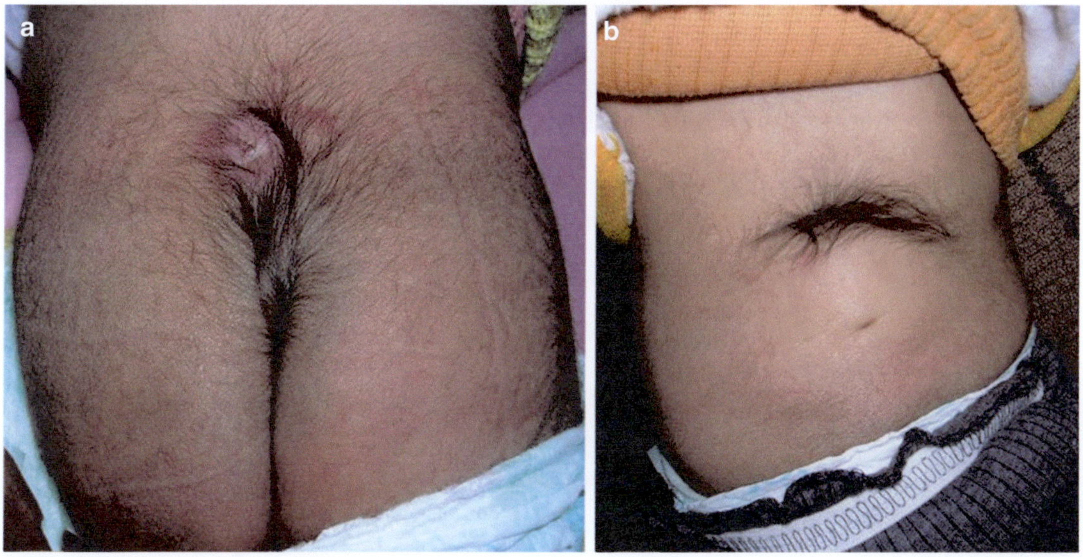

Fig. 18.4 (**a**, **b**) Spina bifida occulta with hairy patch

18.1 Classification of Neural Tube Defects

The incidence of NTD in the population is 1–8/1000 population. Around 90% of cases are sporadic; some are familial. The etiology of NTD is multifactorial. An association of low folic acid intake of mothers with higher incidences of neural tube defects in children has been established.

18.2 Embryology

Spina bifida results from the failure of closure of the neural tube. Understanding the embryological development of the neural tube is essential to grasp the embryopathology of spina bifida.

Bending of the neural placode to form the neural tube requires extrinsic and intrinsic mechanical forces in addition to dorsalizing and ventralizing genetic influences. Expansion of the surface epithelium of the embryo is the principal extrinsic force for the folding of the neuroepithelium to form the neural tube. Cells of the neural placode are mobile and migrate beneath the surface ectoderm, which causes the lateral margins of the placode to become raised toward the dorsal midline. The formation of neuronal folds occurs on day 21, and its fusion occurs on day 23.

Neurulation is a multifactorial process controlled by various intrinsic and extrinsic factors. The intrinsic factors are generated by neuroendocrine cells, which cause.

elongation, rearrangement, nonrandomly oriented rostrocaudal division of neuroendocrine cells, shaping of the neural plate, and wedging. The extrinsic factors include changes in epidermal ectoderm cells.

All these factors influence the shape of the neural tube, and this neural tube closes in the dorsal midline first in the cervical region and then extends rostrally and caudally such that the anterior neuropore closes at 24 days (23–26 days) and the posterior neuropore closes at 28 days (26–30 days).

The bending of the neural plate to form the neural tube is termed primary neurulation.

Primary neurulation includes:

1. Formation of the neural plate
2. Shaping of the neural plate
3. Bending of the neural plate
4. Fusion of the neural folds

Secondary neurulation refers only to the most caudal part of the spinal cord, which develops from the neuroepithelium caudal to the site of posterior neuropore closure. Secondary neurulation occurs in three stages:

1. Formation of medullary cord from tail bud
2. Cavitation of the central aspect of the medullary cord results in the formation of multiple lumina
3. Coalescence of the lumina into a single central cavity surrounded by a peripheral layer of radially oriented medullary cord cells.

Failure of closure of the anterior neuropore by 24 days results in anencephaly (Fig. 18.5). Lack of forebrain neuroectoderm results in failure of

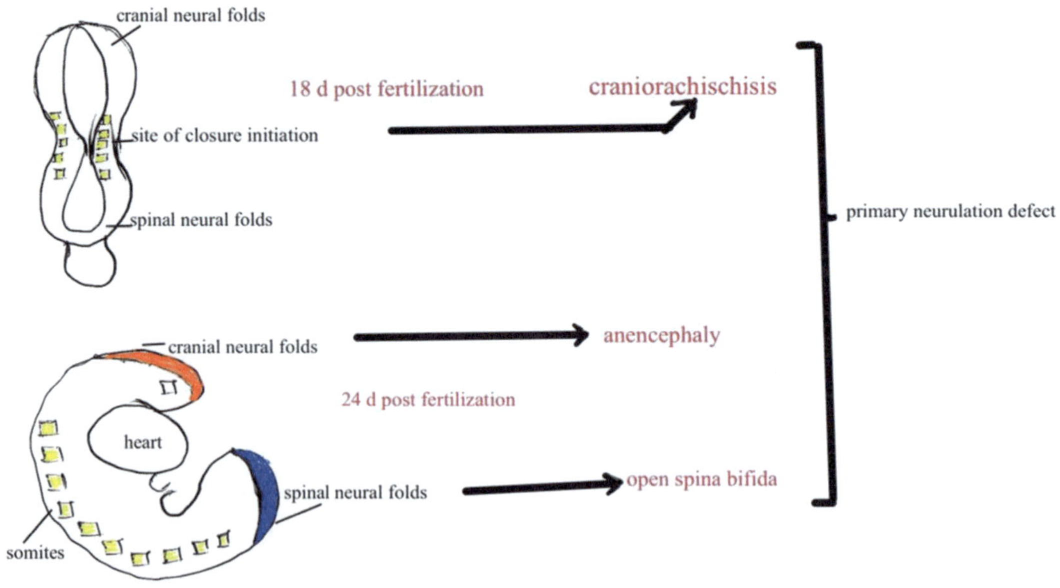

Fig. 18.5 Embryology of defects in primary neurulation

induction of the overlying mesoderm, and the cranium, meninges, and scalp fail to close in the midline.

Failure to close posterior neuropore by 26 days results in open spina bifida/spina bifida aperta or cystica, including myelomeningocele and meningocele (Figs. 18.5 and 18.6). Myelomeningocele consists of an open neural placode surrounded by an intermediate zone of thin epithelium, which is surrounded by normal skin. Meningocele is a skin-covered anomaly characterized by herniation of just meninges through a dorsal bony defect. Myeloschisis refers to a severe form of neural tube defect where the open neural tube appears as a flattened, plate-like mass of nervous tissue with no overlying membrane.

Failure of secondary neurulation results in closed neural tube defects in which the overlying skin is intact, but the caudal neural tube and its membranous coverings develop abnormally (Fig. 18.7).

Development anomalies of the caudal spinal cord include spina bifida occulta:

1. Tight, thickened filum terminale
2. Split cord malformations (diastematomyelia/diplomyelia)
3. Neuroenteric cysts
4. Dermal sinuses
5. Sacral agenesis/caudal regression
6. Lipomatous malformations: lumbosacral lipoma, leptomyelolipoma, lipomyelomeningocele, fatty filum

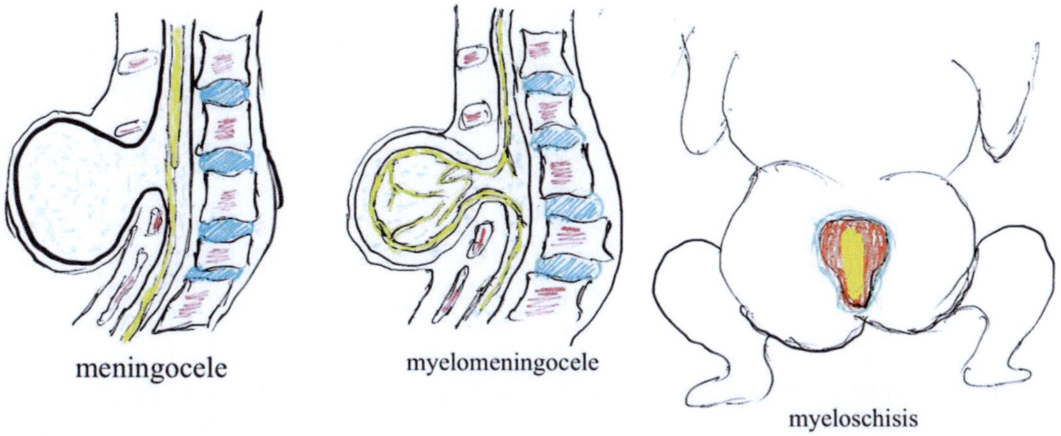

Fig. 18.6 Primary neurulation defects

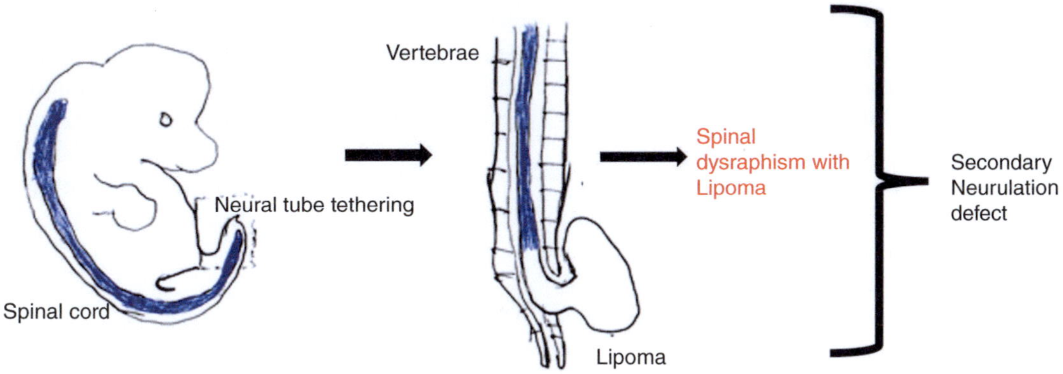

Fig. 18.7 Embryology of secondary neurulation defects

Such anomalies lead to spinal cord tethering, which causes neurological deterioration secondary to traction on the conus medullaris and resultant ischemic injury.

18.3 Prevention

Folic acid (0.4 mg/ day) to expectant mothers has been found to reduce the incidence of neural tube defects. The dose needs to be increased to 4 mg in women with a history of neural tube defects.

18.4 Antenatal Diagnosis and Management

18.4.1 Antenatal Counselling

Antenatal diagnosis allows for counselling of the family regarding the outcome and helps in appropriate decision-making.

- Neural tube defects can be diagnosed by prenatal screening with ultrasonography and maternal serum alpha-fetoprotein (AFP) levels.
- Serum AFP has 75% accuracy in detecting open neural tube defects (NTD) if gestational age is more than 15 weeks. Amniotic fluid AFP is accurate in 98% of cases of open defects.
- Ultrasonography and fetal MRI
  2D ultrasonography has superseded the use of biochemical markers to detect NTD. Ultrasound findings in anencephaly include absent calvarium, reduced crown-rump length, absent neural tissue, and a loss of the normal head contour. Spina bifida is diagnosed by the visualization of the bony defect through which the meningeal sac alone (meningocele) or sac plus neural tissue
  (myelomeningocele) herniates. Spina bifida is also suggested by the scalloping of frontal bones, the "lemon sign," and crescentic deformation of the cerebellum with concavity pointing anteriorly, the "banana sign," seen as a. part of the Chiari type II malformation.
  3D Ultrasonography and fetal MRI provide superior anatomical details of the anomaly.

Parents are overwhelmed by the MMC status and usually follow the lead of the treating physician. The treating physician should resist the urge to share their bias and share an accurate picture. Parents are ultimately responsible for taking care of their children. Issues that require addressing include intellectual performance, continence, mobility level, cognitive functioning, and associated conditions. It should be emphasized that the surgery is a life-saving measure but does not recover the neurological deficits.

All children with MMC will survive initially with proper treatment. Unfortunately, there is a slow attrition to death—Chiari II malformation and shunt obstruction being the common cause. In a 25-year follow-up (Children's Memorial Hospital, Chicago), overall mortality was 24%. In addition, 15% died during the initial 5 years of life. In other series, 1% of patients died yearly (from age 5 to 30 years with an overall mortality of 24–56%).

Approximately 75% will have intelligence quotient >80. Of those with normal intelligence, 60% have learning disabilities. Many of them grow up to become contributing members of society.

Ambulation depends on the sensorimotor level (with L3 being particularly important). Those with lesions above L3 are rarely functional ambulators. A total of 89% of the patients are community ambulators. Beyond adolescence, only 50% are community ambulators, as wheelchair becomes more energy efficient.

Urinary social continence (freedom from incontinence in social situations, with or without clean intermittent catheterization (CIC)) will be achievable in ~80% of school-going children. Chronic constipation is a significant problem in almost 50% of patients. Nearly all the patients have abnormal genital sensations, with at least 64% undergoing one orthopedic procedure.

18.4.2 Antenatal Care

Babies must be preferably delivered in a center with access to neonatal intensive care unit

(NICU) care, with surgeons specialized in operating spina bifida. The fetus usually has a breech presentation (due to lower limb dysfunction and macrocephaly). The mode of delivery for such patients is lower segment cesarean section (LSCS). Evidence suggests that vaginal delivery might cause additional loss of neural function from pressure on the exposed roots in those with vertex presentation, but is insufficient to advocate the universal use of LSCS. Hence, in such cases, the choice is left at the discretion of the obstetrician and the mother.

Parents should also be apprised of the increased risk of MMC in subsequent babies, and folate supplementation (4000 μg daily) should be advised to prevent such recurrences.

18.4.3 Preoperative Care

After birth care: patients with MMC are prone to developing latex allergy, and the reported incidence is high; hence, latex-free gloves are recommended to minimize sensitization. The lesion is covered with sterile saline-soaked dressing (may wrap the dressing in plastic wrapping to prevent dehydration, heat loss, and contamination). The baby should be nursed in a lateral or prone position, with the lesion above the level of the head, to prevent CSF egress.

Most lesions are in the lumbosacral area, followed by the thoracic spine. Other areas involved are frontal, occipital, and nasoethmoidal (Figs. 18.8, 18.9, 18.10 and 18.11) encephalocele.

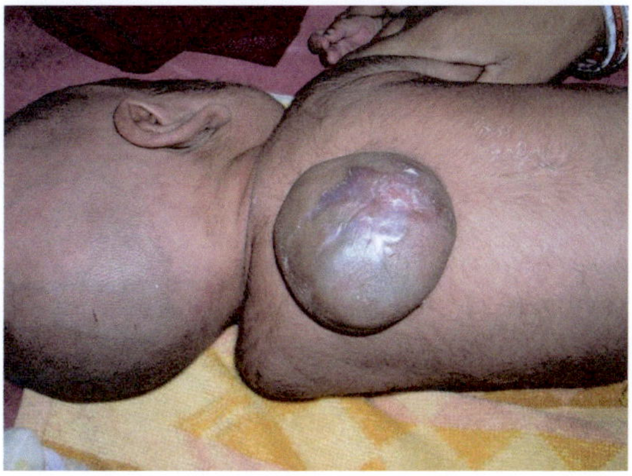

Fig. 18.8 Dorsal meningomyelocele

18.4.4 Examination

- Local examination of the swelling—describes the swelling as size, shape, site, extent, skin coverings, compressibility, cough impulse, and transillumination.
- Physical examination—measure the head circumference, examine the spine and vertebra for kyphoscoliosis, assess the general vigor (cry and suck), anal sphincter tone, upper and lower extremity neurological status, presence of a palpable bladder, orthope-

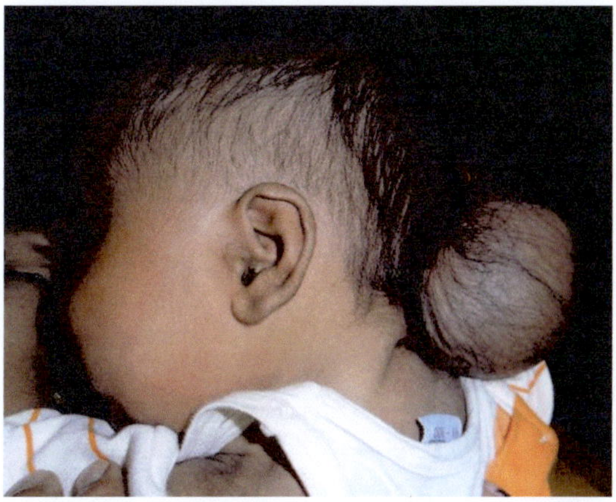

Fig. 18.9 Occipital encephalocele

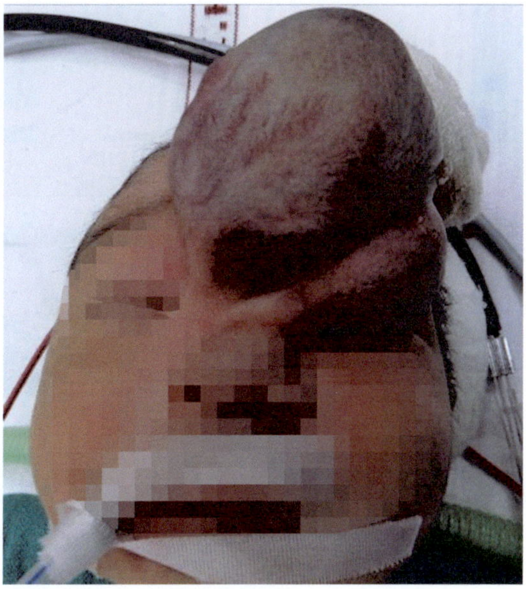

Fig. 18.10 Frontal encephalocele

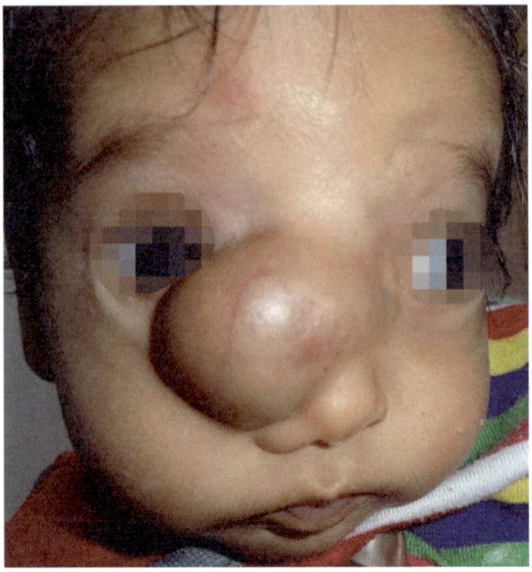

Fig. 18.11 Naso ethmoidal encephalocele

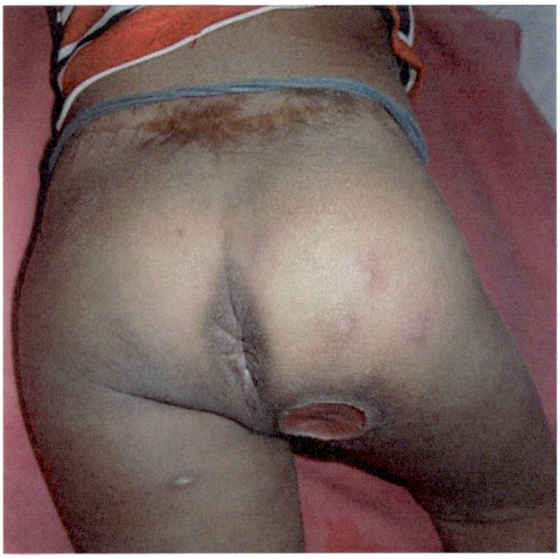

Fig. 18.12 Trophic ulcer in an operated case of spina bifida

dic deformities like clubfeet, and trophic ulcers (Fig. 18.12). These may not be apparent early in life.

- Thorough neurological examination (Tables 18.2 and 18.3)—assessment of fontanelle, cranial sutures, cranial nerve examination, fundoscopic examination, observation of spontaneous activity, degree of activity in response to noxious stimuli, deep tendon reflexes, and anocutaneous reflex.

Table 18.2 Assessment of motor function in patients of spina bifida

	Motor function
L2, L3	Flexion at hip joint
L3, L4	Extension at knee joint
L4, L5	Dorsiflexion at ankle joint
L5, S1	Flexion at knee joint, extension of hallux
S1, S2	Plantar flexion at ankle joint
S2, S3	Flexion of hallux and toes
S2, S3, S4	Anal sphincter tone

Table 18.3 Spectrum of clinical presentation of patients with neural tube defects according to the level of involvement

Paralysis below	Findings
T12	Complete paralysis of lower extremities
L1	Weak to moderate hip flexion, palpable contractures in sartorius
L2	Moderate hip adduction
L3	Almost normal knee extension
L4	Some hip abduction in flexion
L5	Hip extension absent, dorsiflexed foot with flexed thigh
S1	Moderate plantar flexion of foot, extension of all toes with extension in terminal phalanx of great toe, clawing of toes, and flattening of the sole of the foot
S2	Clawing of toes due to weakness of muscles of the sole of the foot

The upper lumbar lesions produce iliopsoas/gluteal imbalance and hip flexion posture. Mid-lumbar lesions affect the quadriceps/hamstring imbalances and knee extension, while the low lumbar lesions cause foot dorsi/plantar flexion imbalance and dorsiflexed ankle deformity.

Brainstem function assessment (usually nurses can identify these)—these may present as apneic spells or poor or dysfunctional swallowing, high-pitched or weak cry, vocal cord palsies, or hypotonia might be noticed.

Odd facial features, low-set ears/malformed ears, abnormally high palate, widened/short neck, low hairline, and simian creases may be noted on physical examination.

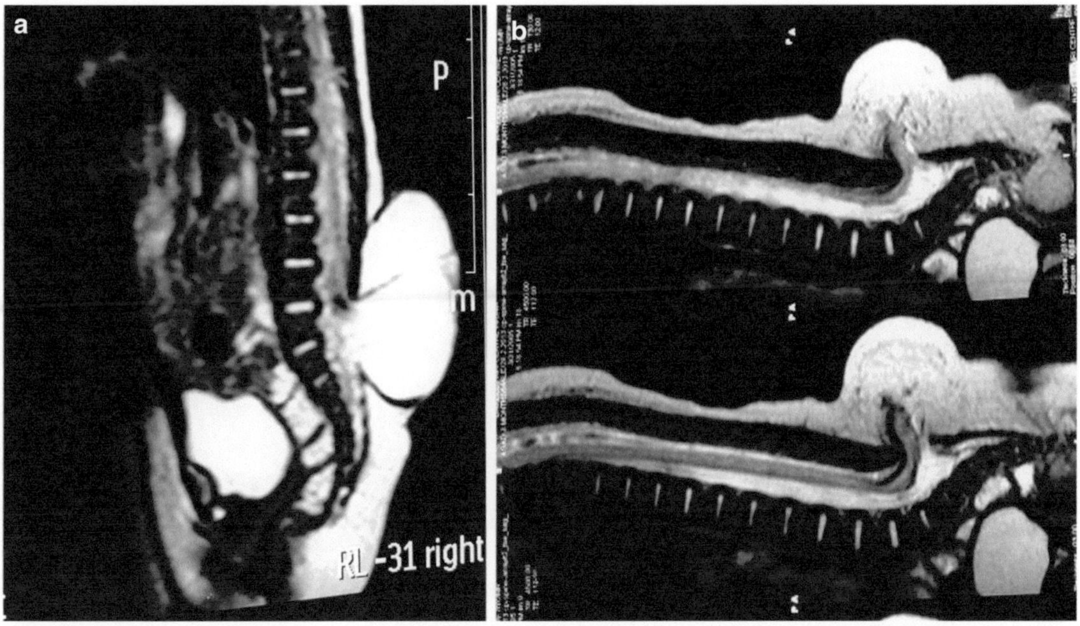

Fig. 18.13 MRI spine, (**a**) Lumbar meningomyelocele; (**b**) Lipomeningocele

18.5 Preoperative Care

Clean intermittent catheterization should be initiated for patients who cannot spontaneously urinate. Head circumference should be measured. Ultrasound of the cranium and KUB is done for baseline information. Blood cultures should be sent, and broad-spectrum antibiotics (ampicillin/gentamicin) must be started. Imaging may be done with an X-ray spine and MRI spine (Fig. 18.13a, b).

18.6 Surgical Treatment

Perhaps the most remarkable change has been the attitude towards MMC patients. In the past, many physicians regarded the treatment of MMC cruel, considering it is more merciful to allow them to die. In 1971, Lorber criteria were formed to decide which patients NOT to be operated on: severe hydrocephalus at birth, total paraplegia, spinal kyphosis at birth, or any additional congenital anomalies. Now, surgery is offered to all patients; however, in case of potentially fatal congenital malformation or chromosomal abnormalities, decisions should be made only after parents have been counselled about the chances of meaningful survival.

18.7 Surgical Management

The timing of surgery has always been a matter of controversy. It has been noted that early closure is not associated with improved neurological outcome, though lower infection rates have been seen. Hence, it is recommended that closure should be done within 24–48 hours of birth. Delay in surgery can lead to colonization of bacteria in the lesion and increase the risk of postoperative infection.

18.8 Surgical Aspects

The infant is kept in a lateral decubitus position or supported supine, and any pressure over MMC during induction should be avoided. Latex-free foley's catheter is inserted for urinary drainage. A prophylactic intravenous antibiotic is given, and the child is then changed to a prone position with bolsters support under the chest and hips ensuring the abdomen is freely hanging and all the pressure points are padded with cotton. Careful aseptic preparation and draping are done. Use of surgical loupes for magnification is useful.

18.9 The Surgical Procedure Is Excision and Repair of the Defect (Fig. 18.14a, b)

An elliptical incision is made on the skin just outside the junction of normal skin and zona epitheliosa. The incision is carried on to the subcutaneous fatty layer until the dura or fascia is encountered. The plane of dissection is developed, and the base of the sac is mobilized medially until it is seen entering the fascial defect. The placode is freed by cutting radially into the cuff of the dystrophic epidermis or arachnoid, excising it circumferentially. Nerves exiting from the placode and terminating in zona epitheliosa or further laterally can be sacrificed (usually non-functional); however, preserve all other nerves. Small feeding vessels or veins should be spared (to avoid vascular injury). Diligently remove all other dermal remnants (prevents the possibility of future lipoma/dermoid formation).

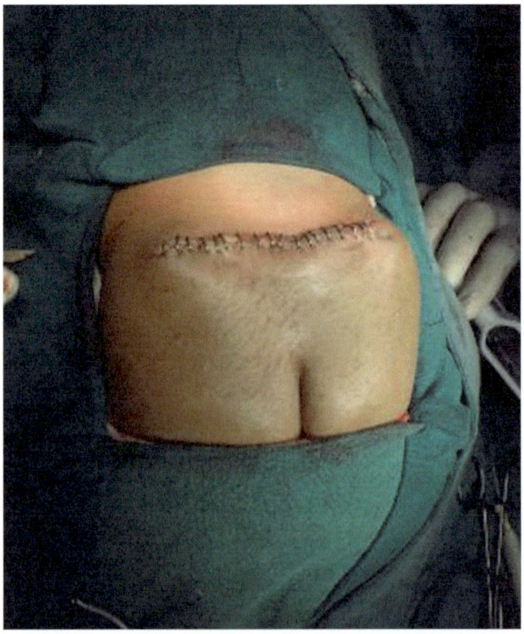

Fig. 18.14 (**a**) Lumbar MMC. (**b**) After surgical excision and repair

Tethered cord requires untethering of the cord with laminectomy, removal of lipomatous mass, diastematomyelia (bony spur), dermal sinus and neuroenteric cyst, release of conus and sectioning of filum terminale.

Patulous but watertight dural closure is performed, followed by an approximation of muscles, fascia, and skin. Associated hydrocephalus may require a ventriculoperitoneal shunt or other drainage procedure.

18.10 Postoperative Care

There are no particular guidelines for the postoperative care of these neonates. The preferences are individual. Generally, postoperative antibiotics are given for 24 hours or until the blood cultures are sterile. The baby is nursed in a prone or lateral position. The area of defect is kept above the level of the head (minimizes CSF leak). A plastic drape is placed above the gluteal folds to protect the wound from soilage.

Postoperatively, the neonate should be monitored for apnea or bradycardia. The head circumference should be measured daily. Clean intermittent catheterization should be initiated at the earliest possible on a regular basis (in addition to spontaneous voiding).

18.11 Postoperative Complications

- Wound disruption
- CSF leak—associated with larger defects (more risk) and may be a sign of worsening hydrocephalus. It is treated with a prone head-down position, oral acetazolamide (Diamox), and may need insertion of a ventriculo-peritoneal shunt (VP) shunt.
- Wound infection—abscess at the wound site may cause ascending infection. Treatment includes broad-spectrum antibiotics, ventricular tap for cultures, and antibiotic sensitivity. Some patients may require reoperation.

18.12 Hydrocephalus in MMC

Hydrocephalus in MMC patients is multifactorial. The most common cause is noncommunicating hydrocephalus. The causes include fourth ventricular outlet obstruction (Chiari II malformation) or aqueductal stenosis. Communicating hydrocephalus may exist due to underdevelopment of arachnoid granulations or scars at arachnoid granulations. A total of 60–80% of the patients will require shunt by the end of 1 year. Hence, a baseline ultrasound head is done for all patients. CT or MRI may be done as and when required. Head circumference is monitored in the postoperative period. Signs of raised intracranial tension (ICT) or bulging at the MMC site or brainstem signs should be looked for. Ventriculoperitoneal shunt is the procedure of choice. Alternatively, endoscopic third ventriculostomy (ETV) with choroid plexus cauterization may also be attempted.

18.13 Management of Myelomeningocele Study (MOMS) Trial

Management of Myelomeningocele Study (MOMS) by Adzick et al. is the largest multi-institutional randomized controlled trial (2003–2010) conducted at three maternal-fetal surgery centers in the USA for prenatal versus postnatal surgical repair. All mothers with singleton pregnancies and fetuses with open spinal dysraphism with an upper level of defect between T1-S1 and evidence of hindbrain herniation (on antenatal imaging) with a gestational age of 19–26 weeks were included in the trial. Patients were randomized into two groups: i) early fetal surgery, ii) standard postnatal surgery.

The study concluded that prenatal surgery reduced the need for shunt placement (40% vs. 82%) and reduced the incidence of hindbrain herniation (64% vs. 96%). There was significant improvement in motor functioning (ambulatory status, neuropsychomotor development tests) in the prenatal surgery group at 30 months of age. However, the prenatal surgery group had an increased rate of preterm delivery and intraoperative complications.

18.14 Tethered Cord

The lower tip of the spinal cord normally lies opposite the disc between the 1st and 2nd lumbar vertebra. In spina bifida patients (meningomyelocele, lipomyelomeningocele), the cord is adhered to the overlying skin and lies lower than normal (low-lying cord). For those with previously repaired defects, with the child's growth, the tethered or fixed cord can get stretched, causing further damage and interfering with vascular supply. The other causes of tethered cord are:

- Dermal sinus tract
- Diastematomyelia
- Lipoma
- Tumor
- Thickened/tight filum terminale (a delicate filament near the tailbone)
- Spine trauma/spinal surgery

Treatment: surgical treatment of untethering of the cord by freeing it from all the surrounding adhesions is required for symptomatic patients. A laminectomy may be necessary to accomplish the procedure. A thickened filum terminale may require division.

Suggested Reading

Albright AL, editor. Principles and practice of pediatric neurosurgery. 3rd ed. New York/Stuttgart: Thieme; 2015. p. 111.

Di Rocco C, Pang D, Rutka JT, editors. Textbook of pediatric neurosurgery. Cham: Springer; 2020.

Ozek MM, Cinalli G, Maixner J. Spina Bifida—management and outcome. Am J Neuroradiol. 2009;30(3):e49.

Partin AW, Dmochowski RR, Kavoussi LR, Peters CA, Campbell MF, Walsh PC, et al., editors. Campbell-Walsh-Wein Urology. 12th ed Philadelphia: Elsevier; 2021. 2345

Sarnat HB, Flores Sarnat L, Pinter JD. Neuroembryology. In: Winn HR, Youmans JR, editors. Youmans & Winn neurological surgery. 8th ed. Philadelphia: Elsevier; 2023. p. 466.e1–e29.

Smith JL. Management of neural tube defects, hydrocephalus, refractory epilepsy, and central nervous system infections. In: Coran AG, Caldamone A, Scott Adzich N, Krummel TM, Laberge JM, editors. Pediatric surgery. 7th ed. Oxford: Elsevier Limited; 2012. p. 1673–80.

19 Cleft Lip and Palate

Jai K. Mahajan and Palak Singhai

19.1 Incidence

Cleft lip with cleft palate occurs in 1:800 to 1000 live births. Isolated cleft palate occurs in 1:1000 to 2500 live births. The relative incidence of various cleft types is:

- Cleft lip alone: 15%
- Cleft lip with palate: 45%
- Isolated cleft palate: 40%

Cleft lip with palate is more common in males than females (2:1), whereas the reverse is true for isolated cleft palate (1:2). Among the unilateral cleft lip, 60% are left-sided. The incidence of cleft lip and palate differs between ethnicities, with Asians being affected more often than Caucasians and Africans. In India, the reported incidence of cleft lip with palate is around 1:1000, whereas the cleft lip alone is 0.1–0.2 per 1000.

19.2 Etiology

Both genetic and environmental factors play a role in the etiopathogenesis of orofacial clefts. Over 60% of cleft patients have associated anomalies or syndromic associations. Associated anomalies such as congenital heart diseases, hydrocephalus, and urogenital defects are commonly associated. Positive family history is a high-risk factor for the occurrence of anomaly in subsequent children (1:25 live births). Monozygotic twins (60%) have a considerably higher incidence than dizygotic twins and siblings (5–10%). More than 400 syndromes have been described in association with orofacial clefts, including Stickler (ophthalmic and musculoskeletal abnormalities), Down, Waardenburg, Apert, and Treacher Collins syndrome (Fig. 19.1). In nonsyndromic cases, several genetic mutations have been identified, such as transforming growth factor-alpha (TGF-α), TGF-β2, TGF-β3, MSX-1, RARA, and BCL3.

Maternal smoking and alcohol consumption increase the risk of orofacial cleft anomalies in a dose-dependent manner. Maternal diabetes, epilepsy, drugs-like steroids, diazepam, and phenytoin and deficiency of vitamin B_6, B_{12}, and folate have all been associated with an increased risk of cleft anomalies.

J. K. Mahajan (✉) · P. Singhai
Department of Pediatric Surgery, Advanced Pediatric Centre, Postgraduate Institute of Medical Education and Research, Chandigarh, India

© The Author(s), under exclusive license to Springer Nature Singapore Pte Ltd. 2025
S. Roy Choudhury (ed.), *Pediatric Surgery*, https://doi.org/10.1007/978-981-96-1257-4_19

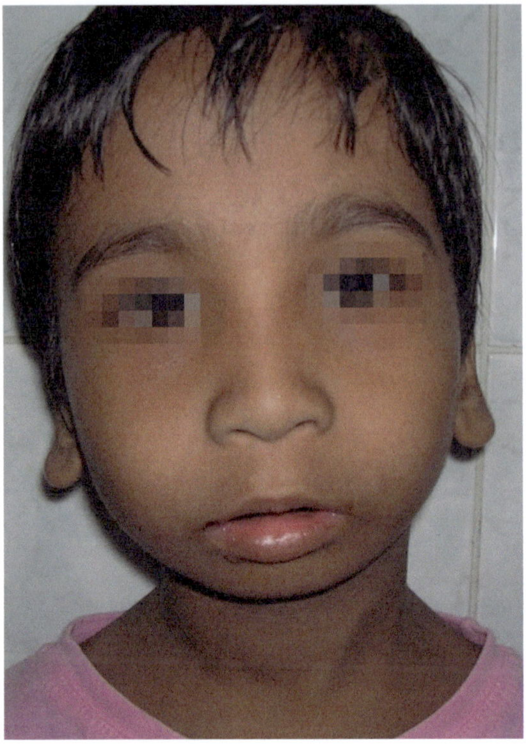

Fig. 19.1 Treacher Collin syndrome (micrognathia, underdeveloped zygoma, malformed ears, downward slanting eyes)

19.3 Embryology

The gestational period from 4 to 7 weeks is critical for the development of cleft lip and palate. The frontonasal, maxillary, and mandibular prominences develop from first 2 pharyngeal arches during 3rd and 4th week of gestation. The lateral and medial nasal prominences are formed at the end of 4th week and develop into nasal ala and tip, columella, philtrum, and the premaxilla, respectively. The maxillary prominences will fuse with the medial nasal process in the next 2 weeks. The failure of this fusion results in a cleft lip.

The palate formation begins at 6th week of gestation with fusion of both the medial nasal prominences and formation of the intermaxillary segment. The intermaxillary segment form the primary palate anterior to the incisive foramen. The lateral palatine shelves arise from the paired maxillary prominences and fuse in the midline. The fusion of the hard palate is completed by the 10th week and soft palate by 12th week of gestation. Failure of this fusion will result in a variety of cleft palate anomalies.

19.4 Classification

Orofacial clefts can be categorized anatomically either as unilateral and bilateral, or complete and incomplete.

Cleft Lip (Fig. 19.2)

- Unilateral: a unilateral cleft lip is characterized by separation of medial and lateral lip elements on one side.
- Bilateral: it refers to the separation of the premaxillary and central prolabium from the two lateral segments on both sides.
- Incomplete: an incomplete cleft lip is a partial defect without extension across the nasal sill.
- Complete: a complete cleft of the lip extends into the nasal floor.

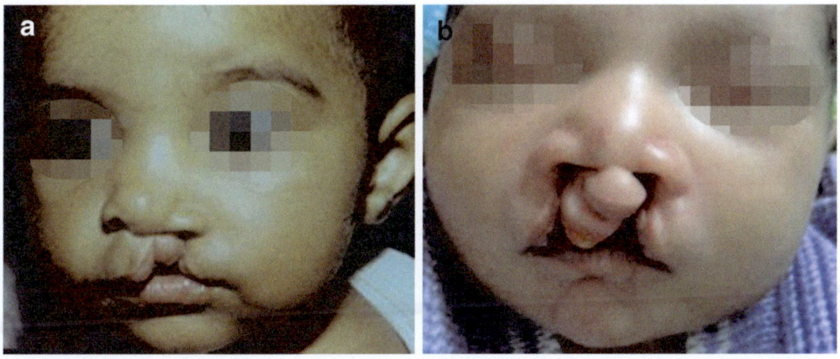

Fig. 19.2 (**a**) Unilateral incomplete cleft lip (**b**) Bilateral cleft lip

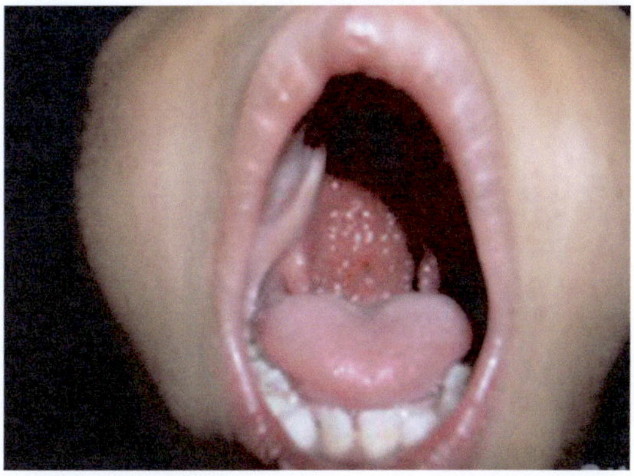

Fig. 19.3 Cleft palate

Cleft Palate (Fig. 19.3)

- The cleft of the primary palate is anterior to the incisive foramen.
- The cleft of the secondary palate extends from the incisive foramen to the uvula.
- Complete: a cleft involving the entire primary and secondary palate length.
- Incomplete: partial cleft of the soft palate or the secondary hard palate alone.
- Submucous cleft palate: an apparently intact palate which is associated with muscular diastasis of the velum.
- Bilateral cleft lip and palate.

Veau Classification categorizes orofacial clefts into four classes:

- Class I: soft palate cleft
- Class II: soft and hard palate cleft up to the incisive foramen
- Class III: soft and hard palate cleft extending through the alveolus unilaterally
- Class IV: soft and hard palate cleft extending through the alveolus bilaterally

The Veau classification does not include isolated cleft lip.

Kernahan striped Y classification and the *Kriens LASHAL classification* are pictorial systems of representation of the entire extent of orofacial cleft anomalies (Fig. 19.4).

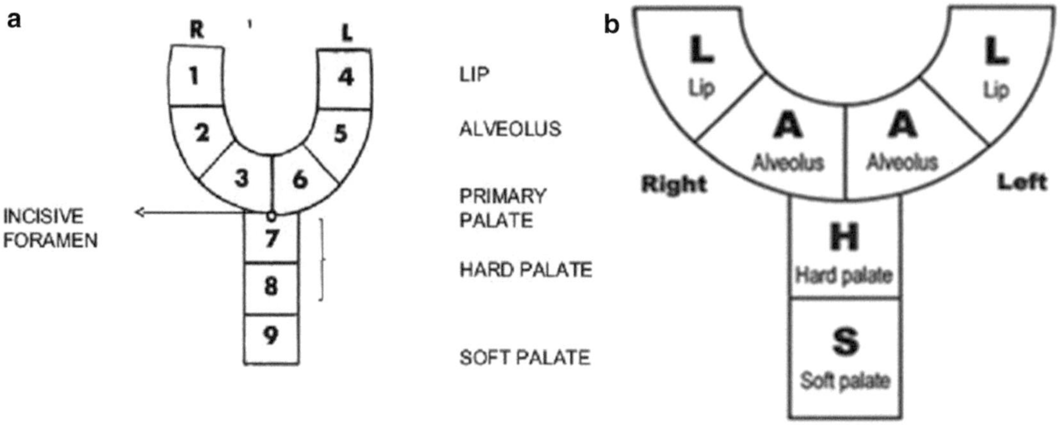

Fig. 19.4 (**a**) Kernahan striped Y classification (**b**) Kriens LASHAL classification

19.5 Anatomy of Defects

Cleft Lip

- Cleft lip is associated with disruption of the muscles of the upper lip and nasolabial region groups (Rings of Delaire).
- A unilateral cleft lip is associated with nasal deformity, lip retraction, and vermillion and lip mucosa changes.
- A bilateral cleft lip is associated with protrusion of the premaxilla, the posterior displacement of the lateral segments, flaring of the nose with flat nasal alar domes, and foreshortening of the columella.
- A complete cleft lip has a pathological insertion of orbicularis oris into the alar base on cleft's side and base of the columella on the noncleft side.

Cleft Palate

- Soft palate clefts have anomalous insertion of the tensor veli palatini and the levator veli palatini muscles. Consequently, there is an inability to close the velopharyngeal opening and impairment of the eustachian tube function. In submucus cleft palate, an apparently intact palate is associated with muscular diastasis of the velum, bifid uvula, and posterior notching of the hard palate.

19.6 Antenatal Diagnosis

All cleft defects except isolated palate can be diagnosed antenatally after 16 weeks of pregnancy. The diagnostic accuracy of ultrasonography for detecting orofacial clefts is highly variable, ranging from 0% to 70%. Use of 3-D ultrasound increases the diagnostic yield. A cleft lip appears as a linear defect running from the lip towards the nasal floor, with distortion of nasal anatomy. The sonographic hallmark of bilateral cleft lip and palate is a protruding maxillary process, seen as an echogenic structure below the alar base. Isolated palate anomalies are difficult to diagnose prenatally as the palate is surrounded by osseous structures. An unremarkable uvula described as an *equals sign* is, however, suggestive of an intact palate. Antenatal diagnosis allows time for parental counseling and the postnatal support. The parents are thus better prepared to accept the waiting time between birth and the first surgical intervention.

19.7 Clinical Features

Besides obvious facial cosmetic defects, the patients with orofacial clefts may have various associated dental conditions. These children also have phonation dysfunction due to abnormal levator veli palatini insertion and often have a nasal twang in their voice. Eustachian tube dysfunction predisposes these children to frequent otitis media and subsequent hearing loss.

19.8 Management

1. *Feeding*
   Most of the babies feed well and thrive. Typically, patients with a cleft lip can breastfeed, whereas those with a cleft palate may require additional assistance. Patients with cleft lip and palate have an open communication between the oral and the nasal cavities. As a result, they cannot generate sufficient negative intraoral pressure for suckling. Moreover, there is excessive aerophagia during nursing. Specially designed bottles like Haberman feeder, Mead Johnson cleft palate nurser bottle, and Pigeon bottle are available to facilitate the feeding. These bottles are made up of soft, squeezable plastic and a long nipple with a cross cut at the tip to help draw milk from the bottle with very little pressure. Feeding with a spoon or a *paladai* in an upright position is recommended.
2. *Management of Respiratory Problems*
   Airway and respiratory problems may occur in patients with syndromic cleft anomalies. Patients with Pierre Robin Syndrome have early life-threatening respiratory difficulties (Fig. 19.5). The following steps may be necessary depending on the severity of the condition.

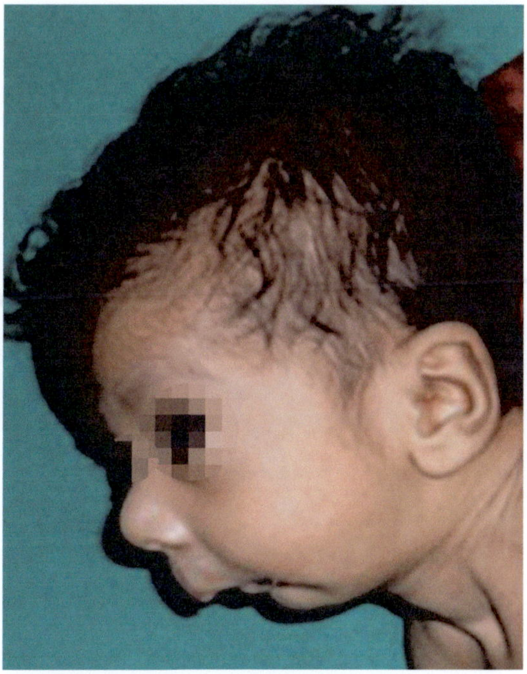

Fig. 19.5 Pierre Robin Syndrome

   - Nursing the baby prone
   - Nasopharyngeal airway tube insertion
   - Intubation of the airway
   - Surgical fixation of lower lip to tongue (labioglossoplasty) to prevent tongue from falling back
3. *Presurgical Orthopedics and Molding*
   The developing facial tissues of a newborn are plastic, and hence can be molded. An appropriately performed molding can aid in the partial correction of the wide cleft deformity before the definitive surgery. Passive molding methods include lip taping, nasoalveolar molding, and surgical lip adhesion. While the active methods of molding use surgical implants that are manipulated to reduce the size of the defect (Fig. 19.6). However, the critics of active molding have raised concerns

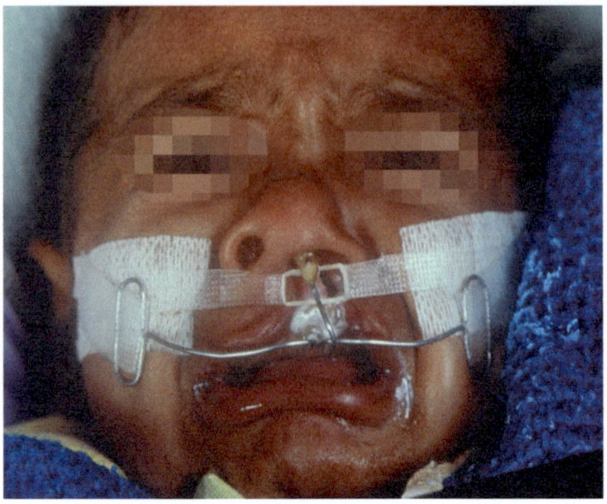

Fig. 19.6 Active presurgical molding

regarding subsequent secondary growth disturbances of the face.

4. *Principles of Surgery*
   The surgery aims to achieve a normal lip, nose, and face appearance with normal speech and dentition.
   (i) Cleft lip surgery attaches and reconstructs the muscles around the nasal aperture and oral sphincter thus creating normal appearance of lip-vermillion border, cupids bow, and nose.
   (ii) Cleft palate surgery aims to bring together muscles to separate the oral and nasal cavities and create a competent velopharyngeal port with minimum scarring.

An in-depth understanding of the anatomy is invaluable for achieving the above-mentioned aims.

19.9 Timing of Surgery

Cleft lip is operated between 3 and 6 months of age. A rule of 10 as applied includes at least 10 weeks of age, 10 pounds body weight, hemoglobin of 10 gm%, and a total leucocyte count <10,000/mm^3 before surgery. However, with advances in both pediatric anesthesia and surgical technique, earlier cleft repairs are being undertaken successfully. Cleft palate surgery is performed between 6 and 18 months of age.

Table 19.1 Suggested timeline of interventions for cleft lip and palate

Age	Medical treatment	Surgery
Prenatal to birth	Genetic counselling SLP (?) consultation for feeding	–
0–5 months	SLP for feeding and growth Monitor hearing Nasoalveolar molding (if indicated)	Cleft lip repair Ear tubes (if chronic otitis media)
9–18 month	–	Palatoplasty Ear tubes (if chronic otitis media)
1–4 years	Introduction to pediatric dentist Assess language development	–
4–6 years	Assess for VPD	Corrective speech surgery Revision lip repair (if indicated) Minor nasal surgery (if indicated)
6–12 years	Orthodontics Assess school and psychosocial development	Alveolar bone grafting
12–21 years	Orthodontics	Orthognathic surgery Definitive rhinoplasty

Adapted from Worley et al. (2018)

Secondary orthodontic surgeries are carried out from 5 to 12 years of age.

A timeline for orofacial cleft management is summarized in Table 19.1.

19.10 Techniques of Cleft Lip Repair

All techniques of cleft lip repair increase the vertical lip height using principles of Z-plasty, geometric flaps, and curvilinear incisions. Various techniques like the Rose Thompson procedure, the LeMesurier Z-plasty, the Millard rotation advancement technique, and the Fisher technique of geometric flaps have been described for the treatment of cleft lip.

The Millard Rotation advancement operation and its modifications are the most commonly performed cleft lip repair. The Millard technique elevates a traditional Z-plasty to just below the nasal sill, with simultaneous downward rotation of the central lip element. The advancement of the lateral lip flap into the rotation defect so created reconstitutes the nasal sill and corrects the nasal flaring (Fig. 19.7).

Postoperatively, the cheiloplasty wound is managed with gentle lip cleaning to avoid

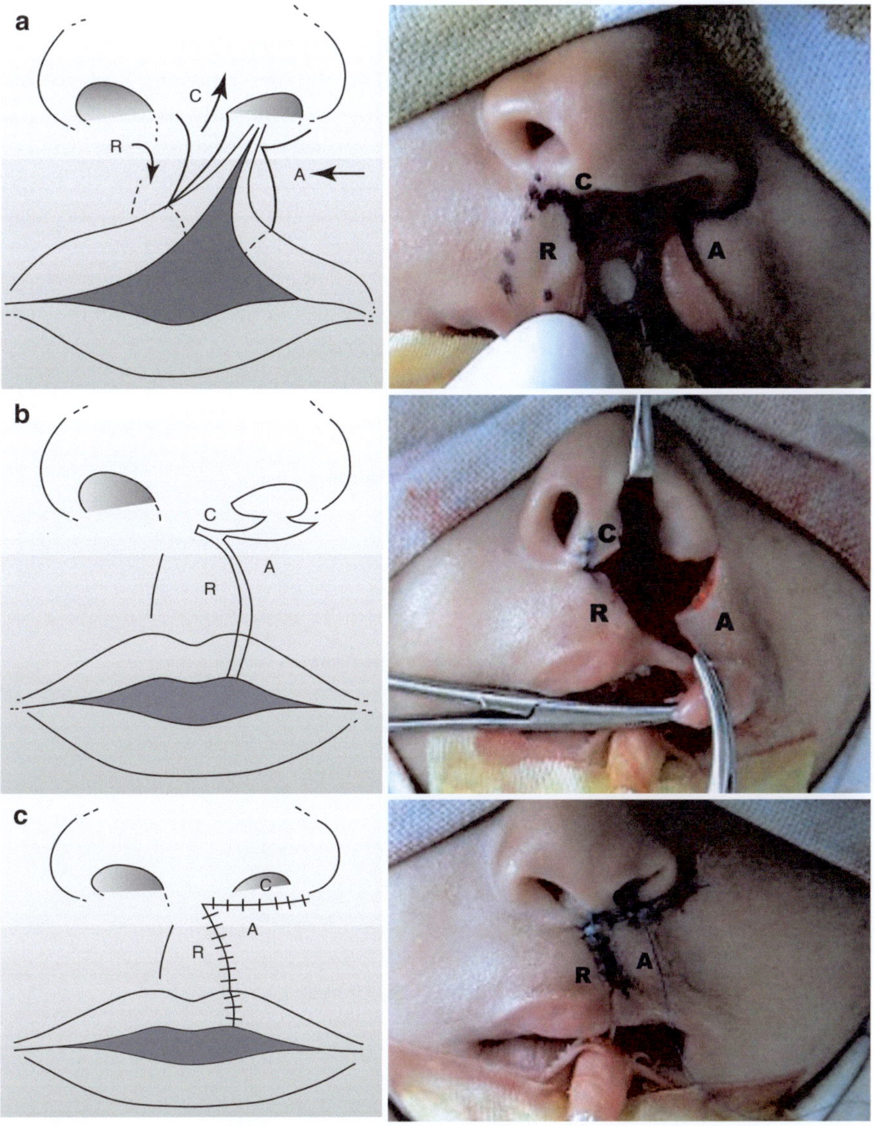

Fig. 19.7 Millard Repair of unilateral cleft lip. (**a**) Medial flap R for downward rotation, Lateral flap A for advancement and to restore nostril sill or lengthening of columella flap C marked (**b**) Flaps mobilized (**c**) Repair completed with final position of flaps

crusting. An antibiotic ointment is applied to keep the suture line moist. Any direct trauma to the surgical site should be avoided.

19.11 Techniques of Cleft Palate Repair

The main objectives of palatoplasty are functional, including correction of the feeding difficulties, phonation defects, and the velopharyngeal insufficiency. Intravelar veloplasty or Furlow's palatoplasty (42%) is commonly performed for soft palate repair. For hard palate repair, the selection of repair technique is dictated by the type of the anatomical defect, and Bardach 2-flap palatoplasty (45%) is the most commonly used technique.

Submucosal and Veau-I defects may require no intervention on the hard palate. Veau-II clefts are managed by using von-Langenback, VY pushback, or Bardach-2 flap palatoplasty. Veau-III and IV clefts are best managed using Barchach 2-flap technique. Veau-IV cleft may additionally require vomerine flaps raised from two sides of vomerine plate.

In Bardach-2 flap palatoplasty, lateral releasing incisions are placed around the alveolar margin, continuous with the cleft margin. Mucoperichondrial flaps based on the greater palatine neurovascular bundles are raised and mobilized to the midline to provide oral closure of the cleft (Fig. 19.8).

The double opposing Z-plasty technique of Furlow is commonly used for soft palate repair. The Z-plasty consists of anteriorly based mucosal and contralateral posteriorly based musculocutaneous flaps, one pair on the nasal and oral side each. The nasal and the oral side flaps are transposed and inset, with an overlap of the levator muscles in the midline and the creation of the levator sling .

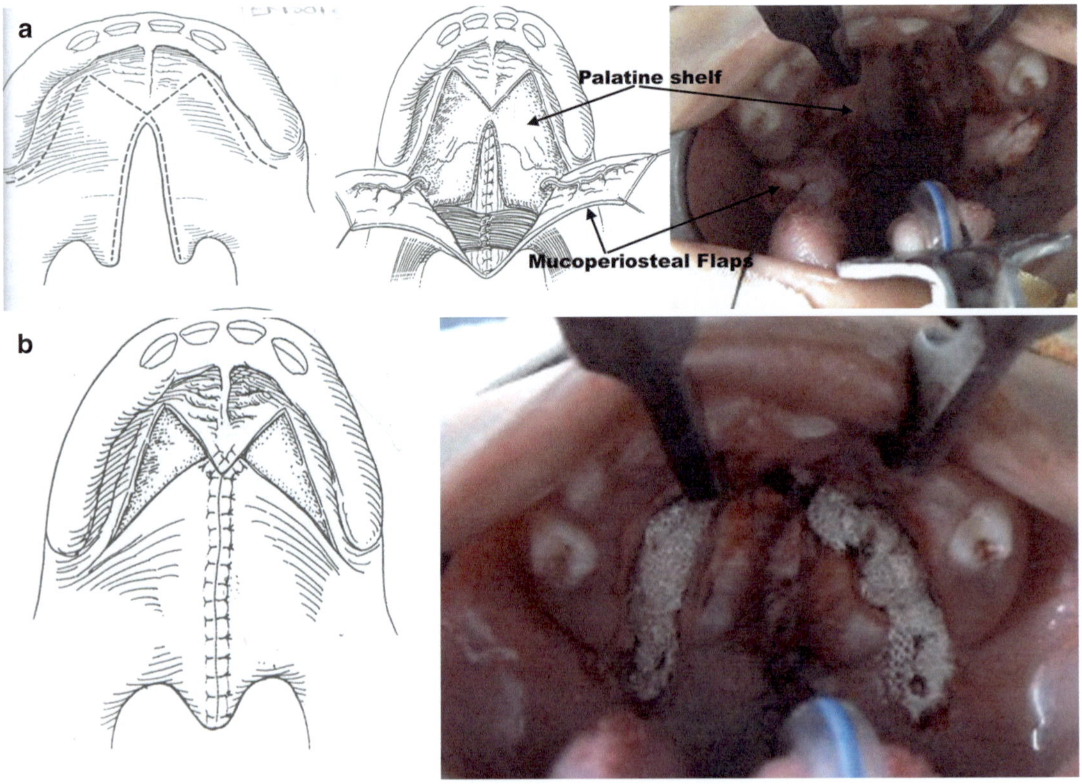

Fig. 19.8 Bardach-2 flap palatoplasty (**a**) Incision lines and mobilization of full-thickness mucoperiosteal flaps based on palatine artery (**b**) Flaps sutured in midline after repair of nasal mucosa

After palatoplasty, the patient should always be nursed in a lateral or prone position to prevent aspiration. In the early postoperative period, patients are started on a clear liquid diet, which is gradually advanced. A medicated mouthwash is added to ensure oral hygiene and prevent the accumulation of debris over the suture line.

19.12 Secondary Procedures for Cleft Management

Speech, dental, and facial growth management requires a multidisciplinary team approach. Due to the high incidence of sensorineural and conductive hearing loss, cleft patients require regular hearing tests for proper speech development. The associated velopharyngeal dysfunction needs detailed evaluation. Speech impairment can occur due to velopharyngeal insufficiency, velopharyngeal incompetence, or velopharyngeal mislearning.

- Velopharyngeal insufficiency is characterized by insufficient palatal length for velopharyngeal port closure and requires secondary surgery such as Furlow conversion, posterior pharyngeal fat grafting, and dynamic sphincter pharyngoplasty.
- Velopharyngeal incompetence (aberrant palatal elevation hampering the closure of the velopharyngeal port despite adequate length of the palate) can usually be managed with speech therapy alone.
- When a patient continues to produce abnormal speech patterns despite a normally functioning palate with adequate length, elevation, and closure, it is called velopharyngeal mislearning. It is managed with speech therapy.

Dental and orthodontic management with alveolar bone graft at 5–10 years of age eliminates oronasal fistula and promotes normal eruption of canine and other teeth.

Secondary orthognathic surgery may be required in up to 25% patients to address maxillary hypoplasia and narrowing of the maxillary arch in teenage years. The LeFort I maxillary advancement with palatal osteotomies is the most commonly performed surgery.

19.13 Complications

The complications of cleft lip and palate repair include bleeding, infection, misalignment, partial or complete dehiscence, scarring, abnormalities of secondary dentition, and facial growth defects. Long-term complications of palatoplasty include palatal fistula, obstructive sleep apnea, and velopharyngeal dysfunction. Postoperative fistula is associated with poor speech and feeding difficulties. Bilateral cleft and older age are the risk factors for fistula formation. Maxillary growth can be impaired in all the patients despite early surgery. Low-resource settings have higher postoperative complication rates following cleft lip or palate repair.

Complications can also occur during orthognathic surgery, such as improper fracture, inferior alveolar and lingual nerve injury, delayed union, or nonunion.

19.14 Advancements in Cleft Management

In the past two decades, three-dimensional computer graphic animation and interactive simulators for safe training have revolutionized the cleft lip and palate surgery. Artificial intelligence-enabled software facilitates accurate detection of the anatomical landmarks, rapid digital cephalometric analysis, prediction of outcomes, and the future need for orthognathic surgery.

19.15 Summary

Cleft lip and palate are the most prevalent congenital anomaly affecting the head and neck region. Management of cleft anomalies requires a multidisciplinary team of specialists to address all aspects of treatment. Before surgery, each patient should undergo a comprehensive assessment to identify any accompanying anomalies, developmental delay, along with psychosocial considerations of the family.

Suggested Readings

Arosarena OA. Cleft lip and palate. Otolaryngol Clin N Am. 2007 Feb;40(1):27–60.

Kernahan DA. The striped Y—A symbolic classification for cleft lip and palate. Plast Reconst Surg. 1971;47(5):469–70.

Kriens O. LAHSHAL: a concise documentation system for cleft lip, alveolus and palate diagnosis in what is a cleft lip and palate?: a multidisciplinary update. New York: Thieme Medical Publishers; 1989. p. 30–4.

Vyas T, Gupta P, Kumar S, Gupta R, Gupta T, Singh H. Cleft of lip and palate: a review. J Fam Med Prim Care. 2020;9(6):2621.

Worley ML, Patel KG, Kilpatrick LA. Cleft lip and palate. Clin Perinatol. 2018 Dec;45(4):661–78.

20 Neck Cysts, Sinuses, Lymphadenopathy, and Torticollis

Vikram Khanna and Subhasis Roy Choudhury

20.1 Introduction

Neck masses in children can arise from various causes, including congenital anomalies and acquired conditions. Accurate diagnosis is crucial for appropriate management. This chapter provides an overview of common neck masses in children, focusing on their clinical presentation, embryology, anatomy, and surgical management.

20.2 Congenital Neck Masses

Congenital neck masses often stem from developmental abnormalities of the thyroglossal duct and branchial arches.

- *Thyroglossal duct cysts and sinuses*: these are the most common congenital neck masses, resulting from incomplete closure of the thyroglossal duct during embryonic development. They typically present as a midline neck swelling that moves with swallowing.
- *Branchial arch anomalies*: these arise from remnants of the branchial arches (particularly second cleft), which are structures present during embryonic development. Branchial cleft cysts and sinuses are the most common type, presenting as lateral neck masses.
- *Lympho-vascular malformations*: these involve abnormal development of lymphatics and blood vessels and can present as various types of neck masses. These may be evident at birth or later in life.

20.3 Acquired Neck Masses

- *Lymphadenopathy*: enlarged lymph nodes can be caused by various infections (e.g., bacterial, viral), inflammatory conditions, or underlying systemic diseases.
- *Tumors*: while less common, various types of tumors can occur in the neck region of children.

20.4 Diagnostic Approach

A thorough history and physical examination are essential for diagnosing neck masses. Key factors to consider include:

- Age of onset
- Location and size of the mass
- Presence of pain, tenderness, or drainage
- Associated symptoms

Imaging studies such as ultrasound, computed tomography, and magnetic resonance imaging

V. Khanna (✉)
Pediatric Surgery, LHMC, New Delhi, India

S. Roy Choudhury
Pediatric Surgery, Lady Hardinge Medical College and Associated Kalawati Saran Children's Hospital, New Delhi, Delhi, India

© The Author(s), under exclusive license to Springer Nature Singapore Pte Ltd. 2025

S. Roy Choudhury (ed.), *Pediatric Surgery*, https://doi.org/10.1007/978-981-96-1257-4_20

can provide valuable information about the nature and extent of the mass.

Fine-needle aspiration cytology (FNAC) may be helpful in some cases to obtain a sample for analysis.

20.5 Management

The management of neck masses depends on the underlying cause. Treatment options may include:

- *Antibiotics*: for infectious causes.
- *Surgery*: for removal of cysts, sinuses, and certain tumors. When surgical removal is necessary, a thorough understanding of the relevant anatomy is crucial to ensure complete excision and minimize complications.
- *Observation*: for some benign, slowly growing masses.

20.6 Branchial Anomalies

- *Origin*: congenital
- *Embryological basis*:
  - The development of these anomalies is linked to the branchial arches, which are structures present during embryonic development.
  - There are six pairs of branchial arches in the human embryo.
  - Each arch has a specific structure:
    - Externally covered by ectoderm
    - Internally lined by endoderm
    - Filled with mesoderm, containing an artery, nerve, cartilage, and muscle.
- *Cleft and pouch formation*:
  - Depressions between the arches are called:
    - *Clefts* externally (lined with ectoderm)
    - *Pouches* internally (lined with endoderm)

The development of neck cysts and sinuses is related to the embryonic processes of fusion, closure, and development of these neck structures (Table 20.1).

Table 20.1 Derivatives of branchial arches, clefts, and pouches

1st Arch:
Cartilage: incus, malleus, sphenomandibular ligament, part of the mandible
Muscles: muscles of mastication, tensor tympani, tensor veli palatini, mylohyoid, and anterior belly of digastric
Nerve: trigeminal nerve (CN V)
Cleft: external auditory canal
Pouch: eustachian tube, middle ear cavity, mastoid air cells
2nd Arch:
Cartilage: stapes, styloid process, stylohyoid ligament, part of the hyoid bone
Muscles: muscles of facial expression, stapedius, stylohyoid and posterior belly of digastric
Nerve: facial nerve (CN VII)
Pouch: palatine tonsil, supratonsillar fossa
3rd Arch:
Cartilage: greater horn and part of the hyoid bone
Muscles: stylopharyngeus
Nerve: glossopharyngeal nerve (CN IX)
Pouch: thymus, inferior parathyroid gland
4th Arch:
Cartilage: thyroid cartilage, cuneiform cartilage, part of the epiglottis
Muscles: constrictors of the pharynx, cricothyroid, levator veli palatini
Nerve: vagus nerve (CN X)
Pouch: superior parathyroid gland
5th Arch:
Pouch: ultimobranchial body (lateral anlage of the thyroid gland)
6th Arch:
Cartilage: cricoid, arytenoid, corniculate cartilages
Muscles: intrinsic muscles of the larynx
Nerve: vagus nerve (CN X, recurrent laryngeal branch)
Artery: pulmonary artery and ductus arteriosus

20.6.1 Branchial Cleft and Arch Formation

- *Development*: branchial clefts and arches form during the 4 to seventh week of intrauterine life. The first branchial cleft becomes the external auditory meatus.
- *Cervical Sinus of His*: the second to fourth branchial arches are normally covered as the second arch overlaps the others to fuse with the fifth arch, thus closing an ectodermal area

superficial to the sternocleidomastoid muscle called the cervical sinus of His.

20.6.2 Branchial Cyst

- *Origin*: develops from the vestigial remnant of the second branchial cleft.
- *Contents*: contains fluid and a tooth-paste-like material.
- *Presentation*: usually presents in the adult age group.
- *Pathology*:
  - Lined by squamous epithelium.
  - Surrounded by lymphoid tissue which may cause recurrent inflammation.
  - Aspirate fluid from the cyst contains cholesterol crystals.
- *Clinical features*:
  - Most common location is under the upper third of the sternocleidomastoid muscle (Fig. 20.1).
  - May show positive transillumination.
- *Treatment*: surgical excision (see below).

20.6.3 Branchial Fistula

- *Presentation*: more common in the pediatric age group.
- *Etiology*:
  - *Congenital*: due to persistence of the second branchial cleft, where the occluding membrane has broken down (persistence of the cervical sinus of His).
  - *Secondary*: following incision of an infected branchial cyst.
- *Clinical features*:
  - *External opening*: located at the anterior border of the lower third of the sternocleidomastoid muscle (Fig. 20.2).
  - *Internal opening*: usually near the posterior tonsillar fossa.
  - *Discharge*: may discharge mucus or mucopus.
- *Histology*: lined by ciliated columnar epithelium and the wall contains muscles.
- *Treatment*: surgical excision.
- *Procedure*:
  - Initial incision is taken around the external fistula opening.
  - Dissection of the fistula tract continues upwards, which may require one or two additional incisions in a step-ladder pattern (Fig. 20.3a, b).
  - The course of the track may be probed through the opening or delineated by injecting methylene blue through the opening.
  - The tract passes through the fork of the common carotid artery, superficial to the hypoglossal and glossopharyngeal nerves, but deep to the posterior belly of the digastric muscle.

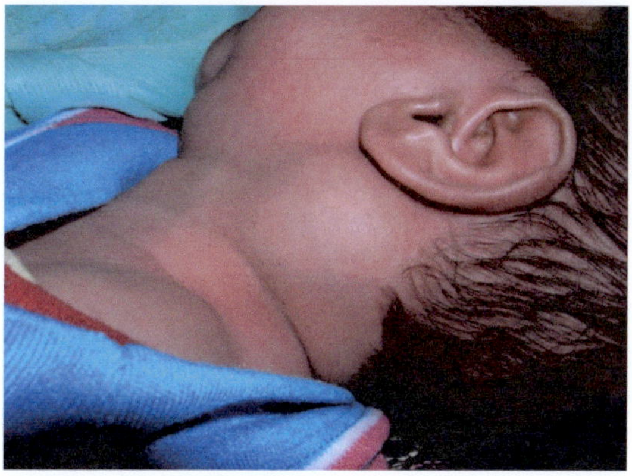

Fig. 20.1 Branchial cyst left side

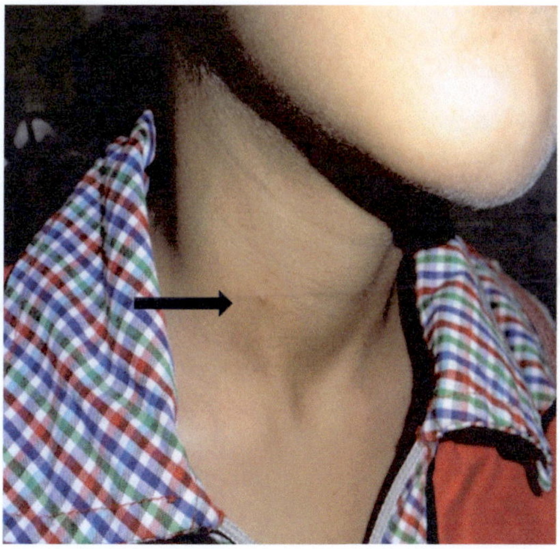

Fig. 20.2 Branchial fistula, note the site at lower one third of anterior border of sternomastoid muscle

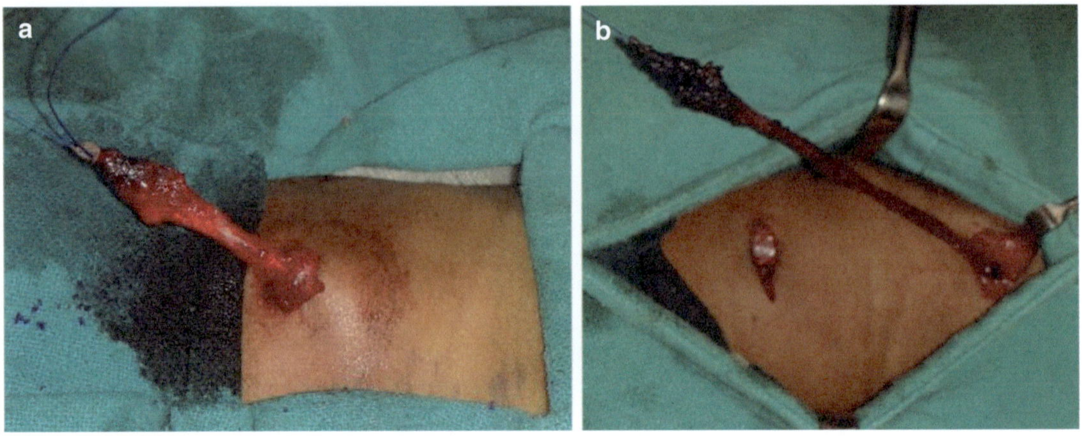

Fig. 20.3 Surgical excision of branchial fistula (**a**) lower end (**b**) stepladder incision for gaining access to the upper end

20.7 Thyroglossal Cyst and Fistula

Embryology

- The thyroid gland originates from the *thyroglossal duct*, a median bud that descends from the foramen cecum at the base of the tongue.
- Incomplete closure or remnants of this duct can lead to the formation of a thyroglossal cyst.

Pathology

- *Cyst lining*: lined by columnar epithelium.
- *Discharge*: can discharge mucus.
- Inflammation: often associated with recurrent inflammation due to the presence of lymphoid tissue in the cyst wall.

Clinical Features

- *Movement with swallowing*: a key characteristic of a thyroglossal cyst (Fig. 20.4) is that it moves with swallowing and protrusion of the tongue.
- *Ectopic thyroid tissue*: in a small percentage of cases (1–2%), the cyst may contain functioning thyroid tissue.
  - This requires screening with thyroid stimulating hormone (TSH) and/or neck ultrasound to assess thyroid function.
  - If the cyst is the only functioning thyroid tissue, thyroid hormone replacement therapy can cause the cyst to regress.

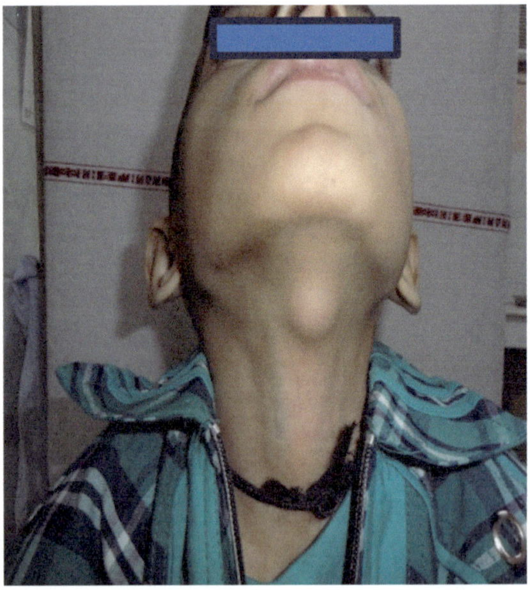

Fig. 20.4 Thyroglossal cyst

Differential Diagnosis

- Dermoid cyst
- Lymph node swelling
- Hemangioma/vascular malformations
- Median ectopic thyroid
- Sublingual bursa

Treatment

- *Sistrunk's operation*: the standard surgical treatment.

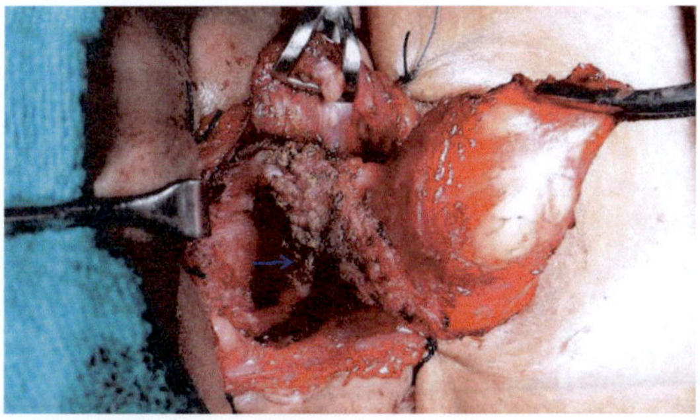

Fig. 20.5 Sistrunk operation: cyst is excised with body of hyoid bone (blue arrowhead)

- Involves removal of the body of the hyoid bone, the cyst tract, and a central core of tongue muscles.
- This approach is necessary because the tract has a close relationship with the hyoid bone and branches into multiple ductuli near the foramen cecum (Fig. 20.5).
- An assistant pushing the tongue down aids in the dissection.

Key Points

- Thyroglossal cysts are congenital anomalies arising from incomplete closure of the thyroglossal duct.
- They are typically located in the midline of the neck and move with swallowing.
- Sistrunk's operation is the standard surgical treatment to prevent recurrence.

20.8 Cystic Hygroma (Lymphatic Malformation) (See Chap. 9)

20.9 Cervical Lymphadenopathy

It refers to the enlargement of lymph nodes in the neck region. It is a matter of concern for both parents and physicians as it can be a sign of various underlying conditions, inflammatory or neoplastic.

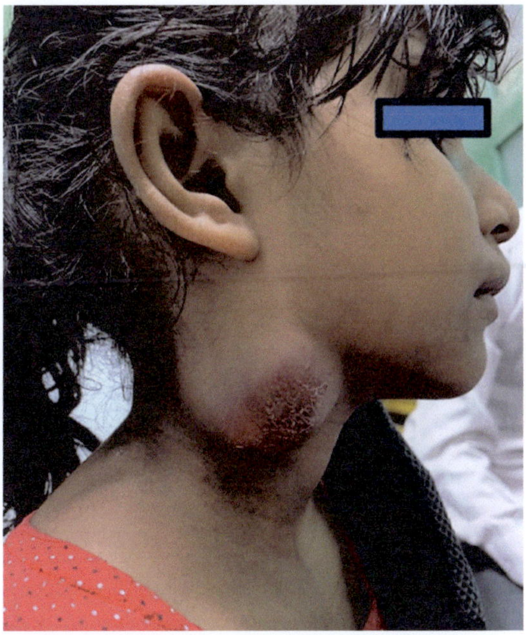

Fig. 20.6 Suppurative lymphadenitis of neck

20.9.1 Causes

- *Acute lymphadenitis*:
  - Often presents with fever, malaise, and tender neck masses.
  - Short duration.
  - Common causes include tonsillitis or dental abscess.
  - Management involves antibiotics, anti-inflammatory, and antipyretic medications.
  - If suppuration occurs, incision and drainage may be necessary (Fig. 20.6).
- *Asymptomatic enlargement*:
  - The most common presentation in outpatient settings.
  - Often no specific cause is identified.
  - Generally attributed to scalp infections.
  - Management includes treating any underlying infection, reassurance to parents, and head shampoo to address scalp issues.

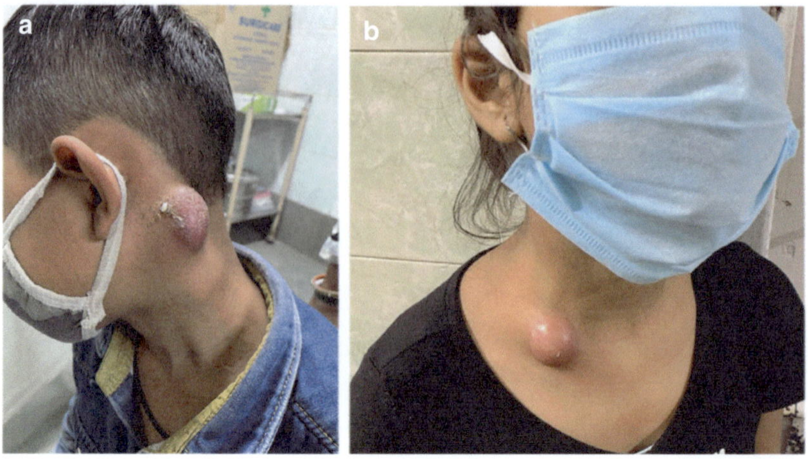

Fig. 20.7 (**a**) Posterior cervical chain of matted lymph nodes with cold abscess. (**b**) Cervical tubercular lymphadenitis with cold abscess

- *Chronic painless lymphadenopathy*:
  - May be due to tuberculosis (Fig. 20.7a), lymphoma, or leukemia.
  - Often involves deep cervical lymph node groups.
  - Lymph nodes may be adhered or matted together.
  - Suppuration can lead to cold abscesses.
  - "Collar stud" abscesses (Fig. 20.7b) can occur when the abscess penetrates through the deep fascia.
  - Management should avoid incision and drainage of cold abscesses to prevent non-healing sinuses.
  - Antigravity needle aspiration can be performed for diagnosis.
  - Rupture can lead to chronic discharging sinuses (Fig. 20.8).
  - Large lymph node masses due to Hodgkin's lymphoma can cause a "bull neck" appearance (Fig. 20.9).

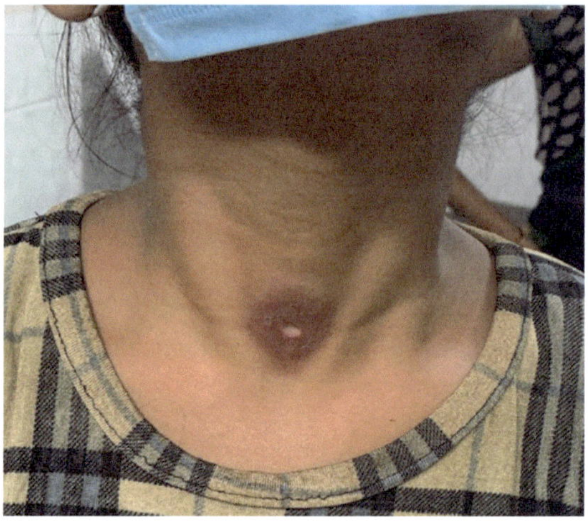

Fig. 20.8 Tubercular sinus neck

20.9.2 Management

- *Investigations*:
  - Complete blood count
  - Erythrocyte sedimentation rate (ESR)
  - Chest X-ray
  - Mantoux test
  - Fine-needle aspiration cytology, lymph node biopsy. Histological features of tuberculosis are caseating on necrotizing granuloma with Langhans -type giant cells and indentification of acid fast bacillus (Fig. 20.10).
- *Treatment*:
  - Antitubercular therapy for tubercular lesions.
  - Surgical excision biopsy for indeterminate or suspicious lesions.
  - Treatment for infections due to atypical mycobacteria or drug-resistant tuberculosis may require surgical excision.

Key Points

- Cervical lymphadenopathy is a common clinical presentation.

- Thorough evaluation is crucial to determine the underlying cause.
- Management strategies vary depending on the cause and severity of the lymphadenopathy.

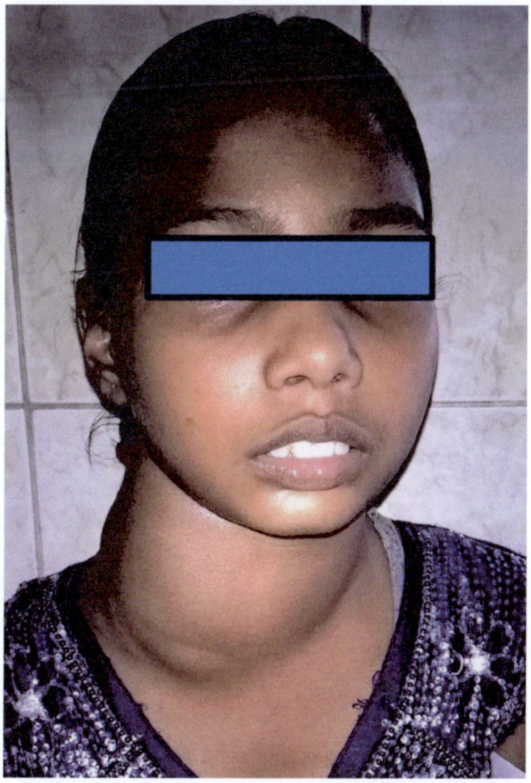

Fig. 20.9 Bull neck due to Hodgkin lymphoma

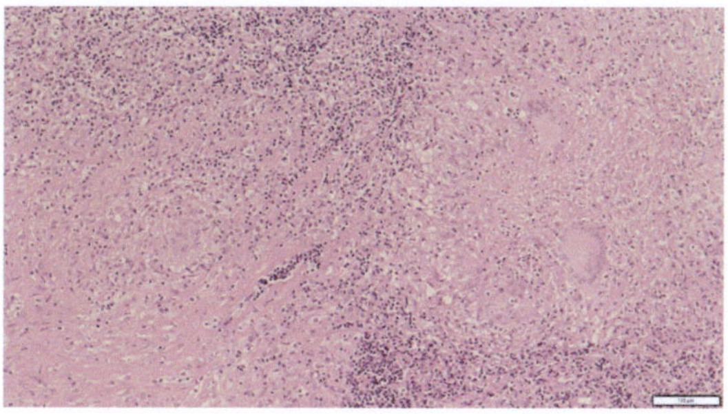

Fig. 20.10 Necrotizing lymphadenitis (tubercular): excision biopsy of lymph node showing necrotizing granulomas with Langhans-type giant cells (H&E10×). (Courtesy Dr. Lavleen Singh, AIIMS, New Delhi)

20.10 Sternomastoid Tumor

- *Presentation*:
  - Typically appears within the first few weeks of life.
  - Presents as a firm mass of 1–3 cm in size within the substance of the sternocleidomastoid muscle (Fig. 20.11).
- *Etiology*:
  - The exact cause is uncertain.
  - Possible causes include:
    - Intrauterine postural disorders leading to sternocleidomastoid compartment syndrome and ischemia.
    - Trauma during delivery resulting in hematoma within the muscle.
- *Clinical features*:
  - *Torticollis*: visible head tilt or torticollis develops later.
  - *Head position*: infants tend to rotate their head to the opposite side of the tumor with only slight flexion of the head towards the affected side.
- *Management*:
  - *Conservative*: gentle neck exercises and reassurance to the family are typically the recommended management approach.

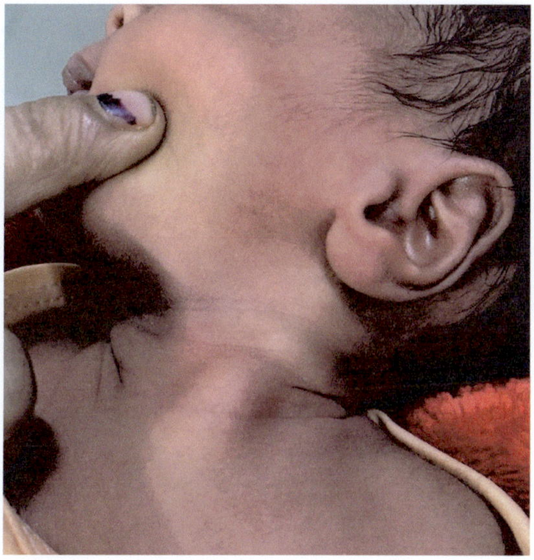

Fig. 20.11 Sternomastoid tumor

  - *Resolution*: the lesion usually resolves spontaneously within a few weeks.
- *Unrecognized tumors*:
  - In older children, unrecognized sternomastoid tumors can present with a fibrotic, shortened sternocleidomastoid muscle, leading to persistent torticollis.

Key Points
- Sternomastoid tumors are benign and typically resolve without specific intervention.
- Conservative management with reassurance and gentle stretching is usually sufficient.
- Persistent torticollis in older children may be due to unrecognized and untreated sternomastoid tumors.

20.11 Congenital Torticollis (Wry-Neck)

It refers to the abnormal twisting or tilting of the head to one side.

- *Causes*:
  - *Most common*: shortening and tightening of the sternocleidomastoid muscle (SCM) on one side.
  - *Other causes*: cervical hemivertebrae, pyogenic cervical spondylitis, cervical/retropharyngeal abscess, atlanto-axial subluxations, posterior fossa tumors, spasmodic torticollis, and postural torticollis.
- *Pathophysiology*:
  - Fibrosis and contracture of the sternocleidomastoid muscle lead to torticollis. SCM appears thickened and tightened along its whole length.
  - *Fibromatosis colli*: histology shows replacement of muscle bundles by fibrous tissue which undergoes atrophy.
  - This process may begin before birth, as suggested by the maturity of fibrous tissue in neonates.
- *Clinical features and examination*:
  - Head tilt to the opposite side of the affected muscle (Fig. 20.12a, b).
  - Restricted rotation and lateral flexion of the head.
  - Infants may compensate by elevating one shoulder to keep their eyes level, more pronounced in older children.
  - Higher frequency of obstetric difficulties reported incidence of breech deliveries up to 20–30%.
  - Rotational movement of SCM is assessed by standing behind the child's head and passively rotating it in between both hands. The rotation to the ipsilateral side is restricted when the muscle is fibrotic.
  - Associated problems include facial asymmetry (hemihypoplasia), scoliosis, craniofacial deformity, and atrophy of the ipsilateral trapezius muscle.

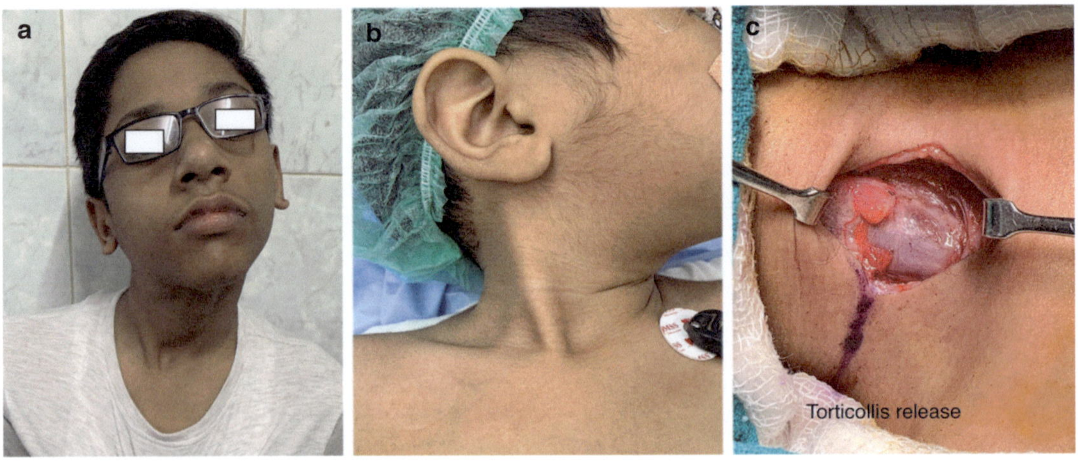

Fig. 20.12 (**a**) Torticollis with facial asymmetry, (**b**) right torticollis, (**c**) Release of torticollis, right side of the neck

- Eye checkup and cervical spine X-ray to rule out squint and bony vertebral anomaly, respectively, are mandatory.
- *Natural history*:
  - Spontaneous resolution occurs in 50–70% of cases by 6 months of age.
  - USG appearance may help predict spontaneous resolution. Localized lesions are more likely to resolve than those involving the whole muscle.
  - Persistence beyond 12 months is seen in about 10%.
- *Management*:
  - *Conservative*: neck physiotherapy is the initial treatment, 90% resolution if started early.
  - *Botulinum toxin*: can be used in younger children with encouraging results.
- *Surgical indications*:
  - Persistent deformity limiting head rotation after failed conservative treatment.
  - Plagiocephaly, facial asymmetry, and hemifacial hypoplasia.
  - Older patients (above 1 year of age).
- *Surgical procedure*:
  - Involves dividing the sternal and clavicular heads of the sternocleidomastoid muscle.
  - A 3–4 cm incision given 1 cm above the clavicle, dividing the muscle (unipolar release) at lower third.
  - Divide the thickened investing cervical fascia from midline extending posteriorly till the anterior border of the Trapezius muscle (Fig. 20.12c).
  - The procedure can also be performed endoscopically (stealth surgery).

Suggested Reading

Acierno SP, Waldhausen JH. Congenital cervical cysts, sinuses and fistulae. Otolaryngol Clin N Am. 2007;40(1):161–76, vii–viii. https://doi.org/10.1016/j.otc.2006.10.009. PMID: 17346566.

Coran AG, Caldamone A, Scott Adzich N, Krummel TM, Laberge JM, editors. Pediatric surgery. 7th ed. Oxford: Elsevier Limited; 2012.

Holcomb GW III, Murphy PJ, Ostile DJ, editors. Ashcrafts pediatric surgery. 6th ed. Philadelphia: Saunders/Elsevier; 2014.

Part V

Thorax

---

21 Chest Wall Deformities

Vishesh Jain and Subhasis Roy Choudhury

21.1 Introduction

Congenital chest wall deformities are common, with an incidence of 1 in 1000 people. There is a higher preponderance for males with a male to female ratio of 5:1. In addition to the cosmetic appearance, they can cause physiologic alterations in the form of restrictive pulmonary function, exercise intolerance, and impaired cardiac filling function. Surgical correction is often deemed necessary based on the age of the patient, degree of deformity, and alteration of the physiological functions.

The common varieties are:

- Pectus excavatum
- Pectus carinatum
- Sternal defects
- Poland syndrome
- Diffuse skeletal disorders with thoracic involvement

V. Jain (✉)
Department of Pediatric Surgery, AIIMS,
New Delhi, India

S. Roy Choudhury
Pediatric Surgery, Lady Hardinge Medical College
and Associated Kalawati Saran Children's Hospital,
New Delhi, Delhi, India

21.1.1 Pectus Excavatum (Funnel Chest)

Pectus excavatum is the most common of all chest wall deformities, accounting for nearly 90% of all chest wall anomalies. In this condition, there is a depression of the central chest wall as compared to the remainder of the chest wall (Fig. 21.1).

A family history is present in nearly one-third and associated scoliosis is present in one-fourth. The etiology is not clear, but aberrant overgrowth of costal cartilages during development results in this abnormality. Family history is often present,

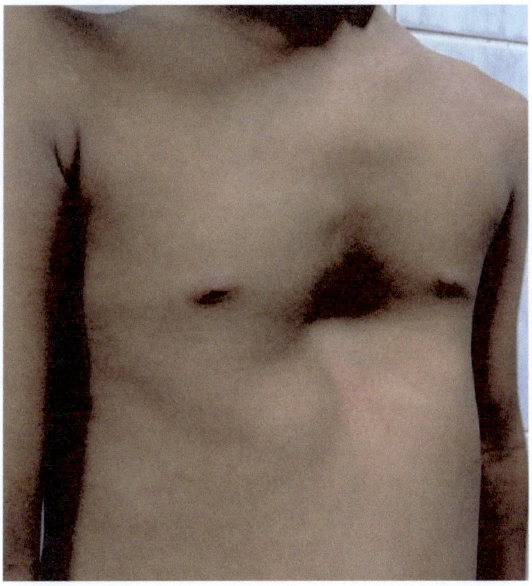

Fig. 21.1 Pectus excavatum

© The Author(s), under exclusive license to Springer Nature Singapore Pte Ltd. 2025
S. Roy Choudhury (ed.), *Pediatric Surgery*, https://doi.org/10.1007/978-981-96-1257-4_21

suggesting an autosomal dominant inheritance with variable penetration. Association with connective tissue disorders like Marfan syndrome and Noonan syndrome has been documented. Disturbances in chondrocyte proliferation and biomechanical factors during chest wall embryogenesis have also been implicated.

A decrease in the anteroposterior diameter of the chest can cause cardiac compression and limitation of lung expansion. Mitral valve prolapse is common in these patients (17%). Though it is usually well tolerated in infancy, many patients experience precordial pain with exertion or even pain at the site of deformity. Others experience palpitations and syncope.

On clinical examination, the depression is often symmetrical but can be asymmetrical also. Identification of asymmetry and its subtype is important in planning surgical management in these patients.

There are essentially two components of the deformity: a. sternal depression at the second and the third costal cartilage and posterior depression of the costal cartilages and ribs extending from the second to the seventh rib.

Park et al. classified pectus excavatum into two main categories. Type 1 encompasses symmetric defects, which may be further designated as typical or broad. Type 2 comprises asymmetric defects, where the deepest point of the chest depression is off-center relative to the sternum. Type 2 is subdivided into:

2A (Eccentric): The sternum remains centered while the maximal depression of the costal cartilage is shifted to one side.
2B (Unbalanced): Although the maximal depression is in midline, one side of the chest exhibits a more pronounced depression than the other.
2C: A mixed pattern displaying features of both 2A and 2B.

These patients are investigated with the following investigations:

- Chest Radiograph.
- CT scan: will show the severity of the defect and the compression of the heart. It is helpful in calculating indices that document the severity of the defect and may be helpful in treatment planning. The two most common indices used are the Haller index and Pectus Correction Index (PCI). The Haller index is given in Fig. 21.2. It is calculated as the transverse diameter of the thoracic cavity divided by the distance between the sternum and the vertebrae at the level of maximal defect. A value of >3.25 is considered a candidate for surgery. The Pectus Correction Index (PCI) represents the percentage deviation from the expected normal chest contour. On a CT scan at the level of maximum deformity, measure the distance (C) from the posterior vertebral body to the anterior chest wall and the distance (A) from the posterior vertebral body to the deepest point of the sternal depression. The correction index is calculated as CI = ((C − A)/C) × 100. For diagnosis, a value of 10% or more is considered suggestive of pectus excavatum. Studies have suggested that a PCI

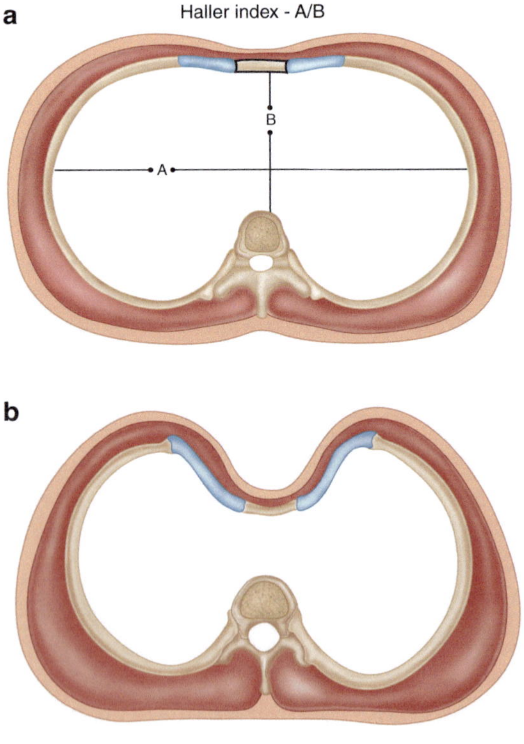

Fig. 21.2 Haller index, (**a**) normal, (**b**) severe pectus deformity

value of >28% corresponds with a Haller index of >3.25.

- Echocardiography: The stroke volume is decreased. Echo will also demonstrate mitral valve prolapse. Congenital heart defect may be present in 2% of patients.
- Pulmonary function tests: All parameters are decreased to about 80% of the normal predicted values.

Patients with mild to moderate deformity are started on deep breathing, aerobic exercise, and a posture program and evaluated yearly. Patients with severe chest deformities are evaluated further with CT chest, cardiac, and pulmonary function tests. Surgery is indicated if 2 or more of the following criteria are positive.

- Evidence of cardiac or pulmonary compression on CT and a Haller index of >3.25.
- A cardiac evaluation demonstrating displacement/ compression/murmur/conduction defects/mitral valve prolapse/significant fall in cardiac output from supine to the sitting position.
- Pulmonary function test demonstrates any sign of obstructive/restrictive lung disease.
- Progressive and symptomatic deformities.
- Recurrent deformities following a failed repair.

The ideal age for surgery is gradually increasing, with a median age of surgery being around 14 years.

Open surgical repair is a modified version of the traditional Ravitch technique and involves the following steps:

- A transverse or chevron incision is made across the chest.
- The pectoral and abdominal wall muscles are elevated off the sternum and deformed ribs up to the costochondral junction.
- The perichondrium covering the deformed ribs is carefully separated.
- The deformed portions of the ribs are excised, starting at the sternum and extending to a few millimeters before the costochondral junction.
- An anterior osteotomy is performed on the sternum, and the posterior table is fractured.
- A support strut is placed to maintain the sternum in its forward position.
- Finally, the muscle layers and overlying tissues are closed.

21.2 Nuss Procedure

The Nuss procedure is a minimally invasive technique for correcting pectus excavatum, where one or more curved metal bars are inserted under the sternum to elevate the depressed chest wall. The shaping of the bars is done depending upon the shape and symmetry of the defect. Using thoracoscopic guidance, the bars are accurately positioned and rotated into place, reducing the need for extensive incisions (Fig. 21.3a, b). The procedure typically takes about 1–2 h, depending on the case complexity and the number of bars required. The bar is subsequently removed after 2–4 years. Overall, it offers a less invasive alternative to traditional open repair, with the benefits of reduced operative time and shorter recovery.

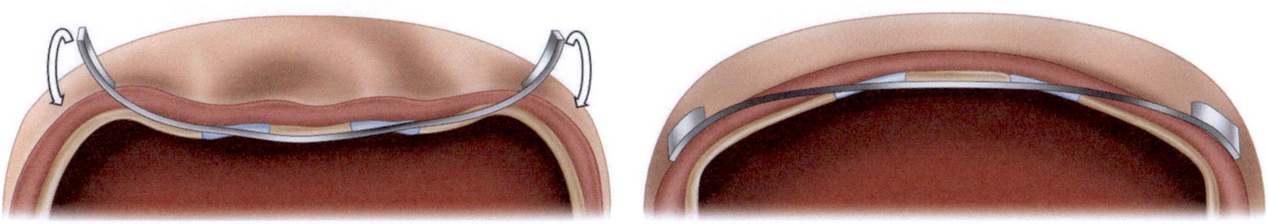

Fig. 21.3 The pectus strut in position (**a**) prior to rotation and (**b**) final position after rotation

21.3 Vacuum Bell Therapy

Gradual reduction in the correction of pectus excavatum with vacuum bell application (Fig. 21.4) is a novel nonoperative management of it. The potential for improvement depends on the depth of the defect, age of the patient, and duration of the therapy. The procedure has the best results in patients of age 10–12 years who have pliable chest wall and a defect of 1.5 cm or less. The family and child needs to be motivated for this treatment. The bell is applied twice a day and needs to be applied for 4 h in a day. The treatment often lasts for 12–18 months.

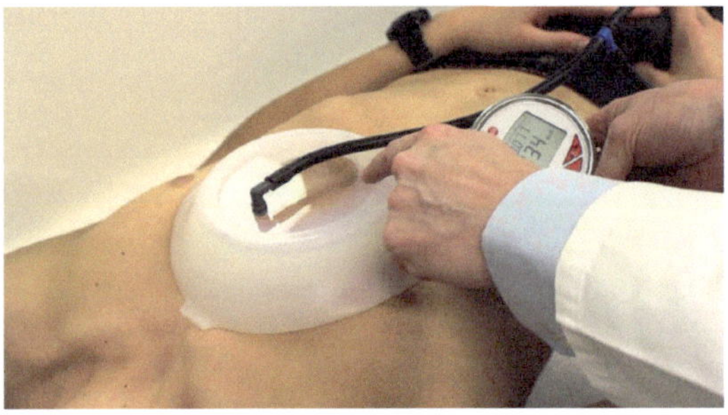

Fig. 21.4 Vacuum bell application for correction of pectus excavatum by negative suction

21.4 Pectus Carinatum

It is an abnormal protrusion of the sternum and the costal cartilages. The treatment if needed is similar to that in pectum excavatum with the excision of deformed cartilage and osteotomy of the sternum, placing it in a normal position. Surgical correction, which is rarely required, consists of a muscle flap, breast augmentation, and bone graft in the case of sternal and rib defects.

21.5 Poland Syndrome

The most consistent feature of this syndrome is the absent or attenuated sternocostal component of the pectoralis major muscle. There is associated variable involvement of the hand, breast, or the chest wall (ribs, Fig. 21.5a, b). No clear genetic association has been found.

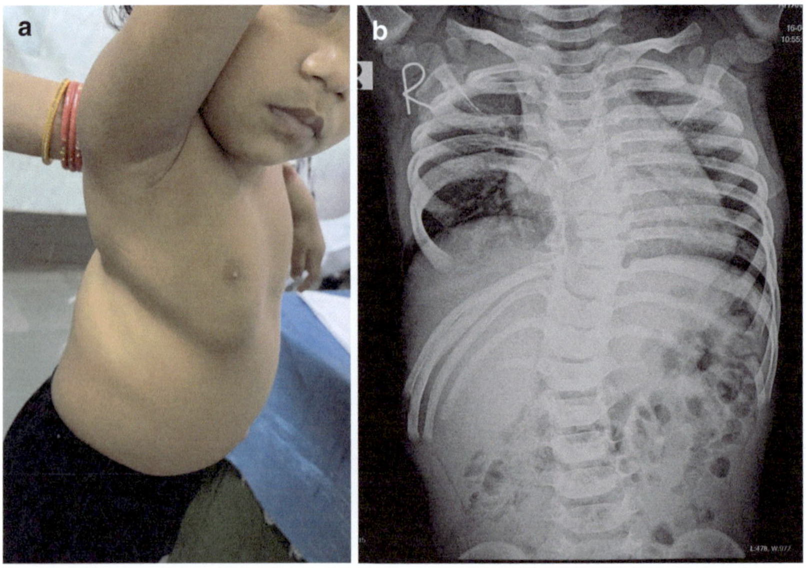

Fig. 21.5 (**a**) Congenital absence of ribs, (**b**) chest x-ray showing left sided rib and vertebral anomalies

21.6 Sternal Defects

Include defects like ectopia cordis, cleft/ bifid sternum.

21.7 Diffuse Skeletal Disorders with Thoracic Involvement

It includes syndromes like asphyxiating thoracic dystrophy and spondylothoracic dysplasia.

21.8 Summary

Correction of pectus deformity is required in children for either cosmetic and psychological reasons or physiological limitations of chest movement. The results of repair by both the open technique and Nuss procedure are comparable, with the additional advantage of the latter for cosmetic scar. The commonest complication following repair is recurrence in the tune of 10–15% cases as reported.

Suggested Reading

Coran AG, Caldamone A, Scott Adzich N, Krummel TM, Laberge JM, editors. Pediatric surgery. 7th ed. Oxford: Elsevier Limited; 2012.

Holcomb GW III, Murphy PJ, St Peter SD, editors. Holocomb and ashcraft's pediatric surgery. 7th ed. Philadelphia: Elsevier; 2020.

Puri P, Hollwarth ME, editors. Pediatric surgery. 2nd ed. Heidelberg: Springer-Verlag; 2019.

22 Mediastinal Masses in Children

Nidhi Sugandhi and Subhasis Roy Choudhury

22.1 Introduction

The mediastinum is the most common site of chest mass in a child, but mediastinal masses often pose a management challenge to the clinician. Due to the difficulty in access and the well-ensconced position of the masses, they pose diagnostic and therapeutic challenges. They may be incidentally detected on plain radiographs or can be symptomatic and present with respiratory distress and other symptoms. About 30–40% of mediastinal masses in children are malignant.

The mediastinum is a potential space bound by the following boundaries

- Superior-thoracic inlet
- Posterior-vertebral column and spine
- Anterior-sternum
- Inferior-diaphragm
- Lateral-visceral pleura

Eighty percent of all mediastinal masses are constituted by

- Neurogenic tumors, including neuroblastoma, ganglioneuroma, and paraganglionoma
- Lymphomas, leukemias, and other LN masses
- Germ cell tumors (GCTs)
- Mesenchymal tumors

Unlike adults, where only 40% of masses may be symptomatic, in children most mediastinal masses present with early symptoms related to airway compression, infection, or invasion of surrounding structures.

Unlike abdominal masses, USG and histopathology are not always possible or contributory when dealing with mediastinal masses in children, and one needs to rely on many supportive investigations like tumor markers for diagnosis. Clinical correlation in terms of age, specific symptoms, and signs is also important in the diagnostic algorithm. Also, surgical access is difficult and needs to be tailored according to the diagnosis and location.

22.2 Anatomical Classification of Mediastinal Masses

For ease of diagnosis and management, the mediastinum is anatomically divided into superior, anterior, middle, and posterior compartments (Fig. 22.1).

N. Sugandhi (✉)
Department of Pediatric Surgery, VMMC and Safdarjung Hospital, New Delhi, India

S. Roy Choudhury
Pediatric Surgery, Lady Hardinge Medical College and Associated Kalawati Saran Children's Hospital, New Delhi, Delhi, India

© The Author(s), under exclusive license to Springer Nature Singapore Pte Ltd. 2025

S. Roy Choudhury (ed.), *Pediatric Surgery*, https://doi.org/10.1007/978-981-96-1257-4_22

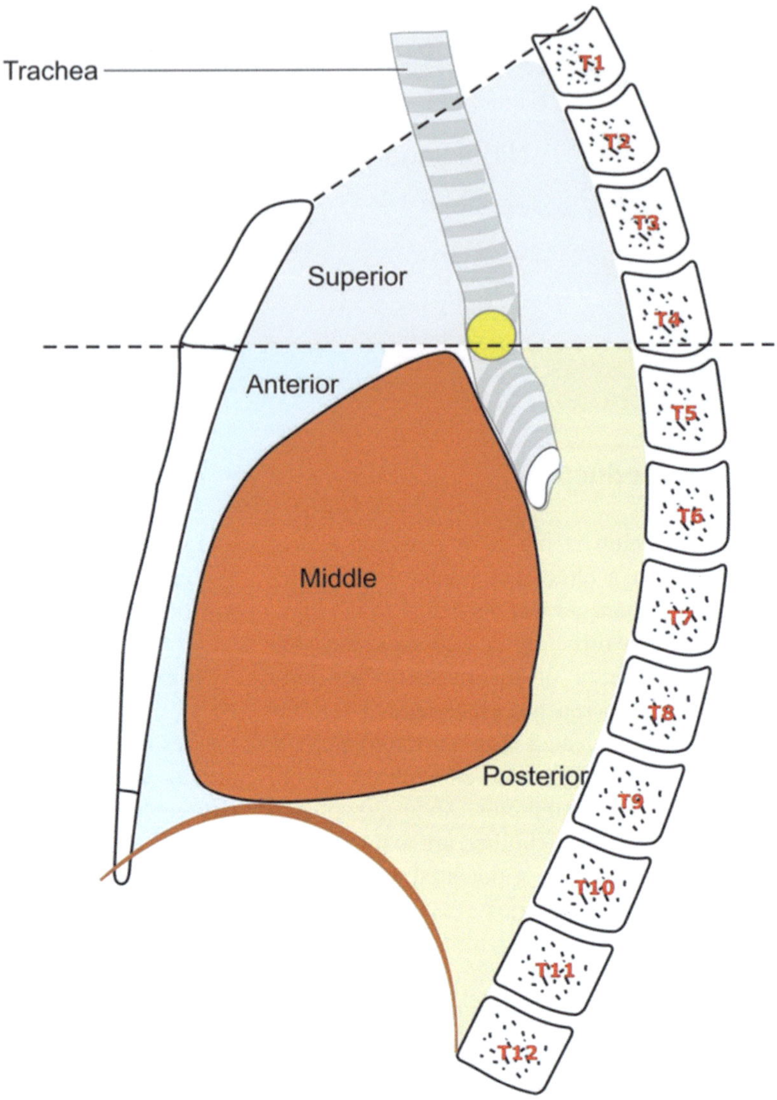

Fig. 22.1 Anatomical divisions of the mediastinum

Anterior mediastinum is the most common site of mediastinal mass in a child (50%), followed by equal incidence in the middle and posterior mediastinum (25% each).

The anatomical location of masses in the mediastinum provides clues to the diagnosis. The most common mediastinal masses according to location are listed below (Table 22.1).

Table 22.1 Anatomical division and boundaries of the mediastinum with normal contents and benign and malignant masses in each compartment

Felson's division	Japanese classification	Boundaries	Normal contents	Common benign masses	Common malignant masses
Anterior mediastinum	Prevascular compartment	Superior: Thoracic inlet Inferior: Diaphragm Anterior: Sternum Lateral: Parietal pleural reflections; lateral margin of the bilateral internal thoracic arteries and veins, and superior and inferior pulmonary veins Posterior: Anterior aspect of the pericardium and the lateral rim of the aortic arch, superior, and inferior pulmonary veins	Thymus Fat Lymph nodes Left brachio-cephalic vein	Teratoma Cystic Hygroma Vascular masses Thymic cysts	Teratoma Germ cell tumors Desmoid Sarcoma Thymoma Lymphomas
Middle mediastinum	Visceral compartment	Superior: Thoracic inlet Inferior: Diaphragm Anterior: Posterior boundaries of the prevascular compartment Posterior: Vertical line connecting a point on each thoracic vertebral body at 1 cm posterior to its anterior margin	Nonvascular: Trachea, carina, esophagus, lymph nodes Vascular: Heart, ascending thoracic aorta, aortic arch, descending thoracic aorta, superior vena cava, intra-pericardial pulmonary arteries, thoracic duct	Bronchogenic cysts Cardiac masses, Rhabdo-myoma	Lymphomas Sarcomas Rhabdo-myosarcoma

(continued)

Table 22.1 (continued)

Felson's division	Japanese classification	Boundaries	Normal contents	Common benign masses	Common malignant masses
Posterior mediastinum	Paravertebral compartment	Superior: Thoracic inlet Inferior: Diaphragm Anterior: Posterior boundaries of the visceral compartment Posterolateral: Vertical line against the posterior margin of the chest wall at the lateral margin of the transverse process of the thoracic spine	Paravertebral soft tissues, Exiting nerves and ganglia	Ganglio-neuroma Duplication cysts	Neuroblastoma Leio-myosarcoma Liposarcoma
Superior mediastinum		Superior-thoracic inlet Inferiorly: Line joining angle of his to T4		Thymoma	Teratoma

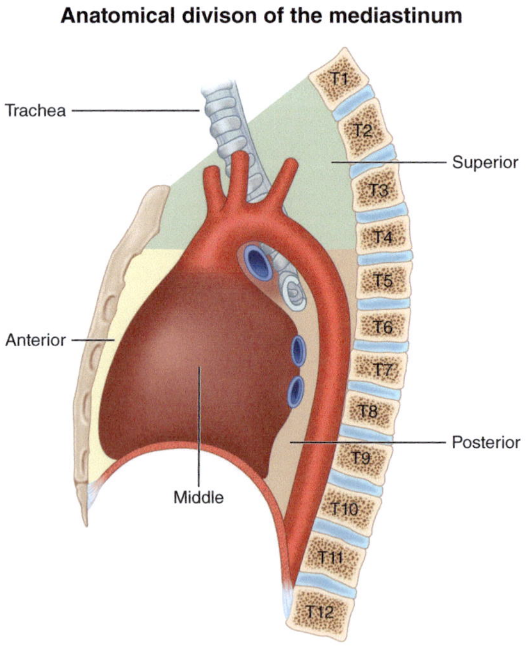

22.3 Epidemiology

The spectrum of masses undergoes a change with age (Fig. 22.2), more likely to be malignant in children. Lymphoma is the commonest anterior mediastinal mass in children, followed by germ cell tumors like teratoma and dermoid. In infants, thymic masses are also common.

Neurogenic tumors are the most common mass in the posterior mediastinum. Neuroblastoma is common in young children. Ganglioneuroma is common in older children. Approximately 50% of mediastinal masses are malignant in children compared to 15% in adults.

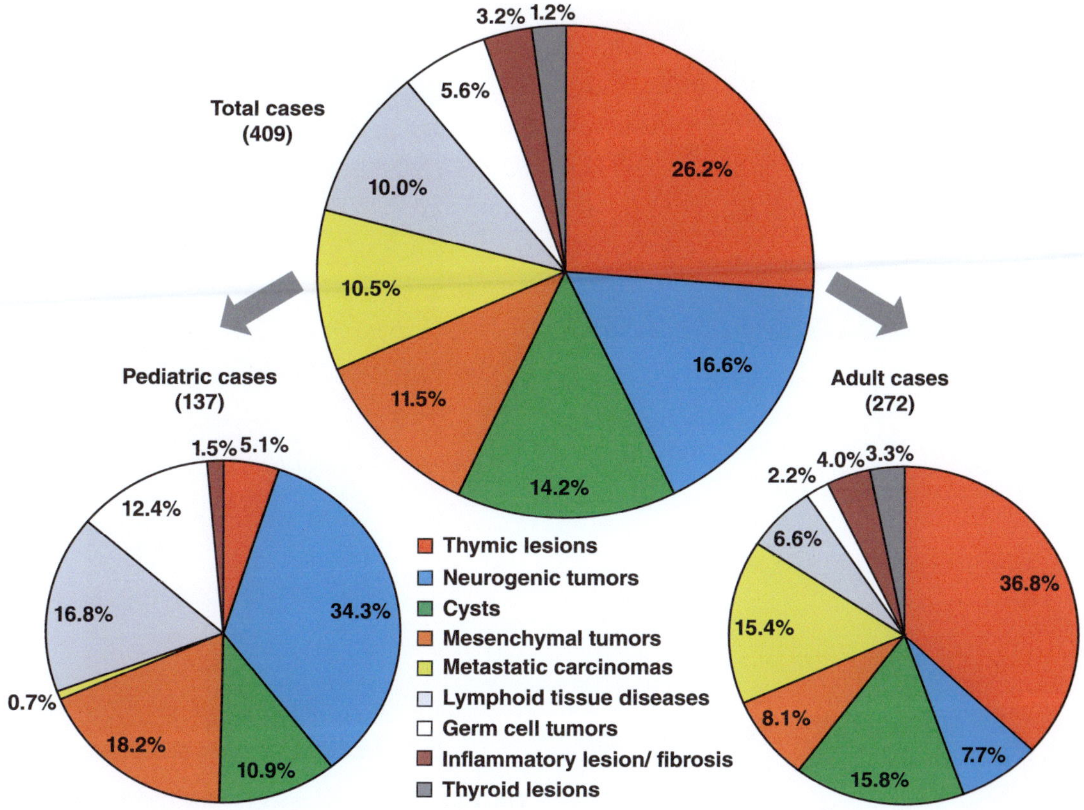

Fig. 22.2 Spectrum of mediastinal masses in different age groups

22.4 Clinical Presentation

Antenatal detection of some lesions is possible with fetal ultrasound. These may include duplication cysts, bronchogenic cysts, lymphangiomas, and vascular masses.

Anterior/Middle Mediastinal Masses: Nearly half of these children are asymptomatic, and the diagnosis is incidental upon imaging for nonspecific symptoms. If symptomatic anterior and middle mediastinal masses in infants present with respiratory distress, stridor, cyanosis, and even superior vena cava syndrome (Figs. 22.3, 22.4 and 22.5). Older children present with cough, dyspnea, orthopnea, and rarely hemoptysis. Infants may also present with sternal bulging, especially if a large mass like teratoma is present (Fig. 22.6).

A middle mediastinal lymphangioma is seen in Fig. 22.7.

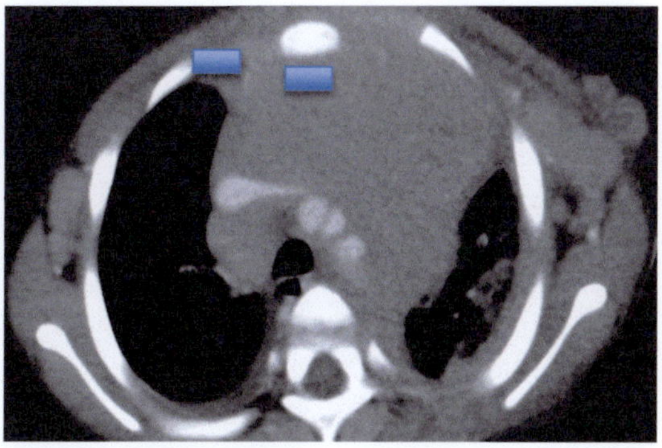

Fig. 22.3 Anterior mediastinal mass (acute lymphatic leukemia)

Posterior mediastinal masses can be quite large yet asymptomatic, often discovered in a chest radiograph done for other indications (Figs. 22.8 and 22.9). Some children may present with dyspnea, cough, dysphagia, pain, or respiratory distress secondary to compression by the

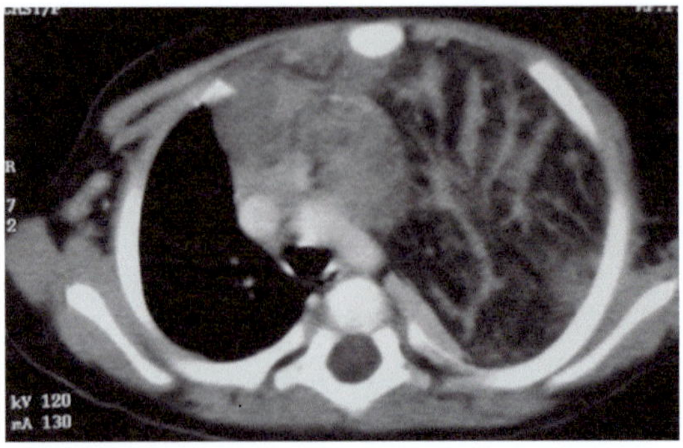

Fig. 22.4 CT scan: thymolipoma

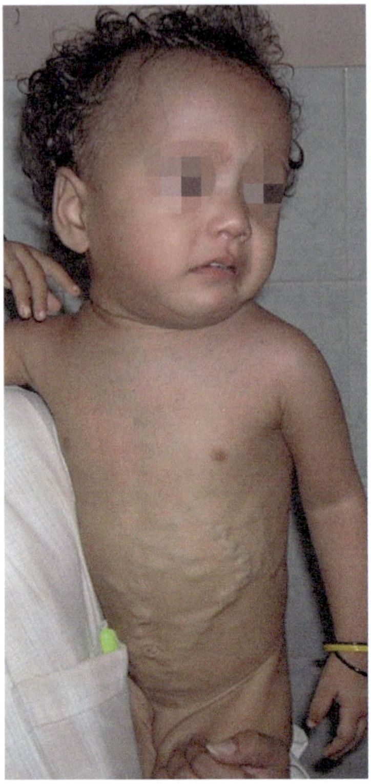

Fig. 22.5 Mediastinal mass causing respiratory distress with features of superior vena caval obstruction

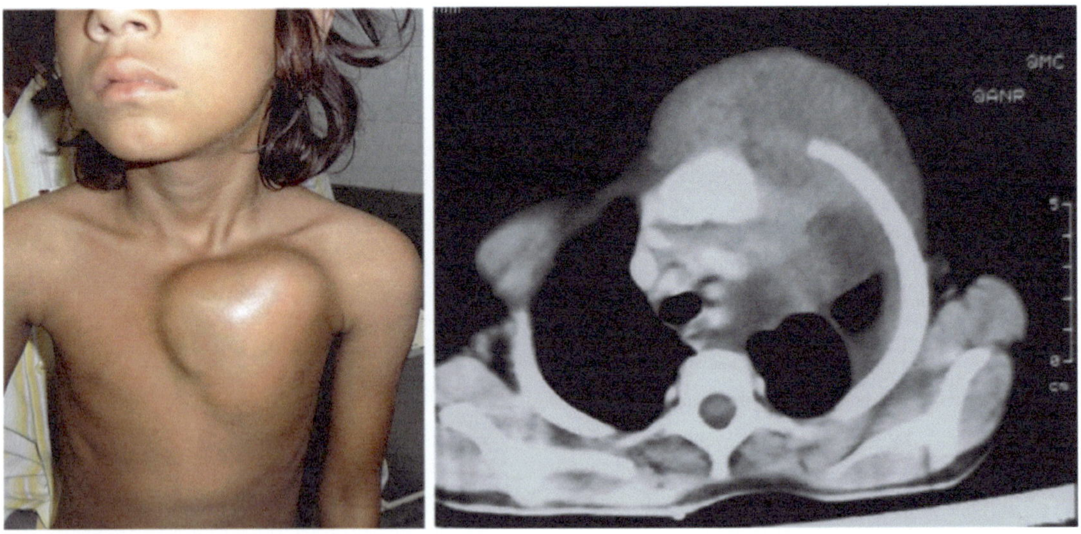

Fig. 22.6 Mediastinal mass with chest wall extension, acute lymphatic leukemia. (**a**) Clinical and (**b**) CT scan

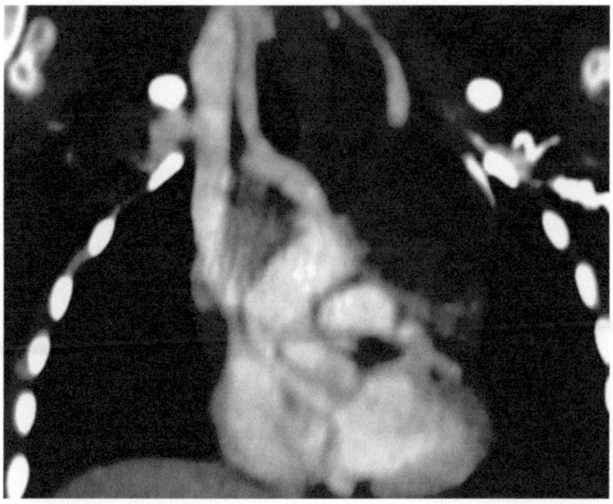

Fig. 22.7 Lymphangioma neck with mediastinal extension

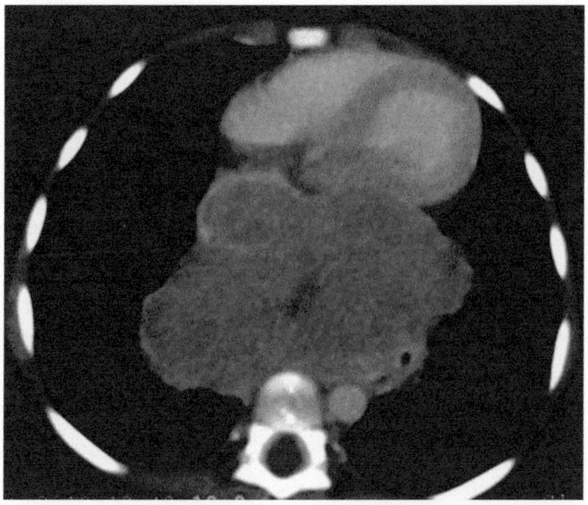

Fig. 22.8 Posterior mediastinal mass (neurogenic tumor)

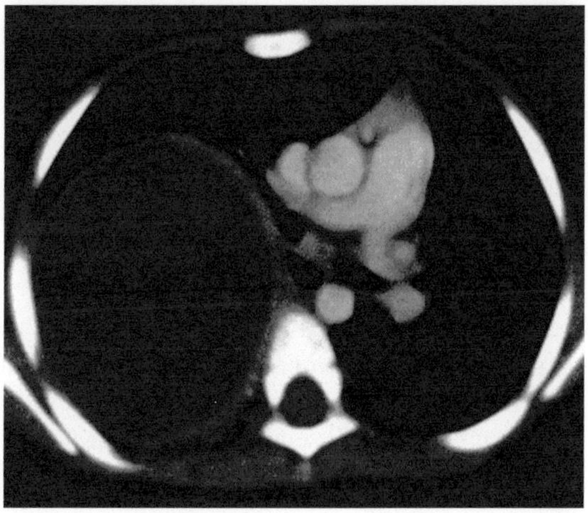

Fig. 22.9 CT scan showing an esophageal duplication cyst

mass. If the tumor extends through the spinal foramina, then features of spinal cord compression may be present. Horner's syndrome (miosis, ptosis, enophthalmos, and anhidrosis) can be present if there is an involvement of the sympathetic ganglia chain. Few cases of neuroblastoma can present with paraneoplastic syndrome (opsoclonus-myoclonus, hypercalcemia, etc.).

22.5 Evaluation/Imaging

- Chest-X ray can reveal widening of the mediastinum with a deviation of the trachea or bronchus. Calcification may be noted in teratoma or neuroblastoma. Bony destruction can be seen in malignant infiltrative tumors. Vertebral abnormalities may suggest a foregut duplication cyst.
- Ultrasound is useful in detecting the nature of the mass (solid or cystic) and vascularity of the lesion. It can also indicate the involvement of pleura, pericardium, and esophagus. A major limitation in ultrasound for mediastinal masses is the inadequate window, especially for deep-seated masses.
- Contrast-enhanced computed tomogram (CECT) is the investigation of choice, which gives important information about the lesion, like extent, organ of origin, calcification, and lymphadenopathy.
- MRI is an excellent investigation for soft tissue details of the masses with its spontaneous tissue± vessel contrast and direct multiplanar capabilities. It is very useful to see the extent of vascular lesions, spinal extension, vascular involvement, and assessment of the relationship with the pericardium and heart cavities.
- PET scan is useful to determine the extent of disease, metastasis, response to therapy, and recurrence from various primary tumors.
- Specific investigations may be required for diagnosing certain masses, e.g.,
  - Duplication cyst:Tc 99 scan for ectopic mucosa.
  - Germ cell tumors: alfa feto protein (AFP), human horionic gonadotrophin (HCG), and lactate dehydrogenase (LDH).
  - Neuroblastoma: MIBG scan and urinary metanephrines.

- Bronchoscopy/esophagoscopy with lavage cytology or guided biopsy may be useful for a limited set of lesions either arising from or in close proximity to the trachea and esophagus.
- Tissue diagnosis: A decision to biopsy or fine needle aspiration cytology (FNAC) in mediastinal masses has to be taken after very careful consideration. Approaching a mediastinal mass for tissue diagnosis can pose danger to surrounding vessels, heart, trachea, and esophagus. The mass may also be present in an area that makes it inaccessible to a biopsy needle. Almost all biopsies would need image guidance under CT, as USG has limited usefulness in the chest cavity. If definitely indicated for some lesions but inaccessible to image-guided techniques, then open surgical or laparoscopic biopsy under general anesthesia may be indicated.

For this reason, biopsy is done in only certain masses like:

- Lymphoma
- Neuroblastoma if not diagnosed by bone marrow or urinary metanephrines
- Other neurogenic tumors: benign or peripheral neuroectodermal tumour (PNET)
- Any other lesion where diagnosis is not possible by CT/MRI/tumor markers, etc.
  Despite the best planning, biopsy still carries a complication rate of 10% and hence needs to be carried out very carefully.
  Various routes can be used for biopsy like:
- CT-guided transthoracic
- Bronchoscopic
- Esophagoscopic
- Thoracoscopic
- Parasternal mediastinotomy (Chamberlain's procedure)
- Cervical mediatinoscopy

22.5.1 Management

Management of mediastinal masses can be medical and surgical. Almost all mediastinal masses require surgical removal, except a few, like lymphomas, which can respond to chemotherapy. Immediate surgery is the treatment for duplication cysts, neurenteric cysts, and benign lesions like ganglioneuroma. Chemotherapy followed by surgery is the usual approach for tumors like neuroblastoma and germ cell tumors. Certain vascular lesions may respond to conservative management like sclerotherapy, but most require surgical removal. Lymphomas, on the other hand, may completely respond to chemotherapy, and surgery may be avoided.

A very careful perioperative planning and consideration are required, and many anesthetic and surgical concerns need to be addressed before embarking on surgery to remove a mediastinal masses as there can be high morbidity associated in terms of prolonged ventilation, injury to vital structures, etc.

A large mediastinal mass poses significant anesthetic challenges. There is a potential for respiratory and cardiovascular compromise on induction as respiratory and airway muscle tone may fall suddenly with muscle relaxants, leading to a sudden collapse of the patient. Children are more susceptible to this due to the more compressible nature of the pediatric airway and smaller lumen. Hence, even small paratracheal masses should not be underestimated.

A mediastinal mass may extend across the anatomical compartments into the spine and abdomen. In such a case the spinal component will be prioritized over the mediastinal compartment, which in turn will get priority over the abdominal part. This is because of possible deterioration due to post-operative edema in the residual lesion.

A thorough preoperative clinical and radiological assessment needs to be carried out, noting especially any signs of superior vena cava, a compression-like upper body edema, syncopal symptoms, or orthopnea. Radiological evidence of the reduction (<70%) in tracheal cross-sectional area, carinal or bronchial compression, great vessel compression, and pericardial effusion should entail proper preparation.

During induction, sedation is avoided to prevent collapse of airways. Flexible intubation in lateral or head-up position is helpful in large masses compressing the airways.

Many surgical approaches have been described for excising a mediastinal mass, as the approach to these deep-seated masses surrounded by vascular structures is difficult, and a single approach cannot suffice for the different locations and extent of involvement of these masses. Following are a few of the described approaches

- Postero-lateral thoracotomy (Fig. 22.10): Most common approach in children, with the advantage of good access to almost the entire mediastinum and thoracic apex. However, it gives poor access to the thoracic apex or the superior mediastinum, especialy in cases of encasement of the vital vascular structures. Also the division of major muscles of the chest can lead to prolonged ipsilateral shoulder and arm dysfunctions as well as compromised pulmonary function and chronic post-thoracotomy pain syndrome.
- Extended lateral thoracotomy: The posterolateral thoracotomy incision can be extended posteriorly by dividing the trapezius and rhomboid muscles. If an additional anterior extension is required, the skin incision is extended to the lateral edge of the sternum, and the serratus anterior and pectoralis major muscles are divided.
- Double lateral thoracotomy: This may be useful in large tumors with multiple adhesions extended bilaterally across the midline, like neuroblastoma and PNET.
- Thoracoscopy: Introduced in 1976, thoracoscopic surgery can be very helpful in minimizing morbidity in skilled hands.
- Median sternotomy: This is not very popular for mediastinal masses as it offers limited exposure to only the cardiac chambers. It is used for pericardial cysts and masses.
- Clamshell sternotomy (Fig. 22.11): This is a transverse incision extending across the entire chest and provides excellent exposure of the mediastinum and anterior cervicothoracic junction. It is especially useful for anterior mediastinal masses extending across both hemithoraces and facilitates single-step complete resection, including pulmonary resections.
- Trapdoor thoracotomy (Fig. 22.12) was described by Grunewald wherein access is obtained by dividing the manubrium and the first costal cartilage. Dartevelle further modified it by resecting the medial clavicular head. It is very useful for superior mediastinal lesions extending across the compartment into the neck, for example, neuroblastomas, vascular malformations, etc.
- Posterior thoracotomy.

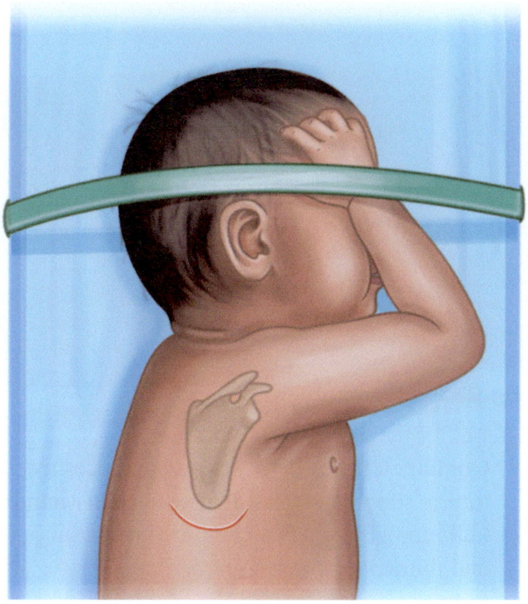

Fig. 22.10 Posterolateral thoracotomy

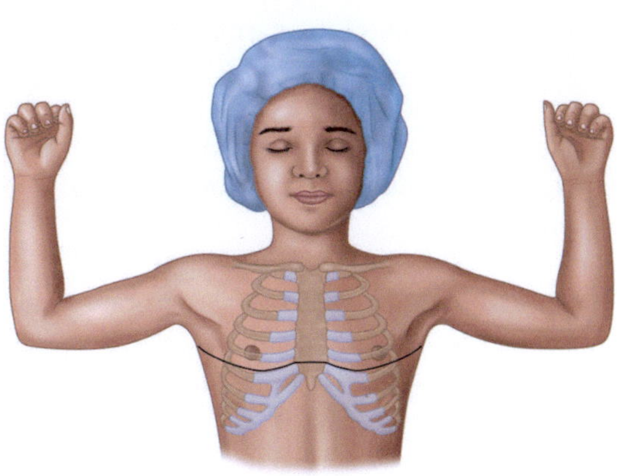

Fig. 22.11 Clamshell thoracotomy

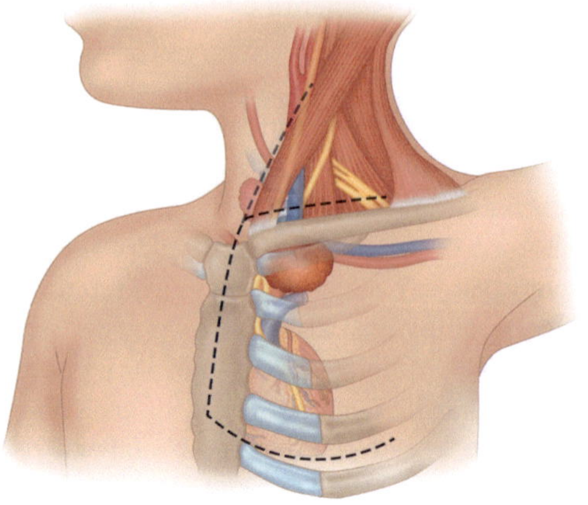

Fig. 22.12 Trapdoor thoracotomy

- Cervical mediastinoscopy: A minimally invasive approach, it entails access to the superior mediastinum through a scope and gives a very clear vision of the superior and anterior mediastinum. It can be used for masses, particularly in paratracheal, pretracheal regions, anterior precarinal and subcarinal space, and the tracheobronchial angles where it enables careful dissection between the great vessels, trachea, esophagus, and nerves.
- Anterior mediastinotomy (Fig. 22.13): Chamberlain procedure. This is a popular procedure, especially for open biopsies of anterior mediastinal masses or for the resection of small masses. It entails a transverse incision over the second or third costal cartilage, excision of the cartilage for exposure purposes, and the option of an intrapleural or extrapleural approach. It is used for masses in the anterior mediastinum, and the right paratracheal and aortopulmonary window areas.
- Thoracoabdominal approach (Fig. 22.14). This is a midline abdominal incision extending across the 7/8th intercostal space by incising the diaphragm. It is the approach for tumors extending across the diaphragm, like neuroblastoma, PNET, and vascular malformations.

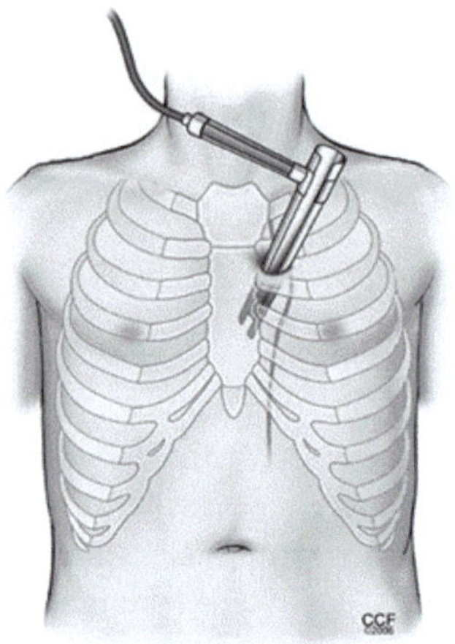

Fig. 22.13 Anterior mediastinostomy or Chamberlain's procedure

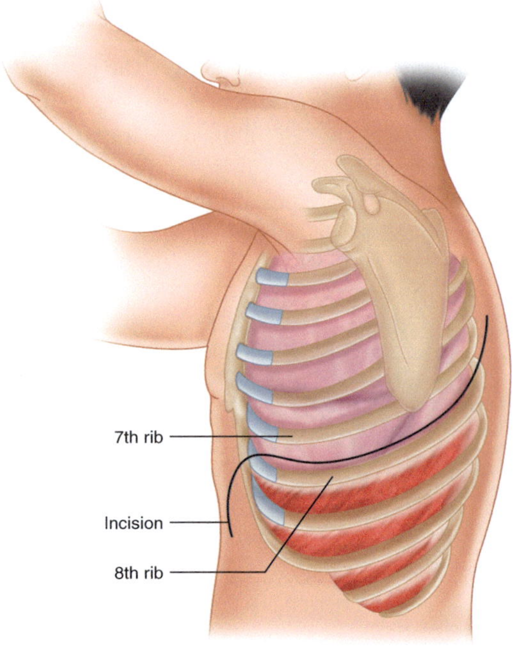

Fig. 22.14 Thoracoabdominal incision

- Combined thoracotomy with laminectomy: A tumor showing intraspinal extension (dumbbell tumor) requires a combined neurosurgical and thoracic approach via laminectomy.

22.6 Common Individual Mediastinal Masses in Children

22.6.1 Lymphomas

Lymphomas are most common anterior mediastinal masses in infants, and overall the most common mediastinal mass in older children. The common forms in children, like Hodgkin's lymphoma and T-lymphoblastic lymphoma (T-LBL), have a good prognosis with cure rates greater than 90%. These respond well to nonsurgical treatment with chemotherapy but need to be biopsied for arriving at an accurate diagnosis by immunophenotyping and histopathologic and cytogenetic studies.

22.6.2 Germ Cell Tumor (GCT)/Teratomas

Primary mediastinal teratomas are located in the anterior mediastinum. They have a bimodal age distribution with the first peak in infancy and then again in the second decade of life. Though difficult to differentiate histopathologically from testicular GCT, testicular or ovarian GCT rarely metastasize to the anterior mediastinum. Nevertheless, any patient who presents with mediastinal GCT needs the exclusion of testicular and ovarian primary. Teratomas are diagnosed by the typical appearance on CT showing a mixture of fat, fluid, and calcification along with raised tumor markers AFP and HCG, seen in malignant GCTs. Babies present with chronic cough, chest pain, wheezing, and, rarely, acute respiratory distress. Occasionally, they may have dysphagia. In rare cases, the tumor may rupture into a bronchus, resulting in expectoration of the contents.

Malignant GCTs respond to chemotherapy with Bleomycin, etoposide, and Cisplatin and may disappear completely. They need close follow-up and monitoring with tumor markers and imaging for recurrence.

Benign teratomas need to be surgically excised. Though benign, they can present as huge life-threatening masses and may require all surgical and anesthetic skills to be excised safely.

22.6.3 Thymic Cyst

It is a rare condition that is a remnant of the thymo-pharyngeal duct. It presents as a fluid containing an anterior mediastinal mass.

22.6.3.1 Thymoma

These are neoplasms of epithelial origin, containing a variable number of lymphocytes, arising from the thymus but can extend to the neck, thyroid, pulmonary hilum, lung, pleura, and pericardium. Thymomas are an infrequent cause of mediastinal tumors in the pediatric age group. Apart from cough, chest pain, and compressive symptoms, around half of the patients present with paraneoplastic syndrome like hypogammaglobulinemia, pure red cell aplasia, or myasthenia gravis. Surgical excision is required along with chemotherapy and radiotherapy.

22.6.3.2 Vascular Lesions

Arising from the middle mediastinum, these lesions include lymphangiomas, arterio-venous malformations, and hemangiomas. These cause symptoms like dyspnea and dysphagia due to compression, and rarely can cause bleeding and hematemesis/hemoptysis due to the erosion of adjacent structures. Hemangiomas may respond to treatment with propranolol and steroids, but all others require excision.

22.6.4 Neuroblastomas

It is the most common posterior mediastinal mass in infants and younger children. Thoracic neuroblastomas are usually diagnosed earlier than abdominal neuroblastomas, presenting with cough, breathlessness, weight loss, and fever. Neurological involvement may lead to paraparesis and even bladder and bowel involvement. Horner's syndrome may also occur due to the involvement of the stellate ganglion. Though diagnosed conclusively by a tissue biopsy, they can also be diagnosed by a combination of positive bone marrow and raised urinary metanephrines. Multimodality treatment, including chemotherapy, radiotherapy, and surgery, is required for the treatment.

22.7 Neurenteric Cysts/ Duplication Cysts/ Bronchogenic Cysts

These present as cystic masses in the middle or posterior mediastinum. They may be detected antenatally. Usual symptoms are dysphagia or dyspnea due to proximity to esophagus or trachea. Diagnosis is based on CECT findings, and treatment is complete surgical excision.

22.8 Summary

Mediastinal masses in children are responsible for great morbidity. They have a unique diagnostic and therapeutic requirement in view of the limited access and concentration of vital structures in the area. Though CECT is a basic investigation to diagnose these masses, a combination of clinical, radiological, and ancillary tests may be needed to conclusively reach a diagnosis. The decision to biopsy a mediastinal mass needs careful consideration of risks and benefits, and also careful planning of the route and image guidance. Except for a few masses like lymphomas, most masses require complete surgical excision. Perioperative risk assessment and management are important for safe surgery and anesthesia. Surgical approach can be difficult due to close proximity of multiple vital structures and needs to be tailored according to location, size, and type of mass.

Suggested Reading

Ahmed G, Hegazy MM, Raafat T, Hafez H, Fadel S, Elshafiey M. Surgical approaches, anaesthetic management and outcome in pediatric superior mediastinal tumors. J Egypt Nat Cancer Instit. 2017;29(3):147–53. https://doi.org/10.1016/j.jnci.2017.08.001.

Carter BW, Marom EM, Detterbeck FC. Approaching the patient with an anterior mediastinal mass: a guide for clinicians. J Thorac Oncol. 2014;9:S102–9. https://doi.org/10.1097/JTO.0000000000000294.

Carter BW, Benveniste MF, Madan R, et al. ITMIG classification of mediastinal compartments and multidisciplinary approach to mediastinal masses. Radiographics. 2017;37:413–36. https://doi.org/10.1148/rg.2017160095.

Coran AG, Caldamone A, Scott Adzich N, Krummel TM, Laberge JM, editors. Pediatric surgery. 7th ed. Oxford: Elsevier Limited; 2012.

Laurent F, Latrabe V, Lecesne R, et al. Mediastinal masses: diagnostic approach. Eur Radiol. 1998;8:1148–59. https://doi.org/10.1007/s003300050525

Empyema Thoracis

23

Subhasis Roy Choudhury and Partap Singh Yadav

23.1 Introduction

Empyema thoracis refers to the accumulation of pus in the pleural cavity, typically resulting from the infection of parapneumonic effusions (PPEs) and subsequent deposition of fibrinous exudates in the pleural space. Its management is dictated by the patient's clinical condition and the disease stage.

23.2 Pathology

Empyema thoracis most commonly arises as a complication of bacterial pneumonia, though it may occasionally follow viral pneumonia. Other, less common causes include:

- *Thoracic trauma:* Penetrating injuries to the chest.
- *Esophageal perforations:* Resulting from iatrogenic injury, ingestion of corrosive substances, or foreign bodies.
- *Post-surgical infections:* Following thoracotomy or esophageal anastomotic leaks.
- *Abscess extension:* From subdiaphragmatic sources such as liver or paravertebral abscesses.

S. Roy Choudhury
Pediatric Surgery, Lady Hardinge Medical College and Associated Kalawati Saran Children's Hospital, New Delhi, Delhi, India

P. S. Yadav (✉)
Department of Pediatric Surgery, LHMC, New Delhi, Delhi, India

23.2.1 Predisposing Conditions

- Chronic pulmonary diseases
- Diabetes mellitus
- Long-term corticosteroid use
- Immune suppression
- Congenital heart disease
- Recurrent aspiration pneumonia

23.3 Pathophysiology

The pleural space contains minimal fluid under normal conditions, maintained by a balance of production and absorption. An inflammatory process in the lung or surrounding areas disrupts this equilibrium, increasing fluid secretion through enhanced vascular permeability and the action of inflammatory cells and cytokines.

1. *Parapneumonic Effusion (PPE):*
   - Fluid accumulates in approximately 50% of pneumonia cases due to excess pulmonary interstitial fluid transudating across the visceral pleura.
   - Initially sterile, this fluid can become infected, leading to complicated PPE and eventually empyema.
2. *Progression to Empyema:*
   - Bacterial infection triggers coagulation cascade activation and reduced fibrinolysis, causing fibrin deposition.

© The Author(s), under exclusive license to Springer Nature Singapore Pte Ltd. 2025

S. Roy Choudhury (ed.), *Pediatric Surgery*, https://doi.org/10.1007/978-981-96-1257-4_23

- Loculations and septations form as fibrin strands compartmentalize the fluid.
- Over time, fibroblasts proliferate, forming a fibrous peel that traps the lung and prevents re-expansion.

3. *Differentiation Between Simple and Complicated PPE:*
   - Fluid analysis is used to distinguish transudates from exudates and detect signs of bacterial infection:
     - *Transudate* vs. *Exudate:* Determined by protein levels and Light's criteria:
       - Pleural fluid protein/serum protein ratio > 0.5
       - Pleural fluid LDH/serum LDH ratio > 0.6
     - Bacterial infection: Low pH, reduced glucose, elevated LDH, or positive Gram stain.

23.4 Stages of Empyema Thoracis

The *American Thoracic Society* recognizes three stages of empyema thoracis:

1. *Stage I (Exudative Phase):*
   - Early bacterial infection of a parapneumonic effusion marks this stage
   - Duration: 24–72 hours before progression to the next stage
2. *Stage II (Fibrinopurulent Phase):*
   - A pyogenic membrane forms, and fibrin strands create septations and loculations
   - This is the most common pathological stage in children
   - Duration: 7–10 days
   - Treatment: Intercostal tube drainage (ICD) with fibrinolytics or video-assisted thoracoscopic surgery (VATS)
3. *Stage III (Organizational Phase):*
   - A thick fibrous rind encases the lung, preventing re-expansion
   - Onset: Typically, 2–4 weeks after initial presentation
   - Treatment: Often requires surgical intervention

23.5 Microbiology

In developing countries, *Staphylococcus aureus* is the most common pathogen associated with empyema thoracis. Other causative organisms include:

- *Streptococcus pneumoniae*
- Various Gram-negative bacteria, such as:
  - *Enterobacteriaceae* (e.g., Klebsiella)
  - *Haemophilus influenzae*
  - *Pseudomonas aeruginosa*
- *Bacteroides*
- Less frequent species, *including Proteus*, *Salmonella*, *Yersinia*, and rare Streptococci. Rare pathogens include tuberculous empyema, fungal pathogens, Mycoplasma, *Legionella pneumophila*, adenovirus, and influenza virus.

23.6 Clinical Features

The initial presentation resembles pneumonia, with symptoms such as

- Cough, fever, breathlessness, malaise, fetor, loss of appetite, lethargy, pleuritic chest pain, and abdominal pain.
- Parapneumonic effusion should be suspected if there is:
  - Tachycardia and tachypnea
  - Decreased chest expansion
  - Stony dullness on percussion
  - Reduced or absent breath sounds
  - Tracheal deviation

Failure to improve with appropriate antibiotics should raise suspicion of an underlying effusion.

23.6.1 Investigations

1. *Blood Tests*
   (a) Complete Hemogram
       - Shows leukocytosis with neutrophilia and elevated erytherocyte sedimentation rate (ESR)

- Persistently high leukocyte counts may indicate residual fluid collection or complications like lung abscess
- C-reactive protein (CRP) levels are elevated and decrease with effective treatment
- Chronic empyema may result in thrombocytosis, though it rarely requires intervention
- Anemia and thrombocytopenia may signal severe disease, while lymphocytosis may point toward tubercular empyema

(b) *Blood Culture*
- Blood cultures are often sterile due to prior antibiotic use, but are crucial for guiding therapy in positive cases

(c) *Coagulation Profile*
- Coagulation studies are necessary before surgical interventions

(d) *Serum Electrolytes and Renal Function Tests*
- Baseline tests are essential and must be monitored in patients with complications like hemolytic uremic syndrome or syndrome of inappropriate antidiuretic hormone secretion (SIADH)

2. *Mantoux Test*
   - Recommended in cases where tuberculosis is suspected
3. *Pleural Fluid Analysis*

(a) *Biochemistry*
- Analyze pleural fluid for pH, glucose, LDH, and adenosine deaminase (ADA) levels

(b) *Microbiology*
- Pleural fluid aspirates should undergo
  - Microscopy
  - Gram staining
  - Culture (bacterial and tubercular)
  - Differential cell count (polymorphonuclear leukocyte predominance is common)

Culture positivity rates for pleural fluid are variable, and samples are frequently sterile. Advanced techniques like 16S rDNA PCR offer rapid and accurate identification of pathogens in culture-negative cases.

4. *Sputum Analysis*
   - If the child can expectorate, send sputum for Gram stain and culture to aid in diagnosis.

23.7 Radiological Investigations

23.7.1 Chest Radiograph

- *Minimal Effusion:* Blunting of the costophrenic angle is observed.
- *Progressive Fluid Accumulation:* Increased haziness in the hemithorax, with tracheal deviation toward the opposite side (Figs. 23.1 and 23.2). Rib crowding and secondary scoliosis are effects of long-standing empyema.
- *Consolidation* vs. *Effusion:* A mediastinal shift toward the affected side on a radiograph often suggests consolidation rather than effusion.

23.7.2 Chest Ultrasonography (USG)

- *Differentiation of Fluid and Consolidation:* USG can distinguish between chest fluid and lung collapse or consolidation, where radiographs show both as haziness.
- *Staging Empyema:* It identifies features like:
  - Echogenicity in the fluid
  - Presence of loculations and pleural thickening

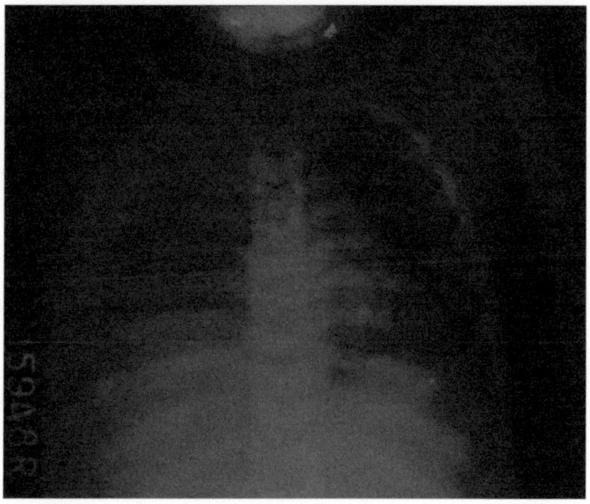

Fig. 23.1 X-ray chest, right empyema

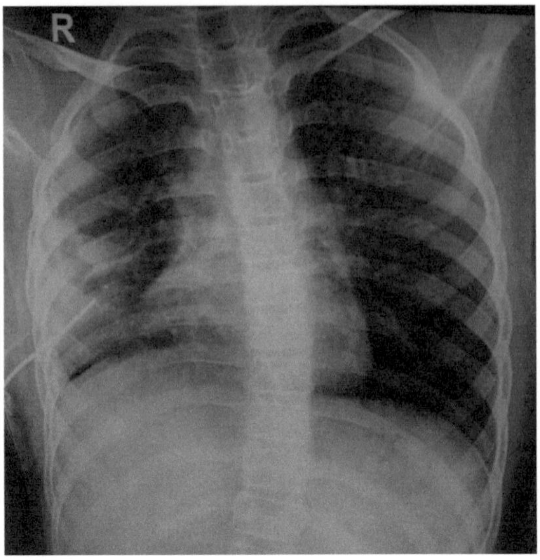

Fig. 23.2 X-ray chest, right empyema with intercostal tube in situ, demonstrating rib crowding and secondary scoliosis

- *Quantitative and Qualitative Fluid Assessment:*
  - Empyema volume can be estimated as mild, moderate, or severe
  - Quantitative measurement uses formulas based on the maximum perpendicular interpleural distance in sitting and supine positions
- *Guided Procedures:* USG assists in:
  - Thoracocentesis
  - Chest drain placement into the pus collection area
- *Monitoring Residual Fluid:* Useful for evaluating residual collections post-treatment
- *Key Advantages:* USG is portable, readily available, and can be repeated as needed for the bedside evaluation of empyema.

23.7.3 Contrast-Enhanced CT (CECT) Chest

- *Indications:* Recommended when surgical intervention, such as decortication, is being considered.
- *Key Features:*
  - *Pleural Split Sign:* Thickening of the parietal and visceral pleura with intervening fluid collection, suggestive of chronic empyema (Fig. 23.3a, b).
  - *Subcostal Fat Findings:* Increased fat and fat stranding.
  - Better visualization of a thickened pleural peel (Fig. 23.4a, b), pus collection, consolidated lung (Fig. 23.5a, b), and associated lung abnormalities (e.g., lung abscess or tumors).
- *Complications:* High-resolution CT (HRCT) can identify complications such as necrotizing pneumonia and bronchopleural fistulas.

23.7.4 Management

The primary goal of empyema management is to clear the pleural cavity of collections, break loculations, and allow lung re-expansion. For advanced-stage empyema, surgical excision of the thickened pleural peel may be required. Management *includes treatment of underlying pneumonia with antibiotics and, for empyema, drainage is a key component.*

23.7.5 Supportive Therapy

Supportive care is essential and includes:

- *Oxygen supplementation:* For respiratory distress with SpO2 < 95%.
- *Intravenous fluids and nutrition:* To maintain hydration and caloric intake.
- *Analgesia and antipyretics:* For pain relief and fever control.
- *Early ambulation and deep breathing:* To improve lung function.
- *Antibiotics:* Empiric therapy with amoxicillin-clavulanic acid or a cephalosporin (e.g., cefotaxime, ceftriaxone) until culture and sensitivity results are available.

23.7.6 Drainage

Pleural space drainage is critical in empyema management and may include the use of fibrinolytics:

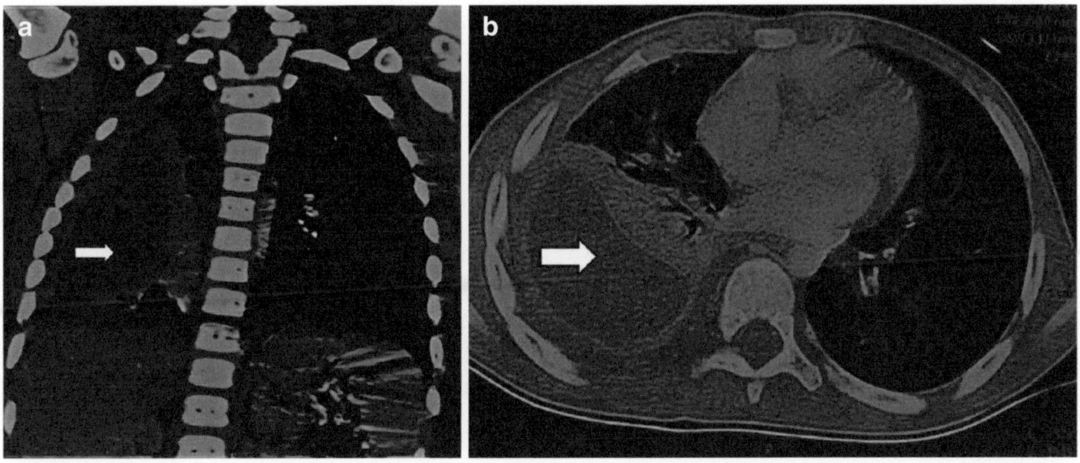

Fig. 23.3 (**a**, **b**) CT scan chest showing pleural collection with the split pleural sign (block arrow)

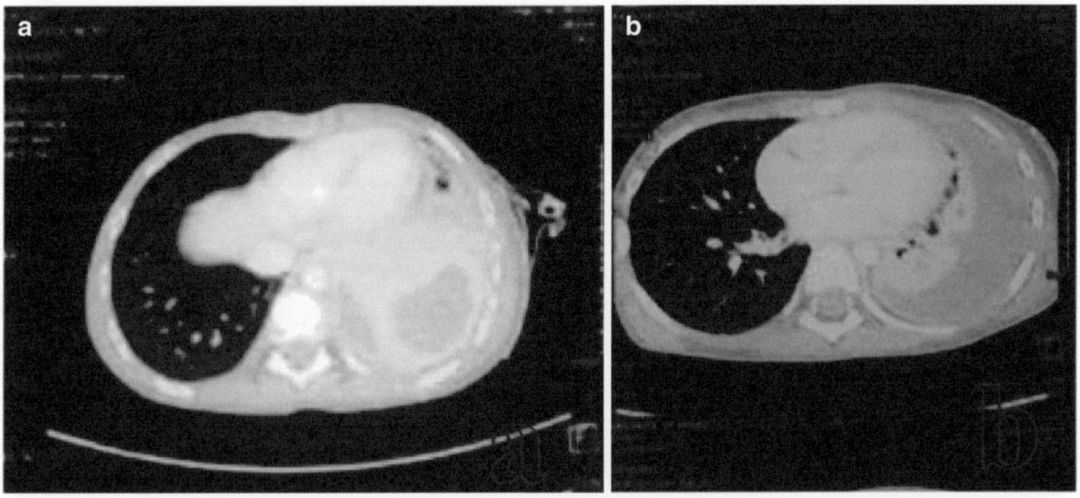

Fig. 23.4 CT chest showing organized empyema with (**a**) left thick pleural peel and (**b**) collapsed left lung

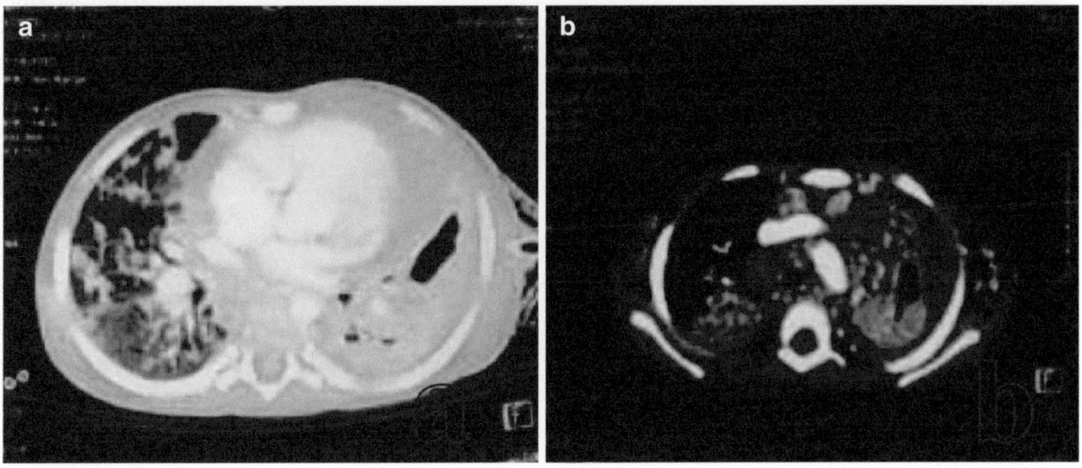

Fig. 23.5 (**a**) Consolidation of lung right side, left empyema. (**b**) Note air-bronchogram within the consolidation (cf. empyema on the left side)

1. *Intercostal Tube Drainage (ICD):*
   - Inserted under local anesthesia or sedation using an appropriately sized tube (16–24 Fr) in the fifth intercostal space at the mid-axillary line
   - Bubbling in the chest drain indicates a bronchopleural fistula, and low-pressure suction may be applied if accompanied by residual pneumothorax
2. *Fibrinolytics:*
   - Fibrinolytic agents, such as urokinase or tissue plasminogen activator (tPA), help break loculations and fibrin deposition
   - *Urokinase Dose:*
     - Children >10 kg: 40,000 IU in 0.9% normal saline, instilled through the chest tube and clamped for 3–4 h
     - Children <10 kg: 10,000 IU
   - Instillations are done twice daily for up to 3 days.

23.7.7 Guidelines for Managing the Intercostal Tube

- *Positioning:* The underwater seal bottle must be upright and placed below chest level.
- *Monitoring:* Keep records of drained fluid volume, temperature, pulse, and fluid balance.
- *Clamping Instructions:*
  - Bubbling chest drains should never be clamped.
  - If chest pain or breathlessness occurs, unclamp the chest drain immediately.
- *Removal of the Chest Tube:*
  - Remove the tube once fluid drainage reduces to <1–2 mL/kg/24 hours.
  - During removal:
    - Older children: Perform Valsalva's maneuver.
    - Younger children: Remove during expiration to prevent air entry.
  - Apply a sterile occlusive dressing and leave it undisturbed for 48 h.
  - A post-removal chest radiograph ensures no pneumothorax.

23.7.8 Surgical Management (Table 23.1)

23.7.8.1 Indications

Surgical intervention is necessary in the following cases:

1. Lack of improvement after adequate antibiotic therapy and drainage
2. Thick, septate pleural collections that cannot be aspirated or drained with a chest tube
3. Advanced-stage empyema (stage III)

23.7.9 Types of Surgical Management

1. *Debridement*
   - Open surgical debridement or VATS (video-assisted thoracoscopic surgery) is effective in the fibrinopurulent stage (stage II)
   - Early debridement is associated with shorter hospital stays and quicker recovery
2. *Decortication*
   - Performed in the organized (stage III) phase of empyema (Fig. 23.6a, b)
   - Involves removing the thickened parietal and visceral pleura encasing the lung, allowing for re-expansion
   - *Procedure:*
     - Access via a posterolateral thoracotomy
     - Muscle-sparing techniques (e.g., between latissimus dorsi and serratus anterior) minimize chest wall deformities
     - Avoid entering the empyema cavity if possible, but ensure removal of the pleural peel
     - Take care to avoid mediastinal and subclavian vessels
     - A wide-bore chest drain is placed postoperatively, and epidural analgesia is provided for pain relief
   - *Contraindications:*
     - Severely damaged lung parenchyma or necrotizing pneumonia
     - Coagulopathy or hemodynamic instability (relative contraindications)

Table 23.1 Management of empyema (*VATS* video-assisted thoracoscopic surgery, *HRCT* high-resolution contrast CT)

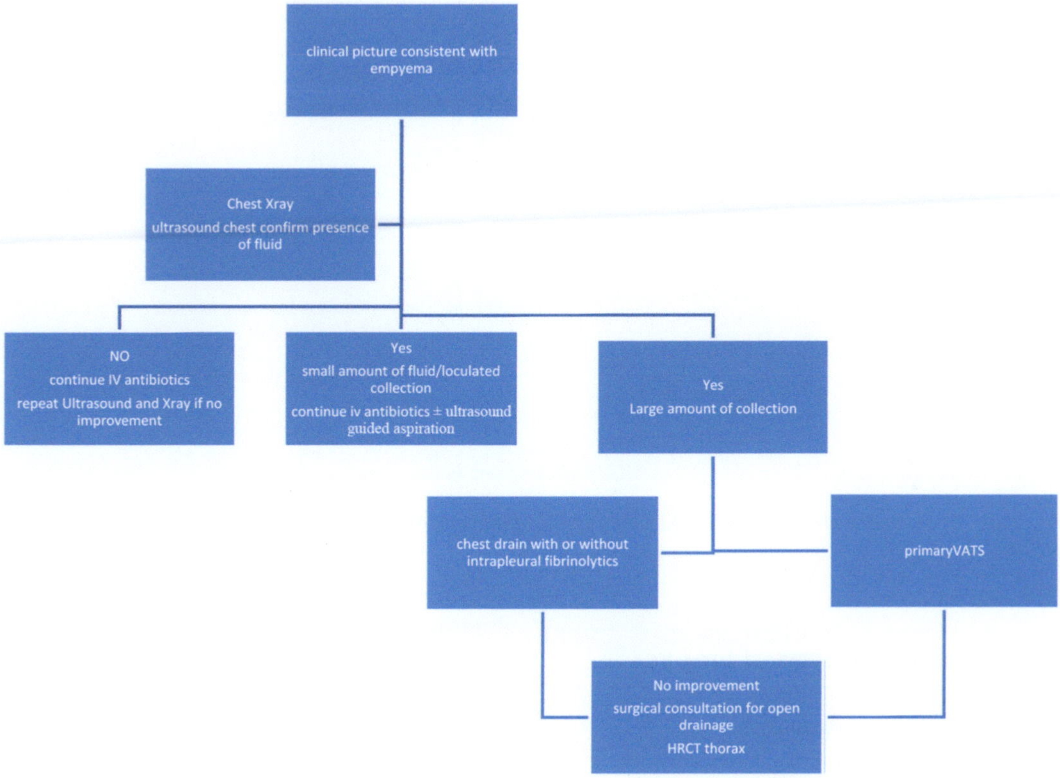

3. *VATS for Empyema*
   - Best suited for early empyema (within 1–2 weeks)
   - Advantages:
     - Reduced pain
     - Better cosmetic outcomes
     - Shorter hospital stays
   - Challenges: Thoracoscopic decortication of thick pleural peels is technically demanding
4. *Management of Bronchopleural Fistula*
   - Persistent fistulas, often due to necrotizing pneumonia or lung abscesses, require:
     - Adequate chest drainage
     - Decortication with suture closure of the fistula or muscle flap thoracoplasty (e.g., from serratus anterior or latissimus dorsi)

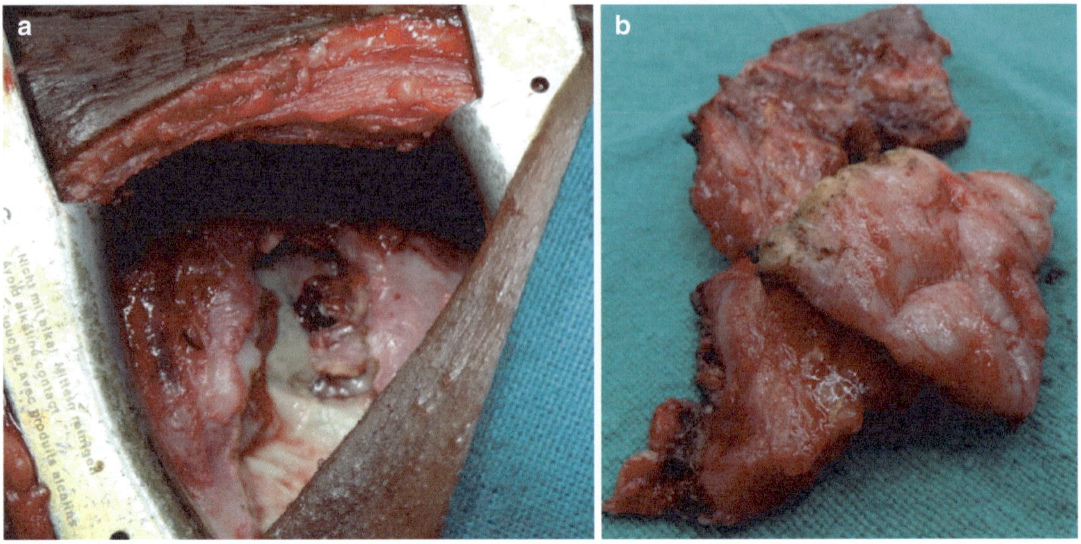

Fig. 23.6 Open decortications (**a**) thickened parietal pleura with underlying pus collection. (**b**) Removed thick parietal pleura

23.8 Complications of Empyema

1. *Empyema Necessitans*
   - Pus can extend along a vessel to the chest wall, forming a fluctuating chest swelling known as empyema necessitans
2. *Rupture into Adjacent Structures*
   - Empyema may rupture into the following areas:
     - *Airway:* Causing bronchopleural fistula and potential respiratory complications
     - *Pericardium:* Leading to life-threatening purulent pericarditis
3. *Spread to Distant Sites*
   - The infection can spread to:
     - *Brain:* Resulting in intracranial complications such as brain abscess
     - *Bone:* Leading to osteomyelitis
4. *Chronic Changes*
   - *Decreased functional lung volume:* Persistent loss of lung function due to incomplete re-expansion
   - *Chest wall collapse:* Accompanied by rib crowding, commonly seen in chronic empyema cases

Summary

1. *Definition:* Empyema thoracis refers to the accumulation of pus within the thoracic cavity, typically caused by pneumonia or extensions from surrounding structures such as the esophagus or liver.
2. *Stages:* The disease progresses through three distinct stages:
   - *Exudative phase (Stage 1):* Initial inflammation with sterile effusion.
   - *Fibrinopurulent phase (Stage 2):* Formation of fibrin, loculations, and pyogenic membranes.
   - *Organization phase (Stage 3):* Development of a fibrous peel that restricts lung expansion.

   The first two stages last from a few days to weeks.
3. *Investigations:* Hematological, biochemical, and microbiological tests are vital for diagnosis, tracking disease progression, and evaluating therapeutic response.
4. *Imaging:* Radiological tools such as ultrasonography and CT scans assist in diagnosis and help plan management strategies.

5. *Medical Management:* The primary approach includes supportive care, appropriate antibiotics, and pleural space drainage to halt disease progression.
6. *Surgical Intervention:* Persistent symptoms or the presence of a thick pleural peel with pleural collection preventing lung re-expansion necessitate surgical intervention, which may include VATS (video-assisted thoracoscopic surgery) or open decortication.

Suggested Reading

Coran AG, Caldamone A, Scott Adzich N, Krummel TM, Laberge JM, editors. Pediatric surgery. 7th ed. Oxford: Elsevier Limited; 2012.

Parikh DH, Crabbe DCG, Auldist AW, Rotherberg SS, editors. Pediatric thoracic surgery. 1st ed. London: Springer-Verlag; 2009.

St Peter SD, Holcomb GW, Murphy JP, editors. Holcomb and ashcraft's pediatric surgery. 7th ed. Elsevier Limited; 2019.

Congenital Diaphragmatic Hernia and Eventration

24

Subhasis Roy Choudhury and Vishesh Jain

24.1 Introduction

Congenital diaphragmatic hernia (CDH) is defined as a defect in the diaphragm during its development which allows herniation of abdominal contents into the thoracic cavity. CDH occurs in 1 per 2000–5000 live births, and one-third remains stillborn. Associated anomalies are a significant cause of poor outcomes. Antenatal diagnosis helps in prognostication and planning the management. Current management strategies have resulted in 70–80% survival of live-born babies. A significant proportion of 25–35% of prenatally diagnosed CDH remains unborn, representing the most severe disease with hidden mortality.

24.1.1 Site of Defect

Left-sided defect occurs in 80%, right-sided defect in 20%, and bilateral CDH cases are rare.

24.1.2 Associated Anomalies

Non-hernia-related anomalies occur in 40% of the cases of postnatally diagnosed CDH, which include congenital heart defects, chromosomal anomalies, tracheobronchial anomalies, musculoskeletal, and neural tube defects. CDH cases have abnormal intestinal rotation and fixation. The survival of isolated CDH cases is significantly better than those with associated non-hernia-related anomalies. All antenatally diagnosed cases merit detailed chromosomal analysis, microarray, and genetic studies in order to prognosticate and counsel the family.

S. Roy Choudhury
Pediatric Surgery, Lady Hardinge Medical College and Associated Kalawati Saran Children's Hospital, New Delhi, Delhi, India

V. Jain (✉)
Department of Pediatric Surgery, AIIMS, New Delhi, India

24.2 Embryology of Congenital Diaphragmatic Hernia (CDH) (Fig. 24.1)

- Anterior central tendon develops from the septum transversum

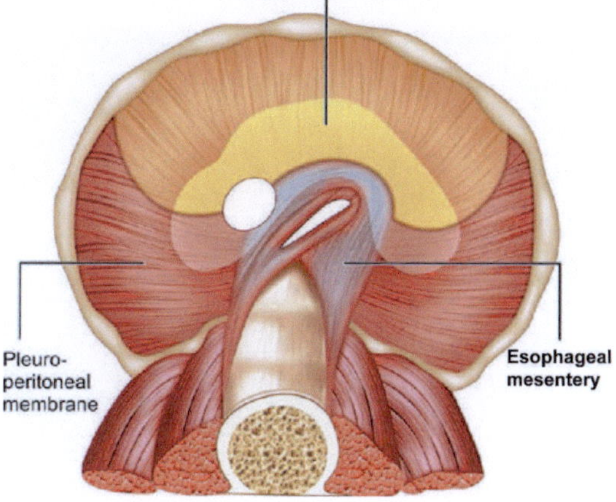

Fig. 24.1 Development of the diaphragm

© The Author(s), under exclusive license to Springer Nature Singapore Pte Ltd. 2025

S. Roy Choudhury (ed.), *Pediatric Surgery*, https://doi.org/10.1007/978-981-96-1257-4_24

- The crura evolve from the esophageal mesentery
- The dorsolateral portion develops from the pleuroperitoneal membranes
- Muscular portion develops from the thoracic intercostal muscle group

Complete closure of the pleuroperitoneal canal occurs by the eighth week of gestation. The midgut returns to the abdomen by the ninth to tenth week. If the canal remains patent during this period (failure of muscular fusion), then CDH occurs. Experimental nitrofen-induced CDH models in mice closely represent the defects seen in human fetuses.

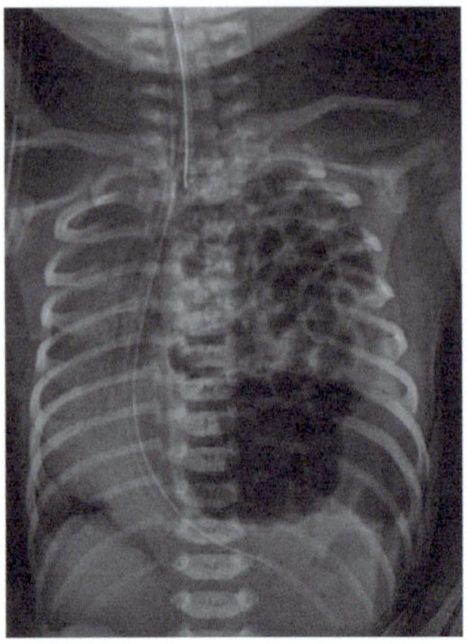

Fig. 24.2a Chest x-ray, left congenital diaphragmatic hernia

24.3 Types of Diaphragmatic Hernia

- Posterolateral foramen of Bochdalek hernia (most common) (Figs. 24.2a and 24.2b)
- Foramen of Morgagni hernia (between sternal and costal attachment) (Fig. 24.3a, b)
- Esophageal hiatus hernia (discussed in Chap. 38)
- Acquired/Traumatic

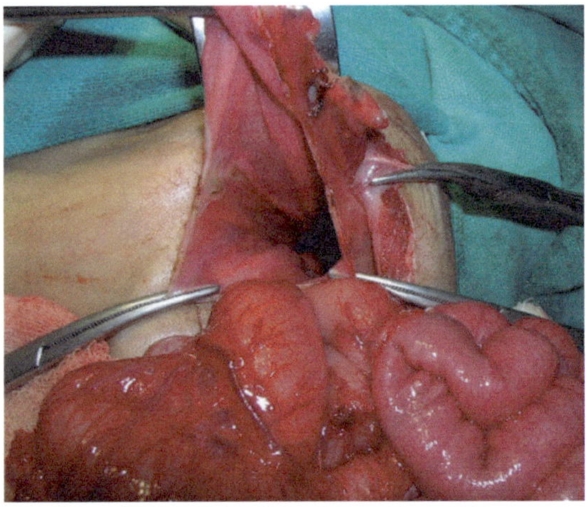

Fig. 24.2b Left CDH with sac at surgery

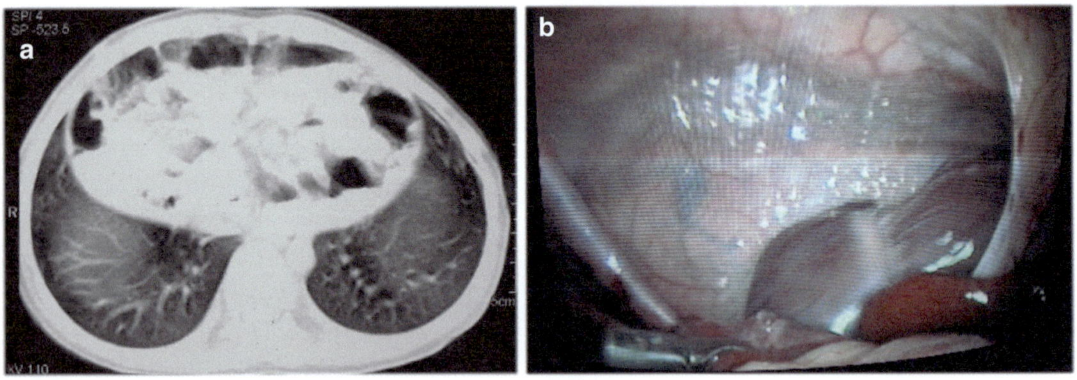

Fig. 24.3 Intrapericardial hernia through the foramen of Morgagni, (**a**) CECT scan and (**b**) laparoscopic view

24.4 Pathology

In 90% of cases, CDH occurs without a hernia sac, while a sac is present in 10% of cases. This sac is evident as a thin membrane between the herniated contents and the lung. The contents of the hernia will depend on the laterality of the defect. The more common left-sided CDH usually contains the stomach, bowel, spleen, and the left lobe of the liver.

24.5 Pathophysiology

Lung development (see Chap. 25) determines prognosis in CDH patients. Pulmonary hypoplasia and decreased pulmonary vascular bed led to pulmonary hypertension, persistence of fetal circulation with right-to-left shunt and desaturation. Factors that predispose to respiratory distress are hypoxia, acidosis, hypothermia, and stress.

24.6 Pathogenesis of Respiratory Distress in CDH

- *Pulmonary hypertension*
  - Extensive muscularization of the pulmonary vessels causes persistent pulmonary hypertension (PPH of the newborn)
  - Decreased cross-sectional area of the pulmonary vascular bed
- *Pulmonary hypoplasia*
  - Reduced airway branching
  - Reduced number of alveoli
- *Compression* of ipsilateral and contralateral lung by herniated contents.

Pulmonary hypertension results in a right-to-left shunt, which results in poorly oxygenated blood reaching peripheral circulation and ultimately the lungs. This causes further constriction of pulmonary arterioles, resulting in increased pulmonary vascular resistance. This results in a vicious cycle with rapidly deteriorating hypoxia, hypercarbia, and acidosis.

24.6.1 Diagnosis

Antenatal diagnosis can be made with an ultrasound scan in 40–90% cases, showing the presence of bowel loops at the level of the heart compressing on the lung (see Chap. 7). Polyhydramnios is present in 80% of cases. The presence of the liver in the chest and severe mediastinal compression with hydrops fetalis are poor prognostic signs. MRI can offer better visualization of the structural anatomy, including a volumetric measurement of the lung; total fetal lung volume (TFLV), which has been correlated with survival.

24.6.2 Antenatal Management

Discussed in Chap. 7.

24.6.3 Postnatal Presentation

The clinical presentation is with different degrees of respiratory distress and a scaphoid abdomen. In newborn patients, the delayed appearance of symptoms indicates better lung reserve and hence better prognosis.

X-ray chest is useful for the diagnosis, which shows bowel loops in the thoracic cavity and mediastinal shift with paucity of abdominal gas shadow (Fig. 24.2a). Other imaging studies, like oral contrast study, ultrasonography, or CT scan, are occasionally required to differentiate CDH from any cystic lung diseases. Echocardiography is essential to assess the degree of pulmonary hypertension and any associated cardiac anomaly.

24.6.4 Eventration of the Diaphragm

Eventration of the diaphragm refers to elevation of the dome of the diaphragm into the thoracic cavity (Fig. 24.4). In contrast to CDH, the diaphragm retains its attachment to the costal margins with the absence of any definite defect in the diaphragm. Eventration of the diaphragm can be

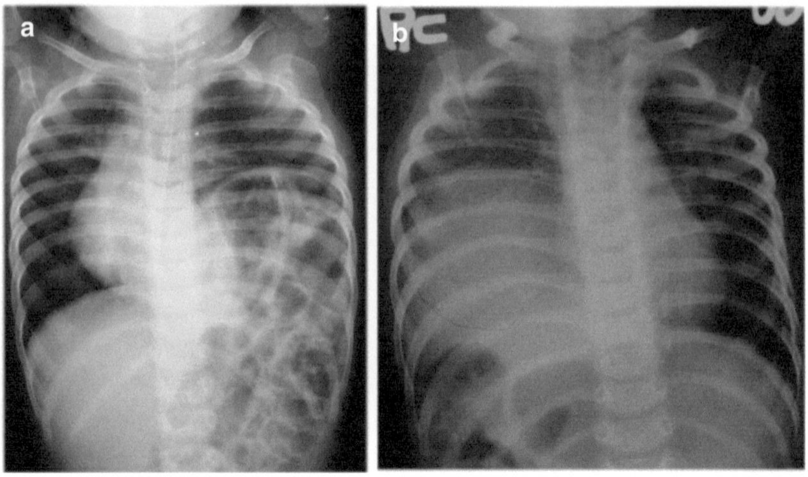

Fig. 24.4 (**a**) Chest X-ray, left eventration of the diaphragm, (**b**) Right eventration of the diaphragm

congenital or acquired due to injury to the phrenic nerve. The clinical presentation is with respiratory symptoms. Symptomatic patients require surgical repair, generally in the form of plication or excision of the sac and repair of the diaphragm using a nonabsorbable suture, either by open or thoracoscopic approach.

24.7 Postnatal Management of CDH (Fig. 24.5)

Initial stabilization: Bag and mask ventilation is to be avoided as it will distend the stomach or bowel present in the thoracic cavity.

- CDH is a *Physiological emergency* and not a surgical *emergency*. Delayed surgical repair after stabilization (resolution/stabilization of pulmonary hypertension) is the preferred treatment.
- *Preoperative Strategy*
  - Resuscitation: endotracheal intubation for ventilation in symptomatic patients.
  - Nasogastric aspiration to decompress the abdominal contents.
  - Establish umbilical venous and arterial lines.
  - Principles of ventilation are pressure-limited ventilation to minimize lung injury. Conventional mechanical ventilation initiated with a peak inspiratory pressure of <25 cm H2O, PEEP: 3–5 cm H2O, and a ventilatory rate of 40–60/min. The goal is to maintain preductal $PaO_2 > 60$ mmHg and $PaCO_2 < 60$ mmHg. Failure to maintain these goals may require the ventilation to be converted to high-frequency ventilation mode.
  - Sedation and reduced handling to prevent sudden reactive pulmonary hypertension.
  - Muscle paralysis is not always indicated.
  - Adequate fluid balance to maintain peripheral perfusion. Vasoactive drugs like dopamine, dobutamine, epinephrine, and milrinone can be added if needed.
- *Pharmacological Therapy*

Currently used drugs in CDH with the aim of decreasing pulmonary hypertension:

- Phosphodiesterase 5 inhibitors: sildenafil
- Calcium channel blockers
- Prostacyclin derivatives
- Endothelin receptor antagonist
- Nitric oxide (inhaled nitric oxide, iNO) for persistent pulmonary hypertension of neonates (PPHN)

Inotropes are not routinely indicated and are used if there is shock or poor perfusion.

Failure to stabilize on conventional ventilation will require the following measures in sequence (Fig. 24.5):

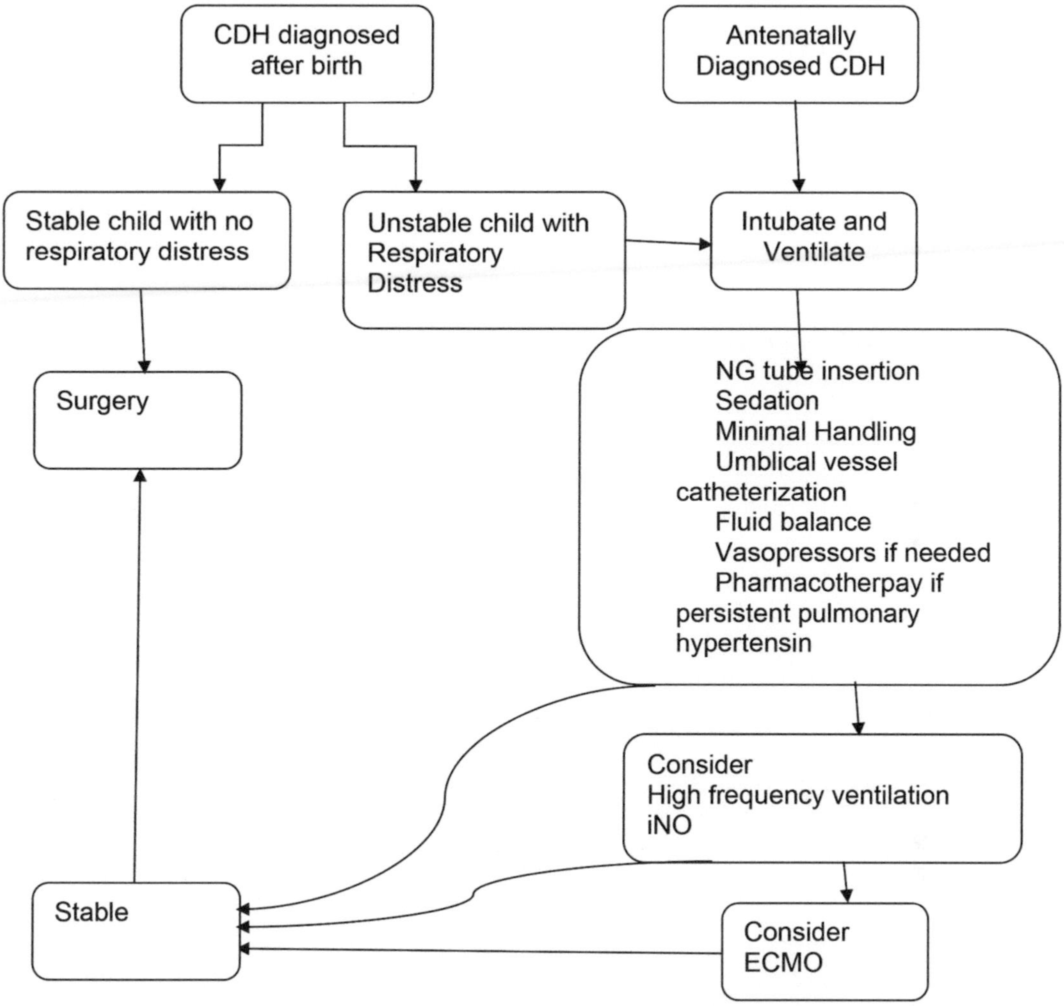

Fig. 24.5 Management algorithm for CDH

(a) Inhaled nitric oxide (iNO) causes pulmonary vasodilatation
(b) High-frequency ventilation (HFV) avoids barotrauma
(c) Extracorporeal membrane oxygenation (ECMO) helps by resting the lungs

The CDH EURO Consortium consensus is as follows.

Physiological stabilization, which is loosely defined as 24 h of the following:

- Mean arterial blood pressure is normal for gestational age, off inotropes
- Preductal saturation levels of >85% SaO_2 in an FiO_2 of <50% off iNO
- Lactate <3 mmol/L
- Urine output >2 mL/kg/hr
- No signs of PH

24.7.1 Operation

Surgical approach for repair of CDH may be abdominal or thoracic. Both open and minimally invasive thoracoscopic, laparoscopic, and robotic techniques are performed. The herniated contents are reduced back into the abdominal cavity. If a hernia sac is present, it should be excised. The diaphragm should be repaired with nonabsorbable suture after defining the edges of the defect. In case of a very large defect, synthetic patch repair (PTFE or Prolene mesh) may be appropriate. The abdominal wall muscle flap may also be considered to cover the defect. Insertion of an intercostal drainage tube is not mandatory.

24.8 Prognostic Factors (Fetal and Postnatal)

- Lung-to-head ratio (LHR in fetus) is calculated as the area of the contralateral lung in mm divided by the head circumference at the level of the four-chamber view of the heart. LHR less than one carries a poor prognosis, and >1.6 has a good survival rate. There is disproportionate growth of the chest in the later part of gestation, resulting in spontaneous improvement in LHR. To account for this observed/expected LHR is used. O/E LHR <25% has 12–30% survival, whereas value <35% has 65–88% survival. The liver position in the chest is associated with poor outcome.
- Gestational age: early herniation is associated with poor prognosis.
- Stomach position: in the chest is associated with poor prognosis.
- Polyhydramnios: associated with poor prognosis.
- Cardiac anomaly: associated with poor prognosis.
- Defect size: larger is associated with poor outcome.

24.8.1 Outcome

Long-Term Morbidity

Chronic lung disease, neurocognitive delay, hearing impairment, musculoskeletal deformities, gastroesophageal reflux disease, operative complications, including intestinal obstruction and recurrence of hernia. A post-operative follow-up protocol for CDH patients is essential.

24.9 Summary

Antenatal diagnosis has a high accuracy rate of diagnosis of CDH. Fetal LHR (observed versus expected O/E LHR) has a good prognostic value. Low LHR, maternal polyhydramnios, associated anomalies, stomach and liver herniation are poor prognostic factors. The current strategy of postnatal management is initial stabilization followed by surgical repair. A Long-term follow-up is necessary to address multi-system problems in the survivors of CDH patients.

Suggested Reading

Coran AG, Caldamone A, Scott Adzich N, Krummel TM, Laberge JM, editors. Pediatric surgery. 7th ed. Oxford: Elsevier Limited; 2012.

Holcomb GW III, Murphy PJ, Ostile DJ, editors. Ashcrafts pediatric surgery. 6th ed. Philadelphia: Saunders, Elsevier; 2014.

Lally PK. Congenital diaphragmatic hernia—current status. Seminar Pediatr Surgery. 2007;16(2):79–134.

25 Congenital Lung Lesions

Sujoy Neogi and Subhasis Roy Choudhury

25.1 Introduction

Congenital lung lesions are a spectrum of developmental anomalies involving the lung and the airway with overlapping pathological features and varying clinical presentations. The pathological types are related to their occurrence at different embryonic stages of development. Pre- and post-natal management of these lesions requires a thorough understanding of the evolution and progress, and working out an appropriate plan.

25.2 Commonly Used Terminologies for Congenital Lung Lesions

Congenital cystic adenomatoid malformation (CCAM)/Congenital pulmonary airway malformation (CPAM)
Congenital lobar emphysema (CLE)
Broncho-pulmonary sequestrations (BPS)
Foregut duplication cysts/bronchogenic cysts

All these lesions are now grouped under one broad name, bronchopulmonary foregut malformation (BPFGM). Hybrid lesions are a mixture of CPAM and BPS. Out of all these, CPAM is the most common lesion, followed by BPS. Other rare lesions are bronchial atresia, lymphangiomas, bronchogenic cysts, and pleuro-pulmonary blastema.

25.3 Embryology

The development of the lungs starts from the third week of gestation till eight years. The development goes through these five stages. (1) The *embryonic stage* starts from the third week of gestation when the lung starts to grow as a diverticulum from the foregut at the level of the laryngotracheal groove, which continues till the 6th week. (2) The *pseudoglandular stage* extends from the 7th to 16th week of gestation when bronchial airways develop. Conducting airways, i.e., trachea to terminal bronchiole, grow till 16 weeks. (3) The *canalicular stage* extends between 16 and 24 weeks when alveolar airspaces develop. Type 1 and type 2 pneumocytes (precursor of surfactant) begin to differentiate, and gas exchange becomes functionally possible at the end of this stage. (4) The *saccular stage* happens between 24 weeks to term when the maturation of alveoli and development of pulmonary vasculature occur. (5) The *alveolar stage* extends from birth to 8 years, when alveolar maturation and multiplication continue.

At the end of six weeks, tracheoesophageal separation starts. The primitive lung bud form by

S. Neogi (✉)
Department of Pediatric Surgery, MAMC, New Delhi, India

S. Roy Choudhury
Pediatric Surgery, Lady Hardinge Medical College and Associated Kalawati Saran Children's Hospital, New Delhi, Delhi, India

© The Author(s), under exclusive license to Springer Nature Singapore Pte Ltd. 2025

S. Roy Choudhury (ed.), *Pediatric Surgery*, https://doi.org/10.1007/978-981-96-1257-4_25

the end of the seventh week with 5 major lobes, 3–5 orders of bronchi. There is embryological, clinical, and histopathological overlap between these anomalies. This leads to a possible shared etiology between these anomalies, like the obstruction of the fetal airway. The various lesions may vary due to severity, timing, and duration of obstruction.

Recently, there has been an increased rate of antenatally diagnosed lung lesions due to advancements of prenatal ultrasonography.

Table 25.1 Classification of CCAM

	Stocker	Adzick
Cyst size	I > 2 cm II <2 cm III solid	Macrocystic >5 mm Microcystic <5 mm
Associated anomalies	II	Microcystic
Prognosis		
Favorable Unfavorable	I III	Macrocystic Microcystic
Echogenicity		
Solid (echogenic) Cystic (echolucent)	III I, II	Microcystic Macrocystic

25.4 Antenatal Diagnosis and Treatment

25.4.1 Congenital Pulmonary Airway Malformation (CPAM) (Formerly Known as Congenital Cystic Adenomatoid Malformation)

The recent data from United States shows the probable incidence is 1.5 per 10,000 live births.

25.4.1.1 Embryo-Pathology

Excessive proliferation of terminal respiratory bronchioles, thus forming cysts of various sizes, results in the formation of CPAM. CPAM, on gross examination, is a discrete intrapulmonary mass that contains cysts ranging in diameter from 1 mm to over 10 cm. There may be multiple small connections with the tracheobronchial tree. It generally involves one lobe of the lung with a preference for the lower lobes. Stoker classified them into three types based primarily on the cyst size, but this classification has little clinical significance. Adzick classified these antenatally detected lesions into two types: macrocystic type (Cyst >5 mm) and microcystic type, which appear as a solid echogenic mass on sonography (Table 25.1).

25.4.1.2 Antenatal Diagnosis

These lesions can be diagnosed on routine antenatal sonography. There can be fetal hydrops associated with large lesions. For better delineation of them, fetal MRI can be beneficial (see Chap. 7).

25.4.1.3 Prognosis

The large microcystic (solid) varieties are more often associated with hydrops and are therefore a bad prognosis. Other prognostic factors identified are the lung-to-thorax transverse ratio (L/T) and CPAM volume ratio (CVR), which is derived from the CPAM volume/head circumference. The CVR is more commonly used for prognostication, and a CVR >1.6 carries an 80% chance of developing hydrops.

25.4.2 Management of CPAM

The outcome of antenatally diagnosed CPAM varies from fetal demise to spontaneous regression in 40% of cases. If the presentation is early gestation at 24–32 weeks with symptomatic lesions, fetal surgery can salvage (Chap. 7). For asymptomatic and late gestation fetuses, treatment after delivery is recommended. Chest x-ray may pick up the lesion; however, chest CT scan is more accurate in the diagnosis (Figs. 25.1, 25.2 and 25.3). A close differential diagnosis for some of the large macrocystic lesions is a pneumatocele arising from staphylococcal pneumonia. Sometimes they are confused with pneumothorax and managed with inadvertent intercostal tube insertion (Figs. 25.1 and 25.2) that results in the persistence of the lesion with air leak. Surgical treatment is by lobectomy of the involved lobe (Figs. 25.4, 25.5 and 25.6). A big and intense debate exists nowadays for the management of asymptomatic lesions postnatally. One group supports conservative management with follow-up based on the observation of

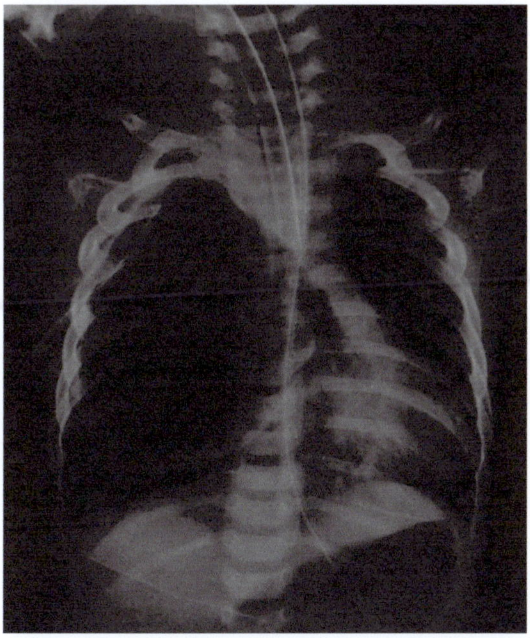

Fig. 25.1 CXR, Macrocystic CPAM right upper lobe, note the intercostal tube in place

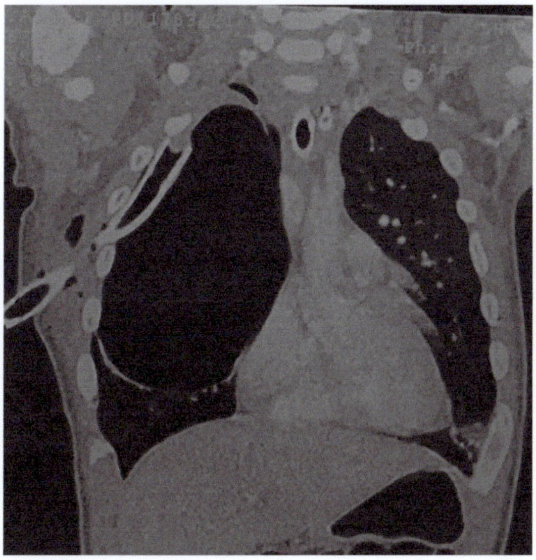

Fig. 25.2 CT CPAM right upper lobe

spontaneous resolution that has been reported with the maturity of the lung. On the other hand, many advocate early surgery between 3 and6 months due to the following reasons: (1) recurrent infections making resections difficult later on, (2) chances of developing malignancy (bronchoalveolar carcinoma and rhabdomyosarcoma), and (3) nonexistent upper limit of follow-up.

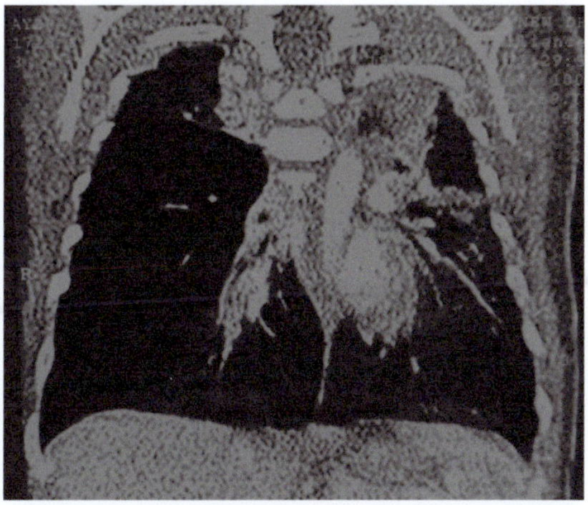

Fig. 25.3 CT Right middle lobe CPAM

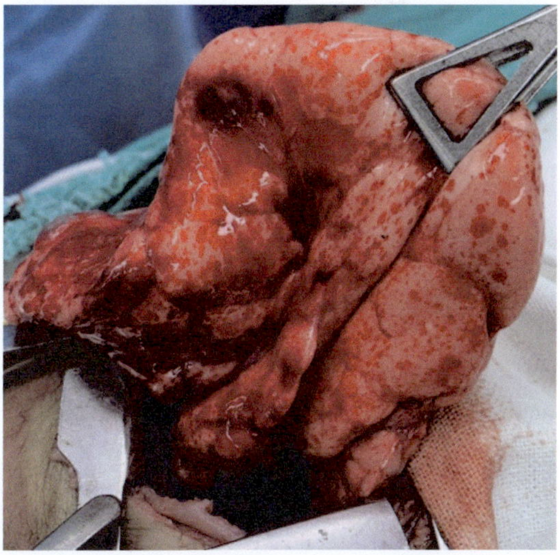

Fig. 25.4 Rt middle lobe CPAM at surgery

25.4.3 Congenital Lobar Emphysema (CLE)

The incidence of CLE in children is 1 per 20,000 to 1 per 30,000. The hallmark feature of CLE is hyperinflation of a pulmonary lobe due to air trapping, also called congenital lobar overinflation (CLO). This leads to concomitant compression of the remaining lung tissue and displacement

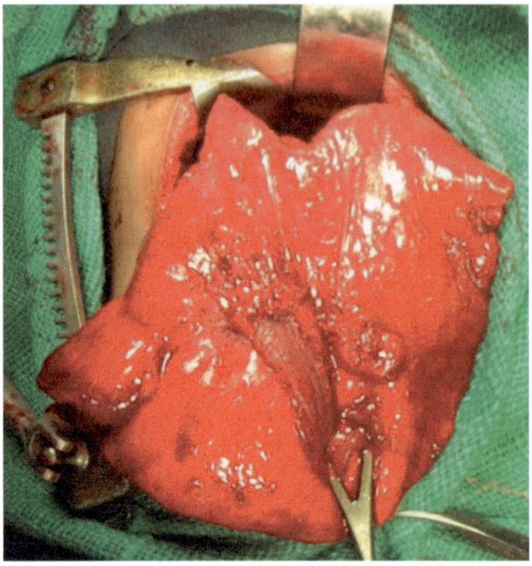

Fig. 25.5 Microcystic CPAM at surgery, solid appearance

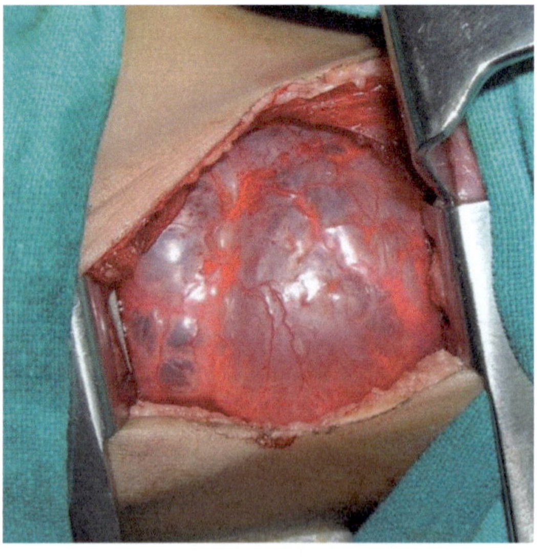

Fig. 25.6 Macrocystic CPAM (large cyst) at surgery

of the mediastinum by herniation of the affected lobe into the opposite side of the chest.

25.4.4 Embryo-Pathology

The primary pathology of CLE could be bronchomalacia with focal cartilaginous deficiency leading to valvular type of action, which thereby leads to air trapping. The patency of the airways is still present. The different etiologies of CLE are given in Table 25.2.

Table 25.2 Etiology of CLE

1	Idiopathic 50%
2	Bronchial cartilage absence, hypoplasia, dysplasia 25%
3	Panrenchymal disease Polyalveolar lobe Pulmonary alveolar glycogenosis
4	Internal bronchial obstruction Bronchial stenosis Bronchomalacia Meconium aspiration Hypertrophic mucosa membrane Mold mucus plaques Foreign body aspirations Bronchial polyps
5	External bronchial obstruction Pulmonary artery sling anomaly Pulmonary rotation anomaly Bronchogenic cyst Lymphadenopathy Mediastinal mass Duplication of esophagus

Clinical Presentation CLE presents with pediatric surgical emergency. One-fourth present at time of birth with respiratory distress**,** 50% present by one month**,** *and almost all* cases present by 6 months of age. There is associated congenital heart disease in 15% of cases; hence, echocardiography is recommended for all cases. Left upper lobe (LUL –40-50%) is the most commonly affected, followed by right middle lobe (RML 30–40%), and then followed by right upper lobe(RUL 20%).

Investigations Skiagram of chest reveals hyperinflated affected lobe**,** mediastinal shift to the opposite side, compression or atelectasis of rest of the lung, and chest opacity due to reduced clearance of lung fluid from the affected lobe after birth. The presence of scant lung markings within the radiolucent with collapse of the adjacent lobe differentiates CLE from pneumothorax (Figs. 25.7 and 25.8). A CT chest is often done for the diagnosis and identification of any possible causes leading to the CLE.

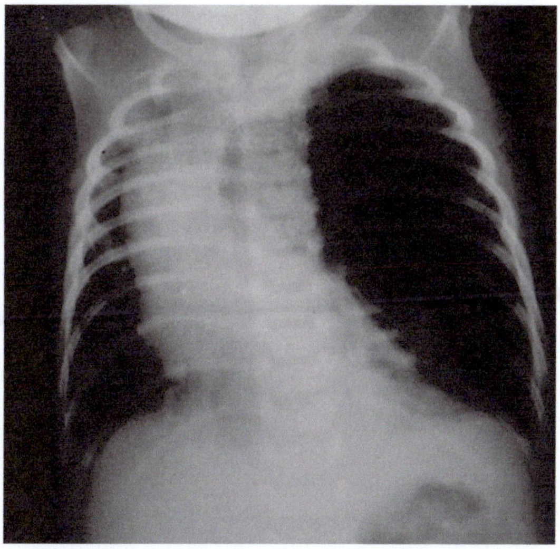

Fig. 25.7 Chest X-ray LUL CLE, note mediastinal herniation to the opposite side

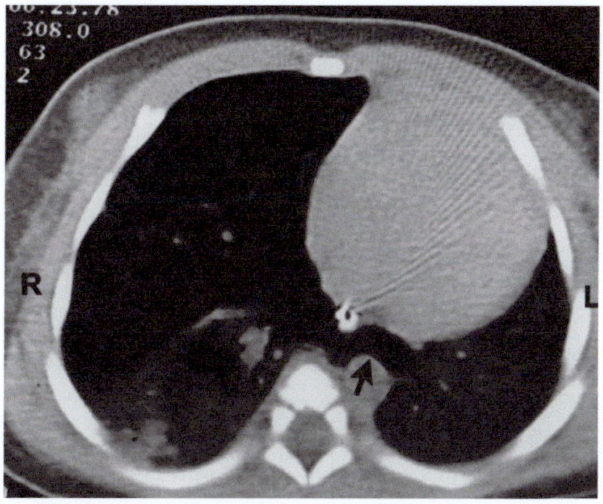

Fig. 25.8 CT (right upper lobe) RUL CLE

25.4.5 Management

CLE is a surgical emergency, and lobectomy of the affected lobe is the surgical treatment of choice. Open is preferred as thoracoscopy is difficult due to limited space. Induction and maintenance of anesthesia should be done through a single lumen tube. Post-induction, the thoracotomy should be done very quickly to reduce cardiac complications due to overinflation of the affected lung. The involved lobe herniates out of the incision as soon as the thorax is opened (Fig. 25.9). Prognosis is excellent with complete recovery of lung volume

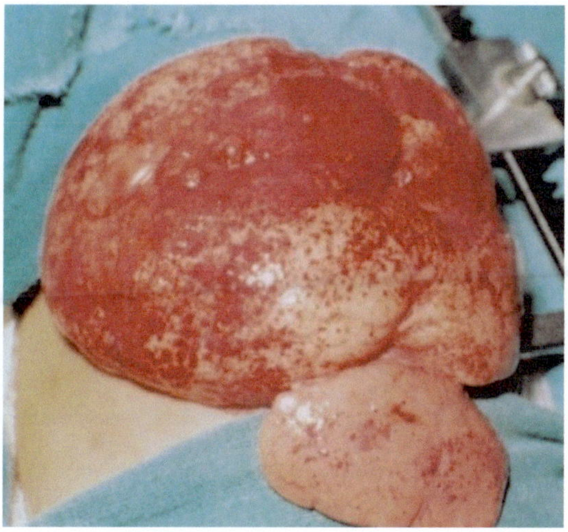

Fig. 25.9 CLE appearance at surgery

and function, on long-term follow-up. Conservative management may be reserved for older infants with minimal symptoms showing radiological improvement over time.

25.4.6 Pulmonary Sequestration

25.4.6.1 Definition and Types

They are lesions of the nonfunctioning lung tissue, which lacks communication with the tracheobronchial tree and are supplied by an anomalous systemic artery. They rarely occur in 10–30% of the cystic bronchopulmonary foregut malformations. In intralobar pulmonary sequestration (ILPS), the aberrant lung tissue is localized within the normal lung, with common visceral pleura (Fig. 25.10). An extralobar pulmonary sequestration (ELPS) is separated from the rest of the lung and has its own visceral pleura. The incidence of ILPS is two to three times more frequent than ELPS. ILPS occur more frequently in males and are more localized to the left posterior mediastinum. ELPS can occur anywhere in the mediastinum, even intra-abdominal lesions are well documented.

Diagnosis ILPS frequently presents with recurrent pulmonary infection, while ELPS is usually an incidental finding on chest x-rays. Few cases

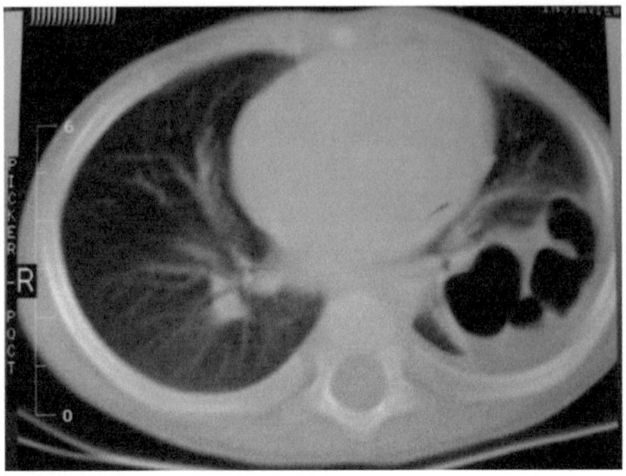

Fig. 25.10 CT intralobar sequestration left lower lobe

can also present with high-output cardiac failure due to hyperdynamic circulation through the anomalous systemic blood supply. ELPS can be confused with neuroblastoma, and in some cases, excision and biopsy are needed for definitive diagnosis. ELPSs are frequently associated with many congenital anomalies like congenital diaphragmatic hernia, tracheoesophageal fistula, pectus excavatum, and congenital heart disease. Contrast-enhanced CT scan is therefore the imaging of choice and has two main aims: (1) to exclude other thoracic pathologies and (2) to demonstrate the presence of anomalous arterial supply.

Treatment The surgical treatment for ILPS involves a lobectomy, while ELPS requires a sequestrectomy. Identification of the supplying systemic artery is important during surgical removal. Few cases of asymptomatic ELPS with the absence of a significant systemic blood supply can be given a trial of observation. Video-assisted thoracoscopy (VAT) has comparable results to open thoracotomy.

25.5 Bronchopulmonary Foregut Malformations (Bronchogenic Cysts, Esophageal Duplication Cysts, and Neuroenteric Cysts)

They are usually single unilocular cysts present in the mediastinum, with no contact with the airway. The presence of cartilages on histopathological examination differentiates these from CPAM, which, on the other hand, has abundance of smooth muscle and elastin fibers in its walls. There is a considerable histopathological overlap between the different congenital cystic lung lesions as they probably represent a spectrum of similar developmental anomalies.

25.5.1 Embryo-Pathology

These lesions result from an abnormal budding of the ventral foregut at 4–8 weeks of gestation. They arise from the trachea, bronchus, or other airways. Connection with the parent structure is lost. In neuroenteric cyst, concomitant vertebral deformities are present (Fig. 25.11).

Diagnosis These are diagnosed by x-ray chest or CT scan of the chest (Fig. 25.12). The findings are smooth, spherical, paratracheal or hilar solid mass lesion, presence of air fluid level, mediastinal shift, absence of calcifications, and rarely honeycombing in case of multilocular cysts.

Treatment Treatment is by thoracotomy or thoracoscopic excision of the lesion. Care should be taken to prevent injury to the adjacent airway or esophagus, as they may share a common muscular wall.

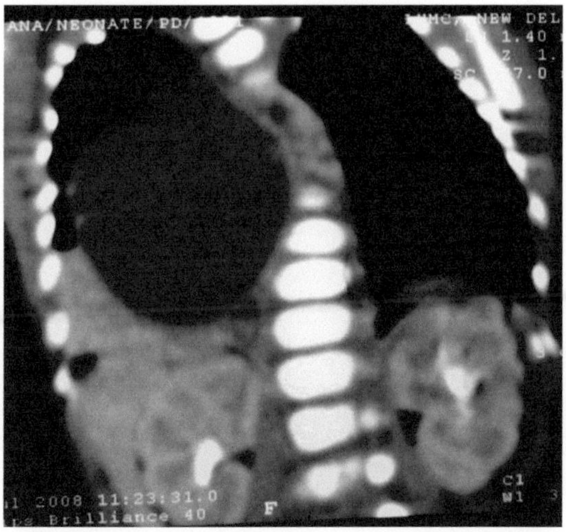

Fig. 25.11 CT neuroenteric cyst, note vertebral abnormality

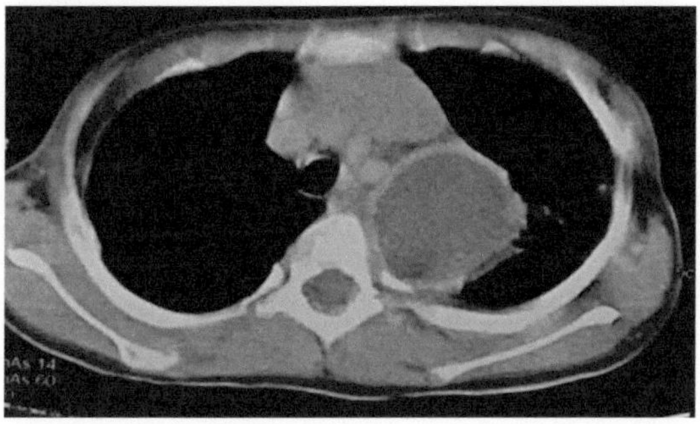

Fig. 25.12 Chest CT bronchogenic cyst

25.5.2 Principles of Lung Lobectomy in Children

Undertaking lung lobectomy by open or thoracoscopy requires a detailed knowledge of the anatomy of the lung, its blood vessels, and the bronchial tree. The lobectomy procedure involves the removal of an anatomical lobe of the lung. The right lung has upper, middle, and lower lobes, and the left lung has upper (along with lingula) and lower lobes, each having segmental arterial supply, venous drainage, and bronchial communications. Generally, the sequence of divisions is the artery first, the vein second, and the bronchus last. A single-lung ventilation is preferred. Children tolerate lobectomies well. Thoracoscopic lobectomy offers the advantages of minimally invasive surgery with a cosmetic scar, less pain, and early recovery.

25.6 Summary

Congenital cystic lesions of the lung and mediastinum covers a wide spectrum of lesions with an embryological basis of their origin. Some of them can be detected antenatally. Management is guided by their effect on the anatomy and function. Symptomatic lesions require surgical removal, whereas some asymptomatic lesions can be initially observed. The operative results for cystic lesions of the lung and mediastinum are satisfactory and long-term relapse-free life can be expected.

Suggested Reading

Chakraborty RK, Modi P, Sharma S. Pulmonary sequestration. 2022 Jul 25. In: StatPearls [Internet]. Treasure Island: StatPearls Publishing; 2023. PMID: 30335347.

Choudhury SR, Chadha R, Mishra A, Kumar V, Singh V, Dubey NK. Lung Resections in children for congenital and acquired lesions. Pediatr Surgery Int. 2007;23:851–9.

Coran AG, Caldamone A, Scott Adzich N, Krummel TM, Laberge JM, editors. Pediatric surgery, vol. 7th. Oxford: Elsevier Limited; 2012.

Demir OF, Hangul M, Kose M. Congenital lobar emphysema: diagnosis and treatment options. Int J Chron Obstruct Pulmon Dis. 2019;14:921–8. https://doi.org/10.2147/COPD.S170581. PMID: 31118601; PMCID: PMC6507121

Fauroux B. Congenital cystic adenomatous malformation (CPAM): remove or not, how can we progress? Paediatr Respir Rev. 2013;14(3):168. https://doi.org/10.1016/j.prrv.2013.06.001. Epub 2013 Jul 17. PMID: 23871554

Holcomb GW III, Murphy PJ, Ostile DJ, editors. Ashcrafts pediatric surgery. 6th ed. Philadelphia: Saunders, Elsevier; 2014.

Leblanc C, Baron M, Desselas E, Phan MH, Rybak A, Thouvenin G, Lauby C, Irtan S. Congenital pulmonary airway malformations: state-of-the-art review for pediatrician's use. Eur J Pediatr. 2017;176(12):1559–71. https://doi.org/10.1007/s00431-017-3032-7. Epub 2017 Oct 19. PMID: 29046943

Esophageal Atresia

26

Muffazzal Rassiwala and Subhasis Roy Choudhury

26.1 Introduction

Since the first successful repair of esophageal atresia (EA) and tracheoesophageal fistula (TEF) in 1941 by Cameron Haight, the survival of patients progressively improved with the current survival rate exceeding 90% due to advancements in anesthesia and neonatal intensive care. The precise surgical anastomosis of the esophageal segments in a newborn is a critical test of a pediatric surgeon's expertise.

> To anastomose the ends of an infant's esophagus, the surgeon must be as delicate and precise as a skilled watchmaker. No other operation offers a greater opportunity for pure technical artistry. Willis J Potts

The *incidence* of EA/TEF ranges from 2 to 4 per 10,000 live births, with a higher prevalence in males. It typically occurs sporadically without a clear hereditary pattern.

26.2 Embryology

Esophageal atresia (EA) and tracheoesophageal fistula (TEF) arise from the incomplete separation of the tracheobronchial tree and the esophageal tube during development. Both structures originate from the embryonic foregut.

Associated anomalies occur in 50–70% of cases.

VACTERL association includes vertebral, anorectal, cardiac, tracheoesophageal, renal, and radial anomalies, as well as limb defects, and is observed in 15% of cases. To meet the criteria for VACTERL association, at least three of the aforementioned anomalies must be present. An additional frequently associated condition is hydrocephalus, referred to as VACTERL-H.

Prenatal ultrasonographic diagnosis is primarily based on the presence of polyhydramnios and a small or absent stomach bubble, though its sensitivity is low. Identifying a dilated cervical esophagus can also be challenging.

26.2.1 Brief History

The history of surgery for esophageal atresia (EA) is a testament to the resilience and dedication of pediatric surgeons. As Confucius said, "Our greatest glory is not in never falling but in rising every time we fall." The earliest recorded description of EA dates back to 1670, in "A Narrative of a Monstrous Birth in Plymouth,"

M. Rassiwala (✉)
Department of Surgery, Index Medical College & Shalby Hospital, Indore, India

S. Roy Choudhury
Pediatric Surgery, Lady Hardinge Medical College and Associated Kalawati Saran Children's Hospital, New Delhi, Delhi, India

© The Author(s), under exclusive license to Springer Nature Singapore Pte Ltd. 2025
S. Roy Choudhury (ed.), *Pediatric Surgery*, https://doi.org/10.1007/978-981-96-1257-4_26

where Durston detailed a blind-ending upper esophageal pouch in a right infant of female thoracopagus-conjoined twins. In 1697, Thomas Gibson documented EA with the typical tracheo-esophageal fistula (EA-TEF) in *The Anatomy of Humane Bodies Epitomized*. Despite these early descriptions, it was not until 1888 that Charles Steel made the first attempt to surgically correct EA without TEF, publishing his findings in *The Lancet* under the title "Case of Deficient Oesophagus." Other key milestones in EA surgery are as follows:

- 1899: Hoffman performed the first permanent gastrostomy in an infant with EA.
- 1925: Lilienthal suggested that the surgical treatment of EA could involve the "division of the tracheoesophageal fistula and anastomosis of the atretic esophagus by tying each pouch over a rubber tube stent."
- 1929: E.C. Vogt, a radiologist, recognized and classified the types of anomalies associated with EA.
- 1941: Cameron Haight conducted the first successful primary repair of EA and published the results in 1943, reporting a 52% overall survival rate.
- 1944: Ladd introduced a five-type numeric classification system for EA.
- 1953: Gross revised the classification system from numeric to alphabetic, which is still in use today.
- 1962: Swenson returned to a numeric classification, replacing Roman numerals with Arabic numbers.
- 1963: Prof. Subir K. Chatterjee reported the first successful TEF repair in India from Kolkata.
- 1976: Kluth published a comprehensive list of EA variations, including 10 main classes and additional subclasses.
- 2000: Rothenberg performed the first successful thoracoscopic repair, with the results published in 2002.

Each of these milestones has significantly contributed to the refinement of EA/TEF management, improving survival and outcomes.

26.2.2 Types of Esophageal Atresia (Gross, Fig. 26.1)

A. Esophageal atresia without fistula (EA)
B. Esophageal atresia with upper pouch fistula (TEF)
C. Esophageal atresia with lower pouch fistula (commonest)
D. Esophageal atresia with upper and lower pouch fistula
E. H-type trachea-esophageal fistula

26.2.3 Clinical Presentation

- *Excessive salivation* in a newborn.
- *Feeding difficulties,* including regurgitation, choking, coughing, cyanosis, and respiratory distress.
- *Failure to pass a nasogastric tube* into the stomach.

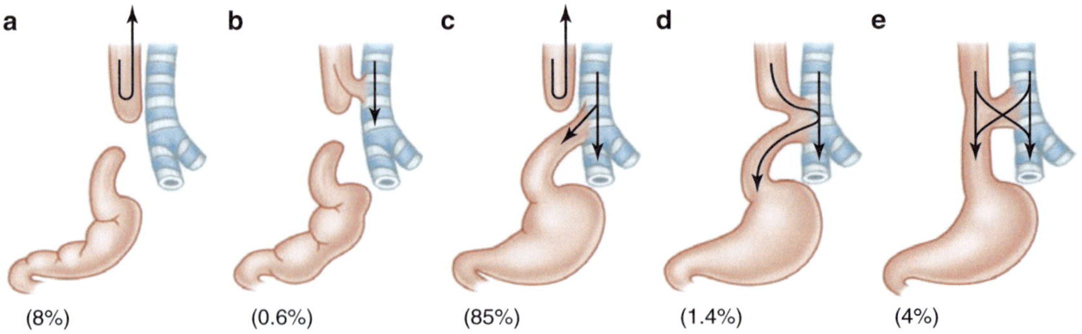

Fig. 26.1 Types of esophageal atresia (gross)

- *Abdominal distension,* particularly in cases with a tracheoesophageal fistula.
- *Risk of aspiration,* leading to pneumonia due to saliva and gastric contents entering the respiratory tract.

26.2.4 Diagnosis

Chest X-ray with a No. 8 or 10 feeding tube, passed either orally or via the nasal route, typically shows an arrest at the T3-T4 vertebral level, approximately 10 cm from the mouth. The presence of air in the abdomen suggests a tracheoesophageal fistula (TEF) (Fig. 26.2).

The level of the nasogastric (NG) tube's arrest relative to the thoracic vertebrae (T1-T4) helps assess the length of the esophageal gap, which is crucial for management planning and prognostication. Radiographic preoperative assessment using a feeding tube in the upper esophagus, showing the arrest level (T1-T4), correlates well with intraoperative findings. Coiling of the NG tube at higher levels (T1-T2) typically indicates a longer gap between the esophageal ends, whereas coiling at lower levels (T3-T4) is often associated with shorter gap lengths. Longer gap lengths generally require postoperative ventilation and may result in poorer outcomes.

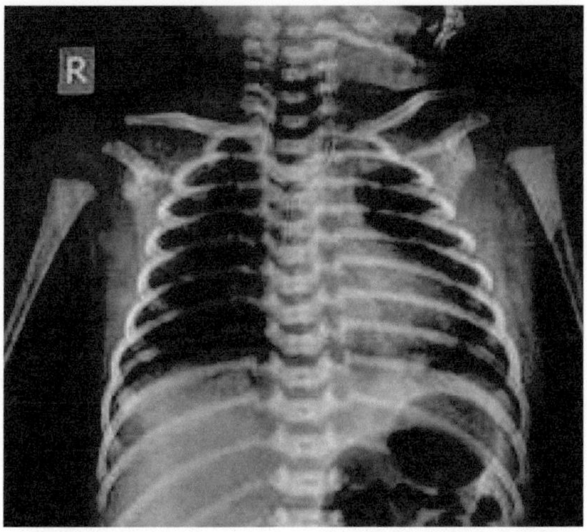

Fig. 26.2 TEF, note the coiled feeding tube in the upper esophagus

Magnetic resonance imaging (MRI) has been proposed for more accurate gap length assessment; however, motion artifacts from infants who cannot stay still and suboptimal scans limit its utility. MRI under anesthesia adds anesthetic risks shortly before surgery, leading many centers to discourage its use since surgery must be performed promptly after diagnosis.

A gasless abdomen on X-ray is suggestive of pure esophageal atresia without TEF (EA). Some centers use an oral contrast study for diagnostic confirmation, but this is discouraged due to the risk of aspiration, which can lead to pneumonia and worsen the patient's condition, especially in cases involving TEF.

26.2.5 Other Investigations

- Echocardiography to rule out cardiac anomalies
- Ultrasonography to assess renal anomalies

26.2.6 Features of Esophageal Atresia (EA) Without TEF (Pure Esophageal Atresia)

- Clinically, a flat-looking abdomen and a gasless abdomen on plain X-ray (Fig. 26.3a, b). A gasless abdomen can also occur with a small distal TEF blocked by a mucous plug.
- The gap between the esophageal ends is typically long (more than two vertebral bodies).
- Staged operations are often required to restore esophageal continuity.
- The stomach size is usually small. A large stomach with bile may indicate an associated duodenal atresia.

26.2.7 Management

The management algorithm is shown in Table 26.1.

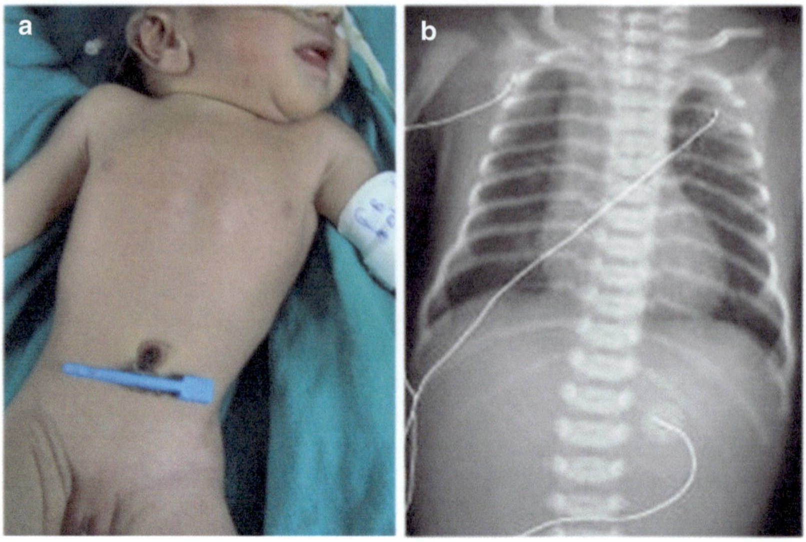

Fig. 26.3 Esophageal atresia (**a**) Flat abdomen (**b**) Gasless abdomen on X-ray

26.2.8 Preoperative Treatment

- A double-lumen Replogle tube (sump catheter) is inserted nasally or orally for continuous drainage of saliva from the upper esophageal pouch, helping reduce the risk of tracheal aspiration.
- Nursing should be done with the infant in a head-up position to minimize gastric juice reflux. Ensuring optimal temperature control is also crucial.
- Initiate intravenous fluids, broad-spectrum antibiotics, and vitamin K as part of the preoperative regimen.
- Special attention must be given to chest care, including physiotherapy.

26.2.9 Role of Preoperative Bronchoscopy

Preoperative bronchoscopy is particularly beneficial in the following scenarios:

(a) Identification of an upper pouch fistula
(b) Low-level TEF (when the fistula is near the carina)
(c) Pre-existing tracheomalacia
(d) Thick mucus requiring suctioning
(e) Detection of tracheal stenosis or a tracheal bronchus to the right upper lobe
(f) Diagnosis of H-type TEF

26.2.10 Surgical Management

Surgical intervention can be performed using either thoracoscopy or thoracotomy. The open technique typically involves a right posterolateral thoracotomy with an extrapleural approach, where the fistula is divided, and a primary end-to-end esophageal anastomosis is performed (Fig. 26.4). In neonates with a right aortic arch, as identified through echocardiography, some surgeons may prefer a left-sided thoracotomy.

26.2.11 Steps of Thoracotomy Surgery

- The approach involves a right posterolateral thoracotomy through the fourth or fifth intercostal space, just below the tip of the scapula. A muscle-sparing technique is employed by retracting the latissimus dorsi muscle posteriorly and the serratus anterior muscle anteriorly, opening the auscultatory triangle. This

Table 26.1 Management algorithm of EA/TEF

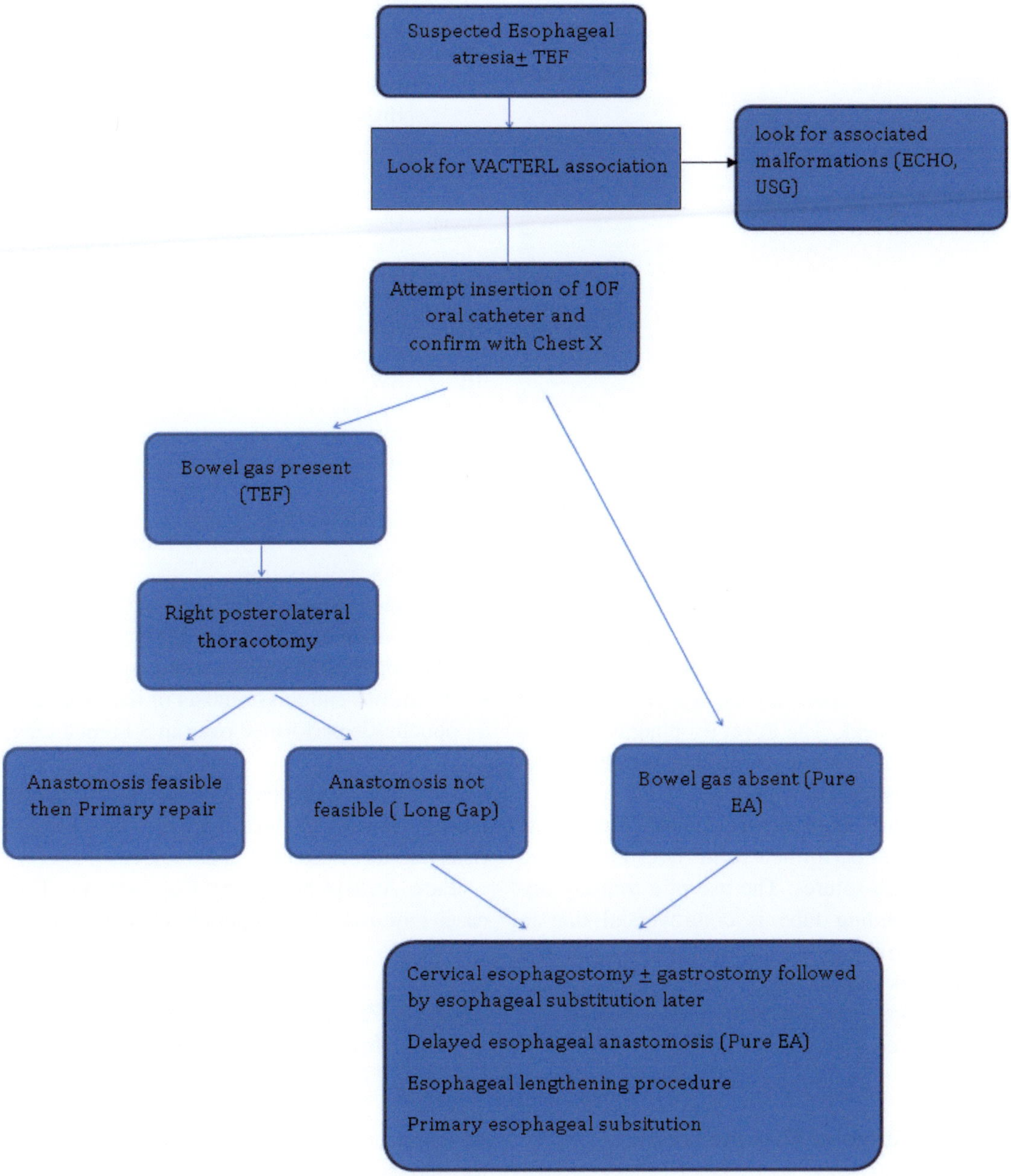

approach helps reduce the likelihood of future chest wall deformities.

- An extrapleural approach is preferred, with the pleura reflected medially to aid in lung retraction.
- Typically, the azygous vein is ligated and divided.
- The tracheoesophageal (TE) fistula is identified and slung. It is usually located at the level of the azygous venous arch and shows distension with ventilation. The vagus nerve, running alongside the lower esophagus, also serves as a landmark. Ligation and division of the TE fistula (Fig. 26.4) are performed close

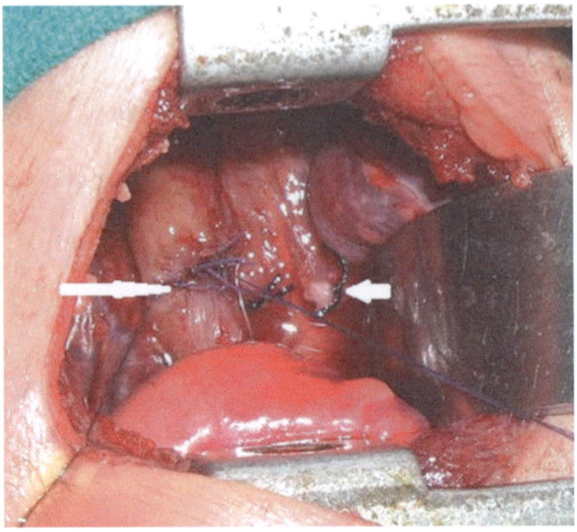

Fig. 26.4 Surgical division of fistula (short arrow) and esophageal anastomosis (long arrow)

Table 26.2 Survival of esophageal atresia/tracheoesophageal fistula

Group	Waterston	Survival
A	B.W. > 2500 gm, otherwise well	100%
B	B.W. 2000–2500 gm and well or Higher weight with moderate associated anomalies	85%
C	B.W. < 2000gm or higher with severe congenital anomalies	65%
Group	Okamoto modification of Spitz classification	Survival
I	BW >2000gm, no major cardiac anomaly	100%
II	BW < 2000 gm, no major cardiac anomaly	81%
III	BW > 2000 gm and major cardiac anomaly	72%
IV	BW < 2000gm and major cardiac anomaly	27%

to the trachea. A delayed absorbable suture, such as PDS (Ethicon), is preferred for fistula ligation.

- Generous mobilization of the upper esophageal pouch is performed to reduce the gap and facilitate the anastomosis, which may extend up to the neck. The lower esophagus can also be mobilized while preserving the segmental blood vessels that supply it.
- End-to-end anastomosis of the esophageal pouches is performed using fine, interrupted absorbable sutures. The use of a transanastomotic feeding tube is controversial due to reports of increased incidence of leaks and strictures with its use.
- Chest closure is completed with the placement of an intercostal drainage tube.

26.2.12 Steps of Thoracoscopic Surgery

- The patient is positioned in a modified prone position, with the right side elevated at approximately 30°.
- The initial port (3 mm or 4 mm) is placed in the fifth intercostal space, just behind the tip of the scapula, and this serves as the camera port.
- One working port is inserted along the mid-axillary line.
- A second working port is introduced in the posterior axillary line.
- The tracheoesophageal (TE) fistula is ligated and divided using a 5 mm clip.
- The upper esophageal pouch is mobilized.
- An end-to-end anastomosis of the esophageal pouches is performed over an 8 French tube.

However, the scope of thoracoscopic surgery is still limited by increased anesthesia-related risks and its availability at all centers.

Pure Atresia and Long Gap Atresia: These cases require a staged operation (see below).

26.2.13 Prognostic Factors for Esophageal Atresia (Table 26.2)

Appropriate postoperative management is crucial for the successful outcome of these patients. Elective postoperative ventilation is followed in some centers, especially with a tight anastomosis.

26.2.14 Postoperative Complications

Common postoperative complications include anastomotic leaks, stricture (Fig. 26.5), recurrent tracheoesophageal fistula (TEF), gastroesopha-

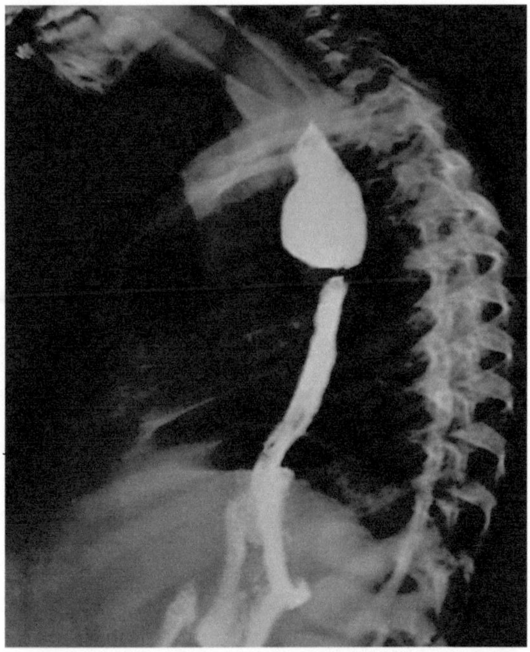

Fig. 26.5 Anastomotic stricture post TEF repair

geal (GE) reflux, disordered esophageal motility, tracheomalacia, and late respiratory morbidity.

- *Anastomotic Leak:* A minor leak may resolve with observation. However, a major anastomotic leak may require surgical intervention, such as re-anastomosis in early cases, or more frequently, diversion via esophagostomy and gastrostomy.
- *Tracheomalacia:* This condition results from the softening of the tracheal cartilage, leading to expiratory collapse and expiratory stridor. It can be diagnosed on bronchoscopy, where collapsing of the tracheal wall is observed even during ventilation. The management is generally expectant, but life-threatening events or recurrent cyanotic spells may necessitate surgical intervention, such as aortic suspension (aortopexy). The principle of aortopexy involves anterior suspension of the aortic arch by stitching it to the posterior surface of the sternum, which elevates the anterior wall of the trachea and widens its lumen. Thoracoscopic posterior tracheopexy, where the membranous posterior wall of the trachea is fixed to the anterior longitudinal spinal ligament with non-absorbable sutures during primary esophageal atresia repair, may prevent life-threatening complications of tracheomalacia.

Laryngeal-Tracheo-Esophageal Cleft (LTEC) Also known as laryngeal cleft (LC), this is a congenital malformation of the posterior part of the larynx, possibly extending to the trachea, creating an abnormal communication between the laryngo-tracheal and pharyngo-esophageal axes.

Over the last 50 years, several classifications of LC have been proposed, focusing on the downward extension of the cleft. These include classifications by Petterson (1955), Armitage (1984), Evans (1985), Benjamin (1989), Meyer (1990), DuBois (1990), and Sandu (2006). These classifications have three main objectives:

- *Descriptive:* To allow comparison of patient series in the literature
- *Therapeutic:* To influence the choice of the reconstructive technique and surgical approach
- *Prognostic:* As success and survival rates are highly correlated with the extension of the LC

The Benjamin and Inglis classification, modified by Sandu in 2006, is the most commonly used and differentiates partial and total clefts of the cricoid cartilage, as well as cervical and tracheo-thoracic clefts. These elements are crucial in determining the appropriate therapeutic strategy.

26.2.15 Classification of Laryngeal Cleft (LC): (Fig. 26.6)

- *Type 0:* Submucosal cleft
- *Type I:* Supraglottic, interarytenoid cleft, above the vocal fold level
- *Type II:* Cleft extending below the vocal folds into the cricoid cartilage
- *Type III a:* Cleft extending through the cricoid cartilage but not into the trachea

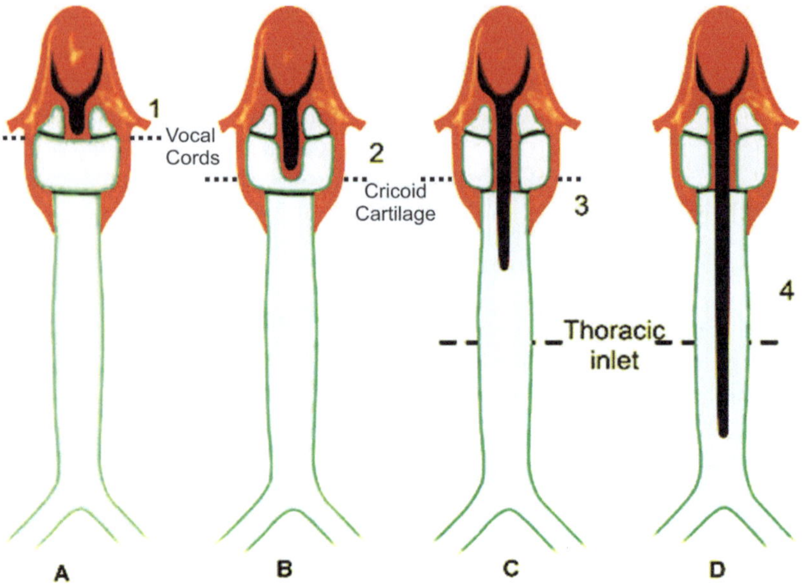

Fig. 26.6 Benjamin-Inglis classification of laryngeal clefts

- *Type III b:* Cleft extending through the cricoid cartilage and into the cervical trachea
- *Type IV:* Cleft extending into the thoracic trachea, potentially down to the carina

26.3 Management of LTEC (Laryngeal-Tracheo-Esophageal Cleft)

A. *Endoscopic Management*

For patients with shorter clefts who are able to tolerate general anesthesia with spontaneous breathing, treatment can be performed using suspension laryngoscopy and CO2 laser ablation. This involves the separation of the cleft's common wall and suturing of the esophageal and laryngeal mucosa to close the cleft.

B. *Open Surgical Management*

For longer clefts (Types 3 and 4), an open surgical approach may be necessary, either through a cervical or a combined cervical and thoracic approach. This involves separating the common wall and performing a suture repair of the cleft, followed by the use of an interposition graft with cartilage. The graft helps prevent the recurrence of the cleft.

26.3.1 TEF Without Atresia (H-Type TEF)

H-type TEF typically presents with a history of coughing, choking during feeding, and recurrent pneumonia. Diagnosis can be confirmed using contrast swallow esophagography (Fig. 26.7) and bronchoesophagoscopy. During a contrast esophagogram, the child is placed in a prone position, and contrast is injected into the distal esophagus via a feeding tube. The contrast is gradually injected while the tube is slowly withdrawn. Surgical treatment involves the ligation and division of the fistula (Fig. 26.8), typically performed through a neck incision approach, though in rare cases, a thoracotomy may be necessary.

26.3.2 Long Gap Esophageal Atresia

- All isolated cases of esophageal atresia without TEF are typically classified as long gap.
- EA/TEF with a long gap is diagnosed when primary esophageal anastomosis is not possible, even after extensive mobilization of the esophageal segments.

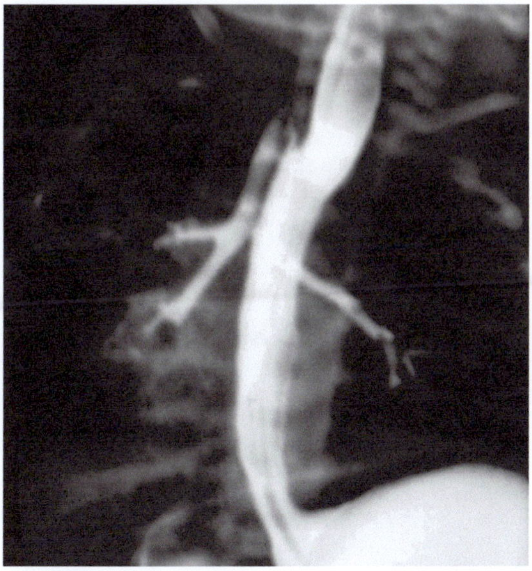

Fig. 26.7 H-type TEF

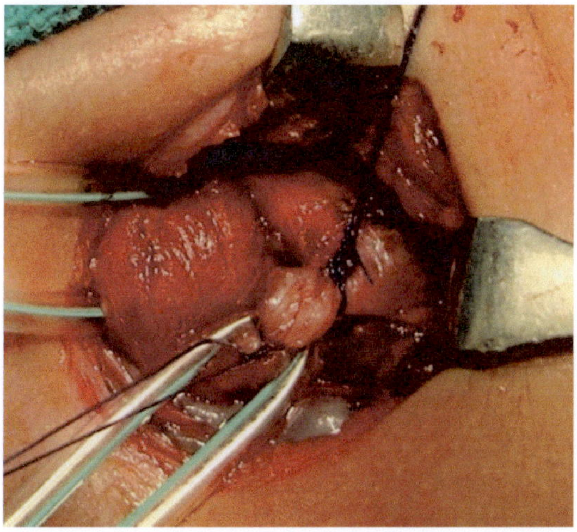

Fig. 26.8 Cervical ligation of H-type TEF

26.3.3 Management Options for Long Gap Esophageal Atresia

- *Primary Anastomosis:* Involves extensive mobilization of the esophageal pouches. While both pouches can be mobilized, performing the anastomosis under tension carries a risk of disruption and leakage.
- *Delayed Primary Anastomosis:* This approach relies on the rapid spontaneous growth of the esophageal ends, making an end-to-end anastomosis feasible after 4–6 weeks (as proposed by Prem Puri). This technique is currently considered the standard procedure. Thoracoscopic mobilization of the pouches, along with initial approximation sutures and delayed anastomosis, may also provide a successful alternative.
- *Intraoperative Myotomy and Flap Techniques:* Techniques such as Livaditi's myotomy and Gough's flap procedure from the upper pouch can help gain additional length for anastomosis.
- *Scharli's Lesser Curve Elongation Technique:* A method to increase the length of the esophagus.
- *Intra-Extra Thoracic Suture Traction Elongation Technique (Focker):* A technique to stretch the esophagus using sutures in both intra- and extrathoracic segments.
- *Multistage Extra Thoracic Elongation Technique (Kimura):* A staged procedure for elongating the esophagus using extrathoracic traction.
- *Magnetic Compression Anastomosis Technique (Liu):* A newer method involving magnetic forces to aid in the anastomosis of the esophagus.
- *Esophagostomy and Gastrostomy in the Newborn:* A temporary solution, followed by delayed bridging of the esophagus using the stomach or colon (Figs. 26.9a and 26.9b).
- *Primary Gastric Transposition:* While not ideal for newborns, this technique may be considered in certain cases.

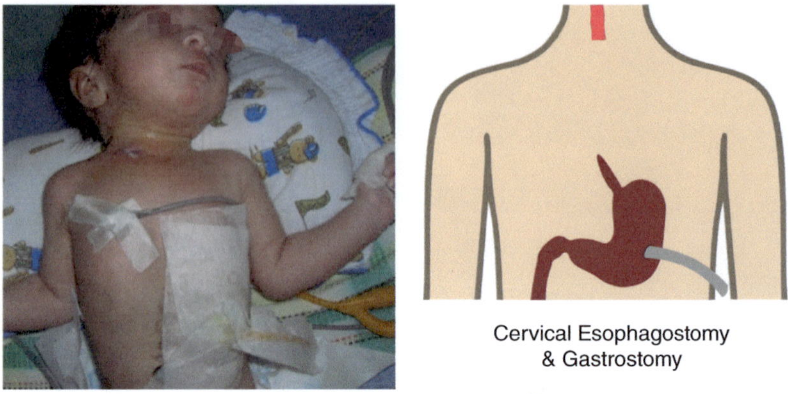

Fig. 26.9a Cervical esophagostomy with feeding gastrostomy

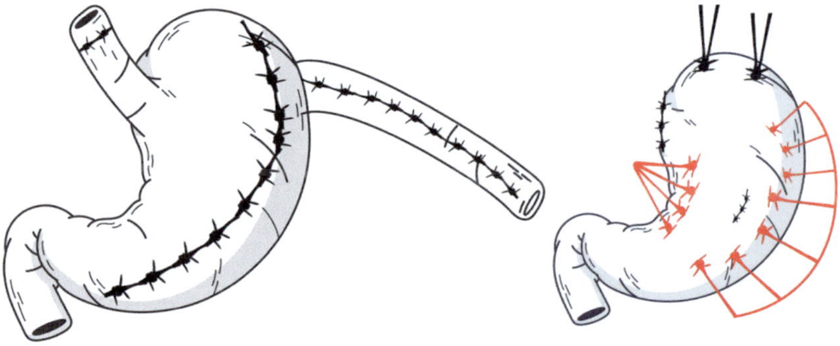

Fig. 26.9b Gastric tube and gastric transposition for esophageal replacement

26.4 Summary

The chance of survival of patients with esophageal atresia is above 90%. VACTERL association is seen in 15% cases. Low birth weight, associated cardiac anomaly or poor lung condition are causes of poor outcome. Repair by open or thoracoscopic technique are both practiced. Long gap esophageal atresia may require a staged approach including the need for esophageal substitution.

Suggested Reading

Benjamin B, Inglis A. Minor congenital laryngeal clefts: diagnosis and classification. Ann Otol Rhinol Laryngol. 1989;98:417–20.

Choudhury SR. Surgical diseases of the esophagus in children. J Indian Assoc PediatrSurg. 2016;21:96–7.

Coran AG, Caldamone A, Scott Adzich N, Krummel TM, Laberge JM, editors. Pediatric surgery. 7th ed. Oxford: Elsevier Limited; 2012.

Leboulanger and Garabédian. Laryngo-tracheo-oesophageal clefts. Orphanet J Rare Dis. 2011;6:81.

Muffazzal R, Roy Choudhury S, Yadav PS, Jhanwar P, Prakash R, Chadha R, Debnath PK. Determinants of gap lengthin esophageal atresia with tracheoesophageal fistula and the impact of gap length on outcome. J Ind Assoc Pediatric Surg. 2016;21:126–30.

Pierro A. Oesophageal Atresia. Seminar Pediatric Surgery. 2009;18(1):1–57.

Roy Choudhury S, Ashcraft KW, Sharp RJ, Murphy JP, Snyder CL, Sigalet DL. Survival of esophageal atresia patients: influence of birth weight, cardiac anomaly, and late respiratory complications. J Pediatric Surgery. 1999;34:70–4.

Sandu K, Monnier P. Endoscopic laryngotracheal cleft repair without tracheotomy or intubation. Laryngoscope. 2006;116:630–4.

Esophageal Replacement in Children

27

Anthony Lander and Subhasis Roy Choudhury

Esophageal replacement substitutes a missing or damaged portion of the esophagus with a conduit that aims to allow the passage of food and liquid from the mouth to the stomach to enhance a child's quality of life and take them into adulthood.

A functioning esophagus facilitates pain-free, safe swallowing of saliva and, ideally, solid and liquid food to meet nutritional needs. The normal esophagus also allows the safe expulsion of swallowed air, proximal intestinal gas, and, when needed, vomitus. When the native esophagus has failed, esophageal replacement may be considered in preference to a permanent esophagostomy and gastrostomy, though supplemental enteral tube feeding may still be needed in some. Interpositions are currently fashioned from the stomach, jejunum, or colon and can be challenging for the patient and the surgeon. A modestly dysfunctional esophagus is generally better than having a troublesome replacement, and the risks and benefits are challenging to assess. Interpositions are not commonly performed, and this is reflected in surgeons often having a preferred organ and technique. The spectrum of operations also reflects that no organ or technique is ideal, and complications can be common and sometimes serious. Specialist centers should discourage occasional practice and develop a team-based approach.

The history of esophageal replacement in children includes a colonic interposition in a 3-year-old in 1921, Swenson and Sweet reporting gastric transpositions in the 1940s, and in 1978 Ein and Shandling reporting on gastric tubes.

27.1 Indications

27.2 Esophageal Atresia

Most children born with esophageal atresia have a repair that unites the upper pouch and the lower esophagus at a functioning anastomosis. Options for the long-gap esophageal atresia (born with or without a fistula) include (1) delayed primary anastomosis after 6–12 weeks with Replogle or intermittent suction of the upper pouch and gastrostomy feeding or (2) serial traction approaches. If these fail, replacement is offered in later infancy or early childhood with an esophagostomy allowing sham feeding in the interim.

Disappointingly, some seemingly satisfactory anastomoses fail, and occasionally, recalcitrant strictures result in the native esophagus being abandoned, and replacement is then an option.

When resources are limited, replacement may be a more viable option than struggling to pre-

A. Lander (✉)
Birmingham Women's and Children's Hospital, Birmingham, UK

S. Roy Choudhury
Pediatric Surgery, Lady Hardinge Medical College and Associated Kalawati Saran Children's Hospital, New Delhi, Delhi, India

© The Author(s), under exclusive license to Springer Nature Singapore Pte Ltd. 2025

S. Roy Choudhury (ed.), *Pediatric Surgery*, https://doi.org/10.1007/978-981-96-1257-4_27

serve the native esophagus. In low- and middle-income countries, the delayed primary repair is often unsuccessful as it requires an extended hospital stay, and chest infections are to be expected if the upper pouch is not well managed. Serial traction approaches in the neonatal period require robust intensive care support between operations, which is expensive and demands expertise that might not be available.

27.3 Caustic Ingestion

Household bleach, oven, and drain cleaners contain sodium and potassium hydroxides, while laundry and dishwasher detergents contain sodium phosphate, sodium carbonate, and ammonia. These can all cause esophageal strictures if ingested; most are managed nonoperatively with serial dilatations, but replacement is occasionally needed. Most ingestions are small volume and accidental, but self-harm in adolescents is on the rise, and ingested volumes can be large and cause severe and extensive damage.

27.4 Reflux Ulceration and Strictures

Poorly managed and protracted acid reflux can damage the lower esophagus. Treatment is usually pharmacological and supported by fundoplication if needed. Only occasionally is a replacement indicated.

27.5 Button Battery Damage

Batteries moving freely in the intestine or immersed in a significant fluid volume do not cause local tissue damage since electrolytic products do not accumulate. However, button batteries can easily lodge in the esophagus at its areas of narrowing, and if they retain a voltage over 1.23 V, electrolysis occurs. The local tissue pH can rise to 10 at the negative pole, causing liquefactive necrosis. Acid is produced at the positive pole. Severe esophageal, tracheal, and even aortic injuries are well described and can result in the esophagus being abandoned. Esophageal replacement may have a role in rehabilitating survivors.

27.6 Rare Indications

Other causes of esophageal failure include achalasia, diffuse leiomyoma, complications of esophageal duplication, scleroderma, epidermolysisbullosa, doxorubicin-induced esophagitis, and Barrett's esophagitis.

27.7 Properties of a Replacement

At the very least, the replacement should provide an efficient conduit for saliva, which functions better than an esophagostomy, improving the quality of life even if food and fluids still require a gastrostomy. Natural tissue should grow with the child and last a lifetime. The operative technique should be simple and applicable to complex patients, some of whom may have hostile chests. If there is an anastomosis to the stomach, this should have minimal reflux. The interposition should tolerate ingested food and any refluxed acid. Respiratory and cardiac embarrassment should be tolerable.

27.8 Planning

Esophagostomies placed on the right are preferable if the colon is the planned interposition and on the left if the stomach is to be used. In neonates where a replacement is anticipated, most surgeons wait until the child is at least six months of age and is well nourished with good respiratory function. Many conduits benefit from gravity to assist clearance, as peristalsis can be poor or disordered.

A gastrostomy is nearly always required to feed the child until definitive surgery is performed, and this is best placed in the antrum of the stomach and away from the greater curvature if a gastric tube is a possible option. Most gastric tubes are fashioned from the greater curvature.

Patients with an esophagostomy should be encouraged to feed by mouth as this facilitates early recovery of feeding and swallowing after the interposition. The input of a specialist feeding team or speech and language therapist may be helpful.

Having more than one experienced surgeon available and familiar with the case is helpful since an alternate procedure may be needed. A "plan B" should be mentally rehearsed and discussed with the parents in advance; for example, the preferred conduit may be unsuitable, have a poor blood supply once mobilized, or be unsatisfactory when brought into the chest.

27.9 The Route from the Abdomen to the Neck

There are three principal routes: retrosternal, transpleural, and posterior mediastinal. If there is to be a passage through the colonic mesentery, this needs to be considered and accurately documented. The characteristics of the three routes are compared in Table 27.1.

Table 27.1 Comparison of three routes of esophageal replacement

Route	Advantage	Disadvantage
Retrosternal	No major structures encountered in this route. Ease of procedure when other routes are compromised by fibrosis.	Longest route from neck to the abdomen Angulation of the graft Problems with access if cardiac surgery is required
Transpleural	Convenience, and often required in a hostile chest	Displacement of the lung Requires thoracotomy
Posterior mediastinal	Most direct route Graft contained in the mediastinum Little or no lung compression Thoracotomy is not always required	Mediastinum may be unavailable because of previous surgery, fibrosis, or inflammation

27.10 Procedural Options

No randomized trials help us choose the best option from (1) gastric transposition, (2) gastric tube, (3) colon interposition, (4) jejunal interposition, and (5) fundal tube esophagoplasty. An examination of the literature finds no significant difference in graft necrosis, anastomotic leaks, late strictures, poor feeding, reflux, graft tortuosity, or Barrett's esophagus in children. Extensive series report fewer complications than small series, suggesting a volume-outcome relationship. Some advantages and disadvantages appear in Table 27.2.

Table 27.2 Advantages and disadvantages of various procedures

Method	Advantages	Disadvantages
Colon	Adequate length Reflux rare	Precarious blood supply Graft necrosis High incidence of leaks and strictures Multiple anastomoses Redundancy long term Slow transit of food
Gastric tube	Adequate length Good blood supply Size of conduit appropriate Rapid transit	Very long suture line High incidence of leaks and strictures Reflux leading to Barrett's esophagus
Jejunum	Appropriate size	Poor blood supply at the top of the graft Retention of peristaltic activity Length can be a problem Three anastomoses
Free jejunal graft	Appropriate size Good peristaltic activity	Microvascular skills needed Prolonged operating time Precarious blood supply High failure rate

27.11 Gastric Transposition

The child is positioned on the operating table in a supine position with arms by the side. The head is slightly elevated, with the neck modestly extended to facilitate access to the esophagostomy. Cervical anesthetic lines are avoided. Unless previous incisions dictate otherwise, a midline incision is made from the sternal notch to the umbilicus, or an oblique incision is made on the left side of the abdomen.

In a gastric transposition, the gastrostomy is closed, and the right gastric and right gastroepiploic vessels are identified and preserved; only then is the stomach isolated and mobilized. The stomach is separated from the left lobe of the liver, the spleen, and the omentum. The short gastric vessels are divided away from the stomach. The left gastric vessels are divided close to the stomach. Any esophageal remnant at the gastroesophageal junction is transected and closed. The vagi will be divided at this time. The most superior region of the fundus is identified for the top of the transposition, as this will provide the greatest length. The second part of the duodenum is Kocherized, and a pyloromyotomy or a Heinecke-Mikulicz pyloroplasty is performed if desired. The stomach should look well perfused and have adequate length when laid on the chest (Fig. 27.1).

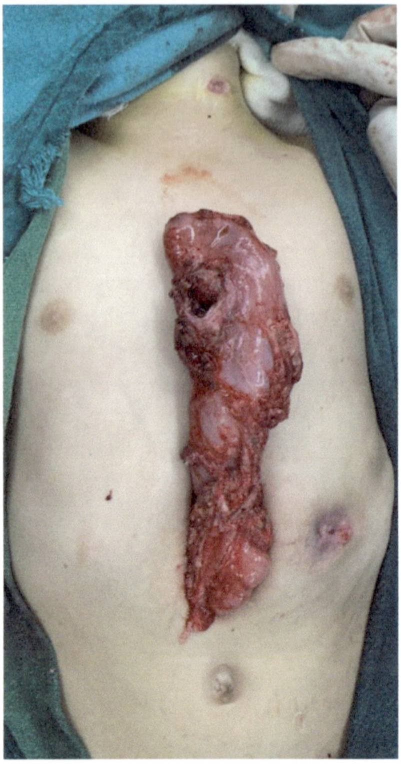

Fig. 27.1 Gastric transposition; note the cervical esophagostomy

For a trans-hiatal route, a posterior mediastinal tunnel is made. The cervical esophagostomy is mobilized, taking care to protect the recurrent laryngeal nerve, and a posterior mediastinal tunnel is fashioned digitally from above and below just in front of the prevertebral fascia, keeping fingers in contact with the vertebrae throughout the blunt dissection. The abdominal and neck dissections are advanced till the fingers meet. The tunnel is then widened until it accepts two or three finger breadths. For a retrosternal dissection, the technique is similar (Fig. 27.2).

The stomach is pulled through the thorax into the neck through the desired route using a tube sutured to it for gentle traction. The cervical anastomosis is to the pharynx or the cervical esophagus. A transanastomotic nasogastric tube is passed to keep the stomach empty. The pyloric antrum can be fixed to the diaphragm. It is essential to have nearly all of the stomach in the chest, avoiding a portion in the abdomen. If part of the stomach is in the abdomen, there can be troublesome shifts in gastric content during respiration when the thoracic pressure falls during inhalation and rises during expiration. A temporary feeding jejunostomy is an option to allow post-pyloric feeding until the new physiology is assessed and can sustain oral nutrition, though jejunostomies are not without their complications. Postoperative care typically includes elective ventilation for 24–48 hours, with assiduous gastric decompression to avoid acute gastric distension, which can compromise ventilation. There is only one anastomosis to worry about in a gastric transposition, and the blood supply should be good. Late complications include anastomotic stricture, dysphagia, delayed gastric emptying, dumping syndrome, reflux, and aspiration. Most will achieve full oral feeds, but a nasogastric tube is ideal if oral feed-

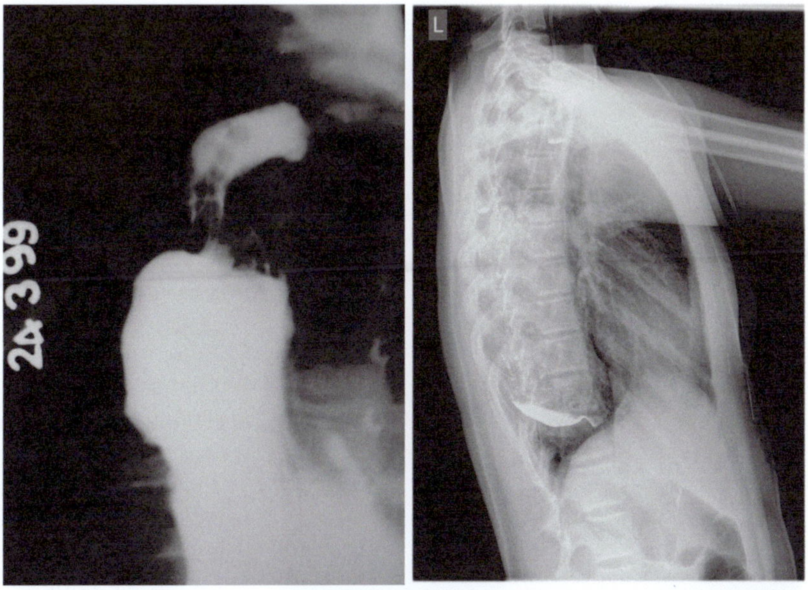

Fig. 27.2 Contrast studies following gastric transpositions

ing is suboptimal. If intake is poor, a gastric transposition will not stop the occasional pediatrician from requesting a gastrostomy!

27.12 Gastric Tube Interposition

There are two options: (1) an antiperistaltic tube based on the left gastro-epiploic artery, which is also known as a reverse gastric tube (Fig. 27.3), and (2) an isoperistaltic tube based on the right gastro-epiploic artery. The tube can also be constructed from the fundus of the stomach, including the esophageal stump as described by Rao (Fig. 27.4).

These tubes are constructed from a rectangle of gastric tissue starting at about 2.5 cm above the pylorus and made around a 22–28 Fr tube. After preparation, the conduit is pulled up retrosternal or through the posterior mediastinum, and the cervical anastomosis is made at the same time or delayed. Complications include anastomotic leaks, mediastinitis (because of the long suture line), reflux, and ulceration. A contrast study is shown in Fig. 27.5.

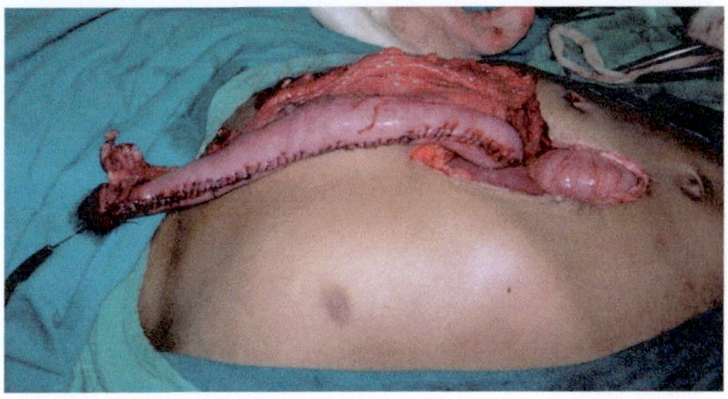

Fig. 27.3 Reverse gastric tube

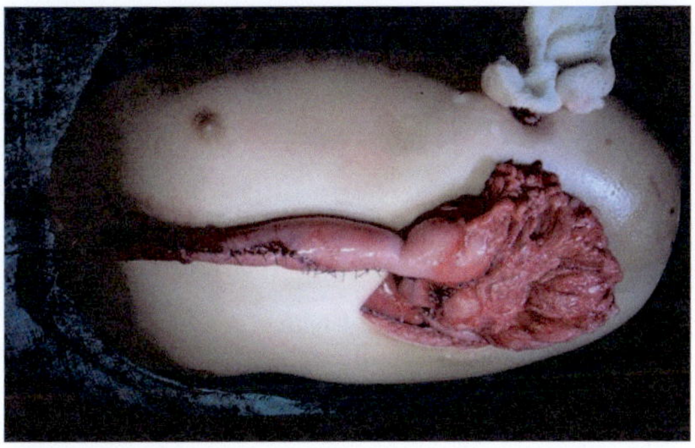

Fig. 27.4 Gastric fundal tube (Rao)

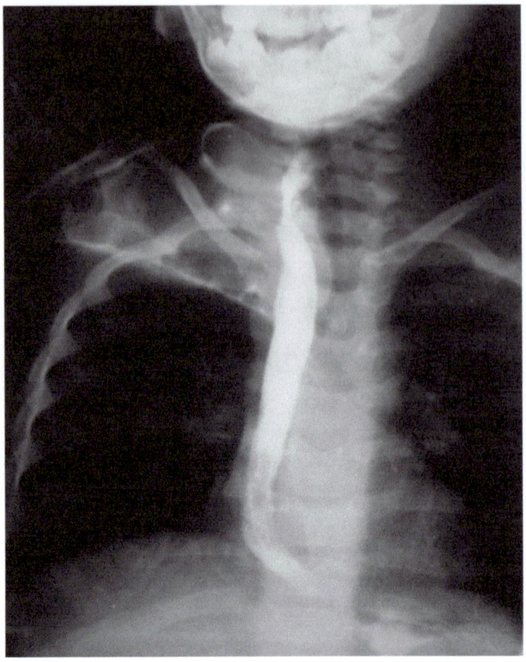

Fig. 27.5 Contrast study of a left-sided gastric tube

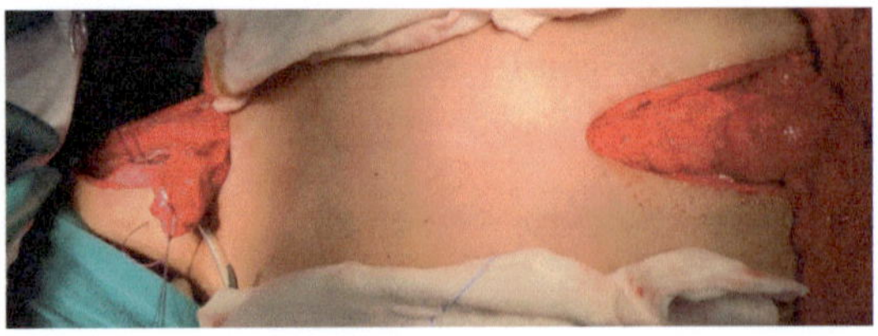

Fig. 27.6 Retrosternal left colonic substitution for corrosive stricture esophagus ↓, note the curved neck incision to reach up to hypopharynx for the anastomosis

27.13 Colonic Interposition

Though the colon is rarely used in adults, it remains popular worldwide in children, as the blood supply is more favorable in children than in adult. Importantly, it would be inappropriate in the presence of an anorectal malformation (often associated with esophageal atresia) or other colonic pathology. In the context of microgastria, the colon can be ideal.

Preoperative bowel preparation and on-table irrigation are required. Different regions of the colon can be used. The right colon can be used isoperistaltic or retroperistaltic, but since its peristalsis is poor, this may make little difference. The right colon graft can be based on the right or left colonic vessels, with the middle colic divided. The left or transverse colon can also be used, either through the retrosternal or posterior mediastinal route (Fig. 27.6). The cervical anastomosis can be end-to-side or end-to-end. The cologastric anastomosis is usually made at the cardia with an anti-reflux partial anterior gastric wrap to limit reflux. Some surgeons place the cologastric anastomosis on the posterior wall of the stomach such that the colon is compressed when the stomach is full. Laparoscopic and thoracoscopic approaches are common in adults and will become more commonly applied in children.

Complications include early graft necrosis, leaks, and strictures. Redundancy and dilatation can cause stasis, halitosis, and dysphagia. When placed in the posterior mediastinum, the shorter and straighter course of the colon may be preferable. Ulceration, colitis, hemorrhage, and polyps are also reported.

27.14 Jejunal Interpostition

The jejunum has an ideal luminal diameter and can retain peristalsis, but it is often not as straight a conduit as one might imagine, and its blood supply can be precarious, especially at the neck. Some surgeons supercharge the graft with a cervical arterial anastomosis, something commonly performed in adults. The marginal vessels can be ligated near the graft's anticipated proximal cervical anastomotic site at a preparatory operation, perhaps six weeks or more before the interposition, so the chosen segment will develop a robust distally based arterial supply and venous drainage. Importantly, there is plenty of jejunum, so removing a section does not affect digestion. In addition, the jejunum is relatively acid-resistant, limiting reflux damage.

Many surgeons open the chest and the abdomen and use a pedicled graft. During the procedure, the child may need to be moved from a supine position to a left lateral position. The first mesenteric vessels are divided close to the base of the mesentery, and the jejunum is divided in two places: 15–20 cm from the ligament of Treitz and at the level of the third mesenteric branch. The uppermost part of this segment is checked for length, and the remainder is excised, leaving just the vascular pedicle. The space for the conduit through the transverse colon's mesentery and the hiatus must be adequate. Delivering the graft to the chest without a twist or undue tension is not easy; one can compromise the jejunum or its blood supply unless very careful. The anastomosis to the upper esophagus occurs in the chest or the neck over a transanastomotic tube. The gastric anastomosis is made, and intestinal continuity is restored with a jejuno-jejunal anastomosis.

Free grafts or supercharging the upper end of the jejunum requires microvascular anastomoses. Tortuosity does not always preclude good function, see Fig. 27.7.

Complications related to the different techniques are listed in Table 27.3.

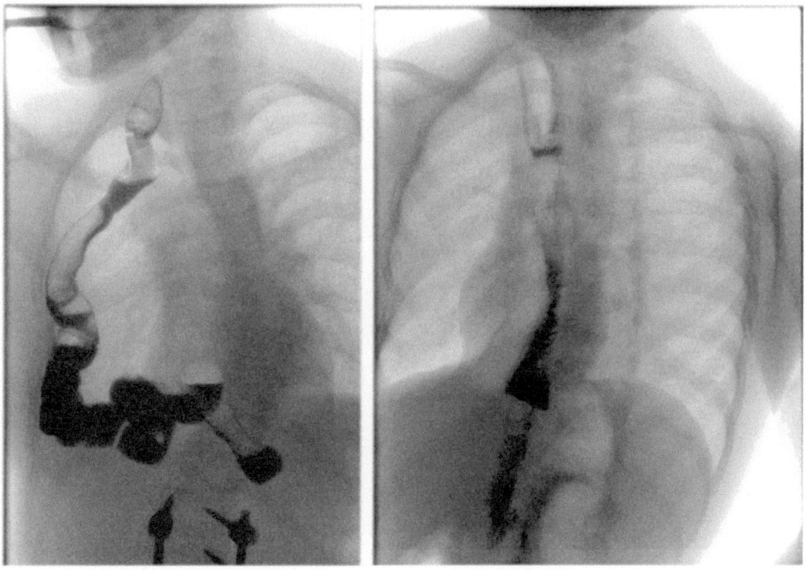

Fig. 27.7 Left shows a tortuous jejunal interposition placed in a hostile and scoliotic chest after a failed Foker with surprisingly good function 6 years after interposition, and right shows a straighter interposition placed in a good chest with excellent function

Table 27.3 Complications of different esophageal replacement procedures

Gastric Transposition	Gastric tube	Colonic interposition	Jejunal interposition
The early complications Pneumothorax Tracheal, major vessel injury Severe tachycardia Respiratory compromise Venous compression Acute gastric dilatation Anastomotic leak Cardiac Arrythmia *Late complications* Anastomotic stricture Swallowing problem Delayed gastric emptying Jejunostomy tube complications Dumping syndrome Anaemia Gastroesophageal reflux	Early Pneumonitis Mediatinitis may occur because of leak from long suture line Cervical *anastomotic leak* Late Stricture (30–40%) GER Ulcer Bleeding Barrett's esophagus	Necrosis of graft Anastomotic leak (30%) Esophago-cutaneous fistula Transient malabsorption Strictures (20%) Gastric outlet obstruction Mediastinitis, empyema Redundancy Halitosis Graft related complications: Ulcer, colitis, hemorrhage, polyp	Problems related to the blood supply of the jejunum Anastomotic complications

27.15 Long-Term Follow-up

Long-term follow-up is wise as late strictures, excessive tortuosity, and Barrett's esophagus may be problematic. However, assessing the lower end of the graft could be difficult with a tortuous interposition.

27.16 The Future

Combining decellularized or synthetic scaffolds with autologous muscle, epithelial cells, and neural crest cells may facilitate the engineering of a peristalsing conduit. Since the esophagus has a precarious intrinsic vascular anatomy and is easily stenosed when poorly perfused, vascularity must be addressed. Cell-scaffold interactions and motility are also a concern.

Xenotransplants, or xenografts, from genetically modified pigs may be attractive once the techniques have been mastered for high-volume transplantations, such as kidney, heart, liver, and lung.

Suggested Reading

Choudhury SR, Yadav PS, Khan NA, Shah S, Debnath PR, Kumar V, Chadha R. Pediatric esophageal substitution by gastric pull-up and gastric tube. J Indian Assoc Pediatr Surg. 2016;21:110–4.

Coran AG, Caldamone A, Scott Adzich N, Krummel TM, Laberge JM, editors. Pediatric surgery. 7th ed. Oxford: Elsevier Limited; 2012.

Holcomb GW III, Murphy PJ, St Peter SD, editors. Holocomb and ashcraft's pediatric surgery. 7th ed. Philadelphia: Elsevier; 2020.

Soccorso G, Parikh D. Esophageal replacement in children: Challenges and long-term outcomes. J Indian Assoc Pediatr Surg. 2016;21:98. https://doi.org/10.4103/0971-9261.182580

Spitz L, Coran C, Teitelbaum DH, Pierro A, Tan HL. Operative pediatric surgery. 7th ed. CRC Press; 2013.

Airway and Esophageal Foreign Bodies, Injuries, and Perforations

28

Palak Singhai, Jai K. Mahajan, and Subhasis Roy Choudhury

28.1 Introduction

Aspiration and ingestion of foreign bodies are one of the frequently encountered pediatric emergencies. The incidence peaks between 1 and 2 years of age due to factors like oral fixation, development of fine motor skills, increased mobility, incomplete dentition, immature swallowing, and a superiorly placed larynx in this age group. Foreign body aspiration (FBA) and esophageal impaction carry a significant risk of morbidity and mortality.

28.2 Airway Foreign Bodies

FBA is one of the most common causes of unintended deaths in infants. As per the WISQARS leading cause of death report (2019) by the Centers for Disease Control and Prevention (CDC), it is the fifth most common cause of death in children aged 1–3 years. Over 80% of affected children are under the age of 3 years. Males are more commonly affected than females.

The most commonly aspirated items are organic such as nuts, seeds, pulses, and corn kernels. They are usually radiolucent but produce other secondary signs on chest X-ray. Older children are more likely to aspirate inorganic items such as beads, coins, pen caps, and whistles. Inorganic foreign bodies are more frequently radiopaque and easier to diagnose on chest X-ray (Fig. 28.1). An aspirated foreign body can lodge anywhere from the hypopharynx, larynx, trachea, and mainstem bronchi to the distal airways. The most common site is the right main bronchus, owing to its wider lumen and straighter course.

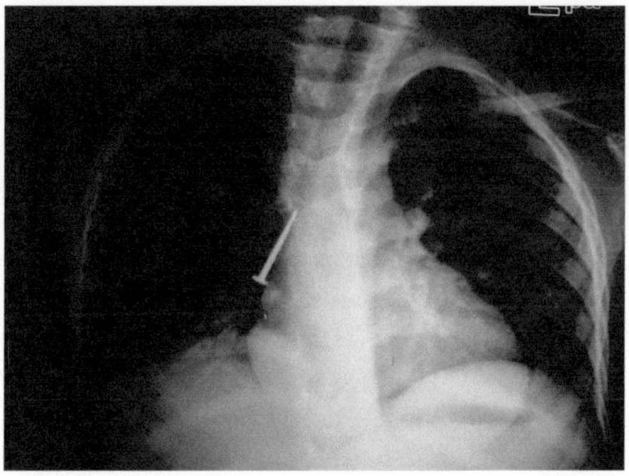

Fig. 28.1 A radiopaque foreign body in the right main bronchus

P. Singhai · J. K. Mahajan (✉)
Department of Pediatric Surgery, Advanced Pediatric Centre, Postgraduate Institute of Medical Education and Research, Chandigarh, India

S. Roy Choudhury
Pediatric Surgery, Lady Hardinge Medical College and Associated Kalawati Saran Children's Hospital, New Delhi, Delhi, India

© The Author(s), under exclusive license to Springer Nature Singapore Pte Ltd. 2025

S. Roy Choudhury (ed.), *Pediatric Surgery*, https://doi.org/10.1007/978-981-96-1257-4_28

28.2.1 Clinical Presentation

Several factors, such as the size, shape, type, site of the foreign body, and the time elapsed since aspiration, determine the clinical presentation of FBA. The classic triad of choking/coughing, wheezing, and asymmetric air entry on auscultation is observed in 15–57% of the patients.

Organic foreign bodies are more likely to produce cough, wheeze, dyspnoea, and fever. A foreign body in the hypopharynx and larynx produces abrupt and severe symptoms like acute onset of cough, drooling, and voice changes. While the upper tracheal foreign bodies produce inspiratory stridor and expiratory wheeze, the distal tracheal and bronchial foreign bodies present with cough, tachypnea, and wheeze and are often misdiagnosed as croup, asthma, or infectious pneumonia.

Temporally, there are three distinct phases in the clinical manifestations of FBA. The initial phase of foreign body impaction is characterized by the acute onset of respiratory symptoms. Gradually, as the foreign body settles in the tracheobronchial tree and the respiratory tract reflexes ebb, the patient enters into an asymptomatic phase. Chronic impaction results in the third phase of complications, presenting as chronic cough, recurrent pneumonias, bronchiectasis, and asthma-like symptoms.

28.2.2 Diagnostic Evaluation

A chest radiograph is the first investigation ordered for diagnosing FBA. Although less than 10% of aspirated foreign bodies are radiopaque, the X-ray chest can show several secondary signs of FBA. Several indirect signs like overdistension of the hypopharynx and swelling of prevertebral soft tissues are seen in foreign body impaction in upper airways, while a foreign body in the lower airways will show hyperinflation, air trapping, mediastinal shift, pneumonia, atelectasis, pneumothorax, and opacification of the whole lung on X-ray of the chest (Fig. 28.2). The cumulative sensitivity of chest radiographs for diagnosing FBA ranges from 60% to 85%, and the specificity ranges from 32% to 71%. It can be normal in up to 50% of patients with laryngotracheal and 25% of bronchial foreign bodies.

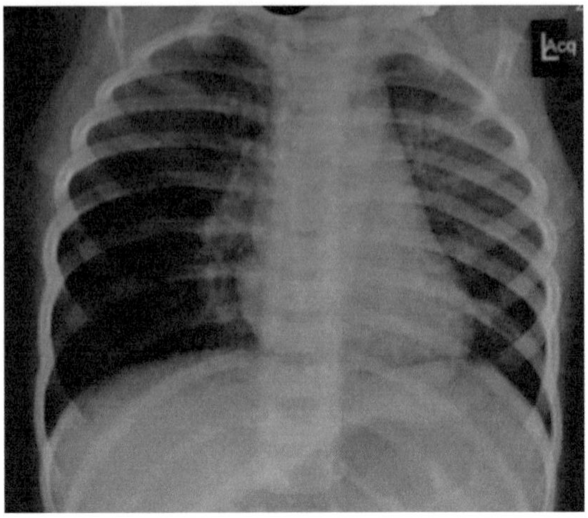

Fig. 28.2 Hyperinflation of the right lung indicating the presence of a foreign body in the right bronchus

Fluoroscopy can be used as an adjunct to the chest radiograph to demonstrate mediastinal shift and paradoxical diaphragmatic movements representing air trapping. However, it is a highly operator-dependent, time-consuming investigation and may be challenging to acquire in an uncooperative and irritable child. Multidetector computed tomography (MDCT) can detect even small and radiolucent foreign bodies, with information on the shape, form, and location within the airway. CT scan is superior to a chest X-ray in demonstrating the secondary signs and complications of FBA, and virtual bronchoscopy generates a 3-D reconstruction of the images. The sensitivity and specificity of CT for detecting airway foreign bodies are >99%.

In a sick child with a strong history and clinical examination suggestive of FBA, no diagnostic investigation is compulsory before taking up rigid bronchoscopy, which is the gold standard investigation. In the absence of a standard protocol, the rate of negative bronchoscopy ranges between 15% and 45%. Several scoring systems have been devised to facilitate decision-making and reduce the number of negative bronchoscopies. In a retrospective observational study of 300 patients with suspected FBA, Janahi et al. noted

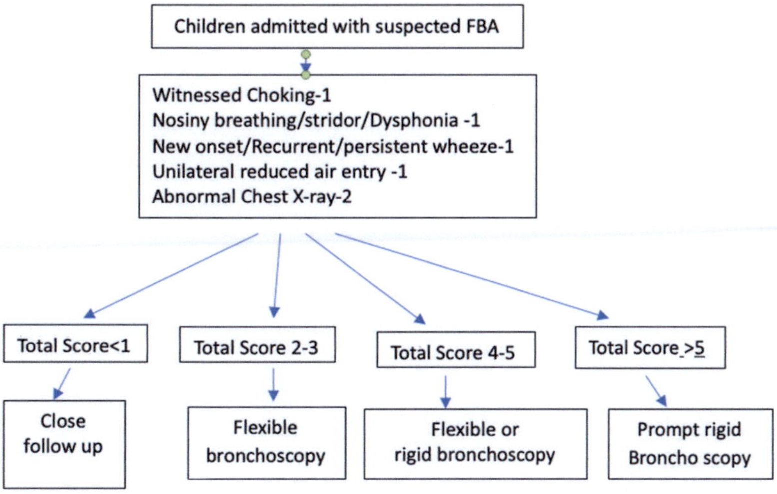

Fig. 28.3 Algorithm for the management of patients with suspected foreign body aspiration. (Adapted from Janahi et al. 2017)

that a history of sudden choking, noisy breathing/stridor, new onset/persistent/recurrent wheeze, reduced unilateral air entry, and abnormal radiographic findings were significant predictors of FBA. The authors proposed a management algorithm to predict patients having a high likelihood of FBA (Fig. 28.3). In patients with an uncertain diagnosis, flexible bronchoscopy is performed first, if the expertise is available. Its smaller diameter allows the distal tracheobronchial tree to be evaluated.

28.2.3 Management

The management of acute airway obstruction due to FBA begins at home. The Australian Resuscitation Council has issued guidelines for caregivers on first aid management of airway obstruction secondary to FBA. In acute choking with an unresponsive child, an oral cavity sweep followed by cardiopulmonary resuscitation should be initiated. If the child is conscious and has complete airway obstruction with cyanosis, five alternating back blows and chest thrusts are performed until emergency medical help arrives.

An immediate airway, breathing, and circulation assessment is performed at the hospital. A patient with hypoxemia may require endotracheal intubation and stabilization before bronchoscopy. Endoscopic retrieval of the foreign body is the treatment modality of choice. The patient is well oxygenated, direct laryngoscopy is performed under general anesthesia, and an appropriate-sized ventilating bronchoscope is inserted into the airway. The foreign body is removed using optical forceps. Smooth, rounded foreign bodies with a central hole, such as necklaces or toy beads, are challenging to grasp and can be retrieved with the help of Fogarty catheters.

The complications of rigid bronchoscopy include laryngeal edema, bronchospasm, pulmonary infiltrates, and atelectasis. Rarely, patients may develop airway perforation, pneumothorax, pneumomediastinum, respiratory failure, and cardiopulmonary arrest, and the incidence ranges from 1 to 8. Perioperative mortality after rigid bronchoscopy is currently <1%.

Recently, fibreoptic bronchoscopy for therapeutic purposes has gained popularity with variable success. A fibreoptic bronchoscope can provide access to more distal airways, but is limited by a small channel diameter and instruments for grasping the foreign body. A backup of rigid bronchoscopy must always be available when taking a patient for therapeutic fibreoptic bronchoscopy.

Postoperatively, a short course of steroids is helpful in selected cases with significant airway edema. Routine use of antibiotics is not indicated, but they are advised in patients with purulent secretions and pneumonia. Successful bronchoscopic removal of foreign bodies is achieved in 97–99% of the patients, with complete retrieval at first attempt in 86% of the patients. Long-standing foreign bodies can be associated with inflammatory bronchial mucosa and obstructive granuloma, which impedes identification and retrieval. If repeated attempts fail to retrieve the foreign body due to poor vision, the procedure can be completed in a staged manner after patient stabilization. Inorganic foreign bodies that are smooth and rounded may be challenging to grasp, and the retrieval of pen caps with distally facing open ends is often unsuccessful. In cases of failed endoscopic extractions, open surgical intervention such as tracheostomy, thoracotomy, bronchotomy, and pulmonary resection may be required in 0.3–4% of patients.

28.2.4 Complications

Late diagnosis of FBA can result in severe acute and chronic complications. In the short term, there is a risk of atelectasis, airway edema, pneumothorax, pneumomediastinum, subcutaneous emphysema, and cardiopulmonary arrest. Following FBA, a delay of more than 4 weeks is associated with a high risk of complications like recurrent pneumonia, bronchiectasis, lung abscess, and empyema.

28.3 Esophageal Foreign Bodies

Ingestion of foreign bodies is a common problem in the pediatric population. Over 100,000 accidental foreign body ingestion (FBI) cases are reported annually in the United States. Most ingested foreign bodies pass uneventfully through the alimentary tract, but a few may cause significant morbidity. Children aged 1–3 years are most commonly affected. The presentation and course of management are determined by the age of the patient, time since ingestion, and the foreign body's type, size, shape, and location. Since most ingested foreign bodies are inorganic metal objects, they are easily diagnosed on plain radiographs, and over 75% of these will present within 24 h of ingestion.

The patients with pre-existing esophageal anomalies or surgery, children with attention deficit hyperactivity disorder, and those facing abuse or neglect are at a higher risk of FBI. Pre-existing esophageal abnormalities can be present in up to 4–14% of patients with FBI.

Commonly ingested foreign bodies include coins, metal objects, plastic toy pieces, button batteries, fish bones, and food boluses. The most common site of the FBI is the first esophageal constriction, the narrowest part of the gastrointestinal tract.

28.3.1 Clinical Presentation

The clinical features of the FBI vary with the age of the patient, type, and location of the foreign body. Infants have nonspecific symptoms like drooling, poor feeding, gagging, and respiratory distress. Older children complain of odynophagia, chest pain, and dysphagia. Large foreign bodies in the esophagus can cause airway obstruction. Drooling, regurgitation, and dysphagia are common complaints when the foreign body is impacted in the upper esophagus. On the contrary, the foreign bodies in the distal esophagus present with chest pain and vomiting. The physical examination includes assessing the vital signs, airway, and oropharynx. The neck and upper thorax are palpated for the presence of subcutaneous emphysema, and the lungs are auscultated to check for air entry.

28.3.2 Diagnostic Evaluation

Over 80% of the ingested foreign bodies are radiopaque, and suspected FBI is evaluated using plain X-rays of the neck, chest, and abdomen in anteroposterior and lateral views. On frontal chest X-rays, esophageal coins appear effaced, while the tracheal coins appear tangential because of a gap in the tracheal rings posteriorly. Double rim or halo sign caused by the bilaminar structure

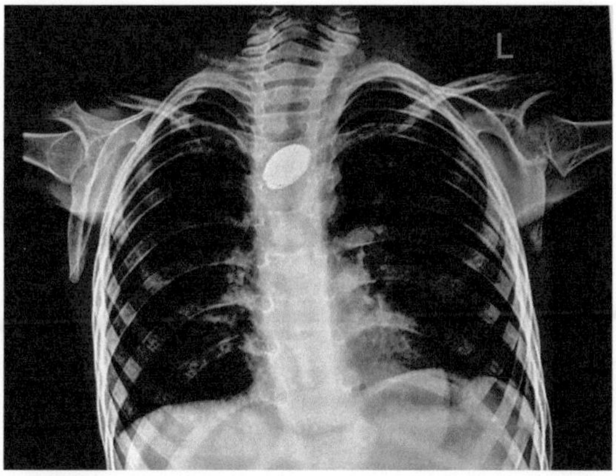

Fig. 28.4 Xray chest showing button battery impaction in the upper esophagus

of the button battery on an anteroposterior view and the step-off sign at the junction of cathode and anode on a lateral view helps distinguish button batteries from the coins (Fig. 28.4). In chronic FBI, there is a thickening of the tracheoesophageal interface or compression of the trachea posteriorly.

A contrast esophagogram is performed if the clinical suspicion is high and the X-ray is negative. It can show esophageal lumen obstruction and detect complications like esophageal perforation or fistulas. MDCT of the chest and the abdomen is a highly accurate investigation for identifying even radiolucent foreign bodies, with detailed information on the size, shape, and location. It has a high negative predictive value and a specificity of 96% in detecting ingested foreign bodies. CT is beneficial when the esophagoscopy is negative, but the symptoms suggest FBI. It also detects complications like abscess, perforation, and fistula formation.

28.3.3 Management

Eighty to ninety percent of ingested foreign bodies pass spontaneously with stool uneventfully, 10–20% may require endoscopic removal, and <1% require open surgery for retrieval.

Flexible endoscopy is the most commonly used modality but may not be successful in cases of complicated impaction. Rigid endoscopy is the gold standard, with an 86% foreign body retrieval success rate. Rigid endoscope has a wider lumen with a broader working channel. The principles of endoscopic removal are to protect the airway, control the object during extraction, and avoid additional damage to the esophageal mucosa. Fixing the endotracheal tube to the left and placing the neck in slight extension with a bolster under the shoulders facilitate the procedure. The esophagoscope is advanced under vision, and the foreign body is retrieved using optical forceps. Large objects may require the removal of the forceps, the foreign body, and the esophagoscope together as a unit. Check esophagoscopy should be performed to look for any residual foreign body and esophageal mucosal injury.

Rigid esophagoscopy is safe, with a complication rate of only 0.2–5% and mortality being <1%. The common intraoperative complications include failure to retrieve, dislodgement of the endotracheal tube, arrhythmia, aspiration, cricopharyngeal, and laryngeal spasm. Postoperative complications are stridor, laryngospasm, and cough.

Coins are the most commonly ingested foreign bodies, and 25–30% pass spontaneously with stool (Fig. 28.5). The presence of symptoms warrants urgent endoscopic removal irrespective of the time elapsed. An asymptomatic patient can be observed for spontaneous passage and repeating the X-ray after 12 h. The coins that are impacted for >24 h in the esophagus should be removed endoscopically. Disimpaction of the coins with a Foley catheter and removal under fluoroscopic guidance has also been reported. The catheter is advanced beyond the coin, and the balloon is inflated. With the patient in the trendelenberg position, it is slowly withdrawn under fluoroscopy guidance. Bougienage can also be employed for uncomplicated coin ingestion. The reported efficacy and safety of all three methods of coin removal vary across the literature. Bougienage and Foley catheter removal is simple, easily accessible, cost-effective, and do not require general anesthesia. However, there are concerns regarding aspiration, acute airway obstruction, and esophageal perforation if these procedures are not performed with dexterity.

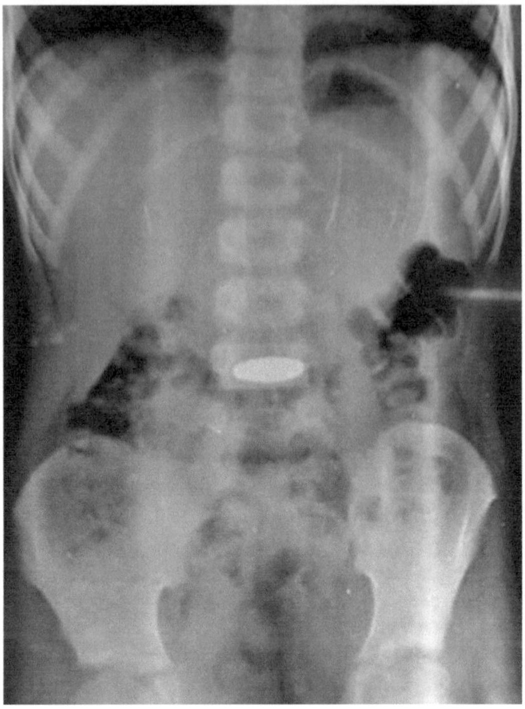

Fig. 28.5 X-ray of the abdomen shows an ingested coin in the stomach

The incidence of button battery ingestion has increased over the past few decades with the growing availability of battery-powered toys and devices. Button batteries cause esophageal wall necrosis due to hydroxide alkaline injury generated by the electric current, leakage of chemicals, and pressure necrosis. They cause significant esophageal damage as early as 2 h after ingestion, which can rapidly progress to esophageal perforation, mediastinitis, tracheoesophageal fistula, and erosion into the great vessels. The North American Society for Pediatric Gastroenterology, Hepatology, and Nutrition (NASPGHAN) Endoscopy Committee recommends that button batteries in the esophagus, whether symptomatic or not, warrant immediate endoscopic removal within 2 h from ingestion. Button batteries in the stomach are observed, if they are asymptomatic, but should be followed with serial X-rays. Nonprogression of the battery even after 2 days since ingestion, size of the battery >15 mm, co-ingestion of a magnet, and age of the patient less than 6 years are indications for the removal of asymptomatic gastric batteries.

Ingestion of multiple magnets or a magnet with a metallic foreign body can cause mucosal pressure necrosis, perforation, obstruction, or fistula formation, and they are removed even if asymptomatic. However, a single magnet, which is not too large, is expected to pass spontaneously.

Impaction of sharp and pointed foreign bodies like safety pins, nails, hairpins, and glass shards is known to have high morbidity and mortality. If the sharp end of the object is facing proximally, it is safer to push the foreign body into the stomach, rotate it, and grasp it with the pointed end being directed distally. Rigid endoscopy should be preferred to remove sharp foreign bodies to prevent mucosal injury during retrieval.

Food bolus impaction is seen in patients with pre-existing esophageal abnormalities, such as caustic, peptic, or postoperative stricture, esophageal stenosis, eosinophilic esophagitis, and dysmotility disorders. Bouginnage is contraindicated in such patients, and esophagoscopy should be performed within 12 h. Retrieval nets, tripod, or pentapod forceps are useful instruments for removing impacted food boluses.

Some newer techniques to remove challenging foreign bodies are the double snare technique for long foreign bodies, the combined forceps and snare technique for safety pins, and the suture technique for any foreign body with a hole.

Surgical removal of foreign bodies is required when there is failure of rigid esophagoscopy, lumen perforation, or associated congenital anomalies. In patients with esophageal perforation secondary to foreign body impaction, it is preferable to remove the foreign body endoscopically, as the esophageal perforation will invariably be smaller than the size of the object. An impacted foreign body in the cervical esophagus is approached via a cervical esophagotomy, while a thoracic foreign body requires a thoracotomy. The esophageal repair can be buttressed with a layer of local muscle or pleural flap. A proposed algorithm for managing impacted foreign bodies in the esophagus is shown in Fig. 28.6. Endoscopic retrieval of the foreign body may be followed by a waiting period to allow for the spontaneous healing of the esophagus.

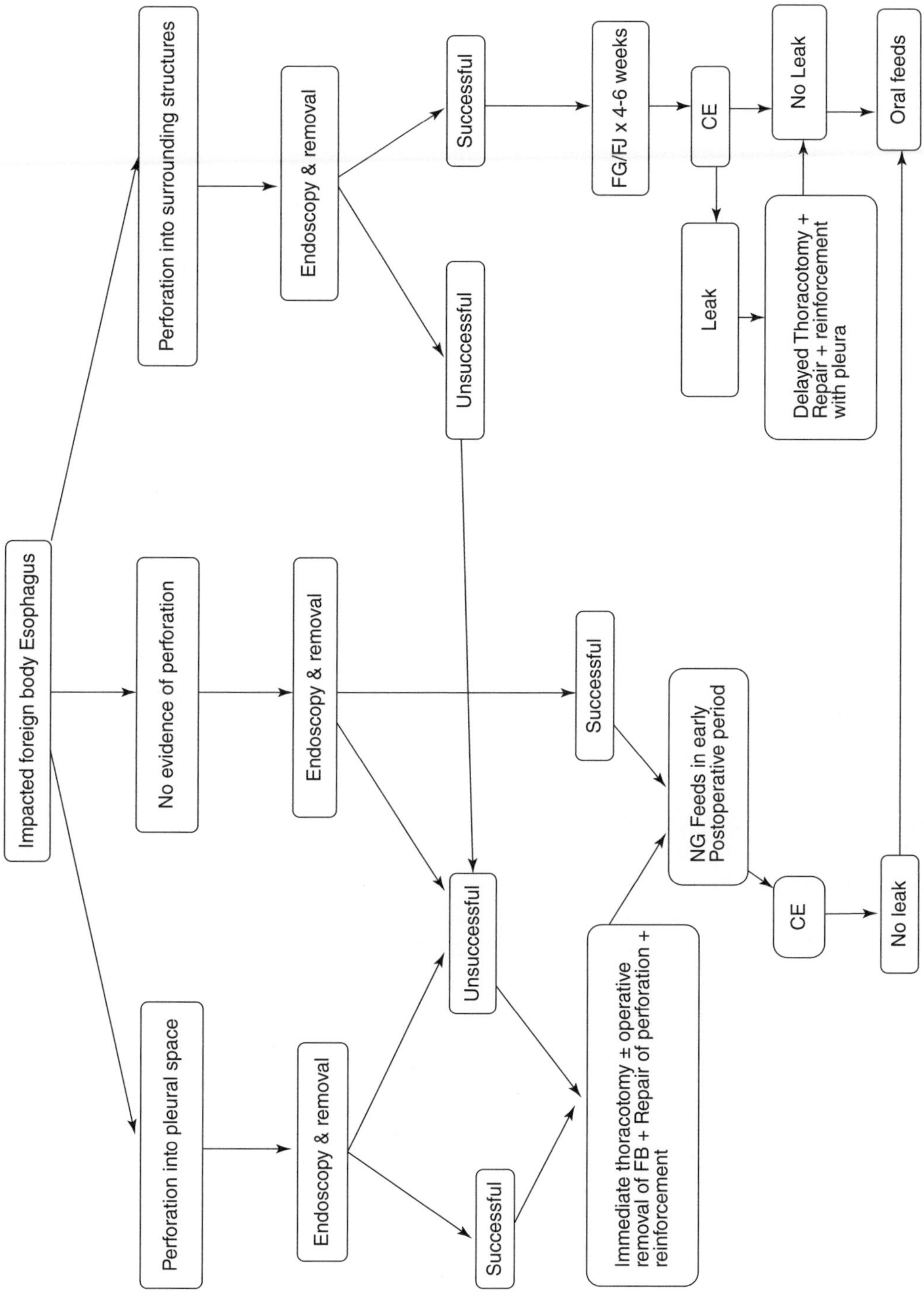

Fig. 28.6 Algorithm for the management of patients with foreign body impaction in the esophagus. (Adapted from Peters et al. 2015)

28.3.4 Complications

Long-standing impacted foreign bodies are at a higher risk of esophageal perforation, periesophageal collection, mediastinitis, neck abscess, tracheoesophageal fistula, aortoesophageal fistula, and esophageal stricture formation. In operated patients of esophageal atresia with tracheoesophageal fistula, unrecognized foreign body impaction can result in late fistula recurrence. Esophageal perforation presents with chest pain, fever, tenderness over the chest, and subcutaneous and mediastinal emphysema.

28.3.5 Prevention

The American Academy of Pediatrics recommends that education regarding aspiration and choking be provided to all caregivers of children aged >6 months. Parental education should include information on age-appropriate foods, encouraging the child to sit quietly while eating, cutting food items into large pieces, and offering one piece of food at a time. All small and hazardous items in the house, which can be potentially aspirated or ingested, should be kept out of reach of children. Consumer protection guidelines, community group efforts to influence strict manufacturing legislation, and product innovation and redesign can make toys safer for toddlers. Caregivers must be educated regarding appropriate first aid measures and need to seek timely medical help to prevent complications.

28.4 Esophageal Injuries and Perforations

The causes of esophageal injuries or perforations are foreign bodies, stricture with attempted dilatation, trauma, caustic infections, and battery-induced injuries. Chest x-ray findings in esophageal perforation include the pneumothorax, subcutaneous emphysema, pneumomediastinum, pleural, and pericardial effusion. A contrast study will generally determine the leak. CT with contrast study has a high percentage of yield.

28.4.1 Management of Esophageal Injuries and Perforations

Conservative management includes nil per oral, intravenous hydration, total pareneteral nutrition if required, and antibiotics. Perforations with free fluid in the thorax mandated intercostal tube drainage. Indications for surgery include perforation into the peritoneal cavity and patients not responding to initial conservative management. Direct repair with a tissue patch from the surrounding structures can also be carried out if presentation is early.

Caustic ingestion, which causes esophageal injuries, is not an uncommon problem. Acid injury results in pain and locally coagulative necrosis which prevent further extension of tissue injury. Alkali ingestion results in liquefactive necrosis and further penetration deeper in the tissues, therefore causing more extensive injury. Acid ingestion most commonly causes gastric and antral injuries, whereas alkali ingestion causes extensive esophageal injury. The duration of contact with the tissue is directly related to the extent of the injury.

Chest x ray and CT scan should be done within the first 24–48 h of injury to look for perforation. UGI endoscopy should be performed within the first 48 h to look for the extent of the injury (Table 28.1).

Patients with grade 1 to 2a injuries are allowed oral liquids and observed for 24–48 h. Those with 2b or 3 are kept NPO, and initial endoscopic placement of an NG tube may be used for feeding. Antibiotics, antifungal, and proton pump inhibitors or H2 receptor blockers are given. The role of systemic steroids is controversial. Patients with higher grade injuries should have a barium

Table 28.1 Classification of caustic esophageal injuries

Grade	Endoscopic findings
1	Mucosal edema and erythema
2a	Friability, hemorrhage, blisters, erosions, erythema, white exudate
2b	Findings of grade 2a plus deep or circumferential ulceration
3a	Small and scattered area of necrosis
3b	Extensive necrosis

swallow after 3 weeks to look for any stricture formation. Strictures are initially managed with serial esophageal dilatations at intervals of 2–4 weeks, and the duration varies depending on their requirement. Local injection or the application of steroids and mitomycin-c is associated with a higher success rate. A feeding jejunostomy may be required for maintaining nutritional requirements. Gastric antral strictures are managed with antro-pylotoplasty or gastrojejunostomy. Long and recalcitrant esophageal strictures may require esophageal replacement. Colonic substitution can be preferred, especially when the stomach may also have scarring. There is a definite high incidence of esophageal carcinoma following extensive alkali-induced injury, which should be kept in mind in the management with the institution of an appropriatre long-term surveillance program.

Suggested Reading

Australian Resuscitation Council. ANZCOR guideline 4—airway: subsection 4 –management of foreign body airway obstruction (choking). East Melbourne: ARC; 2016. Available at https://resus.org.au/

Berdan EA, Sato TT. Pediatric airway and esophageal foreign bodies. Surg Clin North Am. 2017;97(1):85–91.

Janahi IA, Khan S, Chandra P, Al-Marri N, Saadoon A, Al-Naimi L, et al. A new clinical algorithm scoring for management of suspected foreign body aspiration in children. BMC Pulm Med. 2017;17(1):61.

Laya BF, Restrepo R, Lee EY. Practical imaging evaluation of foreign bodies in children. Radiol Clin North Am. 2017;55(4):845–67.

Lee JH. Foreign body ingestion in children. Clin Endosc. 2018;51(2):129–36.

Peters NJ, Mahajan JK, Bawa M, Chabbra A, Garg R, Rao KLN. Esophageal perforations due to foreign body impaction in children. J Pediatr Surg. 2015;50(8):1260–3.

29 Airway Anomalies in Children

Sanjay Rao

Airway anomalies in children are infrequent, but potentially life threatening. If undiagnosed, they can cause significant morbidity and mortality. Hence, a high index of suspicion is necessary when dealing with these children.

Classically, the airways in children can be divided into three levels—for purposes of understanding the various pathologies and their presentation:

1. Upper Airway: This extends from the external nares to the oropharynx.
2. Central Airways: This extends from the supraglottis to the ostia of the secondary bronchi.
3. Distal Airways: This is the part of the airway distal to the ostia of the right and left secondary bronchi.

It is useful to describe the anatomy in this fashion, as there are typical presentations and pathologies that afflict each of these levels.

Airway level	Typical pathology	Typical presentation	Ideal access
Upper	Choanal atresia Pierre Robin	Stertor, feeding difficulty	Trans nasal flexible scope (TNFL)
Central	Laryngomalacia Subglottic stenosis, tracheal stenosis	Stridor	TNFL, rigid bronchoscope and telescope
Distal	Asthma, hyper-reactive airways	Wheeze	Bronchoscope

29.1 Recognising Common Symptoms

Children with airway obstruction most commonly present with noisy breathing. Some of these noises are typical enough to be recognised easily. It is vital to understand that the 'loudness' of the sound is not proportional to the degree of obstruction—infact, children with severe airway obstruction produce very little sound as there is insufficient air flowing across the block.

S. Rao (✉)
Department of Pediatric Surgery, Division of Solid Organ Transplantation, Narayana Health Hospitals, Bangalore, India

© The Author(s), under exclusive license to Springer Nature Singapore Pte Ltd. 2025

S. Roy Choudhury (ed.), *Pediatric Surgery*, https://doi.org/10.1007/978-981-96-1257-4_29

29.1.1 Stertor

Stertor is a snoring sound that is produced by turbulent airflow within the upper airways-usually the nose or oropharynx. It is exaggerated during sleep as there is a greater degree of tongue fall and worsening obstruction during sleep. It is a more guttural sound.

29.1.2 Stridor

Stridor is a sound that is produced due to turbulent airflow through the central airways. It is usually more pronounced during inspiration—inspiratory stridor—as the active process of inspiration forces greater flow of air across the obstruction. In addition, the child needs to generate exaggerated intrathoracic negative pressures to be able to pull in air across the obstruction; this worsens pre-existing trachea/laryngomalacia, and this too adds to the stridor sound. As expiration is a passive process, the turbulence is less, and therefore, sound too is lower in intensity. Biphasic stridor—where sound is present both during inspiration and expiration is typically seen in static obstructions—where the degree of obstruction and turbulence in airflow do not change very much during inspiration and expiration.

29.1.3 Wheeze

While stertor and stridor are audible to the unaided ear, wheeze requires a stethoscope. Wheeze is typically a sound generated at small distal airways.

While it is useful, for the sake of classification and understanding, to describe airway obstructions and sounds in this manner, in clinical practice, there is often significant overlap. Having pathology at multiple levels is the norm, rather than an exception, especially in younger children. Hence, every child with a suspected airway obstruction MUST have a detailed evaluation of the ENTIRE airway—from external nares to the secondary bronchi ostia.

29.2 Evaluation of a Child with Airway Anomalies

The importance of a detailed history cannot be overemphasised. In the majority, this provides a reliable indicator of the level of obstruction. The temporal sequence of onset of symptoms and their progression also provide vital clues.

It is important to carefully listen to the sounds that the child may be producing and assess if it is stertor, stridor or wheeze. A thorough physical examination must follow. This should quickly assess the degree of distress and determine if any urgent airway support is required. The immediate intervention might be something as simple as placement of a nasogastric tube or oral airway, to as complex as urgent tracheostomy or ECMO.

An examination for signs of genetic/chromosomal anomalies must be included in the clinical evaluation. Respiratory examination must evaluate for any laterality of findings. A cardiac evaluation may reveal murmurs.

Radiological imaging will need to be individualised. It may include chest x-rays, CT scans, scans for gastro-esophageal reflux and swallow studies. Brain imaging may be required for suspected neurological pathology. An echocardiogram may be required.

A detailed airway assessment forms the bedrock of diagnosis and treatment planning. The MLB (micro laryngoscopy-bronchoscopy) is a procedure performed in the OR, with the child sedated but breathing spontaneously. A rigid telescope is an ideal tool as it provides detailed images and also allows the assessment of dynamics. The MLB may be combined with an upper GI scopy and flexible bronchoscopy (the Triple-Scopy) during the evaluation of complex aerodigestive problems. At the end of the MLB, there should be agreement on the diagnosis and the potential treatment plan.

Treatment, obviously, will depend on the diagnosis made. We will now look at some common airway anomalies and their management.

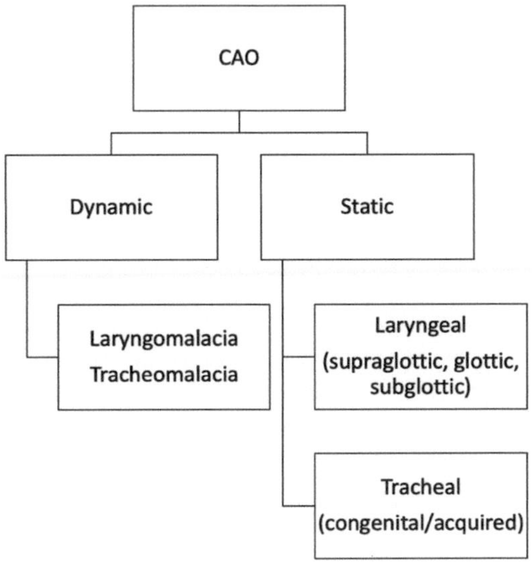

29.3 Laryngomalacia

Laryngomalacia is the commonest cause of stridor in infants. The stridor is predominantly inspiratory. The supraglottic structures prolapse into the glottic inlet, and this results in obstruction during inspiration. During expiration, as the airway pressure turns positive, the prolapse reverses and the stridor disappears. The character and the loudness of the stridor can vary widely between patients, and even in the same baby at different times.

Typically, the stridor begins to appear after the 2-3rd week of life. It reaches its maximum intensity around the 3-4th month and then reduces. In up to 80–85% of infants, the stridor disappears by the 2nd year.

Laryngomalacia is worsened by the presence of gastroesophageal reflux. Similarly, the increased negative intrathoracic pressure the infant must generate to overcome the laryngeal obstruction also results in worsening of the reflux. Hence, every patient with significant stridor must receive aggressive antireflux therapy.

In most children, laryngomalacia is a benign condition and does not cause significant detriment to the child's health. It gradually disappears as the child grows. In this situation, no active treatment is required. Reassurance and anti-reflux therapy are adequate. However, in about 15–20% of children, laryngomalacia can cause problems—significant retractions and distress, failure to thrive and at times acute life-threatening events. In these instances, if aggressive supporting therapy does not work, surgery for correction of laryngomalacia is recommended.

Surgery for laryngomalacia is called supraglottoplasty. It is performed trans-orally with the larynx suspended. The procedure includes the division of short aryepiglottic folds and some debulking of the posterior arytenoid/cuneiform mucosal bulk. Some surgeons prefer to trim the lateral edges of the epiglottis as well—however, this is rarely required. The procedure should be very conservative—the aim should be to relieve the obstruction. Often stridor persists, but will disappear with time. Overcorrection can result in debilitating aspiration and the dreaded problem of supraglottic scarring.

To summarise, laryngomalacia is common and in most cases has a benign course with an excellent chance of spontaneous recovery. Infants who have significant sequelae such as respiratory distress, retractions, failure to thrive and life-threatening events will require aggressive evaluation and treatment. The presence of synchronous lesions in the airway or comorbidities, such as neurological anomalies, may indicate the need for a tracheostomy. However, in most of the others, a well-done supra-glottoplasty spares the child from a tracheostomy.

When the temporal sequence of symptoms is not typical—when the stridor is present at birth or appears later in childhood, one must investigate for other causes. Not every infantile stridor is laryngomalacia. It is reasonable to manage a child with laryngomalacia, exclusively on a clinical diagnosis, only if the history is typical and the child is not severely symptomatic. In the presence of a history that is not typical or when there are the aforementioned red flags, an MLB is mandatory.

29.4 Laryngeal Atresia

Laryngeal atresia is a congenital anomaly due to the failure of recanalisation of the glottis. The vocal cords are fused to varying extents. In milder forms, only the anterior one-third is fused (Grade 1). These children are only marginally symptomatic. In more severe cases, almost the entire length of the vocal cords is fused (Grade 3), leaving only a very small chink in the posterior aspect. These children present with respiratory distress at birth and have a very weak cry. It is important to appreciate that the malformation is not restricted only to the glottis, the cartilages in the subglottic area too are malformed and the stenosis often extends into the subglottis, this is more frequent in the more severe forms of laryngeal atresia (Fig. 29.1).

Management varies depending on the severity of presentation and grade of obstruction. Typically, babies who are symptomatic at birth need a tracheostomy. A formal reconstruction of the glottis and subglottis is performed when the child is older and thriving, usually at about 6–8 months. In milder forms, the child can be managed expectantly, and endo-laryngeal procedures can be carried out when the child is older.

The aim of the surgery must be to minimise scarring and restore the laryngeal anatomy and function. Vocal cord mobility can be restored as there is no ankylosis and the nerve supply is normal. These children have an excellent chance of a normal voice and swallow—a chance that rapidly is lost with the inappropriate use of high-energy devices.

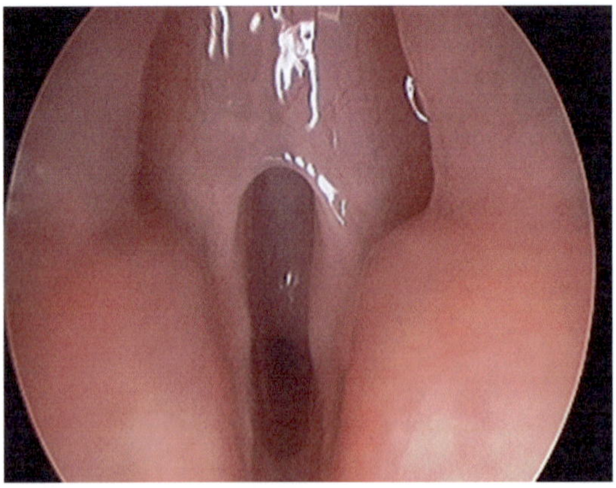

Fig. 29.1 Endoscopic image of laryngeal atresia. Note that the anterior two-third of the vocal cords are fused together. In addition, the airway below the vocal cords also is narrow

29.5 Vocal Cord Palsy

Vocal cord palsy is the second most common cause of neonatal stridor, after laryngomalacia. Typically, these babies have palsy at birth and are symptomatic at birth (unlike in laryngomalacia, where the symptoms begin to appear only by the 2-3rd week). While neurological causes such as Arnold Chiari malformations need to be looked for in these neonates, in the vast majority, no neurological anomaly is detected—i.e. the VC palsy is idiopathic. Spontaneous recovery is the usual course. Hence, in the newborn, attempts to directly interfere with the vocal cords must be resisted.

Unilateral vocal cord palsy is usually asymptomatic—a weak cry being the only symptom. In cases of bilateral vocal cord palsy, the cords are positioned paramedian, and this results in significant respiratory obstruction. A tracheostomy is recommended in this situation as it allows an opportunity for spontaneous recovery, a most desired outcome which leaves the larynx untouched and unscarred. Recovery can be expected even up to 2 years. If the palsy persists beyond 2 years of age, surgery is usually required to allow decannulation. The preferred procedure is a posterior glottic split with costal cartilage augmentation. This allows the arytenoids to be displaced laterally, thus opening the posterior glottic inlet and providing a passage for respiration. There is a slightly higher risk of aspiration in the early post-operative period, however, most children get over this problem in a few weeks.

There is a second peak of idiopathic vocal cord palsy in the late first decade of life—again the aetiology of this is unknown. Children present with late-onset stridor, respiratory distress and poor voice. Again, spontaneous recovery is expected, and hence, irreversible procedures are not recommended at this stage. A unilateral vocal cord lateralisation is adequate and often avoids the need for a tracheostomy. The lateralisation suture can be removed once function returns—a process that could take several months.

Acquired vocal cord palsy can also be iatrogenic—especially after surgical procedures in the neck and upper thorax. Excision of large cystic hygromas, thyroidectomy and patent ductus arteriosus (PDA) ligation are common examples. Violent intubations can also result in direct vocal cord damage. Acquired vocal cord palsy is usually unilateral and presents predominantly with a weak voice and noisy breathing. Again, unless there has been a confirmed severing of the nerve, neuropraxia is presumed and a spontaneous recovery can be expected. If recovery does not occur and the child remains symptomatic due to a paramedian cord, procedures, such as cordotomy or cordectomy, are suggested. However, these are ablative and irreversible procedures and should be options of last resort.

29.6 Laryngotracheal Cleft

Laryngotracheal clefts (LTC) are congenital anomalies where there is a side-to-side communication between the posterior wall of the larynx and trachea and the anterior wall of the oesophagus (Fig. 29.2). This anomaly is thought to occur due to an incomplete separation of the trachea and oesophagus during foregut development. The degree of fusion can vary from remaining above

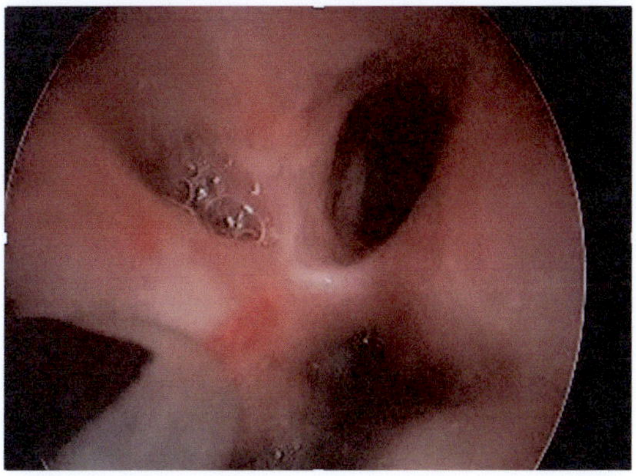

Fig. 29.2 Grade 4 Laryngotracheal cleft. A rigid endoscope allows the airway to stretch, thereby revealing the defect in its posterior wall

the cricoid (Grade 1) to extending up to the intrathoracic trachea and carina (Grade 4) (see Chap. 26). LTC is often associated with other anomalies such as oesophageal atresia. Higher grades of LTC are associated with severe tracheomalacia. LTC presents with features of recurrent aspirations—recurrent pneumonias, secretions, acute life-threatening events and choking while feeding are typical symptoms. Aspiration is confirmed on swallow studies, video fluroscopic swallow study (VFSS) and the diagnosis of LTC are confirmed with MLB.

Treatment is surgical. Grades 1 and 2 LTC can be repaired endoscopically, transorally. However, higher grades require surgery through the neck and chest. The principle is to ensure adequate separation of the oesophageal and tracheal walls and full-thickness repair of the wall of each. A tissue interposition is required to prevent recurrence, as the suture lines overlap. Tibial periosteum, pericardium and strap muscles have all been used for this purpose.

Outcomes vary directly with the extent of the cleft. While lower grades do very well, those with more severe forms have significant morbidity and mortality related to chronic pulmonary complications. Chronic aspiration, recurrent pneumonias, tracheomalacia and prolonged ventilatory requirements all add to pulmonary injury and mortality.

29.7 Subglottic Stenosis

Subglottic stenosis is one of the commonest causes of central airway obstruction in children. The stenosis could be congenital (in about 10%). However, in the vast majority it is iatrogenic, related to intubation and airway handling. Children present with stridor and respiratory distress. More severe grades can present with life-threatening airway obstruction. A high index of suspicion is necessary, especially in someone who develops stridor after intubation in the recent past.

The obstruction occurs in the subglottis, the only area of the entire airway with a complete circumferential ring of cartilage. This area pro-

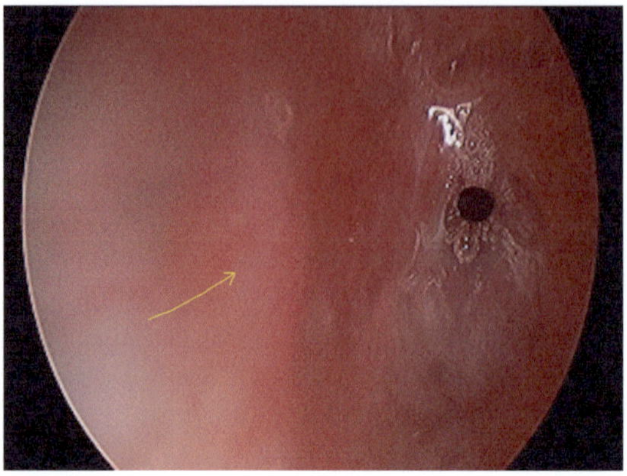

Fig. 29.3 Endoscopic image of a child with severe, Grade 3, subglottic stenosis. The vocal cord can be made out just above the stenosis (arrow)

vides the seal for the uncuffed endotracheal tubes used in children. Prolonged intubation or intubation with larger tubes causes mucosal ischaemia, ulceration and eventual scarring. Perichondritis of the cartilage can deform the cricoid cartilage and worsen the stenosis. There is no correlation between the duration of intubation and the degree of subglottic stenosis.

The Cotton-Myer grading is used to describe the severity: Grade 1 has <50% obstruction, Grade 2 50–90%, Grade 3 > 90% and Grade 4 complete obstruction (Fig. 29.3). However, this system does not account for glottic involvement in the scarring process: an important event that has a significant bearing on the choice of surgery and outcomes.

Congenital subglottic stenosis (SGS) is often not detected early. Typically, the history is of not being able to intubate with an age-appropriate tube when the child comes for an unrelated procedure. More severe forms of congenital SGS present with stridor at birth. Evaluation requires a detailed MLB.

29.7.1 Treatment Options Include

1. Balloon dilatation: Dilation with CRE™ balloons provides good outcomes—up to 70% resolution rates in carefully selected cases. Children with short segment, thin stenosis, presenting within weeks of the inciting event have the best results. Those with thick, established scars, long segment scars respond poorly. If a stenosis does not respond to a maximum of three dilatations, surgery is recommended.
2. Adjuncts to dilatation include the application of mitomycin-c, local injection of steroid, etc. Use of lasers and other energy devices to cut the stricture is often performed in older children and adults—however, in smaller children, this could potentially worsen the injury and scarring.
3. Stenting after dilatation is performed in older children and adults. In younger children, stents result in significant narrowing of the airway, and maintaining them over a period is challenging. Significant complications can occur from stent displacement and blockage.
4. Surgery: Surgical repair is now standard therapy in established SGS, especially in those who have long-segment stenosis or the concomitant involvement of the glottis.

Operations for SGS are of two types: (i) expansion procedures and (ii) resection procedures. The expansion procedures (laryngo-tracheoplasty, LTP) involve the longitudinal opening of the stenotic area and augmenting the diameter with the placement of a cartilaginous keel—usually created from an autologous costal cartilage. The airway is then supported with an endotracheal tube for up to a week. The child is then extubated. This procedure provides excellent results in Grade 2 and early Grade 3 stenosis (Fig. 29.4).

Resection procedures (laryngotracheal resection, LTR) are required for high Grade 3 and Grade 4 stenosis. This procedure partial cricotracheal resection (PCTR) involves the resection of the anterior cricoid arch along with all the scar tissues in the stenotic area. The distal healthy trachea is now anastomosed to the thyroid cartilage. This operation had the advantage of removing all scar tissue and approximating healthy tissues. However, it is a more complex procedure, and complications, such as dehiscence, when they occur, can be challenging.

However, with a proper selection of operative procedures, the majority of children can be

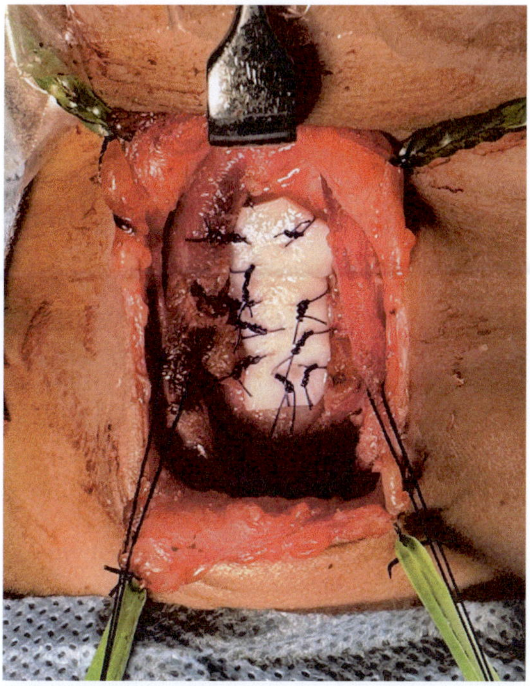

Fig. 29.4 Image showing the anterior costal cartilage graft in place after repair of subglottic stenosis

assured of excellent outcomes with the preservation of all laryngeal functions. The involvement of the glottis is an important factor that can limit functional outcomes—hence every effort must be made to avoid inadvertent secondary injury from energy devices such as lasers and electrocautery—something that is, unfortunately, all too common an occurrence.

29.8 Tracheomalacia

Tracheomalacia is a dynamic obstruction of the trachea, wherein the diameter of the trachea changes during the respiratory cycle. Tracheomalacia is far common in children than tracheal stenosis.

Tracheomalacia could happen due to the intrinsic weakness of tracheal cartilages or as a result of chronic extrinsic compression. Tracheomalacia could also be acquired, typically seen in children with long-term tracheostomy or intubation.

Tracheomalacia, especially in younger children, is associated with laryngomalacia. Laryngomalacia is a lot common than tracheomalacia in many instances, the tracheomalacia is exaggerated by the extremely high negative airway pressures that the baby needs to generate to overcome the obstruction from laryngomalacia. In such an instance, a correction of laryngomalacia improves the tracheomalacia as well. A careful assessment of the airway is essential to understand the dynamics of the entire process in each child. Radiological imaging, such as CT scans, may be required, and echocardiograms and CT Scans would be required to rule out extrinsic compression.

Management is usually directed to aetiological causes if any have been identified. Other management strategies include the use of continuos positive airway pressure ventilation (CPAP), non-invasive ventilation, tracheal stents and operations such as posterior tracheopexy. Often, these babies are sick from comorbidities, and a tracheostomy serves the dual purpose of reducing the work of breathing as well as stenting the tracheomalacia.

Outcomes over the long term depend on coexisting morbidities. A majority of children with tracheomalacia can expect good long-term resolution.

29.9 Tracheal Stenosis

Stenosis of the trachea is less common than subglottic stenosis. In infants and younger children, acquired tracheal stenosis is less common—as cuffed endotracheal tubes are not commonly used. In older children and teenagers, acquired stenosis is more common than congenital ones.

Congenital tracheal stenosis (CTS) occurs due to abnormalities in the tracheal cartilage. Normally, the tracheal cartilages are in the shape of a 'D'. The straight part of the 'D', which is posterior, is formed by the trachealis muscle. This arrangement allows the tracheal lumen to enlarge and constrict based on physiological requirements. In cases of increased demand, such as during exercises, the tracheal diameter and cross-sectional area can increase significantly. In the case of congenital tracheal stenosis, the tracheal rings are complete in the shape of an 'O' rather than 'D'. There is no trachealis component. This invariably results in varying degrees of stenosis, extending to varying lengths. In severe cases, the entire trachea and carina are involved. Unusually, however, the first tracheal ring is almost never involved in CTS.

More than two-thirds of children with CTS have associated malformations in the heart and great vessels. An aberrant take-off of the left pulmonary artery from the right side results in the formation of a pulmonary artery sling. This radiological finding must indicate the presence of CTS in that segment of the trachea. In about 10 to 15% of cases, the right upper lobe bronchus opens directly into the trachea, cranial to the carina (the so-called pig bronchus), requiring reimplantation at the time of tracheal repair (Fig. 29.5).

During the MLB, if CTS is suspected, the telescope should not be passed across the proximal end of the obstruction (Fig. 29.6). Doing so may result in critical airway obstruction. A CT scan of the thorax is performed to assess the length of the stenotic segment, the carinal anatomy and the presence of an aberrant right upper lobe bronchus or anomalies in the great vessels.

As these stenotic segments are long and there is no tracheal substitute, simple tracheal resection and anastomosis are not possible. The optimal operation for correction of CTS is a slide tracheoplasty. This procedure may require being done on cardiopulmonary bypass if the lower trachea or carina is involved or a concurrent cardiac procedure is required.

A slide tracheoplasty results in the doubling of the tracheal diameter, with some concurrent shortening in length. However, it provides a robust, healthy trachea with no tracheomalacia. The trachea will continue to grow and increase in diameter as the child grows. Morbidity and mortality in cases of CTS are related to the concomitant cardiac anomaly rather than the airway obstruction.

Acquired stenosis of the trachea is far common in older children and teenagers. Previous intubation with a cuffed endotracheal tube is often the cause (Fig. 29.7). Less common causes include caustic injury, surgical trauma and complex tracheoesophageal fistulae. Acquired tracheal stenosis is relatively easier to diagnose. There are no associated congenital anomalies and

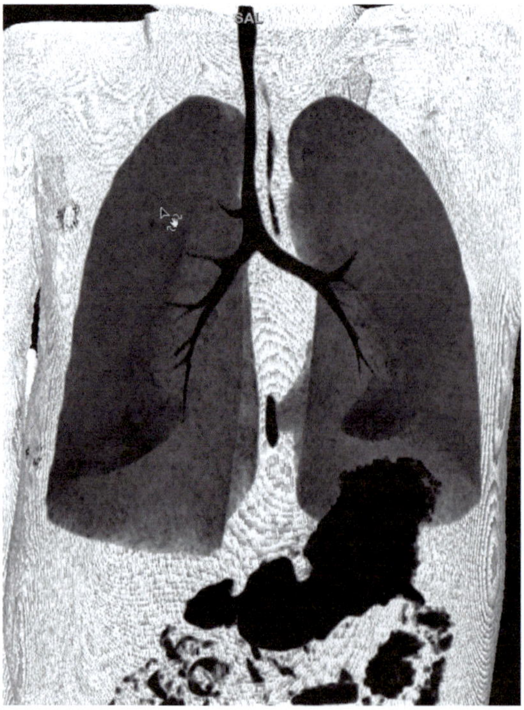

Fig. 29.5 CT scan reconstruction of a child with congenital stenosis of the mid tracheal segment along with an anomalous insertion of the right upper lobe bronchus directly into the trachea, proximal to the carina

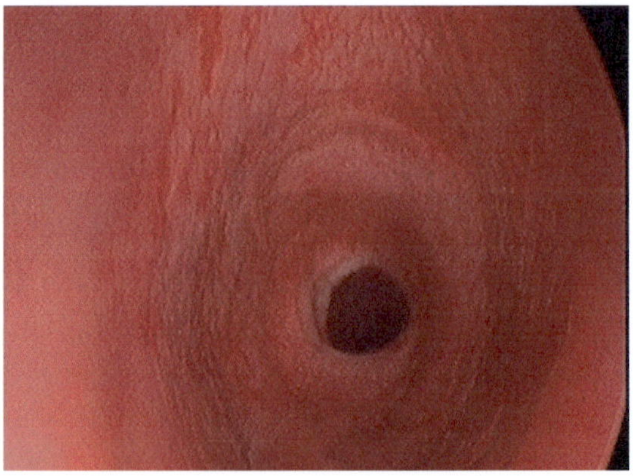

Fig. 29.6 Endoscopic appearance of congenital tracheal stenosis. Note that the narrow segment starts a couple of tracheal rings distal to the vocal cords. Also note the circular shape of the trachea at the level of stenosis

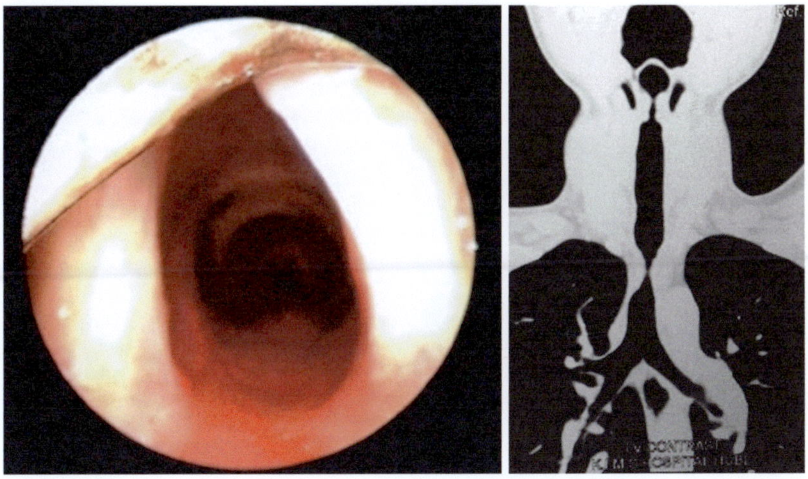

Fig. 29.7 Endoscopic and CT appearance of acquired tracheal stenosis in the case due to injury from a cuffed endotracheal tube

the children are often older. The segment involved often extends to only 2 or 3 rings. As a result, they respond very well to a local resection and anastomosis of the diseased tracheal segment. In early cases, balloon dilatation using CRE balloons is successful in about 40–50% of patients. In case the acquired stenosis involves more than 5 rings, a slide tracheoplasty may be required. A vast majority of these children can be assured of an excellent long-term prognosis.

29.10 Summary

Airway anomalies in children are complex and challenging. A careful history and a well-done MLB clinched the diagnosis in most cases. Further imaging is performed as indicated. A thorough understanding of the anatomy and dynamics of the airway is essential to plan treatment. With proper evaluation and selection of procedures, most children with airway anomalies can be assured of excellent outcomes. Comorbidities, which often coexist, can adversely influence outcomes. Considering the complexities, comorbidities and challenges in these children, specialist multidisciplinary teams are required to ensure optimal outcomes.

Further Reading

Pediatric Airway Surgery, Editor Philippe Monnier, Springer, 2011.

Seminars in Pediatric Surgery, Editors: Bedwell J, Zalzal G; 25(3), June 2016.

Seminars in Pediatric Surgery, Editors: Varela P, Schweiger C; 30(3), June 2021.

Otolaryngology Clinics of North America, 41(5), October 2008.

Part VI
Abdomen

Acute Abdomen in Children

30

Chandra Vibhash, Devprabha Bhagat, and Rahul Saxena

30.1 Introduction

Acute abdomen is defined as the onset of sudden and severe pain in the abdomen due to some intra-abdominal pathology and often requires surgical intervention. The following questions frequently arise while evaluating a child with an acute abdomen:

A. The need for hospital admission versus home treatment
B. When a surgical consultation is mandated
C. Whether analgesics are to be prescribed or not
D. When is the appropriate time for surgical intervention

30.2 Relevant Clinical History in the Evaluation of a Child with Acute Abdomen

- History should be taken from parents in their language, which should be in chronology
- Duration of the current illness
- Periodicity: is the pain constant, getting better, or worse
- Any specific aggravating and relieving factor
- Previous similar episodes
- Associated symptoms: vomiting (? bilious), distension, obstipation fever, diarrhea, or urinary symptoms
- History of trauma or previous surgery/ongoing medications
- Gynecologic history for pubertal girls

30.3 Clinical Examination

1. Need to be patient and gentle with the patient; in the presence of parents, in a comfortable environment
2. It is important to actively look for any signs of dehydration (early decompensation in the pediatric population)
3. Observe the child, his posture, movements, and activity (Fig. 30.1). A child with peritonitis will refrain from movements that aggravate pain

C. Vibhash (✉)
Department of Pediatric Surgery, LHMC, New Delhi, India

D. Bhagat · R. Saxena (✉)
Department of Pediatric Surgery, All India Institute of Medical Sciences, Jodhpur, India

© The Author(s), under exclusive license to Springer Nature Singapore Pte Ltd. 2025
S. Roy Choudhury (ed.), *Pediatric Surgery*, https://doi.org/10.1007/978-981-96-1257-4_30

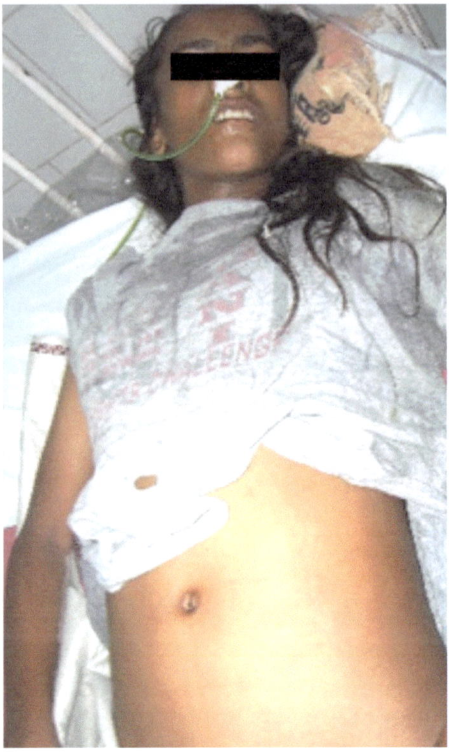

Fig. 30.1 Distended abdomen and bilious NG aspirates Peritonitis facies

30.3.1 Systemic Abdominal Examination

- *Inspection*:
  - Distension (central distension in acute intestinal obstruction)
  - Respiratory movements (reduced with peritonitis)
  - Visible peristalsis
  - Discoloration over the abdomen
  - Hernial orifices
  - Rectal examination: occult blood, red currant jelly (intussusception)
- *Palpation*: The use of the child's hand for palpation is better
  - Hyperesthesia
  - Tenderness: diffuse/localized; pointing sign; rebound tenderness
  - Guarding (voluntary or involuntary)/ rigidity
  - Lump
  - Hernial sites

Tenderness at the Mc-Burneys point, i.e., one third of the distance between the anterior superior iliac spine and the umbilicus, is associated with acute appendicitis. Copes psoas and Copes obturator signs may be elicited for retrocecal and pelvic appendicitis. The Murphy's sign is tenderness in the right mid-clavicular line below the costal margin and is associated with acute cholecystitis.

Tenderness, guarding, rigidity, and rebound tenderness are important signs indicating underlying inflammation. As a general principle, nonspecific abdominal pain is vague, central, and colicky, whereas pain due to appendicitis is localized and worsens over time. Patients presenting in the clinic with doubtful signs merit admission to the hospital with "active observation" and repeat examination. The possibility of child abuse should be kept when the clinical findings are not corroborated by history.

30.4 General Principles of Characteristic of Abdominal Pain

- Visceral pain is dull, poorly localized, and central
- Parietal pain is sharp and localized, cough or movement aggravates pain
- Referred pain follows the same dermatome, e.g., acute appendicitis pain referred to the umbilicus due to the T10 nerve root supply
- Foregut pain is localized to the epigastric region
- Midgut pain is localized to the periumbilical region
- Hindgut pain is localized to the pelvic region

30.5 Red Flag Signs for Acute Abdominal Pain in Children

- History of intra-abdominal surgery
- Bilious vomiting; bilious or feculent output in the nasogastric tube
- Blood in stools or vomitus
- Features of intestinal obstruction (pain, vomiting, distension, and obstipation)
- Features of peritonitis (tenderness, guarding, rigidity, and rebound tenderness)
- Substantial abdominal injury
- Systemic signs of shock or sepsis

30.6 Investigations for Evaluation of Acute Abdomen in Children

(a) Blood Investigations: CBC, Electrolytes, Amylase, Lipase, Liver function tests: Increased leucocyte counts are suggestive of some infective process.

Raised S. Amylase and Lipase for Acute Pancreatitis.

Liver function tests are useful in diagnosing hepatitis/biliary obstruction

(b) Abdominal X-ray: Supine and erect films Both domes of the diaphragm and the pelvis should be included in the films.

Relevant findings are the following:

- Intestinal obstruction: Multiple air fluid levels, dilated bowel loops (Fig. 30.2a, b)
- Necrotizing enterocolitis: Dilated bowel loops, pneumatosis intestinalis, fixed bowel loops, and periportal gas
- Meconium ileus/peritonitis: Right iliac fossa soap bubble appearance and calcification
- Perforation: Pneumoperitoneum (Fig. 30.3)
- Malrotation or volvulus: Paucity of gas in the abdomen (Fig. 30.4)

(c) Ultrasonography: Has the advantage of being readily available and noninvasive without any radiation exposure to children with acute abdomen

- Detection of fluid in abdomen (echogenic fluid suggestive of perforation or pus)
- Intussusception (Fig. 30.5)
- Appendicitis (Fig. 30.6)
- Pathology of the solid visceral organs
- Ultrasound is also useful in assessing genitourinary causes like renal stones, tumor
- Along with Doppler: For vascular status in ovarian or testicular torsion

(d) CT/MRI/contrast enema/swallow is needed in specific cases or when diagnosis is uncertain

(e) Laparoscopy: Significant role when all other investigations are equivocal, but doubt of injury to hollow viscus injury persists (Fig. 30.6)

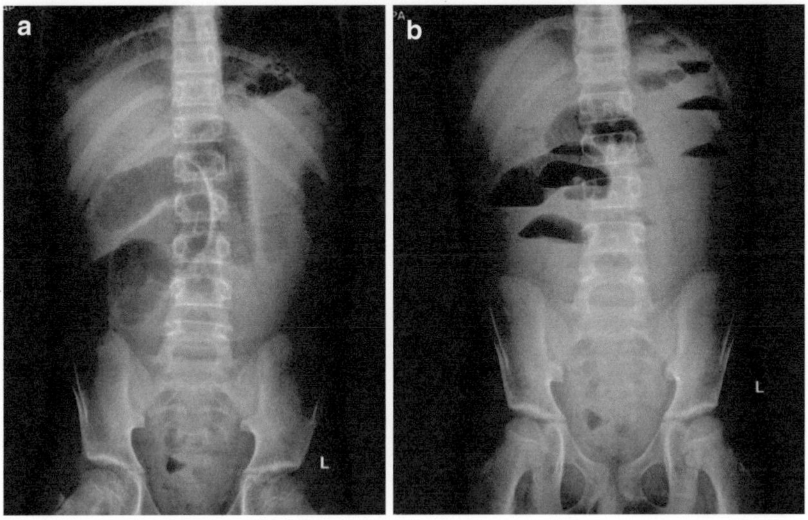

Fig. 30.2 (**a**) Supine: distended bowel loops. (**b**) Erect: multiple air fluid levels

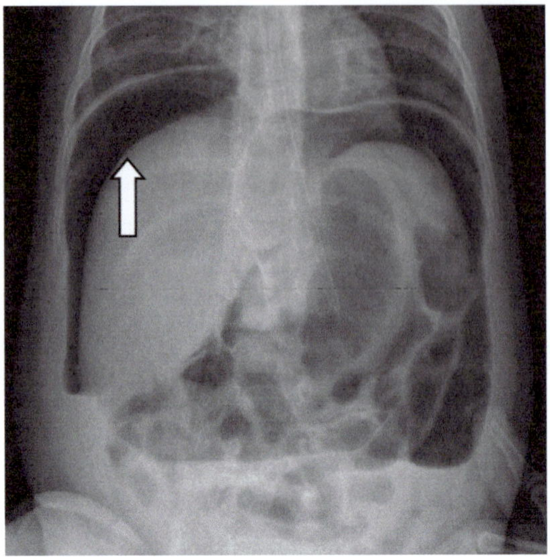

Fig. 30.3 Pneumoperitoneum

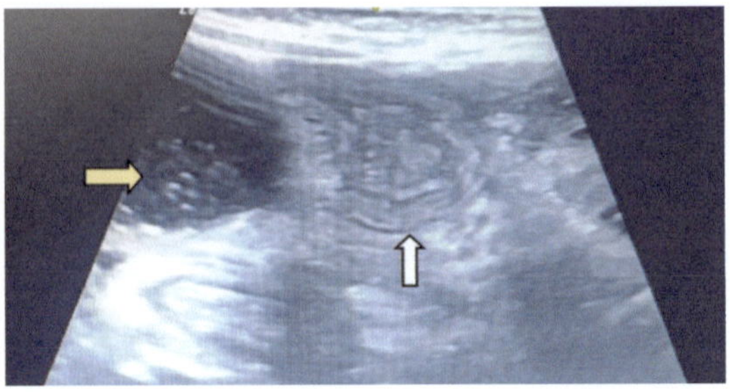

Fig. 30.5 Intussusception: **White** ➔ Target Sign on USG. **Yellow** ➔ Hydrostatic reduction (therapeutic role of USG)

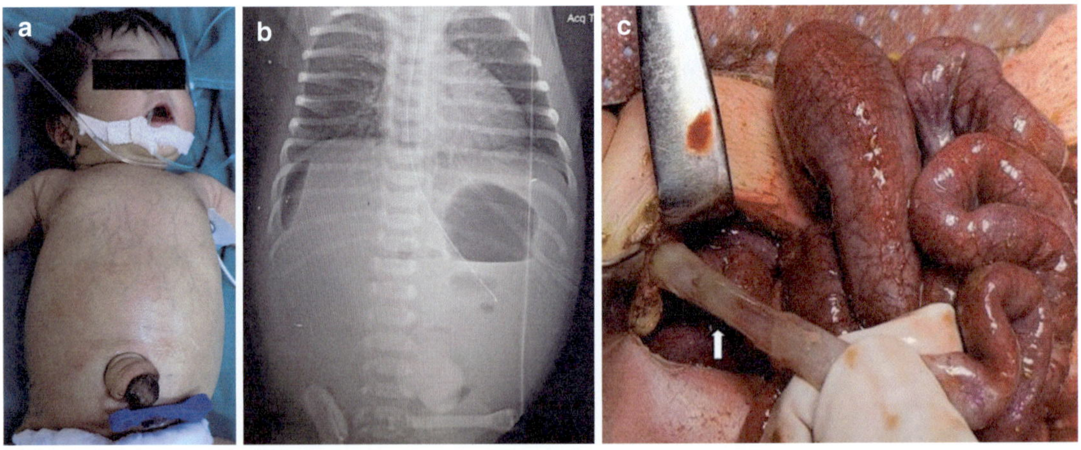

Fig. 30.4 (**a**) Intestinal obstruction in a neonate. (**b**) Paucity of gas with small air-fluid levels in X Ray. (**c**) Etiology: volvulus around vitello intestinal duct

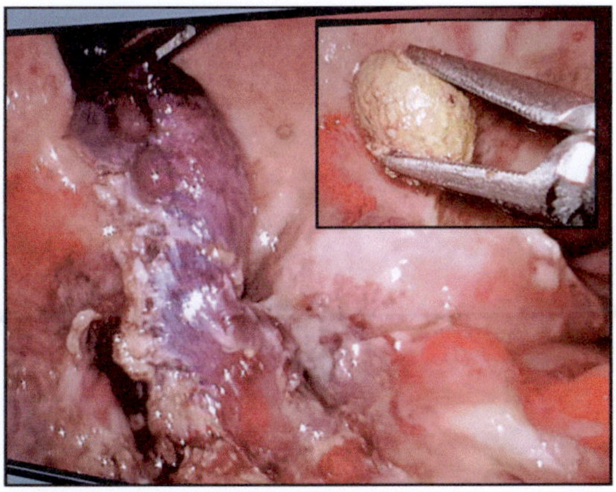

Fig. 30.6 Perforated gangrenous appendicitis with appendicolith (inset)

30.7 Etiology: Points to Remember

- Nonspecific abdominal pain is the commonest cause of acute abdomen in children
- Commonest medical cause of acute abdomen in children is *gastroenteritis*
- Commonest surgical cause of acute abdomen in children is *acute appendicitis*

Causes of Acute Abdomen in Children (Tables 30.1, 30.2)

Nongastrointestinal causes of acute abdomen

- Urinary tract infection and urinary stones
- Typhoid fever, dengue, and pneumonia
- Henoch-Scholein purpura
- Hemolytic disorder
- Diabetic ketoacidosis
- Hepatitis and liver abscess

Summary of Common Differential Diagnoses

Disease	History/examination findings
Intussusception (Fig. 30.5)	Gross/occult blood in stools, palpable lump, ~ 6 months of age Colicky pain, fever/lethargy/ vomiting
Acute appendicitis (Fig. 30.6)	Abdominal pain: migratory (periumbilical ➔ RIF), vomiting
Meckel (Fig. 30.7d)	Bloody stools, Abdominal tenderness/guarding, similar to appendicitis/diverticulitis
Hirschsprung	Abdominal distension, palpable fecal mass, Blast sign, enterocolitis ~1 year of life
Intestinal obstruction	Hyper/hypoactive bowel sounds, pain, distension, bilious vomiting, obstipation
Volvulus (Fig. 30.4)	Diffuse distention, no bowel sound, rigidity like SBO
NEC	Distension, tenderness, abdominal wall erythema, hematochezia, bradycardia, feed intolerance; premature infants
Acute pancreatitis	Epigastric tenderness, tachycardia, irritability, distension, Cullen's sign, Grey Turner's sign
Urolithiasis	Costovertebral/flank tenderness; radiation of pain to groin
Testicular torsion	Tender edematous testis, higher than normal side, absent cremasteric reflex
Ovarian torsion	Tender pelvic mass, cervical motion tenderness
Ectopic pregnancy	Tenderness, vaginal bleeding

Table 30.1 Medical causes of acute abdomen in children

Infants and < 2 years	Children (2–12 years)	Adolescents
Colic	Acute gastroenteritis	Dysmenorrhea
Infantile dyschezia	UTI and urolithiasis	Mittelschmerz
Gastroesophageal reflux	Constipation	Pelvic inflammatory disease
Acute gastroenteritis	Food poisoning	
Constipation	Mesenteric lymphadenitis	
Toxin ingestion	Pneumonia	
	Abdominal migraine	

Table 30.2 Surgical causes of acute abdomen in children

Newborn	Infants and < 2 years	Children (2–18 years)	Adolescents
Malrotation	Malrotation	Urolithiasis	Urolithiasis
Volvulus	Volvulus	Acute appendicitis	Acute appendicitis
Duodenal/intestinal atresia	Intussusception	Perforation peritonitis (Fig. 30.7a, b)	Perforation peritonitis (Fig. 30.7a, b)
Hirschsprung's	Hirschsprung's disease	Intestinal obstruction	Intestinal obstruction
NEC	Incarcerated hernia	Meckel diverticulum (Fig. 30.7d)	Meckel diverticulum (Fig. 30.7d)
Meconium plug syndrome	Infantile hypertrophic pyloric stenosis	Testicular/ovarian torsion	Testicular/ovarian torsion
Meconium pseudocyst	Abdominal trauma	Acute pancreatitis	Acute pancreatitis
		Acute cholecystitis (Fig. 30.7c)	Acute cholecystitis (Fig. 30.7c)
		Worm infestation → IO	Threatened abortion/ectopic pregnancy
		Trauma	Trauma

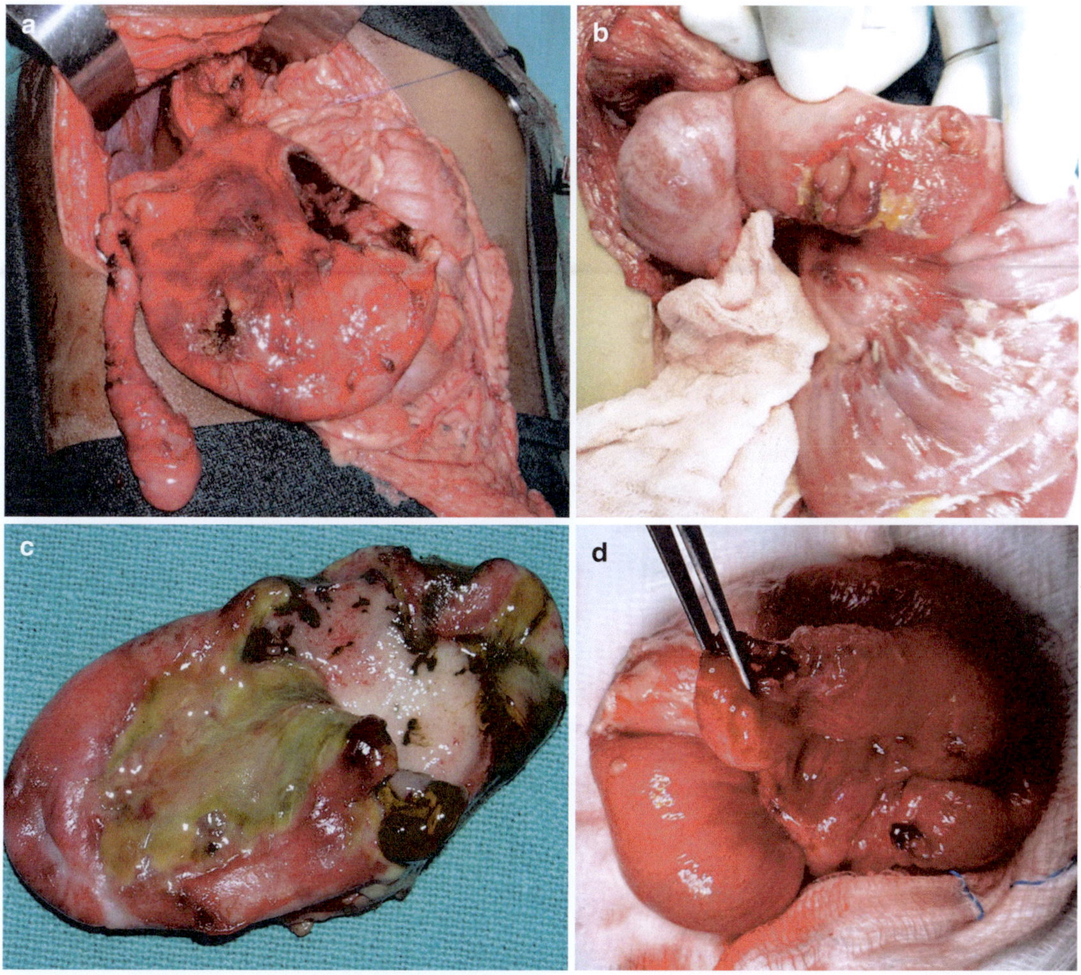

Fig. 30.7 Perforation peritonitis. (**a**) Ruptured choledochal cyst. (**b**) Ileal perforation. (**c**) Perforated gall bladder. (**d**) Perforated Meckel diverticulum

30.8 Surgical Consultation in Cases of Acute Abdomen

30.8.1 Every Patient with an Acute Abdomen Mandates a Surgical Consult

Absolute Indications

- Severe pain with progressive deterioration
- Signs of acute fluid or blood loss
- Bile-stained or feculent vomiting
- Involuntary abdominal guarding, rigidity
- Severe tenderness, and/or rebound tenderness
- Marked distension with diffuse tympany
- Abdominal trauma or history of previous surgery
- Abdominal pain without obvious etiology

Management

The general principles of management include the following:

- Resuscitation of the child
- The initial focus should be on establishing hemodynamic stability:
  - Adequate hydration
  - Abdominal decompression: nasogastric drainage and bladder catheterization
  - Monitoring of urine output: watch for signs of dehydration
  - Analgesics and antibiotics when required according to the provisional diagnosis
- Analgesics

  Morphine (0.1 mg/kg/dose) provides substantial relief in pain without changing the examination findings

  Alternative: fentanyl (0.15–0.2 mg/kg)

  For mild to moderate pain: Paracetamol (15 mg/kg/dose) or other NSAIDS

A Period of Stabilization Is Necessary before any Surgical Intervention

- Identification of cases that need *urgent* surgical intervention.
- In cases requiring surgical intervention but failing to gain stabilization, a *short temporary* procedure (drain placement, diversion) may be indicated.
- Current search of literature does not preclude the use of analgesics in acute abdomen.
- Treatments of different causes of acute abdomen are discussed in the relevant chapters.

30.9 Summary

- Thorough examination coupled with detailed history is key in evaluating children with an acute abdomen.
- Early identification for the need of surgical intervention is crucial.
- Assurance and trust of the child and parents are important in the treatment process.

Suggested Reading

Balachandran B, Singhi S, Lal S. Emergency management of acute abdomen in children. Indian J Pediatr. 2013;80:226–34.

Coran AG, Caldamone A, Scott Adzich N, Krummel TM, Laberge JM, editors. Pediatric surgery. 7th ed. Oxford: Elsevier Limited; 2012.

Hutson JM, O'Brien M, Woodward AA, Beasley SW. Jone's clinical pediatric surgery diagnosis and management. 6th ed. Oxford: Blackwell; 2008.

Williams NS, Bulstrode CJK, O'Connell PR, editors. Bailey & Love's short practice of pediatric surgery. 26th ed. Taylor & Francis Group; 2013.

31 Umbilical Anomalies

Rohit Meshram and Subhasis Roy Choudhury

31.1 Introduction

Umbilical disorders are encountered in general pediatric surgery very frequently. It is important to understand the embryology of the abdominal wall formation and the umbilicus to identify and properly treat these conditions.

31.2 Embryology of the Formation of the Umbilicus

The gastrointestinal tract herniates into the umbilical cord between 6 and 8 weeks of fetal development. This is due to the rapid growth of the bowel, called a physiological midgut hernia, during which the bowel is extracoelomic. By 10–12 weeks, the body wall continues to develop and the intestine returns inside the abdomen, undergoing a 270° counterclockwise rotation and fixation.

Normally, the fibromuscular umbilical ring contracts and closes by birth due to the developing abdominal wall. At birth, the umbilical cord contains two umbilical arteries, one umbilical vein (the right vein is obliterated during fetal life), and fibrous remnants of the urachus and omphalomesenteric duct or the vitellointestinal duct (VID) (Table 31.1).

Care should be taken while placing the umbilical cord clamp, as a small umbilical cord hernia may be present. Clamping should be done a few centimeters away from the base of the umbilical ring. After ligation of the cord, the vessels thrombose and the cord dries and sloughs off (range 3 days to 2 months), leaving a granulating surface that heals by cicatrization and is covered by the epithelium, followed by scar contraction and retraction of the umbilicus. It is a common practice to apply topical antimicrobial agents to prevent infection and bacterial colonization of the umbilical stump, especially when proper cord care is lacking. Delayed cord separation may be due to underlying neutrophil functional disorder, infections or an immunological problem.

A normal umbilicus has a depression with a central eminence and a dense scar.

R. Meshram (✉)
Kalawati Saran Children's Hospital, Lady Hardinge Medical College, New Delhi, India

S. Roy Choudhury
Pediatric Surgery, Lady Hardinge Medical College and Associated Kalawati Saran Children's Hospital, New Delhi, Delhi, India

© The Author(s), under exclusive license to Springer Nature Singapore Pte Ltd. 2025
S. Roy Choudhury (ed.), *Pediatric Surgery*, https://doi.org/10.1007/978-981-96-1257-4_31

Table 31.1 Embryological structures of the umbilicus and their fate

Embryological structure	Fate	Pathologic condition/remnant
Urachus (connects the bladder to the allantois)	Obliterates and forms the median umbilical ligament	Patent urachus, sinus, cyst, diverticulum
Omphalomesenteric duct/ vitelline duct (connects the midgut to the yolk sac)	Obliterates and in 2% of the population, it forms a Meckel diverticulum	Patent/prolapsed omphalomesenteric duct, sinus, cyst, band, or umbilical polyp
Omphalomesenteric arteries	Most regress, fuse to form the coeliac, superior, and inferior mesenteric arteries	Dominant artery may accompany Meckel diverticulum, a fibrous band from the umbilicus to the bowel mesentery
Omphalomesenteric veins	Plexus around the duodenum becomes the superior mesenteric and portal vein	Preduodenal portal vein
Umbilical arteries	Obliterate after birth	Medial umbilical ligaments
Umbilical veins	Right obliterates during fetal life; the left remains and is connected to the ductus venosus, obliterating after birth	Falciform ligament

31.3 List of Anomalies

- Umbilical hernia
- Umbilical granuloma/umbilical polyp
- Umbilical sinus/omphalomesentric duct (OMD) cyst
- Patent vitellointestinal duct (PVID)/omphalomesentric duct, prolapsed VID, Meckel's diverticulum, and fibrous band containing cyst
- Patent urachus, urachal cyst, urachal sinus, and urachal diverticulum
- Exomphalos minor, major
- Gastroschisis
- Exstrophy bladder/cloacal exstrophy
- Acquired (sinus, fistula, infection due to tuberculosis, etc.)

31.4 Common Presentations

31.4.1 Umbilical Hernia

Umbilical hernias are protrusions at the base of the umbilicus with skin lining and generally develop in the first few weeks of life after the cord stump falls off (Fig. 31.1). They occur due to weakness of the umbilical cicatrix. Parents should be reassured and observation is advised for small hernias as they undergo spontaneous closure by cicatrization of the umbilical ring between 2 and 3 years of age. Occlusion of the umbilical defect with a taped coin should be avoided, as there is no benefit. Rarely the hernia can get obstructed.

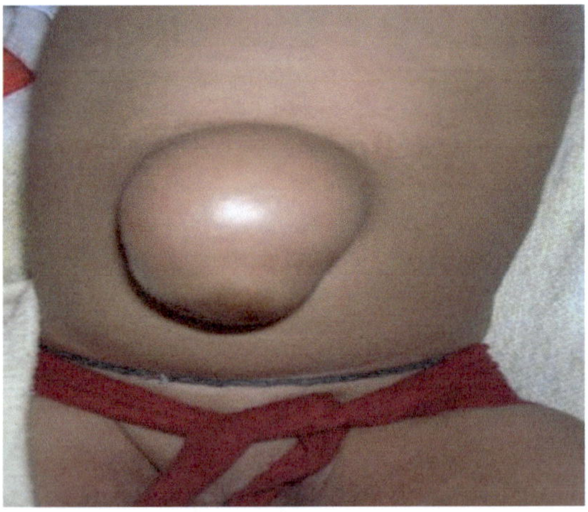

Fig. 31.1 Umbilical hernia

Indications of surgical intervention are:

1. Persistence of the hernia after 2–3 years of age
2. Large defect
3. Obstruction

Surgery involves a small infraumbilical incision with dissection around the neck of the sac, followed by transverse fascial approximation to close the defect, with preservation of the umbilicus.

31.5 Patent Vitellointestinal Duct (PVID)

Depending upon the degree of the obliteration of the vitellointestinal duct, it has various presentations from a discharging sinus to prolapse of the intestine through the duct (Fig. 31.2a, b).

- Umbilical sinus: Usually presents with umbilical discharge and only the part near the umbilicus is patent. Excision is needed.
- Omphalomesentric duct (OMD) cyst: Usually presents with pain with or without discharge at the umbilicus. They are usually single. Ultrasonography (USG) abdomen helps in the diagnosis, and umbilical exploration with cyst excision is needed. They are usually lined by the columnar mucin-secreting epithelium (Fig. 31.3a, b).
- Patent VID: The whole duct is patent. The presentation is with a history of discharge of fecal matter and/or gas from the umbilicus (Fig. 31.4a). Sometimes the small bowel may prolapse from the umbilicus (Fig. 31.2b). Treatment requires surgical exploration, disconnection of the duct remnant from the ileum, and wedge resection and often anastomosis of the native bowel (Fig. 31.4b).
- Umbilical band: These are usually asymptomatic but when symptomatic, the presentation may be abdominal pain, distention and bilious vomiting due to volvulus or obstruction due to twisting of the intestines around the band. Surgical exploration is indicated.
- Meckel diverticulum is discussed in Chap. 43.

If the diagnosis is uncertain, then ultrasonography or sinogram may help. If the diagnosis is still uncertain, umbilical exploration is needed.

31.5.1 Umbilical Mass

The parents may complain of a reddish mass protruding from the umbilicus. The differentials include umbilical granuloma, umbilical the polyp, and rarely patent vitellointestinal duct. The latter is very obvious due to the appearance of intestinal mucosa. Umbilical granuloma is the most common umbilical problem in infants, presenting as an irregular pale mass (Fig. 31.5), ranging from 1 mm to 1 cm. Sometimes they present as bleeding. They are a result of the formation of the granulation tissue at the umbilical stump and have a rough surface, whereas an umbilical polyp represents the remnant of the vitellointestinal duct and has a smooth glistening, red mucosal surface (Fig. 31.6). On histopatho-

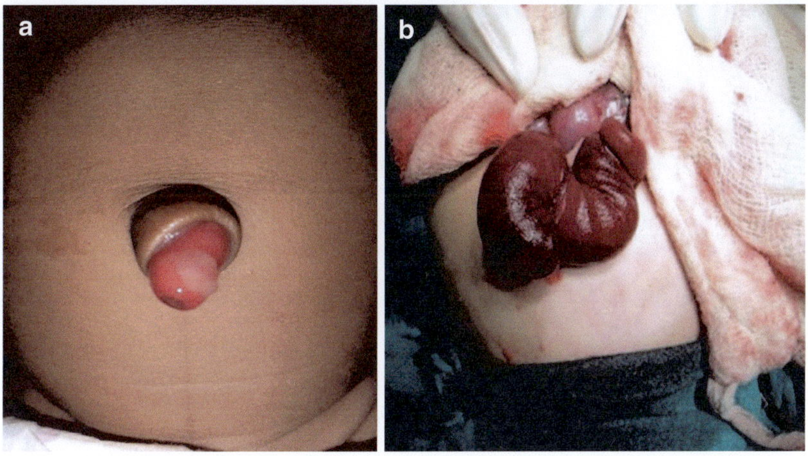

Fig. 31.2 (**a**) Patent VID and (**b**) Prolapsed VID

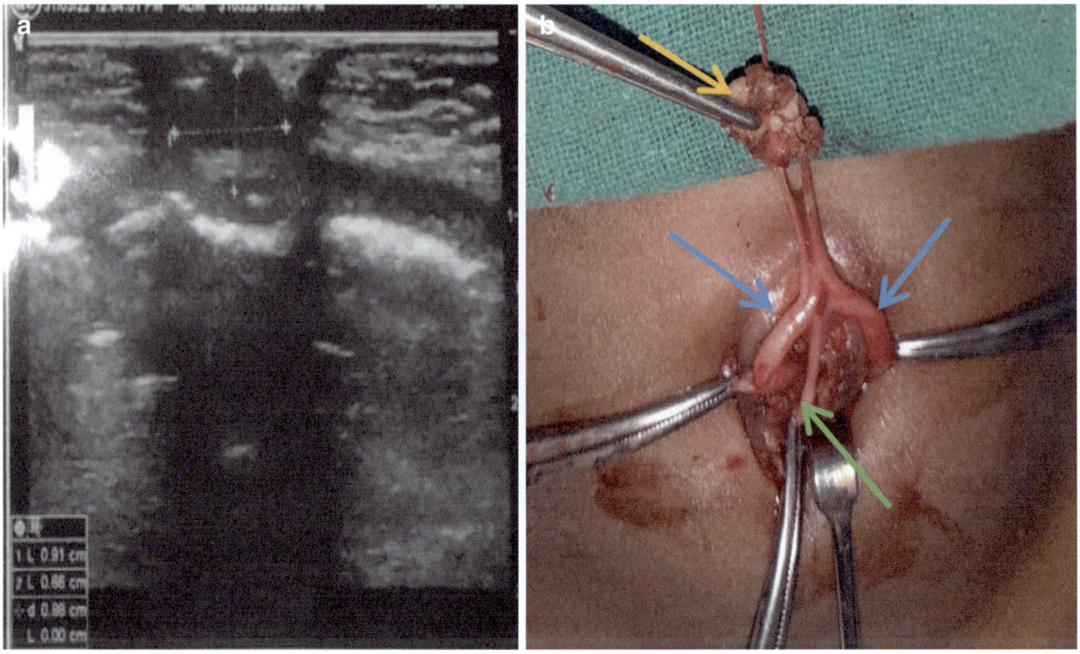

Fig. 31.3 (**a**) USG, cystic lesion (1x1cm) just below the umbilicus (**b**) Intraoperative picture of the OMD cyst (yellow arrow) along with the obliterated umbilical arteries (blue arrow) and obliterated urachus (green arrow)

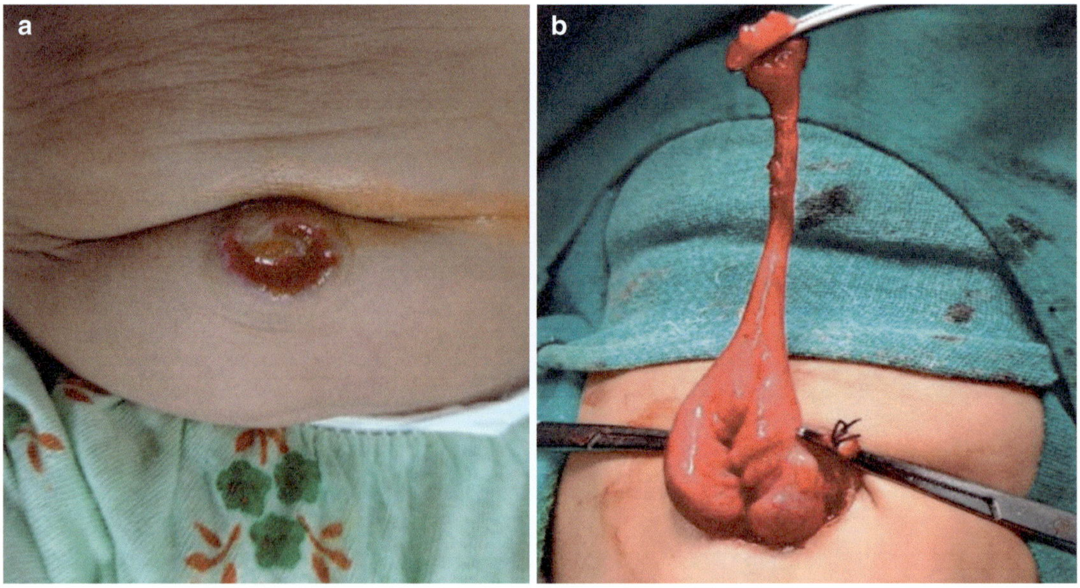

Fig. 31.4 (**a**) Bilious discharge via umbilicus with surrounding redness (**b**) Intraoperative picture of PVID

logical examination, umbilical granulomas consist of true granulation tissue with fibroblasts with abundant capillaries, while umbilical polyps show intestinal epithelium.

31.6 Management

Umbilical granuloma: They are usually managed with a topical application of silver nitrate or trichloroacetic acid (chemical cauterization). Care should be taken to avoid touching any undesired site. More than one application may be required. Pedunculated lesions can be tied off at the base and can be allowed to fall off. Crushing the base of the granuloma with a fine-tip artery forceps is curative and can be done as an outpatient procedure without anesthesia. Sometimes bipolar cauterization in the operating theater may be needed. Persistent discharge should be investigated (USG/sinogram), and surgical exploration may be needed.

Clinical diagnosis of an umbilical polyp warrants an ultrasonography/sinogram as they may be associated with an underlying remnant of the vitellointestinal duct in 30–60% of cases. Surgical exploration and excision of remnants, along with the polyp are curative.

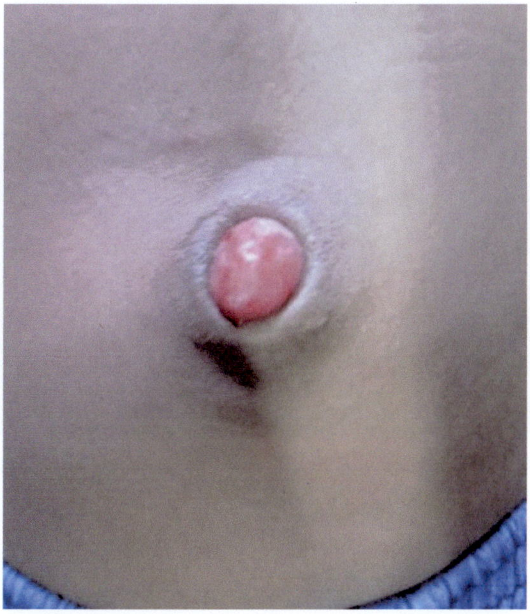

Fig. 31.5 Umbilical granuloma

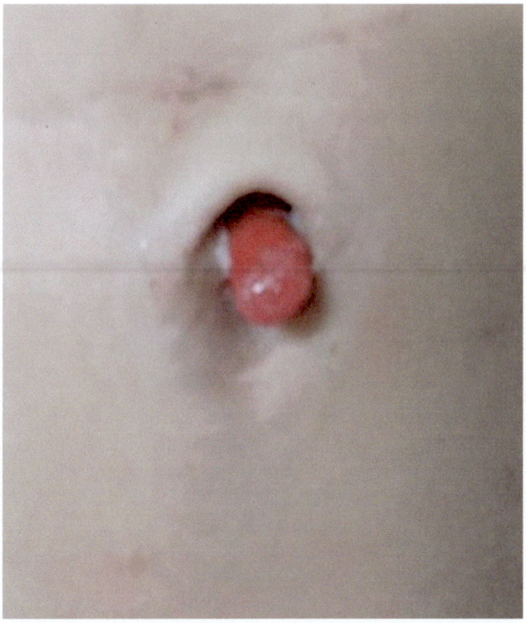

Fig. 31.6 Umbilical polyp

31.7 Infected Umbilical Stump

It presents as redness and purulent discharge from the umbilicus (Fig. 31.7). The infection usually resolves by cleaning of the area with spirit and application of local antiseptic (0.2% mercurochrome lotion). Hospital admission and systemic antibiotics may be necessary. Necrotizing fascitis/umbilical gangrene may occur and requires wide surgical debridement and antibiotics. Rarely, it may be infected with maggots (umbilical myiasis) due to unhygienic conditions that need local turpentine oil application for expulsion of maggots, followed by manual removal and antibiotics.

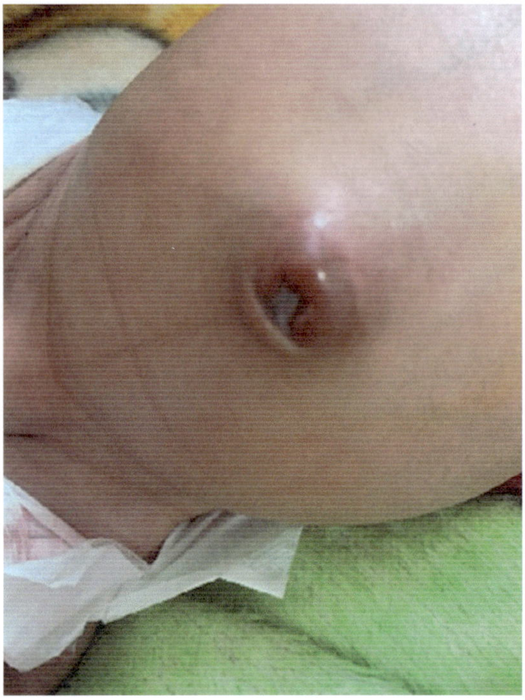

Fig. 31.7 Umbilical infection with abscess

31.8 Urachal Remnants

Urachal sinus can present with umbilical discharge. Initial treatment is antibiotics if infected and then surgical removal.

31.9 Patent Urachus and Urachal Cyst

31.9.1 Patent Urachus

This condition usually presents with the passage of clear discharge (urine) from the umbilicus. Retraction of the umbilicus on passage of urine is also a sign. An ultrasound may detect the patent communication. (Fig. 31.8a) Frank urinary drainage should raise a suspicion of bladder outlet obstruction in which the urachus functions as a popoff valve. Proper history and clinical examination are crucial. USG KUB and a sinogram/dye study are helpful in making diagnosis. (Fig. 31.8b). Micturating cystourethrogram

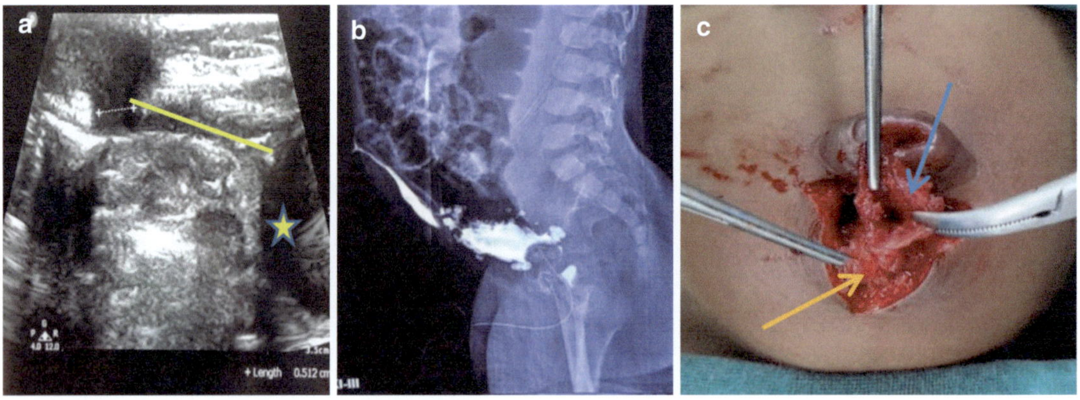

Fig. 31.8 (**a**) USG showing patent urachus up to the bladder (yellow line), star represents the bladder. (**b**) Dye study showing patent urachus in a female patient with watery umbilical discharge. (**c**) Intraoperative image of patent urachus (blue arrow) up to the bladder (yellow arrow)

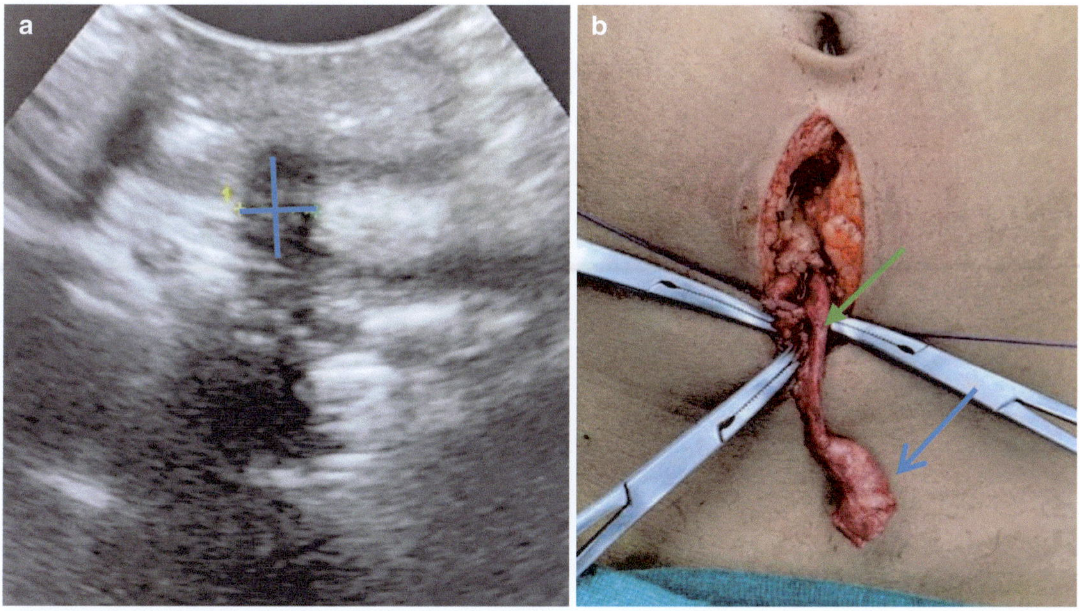

Fig. 31.9 (**a**) USG image showing a 1.5 x1 cm urachal cyst (**b**) Intraoperative image of urachal cyst excision (blue arrow), urachus (green arrow)

(MCU) is indicated if the posterior urethral valve is suspected. Treatment is surgical exploration via umbilical or infraumbilical approach and the excision of the tract along with a bladder cuff and bladder repair in two layers (Fig. 31.8c).

Urachal Cyst Urachal cysts can be an incidental finding on imaging. They usually present with pain in the lower abdomen. An ultrasound examination of the urinary tract can detect an urachal cyst (Fig. 31.9a). Rarely a CT scan is needed. Surgical intervention is necessary as these cysts are prone to getting infected and there is a risk of developing malignancy in the long term (Fig. 31.9b).

For omphalos minor, major and gastroschisis, see Chapter 32 on abdominal wall defects.

31.10 Summary

1. Normally the umbilical cord falls off between 3 days and 2 months (average 14–15 days).
2. Watchful waiting is needed for umbilical hernia for 2–3 years of age.
3. Umbilical granuloma is the most common mass at the umbilicus.
4. Umbilical granulomas usually respond to chemical cauterization by a topical application of silver nitrate or trichloroacetic acid, whereas umbilical polyps do not. Persistence of discharge through the umbilicus along with a suspected internal connection to the intestine, requires surgical exploration.
5. Passage of bilious/fecal discharge via the umbilicus suggests PVID, and surgical wedge resection or resection and anastomosis of the PVID are needed.
6. Patent urachus presents as discharge of clear discharge via the umbilicus and needs surgical excision.
7. Ultrasonography/sinogram and MCU are useful in detecting persistent symptomatic vitellointestinal and urachal remnants.

Suggested Reading

Coran AG, Caldamone A, Scott Adzich N, Krummel TM, Laberge JM, editors. Pediatric surgery. 7th ed. Oxford: Elsevier; 2012.

Partin AW, Dmochowski RR, Kavoussi LR, Peters CA. Campbell-Walsh-Wein. 12th ed. Elsevier; 2021.

32 Abdominal Wall Defects

Shalu Shah and Subhasis Roy Choudhury

32.1 Introduction

Congenital abdominal wall defects occur due to an aberration in the complex embryological process involved in the formation of the abdominal wall. It is, therefore, important to understand the embryology of formation of the abdominal wall in order to identify such anomalies early in the embryonic and fetal period and formulate an appropriate plan of management. The outcome of such anomalies depends on the type, associated anomalies, and quality of available neonatal care. A joint counseling by the perinatology and surgical teams with expert management is associated with better outcomes.

The following abdominal wall defects are discussed below:

- Gastroschisis
- Omphalocele or exomphalos
- Hernia of the umbilical cord
- Exstrophy/cloacal exstrophy
- Prune Belly syndrome

Omphalocele and gastroschisis constitute the two main conditions. *Gastroschisis* has no covering membrane, the defect is usually to the right side of the umbilicus. The bowel is usually thickened, matted, and edematous due to exposure to the amniotic fluid. *Omphalocele or exomphalos* is a large defect >4 cm through the umbilicus, covered with a sac (amniotic membrane) containing intestines, liver, and occasionally spleen and gonad.

Hernia of the umbilical cord or exomphalos minor is a small defect containing only the intestine and covered with a membrane (Fig 32.1).

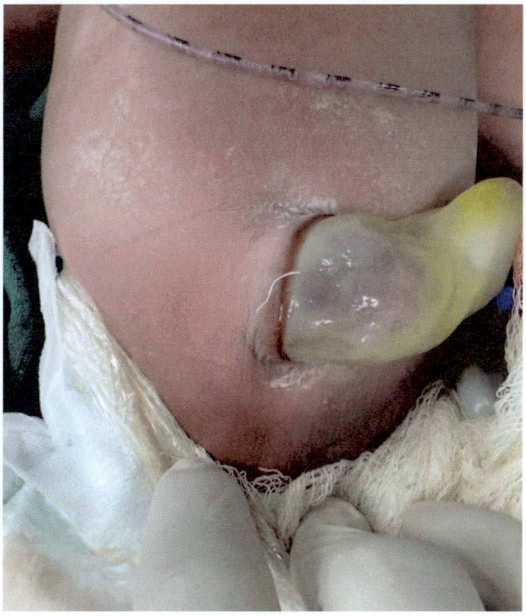

Fig. 32.1 Showing hernia of the umbilical cord

S. Shah (✉)
Pediatric Surgery, ABVIMS and Dr RML Hospital, New Delhi, India

S. Roy Choudhury
Pediatric Surgery, Lady Hardinge Medical College and Associated Kalawati Saran Children's Hospital, New Delhi, Delhi, India

© The Author(s), under exclusive license to Springer Nature Singapore Pte Ltd. 2025

S. Roy Choudhury (ed.), *Pediatric Surgery*, https://doi.org/10.1007/978-981-96-1257-4_32

32.2 Epidemiology of Gastroschisis and Omphalocele (Table 32.1)

The incidence of omphalocele is approximately 1:3000–4000 births as reported from Western countries. The incidence of gastroschisis is higher, with 3–4.5 per 10000 live births. There is an increasing trend in the incidence of gastroschisis in the UK, USA, and Europe. This increase is attributed to young maternal age, low socioeconomic status, nutrient deficiencies, smoking, alcohol, and substance abuse in addition to increased premature deliveries as gastroschisis is more common in preterm babies. There is a male preponderance over females for both diseases. Omphalocele is associated with maternal obesity.

Table 32.1 Epidemiology of gastroschisis and omphalocele

Epidemiology	Gastroschisis	Omphalocele
Incidence:	3–4.5 per 10000 births	1:3000–4000 births
Associations:	Young maternal age Low socioeconomic status Mother's nutrient deficiencies Smoking, alcohol, and substance abuse Environmental toxins and teratogens Premature deliveries	Both young and advanced age mothers Maternal diabetes Genetic and chromosomal anomalies

32.3 Embryology

32.3.1 Embryogenesis of the Defects

During the early embryonic life, the mid-gut herniates through the weakly formed umbilical ring, termed as *physiological umbilical hernia.* Subsequently, the intestines return to the abdominal cavity by the 10th week and undergo *rotation and fixation of the gut.* Failure of the physiological hernia to close results in an exomphalos defect.

There are three body folds, namely caudal, lateral, and cephalic folds, and the anterior body wall is formed by the proper formation and fusion of these folds.

Omphaloceles represent a *lateral fold defect* and are always at the umbilicus. The rectus muscles often insert far apart on the costal margins. The aberrations occur early in embryogenesis, thereby affecting other organ systems as well, so children with omphalocele frequently have associated anomalies. *Cephalic fold* is related to the heart and septum transversum; therefore, defects result in ectopia cordis, diaphragmatic, and pericardial defects named as the *pentalogy of Cantrell.* Similarly, *caudal fold defects* cause bladder and cloacal exstrophy as caudal folds are related to the developing bladder.

There are different theories for the embryogenesis of gastroschisis, the recent one the hypothesized failure of the yolk sac and vitelline structures to be incorporated into the umbilical stalk, leading to gut herniation. The classical location of the defect just to the right of the umbilicus can be explained as this site is relatively unsupported as a result of the resorption of the right umbilical vein. In gastroschisis, the bowel is usually thickened, matted, edematous, and covered with a fibrinous peel, probably due to exposure to the amniotic fluid. Other proposed theories for gastroschisis include partial blockage of the right omphalomesenteric artery and rupture of hernia of umbilical cord.

Umbilical cord hernia is a simple failure of the midgut to return to the peritoneal cavity at 10–12 weeks. This defect contains the midgut and is covered by a membrane. Such hernias are much smaller than omphalocele and have a better outcome.

32.4 Antenatal Diagnosis and Management

Accurate antenatal diagnosis is important for planning subsequent management. An antenatal ultrasound scan in late first and second trimesters can accurately diagnose gastroschisis and omphalocele in over 90% of cases.

The characteristics of the defects on an antenatal ultrasound scan are:

Omphalocele is seen as a protrusion of the viscera, including the liver, from the umbilicus, which is covered by a sac. The sac is composed of peritoneum, Wharton's jelly, and amnion. In gastroschisis, the covering sac is absent. In a hernia of the umbilical cord, there is the absence of the liver in the sac. The sensitivity of ultrasound and maternal serum alpha-fetoprotein screening is approximately 80%. Ruptured omphalocele can be differentiated from gastroschisis by the presence of the liver in the defect and the large size of the defect. Antenatal progressive bowel dilatation has been associated with a poor prognosis for gastroschisis, as it indicates associated bowel atresia. In cases of gastroschisis with severe oligohydramnios, amnioinfusion to restore the amniotic fluid volume can have potential benefits. MRI may accurately measure the size of the defects in omphalocele and pick up pulmonary hypoplasia, which has implications in the formulation of management.

Maternal serum alpha-fetoprotein is elevated. Exomphalos is associated with more than 50% risk of having chromosomal anomalies—trisomy 13, 18, or 21. Cardiovascular and central nervous systems are predominantly involved. Fetal karyotyping and fetal echocardiography should be done in the antenatal period, as the detection of such associations bears a significant influence on the prognosis

Counseling about fetal morbidity and mortality should include details of the type of defect, associated anomalies, and genetic syndromes.

If there are no associated lethal defects, then pregnancy is continued till term with close monitoring by

- Serial ultrasound evaluation every 2–4 weeks to evaluate fetal growth and amniotic fluid volume.
- Fetal physiological assessment by the biophysical profile and nonstress monitoring in the third trimester due to the increased risk of intrauterine death.
- Consultation at a tertiary-level center with maternal fetal medicine, neonatology, and pediatric surgery.

Current evidences support near term delivery by normal vaginal route for gastroschisis and small omphalocele. Caesarian delivery may be considered for a very large omphalocele with the liver in the sac in order to avoid liver injury during delivery. The mode is best decided by the treating obstetrician in consultation with the pediatric surgeon and a multispecialty team.

32.5 Associated Abnormalities Gastroschisis

Prematurity and stillbirth are frequent with gastroschisis. Genetic syndromes and anomalies of other organ systems are rare. The most common bowel abnormalities associated are intestinal atresia, which can occur in up to 30% of patients. Currently, two variants of gastroschisis are identified: *simple and complex*. The complex variety is associated with bowel atresia, stenosis, perforation necrosis, volvulus, bowel loss, and thus results in poor outcome. Gastro-esophageal reflux and undescended testis are also common.

32.6 Omphalocele

Multiple anomalies are seen in 67–88% of fetuses with omphalocele. Cardiac anomalies seen in 50%, gastrointestinal anomalies in 40%, musculoskeletal, genitourinary, and central nervous systems anomalies are commonly associated as well. Chromosomal anomalies are associated in 30–40%, including trisomy 13, 18, and 21; sex chromosome abnormalities such as Turner syndrome (45X0), Klinefelter syndrome (47, XXY), and triploidy (69XXX). Chromosomal anomalies are more likely associated with omphaloceles containing bowel only. Genetic syndromes that are associated with omphalocele are Beckwith-Widemann syndrome (BWS), Pentalogy of Cantrell, and bladder cloacal exstrophy. Half of the fetuses with omphalocele are lost.

The clinical differences of gastroschisis versus omphalocele are shown in Table 32.2.

Table 32.2 Clinical differences between omphalocele and gastroschisis (Figs. 32.2a, b and 32.3a, b)

	Omphalocele	Gastroschisis
Location	Umbilical ring	Lateral to cord right side
Fascial defect	Variable (4–10 cm)	Small (<4 cm)
Sac	Present, may be ruptured	Absent, no remnants
Cord attachment	On to the sac	Normal
Intestinal appearance	Usually normal	Edematous, thickened, peeled
Herniated liver	Often present	Unusual
Abdominal cavity	Small	Usually near normal
Associated anomalies	Common (40–80%)	Rare
Bowel strangulation	Uncommon	Greater risk
Bowel atresia	Rare	Common

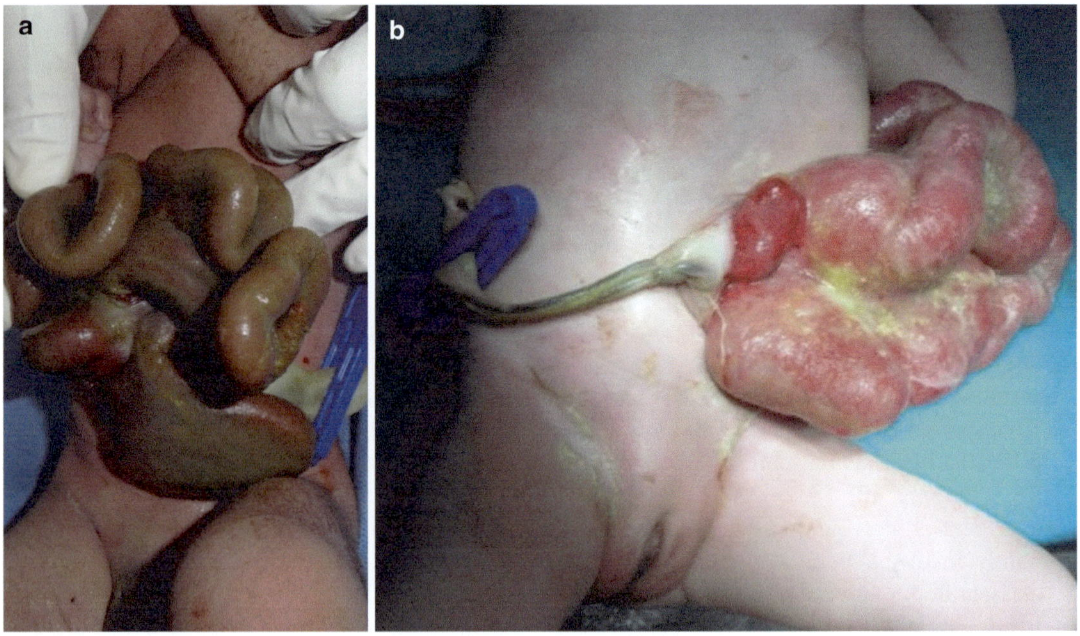

Fig. 32.2 (**a**) Gastroschisis (exposed bowel, no sac) (**b**) Gastroschisis (rare left-sided defect)

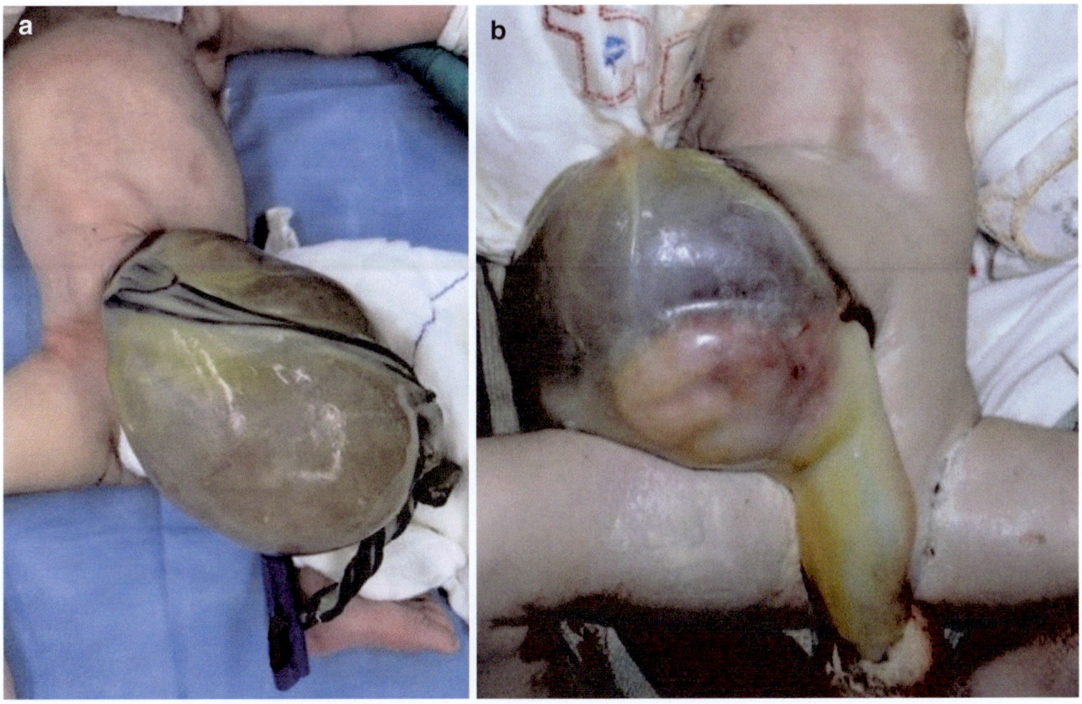

Fig. 32.3 (**a**, **b**) Omphalocele with the sac containing the bowel and liver, note the attached umbilical cord

32.6.1 Newborn Management of Omphalocele and Gastroschisis

The principles of management of abdominal defects are as follows:

- Reduction of the viscera.
- Closure of the abdominal defect.
- Identification and management of associated abnormalities.
- Nutritional support till the child is able to accept full enteral feeds.

32.6.2 Initial Management

- Nasogastric tube decompression.
- Rectal stimulation to evacuate meconium.
- IV hydration (150 ml/kg, larger amount of fluid required for gastroschisis than omphalocele). Babies with BWS require glucose supplementation as they are prone to neonatal hypoglycemia.
- Urethral catheter insertion for urinary output charting.
- Temperature maintenance.
- Antibiotics and vitamin K administration.
- Cardiology evaluation and echocardiography.
- Airway management and ventilation as required.
- The exposed bowel in gastroschisis needs to be covered by a bowel bag, or a makeshift arrangement can be done by using cling film or a urine/blood collection bag.

It is necessary to ensure that the defect in gastroschisis is not very narrow to compromise the vascularity of the eviscerated bowel. It is important to avoid twisting and traction of the intestines and compromising its blood supply by hanging it vertically from above.

32.7 Surgical Repair

The following options can be used for the closure of the defect in patients of omphalocele or gastroschisis:

Reduction and primary closure of defect (Fig. 32.4)

- Primary skin closure is only for large defects
- Sutureless gastroschisis closure with umbilical capping at the bedside without anesthesia
- Primary fascial closure for small gastroschisis (75%) and exomphalos with defect less than 5 cm
- Closure with a prosthetic mesh for large gastroschisis and exomphalos >5 cm

Gradual Reduction of Bowel and Closure of Defect

- Preformed silastic silo (can be applied bedside and is held in place by a preloaded spring)
- Custom-made silo (silo made by a prosthetic mesh sutured to the fascial defect) (Fig. 32.5a)

  The silo is reduced by gravity and/ or by gradually decreasing the size of the silo (Fig. 32.5b). When the bowel can be completely reduced easily, primary closure can be done.

Creation of Ventral Hernia and Delayed Repair

- Only skin closure over the defect
- Eschar formation over the omphalocele sac either spontaneously or by the application of mercurochrome or silver sulfadiazine (Fig. 32.6a, b)

Artificial skin substitute application, like integra, can temporize for a subsequent skin grafting. Tissue expanders may be needed to increase the capacity of the abdomen to accommodate viscera and to achieve proper skin cover.

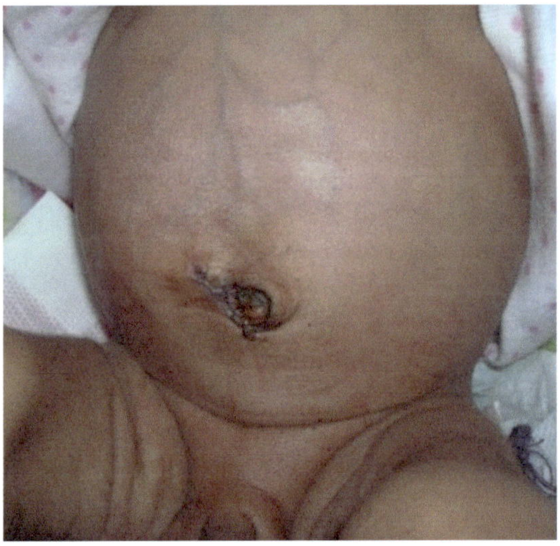

Fig. 32.4 Cosmetic scar following closure of gastroschisis

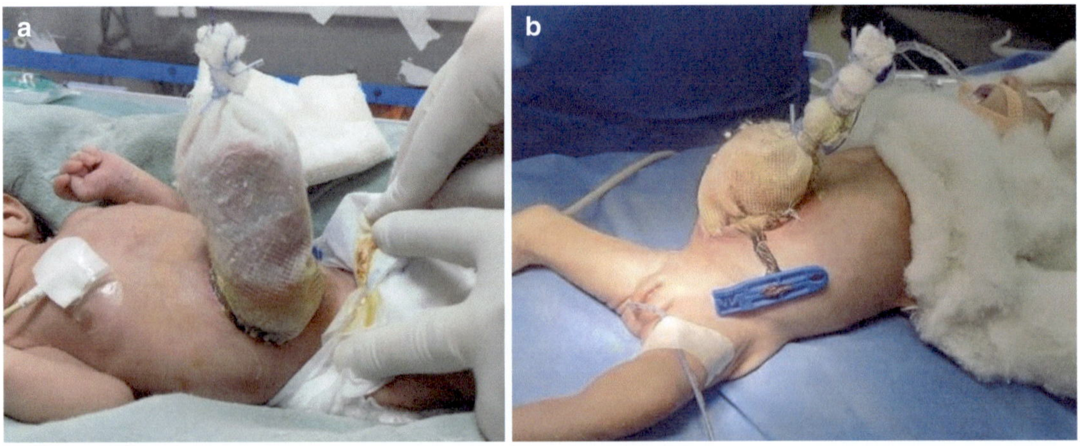

Fig. 32.5 (**a**) Silo closure of gastroschisis (**b**) Serial silo reduction

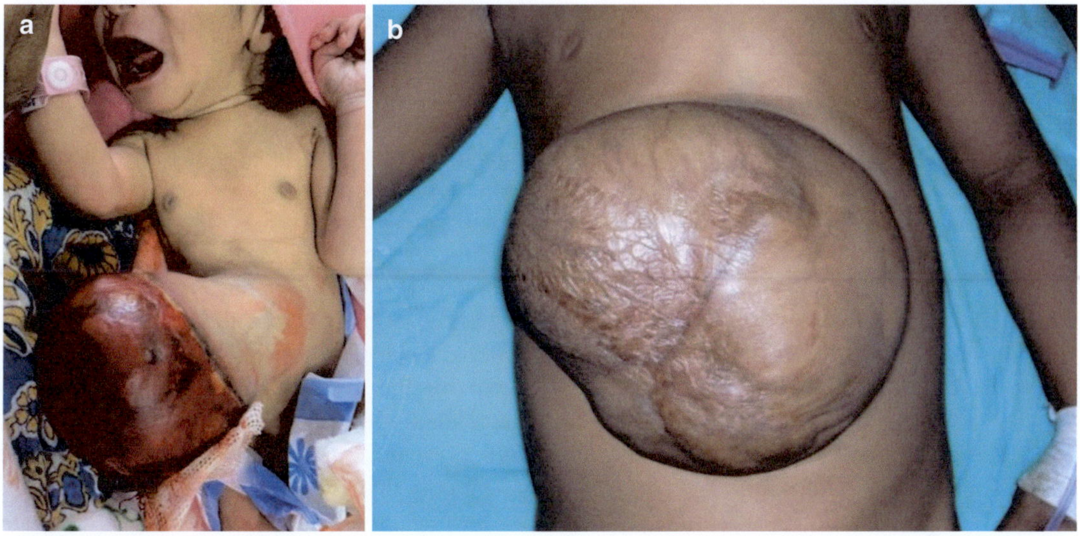

Fig. 32.6 (**a**) Conservative management of large omphalocele (**b**) Healing by epithelization following escharification treatment

32.8 General Principles of Abdomen Closure

Reduction of the bowel first and the liver last, as the liver tends to keep the reduced bowel in place. To aid in reduction, it is helpful if the bowel can be decompressed by gastric aspiration, rectal washes, and compressing the bowel with a warm moist sponge and milking of the bowel. If closure is still difficult, the abdominal wall can be gently stretched by inserting a finger into the defect and stretching the wall by sweeping the finger from posterior to anterior. The defect should be closed with an interrupted suture. Relaxing incisions can be given over the abdominal wall fascia if the closure seems under tension. It is necessary to ensure that the abdominal closure is not under extreme tension; otherwise, abdominal compartment syndrome may result. The following parameters favor silo formation instead of primary closure:

- Mean airway pressure more than 25 cm of water
- Intravesical pressure more than 20 cm of water
- Saphenous intravenous line unable to flow by gravity

Signs of abdominal compartment syndrome, like persistent tachycardia, oliguria, increased ventilator requirements, and a tense abdomen, should be detected early. Such patients need urgent decompression and silo formation.

32.9 Omphalocele Care During Surgical Closure

- Omphalomesenteric duct remnants are frequently present
- Hepatic veins above and the bladder below are at risk of injury
- Kinking of the hepatic veins following forced reduction
- Sac is often adhered to the liver, and the sac over the liver should be left as it is to avoid excessive bleeding
- Any anterior diaphragmatic defect (pentalogy of Cantrell) should be looked for and repaired if present

32.10 Complications Following Surgical Repair

- Decreased venous return
- Abdominal compartment syndrome
- Decreased pulmonary compliance
- Renal failure
- Necrotizing enterocolitis

32.11 Management of Intestinal Atresias with Gastroschisis

Incidence is around 10% of all gastroschisis cases. The different options available are

- Delayed repair of atresia 4–6 weeks after primary abdominal wall closure
- Initial ostomy (for distal atresia or perforation) and delayed bowel anastomosis
- Primary bowel anastomosis for healthy bowel

32.12 Management of Postoperative Dysmotility of Bowel

- Bowel motility may take a long time to recover
- Starting early enteral small-volume (trophic) feeding as tolerated
- Central venous line with total parenteral nutrition (TPN) needs to be instituted and continued as required
- Prokinetic drugs like erythromycin, metoclopramide, and domperidone have variable success rate

Cryptorchidism is associated with gastroschisis, with an incidence of 15–30%. Replacement of the herniated testis into the abdominal cavity will result in normal testicular descent into the scrotum in the majority of cases.

32.13 Beckwith-Wiedemann Syndrome (BWS)

It is characterized by *Macroglossia, gigantism, omphalocele, macrosomia, and visceromegaly* (Fig. 32.7). Incidence is 1 in 13700 births. A small percentage (15%) are familial with a slightly increased inheritance risk, the rest are sporadic. Ultrasound findings for BWS are macroglossia, umbilical anomalies, polyhydramnios, enlarged placenta, omphalocele, visceromegaly involving the liver, kidney, and spleen. BWS is associated with increased risk of birth trauma, hypoglycemia, congestive heart failure, and respiratory distress.

Several tumors have an association with BWS: Wilms' tumor, hepatoblastoma, neuroblastoma,

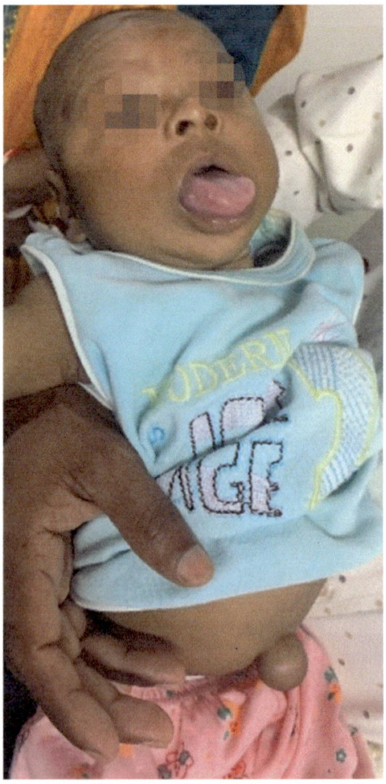

Fig. 32.7 Beckwith-Wiedemann syndrome, note macroglossia with a small umbilical hernia

and rhabdomyosarcoma. The prognosis is generally not bad as most of the associations including tumors are treatable.

32.14 Pentalogy of Cantrell

Omphalocele, ectopic heart, pericardial or pleural effusions, intracardiac abnormalities, sternal cleft, two vessel cord, scoliosis, and craniofacial abnormalities. Chromosomal anomalies such as trisomy 13 and 18, and Turner's syndrome may be associated. Most cases have a fatal outcome.

32.15 Amniotic Band Syndrome

Spectrum of constrictions, amputations, and slash deformities due to amniotic bands. One in 200 births. Sonographic findings: multiple, asymmetric, and bizarre craniofacial, limb, and abdominal wall defects. Large body wall defects omphaloceles, gastroschisis, and bladder exstrophy. Most infants with severe craniofacial deformities have a fatal outcome, while infants with isolated limb defects have a favorable outcome.

32.16 Bladder and Cloacal Exstrophy (Fig. 32.8, see Chap. 70)

This results from caudal fold fusion defects (see embryology), resulting in midline defects of the infraumbilical ventral wall, causing *herniation of the bladder and hindgut. The i*ncidence of bladder exstrophy is 1 in 33,000 live births, and that of cloacal exstrophy is 1 in 200,000 to 400,000 live births. Antenatal sonographic findings include infraumbilical abdominal wall defect with an irregular soft tissue mass, nonvisualization of the normal fluid-filled urinary bladder, and low umbilical cord insertion. There may be association with the *OEIS complex*: omphalocele, bladder exstrophy, imperforate anus, and spinal anomalies. The prognosis of bladder exstrophy is favorable, but cloacal exstrophy is not so favorable due to the complexity of gastrointestinal and genitourinary malformation.

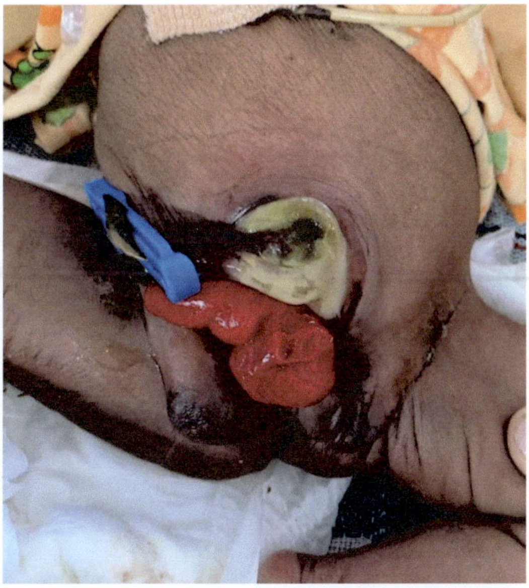

Fig. 32.8 Cloacal exstrophy : prolapsed ileum in the midline (elephant trunk appearance), hemi bladder, bifid scrotum, and exomphalos

32.17 Prune Belly Syndrome

Prune belly syndrome (triad syndrome, Eagle-Barrett syndrome) comprises of deficiency of abdominal muscles, hydroureteronephrosis, and cryptorchidism (Fig. 32.9a). The abdominal skin gives a wrinkled (pruned) appearance. The majority of the patients are male. The mode of inheritance is unknown. The spectrum of the defect varies from severe renal dysplasia leading to stillbirth to minor urinary abnormalities (Fig. 32.9b). Those with severe pulmonary and renal dysplasia are grouped as category 1, and those with minimal dysplasia are category 3, with category 2 having minimal renal dysplasia, which may progress to renal failure. The early management revolves around relieving the obstructive uropathy by establishing adequate urinary drainage. A vesicostomy or inter-

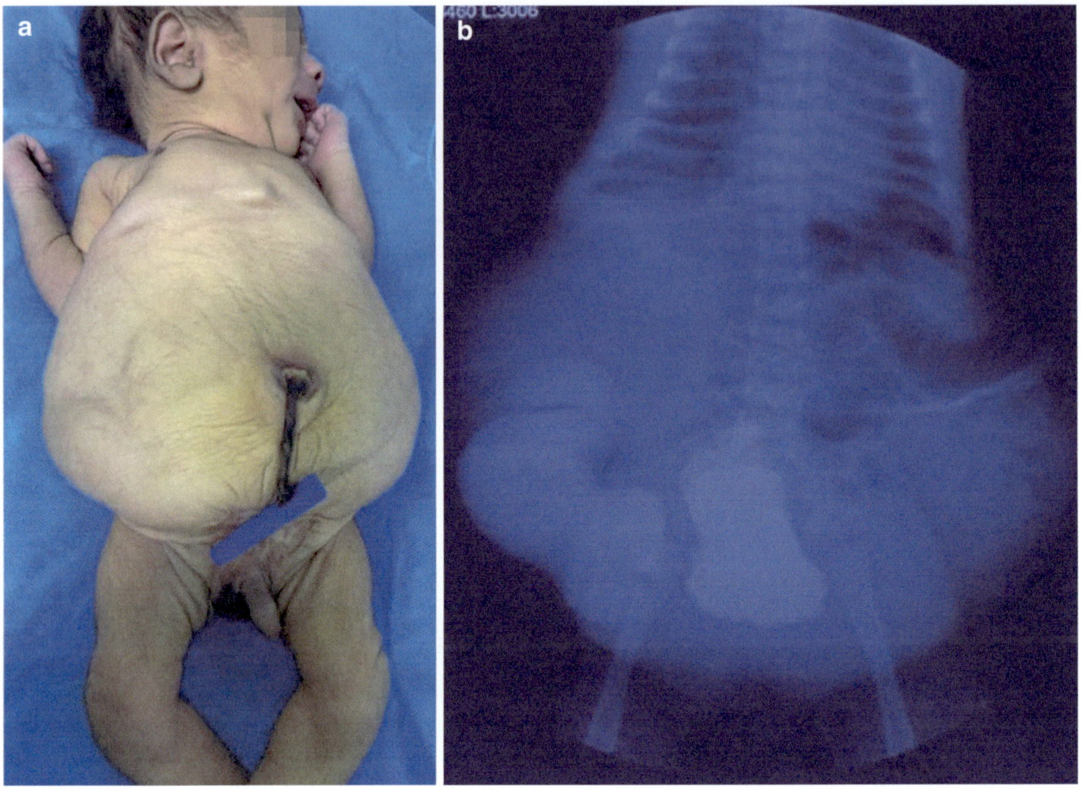

Fig. 32.9 (**a**) Prune belly syndrome (**b**) Micturating cystourethrogram (MCU) showing abnormal shape of the bladder, vesicoureteral reflux (VUR) with dilated tortuous right ureter, and a patent urachus

mittent catheterization may be helpful. Late management consists of the reconstruction of the abdominal wall muscles (Monfort procedure) and orchidopexy. Assisted fertility may help them in reproduction due to associated infertility.

32.18 Outcome

The clinical outcome of antenatally diagnosed abdominal defects appears to be favorable with postnatal treatment (Table 32.3). Those with associated major chromosomal and organ anom-

Table 32.3 Algorithm of antenatal management of abdominal wall defects

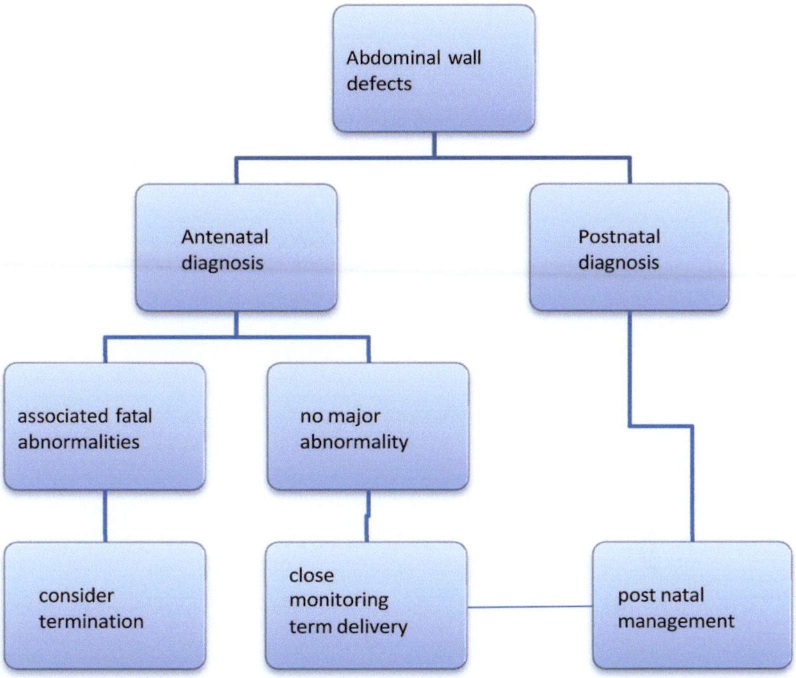

Summary

- Fetal diagnosis is possible and accurate in over 90% of cases of abdominal wall defects. Fetal karyotyping should be offered in all cases. Isolated anomalies have a better outcome.
- Early and close prenatal consultation by the obstetrician, neonatologist, and the pediatric surgeon led to better management and outcome.
- Survival of newborns with gastroschisis is above 90%, with excellent long-term outcomes. Major causes of death are prematurity, sepsis, and bowel ischemia. Staged surgical closure may be needed.
- Omphalocele is associated with higher mortality (30–70%), especially in those with associated chromosomal, cardiac, or other major anomalies.
- Long-term outcome and quality of life in survivors of gastroschisis and isolated omphalocele are excellent.

alies have a poor outcome. Patients with omphalocele or gastroschisis rarely experience severe late cardiorespiratory and pulmonary complications.

Suggested Reading

Coran AG, Caldamone A, Scott Adzich N, Krummel TM, Laberge JM, editors. Pediatric surgery. 7th ed. Oxford: Elsevier Limited; 2012.

Holcomb GW III, Murphy PJ, St Peter SD, editors. Holocomb and Ashcraft's pediatric surgery. 7th ed. Philadelphia: Elsevier; 2020.

Puri P, Hollwarth ME, editors. Pediatric surgery. 2nd ed. Heidelberg: Springer-Verlag; 2019.

33 Lesions of the Pancreas and Spleen

Prabudh Goel, Mehak Sehgal,
and Subhasis Roy Choudhury

Pancreatic lesions in children are diverse and could be due to developmental and acquired conditions affecting the gland. The pancreas originates from the fusion of two endodermal buds. An error in rotation, fusion, development, or endocrinological defects results in congenital anomalies of the pancreas. The acquired anomalies are usually rare, but the causes can be variable. Some of the diseases of the pancreas in children include:

- Annular pancreas (see duodenal obstruction)
- Pancreas divisum and ductal anomalies
- Acute pancreatitis
- Chronic pancreatitis
- Pancreatic cysts and pseudocysts
- Neoplasms
- Endocrine abnormalities (including persistent hyperinsulinemic hypoglycemia of infancy (PHHI))
- Cystic fibrosis

33.1 Acute Pancreatitis

Acute pancreatitis is defined as acute inflammation of the pancreas and is clinically defined as the presence of abdominal pain with elevated pancreatic enzymes. The various possible causes are listed below:

33.1.1 Causes of Acute Pancreatitis in Children

- Idiopathic
- Choledocholithiasis and other obstructive causes
- Infections: mumps, rubella, Coxsackie B virus
- Traumatic, post-liver transplantation
- Congenital anomalies: pancreas divisium, choledochal cyst, pancreaticobiliary malunion
- Drugs: azathioprine, tetracycline, L-asparaginase, valproic acid
- Metabolic: Inborn errors of metabolism, hypercalcemia, hypertriglyceridemia

P. Goel (✉) · M. Sehgal
Pediatric Surgery, All India Institute of Medical Sciences, New Delhi, India

S. Roy Choudhury
Pediatric Surgery, Lady Hardinge Medical College and Associated Kalawati Saran Children's Hospital, New Delhi, Delhi, India

© The Author(s), under exclusive license to Springer Nature Singapore Pte Ltd. 2025
S. Roy Choudhury (ed.), *Pediatric Surgery*, https://doi.org/10.1007/978-981-96-1257-4_33

33.1.2 Diagnosis

The diagnosis largely depends on clinical, biochemical, and radiological investigation. In accordance with the INSPPIRE (International Study Group of Pediatric Pancreatitis; In Search for a Cure) criteria, the diagnosis of acute pancreatitis is considered ***if two of the three*** are suggestive of pancreatitis.

1. *Clinical*: Acute pancreatitis has a wide spectrum of presentation. It usually presents with epigastric pain, which often radiates to the back, nausea, vomiting, anorexia, and abdominal distension. In severe cases, the presentation is that of a multisystem organ failure.
2. *Biochemical*: The most useful test is elevated pancreatic enzymes, amylase, and lipase, which are usually elevated more than 3 times the normal value. Though they are the most reliable biochemical marker still their sensitivities range between 50% and 85%. Complete blood count and kidney function tests should also be obtained. Additionally, levels of liver enzymes, triglycerides, and calcium should be tested to identify the etiology.
3. *Radiological*: Ultrasonography is the initial preferred investigation and will show edema of the pancreas with or without peripancreatic fluid collection. It also detects the presence of dilated pancreatic or biliary ducts and calculi. Magnetic resonance cholangiopancreatography (MRCP), with or without secretin injection, provides better delineation of the anatomy. Endoscopic retrograde cholangiopancreatography (ERCP) is usually reserved for therapeutic interventions like sphincterotomy and stenting.

Imaging is often required only when the diagnosis is not confirmed by the biochemical tests. If the amylase and lipase, along with the clinical symptoms, are suggestive of pancreatitis, imaging is not mandated.

33.1.3 Treatment

Medical management is successful in the majority of patients. Conservative treatment includes keeping nil by mouth, nasogastric aspiration, intravenous hydration, and parenteral hyperalimentation to provide rest to the inflamed gland. As per the recent NASPGHAN (North American Society for Pediatric Gastroenterology, Hepatology and Nutrition) guidelines:

- The initial fluid therapy is based on the clinical status. In most cases, a crystalloid bolus of normal saline or Ringer's lactate can be administered at 10–20 ml/kg. The maintenance fluid is administered at a 1.5–2 times higher rate, especially for the initial 24–48 h, keeping a close watch on the urine output. Children with a mild form of acute pancreatitis can be started on early enteral nutrition, while in those patients where enteral nutrition would not be possible for 5–7 days, parenteral nutrition should be considered to avoid a catabolic state.
- Pain relief is an essential component of management, and graded escalation from acetaminophen and NSAIDS to opioids may be needed in some cases. Prophylactic antibiotics are not recommended and should be used only in infected necrosis. Similarly, there is no role for antiproteases for the management of acute pancreatitis in children. Proton pump inhibitors are administered for stress ulcer prophylaxis and do not have any other definitive role in the management. Octreotide is a powerful inhibitor of exocrine pancreatic secretion; however, its utility in reducing complications of acute pancreatitis is still debatable.
- ERCP is indicated in the management of choledocholithiasis, pancreatic ductal stones, or leak, and depends on the local expertise.
- Surgical intervention is restricted in these settings as it can be associated with morbidity and mortality. Acute intervention may be needed in post-trauma. In case of mild acute

biliary pancreatitis, cholecystectomy can be performed before discharge. However, the management of acute necrotic collections should be avoided and delayed, if possible, until after 4 weeks of onset. If necessary, drainage or necrosectomy should be performed endoscopically or via less-invasive percutaneous routes.

- Anatomical abnormalities may require surgical correction:
  - Biliary pancreatitis: ERCP and stone removal are recommended, followed by cholecystectomy after 2–4 weeks of resolution of the disease.
  - Sphincter of Oddi dysfunction: ERCP and sphincterotomy may be curative.
  - Choledochal cyst and pancreato-biliary malunion (Fig. 33.1): Excision of the cyst and hepaticojejunostomy should be done.
  - Pancreas divisum (described below): The condition can be treated with endoscopic or surgical dilatation of the minor papilla or sphincterotomy.
- Early and late complications are known. Since these children can progress to systemic inflammatory response syndrome and multiorgan failure, close monitoring is essential. Up to 15–35% of cases may recur, hence long-term follow-up is needed.

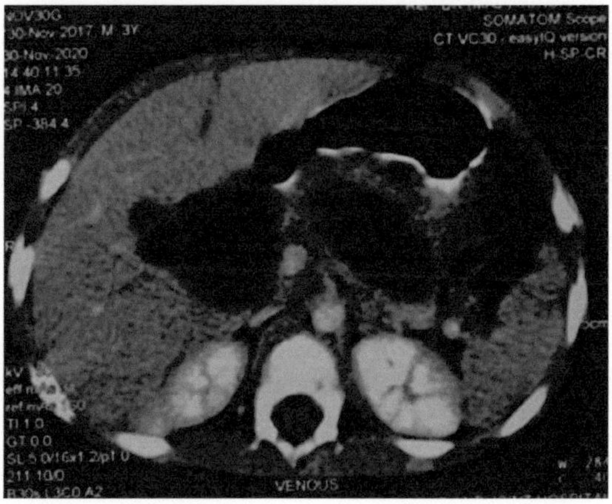

Fig. 33.1 Fusiform dilatation of the cystic duct along with a cystic lesion in the body and tail of the pancreas

33.2 Chronic Pancreatitis

Chronic pancreatitis results from repeated inflammation of the pancreas in individuals with genetic, environmental, or other risk factors, which results in irreversible progressive damage to the pancreas. It may be preceded by acute pancreatitis and/or acute recurrent pancreatitis. This may result in pain syndromes, exocrine or endocrine disturbances, which may be irreversible.

Causes in children can be due to trauma, hereditary and metabolic disorders, congenital anomalies causing obstructive pathology like pancreas divisum and choledocholithiasis, autoimmune, or idiopathic causes.

The most common presentation is with persistent or recurrent abdominal pain. It is a cardinal feature of chronic pancreatitis, typically located in the epigastric region, with radiation to the back. They can be asymptomatic till disease progression to fat and protein malabsorption, or diabetes mellitus. Other uncommon presentations can be due to pseudocyst, portal hypertension due to splenic vein thrombosis, or due to pancreatic pseudoaneurysms resulting in hematemesis, hemobilia, or hemoperitoneum.

33.2.1 Diagnosis

History and examination may help to clinically suspect chronic pancreatitis and help rule out other causes of chronic pain. Investigations like complete blood count, glucose, calcium, and electrolyte levels may be normal. Normal values of serum amylase and lipase do not rule out chronic pancreatitis. Liver enzymes may be elevated in biliary etiology. In addition, tests may be performed for pancreatic insufficiency, such as fecal elastase and levels of fat-soluble vitamins.

Imaging by means of ultrasound (USG), contrast enhanced computed tomography (CECT), and magnetic resonance cholangiopancreatography (MRCP) helps in establishing the diagnosis and describing the anatomical ductal and parenchymal changes. It often reveals a small atrophic pancreas with calcification and a dilated duct. The pancreatic duct may have multiple strictures

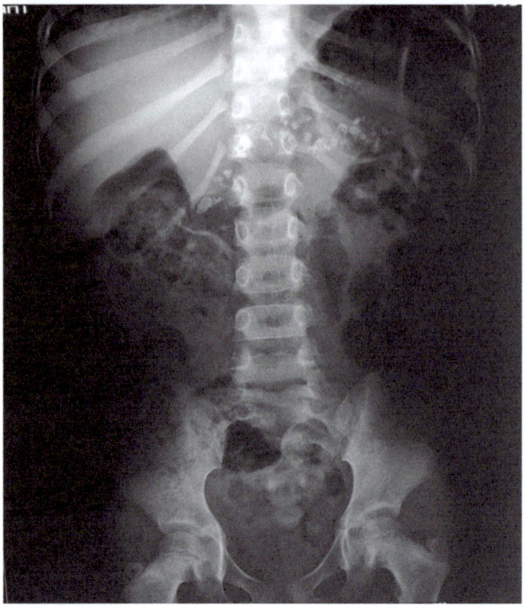

Fig. 33.2 Multiple pancreatic calculi as evident on a plain radiograph

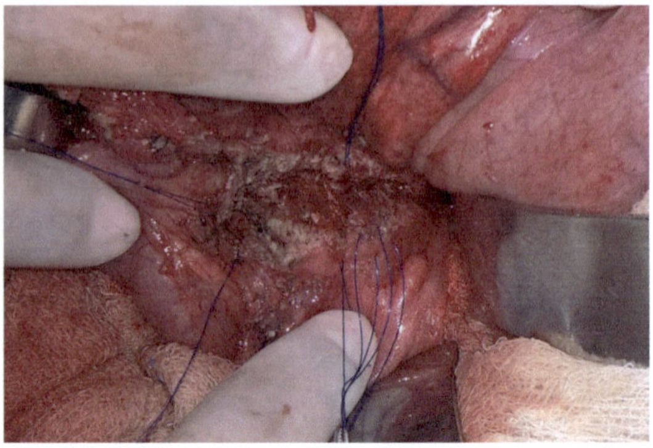

Fig. 33.3 A dilated pacreatic duct containing multiple stones has been laid open between stitches, stones cleared, and being prepared for lateral pancreatico-jejunostomy (Puestow) for chronic pancreatitis

and stones (Fig. 33.2). ERCP may occasionally be required. Genetic evaluation may be carried out to test for mutations in genes such as CFTR, SPINK1, PRSS1, and CPA1.

Management options include pain management, nutritional support, therapeutic ERCP, and surgery. Surgical treatment for chronic relapsing pancreatitis includes:

- Sphincterotomy (pancreas divisum) and sphincteroplasty of the sphincter of Oddi
- Longitudinal pancreatico-jejunostomy (Puestow) (Fig. 33.3) and distal pancreatico-jejunostomy (Duval), with or without localized head resection—done in cases with a dilated duct
- Distal pancreatectomy: if the pathology is limited to the tail of the pancreas
- Pancreatico-duodenectomy or total pancreatectomy, with and without islet cell auto transplantation

33.3 Pancreas Divisum

- Also called "dominant dorsal duct syndrome," it is the commonest ductal variation.
- In this condition, the minor pancreatic duct of Santorini becomes the main drainage for the pancreas, and the major duct of Wirsung becomes attenuated or rudimentary.
- Inadequate drainage causes elevated intraductal pressure and may cause recurrent pancreatitis. While in the normal population it may be found in up to 5–7%, a higher prevalence of 20–25% is found in those with chronic pancreatitis. Only 5% of those with pancreatic divisum are symptomatic.
- Associated with annular pancreas and sphincter of Oddi dysfunction.
- Three subtypes identified: Complete/classic, incomplete, and reverse (Fig. 33.4).
- Evaluation is done by ultrasonography, MRCP, and ERCP. Treatment consists of adequate drainage of the duct of Santorini (minor papilla) by endoscopic sphincterotomy.
- In case of re-stenosis and a dilated pancreatic duct, longitudinal pancreaticojejunostomy should be considered.

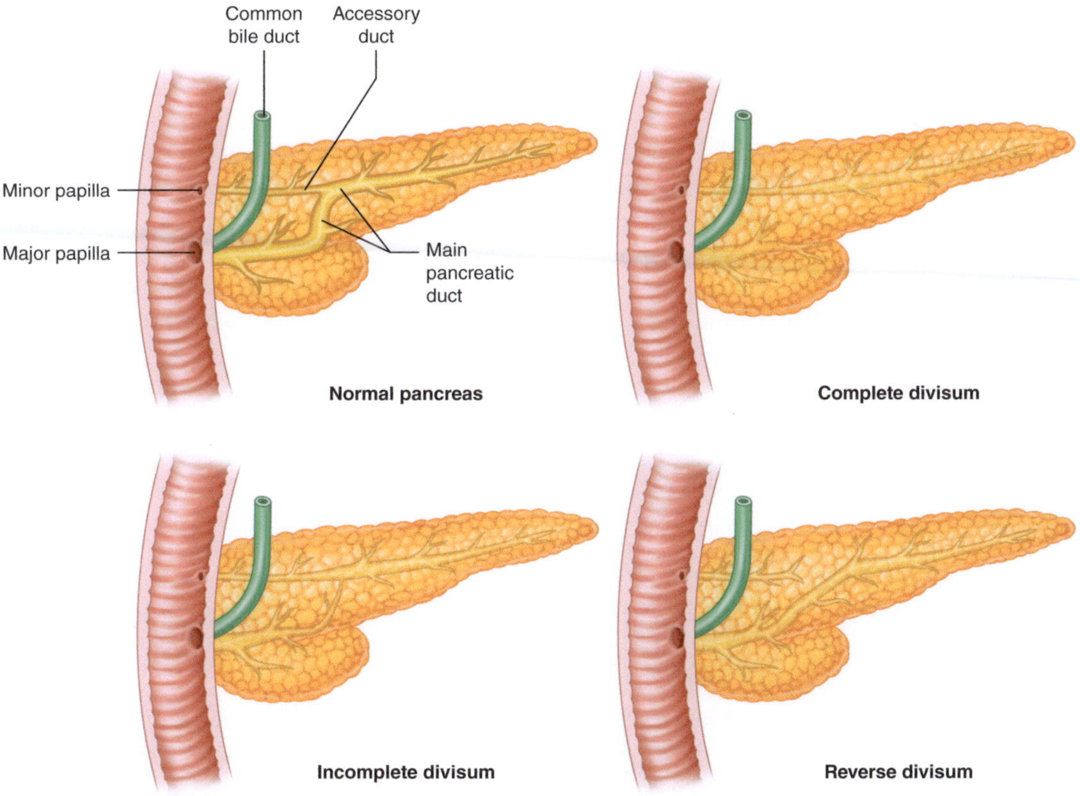

Fig. 33.4 Types of pancreatic divisum

33.4 Pseudocyst of the Pancreas

Pseudocyst of the pancreas is a collection of fluid usually in the lesser sac, walled off by fibrous tissue and lacking an epithelial lining. It often complicates the course of acute pancreatitis, where inflammation and ductal damage lead to extravasation and collection of fluid. The causes in children include trauma, pancreatitis, and obstruction of the duct. It usually develops within 4 weeks of the episode.

An upper abdominal lump is a characteristic presentation (Fig. 33.5). Others may be asymptomatic or may present with nausea, vomiting, early satiety, or jaundice—secondary to compressive effect on nearby structures. On investigation, elevated lipase levels may be found. Ultrasonography and CT scan are useful in making the diagnosis (Fig. 33.6), which may be suggestive of a circumscribed, extra-pancreatic homogeneous collection, with a well-defined wall. In case of a diagnostic dilemma, endoscopic ultrasonography (EUS), with fluid sampling, can be performed for confirmation.

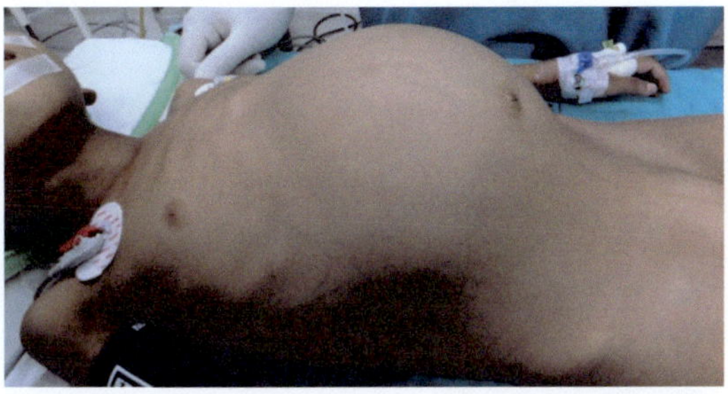

Fig. 33.5 Large upper abdominal lump due to the pseudocyst of the pancreas

Conservative treatment with nutritional care is offered in acute cases. Generally, after a period of 6 weeks, the cyst either disappears or the cyst wall becomes mature. Persistent pseudocysts after 6 weeks and cyst diameters larger than 5 cm require surgical drainage by either cystogastrostomy (open or endoscopic) (Fig. 33.7) or cystojejunostomy, depending on the proximity of the cyst wall to the viscera, which causes collapse of the cyst. Other options include conservative management for asymptomatic patients with small cysts and ERCP stenting. An infected pseudocyst requires external drainage.

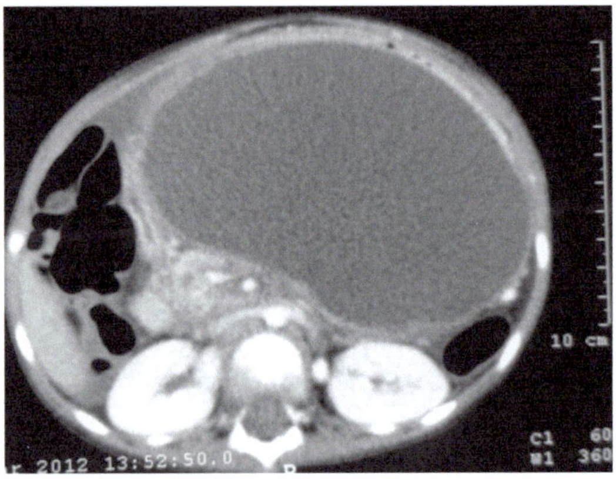

Fig. 33.6 CT scan showing a large pancreatic pseudocyst

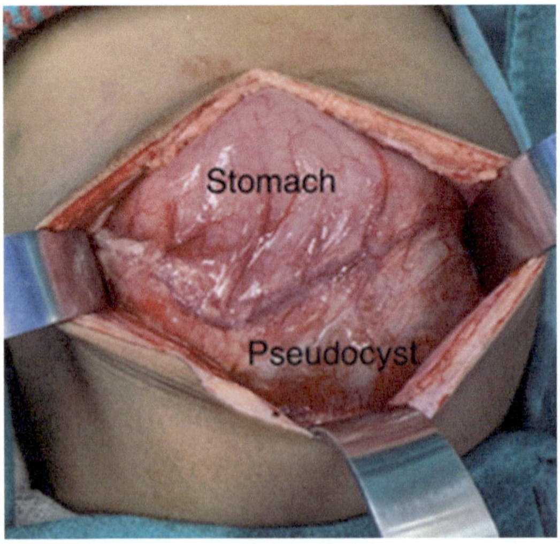

Fig. 33.7 Open cysto-gastrostomy

33.5 Persistent Hyperinsulinemic Hypoglycemia of Infancy (PHHI)

PHHI is a rare but very important cause of severe neonatal hypoglycemia. More common in males, this entity generally presents in the neonatal period or infancy. It should be differentiated from other causes of hypoglycemia in neonates. Timely recognition and treatment of this entity become important since severe and frequent hypoglycemia may lead to severe neurological damage or even a life-threatening event.

33.5.1 Etiopathogenesis

- An excessively high secretion of insulin due to a defect at the level of β cells of the pancreas.
- The most common and severe form occurs due to abnormalities of the K/ATP channel (encoded by the sulfonylurea receptor 1-SUR 1 and Kir6.2 genes), which is responsible for the altered control of insulin secretion and glucose regulation. Clinically, they can be classified as diazoxide responsive and unresponsive. Histologically, it can be either focal (30–50%) or diffuse (50–70%). For the focal form, surgical resection is curative.
- Other causes include mutations in glutamate dehydrogenase, glucokinase, HNF4A, HADH (hydroxyacyl-CoA dehydrogenase), and UCP2.

33.5.2 Clinical Features

These children can be large for gestational age at birth, with higher birth weights. The symptoms of hypoglycemia appear soon after birth, including hunger, jitteriness, lethargy, apnea, and may even progress to seizures. Mild to moderate hepatomegaly may be present due to steatosis. Care must be taken to avoid fluid overload due to high intravenous glucose requirements, anemia secondary to frequent blood sampling, and central line infections.

33.5.3 Diagnosis of PHHI

- Nonketotic hypoglycemia (blood sugar levels less than 36 mg/dL), both fasting and postprandial. The definition of hypoglycemia will depend on the gestational age in the case of neonates.
- Hyperinsulinemia (plasma insulin level >3 mU/L).
- Need for a high rate of glucose infusion (>10 mg/kg/min) to maintain blood glucose levels more than 54 mg/dL.
- Rise in blood glucose levels in response to the administration of glucagon. Usually, the blood sugar levels rise by 18–36 mg/dL following the administration of 0.5 mg of glucagon by subcutaneous or intramuscular route. Most other hypoglycemic conditions in infancy induce a starvation-like state with exhaustion of the liver glycogen. In such situations, there is a failure to increase the blood glucose concentration after the administration of glucagon.
- Supportive findings:
  - Blood β-hydroxybutyrate (BHB) <2 mmol/L (2000 μmol/L)
  - Blood free fatty acids (FFA, NEFA) <1.5 mmol/L (1.5 mEq/L)

33.5.4 Investigations

- Biochemical investigations are done to confirm the diagnosis.
- Another parameter that affects the management of PHHI is whether the disease is local or diffuse. This can be differentiated based on genetic testing, where available. Rarely, an MRI can show the presence of focal disease. Other ways to confirm the presence of focal disease is through interventional radiology, where either the selective sampling of the pancreatic veins (Transhepatic Portal Venous catheterization and Selective sampling of Pancreatic Veins) or by the stimulation of the pancreas by specific cannulation of its artery and detecting insulin in the blood (Arterial Stimulation with Venous Sampling). PET-CT scan using L-DOPA may also help to localize a focal disease.

33.5.5 Management

Medical management includes a high level of glucose infusion along with drugs. Of the following drugs, diazoxide is the first-line drug followed by somatostatin.

Drugs that inhibit insulin secretion (diazoxide, somatostatin, epinephrine, diphenylhydantoin, and calcium channel blockers)
Drugs that antagonize the insulin effect of body tissues (epinephrine, glucagon, and growth hormone)
Drugs that destroy islet cells (alloxan)

Surgical treatment is indicated in

1. Failure of medical management
2. Presence of a focal lesion that is amenable to surgical resection
3. Poor compliance with medical management

For focal lesions, localized excision can be done. For diffuse lesions and for those for patients with intractable hypoglycemia despite medical treatment, a near total pancreatectomy, sparing the pancreas near the bile duct with resection of 95–98% of the pancreas (Fig. 33.8), is recommended wherein all the pancreas barring the pancreatic tissue between the duodenum and the common bile duct is left. A gastrostomy tube is also placed to facilitate postoperative feeding. This may result in diabetes mellitus or recurrent postoperative hypoglycemia. In the long term, these children are predisposed to poorer neurocognitive outcomes.

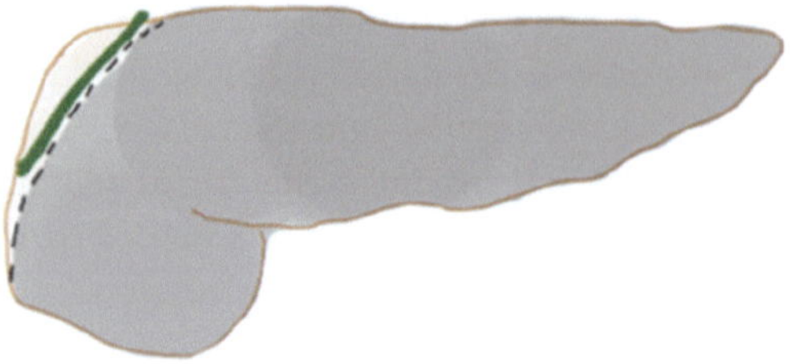

Fig. 33.8 Near total pancreatectomy, sparing the part of the head of the pancreas near the bile duct (green)

33.6 Pancreatic Neoplasms

Neoplasms of the pancreas in the pediatric age group are relatively rare. They are classified as described below (Fig. 33.9). Diagnosis is confirmed by USG and CT. Surgical management is amenable in most cases. Whipple's procedure, extended Whipple's procedure, pyloroduodenectomy, distal, or central pancreatectomy is performed based on extent.

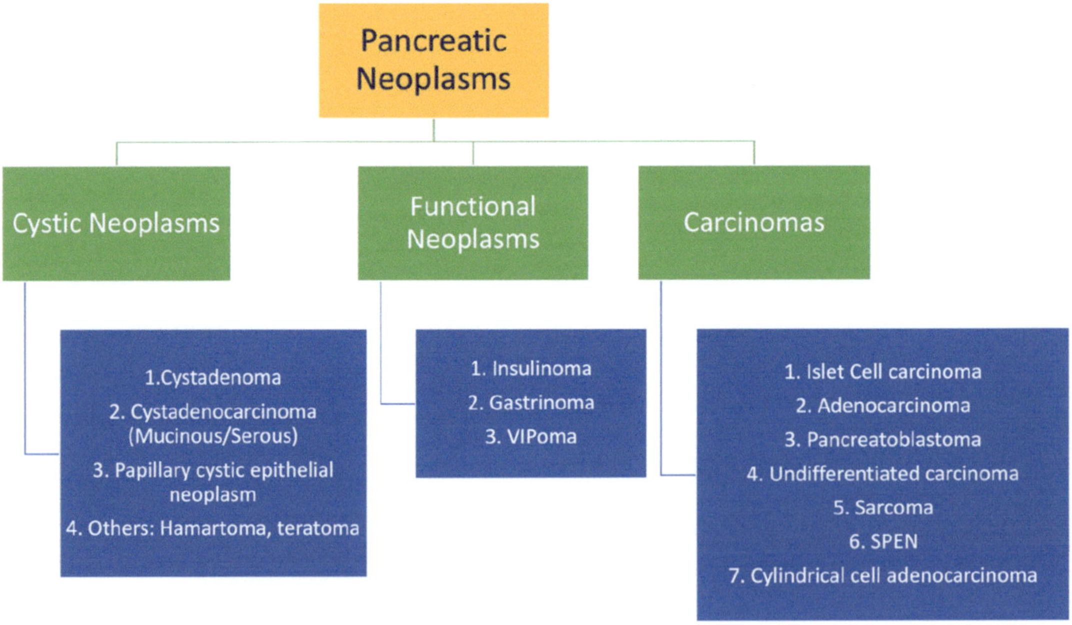

Fig. 33.9 Classification of pancreatic neoplasms

33.7 Splenic Disorders in Children

33.7.1 Splenic Cysts

Splenic cysts are usually asymptomatic, but may present with an abdominal mass and pain, complications such as infection, hemorrhage or rupture, or compressive symptoms. They are classified as described in Fig. 33.10.

33.7.2 Epithelial Cysts

These are epithelial-lined cysts, often called epidermoid cysts, which originate from the inclusion of surface mesothelium. Small cysts <5 cm may be observed. Larger cysts >5 cm or symptomatic cysts require treatment. Aspiration and sclerosis may be successful; however, a better treatment option is the excision of the cyst wall and marsupialization of the remaining cyst either by open or by laparoscopic approach. Partial splenectomy can be done in large cysts. Omentopexy reduces the recurrence rates.

33.7.3 Splenic Abscess (See Chap. 46)

33.7.3.1 Indications for Splenectomy

- Hereditary spherocytosis: Persistence of reticulocyte count more than 10% with moderate to severe anemia
- Immune thrombocytopenic purpura: Symptomatic thrombocytopenia unresponsive to medical management
- Sickle cell disease: Recurrent or single major episode of sequestration
- Thalassemia: Blood transfusion requirement more than 250ml/kg/year
- Gaucher's disease: Associated with massive splenomegaly with hypersplenism
- Trauma (accidental or operative), rare
- Severe hypersplenism with portal hypertension

Vaccination and Prophylaxis Before Splenectomy For elective splenectomy, vaccinations against *Streptococcus pneumoniae,*

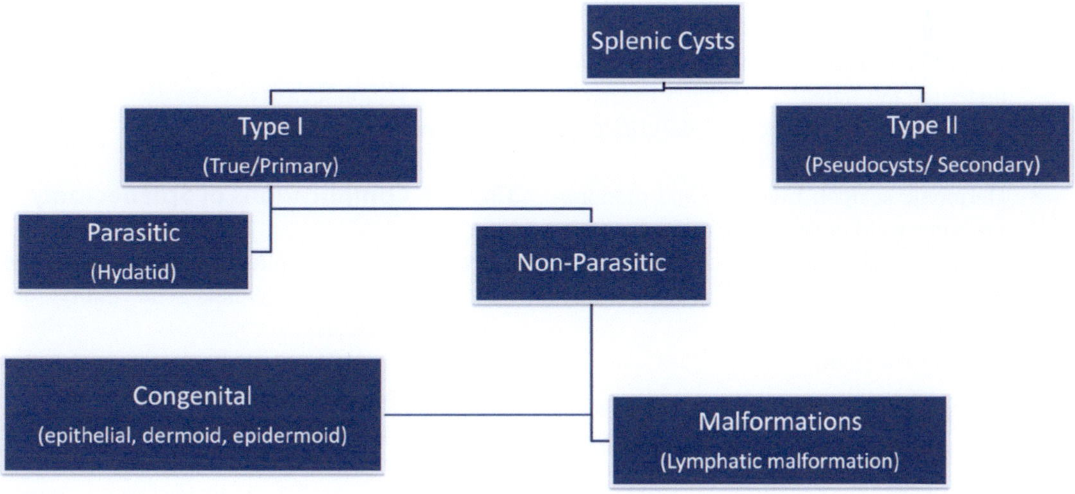

Fig. 33.10 Types of splenic cysts

Haemophilus influenzae, and Neisseria meningitidis are recommended. The annual influenza vaccine is also recommended for asplenic patients. All vaccinations should be completed 2 weeks prior to splenectomy. Ideally, the vaccination schedule should be started 10-12 weeks prior to the planned splenectomy. In an emergency, such as trauma, vaccination can be given 2 weeks after, in the postoperative period.

33.7.3.2 Surgical Approaches to Splenectomy

1. Open Splenectomy:
   - Spleen is approached by a left upper quadrant incision.
   - After identification, the spleen is retracted medially, and the ligaments of the spleen (splenorenal, splenophrenic, and splenocolic) are divided.
   - The lower pole is delivered out of the incision.
   - Gastrosplenic ligament, the short gastric vessels, and hilar vessels are subsequently divided.
   - Accessory spleen should be looked for, which can be found in 15–30% of patients.
2. Laparoscopic Splenectomy
   - Patient is positioned supine with a support under the left flank.
   - The ports are placed as described in Fig. 33.11.
   - Harmonic scalpel, Ligasure, and monopolar cautery aid in splenic dissection.
   - Spleen is retrieved using retrieval bags, morcellation, or mini-laparotomy/Pfannensteil incision.
3. Robotic Splenectomy

33.7.3.3 Hematological Changes Following Splenectomy

1. Erythrocytes
Howell-Jolly bodies (nuclear fragments)
Heinz bodies (hemoglobin deposits)
Pappenheimer bodies (iron deposits)
Target cells
Spur cells (achanthocytes)
2. Platelets
Transient thrombocytosis

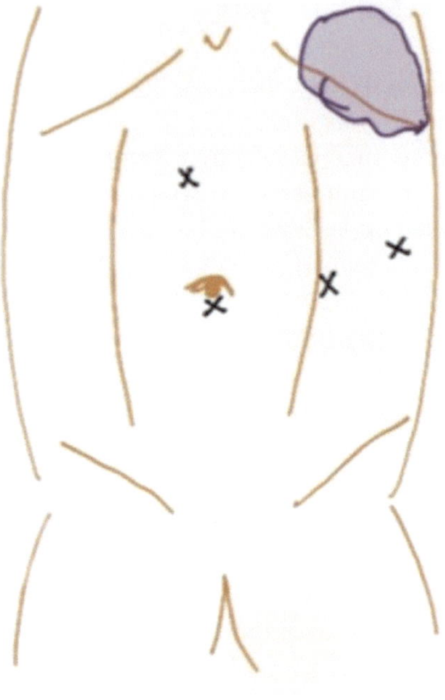

Fig. 33.11 Sites of port placement for laparoscopic splenectomy

3. Leucocytes
Transient leucocytosis
Persistent lymphocytosis
Persistent monocytosis

33.7.3.4 Complications of Splenectomy

- Immediate complications: Hemorrhage, hematemesis, gastric/pancreatic injury, and basal atelectesis.
- Delayed complications: Postsplenectomy septicemia due to bacterial infection from *pneumococcus*, *Haemophilus influenzae type b*, *meningococcus,* and *Escherichia coli*, and overwhelming post-splenectomy sepsis (OPSI).

Overwhelming Post-splenectomy Sepsis (OPSI) is a major concern during the first 2–3 years of splenectomy in children. OPSI presents as fulminant sepsis, meningitis, or pneumonia in an asplenic/hyposplenic patient. The incidence of OPSI is 0.5–2%, and the risk and associated death are the highest in the first year after splenectomy. It is a medical emergency as the mortality rate ranges from 30% to 70%, and most death occurs within the first 24 h.

Postsplenectomy oral antibiotic prophylaxis with penicillin, erythromycin, amoxicillin, or co-amoxiclav is effective and generally indicated for children until the age of 10–15 years. Lifelong prophylaxis is indicated in immunocompromised patients and those with a history of prior sepsis with encapsulated organisms. The recommended emergency standby treatment in children for fever with systemic signs is amoxicillin 50 mg/kg in three divided daily doses.

Suggested Reading

Puri P, Hollwarth ME, editors. Pediatric Surgery. 2nd ed. Heidelberg: Springer-Verlag; 2019.
Zinner MJ, Ashley SW. Maingot's abdominnal operation. 12th ed. McGraw Hill USA; 2013.

Infantile Obstructive Cholangiopathy, Biliary Atresia

34

Rajeev Redkar, Anant Bangar, and Subhasis Roy Choudhury

34.1 Introduction

Physiological jaundice in newborns is a frequent and generally harmless condition that resolves on its own. However, jaundice lasting beyond two weeks of age postnatal, particularly when associated with elevated conjugated bilirubin levels, warrants further investigation. This prolonged jaundice could indicate an underlying pathological issue, requiring differentiation between conditions such as biliary atresia (BA) and neonatal hepatitis (refer to Table 34.1). Landing introduced the term "infantile obstructive cholangiopathy" to describe a spectrum of disorders, including neonatal hepatitis, biliary atresia, and choledochal cysts.

Persistent hyperbilirubinemia, defined as levels exceeding 10 mg/dL and lasting for more than two weeks, requires prompt evaluation. The initial assessment should include a comprehensive medical history, thorough physical examination, and relevant biochemical and hematological tests. Infants presenting with pale stools, yellow discoloration of urine, and predominantly conjugated hyperbilirubinemia (direct/conjugated bilirubin levels exceeding 1.0 mg/dL when total serum bilirubin (TSB) is 5.0 mg/dL, or more than 20% of TSB if TSB is above 5.0 mg/dL) should be further evaluated for potential obstructive cholangiopathy.

34.1.1 Extrahepatic Biliary Atresia

Extrahepatic biliary atresia (EHBA) is a rare condition characterized by the obstruction of the bile ducts, leading to neonatal jaundice. It occurs in approximately 1 in 10,000 to 1 in 16,700 live births and is more common in

Table 34.1 Causes of conjugated hyperbilirubinemia in infancy

Extrahepatic causes	Intrahepatic causes
Extrahepatic biliary atresia (EHBA) Choledochal cyst Bile duct stenosis Spontaneous perforation of the bile duct Cholelithiasis Inspissated bile/mucus plug Extrinsic compression of the bile duct	Idiopathic neonatal hepatitis Toxic: total parenteral nutrition (TPN), drug induced Genetic/Chromosomal: trisomy 18, 21 Infectious: TORCH, hepatitis Metabolic, endocrine disorders Miscellaneous: Alpha-1-antitrypsin deficiency, Alagille syndrome, carolis disease, Byler's disease, congenital hepatic fibrosis

R. Redkar (✉) · A. Bangar
Lilavati Hospital and Research Centre, Mumbai, India

S. Roy Choudhury
Pediatric Surgery, Lady Hardinge Medical College and Associated Kalawati Saran Children's Hospital, New Delhi, Delhi, India

© The Author(s), under exclusive license to Springer Nature Singapore Pte Ltd. 2025
S. Roy Choudhury (ed.), *Pediatric Surgery*, https://doi.org/10.1007/978-981-96-1257-4_34

females, with ratio ranging from 1.4:1 to 1.7:1. Congenital anomalies are associated with EHBA in 11–20% of cases, with polysplenia reported in about 7.5% of cases. Cases involving biliary atresia alongside splenic malformations are classified under the syndromic group known as biliary atresia with splenic malformations (BASM).

34.2 Etiology

Occult Viral Infections Infections with viruses such as reovirus 3, cytomegalovirus (CMV), rotavirus C, human papillomavirus, and retroviruses may trigger an immune response due to viral-induced neoantigens on the biliary epithelium.

Developmental Failure A failure in the recanalization process of the biliary ducts during development.

Ductal Plate Malformation Theory Poorly supported biliary ducts may rupture, leading to intense fibrosis that eventually causes ductal obliteration.

Exposure to Environmental Toxins Contact with environmental toxins may contribute to the condition.

Based on etiopathogenesis, extrahepatic biliary atresia (EHBA) can be categorized into four groups:

1. *Syndromic Biliary Atresia (Embryonic Type)*: This type is associated with congenital anomalies such as an interrupted inferior vena cava, preduodenal portal vein, intestinal malrotation, situs inversus, cardiac defects, and polysplenia. Also known as BASM syndrome (Biliary Atresia Splenic Malformation Syndrome), it accounts for 10–20% of cases and is associated with a poor prognosis.
2. *Cystic EHBA*: This type, observed in 5–10% of cases, involves cystic dilation of the biliary tree.
3. *Cytomegalovirus-Associated EHBA*: Approximately 10% of cases are linked to cytomegalovirus infection, characterized by elevated IgM anti-CMV antibodies.
4. *Isolated (Nonsyndromic) EHBA*: This is the most common type, comprising 70–80% of cases.

The first two types typically develop during the prenatal period, while the latter two may have either a prenatal or postnatal onset.

34.3 Classification

Morphologic classification of biliary atresia (proposed by the Japanese Society of Pediatric Surgeons) Principal types (Fig. 34.1):

- Type I: atresia of common bile duct (approx. 5%), proximal duct is intact.
- Type II: atresia of hepatic duct (approx. 2%). Type IIa is obliteration of the common hepatic duct with intact common bile duct and type IIb is obliteration of the cystic duct, common bile duct and common hepatic duct.
- Type III: atresia of bile duct at the porta hepatis (commonest type >90%). In this type the cystic duct, the common bile duct, the hepatic ducts and intrahepatic ducts are obliterated.

In the early stages of biliary atresia, the liver is typically enlarged, firm, and green in color. The gallbladder may appear small and filled with white mucus (Fig. 34.2a) or may be entirely atretic (Fig. 34.2b). As the disease advances, the liver becomes hard and nodular. Distinct microscopic characteristics are present, which aid in distinguishing biliary atresia from other types of neonatal hepatitis.

Fig. 34.1 Types of EHBA

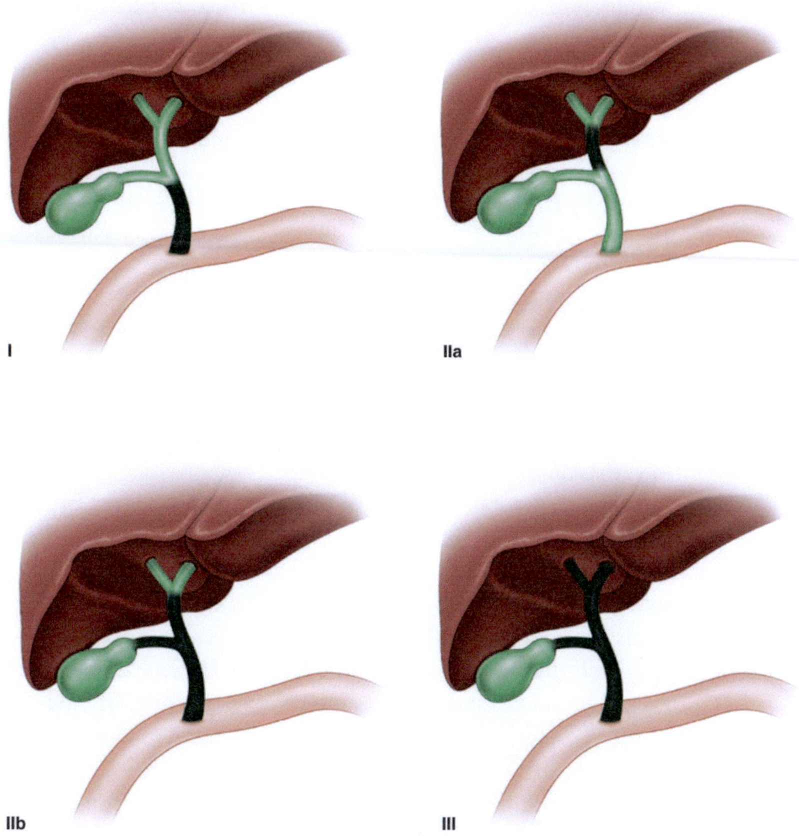

Fig. 34.2 (**a**) Mucous filled gall bladder (arrow) and (**b**) Atretic gall bladder (arrow)

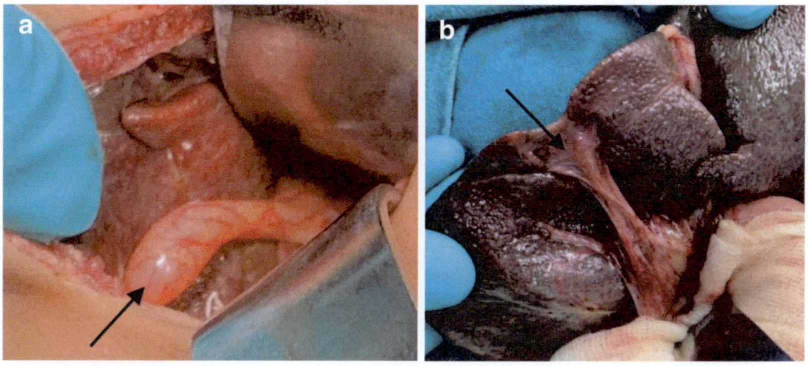

34.4 Diagnosis of Biliary Atresia

34.4.1 Clinical Features

Neonates with biliary atresia typically present with persistent jaundice, pale or acholic stools, dark-stained urine, and hepatomegaly. These infants often appear active, not acutely ill, and maintain a good body weight. Over time, they develop progressive jaundice, acholic stools, and hepatomegaly.

In contrast, infants with cholestasis due to medical conditions such as neonatal hepatitis or prematurity are generally more unwell, have lower body weight, and show signs of jaundice from birth.

34.5 Investigations

34.5.1 Laboratory Investigations as Shown Below

34.5.1.1 Laboratory Investigations for Neonatal Obstructive Cholangiopathy

Liver Function Tests

- *Conjugated Bilirubin*: Levels exceeding 1.0 mg/dL when the total serum bilirubin (TSB) is 5.0 mg/dL or more than 20% of TSB when TSB is above 5.0 mg/dL.
- *Transaminases and Alkaline Phosphatase*: Elevated levels are commonly observed.
- *Gamma-Glutamyl Transpeptidase (GGT)*: Levels above 250 units/L strongly suggest biliary atresia.

Comprehensive Evaluation to Exclude Metabolic Causes

- *Complete Hemogram*: To assess general health and identify potential anomalies.
- *Coagulation Profile (PT/INR)*: To evaluate blood clotting function.
- *Viral Serology*: Testing for Hepatitis A, B, and C.
- *TORCH Panel*: To identify infections from Toxoplasmosis, Rubella, Cytomegalovirus, Herpes simplex, and others.
- *Alpha-1 Antitrypsin Level*: To rule out deficiency-related liver diseases.
- *Serum Lipoprotein-X*: Levels greater than 300 mg% is indicative of cholestasis.
- *Thyroid Function Tests*: To detect any thyroid-related causes.
- *Urine Reducing Sugars*: Screening for metabolic disorders.
- *Urinary Aminoacidogram*: For identifying amino acid metabolism disorders.

34.5.2 Radiological Investigations

34.5.2.1 Ultrasonography

Ultrasound is the first-line imaging modality for evaluating jaundiced infants. It is used to

- Assess the presence and characteristics of the gallbladder.
- Detect intrahepatic or extrahepatic bile duct dilation.
- Evaluate liver parenchymal echogenicity.

Key findings suggestive of biliary atresia include:

- *Triangular Cord Sign*: Atretic bile ducts in the porta hepatis create this characteristic feature.
- *Gallbladder Ghost Triad*: Abnormal gallbladder size, wall thickening, and mucosal irregularity.
- *Hepatic Artery Enlargement*: An increased diameter of the hepatic artery is another indicative feature.

Observation of postprandial gallbladder contraction excludes the diagnosis of biliary atresia. In advanced cases, ultrasound may reveal signs of portal hypertension. USG when done with a skilled radiologist has an accuracy rate exceeding 90%, ultrasonography is highly effective in diagnosing or ruling out biliary atresia.

34.5.3 Magnetic Resonance Cholangio-Pancreatography (MRCP)

MRCP has recently emerged as a reliable diagnostic tool for biliary atresia, providing detailed visualization of the biliary tree and associated abnormalities.

34.5.4 Radionuclide Scintigraphy

34.5.4.1 Hepatic Scintigraphy with Hepatobiliary Iminodiacetic Acid (HIDA) or Diisopropyl Iminodiacetic Acid (DISIDA)

Hepatic scintigraphy using radiotracers such as HIDA (commonly referred to in the context of hepaticobiliary scintigraphy) or more commonly Tc-99 mebrofenin is employed to assess biliary function. Before the procedure, patients are "primed" with oral phenobarbital (5 mg/kg) for up to 5 days to enhance the sensitivity of the test. The absence of a radiotracer in the gastrointestinal tract suggests biliary atresia (Fig. 34.3).

34.5.5 Percutaneous Liver Biopsy

Liver biopsy, with histopathological examination, has a diagnostic accuracy of over 90%. While there are no findings that are absolutely diagnostic of extrahepatic biliary atresia (EHBA), certain features strongly suggest it. Key findings include:

- *Bile Duct Proliferation* (most significant indicator)
- *Portal Fibrosis*
- *Absence of Sinusoidal Fibrosis*

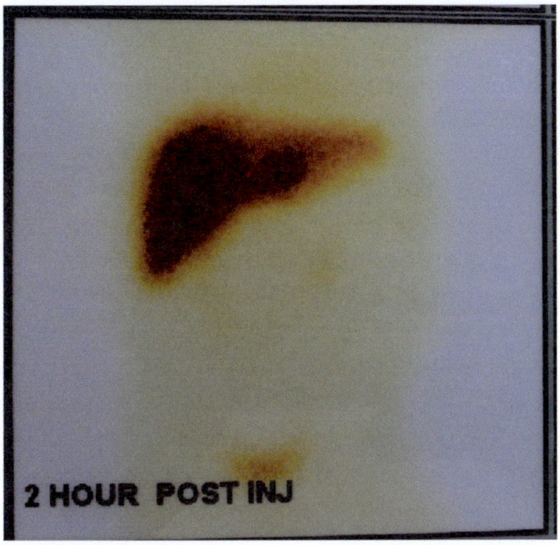

Fig. 34.3 Liver nuclear scan showing nonexcretion of the dye in the gut suggestive of biliary atresia

Additional features may include bile stasis, periportal inflammation, and the presence of giant cells (refer to Table 34.2). A liver biopsy can be very useful in diagnosing EHBA when conducted by an experienced pathologist.

34.5.6 Duodenal Aspiration for Bile

This test involves aspirating the contents of the duodenum to check for the presence of yellow bilirubin pigment. If bilirubin is found, the diagnosis of biliary atresia is excluded. However, this test is not routinely performed.

34.5.7 Endoscopic Retrograde Cholangio-Pancreatography (ERCP)

This procedure is rarely used but can be considered in specific cases for further investigation of biliary structures.

34.5.8 Surgical Cholangiography

Surgical cholangiography is considered the gold standard for confirming the diagnosis of biliary atresia (Fig. 34.4). If radiographic imaging reveals a patent biliary tract, both intrahepatic

Table 34.2 Histopathology of neonatal hepatits and extrahepatic biliary atresia

Idiopathic neonatal hepatitis	Extrahepatic biliary atresia
Intracytoplasmic and canalicular cholestasis Disarranged architecture Giant cell formation Inflammatory infiltrate in the portal space Little fibrosis Extramedullary hematopoiesis	Intracytoplasmic and canalicular cholestasis Preserved architecture Rare giant cells Discrete inflammatory infiltrate Portal and periportal fibrosis Ductal proliferation Bile thrombus in the interlobular ducts

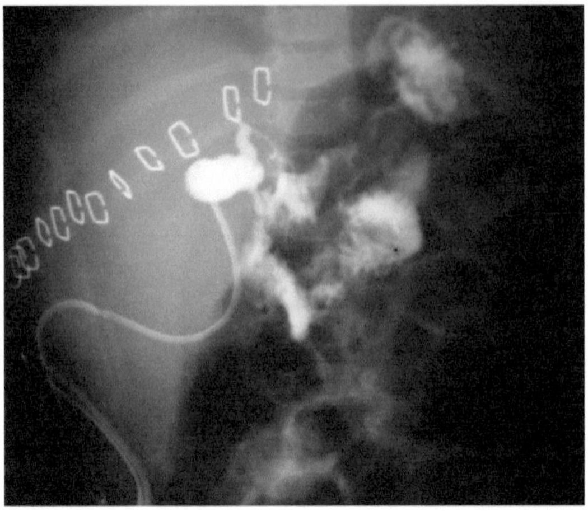

Fig. 34.4 Cholangiogram through the gall bladder showing distal bile duct patency, proximal biliary atresia (absence of intrahepatic biliary radicals, clips are post-open surgery)

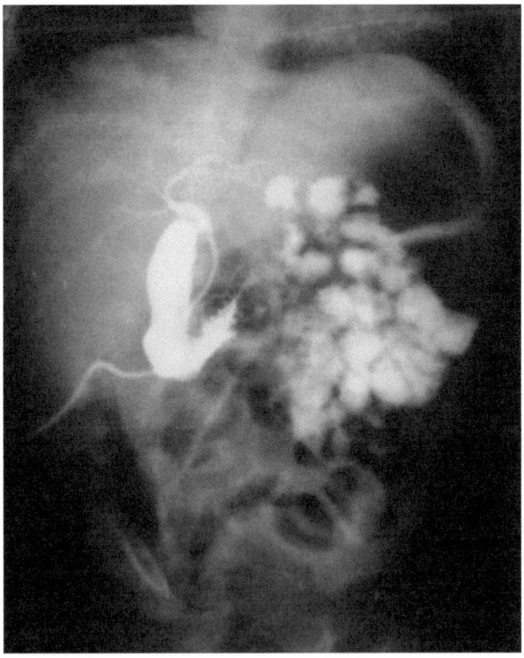

Fig. 34.5 Cholangiogram showing patent biliary tree. Note the patent intrahepatic biliary radicals above and the flow of the dye into the intestine

and extrahepatic, biliary atresia can be excluded (Fig. 34.5).

Laparoscopic operative cholangiography provides a minimally invasive alternative for diagnosing biliary atresia.

34.5.9 Biliary Hypoplasia

Biliary hypoplasia is a rare cause of persistent neonatal conjugated hyperbilirubinemia. Management is generally conservative, as the outcome following a Kasai procedure for biliary hypoplasia is poor.

34.6 Management

34.6.1 Surgical Kasai Portoenterostomy (KPE)

The Kasai portoenterostomy remains the gold standard surgical treatment for biliary atresia. Management is typically guided by the protocol outlined in Fig. 34.6.

Redkar et al. developed a scoring system (Table 34.3) that can be applied to all children diagnosed with biliary atresia. This scoring system helps determine the appropriate surgical treatment based on the patient's score.

34.6.2 Kasai Procedure

The Kasai procedure involves excising the obliterated extrahepatic biliary system (Fig. 34.7) and connecting the proximal portal plate to a Roux-en-Y jejunal loop (Fig. 34.8). The procedure starts with a small incision for intraoperative cholangiography, and the approach is adjusted based on the findings.

Dissection of the fibrous biliary tree should extend to the entry point of the anterior branch of the right hepatic artery on the right side and to the point where the umbilical vein enters the left portal vein on the left side. The fibrous cone is carefully transected up to the posterior surface of the portal vein, ensuring a wide raw surface for anastomosis. Dissection depth should stay limited to the liver capsule, avoiding penetration into the liver parenchyma. Kasai scissors are helpful in this process, as they allow the dissection to remain above Glisson's capsule. Minimal cautery should be used to prevent damage to the bile ductules.

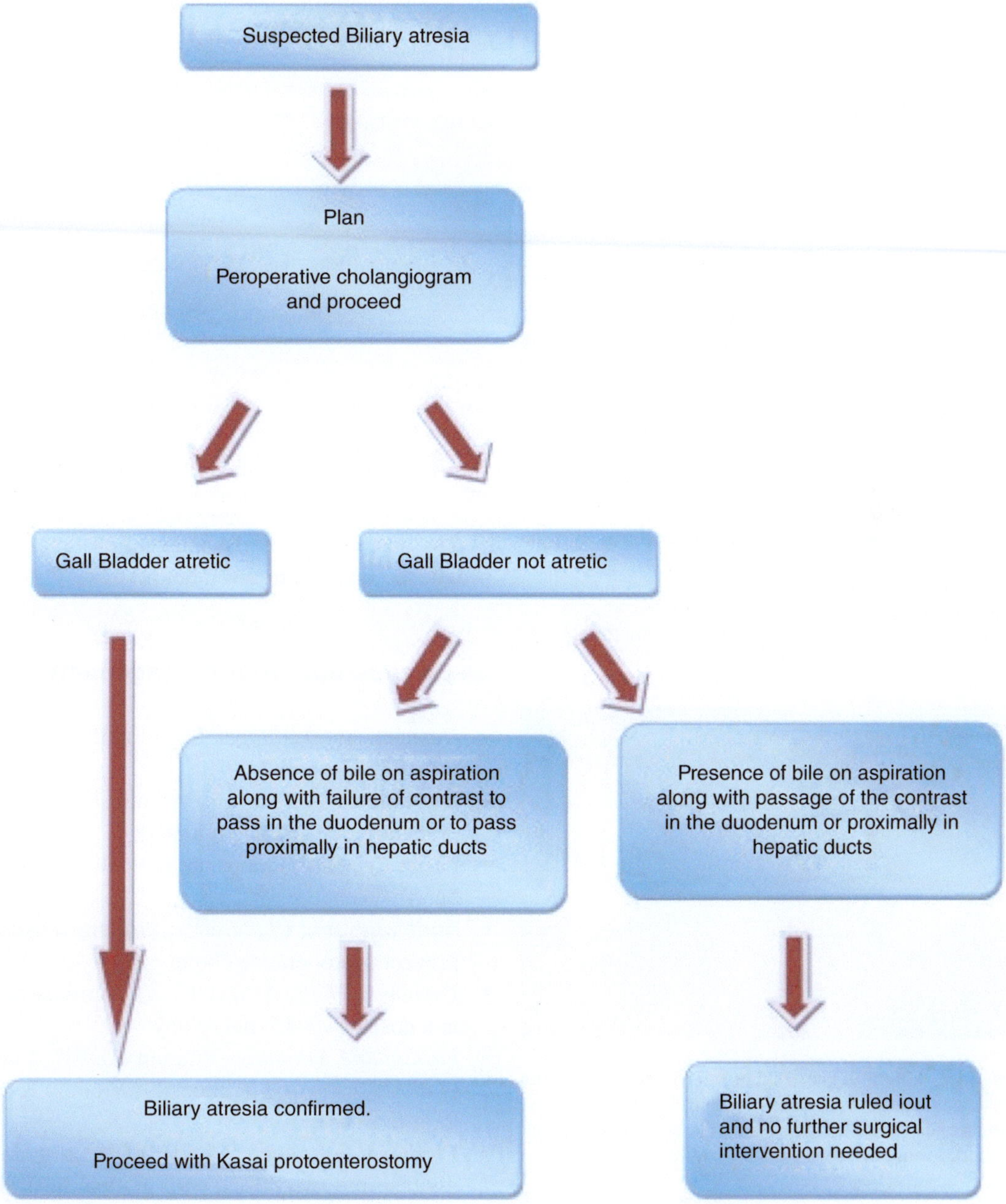

Fig. 34.6 Management of children with biliary atresia

The length of the Roux-en-Y limb should be at least 40 cm to help prevent cholangitis. A liver biopsy is essential to assess the degree of fibrosis present. An abdominal drain is placed before closure.

Minimally invasive laparoscopic techniques can also be used for a successful diagnosis and portoenterostomy.

Table 34.3 Risk prediction scoring system

Grade of fibrosis	Score	Ratio of AST/ALT	Score	APRI index	Score
Grade 1	1	0–1.0	1	0–1	1
Grade 2	2	1.01–2.19	2	1.01–1.8	2
Grade 3	3	2.20–2.39	3	1.81–2.39	3
Grade 4	4	>2.4	4	>2.4	4
Grade 5	10				
Grade 6	12				
Cumulative score			Risk		
3–7			Mild		
8–16			Moderate		
17–20			Severe		

AST Aspartate transaminase, *ALT* Alanine transaminase, *APRI* Aspartate platelet ratio index

Based on the scores, the authors recommend the following:

1. Between 3 and 7: Should perform a Kasai Portoenterostomy (KPE)
2. Between 8 and 16: Could recommend a KPE if the child is not fit for a liver transplant
3. Between 17 and 20: Should recommend a liver transplantation

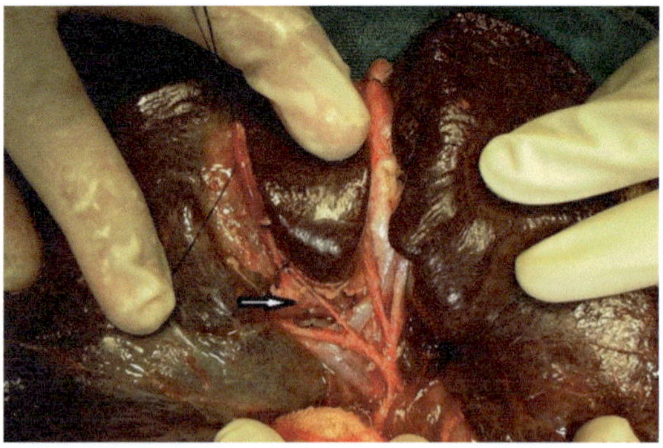

Fig. 34.7 Hilum of the liver in biliary atresia showing atretic gall bladder (silk thread) and atretic bile duct in the portahepatis (arrow). Branches of the hepatic artery and the portal vein have been isolated.

34.6.3 Timing and Prognosis

The best outcomes from the Kasai procedure are seen when performed within the first 60 days of life. Therefore, early identification and referral of suspected cases are crucial. Delayed surgery, particularly beyond 120 days of life, significantly worsens the prognosis, with near-universal poor outcomes after this point.

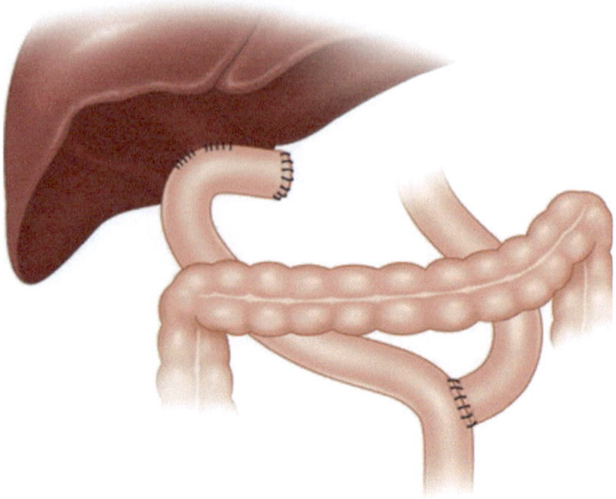

Fig. 34.8 Roux-en-Y hepaticoportoenterostomy (Kasai)

The post-operative management protocol and prognostic factors are given below.

34.6.4 Postoperative Management

- *Nasogastric Drainage*: Used until intestinal function is restored.
- *Intravenous Antibiotics*: Administered until oral antibiotics can be initiated.
- *Drain Removal*: Drains are typically removed before discharge.
- *Antibiotics and Choleretics*: Prolonged use to prevent postoperative cholangitis.
- *Ursodeoxycholic Acid (UDCA)*: Administered at a dose of 10–15 mg/kg/day.
- *Fat-Soluble Vitamins*: Vitamin ADEK drops (1 ml/day) and oral or injectable Vitamin K for long-term use.
- *Prednisolone*: Given at a dose of 2 mg/kg/day, divided into two doses, with gradual tapering over 2–3 weeks.

34.6.5 Complications and Long-Term Outlook

Despite successful postoperative bile flow, almost 75% of patients will develop portal hypertension. They may present with complications such as esophageal varices, hypersplenism, and ascites.

Liver transplantation is considered for patients with failed portoenterostomy, progressive liver failure, or those referred for surgery late in the course. Other potential complications include cholangitis, hepatopulmonary syndrome, and pulmonary hypertension, which may arise due to intrapulmonary shunting.

34.6.6 Survival and Prognosis Following Kasai Portoenterostomy

Results of 121 cases of operated biliary atresia at various ages by Redkar et al. showed the findings given in Table 34.4.

An important finding is that the survival rate is not very poor if the surgery is performed after 3 months of age. In the Indian context, late presentation of biliary atresia is quite common.

- *Initial Good Biliary Drainage*: More than two-thirds of patients show good initial biliary drainage (ranging from 25% to 86%).
- *Sustained Bile Flow*: About one-third (35%) of the total cases (or half of those who achieve good bile drainage) continue to have sustained bile flow and remain free of long-term complications.
- *Progressive Liver Failure*: Another one-third (35%) of patients (half of those achieving good bile drainage) will experience the gradual onset of progressive liver failure, with jaundice returning in the long term.
- *Need for Liver Transplantation*: Approximately 15–30% of patients will never achieve bile drainage after portoenterostomy and will progress to liver failure, requiring early liver transplantation.

Table 34.4 Age of surgery versus survival in biliary atresia

Age (days)	Alive, No. (%)
<60 (*n* = 11)	7 (63.6)
60–90 (n = 31)	16 (51.6)
90–120 (n = 28)	12 (42.9)
120 (n = 19)	7 (36.8)
Total (n = 89)	42 (47.2)

34.6.7 Prognostic Factors for Biliary Atresia

- *Serum Bilirubin Levels*: The serum bilirubin value at 3 months after surgical intervention can be a predictor of long-term survival.
- *Types I and II Biliary Atresia*: These types generally have a good prognosis when treated early.
- *Type III Biliary Atresia*: The presence of larger bile ductules at the porta hepatis (greater than 150 mm in diameter) is associated with a better prognosis.
- *Syndromic Biliary Atresia*: Patients with syndromic biliary atresia tend to have worse outcomes, including difficulty in clearing jaundice and higher overall mortality rates.
- *Cytomegalovirus (CMV) Infection*: Infants with concomitant CMV infection tend to have a less favorable outcome after portoenterostomy.

34.6.8 Liver Transplantation in Biliary Atresia

Biliary atresia is the leading cause of liver transplantation in children, with 70–80% of patients ultimately requiring a transplant.

The indications for liver transplantation in patients with postoperative biliary atresia are:

1. *Complete Absence of Bile Drainage*: This leads to inevitable clinical deterioration.

2. *Developmental Retardation*: If developmental delays or their consequences become uncontrollable, transplantation is required.
3. *Decreased Bile Drainage with Progressive Liver Failure*: This progression necessitates liver transplantation.
4. *High Hepatic Artery Resistance*: A high resistance index in the hepatic artery, measured via Doppler ultrasonography, indicates a need for relatively urgent transplantation.

The five-year survival rate after liver transplantation for biliary atresia currently ranges from 80% to 90%.

34.6.9 Other Rare Causes of Surgical Jaundice in Infants

- *Inspissated Bile Syndrome*: This condition is caused by the impaction of thick, viscid bile or sludge in the bile ducts. It can result from factors such as dehydration, hemolysis, cystic fibrosis, total parenteral nutrition, or defects in bile secretion. It can sometimes be difficult to distinguish from biliary atresia. While it is generally self-limiting, persistent obstruction may require intraoperative cholangiography and biliary tree flushing.
- *Idiopathic Perforation of the Bile Duct*: This rare condition occurs due to a weakness in the bile duct wall, typically at the junction of the cystic duct and the common bile duct. It may be associated with pancreaticobiliary duct malformations. Symptoms include jaundice, clay-colored stools, ascites, and malnutrition.

Summary

The chapter focuses on *infantile obstructive cholangiopathy*, particularly *biliary atresia* (BA), a rare condition in neonates where obstruction of the bile ducts leads to jaundice. BA presents with prolonged jaundice, pale stools, dark urine, and hepatomegaly, and is diagnosed through laboratory tests, ultrasound, MRCP, and liver biopsy. It can be caused by factors like viral infections (e.g., CMV), developmental issues, or environmental toxins. *Extrahepatic biliary atresia (EHBA)* is categorized into four types: syndromic, cystic, CMV-associated, and isolated.

The chapter also discusses diagnostic features such as the *triangular cord sign* on ultrasound, *HIDA scans*, and *surgical cholangiography* for definitive diagnosis. The mainstay of treatment is the *Kasai portoenterostomy (KPE)*, a surgical procedure to bypass the obstructed bile ducts. Early surgery (within 60 days) is crucial for better outcomes, while delayed intervention worsens prognosis.

Prognosis depends on factors like *age at surgery, serum bilirubin levels*, and the type of BA. After surgery, many children develop *portal hypertension* and may need *liver transplantation.* Long-term survival rates post-transplantation are high (80–90%). Additionally, the chapter highlights other rare causes of surgical jaundice, such as inspissated bile syndrome and idiopathic perforation of the bile duct.

Surgical drainage, often through a cholecystostomy, usually promotes healing of the perforation.

Suggested Reading

Coran AG, Caldamone A, Scott Adzich N, Krummel TM, Laberge JM, editors. Pediatric surgery. 7th ed. Oxford: Elsevier Limited; 2012.

Kliegman R, Stanton B, Geme JS, Schor N. Nelson textbook of pediatrics. 20th ed. Philadelphia: Saunders, Elsevier; 2015.

Redkar R, Karkera PJ, Raj V, Bangar A, Hathiramani V, Krishnan J. Outcome of biliary atresia after Kasai's portoenterostomy: a 15-year experience. Indian Pediatr. 2017;54(4):291–4. https://doi.org/10.1007/s13312-0171091-5. Epub 2017 Feb 2. PMID: 28159941.

Redkar R, Agarwal P, Raveenthiran V, Gosavi SJ, Bangar A. Iaps textbook of pediatric surgery. Jaypee Brothers Medical Publishers; 2020a.

Redkar R, Raj V, Chigicherla S, Tewari S, Tampi C, Joshi S. Risk prediction scoring system to predict the postsurgical outcomes of biliary atresia. J Indian Assoc Pediatr Surg. 2020b;25(5):280–5. https://doi.org/10.4103/jiaps.JIAPS_118_19. Epub 2020 Sep 1. PMID: 33343108; PMCID: PMC7732010.

Spitz L, Coran C, Teitelbaum DH, Pierro A, Tan HL. Operative pediatric surgery. 7th ed. CRC Press; 2013.

Portal Hypertension in Children

35

Partap Singh Yadav and Subhasis Roy Choudhury

35.1 Pediatric Portal Hypertension

Portal pressure is directly proportional to the amount of blood flowing through the portal system and the resistance created by hepatic sinusoids and capillaries. Most causes of portal hypertension (PH) are due to increased resistance; a very small decrease in vessel diameter produces a significant increase in the resistance due to their inverse relationship. This increase in resistance could be due to structural factors (thrombosis, fibrosis, and regeneration) or increased vascular tone due to endogenous factors. The second mechanism of increased portal blood flow occurs due to splanchnic arteriolar vasodilatation and activation of the renin–angiotensin mechanism, leading to salt and water retention, which ultimately leads to increased cardiac output and a state of hyperdynamic circulation.

35.2 Pathophysiology of Portal Hypertension (Fig. 35.1)

Portal hypertension is defined as

- Portal venous pressure >11 mmHg
- Splenic pulp pressure >16 mmHg
- Increase in hepatic venous pressure gradient (wedged hepatic venous pressure minus free hepatic venous pressure, normal range is 7–8 mm of Hg)

The investigations to determine the above pressures are not performed clinically, so they are irrelevant for the diagnosis of portal hypertension. Therefore, patients with splenomegaly and the presence of esophageal varices with supportive radiological findings can be labeled as having portal hypertension.

P. S. Yadav (✉)
Department of Pediatric Surgery, LHMC, New Delhi, Delhi, India

S. Roy Choudhury
Pediatric Surgery, Lady Hardinge Medical College and Associated Kalawati Saran Children's Hospital, New Delhi, Delhi, India

© The Author(s), under exclusive license to Springer Nature Singapore Pte Ltd. 2025
S. Roy Choudhury (ed.), *Pediatric Surgery*, https://doi.org/10.1007/978-981-96-1257-4_35

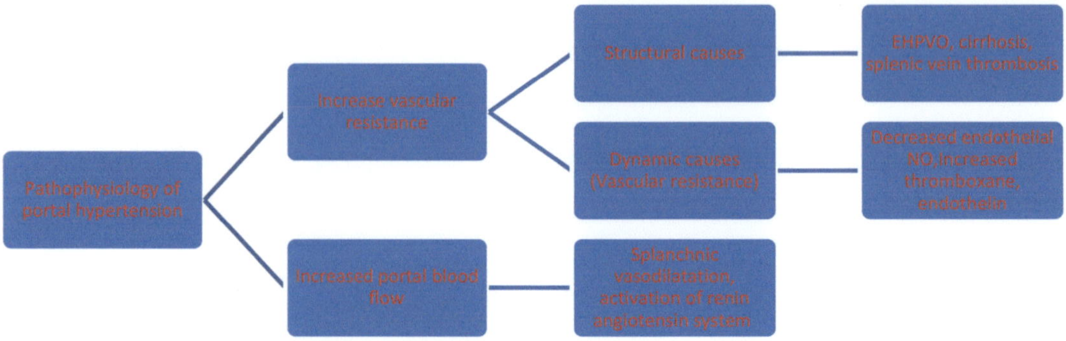

Fig. 35.1 Pathophysiology of portal hypertension

35.3 Etiology and Types of Portal Hypertension (Table 35.1)

Depending on the etiology and the level of obstruction/increased vascular resistance portal hypertension can be classified as

- Cirrhotic
- Noncirrhotic
  - Prehepatic: Extrahepatic portal venous obstruction (EHPVO), common in children
  - Intrahepatic
    - Presinusoidal: Portal vein sclerosis, congenital hepatic fibrosis/noncirrhotic portal fibrosis
    - Sinusoidal: Cirrhosis
    - Postsinusoidal: Veno-occlusive disease
  - Posthepatic: Budd–Chiari syndrome

While intrahepatic causes are more common in developed countries, in a developing country like India, extrahepatic portal venous obstruction (EHPVO) is the commonest cause of prehepatic portal hypertension in children. Portal vein thrombosis is the commonest cause of EHPVO; other less common causes include congenital malformations (stenosis, atresia). In the majority of patients with EHPVO due to portal vein thrombosis, the exact etiology is unknown; it may result from perinatal omphalitis, umbilical venous cannulation, intra-abdominal sepsis, dehydration, multiple exchange transfusions, and prothrombotic states. Initially, after portal vein thrombosis, there is the formation of portal cavernoma and development of portosystemic collaterals (Fig. 35.2). Patients with EHPVO usually have normal liver function but with significant effects of portal hypertension, like variceal hemorrhage and hypersplenism. Biliary atresia, followed by post-total parenteral nutrition induced cholestasis, are the commonest causes of cirrhosis leading to portal hypertension in children. Congenital hepatic fibrosis, focal biliary cirrhosis, alpha1 antitrypsin deficiency, chronic active hepatitis, and cystic fibrosis are other causes of portal hypertension in children. These children with cirrhosis have abnormal liver function with enlarged firm liver, ascites, jaundice, and malnutrition. Budd-Chiari syndrome is due to the obstruction of the hepatic veins. This could be due to webs or in association with coagulation disorders (protein C, protein S, and antithrombin 3 deficiency), malignant disease, oral contraceptives, and autoimmune disorders. Congenital portosystemic shunts (CPSS) – also known as Abernethy malformation is a rare malformation in which there is stealing of blood from the liver due to presence

Table 35.1 Types and causes of portal hypertension in children

Pre-sinusoidal	
Extrahepatic	EHPVO, splenic vein thrombosis, malformations
Intrahepatic	Congenital hepatic fibrosis, Noncirrhotic portal fibrosis
Sinusoidal	Cirrhosis
Postsinusoidal	
Intrahepatic	Veno-occlusive disease
Extrahepatic	Budd–Chiari syndrome, IVC obstruction

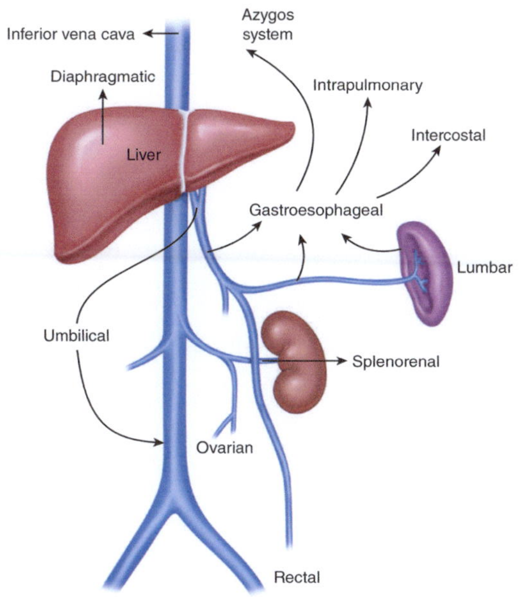

Fig. 35.2 Sites of porto-systemic collaterals

of abnormal communications between the portal circulation and systemic flow. This direct communication, bypassing the hepatic vascular bed creates a natural shunt and presents with hepatic dysfunction and pulmonary complications.

35.4 Presentation

The usual presenting features are bleeding esophageal varices. Cirrhotic patients bleed less frequently, but have high mortality, whereas EHPVO patients bleed earlier and more frequently; however, they tolerate it better. Variceal hemorrhage occurs from the submucosal plexus of the lower esophagus due to portosystemic collaterals around the distal esophagus (Fig. 35.2). Retroperitoneal, periumbilical, and hemorrhoidal collaterals can develop (Fig. 35.3). The collaterals help to reduce the portal hypertension, but can cause variceal bleeding from different sites and lead to splenomegaly. Children tolerate variceal bleeding much better than adults, and the overall outcome in children is much better than in adults.

Splenomegaly and resultant hypersplenism (Fig. 35.4) are characterized by enlarged spleen, multi-lineage cytopenia, and compen-

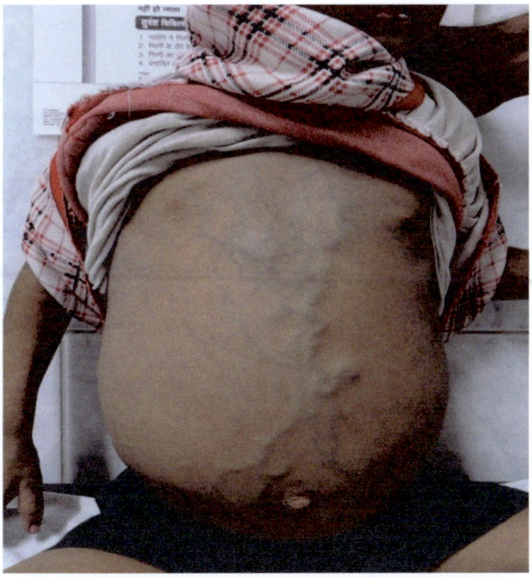

Fig. 35.3 Abdominal wall collateral venous dilatation due to portal hypertension

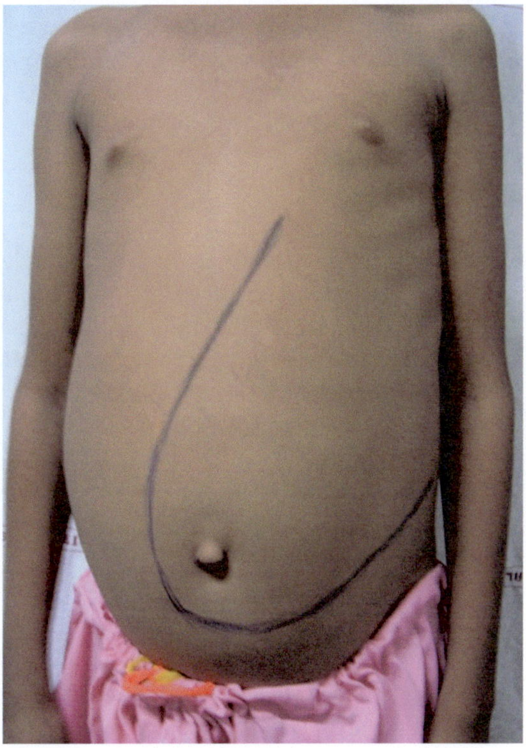

Fig. 35.4 Massive splenomegaly due to EHPVO

satory hypertrophy of bone marrow. Ascites is rare and transient, and associated with hypoalbuminemia. Persistent ascites is seen in late cases with progressive deterioration of liver function.

Growth retardation is seen in nearly half of these children and is due to nutritional, hypersplenism, or growth hormone resistance. Portal biliopathy due to ductal compression by dilated venous collaterals is generally a late presentation of portal hypertension in children (see below). Minimal hepatic encephalopathy is related to poor blood flow to the liver and may be a consequence of nonselective portosystemic shunting. Pediatric portal hypertensive encephalopathy presents with subtle signs like poor concentration, learning difficulties, and behavioral changes. Noncirrhotic patients maintain normal liver function. Deranged synthetic functions of the liver and ascites point to a cirrhotic etiopathology. Parenchymal extinction and hepatocellular dysfunction may occur with a prolonged duration of the disease in noncirrhotic patients. A hyperdynamic circulatory state associated with EHPVO is possibly due to increased nitric oxide levels.

35.5 Diagnosis

- Doppler ultrasonography is accurate in making the diagnosis. It gives information about direction, velocity, and waveform of the portal blood flow. In cases of EHPVO, portal vein cavernoma can be seen. It can also confirm the patency of the inferior mesenteric and splenic veins.
- MRI and CT angiography are more specific in making the anatomical diagnosis. They are also helpful in determining the patency of major vessels before planning shunt procedures.
- Endoscopy is done to visualize, grade, and manage esophageal varices. Management of varices by either sclerotherapy or banding can be done at the same time.

35.5.1 Grading of Varices

- Grade 1: present but small and collapsible
- Grade 2: tortuous vein filling less than one-third of the esophageal lumen
- Grade 3: tortuous vein filling more than one-third of the esophageal lumen
- Grade 4: varices with stigmata (cherry red spots and "varices on varices")

Liver biopsy is generally not indicated in the diagnosis of EHPVO.

Management Management of variceal bleeding

- *Resuscitation includes*
  - Insertion of 2 large-bore iv lines and the commencement of intravenous fluid volume resuscitation
  - Sending investigations (hemogram, coagulation profile, renal, and liver function tests)
  - Transfusion of RBC to maintain hemoglobin of 10 gm/dl, do not over-transfuse.
- *Medical management*
  - Correction of coagulopathy with injection of vitamin K and fresh frozen plasma infusion
  - Starting octreotide: bolus dose of 1μg/kg (max 50μg) followed by infusion of 1-3μg/kg/hr (max 50μg) and continue till 24 h after bleeding ceases and then taper.
  - Keeping nil by mouth
  - If needed, then balloon tamponade with the Sengstaken–Blakemore tube may be applied
  - Histamine 2 receptor blocker drugs
- *Treatment of varices*: Upper GI endoscopy within 24 h to confirm and treat bleeding varices by either endoscopic sclerotherapy or banding.
- For uncontrolled bleeding, TIPS (transjugular intrahepatic portosystemic shunt) or emer-

gency portosystemic shunt should be considered.
- *Pre-primary prophylaxis*: Prevention of variceal formation.
- *Primary prophylaxis* of variceal bleeding: Beta blockers (propranolol), Endoscopic sclerotherapy (EST), and Meso-Rex shunt.
- *Secondary prophylaxis*: Prevention of recurrent bleeding (endoscopic, surgical).

35.5.2 Primary Prophylactic Treatment (Treatment Before Bleed)

- Beta blockers reduce portal venous pressure and decrease the chances of the first episode of bleeding and subsequent bleeding.
- The role of prophylactic banding is unclear in children.

TIPS are also indicated in patients with recurrent variceal bleeding who await liver transplantation. The debate that whether a patient after control of initial variceal bleed is best managed with serial endoscopic variceal management or portosystemic shunt is still ongoing.

35.5.3 Indications of Surgical Intervention

- Failed medical management (failure to achieve control of variceal bleed after 2 sessions of endoscopy)
- Severe symptomatic hypersplenism
- Massive symptomatic splenomegaly
- Lack of access to expert endoscopy therapy
- Bleeding gastric or other ectopic variceal bleeding
- Rare blood group
- Portal biliopathy
- A few selected cases of Budd–Chiari syndrome where obstruction does not extend into the inferior vena cava (IVC)

Intraparenchymal liver disease requires liver transplantation. Hepato-pulmonary syndrome and porto-pulmonary hypertension may require treatment with liver transplantation.

Left-sided portal hypertension: Isolated splenic vein thrombosis leads to the development of portal hypertension with sparing of the superior mesenteric territory, leading to the formation of isolated gastric varices. Causes include pancreatic diseases, including pancreatitis, pseudocysts, and neoplasms. It is a rare condition, and treatment is splenectomy.

35.5.4 Budd–Chiari Syndrome

is the commonest cause of posthepatic portal hypertension. Overall, it is a rare cause accounting for 1–7% of cases of portal hypertension in children, although the incidence may be higher in developing countries. Etiologies include congenital webs in hepatic veins and IVC, prothrombotic states, and neoplasms leading to hepatic venous obstruction. Occasionally, the obstruction extends to the IVC or cavo-atrial junction. This leads to the development of acute portal hypertension; initially, the liver function remains normal, but in chronic cases, cirrhosis develops.

Treatment of Budd–Chiari Syndrome

- Anticoagulation
- Thrombolytic therapy
- Percutaneous baloon angioplasty with or without placement of stents
- TIPS
- Shunt surgery (high risk of postoperative shunt thrombosis)
  - In cases without significant IVC obstruction, portosystemic shunt surgery can be considered.
  - In the presence of significant IVC obstruction, the Meso-atrial shunt becomes an option.

35.6 Surgical Options for Portal Hypertension in Children (Fig. 35.5)

The role of surgical management (shunt surgery) in portal hypertension is guided by the hepatic reserve of the patients and the anatomy of the portal system and other vasculature on imaging studies.

Patients with good hepatic reserve are candidates for shunt surgery if meeting indications; however, if the functional hepatic reserve is poor, then they should be managed with TIPS (if indicated) awaiting liver transplantation.

On imaging (CT/MR portogram), detailed anatomy should be delineated when contemplating shunt surgery. The extent and involvement of thrombosis in the portal, splenic, and mesenteric vasculature, as well as the size of the splenic vein and patency and anatomy of the renal vein, guide the surgical procedure choice. A splenic vein diameter of more than 7 mm is good for consideration of shunt surgery.

- *Shunt operations*
- *Nonshunt procedures*
- *Reconstructive procedures*

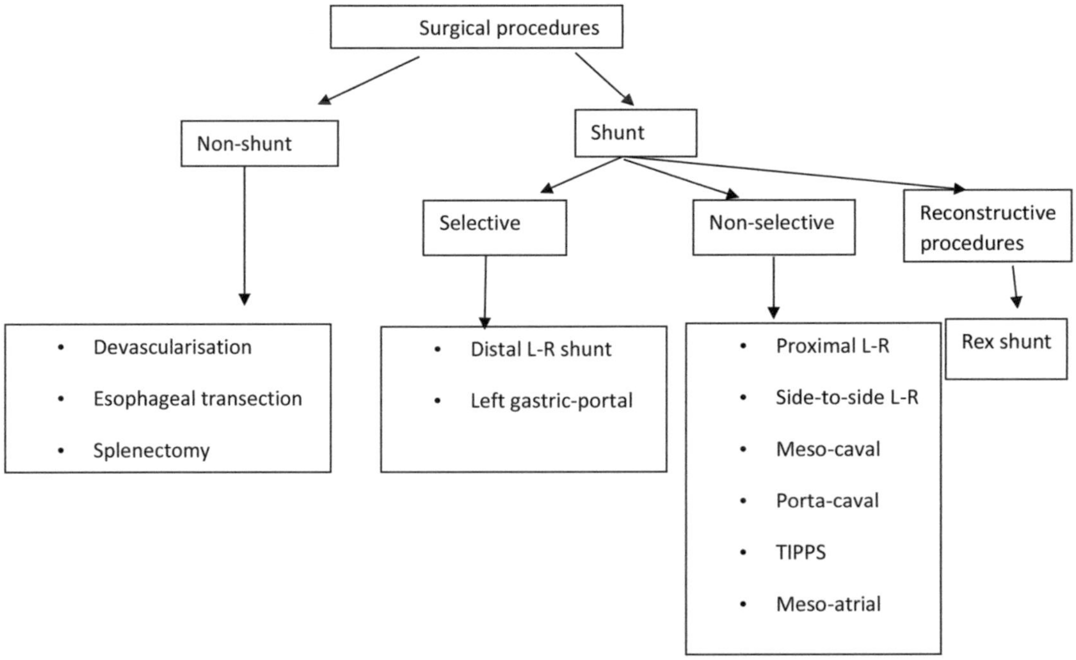

Fig. 35.5 Surgical options for portal hypertension in children

35.7 Shunts

- *Portosystemic shunts (Fig. 35.6)*
  - *Nonselective*: diverts a large portion of mesenteric blood away from the liver, hence prone to long-term complications of encephalopathy.

Total

- *Lienorenal shunt (central):* side-to-side lienorenal shunt (Mitra) has the advantage of preserving the spleen in children with mild to moderate splenomegaly, which may resolve following a patent shunt. End-to-side

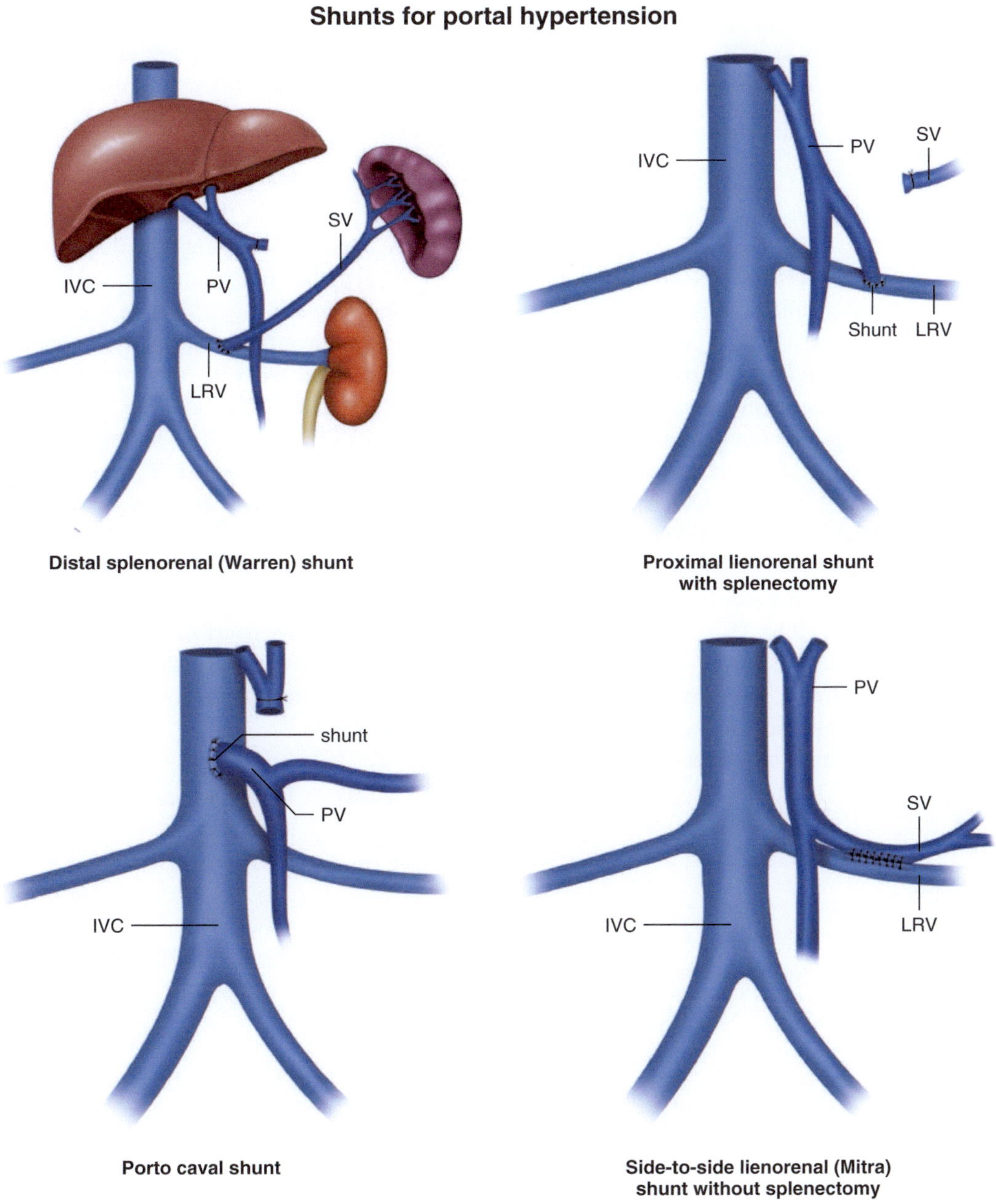

Fig. 35.6 Different shunts for portal hypertension

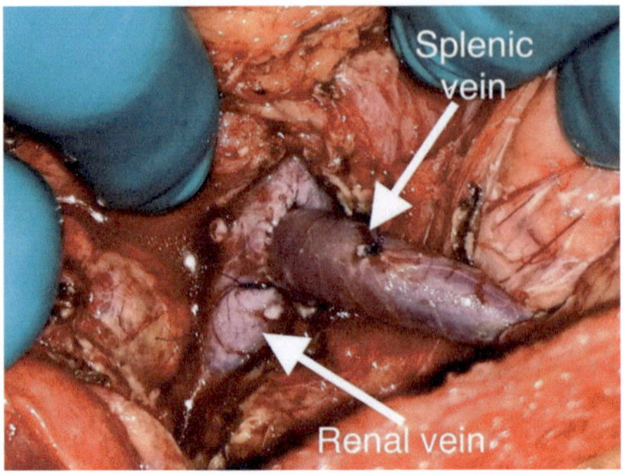

Fig. 35.7 Lienorenal shunt with splenectomy

lienorenal shunt with splenectomy (Fig. 35.7) is a good option in patients with massive splenomegaly and a patent splenic vein.

- Portacaval shunt end-to-side/side-to-side are historic now.
- Mesocaval shunt with a large diameter graft is rarely performed.

Partial

- Sarfeh shunt in which an attempt is made to drop mesenteric pressure below 12 cm of water to decompress varices but still maintain some hepatopetal flow. Usually, a graft of 8 mm diameter is used.

– *Selective shunt*: Preserve the majority of portal/mesenteric flow to liver while shunting blood from high-pressure gastroesophageal varices to low-pressure systemic circulation.

- *Distal splenorenal shunt (Warren shunt Fig. 35.6).* In this operation, the varices are decompressed through the short gastric veins into the splenic vein and then to the left renal vein. The coronary vein is ligated, and splenopancreatic disconnection is done to maintain the selectivity of the shunt. However, over a period of time, the pancreatico-splenic collaterals open up to drain portal blood through the shunt, thereby losing their selectivity, called the "*pancreatic syphon*" effect. In cirrhotic, this can cause deterioration of liver function due to loss of hepatotrophic factors.

– *Rex by-pass shunt*: Using generally an internal jugular venous graft to connect the left portal vein to the mesenteric vein (Fig. 35.8). This can be performed in EHPVO patients. The prerequisites are a normal liver, a patent left portal vein at Rex fissure (umbilical fissure), and a suitable vein in mesenteric circulation to function as an inflow tract. This is a physiological shunt as it maintains portal venous blood flow into the liver; however, this shunt is technically demanding and has a higher rate of complications compared to lienorenal shunts.

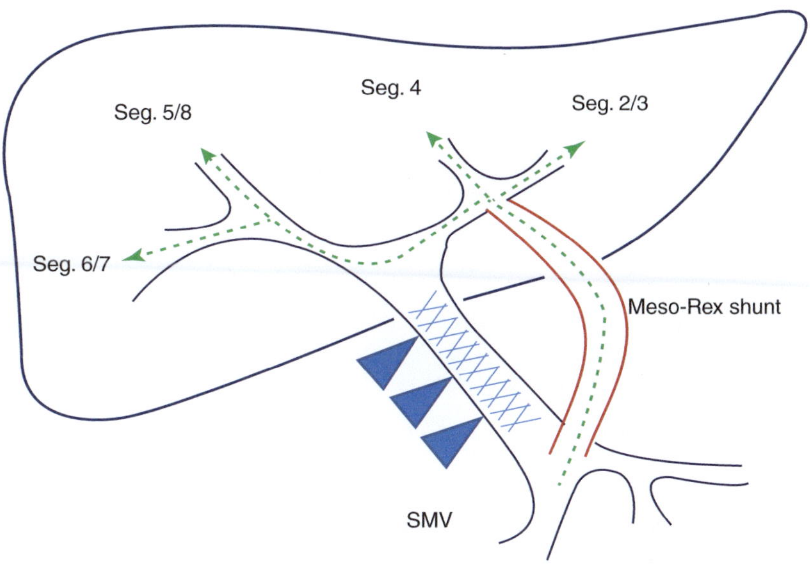

Fig. 35.8 Meso-Rex shunt

35.8 Postoperative Anticoagulation

Various regimes used are:

1. Single intraoperative dose of heparin at 100 IU/kg IV before vessel clamping.
2. Intraoperative heparin at 100 IU/kg IV and continued in the same dose twice a day subcutaneously for 2 weeks.
3. Low molecular weight heparin (Enoxaparin) 1 mg/kg subcutaneous once daily.
4. Postoperatively, oral aspirin/clopidogrel has also been used after heparin is stopped for six months.

   Postoperative Doppler ultrasound should be performed at day 7 to see for blood flow across the shunt. If Doppler study is inconclusive, then a CT/MR portogram should be considered. And shunt patency is assessed during follow-up with Doppler studies. An endoscopy is performed in the follow-up period to document the resolution of varices. Resolution of varices and reduction in spleen size are indirect evidence of shunt function.

Complications of shunt surgery include shunt block and the risk of encephalopathy due to shunting away of blood from the liver.

Nonshunt operations such as the Sugiura procedure (splenectomy with esophago-gastric devascularization with esophageal transaction and anastomosis) are successful for managing variceal bleeding. They are considered particularly when a shuntable splenic or mesenteric vein is not available and in cases of massive splenomegaly with severe hypersplenism where splenectomy becomes necessary. Splenectomy with gastroesophageal decongestion, as originally described by Hassab for managing bilharzial cirrhosis with portal hypertension, has the merits over the Sugiura procedure that thoracotomy and esophageal transaction are avoided, thereby eliminating the possibility of esophageal leakage (Fig. 35.9a,b). Although this is an effective procedure with a minimum complication rate, there are reports of a slight higher incidence of rebleeding.

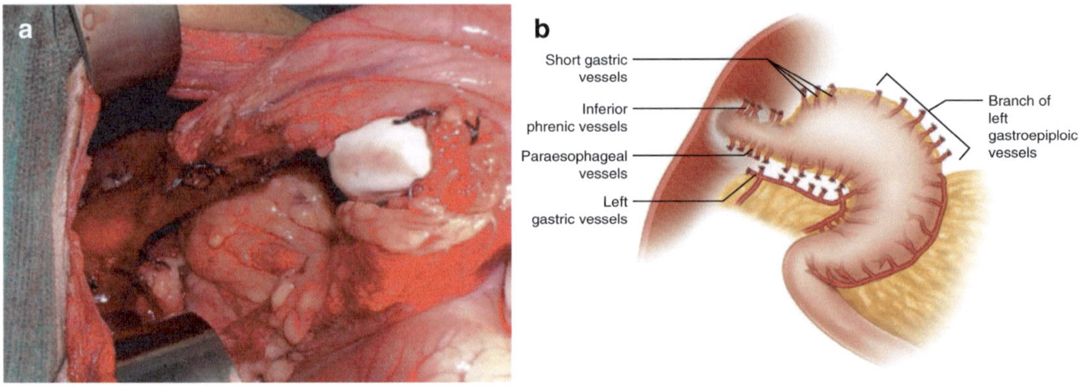

Fig. 35.9 (**a**, **b**) Esophago-gastric devascularization procedure

35.9 Complications of Portal Hypertension

- Ectopic varices
- Growth retardation
- Hypersplenism
- Portal biliopathy
- Ascites
- Hepatorenal syndrome
- Hepatopulmonary syndrome
- Encephalopathy (due to spontaneous porto-systemic shunt)

35.9.1 Portal Billopathy

Portal billopathy occurs in patients with long-standing portal hypertension, it is identified on imaging studies as cholangiographic abnormalities such as indentations and strictures with dilatation of intrahepatic biliary radicals and derangement of liver function tests. The pathophysiological mechanism is the pressure on bile ducts from bridging tortuous paracholedochal, epicholedochal, and cholecystic veins, which results in ischemic strictures over long term. It is a progressive disease, and patients present with cholestasis and cholangitis, and may ultimately lead to cirrhosis. MRCP can detect the changes. Management includes endoscopic therapy (stenting) and shunt surgery.

Summary

Pediatric portal hypertension (PH) is defined as portal pressure more than 10 mmHg or higher hepatic venous pressure gradient. Portal hypertension in children is mostly noncirrhotic with EHPVO being the predominant etiology. In the majority of patients with EHPVO, the exact etiology of portal venous thrombosis is not known; however, neonatal sepsis, portal pyaemia, umbilical vein cannulation, dehydration, and hypercoagulable states have been implicated. Doppler ultrasonography, endoscopic identification of varices, and radiological imaging with CT portography or MR help in clinching the diagnosis and planning management. The clinical presentation is with recurrent variceal hemorrhage, features of hypersplenism and growth retardation with generally preserved synthetic hepatic function. Cirrhotic pathology is associated with altered liver function and ascites. Medical and endoscopic management is the mainstay for variceal bleeding. Surgical management is indicated in selected patients with refractory variceal bleeding and splenomegaly with hypersplenism, with good hepatic synthetic functional reserve. Patients with poor hepatic function are candidates for liver transplant (Fig. 35.10).

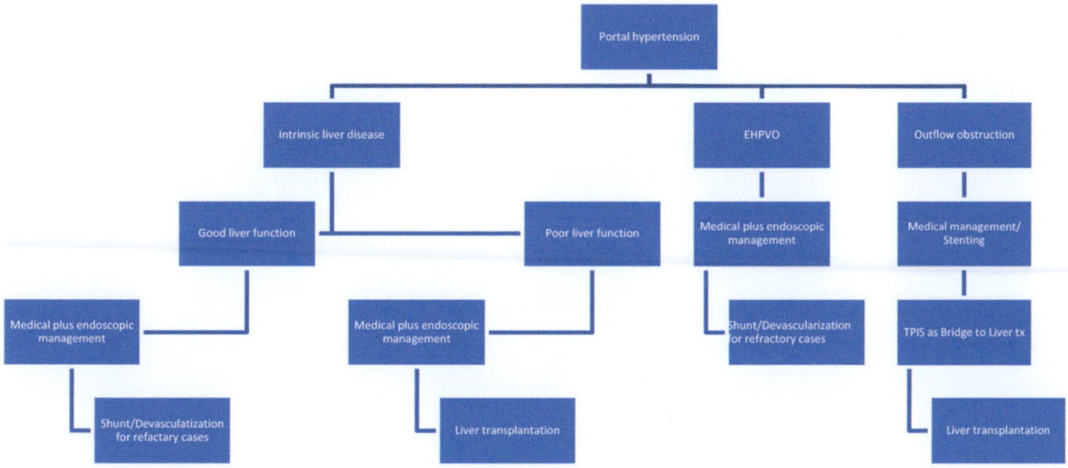

Fig. 35.10 Management algorithm of portal hypertension in children

Suggested Reading

Coran AG, Caldamone A, Scott Adzich N, Krummel TM, Laberge JM, editors. Pediatric surgery. 7th ed. Oxford: Elsevier Limited; 2012.

Roy Choudhury S, Chadha R, Sharma AK, Anand VK, Patwari AK. Surgical management of massive splenomegaly and severe hypersplenism secondary to extrahepatic portal venous obstruction in children. Surg Today. 2007;37:19–23.

Zinner MJ, Ashley SW. Maingot's abdominnal operation. 12th ed. McGraw Hill USA; 2013.

Choledochal Malformations

36

Satya Sree Balija, Enono Yhoshu, and Subhasis Roy Choudhury

36.1 History

The following table highlights the history of choledochal malformations.

Pioneer, year	Area
Abraham Vater (1723)	Earliest description of a choledochal cyst (Germany)
Halliday Douglas (1852)	Earliest detailed report of clinical features and external drainage ofcholedochal cyst in a 17-year-old girl (Scotland)
William Swain (1895)	Earliest operative intervention with creation of an internal fistula withadjacent jejunal loop using a murphy's button (England)
Golder Lewis McWhorter (1924)	Earliest successful operation involving excision of a choledochal cystand restoration of continuity using a hepaticoduodenostomy (USA)
Alonso-Lej et al. (1959)	Classified choledochal cyst into 3 categories based on 96 cases (Spain)
Takuji Todani et al. (1977)	Added 2 more types and reclassified choledochal cysts (Japan)
Gianantonio Farello et al. (1995)	First report of laparoscopic repair in a 6-year-old child (Italy)

S. S. Balija (✉) · E. Yhoshu
Department of Paediatric Surgery, AIIMS Rishikesh, Rishikesh, Uttarakhand, India

S. Roy Choudhury
Pediatric Surgery, Lady Hardinge Medical College and Associated Kalawati Saran Children's Hospital, New Delhi, Delhi, India

36.2 Epidemiology

Choledochal malformations have varied incidence worldwide, ranging from 1:100,000–150,000 in Western populations to 1:1000–13,000 in Asian countries. A female preponderance of 3–4:1 ratio in both children and adults has been well documented. Familial cases have been seen in Caroli's disease, but neither a genetic basis nor association with other anomalies has been seen.

About 20–25% are diagnosed prenatally, an additional 60% become symptomatic by the first decade, and a remaining 20% present later in childhood or adulthood. An increase in prenatal detection and early presentation has been attributed to antenatal supervision with improved imaging techniques.

36.3 Classification

Anatomical classification of choledochal malformations was originally given by Alonso-Lej et al. and modified by Todani et al. after analyzing the cholangiograms and operative findings of their 37 cases. Table 36.1 describes the types of CMs.

A French gastroenterologist first described Caroli disease (Todani type V) in 1958—multiple intrahepatic biliary ductal dilation—which is a rare autosomal recessive disorder. When Caroli disease occurs concomitantly with congenital hepatic fibrosis, renal cystic changes, or fibrosis,

© The Author(s), under exclusive license to Springer Nature Singapore Pte Ltd. 2025

S. Roy Choudhury (ed.), *Pediatric Surgery*, https://doi.org/10.1007/978-981-96-1257-4_36

Table 36.1 Types of choledochal malformation

	Pictorial depiction	Description
I (80–90%)	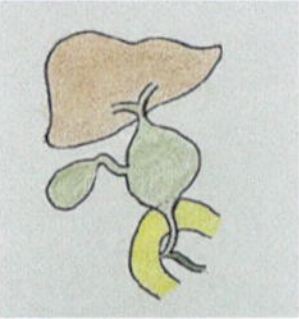 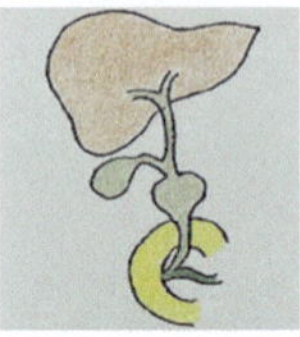 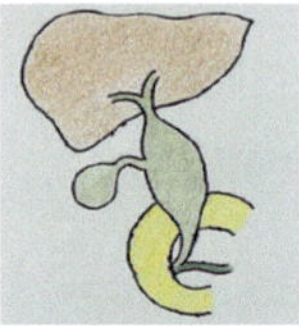	(a) Cystic diffuse dilation of the entire CBD (b) Cystic focal dilation of a segment of the CBD (c) Fusiform diffuse dilation of the CBD
II (2%)	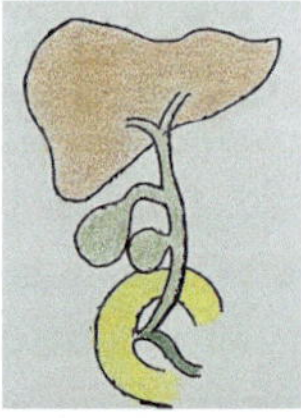	Diverticulum of the extrahepatic duct
III (4%)	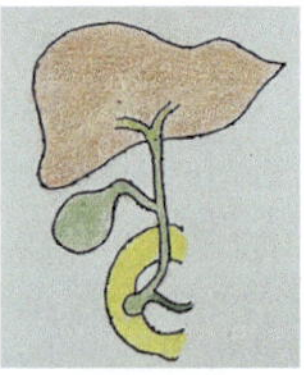	Choledochocele: Cystic dilation of the distal CBD that is either intraduodenal or intrapancreatic
IVa (15–20%) IVb	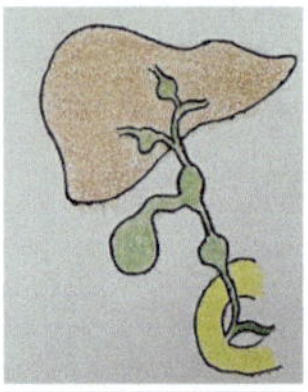 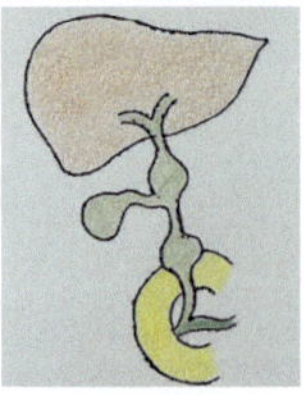	Multiple intrahepatic and extrahepatic cysts Multiple extrahepatic ducts
V	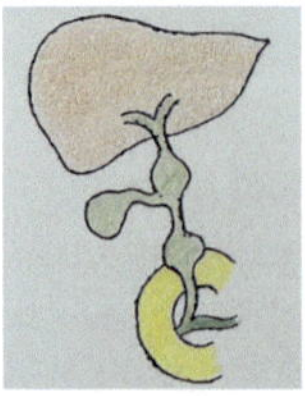	Segmental intrahepatic bile duct cyst Single (true congenital CM) or multiple (Caroli's disease)

Table 36.2 Symptoms in relation to the age of presentation

Prenatal diagnosis	Infants (0–1 year) children	(1–18 years)	Adults(>18 years)
Second and third trimester Usg: Cyst in the porta hepatis Differential diagnosis: Hepatic cyst, intestinal duplication, mesenteric or omental cysts, duodenal atresia, gallbladder duplication, ovarian cysts	Abdominal mass Jaundice Acholic stool Hepatomegaly Rupture and biliary peritonitis (<5%)	Abdominal pain Jaundice Cholangitis Vomiting Asymptomatic	Abdominal pain Jaundice Nausea/vomiting Cholangitis Pancreatitis Malignancy Asymptomatic

the constellation of findings is termed Caroli syndrome.

John Lilly in 1985 described a pancreatobiliary entity known as "Forme Fruste" observed in 4 of his patients. It is used for cases wherein there is minimal or no dilatation of the bile ducts (<10 mm) and a long common channel (>15 mm).

36.4 Etiology and Pathogenesis

Choledochal malformations are thought to be congenital, though the precise etiology remains disputed. The most accepted hypothesis includes the following:

(a) The obstructing segment hypothesis: The presence of a true congenital narrow distal segment, which leads to proximal dilatation of the biliary tracts. This includes abnormal ductal insertion into the duodenum, distal common bile duct stenosis, persistent epithelial webs, valve dysfunction, or neuromuscular irregularity of the sphincter.
(b) The pancreatic reflux hypothesis (Babbitt, 1969): Reflux of the activated proteolytic pancreatic enzymes to the biliary tract via the long common channel of the abnormal pancreaticobiliary junction (APBJ), leading to weakness and dilatation of the walls.
(c) Choledochocele theory: Either due to an obstruction of the ampulla and a low insertion, or a congenital duodenal duplication.
(d) Caroli disease theory: In utero malformation of the ductal plate at the hilum leading to the formation of ectasia of the intrahepatic bile ducts.

36.5 Clinical Presentation

Clinical presentation varies with age, with about 80% becoming symptomatic before 10 years. The infantile form (0–1 year) consists of features of obstructive jaundice similar to biliary atresia. The classic triad of nonspecific pain abdomen, jaundice, and abdominal mass in the right upper quadrant is seen in about 20% only, mainly in the pediatric population (>1 year). About 80% of the children show 2 of the 3 symptoms at presentation (Table 36.2).

Symptoms occur due to the abnormal pancreaticobiliary junction (reflux of biliary and pancreatic juices) and biliary obstruction, which further can cause inflammation, bile stasis, sludge and stone formation, and recurrent superinfection. Hence, besides non-specific abdominal pain, patients can present with complications like ascending cholangitis, obstructive jaundice, cholelithiasis, choledocholithiasis, pancreatitis, and secondary biliary cirrhosis, leading to portal hypertension.

36.6 Diagnosis

Blood investigations should include: Hemogram. Leukocytosis is found in association with cholangitis.

Liver function tests: May be normal or suggestive of obstructive jaundice (raised conjugated bilirubin, alkaline phosphatase, gamma glutamyl transpeptidase). Chronic biliary obstruction can lead to an abnormal coagulation profile. Raised serum amylase and lipase indicated an association with acute pancreatitis.

Imaging Studies (Table 36.3).

Table 36.3 Different imaging studies for making the diagnosis

Imaging	Comments	Function
1. Ultrasound abdomen	Noninvasive Inexpensive Excellent detail of portal structures Sensitivity 71–97%	Cystic mass in the porta hepatis seen separately from the gallbladder, in continuity with the biliary tree. Liver echotexture Intrahepatic ductal dilatation Gallbladder and CBD stones Long common channel
2. Magnetic resonance cholangiopancreatography (MRCP) (Fig. 36.1a, b)	Gold standard Sensitivity 90–100% Improved technology visualizes smaller ducts with finer details Escapes the radiation associated with CT scan and endoscopic retrograde cholangiopancreatography (ERCP)	Type and extent of cyst well visualized Increased diagnosis of accessory and aberrant bile ducts, pancreatic divisum, and APBJ Images can be reconstructed in 3 dimension
3. Abdominal computed tomography (CT) scan	Risk is contrasted toxicity and radiation exposure Sensitivity of CT cholangiography (CTC) for the biliary tree is 93%, for CM 90%, and pancreatic ducts is 64% Multidetector CT (MDCT) allows very thin collimation, detailed information on the pancreatic duct and bile ducts	Conventional CT useful imaging tool for CMs, but difficult to characterize the pancreatic and bile duct union
4. Technetium −99 hepatobiliary Iminodiacetic acid (HIDA) scan	Rarely required Decreased sensitivity for intrahepatic cyst	Shows continuity with bile ducts Differentiating CM from cystic biliary atresia Diagnosis of cyst rupture Beaded appearance in Caroli disease
5. Endoscopic retrograde cholangiopancreatography (ERCP)	Not usually needed Risk of cholangitis and pancreatitis	Gold standard for the diagnosis of APBJ Useful in choledochocele, unroofing, and sphincterotomy

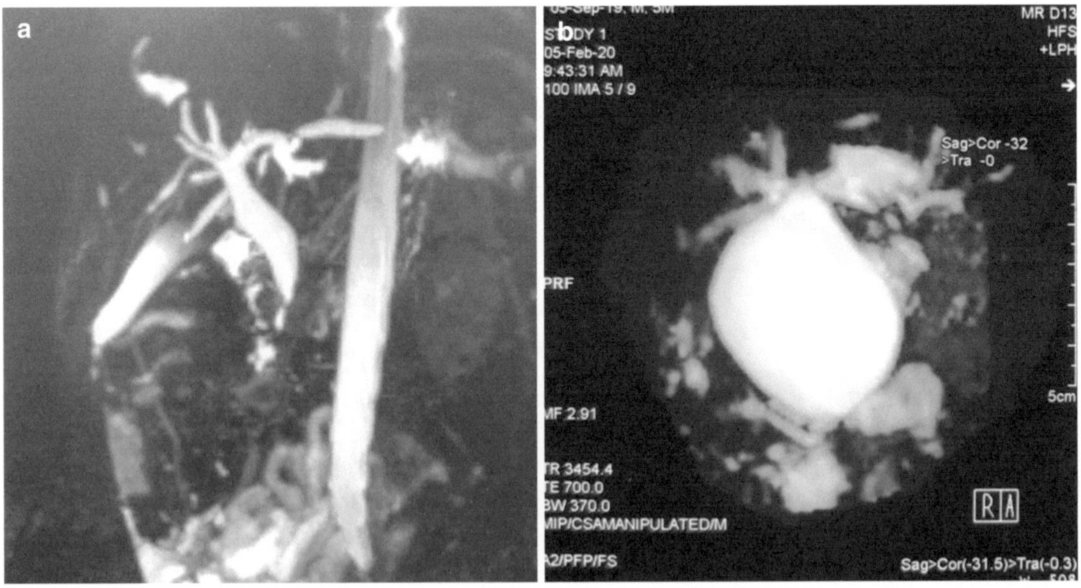

Fig. 36.1 MRCP of choledochal malformation cases. (**a**) Showing a fusiform dilatation of the extrahepatic duct (type 1c) and (**b**) cystic dilatation of the extrahepatic bile duct (type 1a)

36.7 Management

The establishment of CM diagnosis and its type should be followed by planning for definitive surgery in an elective manner, after adequate treatment of any cholangitis or pancreatitis with antibiotics and biliary decompression if present. The surgical technique depends on the type of cyst, but in general entails total excision of the cyst (entire dilated extrahepatic bile duct and gallbladder) and bilioenteric drainage to the duodenum or jejunum. Care should be taken to identify and preserve any aberrant or variant anatomy of vessels and the biliary tract in this area.

CM types 1: Total excision of cyst, cholecystectomy, and hepaticoenterostomy–hepaticoduodenostomy or roux-en-y hepaticojejunostomy. Open Exploration is done with subcostal incision or high transverse incision.

After dissecting and visualizing the portal structures (Fig. 36.2), the CBD is transected as distally as possible without injuring the junction with the pancreatic duct. If the distal duct is dilated, the mucosa should be stripped off. Proximal cyst transection is done at the hepatic bifurcation, followed by good saline irrigation of the proximal tract for protein plugs or calculi or a choledochoscope if available in larger ducts. Also the examination of any proximal stricture is essential as transection has to be more proximal if present. In cases of chronic inflammation leading to dense adhesion with the portal vein, Lilly's technique of incision of the anterior cyst (Fig. 36.3) away from the hepatic artery and portal vein, followed by the removal of the inner epithelial lining of the CM is advocated. A liver biopsy is performed at the end of the surgery to document hepatic histology. A drain is preferably placed in the Morrisons pouch.

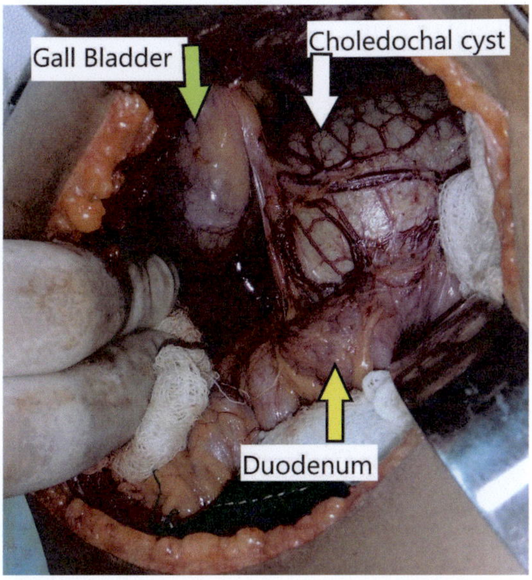

Fig. 36.2 Open exploration finding a choledochal cyst in the porta (white arrow) with blood vessels traversing its anterior wall, gall bladder (green arrow), and duodenum (yellow arrow) inferiorly

CM type 2: They are treated with diverticulectomy or simple cyst excision. Primary closure can be done or over a T-tube, and rarely in the case of significant CBD luminal narrowing, hepaticojejunostomy may be needed.

CM type 3: They are treated by endoscopic sphincterotomy or cyst marsupialization by ERCP. Cysts that are not amenable to the endoscopic approach may be managed with lateral duodenotomy with sphincteroplasty and unroofing or marsupialization of the cavity. Due to the rarity of this type, the incidence of cancer is unclear, and they need close follow-up as there have been reports of malignancy.

CM type 4: Type 4b cysts are managed in the same manner as type 1. However, the treatment of type 4a will be decided by the extent and pattern of the intrahepatic involvement as well as the presence of functional liver disease. An on-table choledochoscopy is recommended to ensure drainage of the entire biliary system, identification and dilatation of strictures, and complete removal of stones. If the intrahepatic dilatation is anatomic and isolated, then a partial liver resection may be needed due to the probable risk of malignant transformation. However, if the distribution of dilatation is more diffuse or imaging is inconclusive, treatment as of type 1 followed by close postoperative surveillance for long term

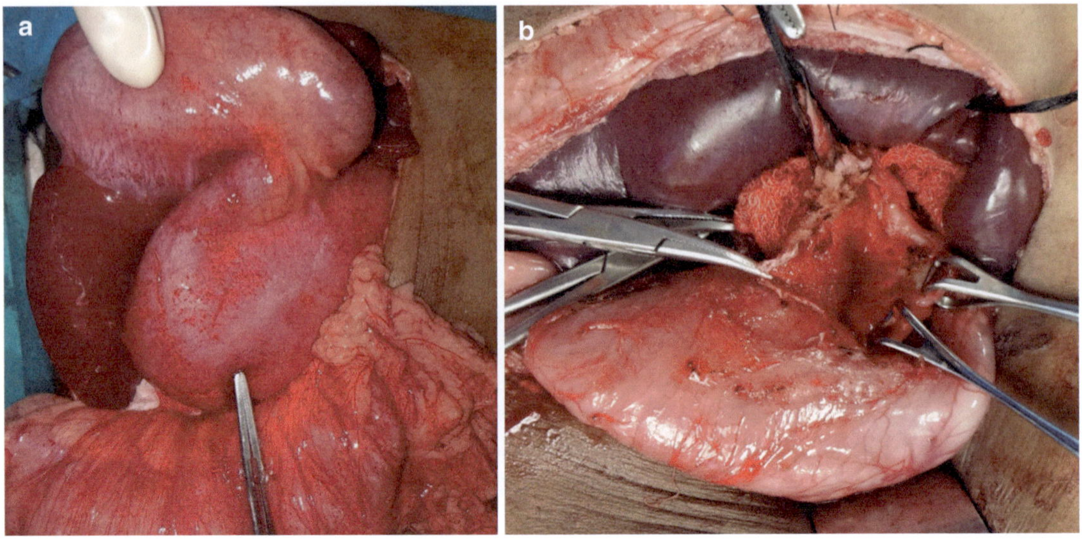

Fig. 36.3 (**a**) Artery forceps pointing out an inflamed choledochal cyst with the gall bladder retracted above by an assistant. (**b**) Anterior wall of the choledochal cyst opened up and held with the artery and Babcock's before stripping off the mucosa from its posterior wall

to monitor the relative intrahepatic duct size and the possibility of lithiasis and cholangitis is preferred.

CM type 5: If asymptomatic, surgery should be delayed in these patients, as surgery is challenging. The type can vary from isolated segmental or unilobar involvement of the liver, or they can have bilobar involvement. Isolated lesions if associated with cholestasis, stone formation or diagnostic concern should undergo anatomic hepatectomy and bilioenteric bypass. There is not much role of surgery in bilobar involvement, and they are usually managed nonoperatively with antibiotics for infection, litholytic agents such as ursodiol, treatment of varices, and percutaneous drainage as needed. Aggressive monitoring for malignant transformation is recommended. Liver transplantation has a role in patients with diffuse bilobar involvement with symptomatic cirrhosis or portal hypertension.

Minimally invasive approaches—Laparoscopy or robotic-assisted laparoscopic surgery—have been done with similar success. The first report in the literature of a pediatric laparoscopic surgery for CM was in 1995 by Farello G. et al. This has been followed by a number of centers adopting a minimally invasive approach for CMs, particularly in Asia. Laparoscopy is now considered at par with an open approach with regard to feasibility, safety, postoperative morbidity, blood loss, and length of hospital stay.

Either 4 or 5 ports are typically used. One 10 mm or 5 mm trochar is inserted through the umbilicus for the camera. Three additional 3 mm or 5 mm trocars are placed for instruments: one at the right and left flanks each for the surgeon's working ports, and one at the left hypochondrium for retracting the gall bladder and liver superiorly. Hepaticoduodenostomy has been preferred by some surgeons, but most series report more bile reflux with this drainage technique.

36.8 Complications and Long-Term Outcomes

Timely diagnosis and cyst excision have been seen to be associated with low complications in most centers. The internal drainage type has not been shown to affect the postoperative complications.

Early Complications include anastomotic leak, postoperative bleeding, acute pancreatitis, wound infection, and biliary or pancreatic fistula.

The anastomotic leak can be at the bilioenteric site or the jejunal anastomosis. The usage of a drain aids in management—decision being based on the content and amount in the drain and the condition of the patient. Conservative management has been successful, with seldom a requirement for re-exploration. Intraoperative and postoperative increased bleeding at the CM site in certain cases has been reported, and optimization of the coagulation profile is essential before an elective surgery.

Late complications include anastomotic stricture (most common, 10–25%), cholangitis, hepatolithiasis (from 3 to 22 years postoperatively), cirrhosis, and malignancy.

The creation of a wide bilioenteric anastomosis is considered essential to prevent stricture. Anastomotic strictures have been managed by endoscopic balloon dilatation or by surgical revision. Postoperative stone formation and cholangitis have been reported more with type IV a CM. Secondary biliary cirrhosis has been seen in 40–50% of patients due to obstruction and inflammation, and has progressed to portal hypertension in a few patients.

Close surveillance is warranted in patients of CM even after surgical excision as biliary cancer risk increased, though the cause remains unclear—related to incomplete excision or inherently greater biliary cancer susceptibility. The development of cancer was predominantly seen in patients with types 1 and IV CM. Although the risk of cancer reduces with total cyst excision, the risk of malignancy does not return to baseline general population levels. The rate of malignant transformation was found to be about 3.4%. Nearly 10% of adult CM series have established malignant change at laparotomy.

36.9 Summary

Choledochal malformations are rare anomalies of the biliary tract that have varied clinical presentations. The management has been more or less standardized with good outcomes. Imaging studies play an important role in clinching the diagnosis. The emerging role of minimally invasive procedures, with their advantages of being feasible and safe, has been proven by surgeons across the globe. However, the standard open technique with proven long-term good outcomes and minimal complication rates needs to be noted.

Acknowledgments Soumya Kashiv has helped with the artwork of types of choledochal malformations.

Suggested Reading

Atkinson J, Davenport M. Controversies in choledochal malformation. South African Medical Journal. 2014;104 (11):816–9.

Friedmacher F, Ford KE, Davenport M. Choledochal malformations: global research, scientific advances and key controversies. Pediatr Surg Int. 2019;35(3):273–82. https://doi.org/10.1007/s00383-018-4392-4. Epub 2018 Nov 7. Erratum in: Pediatr Surg Int. 2018 Dec 19: PMID: 30406431

Soares KC, Goldstein SD, Ghaseb MA, Kamel I, Hackam DJ, Pawlik TM. Pediatric choledochal cysts: diagnosis and current management. Pediatr Surg Int. 2017;33(6):637–50. https://doi.org/10.1007/s00383-017-4083-6. Epub 2017 Mar 31. PMID: 28364277

Hathiramani V, Davenport M. Congenital choledochal malformation. In: Agarwal P, Raveenthiran V, Redkar R, editors. IAPS textbook of pediatric surgery. 1st ed. Jaypee Brothers Medical Publishers; 2020. p. 422–32.

Kumar M, Roy Choudhury S, Singh S, Sarin YK. Liver histopathology in pediatric patients with choledochal cyst. J Ind Assoc Ped Surg. 2024;29:213–8.

Lesions of the Stomach

37

Ankur Mandelia and Subhasis Roy Choudhury

37.1 Peptic Ulcer Disease (PUD)

37.1.1 Definition

Peptic ulcer disease refers to ulceration in the gastroduodenal region due to an imbalance between acid production and protective mechanisms.

37.1.2 Incidence

The incidence of PUD in children is approximately 5 per 100,000, with a higher prevalence in boys.

37.1.3 Pathology

Peptic ulcer disease in children can be classified into *primary* and *secondary* types.

37.1.4 Primary Disease

- Occurs in the absence of systemic illnesses.
- Commonly caused by gastric hypersecretion (excess HCl production and pepsin activity).
- *Genetic predisposition* is frequently noted.
- *Helicobacter pylori* is the primary causative agent.
- Produces urease, hydrolyzing urea into ammonia (cytotoxic) and bicarbonate, disrupting the mucus barrier.
- Produces cytotoxins that directly damage the gastric epithelium.
- Typically presents as a single ulcer in the gastric antrum or duodenum.

37.1.5 Secondary Disease

- Associated with systemic conditions such as trauma, burns (*Curling ulcer*), head injury (*Cushing ulcer*), sepsis, or shock.
- May also result from chemical agents (e.g., NSAIDs or corticosteroids).
- Decreased mucosal blood flow, stress-related hyperacidity, and disruption of the mucosal barrier contribute to ulcer formation.
- Often involves multiple superficial erosions in the stomach, though *Cushing* and *Curling* ulcers may present as single, deep ulcers prone to bleeding or perforation.
- Represents 80% of PUD cases in infants or young children.

A. Mandelia (✉)
Department of Pediatric Surgery, Sanjay Gandhi Post Graduate Institute of Medical Sciences (SGPGIMS), Lucknow, India

S. Roy Choudhury
Pediatric Surgery, Lady Hardinge Medical College and Associated Kalawati Saran Children's Hospital, New Delhi, Delhi, India

© The Author(s), under exclusive license to Springer Nature Singapore Pte Ltd. 2025
S. Roy Choudhury (ed.), *Pediatric Surgery*, https://doi.org/10.1007/978-981-96-1257-4_37

37.1.6 Clinical Presentation

- *Primary PUD:* Typically presents with chronic, recurrent abdominal pain, especially in the epigastric region. Symptoms may include vomiting, refusal to feed (in infants), and nocturnal awakening due to pain, which differentiates it from psychogenic abdominal pain. Gastrointestinal bleeding or perforation is rare.
- *Secondary PUD:* Frequently presents with severe complications such as massive gastrointestinal bleeding, perforation, or shock, often in children with a predisposing systemic condition.

37.1.7 Diagnosis

37.1.7.1 Upper Gastrointestinal Endoscopy

- The standard tool for diagnosis, usually performed with a gastric biopsy to detect *H. pylori*.
- Indications include:
  - Gastrointestinal bleeding.
  - Dysphagia.
  - Persistent vomiting.
  - Recurrent or persistent abdominal pain.
  - Refractory anemia.

37.1.7.2 *H. pylori* Detection

- Biopsy: microscopic evaluation, culture, and urease testing.
- Noninvasive tests:
  - *Urea breath test* using radiolabeled urea.
  - *Stool antigen detection* for *H. pylori*.
- Serum antibody testing via ELISA is unreliable and not recommended in children.

37.1.8 Treatment

37.1.8.1 Primary PUD

H. pylori **eradication**

- The combination of two antibiotics (e.g., amoxicillin, clarithromycin, or metronidazole) for 2 weeks plus a proton pump inhibitor (PPI) for 4 weeks.
- Triple therapy achieves eradication rates of 80–90%.

37.1.8.2 Secondary PUD

- Discontinue causative agents (e.g., NSAIDs, corticosteroids).
- Treat underlying systemic conditions.
- Use acid suppression therapy to manage symptoms and facilitate healing.

37.1.8.3 Surgical Intervention

- Reserved for complicated cases with:
  - Massive, uncontrollable gastrointestinal hemorrhage.
  - Gastroduodenal perforation.

37.2 Foreign Bodies and Bezoars

37.2.1 Foreign Bodies in the Stomach

Foreign bodies in the stomach are commonly encountered in children. Once a foreign body passes through the esophagus (cricopharyngeus), smooth objects usually traverse the remainder of the gastrointestinal tract uneventfully. *Management* generally involves watchful waiting and reassurance.

37.2.1.1 Exceptions

1. Sharp objects.
2. Button batteries.
3. Multiple magnets.

These require prompt removal, typically with *endoscopic assistance*, to prevent complications such as perforation or fistula formation.

37.2.1.2 Bezoars

Bezoars are solid masses of indigestible material that accumulate in the gastrointestinal tract.

Types of Bezoars

1. Phytobezoars: composed of vegetable matter.
2. Trichobezoars: made up of swallowed hair (*Rapunzel syndrome*, Fig. 37.1).
3. Pharmacobezoars: result from the accumulation of poorly soluble drugs.

Risk Factors

- Delayed gastric emptying.
- Reduced acid secretion in the stomach.

Management

- Small bezoars: May pass spontaneously or can be removed endoscopically.
- Large bezoars: Often require surgical removal, either through open or laparoscopic techniques.

37.2.2 Gastric Volvulus

Gastric volvulus in children is rare and may present acutely or chronically. It occurs when the attachments of the ligaments of the stomach are lax or absent. It can be associated with conditions such as eventration of the diaphragm, hiatal hernia, or diaphragmatic hernia. The age group primarily affected includes neonates and young infants. Depending on the axis of rotation, gastric volvulus is classified into two types:

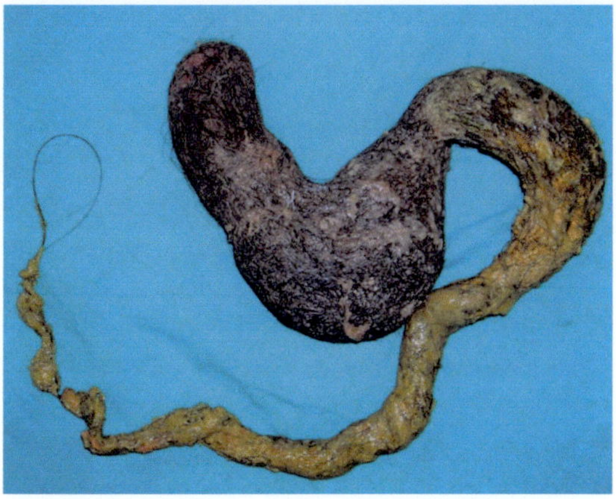

Fig. 37.1 Trichobezoar. (Reprinted with permission from Prof. S Roy Choudhury, Choudhury, S.R. (2018). Lesions of the Stomach. In: *Pediatric Surgery*. Springer, Singapore. https://doi.org/10.1007/978-981-10-6304-6_29)

- *Organo-axial:* The stomach rotates on the longitudinal axis, with the greater curvature usually coming anterior to the lesser curvature. This type is often associated with diaphragmatic defects and has a higher risk of necrosis.
- *Mesentero-axial:* The stomach rotates around the line joining the lesser and greater curvature, with the antrum typically passing anterior. This form tends to present with chronic symptoms, and necrosis is less common.

The classical presentation consists of a triad of symptoms: upper abdominal pain or distension, nonproductive vomiting or retching, and an inability to pass a nasogastric tube. This triad is known as Borchardt's triad. Other features that may be seen include cyanosis or respiratory distress in acute cases and growth failure in chronic cases.

Radiological imaging with an upper gastrointestinal contrast study is essential for diagnosis (Fig. 37.2a,b). It also helps in identifying underlying predisposing conditions like hiatal hernia, diaphragmatic hernia, or eventration.

Acute gastric volvulus is a surgical emergency, as it can rapidly progress to necrosis and gangrene of the stomach. Inserting a nasogastric tube upon diagnosis can relieve symptoms and serve as a temporizing measure. Surgical correction, either through gastrostomy or gastropexy (open or laparoscopic), is generally successful. The underlying diaphragmatic defects should also be repaired during the same surgical procedure to prevent recurrence.

37.2.3 Pyloric Atresia

Pyloric atresia is an extremely rare condition, accounting for only 1% of all intestinal atresias. It presents with features of gastric outlet obstruc-

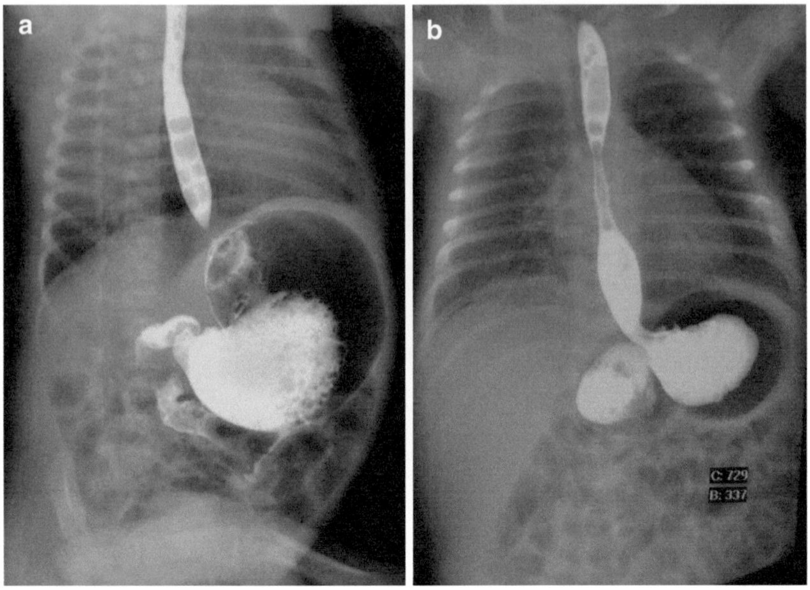

Fig. 37.2 (**a**, **b**) Upper gastrointestinal contrast study showing gastric volvulus. (Reprinted with permission from Prof. S Roy Choudhury, Choudhury, S.R. (2018). Lesions of the Stomach. In: Pediatric Surgery. Springer, Singapore. https://doi.org/10.1007/978-981-10-6304-6_29).

tion. On plain x-ray, a large "single bubble" of a distended stomach is typically seen. The diagnosis is confirmed through a contrast study, which can also help differentiate pyloric atresia from other conditions, such as hypertrophic pyloric stenosis.

Pyloric atresia has been associated with epidermolysis bullosa and other gastrointestinal anomalies, which often result in a poor prognosis. In some cases, the atresia may be partial, presenting as a web rather than complete atresia. Surgical correction involves gastroduodenostomy (Billroth type I anastomosis), which is necessary to establish continuity between the stomach and duodenum.

37.2.4 Gastric Perforation and Necrosis

Gastric perforations are most commonly observed in premature neonates. These perforations can be idiopathic, iatrogenic, or secondary to peptic ulcer disease. The majority of gastric perforations in neonates are idiopathic, often referred to as spontaneous gastric perforations. There have been reports of fungal isolation from perforation sites, suggesting a possible fungal etiology. The most common setting for spontaneous gastric perforations is perinatal stress, where decreased enteric blood supply may lead to ischemia, making the stomach more prone to perforation. Iatrogenic causes of gastric perforation include overzealous bag and mask ventilation, accidental esophageal intubation and ventilation, or injury during the insertion of a nasogastric tube.

37.2.5 Clinical Presentation

The most common presentation of gastric perforation is sudden, severe, rapidly progressive abdominal distension due to massive pneumoperitoneum, which can lead to respiratory distress. Additional findings may include sepsis or peritonitis.

37.2.6 Management

Management begins with resuscitation, followed by surgical repair. If the abdominal distension leads to significant respiratory compromise, free air can be aspirated to relieve pressure. Alternatively, a soft plastic cannula or glove drain can be inserted into the abdominal cavity to stabilize the condition temporarily before definitive surgery. Isolated gastric perforations can be closed primarily, with or without an omental patch. In cases with more extensive necrosis, partial or, rarely, total gastrectomy may be necessary.

37.2.7 Gastric Teratoma

Gastric teratomas are rare, accounting for only 1% of all teratomas. These tumors can present with symptoms such as abdominal mass, vomiting, hematemesis, and melaena, commonly in male infants. Although most gastric teratomas are benign, histological examination may reveal both mature and immature tissues, including neuroglial tissue.

Treatment for gastric teratomas involves complete surgical excision (Fig. 37.3). Even after surgical removal, close follow-up is essential, often with the monitoring of serum alpha-fetoprotein (AFP) levels to detect any potential recurrence.

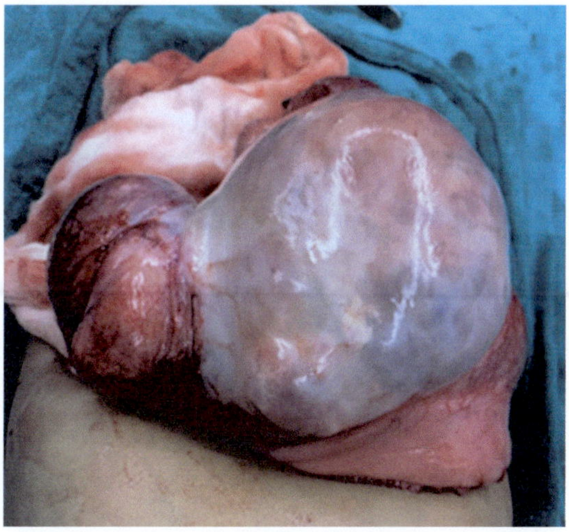

Fig. 37.3 Gastric teratoma. (Reprinted with permission from Prof. S Roy Choudhury, Choudhury, S.R. (2018). Lesions of the Stomach. In: Pediatric Surgery. Springer, Singapore. https://doi.org/10.1007/978-981-10-6304-6_29)

Suggested Reading

Coran AG, Caldamone A, Scott Adzich N, Krummel TM, Laberge JM, editors. Pediatric surgery. 7th ed. Oxford: Elsevier Limited; 2012.

Holcomb G, Murphy JP, St Peter SD, editors. Holcomb and Ashcraft's pediatric surgery. 7th ed. Elsevier; 2019.

Sierra D, Wood M, Kolli S, Felipez LM. Pediatric gastritis, gastropathy, and peptic ulcer disease. Pediatr Rev. 2018;39(11):542–9. https://doi.org/10.1542/pir.2017-0234. PMID: 30385583

Guariso G, Gasparetto M. Update on peptic ulcers in the pediatric age. Ulcers. 2012., Article ID 896509, 2012:9.

Gastroesophageal Reflux, Achalasia Cardia, Congenital Esophageal Stenosis, Barrett's Esophagus

38

Subhasis Roy Choudhury and Anthony Lander

38.1 Introduction

Reflux describes a fluid flowing in the opposite direction to normal flow, often through a valve or sphincter. Reflux is synonymous with a degree of valvular or sphincteric incompetence. Gastroesophageal reflux (GER) is the passage of gastric contents into the esophagus; a reflux event need not result in vomiting and can be innocent. Gastroesophageal reflux can appear asymptomatic or silent yet still cause pathology; its most mild manifestation is considered physiological. The lower esophageal sphincter (LES) is a distinct high-pressure zone in the lower esophagus, and when it transiently relaxes with prograde esophageal peristalsis, it may permit some reflux. In ruminants, reflux is physiological.

38.2 Terminology

Care is needed to determine what a patient, clinician, or writer means by various terms. Commonly but not always, *vomiting* is the expulsion of gastric contents from the mouth. For some people, regurgitation is strictly the expulsion of esophageal contents that have not made it to the stomach, whereas this term for others means mild vomiting or reflux into the oropharynx without expulsion. *Forceful vomiting* describes any violent expulsion of contents, whereas *projectile vomiting* implies that a clinician is considering pyloric stenosis. *Posseting* is the innocent, effortless vomiting of a small quantity of milk shortly after feeding in young infants. *Belching* or *eructation* is the expulsion of gastric air.

38.3 Epidemiology

Almost all newborns vomit due to physiological GER; this posseting may be milk accompanying eructation. Though present from birth, it can become more pronounced over the first few weeks of life before disappearing in most by late infancy. The disappearance is attributed to the maturation of the LES. Persistence beyond 18 months (<2%) is associated with complications. GER is twice as common in boys as in girls. Preterm infants are particularly troubled, and this is attributed to a less mature LES, poorer esophageal clearance, a higher milk intake per unit weight, and slower gastric emptying. Breastfed infants have less GER than formula-fed infants. Cow milk protein allergy can cause vomiting, indistinguishable from GER.

It is essential to differentiate physiological GER from gastroesophageal reflux disease (GERD), which is said to be present whenever

S. Roy Choudhury
Pediatric Surgery, Lady Hardinge Medical College and Associated Kalawati Saran Children's Hospital, New Delhi, Delhi, India

A. Lander (✉)
Birmingham Women's and Children's Hospital, Birmingham, UK

© The Author(s), under exclusive license to Springer Nature Singapore Pte Ltd. 2025
S. Roy Choudhury (ed.), *Pediatric Surgery*, https://doi.org/10.1007/978-981-96-1257-4_38

reflux results in major symptoms or complications. GERD is associated with neurological impairment, chromosomal anomalies, congenital heart disease, congenital diaphragmatic hernia, esophageal atresia, cystic fibrosis, and, in older children, obesity.

38.4 Adjuncts Opposing Gastroesophageal Reflux

The lower esophageal muscles form the LES, which maintains a 5–20 mmHg pressure. Peristalsis in the distal esophagus serves to clear any refluxed gastric fluid. Gravity also helps the esophagus empty and opposes reflux.

Several mechanisms limit fluid reflux, and any one or several of them may fail, leading to GERD. Disappointingly, if surgery is needed, we generally have only one operation with a few variations. The crural ligament, the angle of His, and the phrenoesophageal ligament all limit reflux. Gastric contents and distension trigger transient relaxation of the LES and may allow reflux. Raised intraabdominal pressure causes reflux, and delayed gastric emptying is a factor in some.

38.5 Anatomical Factors

The phrenoesophageal membrane is a structure that encases the lower esophagus and the gastroesophageal junction, together with a little cylinder of fat for a short distance above and below the hiatus. This permits a little movement during breathing and swallowing. Understanding this anatomy helps dissection in both open and laparoscopic fundoplications. The membrane is attached to the diaphragm's superior and inferior surfaces; a hiatus hernia is inevitable without it.

The angle of His creates a valve-like mechanism when the fundus distends; it is thought that the angle becomes more acute in late infancy and early childhood, which may contribute to the resolution of symptoms in some infants.

A good length of the intrabdominal esophagus is perhaps two or more cm long. Such a region is compressed when intraabdominal pressure rises, thus occluding the lower esophagus and opposing reflux. Furthermore, the length of the esophagus is part of the LES and has a distinct muscular tone and innervation.

The junction between the esophagus and the stomach (GEJ) is a poorly defined region at risk of inflammation, metaplasia, and, in adults, neoplasia. Endoscopists try to locate the hiatus in relation to the squamocolumnar mucosal junction. The mucosal palisade veins and the proximal gastric folds form a rosette that opposes reflux.

The right crus of the diaphragm wraps around the esophagus and pinches it during inspiration when the thoracic pressure falls. Lower thoracic pressure encourages reflux, and so this so-called pinch-cock effect opposes reflux.

A hiatus hernia is the herniation of the GEJ, LES, and sometimes the upper stomach into the chest through the hiatus. Numerous mechanisms limiting reflux fail; there is no intraabdominal esophagus, no crural pinch-cock, and no angle of His, and the upper stomach is subjected to reduced intrathoracic inspiratory pressure.

38.6 Physiological Factors

Control of the LES is ill-understood, and currently, much reflux is attributed to transient LES relaxation (tLESR). Timely and effective gastric emptying also reduces reflux, so gastric stasis is a problem in some. GERD is particularly problematic in some neurologically impaired children, and this may be made up of tLESR combined with retrograde gastric peristalsis and anatomical deficiencies at the hiatus.

38.7 Associations of Interest

Reflux is seen in children with congenital diaphragmatic hernias and repaired esophageal atresia, and it is easy to speculate upon potential mechanisms and defects—some need a fundoplication. However, reflux is also associated with malrotation of the duodenojejunal flexure, where potential mechanisms are less clear. Indeed, there are some children investigated for non-bilious vomiting who have a contrast study in a work-up for a fundoplication but are found to have malrotation; in many, the vomiting resolves after a Ladd's procedure and no fundoplication. These individuals are not thought to have been intermittently volving their small bowel, so the mechanism of reflux and its resolution remains a mystery.

38.8 Symptoms of GER

Well-recognized symptoms include vomiting, spitting up, posseting, gagging, and the regurgitation of gastric juice into the oropharynx, which is sometimes called water brash. Grimacing, feed refusal, and some unusual postures are less apparent symptoms. In infants, irritability and excessive crying are non-specific manifestations, while older children may have dysphagia, sore throats, heartburn, retrosternal or epigastric pain, and later dental erosions, halitosis, and a hoarse voice.

Chronic cough, wheezing, and stridor may relate to microaspiration, or esophageal acidity may cause vagal nerve-related bronchospasm. Sandifer syndrome is a classic but uncommon association of marked hyperextension of the head, neck, and spine (opisthotonus) with torticollis.

Acute Life-Threatening Events (ALTEs) with apnoeas and bradycardias may follow aspiration, vagal reflexes, or both. The complications of acid reflux include peptic ulceration, erosive esophagitis, esophageal strictures, and Barrett's esophagus.

Barrett's esophagus refers to premalignant mucosal metaplasia from stratified squamous epithelium to simple columnar epithelium seen in the lower esophagus, with interspersed goblet cells only normally seen in the small intestine or colon. Further transition to esophageal adenocarcinoma is reported.

38.9 Differential Diagnosis

Vomiting due to mechanical, infective, allergic, and neurological causes should be excluded.

Only rarely is GER found to be the cause of severe dehydration in a sick infant who presents to the hospital; in this context, GER is diagnosed after more immediate and serious conditions have been excluded. GER is very low down in the differential diagnosis of an acutely sick infant.

More commonly, GER becomes the working diagnosis for a physiologically stable, apyrexial, well-hydrated child with a history of vomiting; what less common alternatives should we entertain in this differential diagnosis in this context? Some elements of that differential follow:

Pyloric Stenosis This is seen in a child of 3–9 weeks of age. In contrast to GER, symptoms progressively worsen daily and soon affect every feed; there may be a family history, ultrasound scanning is diagnostic, and hypochloramic metabolic alkalosis needs to be excluded and managed. Rarely a child can have both GER and pyloric stenosis.

Overfeeding Determine the feeding volume and check the growth velocity. Adjust feeds and follow up closely. GER and overfeeding can go together if an infant responds to their esophagitis by demanding a lot of milk.

Duodenal Web A web with a hole permits some forward flow but can impair gastric emptying. Antenatal ultrasound scanning may have revealed suspected duodenal atresia that was later dismissed, or there may have been polyhydramnios. A contrast study or endoscopy may be diagnostic.

Malrotation of the DJ Flexure Though classically presenting with bilious vomiting after a few days of life once feed volumes rise, malrotation can be associated with non-bilious vomiting resembling marked reflux and may be found during a contrast study. All contrast studies looking for GER should identify the DJ flexure.

Cow Milk Protein Allergy (CPMA) This allergy involves an atypical IgE response, wheezing, and skin reactions, but it is associated with altered gastric motility and delayed gastric emptying that exacerbate GER.

Achalasia Rarely seen before ten years of age and easily diagnosed on a contrast study and confirmed on manometry.

Raised Intracranial Pressure Intracranial hypertension should be considered if there have been headaches, blurred or double vision, or photophobia. If the anterior fontanelle is still open (up to 18 months), examine for a bulge.

38.10 Investigations

- Upper gastrointestinal (UGI) imaging series.
- Gastric scintigraphic scan.
- Esophagogastroduodenoscopy and biopsies.
- Continuous 24-hour esophageal pH and impedance monitoring.
- Esophageal manometry. Intraluminal esophageal electrical impedance.

An upper gastrointestinal contrast study can demonstrate anomalies such as esophageal strictures, motility disorders, peristalsis, and sometimes ulceration or achalasia may be seen in the esophagus. A hiatus hernia, gastric outlet obstruction, malrotation, or a duodenal web may be found (Fig. 38.1). It is wise for the surgeon to attend the study and see it live as it is a dynamic test, and the images relate to what the child is doing at the time of the study and how they are taking the contrast. Sometimes reflux is seen going high up in the esophagus during a study, and the GEJ looks wide open, and there is no angle of His and no length of intraabdominal esophagus—the decision to operate may then be easy. It is unwise to inform a mother that there is no issue simply because no reflux episode was witnessed during a brief study.

Clues about delayed gastric emptying may be obtained, but if gastric emptying is to be investigated further, radionucleotide scintigraphy can be performed, though normal values are not well-established. Delayed images may show activity in the lungs, suggesting aspiration.

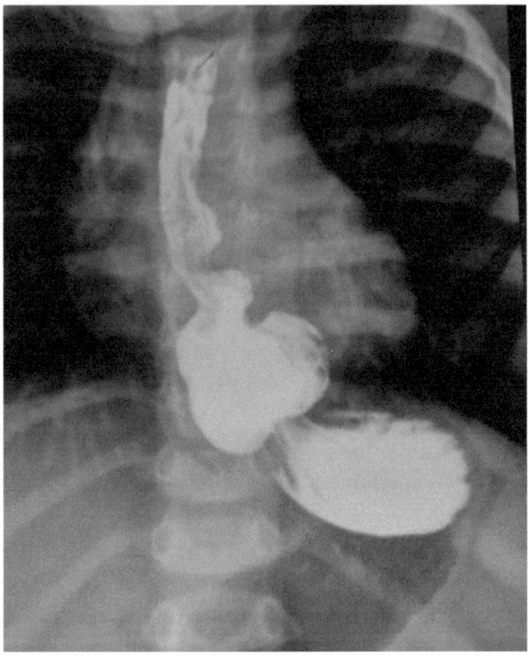

Fig. 38.1 Sliding hiatal hernia with gastroesophageal reflux

Upper gastrointestinal endoscopy may provide macroscopic and histologic evidence of esophagitis, and Barrett's esophagus can be identified. The GEJ, stomach, and proximal duodenum should be inspected. A rapid urease test (CLO test—Campylobacter-like organism) can be performed in the theater, looking for *Helicobacter pylori*. *H. pylroi* secretes urease, which converts urea to ammonia and carbon dioxide, turning the test red.

Twenty-four-hour esophageal pH monitoring estimates the % of time the lower esophagus is exposed to a pH < 4 (typically $<4\%$), called the reflux index. It reports the number of reflux episodes exceeding 5 min, the duration of the longest episode, and the total number of episodes. Antacids must be stopped for the study.

Esophageal manometry is not routinely performed as it requires a cooperative and quiet child. It is still helpful in doubtful cases as it may show tLESR, gives information about LES (length and tone), and also predicts children who may have postoperative dysphagia because of abnormal or inadequate peristalsis.

Intraluminal impedance studies detect non-acid reflux in addition to acid, and so it can be used on children on H2-receptor antagonists.

38.11 Treatment

38.11.1 Medical

Sitting upright during and after feeds reduces reflux since gravity helps keep the stomach contents down and promotes esophageal clearance. Placing the baby in an inclined position, such as using a baby seat or raising the head of the crib, helps.

Feeding techniques: The way infants are fed can affect reflux. Overfeeding or feeding too quickly can increase the likelihood of reflux. Ensuring the baby is appropriately positioned during feeding, with the head slightly elevated, is essential. Burping the baby frequently during and after feeding can also help release trapped air and reduce reflux episodes. Smaller but more frequent meals may help.

Thickened feeds: In some cases, adding a thickening agent, such as rice cereal, to the baby's formula or breast milk can help reduce reflux. The thicker consistency of the feed can make it more difficult for stomach contents to flow back up into the esophagus. However, thickened feeds can cause milk curd impaction in the premature baby, and caution is advised in the neonatal unit.

Avoiding certain foods: If breastfeeding, the mother may try avoiding spicy or acidic foods, caffeine, and chocolate. If the baby is formula-fed, switching to a different type of formula may be recommended.

Pharmacologic agents include gastric acid secretion reduction (H-2 receptor blockers and proton pump inhibitors) and prokinetic drugs (domperidone, metoclopramide, and erythromycin).

38.12 Surgical Treatment

Surgical treatment of GER should be considered for the following patients

- Failure of adequate medical treatment to alleviate symptoms of GER.
- For those with ALTE related to GER, however, a period of medical therapy under close monitoring should be attempted.
- Patients with complications of GER, such as aspiration, stricture, or Barrett's esophagus.
- Patients with neurologic impairment who require a gastrostomy and who have pathologic reflux.
- Patients with chronic reflux and recurrent anastomotic strictures after repair of esophageal atresia.
- Patients with pathological anatomy like a hiatus hernia.

38.13 Fundoplication

The fundoplication operation aims to prevent acid reflux by creating a length of intraabdominal esophagus and a high-pressure zone at the lower esophagus. Additionally, narrowing the hiatus by crural approximation, restoration of the angle of HIS, and reduction of hiatus hernia reduce GER (Fig. 38.2). A fundoplication is best performed laparoscopically as the view is excellent and recovery prompt. An open operation needs a large incision.

The commonly performed fundoplication procedures are shown in Fig. 38.3.

Nissen fundoplication involves a 360° complete wrap of the gastric fundus around the lower esophagus and narrowing the hiatus by crural suturing. In the *Thal fundoplication,* a 270° partial wrap of the gastric fundus around the lower anterior esophagus is created. The *Toupet procedure* uses a 180° posterior wrap. Depending on the patient, the wrap can be tight (neurologically impaired children) or floppy (GER post-esophageal atresia repair). A tight wrap is associated with a higher incidence of gas bloat and dysphagia, whereas a partial or floppy wrap may be associated with vomiting.

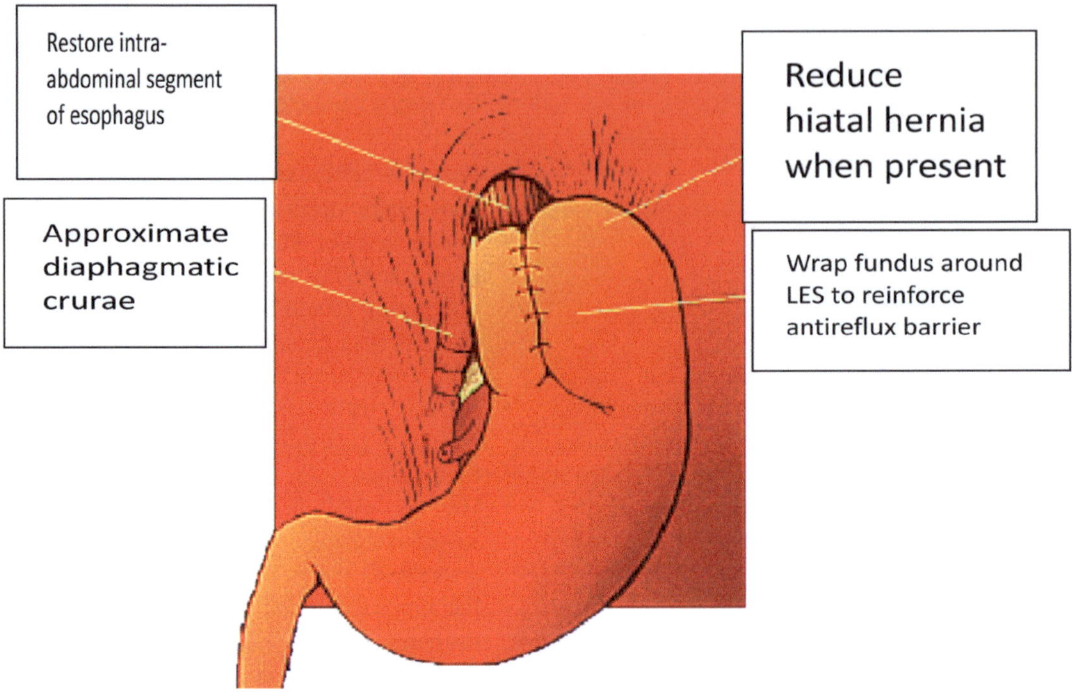

Fig. 38.2 Principles of fundoplication operation

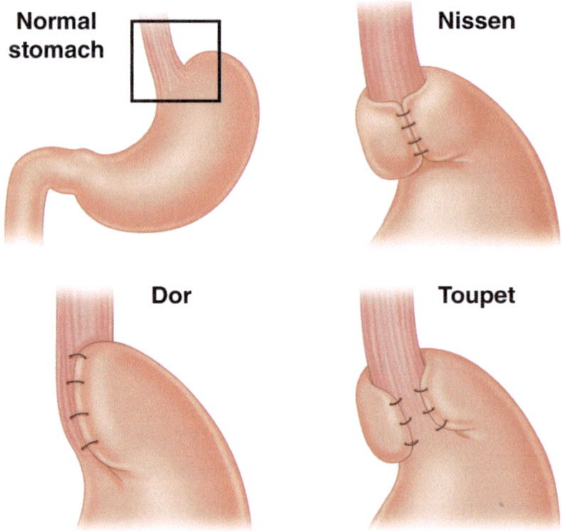

Fig. 38.3 The commonly performed techniques of fundoplication

Other complications of fundoplication include early intussusception, later dumping syndrome, and bowel obstruction, the latter having a higher incidence with open than with laparoscopic surgery.

The chance of failure of surgery is higher in neurologically impaired children than in normal children, so esophagogastric dissociation with esophagojejunostomy can be an option in some neurologically impaired children with severe GER.

Several endoscopic procedures like the Stretta (radiofrequency energy to the esophagogastric junction), endoscopic fundoplication to create mucosal valves, and endoscopic injection at the esophagogastric junction have been proposed, but experience in childhood is limited.

38.14 Achalasia Cardia

Achalasia is not seen in infants and is uncommon in later childhood. The LES fails to relax on swallowing, causing dysphagia and regurgitation of esophageal contents instead of vomiting of gastric contents, as seen in GER. Chest pain can follow esophageal spasms. Progressive dilatation of the esophagus affects peristalsis and leads to further dilatation. Liquid and solids pool in the esophagus and nocturnal aspiration leads to coughing and recurrent chest infections.

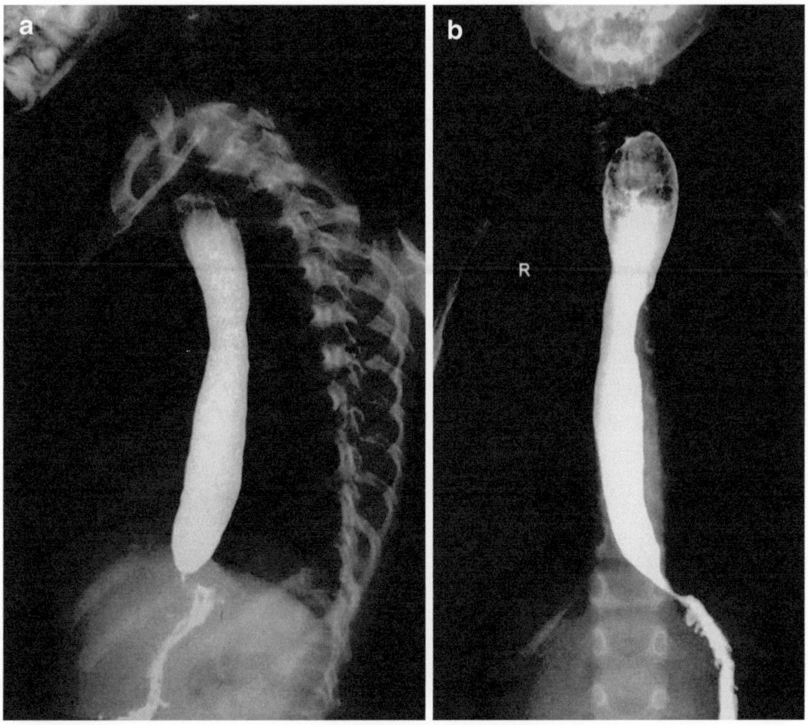

Fig. 38.4 (**a**, **b**) Contrast swallow showing smooth tapering lower end suggestive of achalasia cardia.

Achalasia may follow degeneration of inhibitory (nitric oxide and vasoactive intestinal peptide) myenteric plexus cells, leading to unopposed excitatory (acetylcholine) cells; this causes poor peristalsis and a failure of the LES to relax. Achalasia is very rare in small children who present with difficulty in swallowing along with regurgitation, vomiting, and acute life-threatening events. The differential diagnosis includes congenital esophageal stenosis, gastroesophageal reflux, milk allergy, duplication cyst of the esophagus and the stomach, and diffuse esophageal spasm. The diagnosis is made on a contrast esophagogram showing a dilated esophagus with smooth narrowing of the distal esophagus and esophagogastric junction, also called the "bird-beak" sign (Fig. 38.4). Manometry shows failure of relaxation of the GEJ on swallowing with reduced esophageal peristalsis. Sometimes, it is challenging to differentiate congenital esophageal stenosis from achalasia cardia.

Endoscopic balloon dilatation, pharmacotherapy with isosorbide dinitrate, nifedipine, and local botulinum toxin injections are often unsuccessful. Heller's myotomy is best performed laparoscopically and involves a longitudinal incision in the muscle, taking care to avoid breaching the mucosa. A partial fundoplication (Thal-Dor, Fig. 38.3) is sometimes advocated. Per oral endoscopic myotomy (POEM) is an attractive development. Occasionally, partial or total esophagectomy is needed.

38.15 Congenital Esophageal Stenosis (CES)

Isolated congenital stenoses usually transmit milk adequately but manifest during weaning with dysphagia, food impaction, respiratory distress, or faltering growth. If associated with esophageal atresia, they appear in the lower component and are detected well before weaning on contrast studies or when a trans anastomotic tube proves challenging to pass. There may be tracheobronchial remnants or fibromuscular thickening with or without a membranous web. If balloon dilation fails, excision may be required. Histopathological demonstration of tracheobronchial cartilage supports the diagnosis.

38.16 Barrett's Esophagus

A long-term complication of GERD is Barrett's esophagus, which is defined as replacement of the esophageal mucosa above the GE junction with metaplastic intestinal columnar epithelium. This has five times higher neoplastic potential for the development of adenocarcinoma. Treatment is rarely needed in childhood, but transition to adult care and endoscopic surveillance is required. It is currently advised that adults operated for esophageal atresia in childhood should have endoscopic surveillance every 5 years. The cells are classified as nondysplastic or having low or high-grade dysplasia or carcinoma. High-grade dysplasia and early adenocarcinoma are treated by endoscopic resection or radiofrequency ablation; advanced disease requires resection or palliation.

Suggested Reading

Brunicardi FC, Andersen DK, BilliarTR DLD, Hunter JG, Jeffrey B. Schwartz's principles of surgery. 10th ed. McGraw Hill, USA; 2014.

Coran AG, Caldamone A, Scott Adzich N, Krummel TM, Laberge JM, editors. Pediatric surgery. 7th ed. Oxford: Elsevier Limited; 2012.

Operative Pediatric Surgery 8th Edition Edited by Mark Davenport, James Geiger 2020, CRC Press

Infantile Pyloric Stenosis

39

Ankur Mandelia and Subhasis Roy Choudhury

Infantile hypertrophic pyloric stenosis (IHPS) is characterized by the progressive thickening and enlargement of the gastric pyloric muscles, resulting in gastric outlet obstruction in infants. This condition was first documented by Fabricius Hildanus in 1627, while the modern understanding stems from Harald Hirschsprung's pivotal work in 1888. The incidence is reported to be 1–3 per 1000 live births in Western populations, with significantly lower prevalence among Asian and African populations. IHPS predominantly affects firstborn male infants, with a male-to-female ratio of 4:1. Although it can run in families, the exact inheritance pattern remains unclear, and associated anomalies are infrequent.

The precise cause of IHPS is unknown. One hypothesis suggests that increased gastric acidity triggers pylorospasm, which leads to stasis and further exacerbates the condition. Stasis and alkaline milk feeds may stimulate gastrin production, perpetuating the cycle of acidity and pylorospasm. Other proposed mechanisms include excessive substance P, reduced neurotrophins, deficient nitric oxide synthase, abnormal innervation, and pyloric muscle dysfunction resembling achalasia cardia. Genetic predisposition is supported by the higher prevalence in males and certain ABO blood types. Breastfeeding is considered a protective factor, whereas bottle feeding may increase the risk. Additional risk factors include maternal smoking, alcohol use during pregnancy, and infant exposure to macrolide antibiotics like erythromycin.

39.1 Pathology

In IHPS, there occurs pronounced hypertrophy and hyperplasia of both the circular and longitudinal muscle layers of the pylorus, resulting in a narrowed and elongated pyloric canal. This is accompanied by edema and thickening of the pyloric mucosa, which can severely obstruct the gastric outlet. Such obstruction leads to postprandial, non-bilious projectile vomiting. Over time, the stomach becomes increasingly distended, and stasis can result in gastritis, often causing vomitus to appear blood-tinged.

A. Mandelia (✉)
Department of Pediatric Surgery, Sanjay Gandhi Post Graduate Institute of Medical Sciences (SGPGIMS), Lucknow, India

S. Roy Choudhury
Pediatric Surgery, Lady Hardinge Medical College and Associated Kalawati Saran Children's Hospital, New Delhi, Delhi, India

© The Author(s), under exclusive license to Springer Nature Singapore Pte Ltd. 2025

S. Roy Choudhury (ed.), *Pediatric Surgery*, https://doi.org/10.1007/978-981-96-1257-4_39

39.2 Clinical Features

The classic presentation of IHPS is non-bilious projectile vomiting in a full-term infant aged 3–6 weeks. In preterm infants, symptoms typically appear about two weeks later. Vomiting is forceful and occurs after feeding, sometimes appearing as "coffee ground" due to gastritis. Other associated features include failure to thrive, weight loss, persistent hunger, constipation, and signs of dehydration. Approximately 2% of affected infants may develop jaundice, attributed to reduced hepatic glucuronyl transferase activity, which usually resolves post-surgery.

Key examination findings include the palpation of a mobile, ovoid mass or "olive" in the right upper quadrant, often facilitated by a test feed, and visible gastric peristalsis. Studies indicate that the positive predictive value of palpating the "olive" for diagnosing IHPS can reach up to 99%, with success rates in detecting the mass varying between 40% and 100% in the literature (Fig. 39.1).

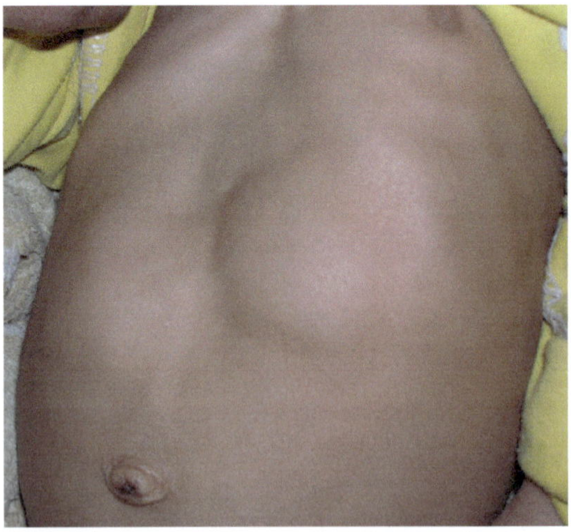

Fig. 39.1 Demonstration of visible gastric peristalsis caused by pyloric obstruction. (Reprinted with permission from Prof. S Roy Choudhury, Choudhury, S.R. (2018). Pyloric Stenosis. In: Pediatric Surgery. Springer, Singapore. https://doi.org/10.1007/978-981-10-6304-6_31)

39.3 Differential Diagnosis

Conditions that mimic IHPS include overfeeding, gastroesophageal reflux, delayed gastric emptying, acute gastroenteritis, raised intracranial pressure, antral web, pyloric or gastric duplication, and extrinsic compression.

39.4 Investigations

39.4.1 Biochemical Alterations

Recurrent vomiting and loss of gastric acid lead to hypokalemic, hypochloremic metabolic alkalosis. The compensatory action of aldosterone causes renal tubular reabsorption of sodium and water in exchange for potassium and hydrogen ions, depleting these further. Bicarbonate reabsorption compensates for low chloride levels, resulting in metabolic alkalosis with paradoxical aciduria. Hence, biochemical testing is essential to identify these changes.

39.4.2 Ultrasonography

Ultrasonography is the diagnostic gold standard, with 100% accuracy reported in skilled hands. Key findings include the "doughnut," "target," or "bull's-eye" sign, pyloric muscle thickness > 4 mm, and pyloric channel length > 17 mm. A pyloric diameter exceeding 14 mm is also diagnostic. Notably, the canal's thickness and length correlate with the infant's age and weight.

39.4.3 Contrast Study

A contrast study is rarely needed, typically reserved for diagnostic uncertainties. Diagnostic signs include a distended stomach with delayed emptying, the "string sign" (thin contrast passage through the pylorus), and the "shoulder sign" (hypertrophied muscle bulging into the stomach lumen).

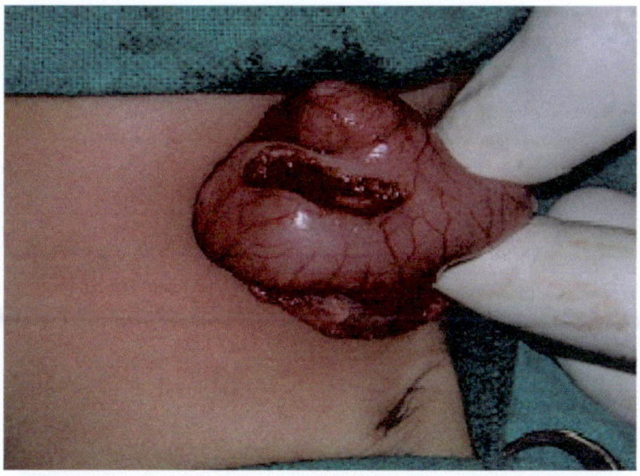

Fig. 39.2 Intraoperative photograph of an open pyloromyotomy procedure. (Reprinted with permission from Prof. S Roy Choudhury, Choudhury, S.R. (2018). Pyloric Stenosis. In: Pediatric Surgery. Springer, Singapore. https://doi.org/10.1007/978-981-10-6304-6_31)

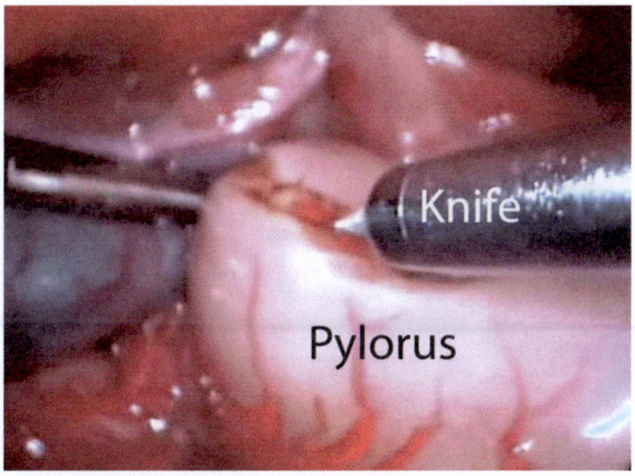

Fig. 39.3a Laparoscopic pyloromyotomy performed using a knife. (Reprinted with permission from Prof. S Roy Choudhury, Choudhury, S.R. (2018). Pyloric Stenosis. In: Pediatric Surgery. Springer, Singapore. https://doi.org/10.1007/978-981-10-6304-6_31)

39.4.4 Management

IHPS is considered a "physiological" emergency rather than a surgical one. Initial resuscitation in severely dehydrated infants involves normal saline boluses of 10–20 mL/kg body weight, followed by 5% or 10% dextrose in 0.45% saline (half-normal saline) at 1.5 times the maintenance rate. Potassium (20–30 mEq/L) is added after confirming adequate urine output. Resuscitation typically takes 24–48 h to correct metabolic and electrolyte imbalances, preparing the infant for safe surgery. Indicators of adequate resuscitation include serum bicarbonate <28 mEq/L, serum chloride >100 mEq/L, moist mucous membranes, good skin turgor, and sufficient urine output.

39.4.5 Surgery

The definitive treatment is pyloromyotomy, first described by Ramstedt in 1912. This procedure involves extra-mucosal longitudinal splitting of the pyloric muscle without suturing (Fig. 39.2).

39.5 Management

Performed under general anesthesia, OP is typically done through a small transverse upper quadrant or circumumbilical (Bianchi) incision. The thickened pylorus is identified by its connections to the omentum and transverse colon and carefully delivered through the incision. An incision is made on the avascular pyloric serosa, and the muscle is split using a spreader, extending from the pyloroduodenal junction (pre-pyloric vein) to the stomach antrum. This allows the intact mucosa to protrude through the incision. The adequacy of the pyloromyotomy is confirmed by ensuring free movement of the split pyloric edges and checking mucosal integrity using air or saline injected into the stomach via a nasogastric tube.

39.6 Outcomes

LP is gaining popularity due to reduced postoperative pain, quicker recovery, and superior cosmetic outcomes (Figs. 39.3a and 39.3b). Although introduced by Alain et al. in 1991, debates still persist about its advantages over OP and its potential risks. A 2021 Cochrane review analyzing seven Randomised Controlled Trial (RCT) concluded that LP may have a slightly higher risk of mucosal perforation compared to OP. It also noted an increased likelihood of incomplete pyloromyotomy with LP, though the evidence was not definitive. Other studies suggest that LP, when performed by experienced surgeons, may result in fewer complications compared to OP.

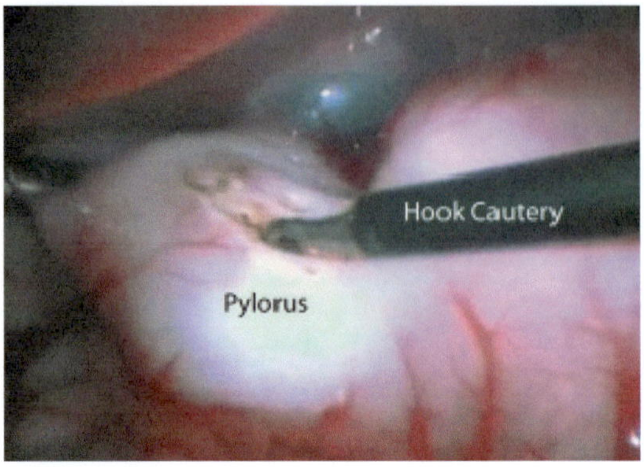

Fig. 39.3b Pyloric incision created with a hook cautery. (Reprinted with permission from Prof. S Roy Choudhury, Choudhury, S.R. (2018). Pyloric Stenosis. In: Pediatric Surgery. Springer, Singapore. https://doi.org/10.1007/978-981-10-6304-6_31)

39.6.1 Outcomes and Complications

The results of pyloromyotomy are highly favorable. Postoperative feeding usually begins 6–8 h after surgery and is gradually increased as tolerated. The overall complication rate ranges from 5% to 12% and may include:

- *Mucosal perforation:* Repairable with a patch of omentum.
- *Incomplete pyloromyotomy:* Requires reintervention.
- *Wound infection:* Managed with standard care.
- *Persistent vomiting:* Often due to gastroesophageal reflux.

Long-term sequelae are exceptionally rare in infants treated for IHPS.

Summary

- Infantile hypertrophic pyloric stenosis (IHPS) involves progressive thickening of the pyloric muscle, causing near-complete obstruction of the pylorus and resulting in non-bilious projectile vomiting.
- IHPS commonly presents between 3 and 6 weeks of age and is more frequently observed in firstborn male infants.
- The hallmark biochemical abnormality caused by repeated vomiting of gastric contents is hypokalemic, hypochloremic metabolic alkalosis with paradoxical aciduria.
- Ultrasonography is the diagnostic gold standard, with near-perfect accuracy. Key diagnostic criteria include a pyloric muscle thickness greater than 4 mm and a pyloric channel length exceeding 17 mm.
- The definitive treatment is Ramstedt's pyloromyotomy, a procedure that involves longitudinal splitting of the pyloric muscle while leaving the mucosa intact. This can be performed using either an open or laparoscopic technique.

Suggested Reading

Coran AG, Caldamone A, Scott Adzich N, Krummel TM, Laberge JM, editors. Pediatric surgery. 7th ed. Oxford: Elsevier Limited; 2012.

Peters B, Oomen MW, Bakx R, Benninga MA. Advances in infantile hypertrophic pyloric stenosis. Expert Rev Gastroenterol Hepatol. 2014;8(5):533–41. 10.1586/17474124.2014.903799. Epub 2014 Apr 10. PMID: 24716658

Aspelund G, Langer JC. Current management of hypertrophic pyloric stenosis. Semin Pediatr Surg. 2007;16(1):27–33. https://doi.org/10.1053/j.sempedsurg.2006.10.004. PMID: 17210480

Staerkle RF, Lunger F, Fink L, Sasse T, Lacher M, von Elm E, Marwan AI, Holland-Cunz S, Vuille-Dit-Bille RN. Open versus laparoscopic pyloromyotomy for pyloric stenosis. Cochrane Database Syst Rev. 2021;3(3):CD012827. https://doi.org/10.1002/14651858.CD012827.pub2. PMID: 33686649; PMCID: PMC8092451

40 Neonatal Intestinal Obstruction

Laura Phillips, Subhasis Roy Choudhury, and Govind V. S. Murthi

40.1 Introduction

Neonatal intestinal obstruction (NIB) presents with the triad of: bilious vomiting, abdominal distension, and delay or failure to pass meconium. Initial resuscitation followed by a systematic approach to investigation, through clinical examination and radiological investigations, is imperative. Plain abdominal x-ray serves to differentiate between proximal and distal obstruction in the majority of cases and directs whether further upper or lower gastro-intestinal (GI) contrast studies are needed. Malrotation with volvulus and bowel perforation evidently need emergency intervention, but consideration of the septic neonate also presenting acutely unwell is necessary, as well as cases of functional obstruction such as Hirschsprung disease. Short gut secondary to loss of bowel is associated with major morbidity, and steps to mitigate this adverse outcome are imperative.

Neonatal intestinal obstruction usually presents with the classic triad of:

- Bilious vomiting.
- Abdominal distension.
- Delay/failure to pass meconium.

Figure 40.1 outlines a practical systematic approach to the management and investigation of a neonate with NIB following initial resuscitation and stabilization. This algorithm demonstrates that sequential examination and investigation determine what further tests and treatment are needed to appropriately manage a neonate with intestinal obstruction.

While most clinicians and radiologists would consider a upper gastro-intestinal (UGI) contrast study to exclude malrotation and volvulus in the presence of bilious vomiting, in certain situations, with obvious distal obstruction, this may not be necessary. Similarly, given that a rectal biopsy is the gold standard for diagnosis of Hirschsprung's disease, if rectal and abdominal decompression are achieved by rectal washouts, a lower GI contrast study is often not necessary, and is commonly only utilized in patients where decompression is not possible, as both a therapeutic and diagnostic study. Similarly, a plain abdominal x-ray (AXR) may itself indicate the need for a laparotomy and no need for further contrast studies. However, clinicians must be flexible in their approach, given unusual or atypical presentations of these conditions that may require further investigation outside of this algorithm.

L. Phillips · G. V. S. Murthi (✉)
Paediatric Surgical Unit, Sheffield Children's Hospital, Sheffield, UK
e-mail: govind.murthi@nhs.net

S. Roy Choudhury
Pediatric Surgery, Lady Hardinge Medical College and Associated Kalawati Saran Children's Hospital, New Delhi, Delhi, India

© The Author(s), under exclusive license to Springer Nature Singapore Pte Ltd. 2025
S. Roy Choudhury (ed.), *Pediatric Surgery*, https://doi.org/10.1007/978-981-96-1257-4_40

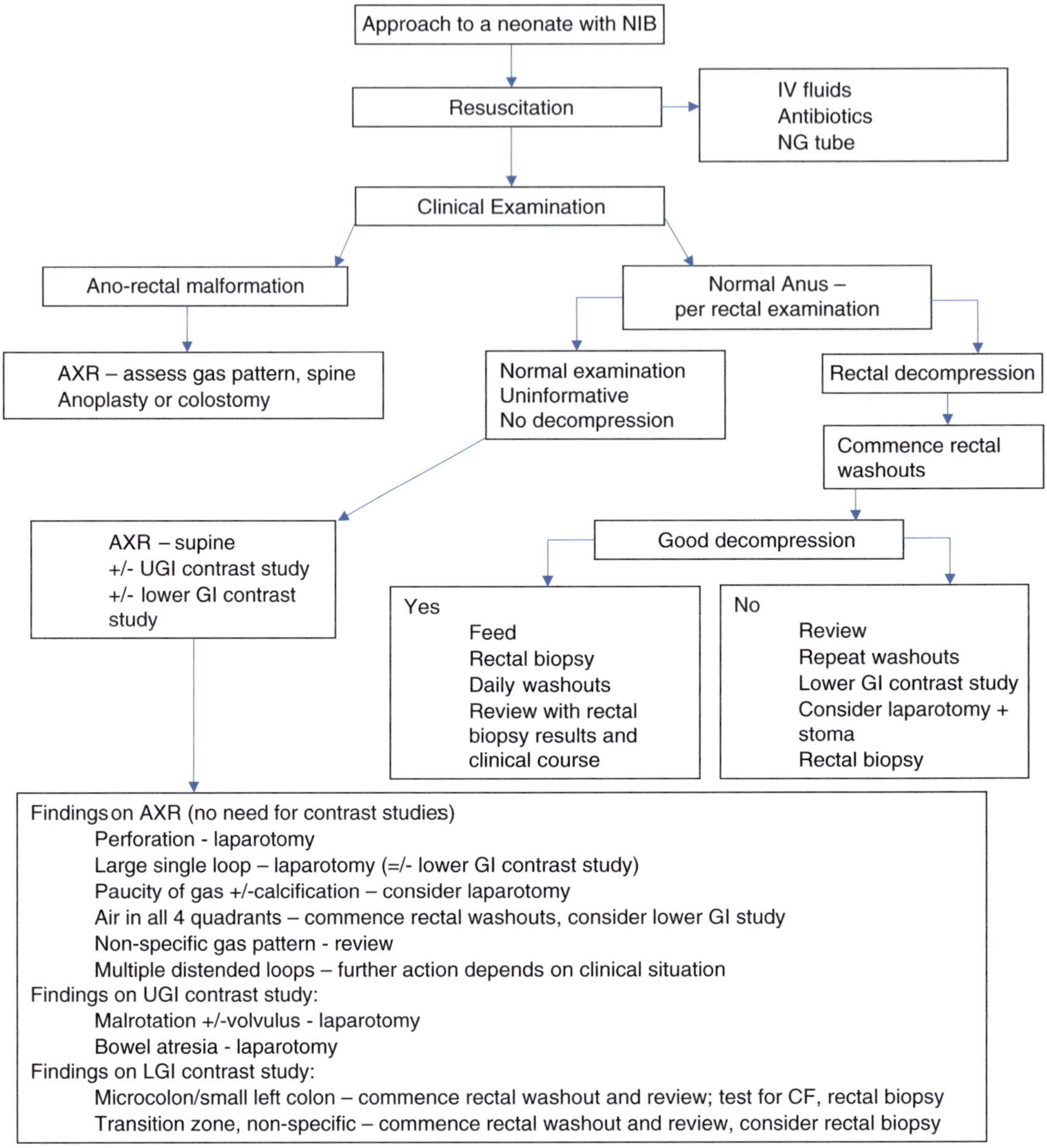

Fig. 40.1 Approach to the management of NIB

Neonatal intestinal obstruction occurs in 1 in 2000 live births.

Congenital atresia and stenosis, which can occur at any point through the small or large bowel or at multiple sites, constitute the majority of cases. Other causes include malrotation with or without volvulus, meconium ileus, Hirschsprung disease, and anorectal malformations. Prenatal sonography showing echogenic bowel, dilated bowel, and polyhydramnios is suggestive of intestinal anomalies.

40.2 Intestinal Atresia and Stenosis

40.2.1 Pyloric Atresia

This rare, familial condition has an association with epidermolysis bullosa. A single large gastric bubble on X-ray is. Surgical reconstruction may be undertaken by a Heinecke-Mikulicz pyloroplasty for a pyloric web or Bilroth 1 gastroduodenostomy for solid pyloric atresia. Gastrojejunostomy should be avoided.

40.2.2 Duodenal Atresia and Stenosis

This group of conditions is caused by failure of recanalization during the embryonic development of the duodenum. Atresia is more common than stenosis (20% of cases).

40.2.2.1 Varieties

Duodena Atresia

- Type I membrane, wind sock with diaphragm (Fig. 40.2).
- Type II atresia with intervening fibrous cord.
- Type III atresia with complete gap.

Duodenal stenosis/partial obstruction (often associated with Down syndrome)

- Web with a hole.
- Annular pancreas (Fig. 40.3).
- Pre-duodenal portal vein.
- Ladd's band in malrotation—occasionally malrotation with volvulus may present with a double bubble sign on AXR; and therefore delay in operating (>24 h) on suspected duodenal atresia without confirmatory upper GI contrast is best avoided.

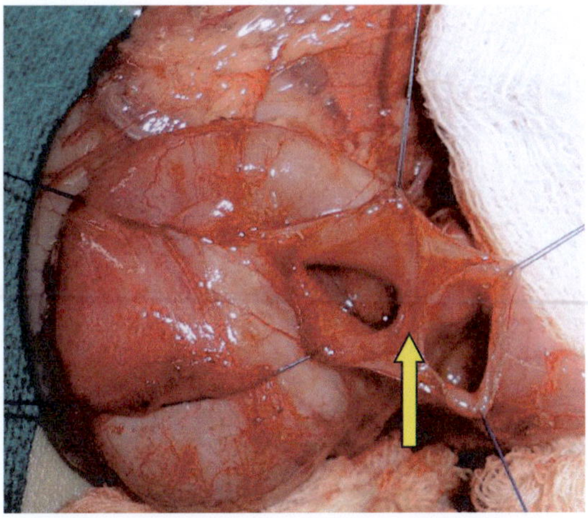

Fig. 40.2 Duodenal web (arrow)

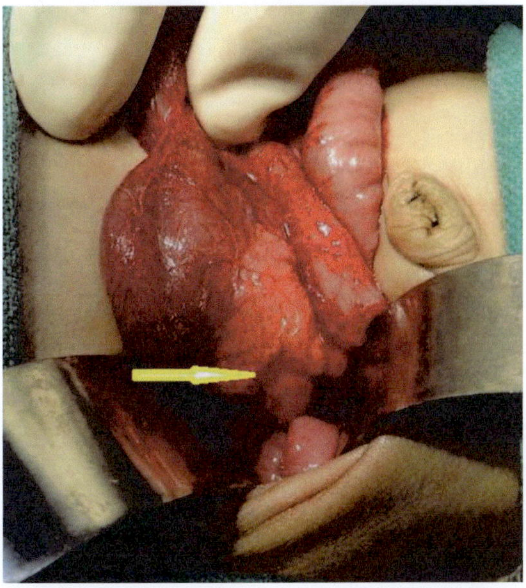

Fig. 40.3 Annular pancreas

40.2.2.2 Associations

Prematurity, growth restriction, other malformations 50% (malrotation, congenital heart disease), Trisomy 21 (35%).

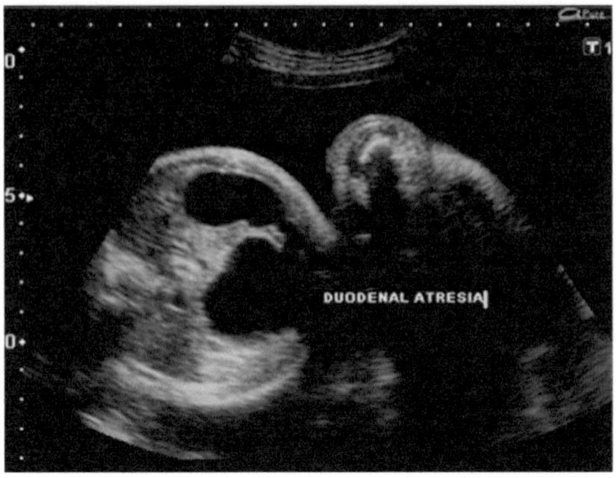

Fig. 40.4 Antenatal scan showing duodenal atresia

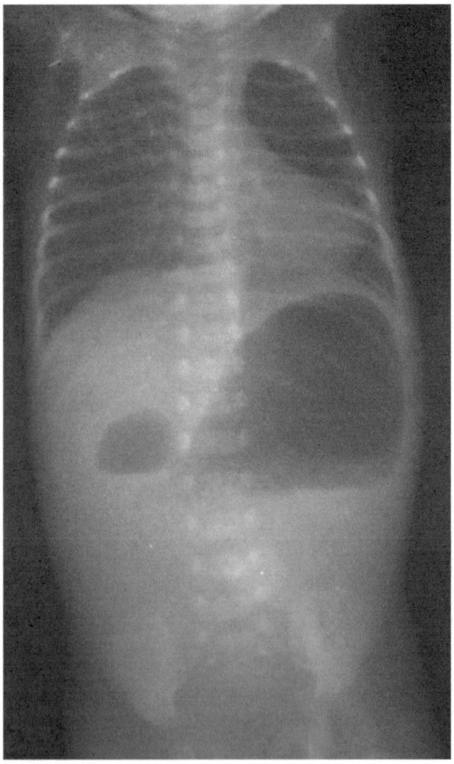

Fig. 40.5 Doudenal atresia (double bubble)

40.2.2.3 Antenatal Diagnosis

Antenatal detection of polyhydramnios (50%), intrauterine growth restriction, and double bubble appearance on ultrasonography (Fig. 40.4) are suggestive of duodenal obstruction and prompt for fetal karyotype study. No further antenatal management is required.

40.2.3 Diagnosis

Clinical presentation includes bilious vomiting, high nasogastric bilious aspirate, electrolyte imbalance, or upper abdominal distension. AXR shows *double bubble* (gastric and duodenal) with distal paucity of gas (Fig. 40.5), although distal gas may be present in cases of stenosis or incomplete web. Atresia generally occurs at the level of the ampulla of Vater. In 15% of cases, the atresia may be preampullary and bilious vomiting is absent.

40.2.4 Treatment

Initial management comprises nasogastric decompression, correction of fluid and electrolyte imbalance and investigation of associated anomalies. Congenital heart disease may have anesthetic implications and is best investigated with early echocardiogram, and later investigation of Trisomy 21 if clinical features are present.

40.2.4.1 Surgery

Duododuodenostomy. A wide diamond-shaped anastomosis between the two ends of the duodenum (Kimura) has a high success rate. Single-layer, full-thickness, interrupted sutures suffice. Division of the intervening membrane is not recommended to avoid injury to the ampulla of Vater. It is imperative to check for a windsock anomaly to ensure anastomosis is undertaken beyond the level of the membrane. Transanastomotic feeding tube placement is useful for starting early enteral feeding, although parenteral nutrition (PN) is another option if a tube cannot be navigated through the pylorus. In extreme prematurity (<1000 g), it may be best to keep the baby on total parenteral nutrition (TPN) and wait for weight gain to at least >1500 g before surgical intervention. Association with jejunoileal atresia is rare (<1%) but may be confirmed by flushing the distal bowel with saline intraoperatively.

40.2.5 Jejunoileal Atresia and Stenosis

The probable etiology is a localized intrauterine vascular accident, as evidenced by the V-shaped defect extending into the adjacent mesentery.

40.3 Diagnosis

40.3.1 Clinical Presentation

40.3.1.1 Antenatal Diagnosis

Presence of polyhydramnios, echogenic bowel, dilated and thickened bowel on antenatal ultrasound are suggestive. One third of cases are suspected antenatally.

40.3.1.2 Postnatal Diagnosis

Clinical presenting features are bilious vomiting, abdominal distension, jaundice and failure to pass meconium, depending on the level of obstruction. Occasionally a small amount of meconium may be passed. Features of intestinal obstruction develop with prominent abdominal wall veins, dilated loops of bowel with visible peristalsis (Fig. 40.6).

40.3.1.3 Radiological Diagnosis

Diagnosis can usually be made on a supine x-ray (XR) of abdomen, erect xrays are not required in neonates and best avoided. Dilated loops of bowel suggest obstruction. More distal obstruction is associated with larger amount of dilated loops (Figs. 40.7, 40.8 and 40.9).

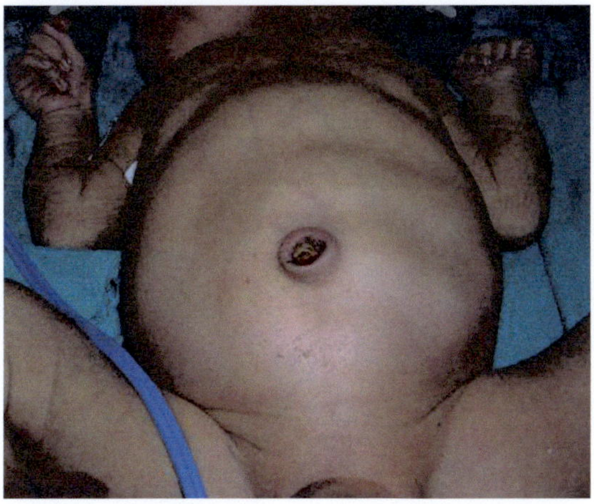

Fig. 40.6 Dilated loops of bowel with visible peristalsis

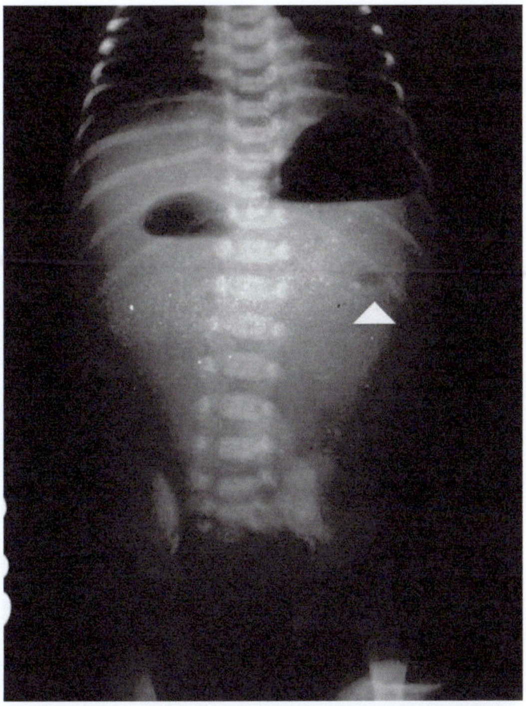

Fig. 40.7 Likely high jejunal atresia (white arrow pointing to a third air-fluid level

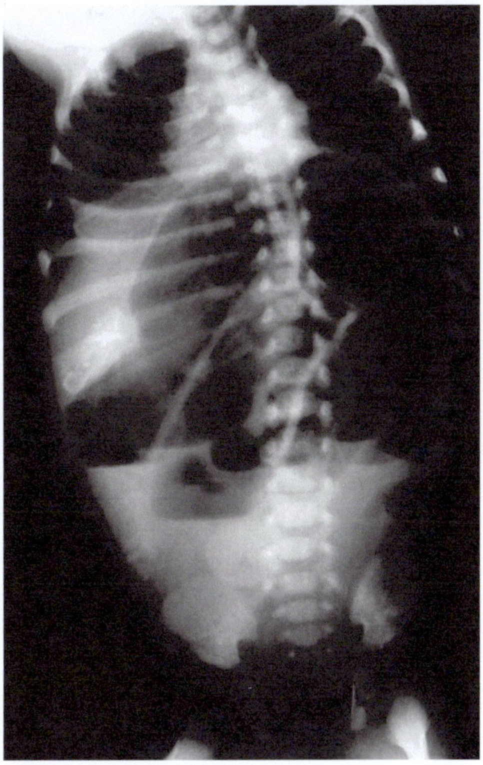

Fig. 40.8 Small bowel obstruction - most likely intestinal atresia given the severely dilated bowel loops

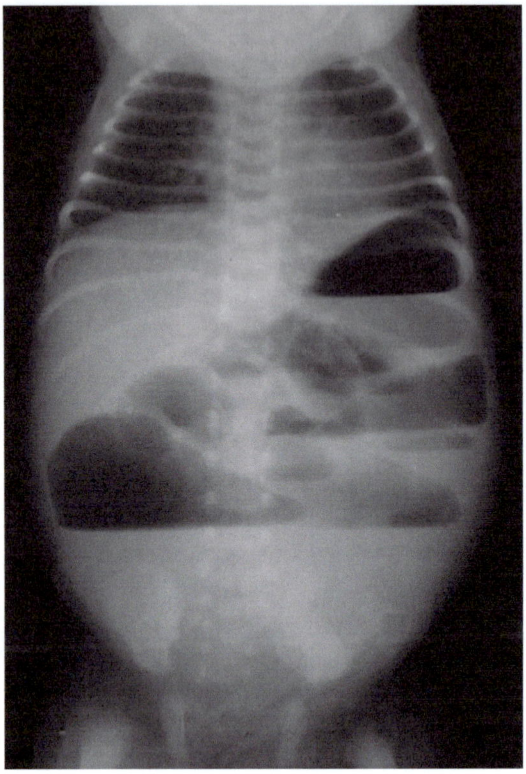

Fig. 40.9 AXR showing multiple dilated bowel loops with air-fluid levels. The air-fluid levels are due to the baby being help upright, but such practice is best avoided

Figures 40.8 and 40.9, abdominal X-ray erect and supine showing dilated small bowel loops with air-fluid levels, note absence of gas in the pelvis. Features are suggestive of intestinal obstruction.

Types (Grosfeld classification): (Fig. 40.10).

- I—Mucosal (membraneous) atresia with intact bowel wall and mesentery (Fig. 40.11).
- II—Blind ends separated by a fibrous cord (Fig. 40.12).
- IIIa—Blind ends are separated by a mesenteric defect (V-shaped gap) (Fig. 40.13).
- IIIb—Apple peel atresia, typically with single vessel (Fig. 40.14).
- IV—Multiple atresia (string of sausages) (Fig. 40.15).

In the neonate, differentiation between large bowel and small bowel on plain x-ray is difficult and best avoided, as typical bowel characteristics, such as haustra, are often absent. A supine AXR is always sufficient for clinical purposes and the current practice of an erect AXR in order

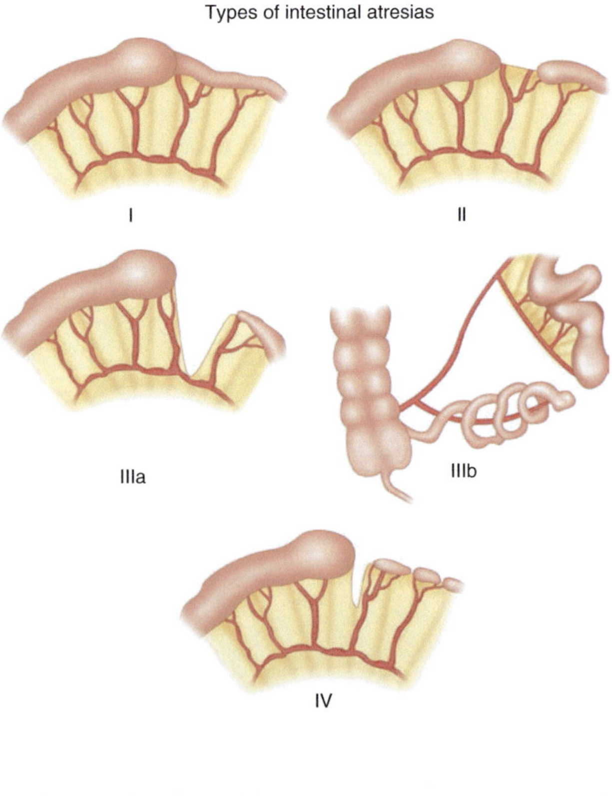

Fig. 40.10 Classification of intestinal atresia

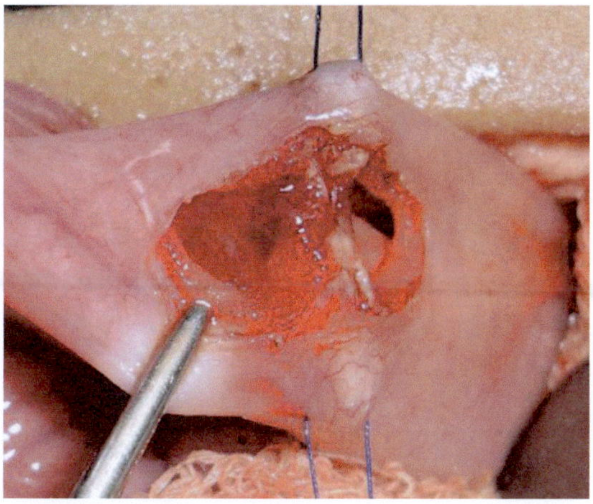

Fig. 40.11 Jejunal web

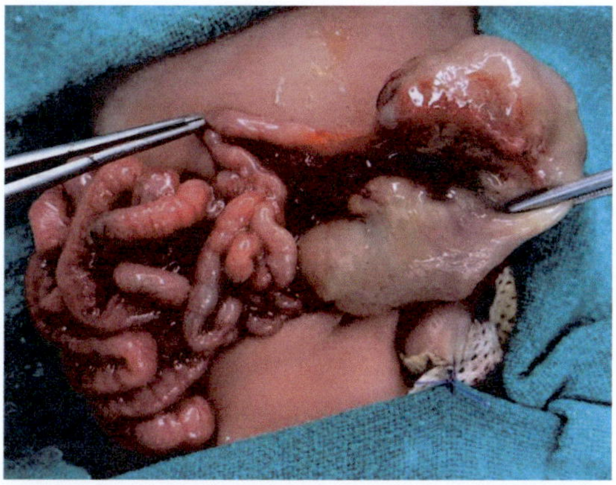

Fig. 40.12 Jejunal atresia type 2

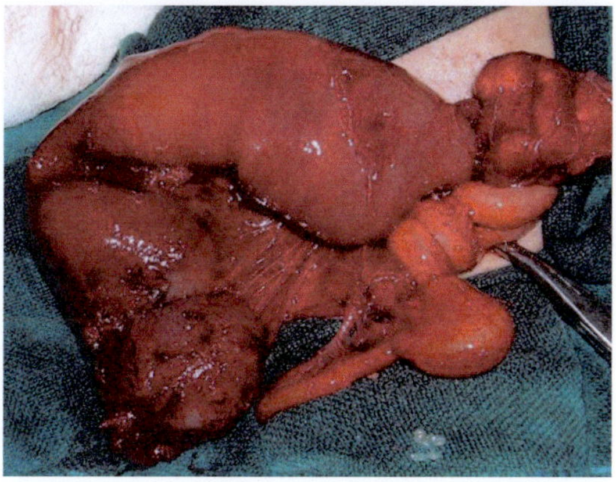

Fig. 40.13 Jejunal atresia type 3a, note V-shaped mesenteric defect

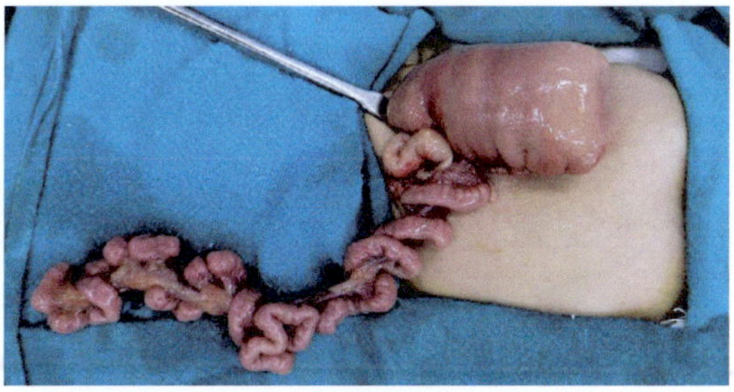

Fig. 40.14 Apple peel jejunal atresia (type 3b)

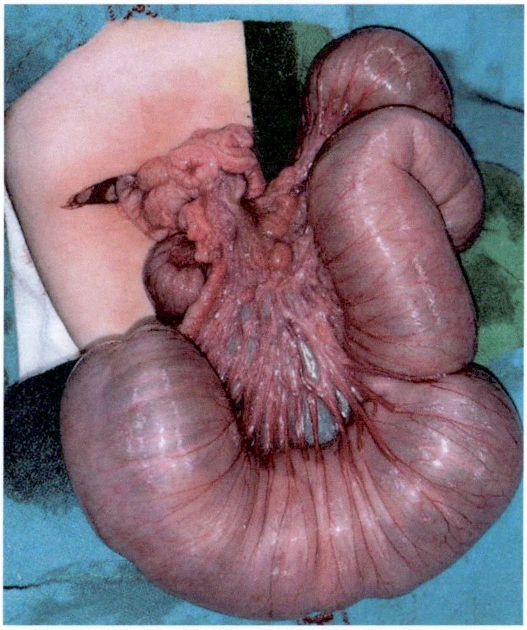

Fig. 40.15 Jejunal atresia multiple (type 4)

to get air-fluid levels is unnecessary and best avoided. Contrast enema may be useful to differentiate low small bowel obstruction from colonic obstruction, depending on how far the contrast progresses. The end point of a lower GI contrast study in such cases is the free flow of contrast into the small bowel.

Differential diagnoses of distal small bowel obstruction include ileal atresia, meconium ileus, and total colonic aganglionosis.

40.3.2 Treatment

Pre-operative management includes nasogastric decompression, intravenous hydration, temperature control and administration of vitamin K.

40.3.3 Surgery

One approaches a laparotomy for small bowel atresia with trepidation—does the child have an adequate length of bowel remaining? While resection and end-to-end anastomosis of a single small bowel atresia is one of the most gratifying operations in pediatric surgery, a full assessment of the length of small bowel, number and location of atresia(s), and discrepancy in bowel lumen across an atresia should be made before any resection is undertaken.

Resection of the atretic part and end-to-end anastomosis are preferably performed. The proximal bowel may be very distended and atonic. This atonic portion needs to be resected with caution, and a conservative resection is recommended, particularly in cases with multiple atresias or shortened bowel length. An end-to-side anastomosis may be considered in a very discrepant anastomosis where cut back or tapering is not feasible. If resection of the dilated segment is not possible then tapering can be considered. It is imperative to rule out any distal obstruction by milking the bowel or flushing with saline through a feeding tube and seeing it pass through the rectum (Fig. 40.16).

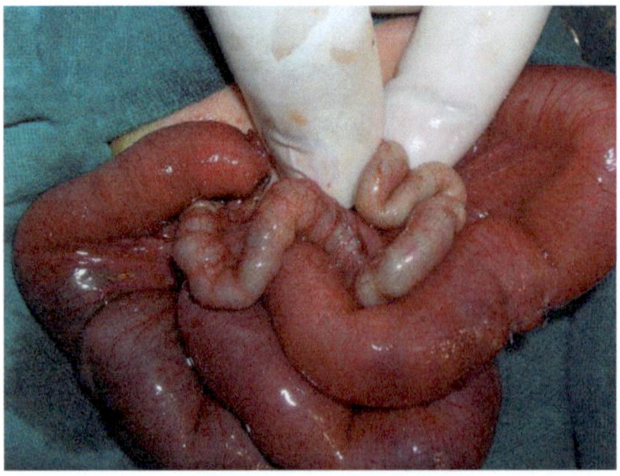

Fig. 40.16 Small bowel atresia with intraluminal pellets, which need emptying by milking or flushing through an enterostomy

Malrotation with Volvulus This is associated with extrinsic duodenal obstruction due to volvulus of (often) the entire small bowel on a narrow mesenteric base, along with a band from the colon (Ladd's band) going across the second part of the duodenum, which may also contribute to the obstruction. This typically presents in the newborn period with bilious vomiting and may have similar X-ray findings to duodenal atresia.

Presentation

- Malrotation without volvulus presents with bilious vomiting in an otherwise normal child.
- Malrotation with acute volvulus (Figs. 40.17 and 40.18): Irritable sick child, abdominal pain, abdominal distension with tenderness and guarding. *This is a surgical emergency due to ischemia and gangrene of the volved bowel.* Bleeding per rectum may be present in late presenters.
- Malrotation with chronic volvulus: chronic abdominal pain, vomiting, and malnutrition.

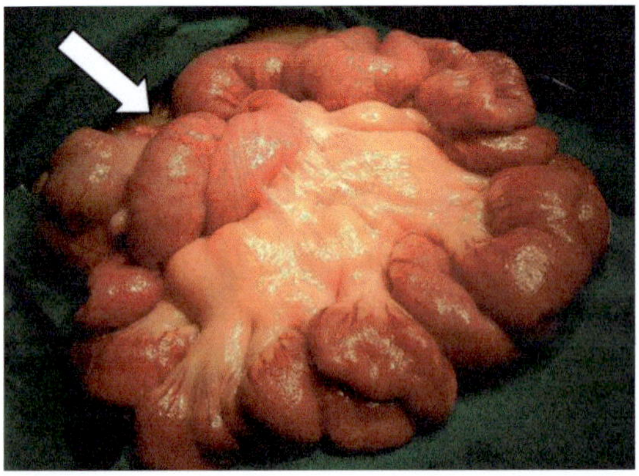

Fig. 40.17 Malrotation with volvulus

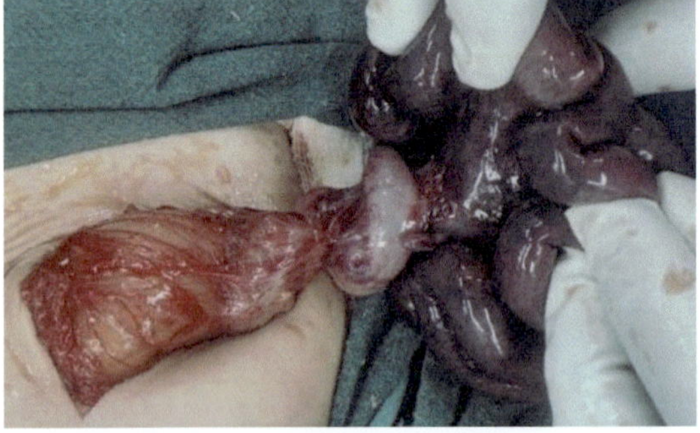

Fig. 40.18 Mid gut volvulus with gangrene

40.3.4 Diagnosis

An urgent UGI contrast study is the gold standard test to exclude malrotation +/– volvulus where there is clinical suspicion, and should not be delayed in preference to either an AXR or a Doppler US as the latter are not conclusive. In situations of the clinically unstable patient, the decision may be to proceed directly to theater with ongoing resuscitation rather than to await a contrast study.

Abdominal X-ray: Double bubble sign will be present in cases with significant duodenal obstruction. Small bowel loops will present primarily on the right side, and a small amount of distal gas may also be present.

USG abdomen can detect the presence of volvulus (whirlpool sign) and also determine the mesenteric axis by examining the relationship of superior mesenteric artery and vein, which are reversed in malrotation i.e. the vein is to the left of the artery.

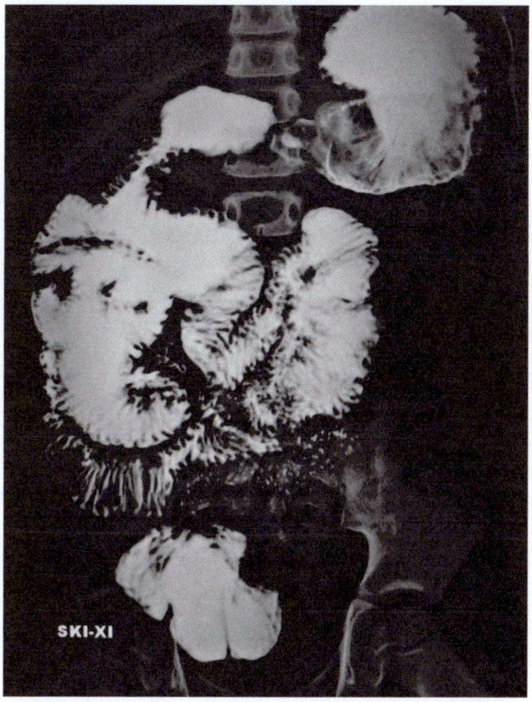

Fig. 40.19 Upper gastrointestinal contrast study showing *Cork screw* appearance of the duodenum suggestive of malrotation with volvulus

Contrast upper GI study: Duodenojejunal junction is present on the right side of the vertebral column. "Z" shaped duodenojejunal loop is frequently present. *Cork screw* appearance is present in case of volvulus (Fig. 40.19).

Operative procedure (Ladd's procedure) involves counterclockwise derotation of bowel, division of Ladd's band, widening the base of the mesentery, placing small bowel on the right side and large bowel on the left side of the abdomen in the non-rotated orientation, and an appendectomy (optional). Resection of frankly ischemic bowel may be necessary, or a "clip and drop" procedure with a plan to return in 24–48 h to assess whether any further bowel is viable and can be salvaged. In well patients or delayed presentation with chronic volvulus, this procedure may also be undertaken laparoscopically with appropriate expertise and skill.

40.3.5 Meconium Ileus

This condition is a neonatal manifestation of cystic fibrosis, inherited as an autosomal recessive genetic defect. The neonate presents with features of intestinal obstruction due to small bowel impaction with thick, viscid, inspissated meconium secondary to lack of pancreatic enzymes

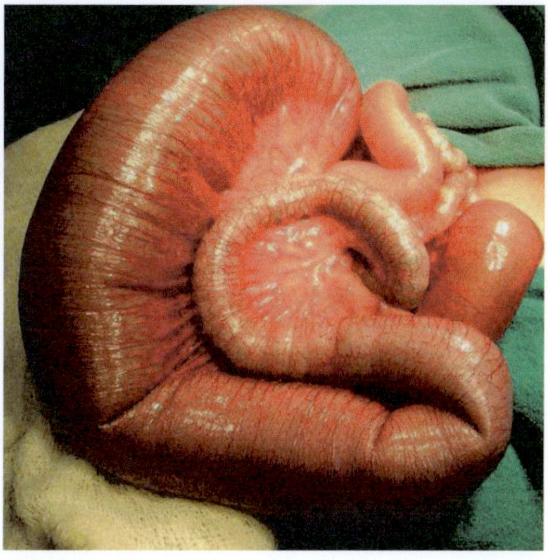

Fig. 40.20 Meconium ileus

(Fig. 40.20). This may be detected antenatally due to echogenic or dilated bowel or postnatally due to intestinal obstruction.

Abdominal X-ray

- Air-fluid levels are generally absent on abdominal X-ray as the thick viscid meconium does not form air-fluid levels.
- Meconium mixed with air can give a ground glass appearance or "soap bubble" appearance in the right lower quadrant.

Contrast enema may show a microcolon of disuse (Fig. 40.21).

Low level of fecal trypsin, high level of sodium chloride in the sweat, and genetic testing or = immunoreactive trypsinogen (IRT) levels on neonatal blood spot testing are suggestive of cystic fibrosis. Of these tests, sweat chloride cannot be performed in a neonate because of insufficient sweat produced for analysis and generally requires infants to be over 3 kg for testing.

Nearly 40% of cases may be complicated with volvulus, atresia, or meconium peritonitis. A contrast enema may be diagnostic (Fig. 40.21) as well as therapeutic, as it may displace the obstructing meconium and relieve the obstruction owing to its high osmolarity and detergent action. Calcification may be noted on X-ray due to antenatal perforation, which may be sealed or associated with atresia if the patient is born in relatively good condition.

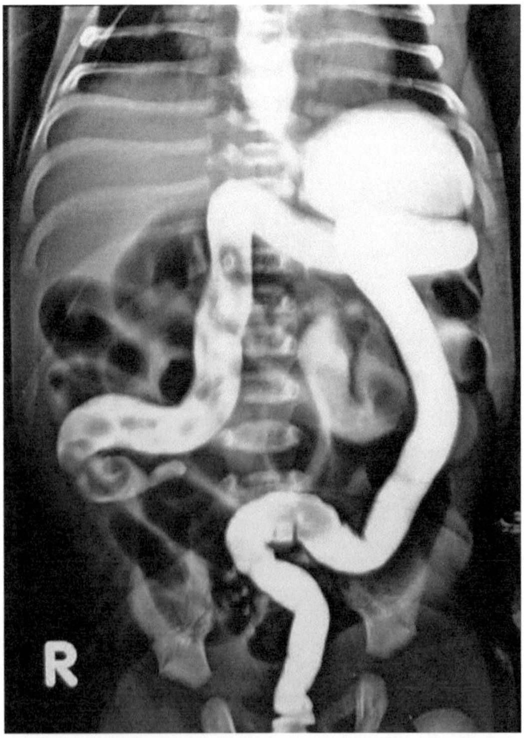

Fig. 40.21 Barium enema showing meconium ileus with microcolon

Surgical treatment is required if conservative treatment fails. An enterotomy with manual evacuation of the meconium, resection of a segment of dilated ileum, and end ileostomy and mucous fistula (option A) or a tube enterostomy (option D) or primary anastomosis are potential surgical options. Stoma variations such as the Bishop-Koop and Santulli stomas (options B and C) are of historical interest and not recommended in current clinical practice because of the high risk of obstruction of the T-junction with inspissated plugs (Fig. 40.22). Additional irrigation with N acetyl cysteine may help in evacuation of viscid meconium and can be given both via naso-gastric (NG) and PR.

40.3.6 Meconium Plug Syndrome

This is a condition where there is delayed or difficult passage of neonatal first meconium due to a thick sticky plug of meconium with a firm head, which often dislodges following rectal stimulation or washout. Once the meconium plug is passed, the obstruction gets relieved. However, persistence of symptoms calls for further investigations as this could be associated with cystic fibrosis, small left colon syndrome (typically in patients with diabetic mothers), Hirschsprung disease, hypothyroidism, or maternal opioid use. Appropriate test to rule out cystic fibrosis and a suction rectal biopsy to exclude Hirschsprung disease are reasonable, as up to 15% of patients may have Hirschsprung disease.

40.3.7 Meconium Peritonitis

Peritoneal calcification on abdominal x-ray indicates intrauterine perforation with meconium peritonitis (Fig. 40.23). Large single air-fluid

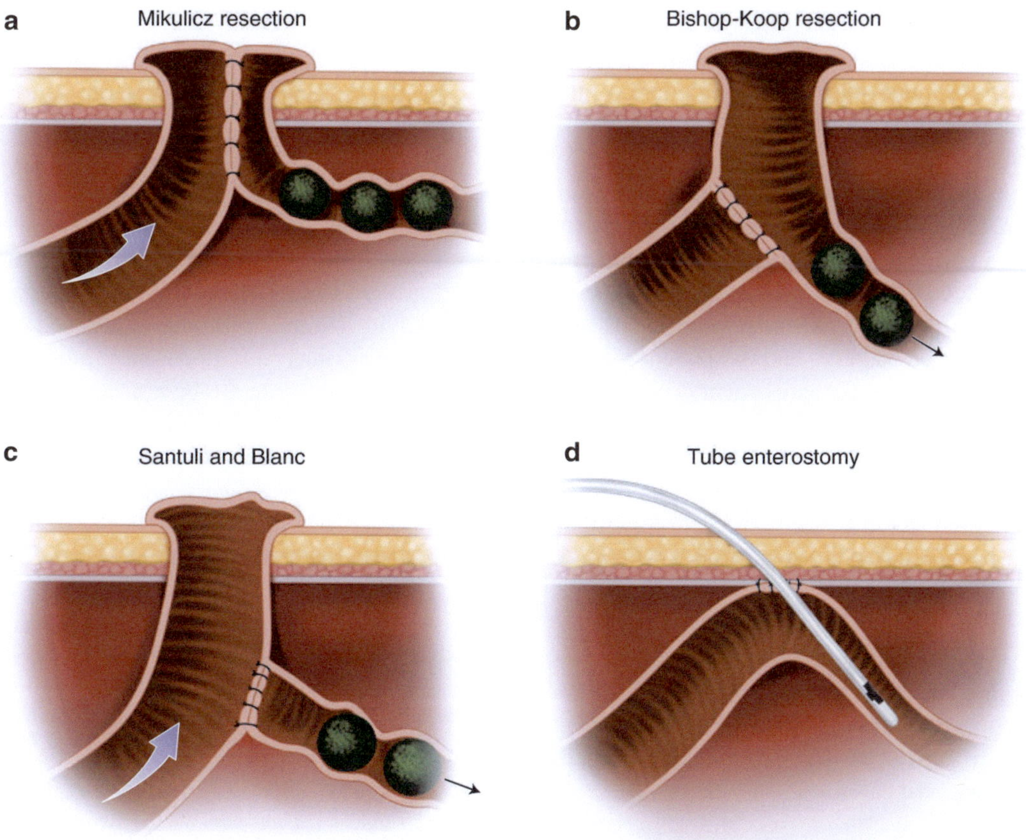

Fig. 40.22 Surgical procedures for meconium ileus

Fig. 40.23 Intra peritoneal calcification due to meconium peritonitis

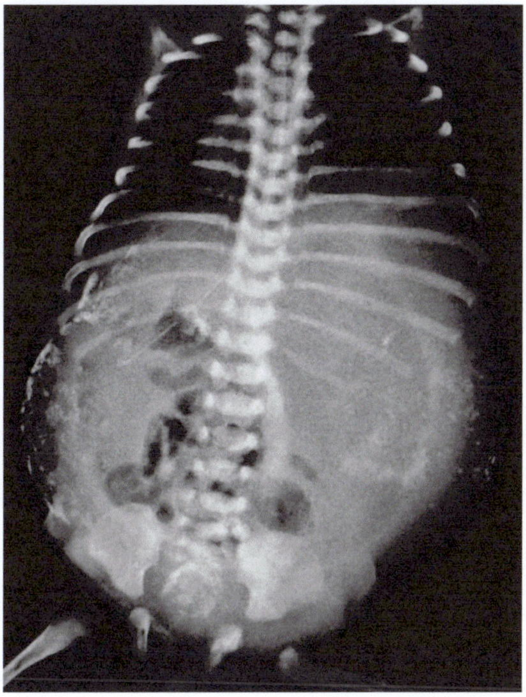

level indicates a giant meconium pseudocyst associated with meconium peritonitis. Treatment is surgical and often challenging due to inflammation and potential foreshortened bowel (see above).

In patients with persistent intestinal obstruction, in which no mechanical cause can be found and in which Hirschsprung disease and meconium ileus have been excluded, a potential diagnosis of pediatric intestinal pseudo-obstruction should be considered, and the patient referred to gastroenterology for assessment.

Summary

- Neonatal intestinal obstruction presents with the triad of bilious vomiting, abdominal distension and delay or failure to pass meconium.
- Following initial resuscitation, a systematic approach to clinical examination and investigation yields a treatment plan (surgery or conservative approach) in most cases.
- It is useful to try and differentiate between upper and lower GI obstruction by means of AXR and contrast studies.
- An "erect AXR" to elicit air-fluid level should never be done on a neonate; a supine AXR is just as informative.
- Calcification indicates antenatal perforation and raises the potential of a difficult laparotomy due to inflammation and the likelihood of short gut syndrome.
- Large, extensive bowel resections are best avoided in order to prevent short gut syndrome.
- Divided stomas are preferred to end-to-side or other variations; very proximal (jejunal) stomas are best treated with a tube enterostomy to gain control of the effluent in order to protect skin and allow appropriate fluid balance monitoring.

Suggested Reading

Coran AG, Caldamone A, Scott Adzich N, Krummel TM, Laberge JM, editors. Pediatric surgery. 7th ed. Oxford: Elsevier Limited; 2012.

Ladd AP, Rescorla SJ, Grosfeld JL. Handbook of pediatric surgical patient care. 1st ed. World Scientific Publishing Company; 2014.

Necrotizing Enterocolitis

41

Subhasis Roy Choudhury, Joshua Rae,
and Govind V. S. Murthi

Necrotizing enterocolitis (NEC) is characterized by varying grades of intestinal injury due to multiple factors.

NEC is the commonest abdominal emergency in newborns. The incidence is 1–3 per 1000 live births. This increases to 30 per 1000 live births for low birth weight neonates, affecting roughly 11% of infants weighing 401–750 g, 9% of infants 751–1000 g, 6% of infants weighing 1001–1250 g, and 4% of infants weighing 1251–1500 g.

41.1 Etiology

NEC pathophysiology is poorly understood; contributing factors are summarized in Fig. 41.1.

Progression of the disease is influenced by numerous mediators such as tumor necrosis factor-α (TNF-α), platelet-activating factor (PAF), and nitric oxide (NO).

Although multiple factors may affect the development of NEC, the final effector pathway remains the same. Immature gut or prenatal

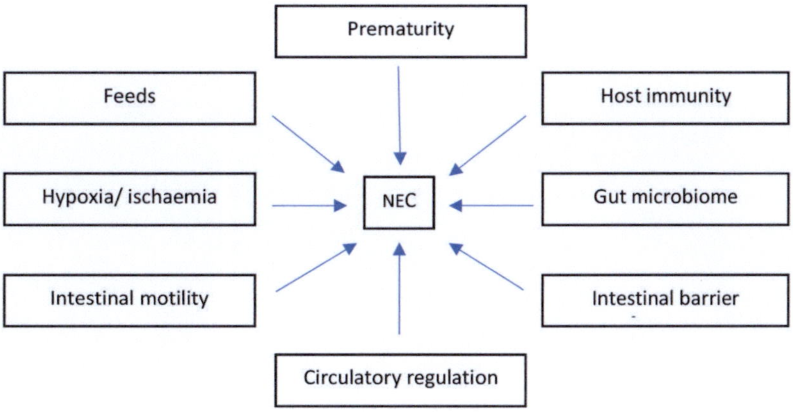

Fig. 41.1 Pathogenesis of NEC

S. Roy Choudhury
Pediatric Surgery, Lady Hardinge Medical College and Associated Kalawati Saran Children's Hospital, New Delhi, Delhi, India

J. Rae · G. V. S. Murthi (✉)
Paediatric Surgical Unit, Sheffield Childrens Hospital, Sheffield, UK

© The Author(s), under exclusive license to Springer Nature Singapore Pte Ltd. 2025

S. Roy Choudhury (ed.), *Pediatric Surgery*, https://doi.org/10.1007/978-981-96-1257-4_41

stressors lead to altered gut barrier or immunity, a virulent organism then takes advantage of this and sets in motion an inflammatory cascade which ultimately results in ischemia and necrosis of the bowel.

NEC most commonly affects the terminal ileum followed by the colon. The disease can involve a single segment or can have multiple skip lesions. The most fulminant form is NEC totalis in which more than 75% of the bowel is involved.

41.2 Presentation

The presentation of NEC can vary from a benign course with non-specific signs to overwhelming systemic shock with multi-organ failure.

Clinical signs may become apparent including abdominal distension, abdominal wall erythema, tenderness, and crepitus (Fig. 41.2).

Radiographic findings include bowel dilatation, bowel wall thickening, portal venous gas, pneumatosis, and pneumoperitoneum (Figs. 41.3a,b, 41.4a, and 41.4b).

Severity of the disease is classified according to Bell's classification as stage I (suspected), stage II (definite), stage III (advanced) (Table 41.1).

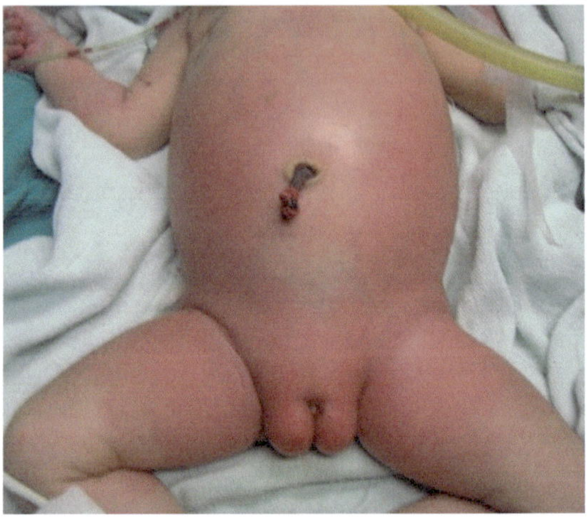

Fig. 41.2 Abdominal wall erythema and gastrointestinal bleeding (NG tube) due to NEC

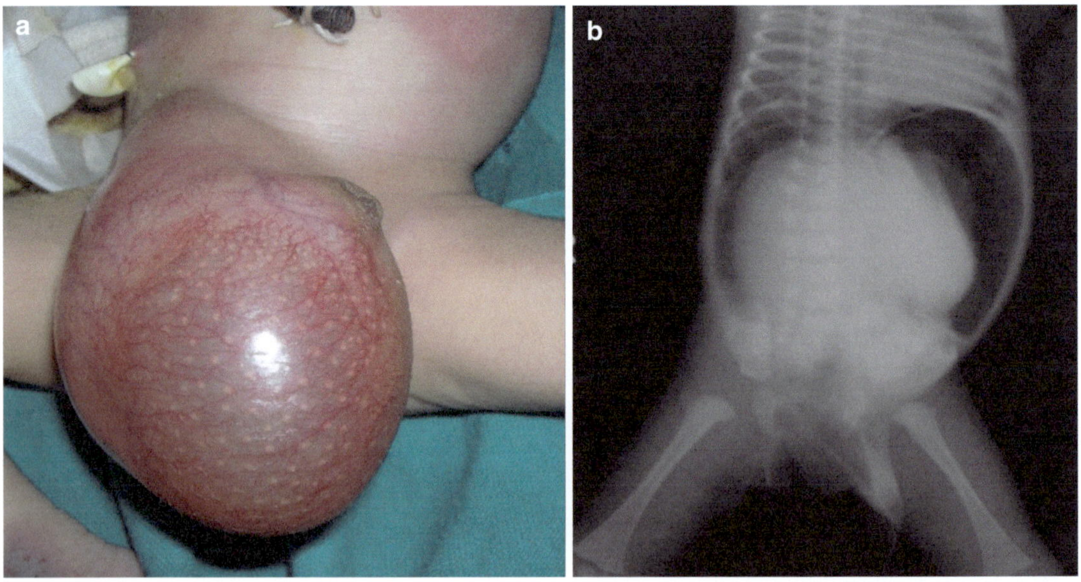

Fig. 41.3 (**a**, **b**) Pneumoperitoneum with scrotal air

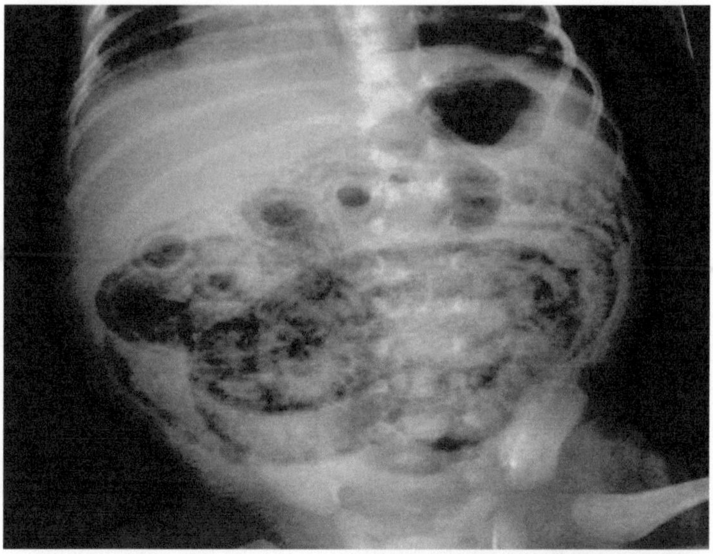

Fig. 41.4a NEC with pneumatosis intestinalis

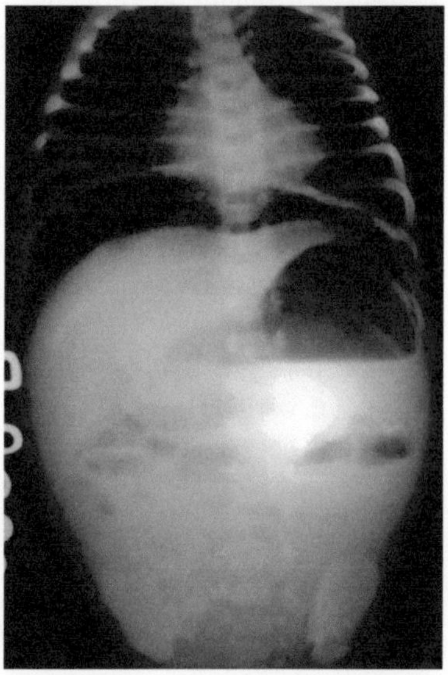

Fig. 41.4b Pneumoperitoneum

Table 41.1 Modified Bell's staging for NEC

Stage	Clinical finding	Radiological finding	Gastrointestinal finding
I—Suspected	Apnea, bradycardia, temperature instability	Gas pattern of mild ileus increased gastric residuals	Occult blood in stool, mild abdominal distention
IIa—Definite	Apnea, bradycardia, temperature instability	Ileus gas pattern with one or more dilated loops, focal pneumatosis	Grossly bloody stools, prominent abdominal distention, absent bowel sounds
IIb	Thrombocytopenia, mild metabolic acidosis	Widespread pneumatosis, ascites, portal venous gas	Abdominal wall edema with palpable loops and tenderness
IIIa—Advanced	Mixed acidosis, oliguria, hypotension, coagulopathy	Prominent bowel loops, worsening ascites, no free air	Worsening wall edema, erythema and induration
IIIb	Shock, deterioration in laboratory values and vital signs	Pneumoperitoneum	Perforated bowel

41.3 Treatment

Initial medical management consists of withdrawal of enteral feeding, nasogastric tube decompression, intravenous fluid, and initiation of parenteral nutrition. Broad-spectrum antibiotics are instituted. Close clinical and biochemical monitoring is necessary, with serial radiographs useful in monitoring disease progression. Once the child stabilizes and an adequate period of bowel rest has passed (7–10 days), oral feeds are initiated and gradually progressed.

41.3.1 Indications for Surgery

The decision to operate an be difficult. Whilst the presence of pneumoperitoneum (indicating perforation) is a clear indication for surgery, in most cases the decision to operate is subjective and depends on various associated factors.

The decision to operate is best reached through, a multidisciplinary team (MDT) approach which takes take the whole clinical picture into context, including:

- Pre-existing morbidity—such as gestation, weight, cardiac, respiratory, neurological, and genetic conditions.
- Clinical signs such as a palpable mass, worsening abdominal wall erythema, and need for inotropes.
- Radiological signs of a fixed loop, portal venous gas, and obstruction.
- Laboratory investigations show worsening thrombocytopenia, neutropenia, or rising inflammatory markers.

41.3.2 Surgical Intervention

Peritoneal drainage (PD) as a temporizing procedure is often beneficial, especially in extremely low birth weight babies (<1000 g) with pneumoperitoneum secondary to NEC. Some neonates may become stable by PD itself and can be managed conservatively, whereas neonates who fail to stabilize within 24–48 h of drainage need a rescue laparotomy.

For focal disease, limited bowel resection with either end-to-end anastomosis or enterostomy (stoma) is done. For extensive bowel involvement, a more conservative approach is followed by second look exploration after a period of 24–48 h, checking for any viable bowel that could be preserved (Fig. 41.5a). Extensive NEC needing massive bowel resection results in short

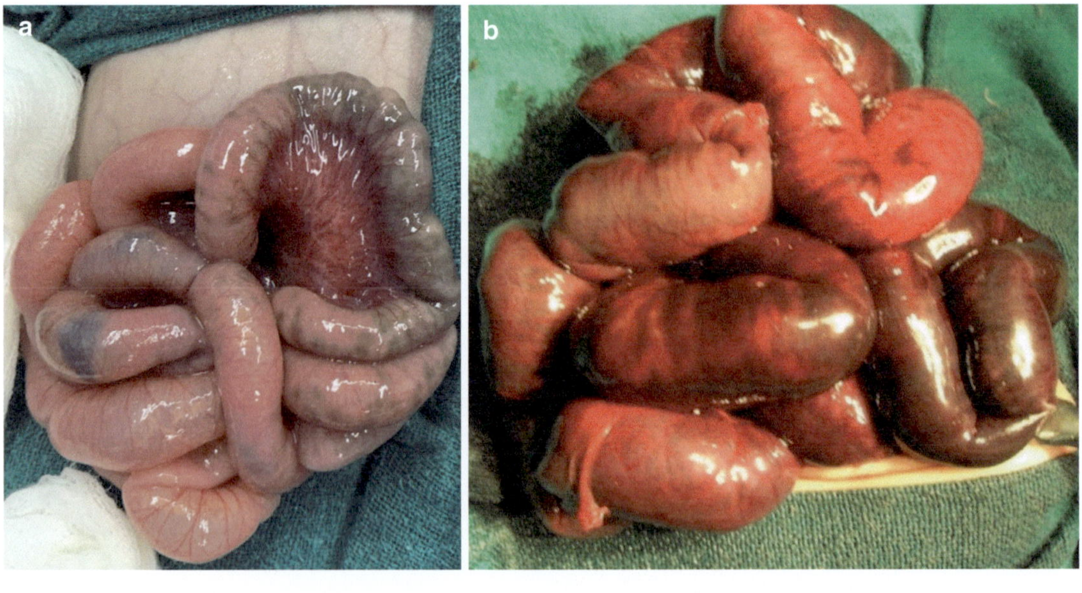

Fig. 41.5 (**a**) Patchy bowel necrosis (**b**) Extensive bowel necrosis

bowel syndrome (Fig. 41.5b). Patients in whom the bowel necrosis is extensive should be discussed with an MDT approach including the parents about implications, and in cases where there is total bowel necrosis, an "open and close" laparotomy with reorientation of care should be considered.

41.3.3 Solitary Intestinal Perforation (SIP)

Solitary or isolated intestinal perforation (SIP) is considered a separate entity from NEC. It is seen in very premature babies with perforation usually involving the terminal ileum, sparing the rest of the bowel (Fig. 41.6). Radiologically prominent pneumoperitoneum and absence of pneumatosis are suggestive of SIP. Surgical treatment includes peritoneal drainage only or drainage followed by laparotomy in unresponsive patients. Intestinal perforation may be managed by repair or resection of the involved segment. The outcome of SIP appears to be better than that of NEC.

Outcome: The mortality rate is high in NEC (15–30%).

41.3.4 Complications

(a) Stoma-related complications.
(b) Post NEC stricture (Fig. 41.7) that may be focal or multiple, occurs as a result of the healing of NEC. Patients present with recurrent abdominal distension and may have multiple episodes of feed intolerance before being diagnosed.
(c) Cholestatic liver disease due to prolonged TPN. This has become less common with strategies such as the use of SMOF (composite lipid emulsion), TPN cycling, and the use of prophylactic antibiotics for bacterial overgrowth.
(d) Short bowel syndrome in cases of extensive bowel loss.
(e) Growth and neuro-developmental problems.

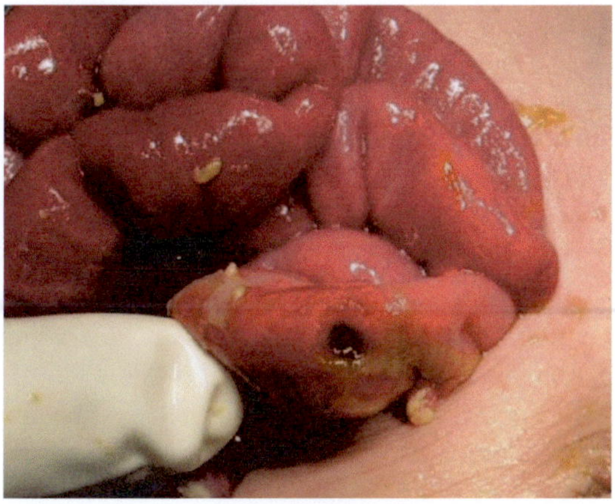

Fig. 41.6 Sigmoid colon perforation

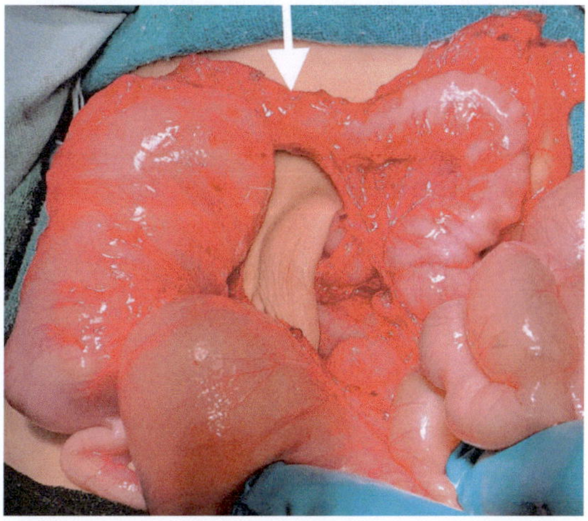

Fig. 41.7 Bowel (transverse colon) stricture due to NEC

41.3.5 Prevention of NEC

- Interventions to increase gut immunity and maturation include maternal glucocorticoid supplementation, administering breast milk (with an estimated threefold to tenfold risk reduction in infants fed human milk compared with formula milk), and oral immunoglobulins.

Measures to prevent injury to the gut mucosa are:

- Feeding regimes:
  - trophic feeds to be initiated early,
  - low volume feeds,
  - gradual increase in feeds.
- Colonization by commensal bacteria through the use of probiotics.
- Controlling inflammation by the use of anti-inflammatory molecules like PAF (Platelet Aggregating Factor) antagonist or degrading enzymes.
- Remote ischemic conditioning (RIC). The aim is to produce a time-limited reversible ischemia in a limb with subsequent reperfusion. This activates endogenous signaling pathways which lead to increased bowel micro-perfusion and has shown promise in animal models of NEC.

41.4 Summary

Necrotizing enterocolitis (NEC) is characterized by varying grades of intestinal injury due to multiple factors namely prematurity, formula feeding and stress with circulatory insufficiency. The incidence is 1–3 per 100 live births and the disease commonly affects the terminal ileum followed by colon. Most babies can be managed conservatively however, some may need surgical intervention. Surgical treatment is guided by the extent and location of the bowel disease and the condition of the neonate. Outcome is variable and depends on the gestation and weight of the neonate and other co-morbidities. Prevention of NEC is based on avoidance of the known precipitating factors, with proper feeding practice.

Suggested Reading

Coran AG, Caldamone A, Scott Adzich N, Krummel TM, Laberge JM, editors. Pediatric surgery. 7th ed. Oxford: Elsevier Limited; 2012.

Puri P, Hollwarth ME, editors. Pediatric surgery, Diagnosis and management. Heidelberg: Springer-Verlag; 2009.

Ganji N, Biouss G, Sabbatini S, Li B, Lee C, Pierro A. Remote ischemic conditioning in necrotizing enterocolitis. Semin Pediatr Surg. 2023;32(3):151312. https://doi.org/10.1016/j.sempedsurg.2023.151312. Epub 2023 Jun 1

Lin PW, Stoll BJ. Necrotising enterocolitis. Lancet. 2006;368(9543):1271–83. https://doi.org/10.1016/S0140-6736(06)69525-1.

Short Bowel Syndrome

42

Ashwin Pimpalwar

42.1 Introduction

Short Bowel Syndrome (SBS) is a condition resulting from the loss of gut tissue, either due to mechanical or functional factors. The intestine serves a vital role in not only processing and absorbing nutrients from our diet but also fulfilling various other functions essential for our well-being. Thus, the loss of the intestine leads to a cluster of altered functions, which has earned it the designation of a syndrome. The length of the remaining gut determines outcome in most patients, and that length has been gradually reducing over the last few decades due to improvements in the prevention and or management of the long-term complications, such as intestinal failure/parenteral nutrition (PN) associated liver disease and central venous catheter infections. Although length is important, it is not the only determinant of outcome in SBS. In fact, the definition of SBS is more functionally oriented, with the outcome being dependent on the amount of absorptive surface available and the efficiency of nutrient absorption. SBS can be described as a condition in which there is an insufficient functional bowel length to adequately absorb micro- and macronutrients, essential for proper growth and weight gain.

Thankfully, with a multidisciplinary team approach, excellent outcomes can be achieved for patients with SBS, allowing 80–90% of them to avoid the need for a small bowel transplant. Advances in medical management, including the development of new drugs and parenteral nutrition options, have significantly transformed the treatment landscape in recent years. Additionally, surgical management has seen improvements, with better-defined criteria for the timing and type of surgery, leading to enhanced outcomes and reduced referrals for small bowel transplant.

Overall, these progressive changes in medical and surgical interventions have contributed to reduced mortality rates, reduced duration of PN, and improved growth and overall quality of life for children living with short bowel syndrome. In this chapter, we will explore the various aspects of SBS, including its etiology, diagnosis, management, and the latest therapeutic options, highlighting the collaborative efforts that have led to enhanced patient care and outcomes.

42.2 Etiology

Based on the data from the pediatric intestinal failure consortium (Fig. 42.1) causes of SBS are necrotizing enterocolitis (26%), gastroschisis (16%), intestinal atresia's (10%), volvulus (9%), combination of these diagnosis (17%) long-segment Hirschsprung disease (4%), other single or multiple diagnoses (18%).

A. Pimpalwar (✉)
Bon Secours Mercy Health Children's, Department of Pediatric Surgery, Richmond, VA, USA

© The Author(s), under exclusive license to Springer Nature Singapore Pte Ltd. 2025
S. Roy Choudhury (ed.), *Pediatric Surgery*, https://doi.org/10.1007/978-981-96-1257-4_42

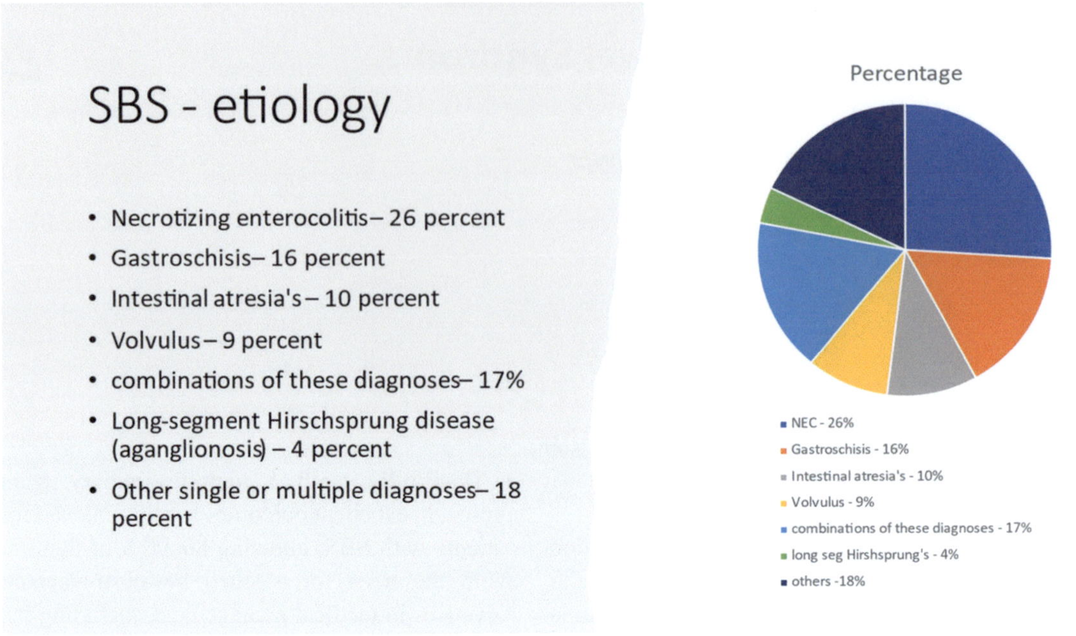

Fig. 42.1 Short bowel syndrome – etiology

42.3 Clinical Presentation of SBS

Diarrhea is often severe, watery, and may be associated with malodor. The reduced length of the small intestine limits the absorption of nutrients and fluids, contributing to increased bowel movements.

Malabsorption is due to the decreased surface area available for nutrient absorption and can manifest as failure to thrive, weight loss, and poor growth.

Abdominal Pain and Distension is due to gas and fluid accumulation.

Dehydration is due to diarrhea and malabsorption and may present with symptoms such as increased thirst, dry mouth, decreased urine output, and lethargy.

Electrolyte Imbalance is due to malabsorption of electrolytes, such as sodium, potassium, and calcium, leading to symptoms like weakness, muscle cramps, and irregular heartbeats.

Nutritional Deficiencies and delayed development are due to loss of absorptive surface and can lead to deficiencies in essential vitamins and minerals.

IFALD is due to prolonged dependence on parenteral nutrition, and this may present with jaundice, hepatomegaly, and elevated liver enzymes.

42.4 How Much Bowel Lost or Remaining

Normal bowel length depends on age. It is about 100–125 cm at 27–29 weeks of Gestation. At term it is about 150–200 cm. Less than 75 cm of bowel remaining is a risk for short bowel syndrome. If the remaining bowel is more than 38 cm, the likelihood of SBS is greater than 60%; however, if the remaining bowel is less than 15 cm, the likelihood of achieving independence from parenteral nutrition drops to 7%.

42.5 What Portion of Bowel Remaining or Lost

42.5.1 Jejunum

Jejunum with its large deep villi and digestive enzymes, serves as the primary site for intestinal absorption of fluids and macro and micronutrients. Loss of jejunum leads to a temporary reduction in the absorption of fluids and nutrients. The jejunal epithelium is leaky because of large gaps in the epithelial cells, allowing for nutrients and water to leak in either direction. However, jejunal function could be easily taken over by the ileum after jejunal loss. Jejunal adaptation mostly occurs via changes in transport protein and enzyme activity, and not by changes in absorptive surface.

42.5.2 Ileum

Ileum is responsible for multiple functions. It is responsible for a significant amount of absorption of water and electrolytes, mainly sodium and fluids secreted by the jejunum. The distal 50–60 cm of ileum serves important functions like vitamin B12, iron, and bile acid absorption. It is also responsible for the ileal brake (delay in gastric emptying due to unabsorbed lipids reaching the ileum). Ileum has a better capacity for adaptation compared to jejunum. The ileum can undergo marked adaptation after small bowel resection, with significant growth in villus surface area, as well as increase in intestinal length, diameter, and motor function. Therefore, loss of distal ileum is worse compared to jejunum.

42.5.3 Ileocecal Valve

The ileocecal valve allows the passage of contents from the ileum to the cecum and prevents backflow. This prevents bacterial overgrowth and delays the transit of contents from ileum to cecum. Loss of ileo-cecal valve is associated with increased intestinal transit and increased incidence of bacterial overgrowth. Loss of the IC valve has been shown to be associated with requiring a longer duration of weaning from PN.

42.5.4 Colon

Colon serves a very important function in children with SBS. Its absorptive capacity is huge, and it can absorb up to 6 liters of fluid every day in an adult. Hence, having a colon could be extremely useful for the prevention of water and electrolyte losses in older children with SBS, but its role is not clear in infants because of the capacity of the small bowel to adapt and take over the function of the colon in this age group. There is no evidence in the literature to suggest that the presence of colon can help weaning from total parenteral nutrition (TPN) in infants to date.

Colon propels food by mass contraction and slows down the transit, which is very helpful for patients with SBS. It can absorb complex and malabsorbed carbohydrates and short-chain fatty acids. Complex carbohydrates have a high osmotic load and can cause diarrhea and hence may not be useful in infants with SBS but could be great source of nutrition for older children and young adults. Retained colon undergoes adaptation after small bowel resection. There is a gradual increase in enterocyte mass and gut hormone-releasing cells like glucagon-like peptide-1 (GLP-1) and peptide YY.

42.5.5 Adaptation

Changes in the remaining bowel after bowel loss are called adaptation. Adaptation is essential for survival in children with SBS, and it entails microscopic and macroscopic changes in the bowel resulting in increased bowel absorptive capacity. Hyperplasia of the epithelial cells, villus lengthening, expansion in microvilli, and an increase in crypt depth are the microscopic changes, and dilatation of the bowel and an increase in length are the macroscopic changes. There is also an increase in gut hormone production and changes in the gut microbiome. The exact mechanisms of how adaptation occurs are not clear yet, but it is well known that the presence of enteral nutrients is essential for adaptation to occur. Other factors such as GI secretions, gut hormones, biochemical factors, growth factors, and genetic factors also contribute to this process. Adaptation is most prominent in the ileum and, to a lesser extent, in the jejunum and colon.

42.5.6 Stimulants for Adaptation

42.5.6.1 Nutrients

- Parenteral administration of Citrulline/arginine has been shown to enhance adaptation and their levels corelate well with the enterocyte mass.
- Enteral Long-chain triglycerides have also been shown to improve intestinal adaptation.
- Glutamine has been trialed in humans and has been found to be only moderately beneficial, but these studies additionally included growth hormone.
- Fish oils (omega-3 fatty acids): Evidence now suggests that parenteral administration of lipids derived from fish oil (Omegaven) may reduce serum bilirubin levels and reverse intestinal failure-associated liver disease, compared with conventional soy-based lipids.

42.5.6.2 Gut Hormones

- GLP2 (glucagon-like peptide) secreted by the enteroendocrine L cells located in the ileum and colon induces adaptation and absorption in animal models. Its long-acting analog, teduglutide, has been shown to improve adaptation in human trials. Treatment with teduglutide (Revestive, Gattex) was associated with a significant reduction in PN requirements compared with untreated children.
- Trials with newer long-acting GLP2 analogs (Glepaglutide, apraglutide) have shown good results in adults, but results in pediatric trials are still awaited.
- Peptide YY (PYY) has been localized to enteroendocrine cells in the mucosa of the gastrointestinal tract and is most highly concentrated in the ileum and colon. PYY is produced predominantly by L cells of the ileum and colon, where it is colocalized with enteroglucagon. PYY is also produced in other enteroendocrine cells throughout the intestine. It is responsible for delayed gastric emptying, “ileal break”.

42.6 Small Intestinal Bacterial Overgrowth (SIBO)

Loss of bowel with adaptation of the remaining bowel is the reason for developing SIBO in children with SBS. Normal intestinal diameter, motility, forward/antegrade peristalsis, with normal gastric acid secretions, pancreatic enzymes, intestinal secretions, enterocyte turnover, and the presence of IC valve are all factors responsible for the prevention of SIBO in normal children. However, in SBS, several of these factors are missing, leading to SIBO. SBS leads to loss of the ileocecal valve, dysmotility/stasis (due to dilatation, stricture formation, multiple anastomosis, and extensive adhesions), acid-suppressing medications (PPIs), and lack of enteral feedings. SIBO leads to bacterial stasis and subsequent translocation of bacteria, which increases the risk of central line infections. SIBO causes malabsorption (deconjugation of bile acids by the bacteria diminishes the intestinal absorption of monoglycerides and fatty acids, leading to steatorrhea/diarrhea and the inflammatory damage of the absorptive surface caused by bacterial overgrowth leading to protein malabsorption). SIBO-related symptoms include bloating, gassiness, abdominal distension, and foul-smelling stool or breath, endotoxemia, and vitamin B12 deficiency. SIBO leads to alteration of the normal microbiome and symptoms related to that.

42.7 Normal Microbiome Alteration in SBS, SIBO, and Subsequent Dysbiosis

The human gut microbiome refers to the complex community of microorganisms, including bacteria, viruses, fungi, and other microbes, that reside within the gastrointestinal tract of a human being. This microbiome plays a crucial role in various aspects of human health and physiology, exerting a profound influence on digestion, metabolism, immune function, and even aspects of brain function and mental health.

The gut microbiome is incredibly diverse, with thousands of different species of microorganisms present. The composition of the microbiome can vary significantly from person to person and is influenced by factors such as genetics, diet, environment, and lifestyle.

The gut microbiome serves several important functions (Fig 42.2):

1. Digestion and Nutrient Metabolism: Many microbes in the gut help break down complex carbohydrates, fiber, and other components of our diet that our own digestive enzymes cannot process. This fermentation process produces short-chain fatty acids and other metabolites that provide energy and support gut health.
2. Immune System Regulation: The gut microbiome plays a critical role in educating and regulating the immune system. It helps distinguish between harmful pathogens and beneficial microbes, ensuring that the immune system responds appropriately.
3. Protection Against Pathogens: Beneficial microbes within the gut can compete with and inhibit the growth of harmful bacteria, providing a protective barrier against potential infections.
4. Synthesis of Vitamins and Nutrients: Some gut bacteria produce vitamins, such as B vitamins and vitamin K, which are essential for human health.
5. Neurological and Mental Health Impact: Emerging research suggests a strong connection between the gut microbiome and the brain, known as the gut-brain axis. Changes in the gut microbiome have been linked to conditions like anxiety, depression, and even neurodegenerative disorders.
6. Metabolism and Weight Regulation: The composition of the gut microbiome has been associated with metabolic health and body weight. Some studies suggest that certain microbes are linked to obesity and metabolic disorders.
7. Influence on Chronic Diseases: The gut microbiome has been implicated in various chronic diseases, including inflammatory bowel diseases (IBD), autoimmune conditions, allergies, and even some types of cancer.

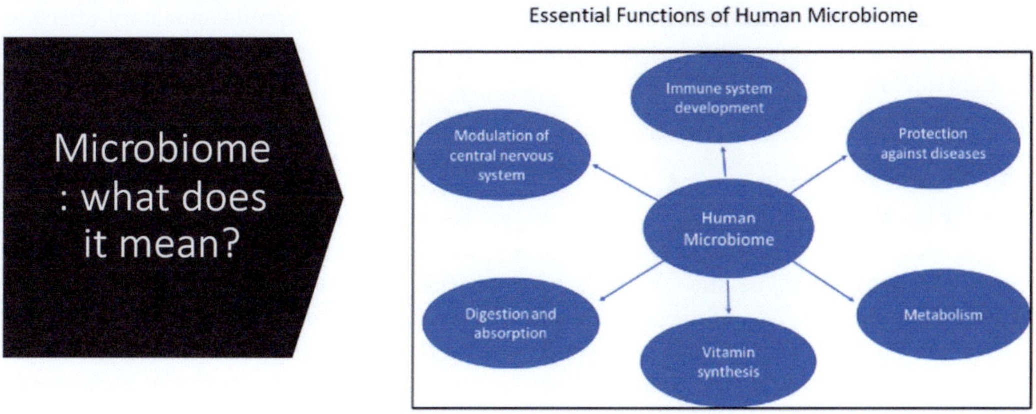

Fig. 42.2 Short bowel syndrome and Microbiome

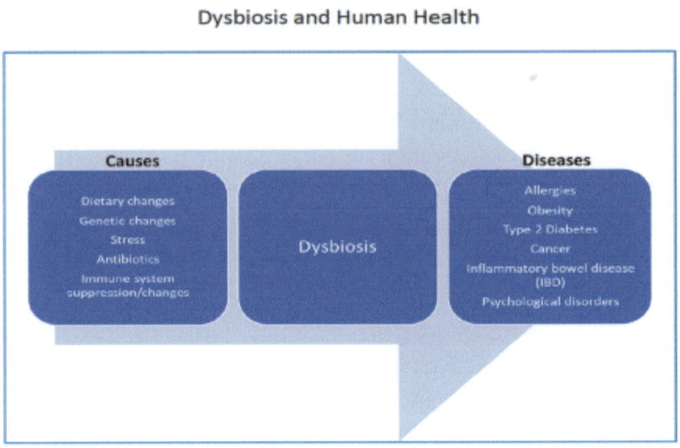

Loss of gut in patients with SBS leads to loss of microbiome. Investigation into the microbiome in SBS patients revealed a significant alteration in the composition of the microbiome. The exact structure, characterization, and anatomical location of small bowel loss hold profound implications for microbial richness and diversity. The composition and bacterial metabolites have also been shown to play a role in SBS. Abnormal bacteria proliferate due to extensive antibiotic usage. Dilation of the gut and reduced motility help the proliferation of pathogenic and harmful bacteria, leading to dysbiosis. Treatment of SIBO with antibiotics and with the replacement of non-pathogenic bacteria that compete with pathogenic bacteria seems to be the way forward. Emerging data also support the use of fecal microbiota transplant as a therapeutic. Uncovering the complex relationships between the gut microbiome, the gut-brain axis, and SBS remains a major focus and opens the potential for personalized medicine approaches based on individual gut microbiome profiles.

42.8 Medical Management (Fig. 42.3)

- **Start with central venous line.**
  Immediately after the loss of gut in an infant or a child, the first goal should be to provide adequate fluids, electrolytes, and nutrition through a central venous line. A tunneled central line or a PICC line is both a good option. The PN catheter should always be managed with a strict aseptic technique by experienced clinicians or carefully trained caregivers. When catheter-related or other infections are suspected, they should be identified and treated promptly. Antibiotic and ethanol locks may be helpful in treating catheter-related sepsis.
- **Total parenteral nutrition (TPN)**
  Parenteral nutrition should be planned by the nutritionist and the gastroenterologist on the team. A balanced TPN with regular monitoring of electrolytes and carbohydrate levels is essential for good outcomes. Long-term intralipids are associated with IFALD (intestinal failure-associated liver disease). Accumulating evidence suggests that soy-based lipid emulsions are important contributors to the pathogenesis of IFALD. Soy-based lipid emulsions may cause liver injury because excessive omega-6 fatty acids have proinflammatory effects and impair triglyceride export. Hepatoprotective lipids like fish oil-based lipids (Omegaven) monotherapy or the newer mixed lipid emulsions (SMOF lipids: Soy, Medium chain triglycerides, Olive oil, Fish oil-based lipids) have been useful in preventing IFALD in many children with SBS because they have omega-3 fatty acids which are anti-inflammatory and have insulin-sensitizing effects, acting through the GPR120 receptor. Studies in infants demonstrate a reversal of IFALD after changing from soy-based to fish oil-based fat emulsions. There are several other causes of IFALD in children

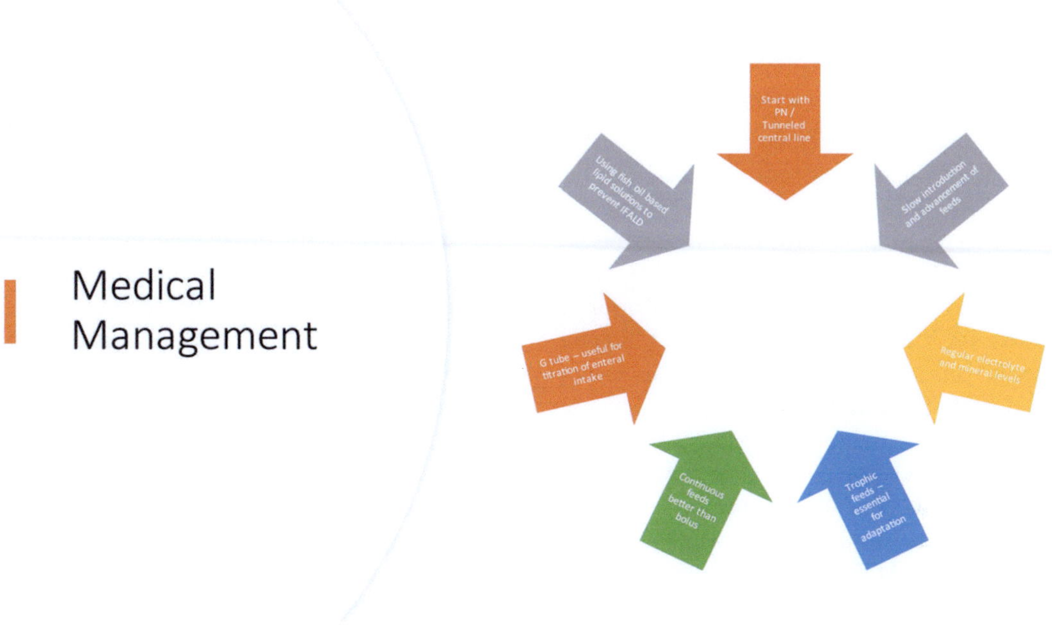

Fig. 42.3 Medical management of SBS

with SBS. The more significant of those are immaturity of the liver in premature babies, central line infection, bacterial translocation, SIBO, alteration of the microbiome and dysbiosis, mediators of inflammation like cytokines, nutrient deficiencies, and trace element excess.

- **Fluid Management**
  Significant fluid depletion resulting from gastric or proximal small bowel secretions is frequently observed in the initial phase. Consequently, patients necessitate robust fluid with electrolyte replenishment comprising sodium, potassium, chloride, and magnesium.

  Measurement and restitution of fluid and electrolyte losses through an enterostomy or in fecal matter are imperative. For the most part, sustained fluid replacement can be efficiently achieved via parenteral nutrition (PN), utilizing a customized solution tailored to the patient's specific fluid and electrolyte requisites. Instances of sudden escalation in enteral losses may demand immediate replenishment. This procedure ought to be carried out using a distinct solution apart from the PN setup to ensure timely and accurate compensation for the losses.

  In cases of high-output ostomy or substantial stool losses, appropriately formulated oral rehydration solutions can be integrated as a supplement to human milk or formula feeds. These solutions typically encompass a well-designed amalgamation of water, electrolytes, and carbohydrates aimed at offsetting the losses incurred due to diarrhea.
- **Treatment of Gastric Hypersecretion**
  Gastric hypersecretion is known after major bowel loss. There is increased gastric acid secretion due to hypergastrinemia. This reduces pH below the optimal level needed for fat absorption (by inactivating pancreatic lipase and deconjugating bile salts), increases intestinal fluid losses, and alters enteral drug absorption. Treated with H2 receptor blockers first and proton pump inhibitors later if adequate control of acid level is not attained by H2 receptor blockers. The gastric hypersecretion typically resolves during the first few months after surgery, and weaning of the acid-

suppressing medications should be attempted a few months after the intestinal resection.

- **Enteral Nutrition**
  Enteral nutrition should be introduced slowly with gradual advancement of enteral feeds. Should be started as soon as possible after bowel loss or resection, once bowel function is confirmed postoperatively. Enteral nutrients are essential for the process of adaptation; without them, the intestine undergoes mucosal atrophy. Even small amounts of feeds called "trophic feeds" are useful to prevent mucosal atrophy and help stimulate the process of adaptation. Human milk is the best for an infant and should be the first choice unless it is not available. Human milk (HM)has several factors and immunoglobulins that help adaptation, reduce the risk of IFALD, and improve mucosal barrier function due to its hypoallergenic nature. Broken down amino acid-based formulas can be used as an alternative to HM when HM is not available or is not tolerated. For later childhood, protein mixed food formulas may be used. NG tubes or gastrostomy tubes are useful for better titration of the diet. Continuous feeds are better than bolus feeds because of the limited absorptive capacity in SBS patients. Oral feeds should not be completely discontinued to prevent oral aversion. The enteral feeds should be gradually advanced and the PN should be gradually reduced keeping the fluid balance in mind. Daily fluid losses from the ostomy less than 2–3 ml/kg/hr or stools less than 20–30 ml/kg/day are acceptable (threshold for enteral tolerance), and enteral feeds could continue to be advanced. Nutrient/carbohydrate requirements could be monitored using the growth as measured by height and weight. Less than 1% reduction in substances in the ostomy or stool output is acceptable, but anything more than that is a "no" for enteral feed advancement. Once the patient is receiving half the energy requirement through enteral feeds, bolus feeds should be tried. Bolus feeds lead to better markers of adaptation compared to continuous feeds. A combination of daytime boluses and night-time continuous feeds is usually successful.

42.9 Medications Useful in SBS

- **Supplements (Minerals and Vitamins)** are needed because of unpredictable absorption from the remnant bowel. These are routinely included in the TPN but are needed separately once they are weaned from the TPN. Vitamin B12 is needed for distal ileal loss. Routine administration of all fat-soluble vitamins needed, as bile acids are lost due to altered bile acid recycling and fat absorption, along with the absorption of fat-soluble vitamins, is altered. Even though energy and growth are normal, micronutrient deficiency may occur in SBS, and this needs to be monitored and replaced.
- **Acid suppression** is needed in the initial management of SBS as there is hypersecretion of acid due to gastrin release. Refer to the gastric hypersecretion section above.
- **Reduction of transit time** is useful in patients with SBS due to inadequate time for absorption as a result of reduced length of the gut. Medications that reduce the transit time and provide more time for absorption are therefore used in SBS patients.
  - **Loperamide** acts directly on circular and longitudinal intestinal muscles, through the opioid receptor, to inhibit peristalsis and prolong transit time; reduces fecal volume, increases viscosity, and diminishes fluid and electrolyte loss; demonstrates antisecretory activity. Loperamide increases tone on the anal sphincter. It is to be used with caution in SBS as it may lead to bacterial stasis and SIBO.
  - **Cholestyramine** is a bile acid chelating agent and is useful in bile acid-related diarrhea.
  - **Octreotide** may be useful in children with excessive diarrhea uncontrolled by the above medications.
- **Adaptation stimulants,** GLP2 analogs like teduglutide, and others are useful for the stimulation of adaptation. Teduglutide has been approved by the FDA for children >1 years of age to promote adaptation in children with

major bowel loss and who remain on TPN for more than 1 year. Refer to the "Adaptation" section.

42.10 Role of Multidisciplinary Bowel Rehabilitation Program

The advantages of incorporating small bowel syndrome (SBS) management within an intestinal rehabilitation program have been substantiated through a plethora of reports. These specialized programs bring together a diverse team of experts within a dedicated center that focuses on SBS, aiming to optimize the administration of enteral feeding, gradual transition away from parenteral nutrition (PN), and the judicious application of pharmacotherapy and surgical interventions. This comprehensive approach is closely linked to enhanced survival rates and the attainment of independence from PN reliance. Clinical directives put forth by the American Society for Parenteral and Enteral Nutrition underline the convincing enhancement in survival for patients under the care of multidisciplinary teams.

42.11 Indications for Bowel Lengthening (BL)

- The decision to pursue bowel lengthening is tailored to each patient's unique circumstances and needs.
- Bowel lengthening criteria are patient-specific and not standardized.
- Bowel lengthening becomes a consideration when enteral autonomy cannot be achieved after conventional medical and nutritional interventions have been exhausted, preferably under the guidance of an established intestinal rehabilitation program.
- In cases where continued total parenteral nutrition (TPN) poses a risk of intestinal failure-associated liver disease (IFALD), BL may be indicated. A prerequisite for bowel lengthening is a bowel diameter equal to or exceeding 4 cm.
- Bowel lengthening may be considered if a child is on full enteral feeds but experiences recurrent small intestinal bacterial overgrowth (SIBO) due to bowel dilation.
- BL should only be done when adequate post-procedure length can be anticipated after AIRS.
- BL is also indicated in babies with congenital intestinal atresia with dilated proximal bowel and a marginal intestinal length.

42.12 Autologous Intestinal Reconstructive Surgery (AIRS)

Involves reconstruction of autologous bowel to increase absorptive surface and improve motility. In the pediatric population, the minimum amount of bowel necessary for nutritional autonomy is a small bowel residual length greater than 25% of the expected for gestational age. There are different ways of achieving this, and all the historic and presently used (in bold letters and underlined) techniques are mentioned below:

- Delaying transit time to improve absorption. (Historical procedures from 1970 to 1985.)
  - Recirculating loop
  - Intestinal pouch
  - Intestinal valves
  - Reversed or anti-peristaltic segments
  - Colonic interposition
- Tapering procedures
  - Tapering
  - Plication
- SB lengthening procedures
  - <u>**Longitudinal intestinal lengthening and tailoring (LILT)**</u>
  - <u>**Serial transverse enteroplasty (STEP)**</u>
  - Spiral intestinal lengthening and tailoring
  - Kimura bowel elongation technique
  - Bianchi composite ileo-colic loops (experimental)

- Small bowel expansion (tissue expansion approach)
  - Intentional SB expansion/distention and delayed correction
  - Controlled Tissue Expansion by formation of an obstructing Nipple valve
  - Controlled Tissue Expansion using occlusion tube jejunostomy
- Duodenal lengthening procedures
  - Serial transverse duodenoplasty
  - Transverse flap duodenoplasty

Of all the procedures mentioned above, lengthening is the most used technique, and we shall discuss the different lengthening techniques below.

42.13 Surgical Bowel Lengthening

- Serial transverse enteroplasty (STEP)
  Of the different lengthening techniques, STEP is the commonly used technique due to its simplicity and reproducibility. STEP procedure increases bowel length, increases absorptive capacity by increasing transit time, and prevents SIBO by reducing dilatation and improving motility. The more the dilation, the greater the length that can be obtained as compared to LILT, where the length can only be doubled. It can be done on variable bowel diameters and can be done after a previous LILT or STEP. STEP procedure does not require any bowel anastomoses. Endo-GIA stapler is applied sequentially, from alternating and opposite directions, in a transverse, partially overlapping fashion, creating a zigzag-like channel of approximately 2 to 2.5 cm in diameter. This requires the creation of a mesenteric defect at each staple line. The staplers were placed from the 90° and 270° positions (Figs. 42.4a, b, c). STEP improves nutritional status, limits bacterial proliferation, and promotes weight gain.

A large meta-analysis on STEP procedure by A. Lauro et al. included 16 studies with a total of 180 pediatric patients. The average age was 2 months to 5 years. The median length of the small bowel remnant was between 18 and 29 cm, with a range from 10 to 145 cm. The pre-STEP length was, and pre-STEP diameter was 4–6 cm and the increase in SB length achieved post STEP was 42–100% over a median follow up of 5 months to 3.9 years. Thirty-two percent of patients achieved enteral autonomy, re-STEP was needed in 17%, mortality was 5.5%, and only 6% patients were referred for SB transplant. As seen from the above data; the STEP procedure represents an essential therapeutic option in SBS cases, and it produces excellent results in terms of enteral autonomy when associated with Intestinal Rehabilitation Programs (IRP).

- **Bianchi procedure/LILT**
  Bianchi in the early 1980s proposed intestinal lengthening; this technique divides the dilated small intestine longitudinally, reconstructs the split intestine into two equal narrow tubes, and re-anastomoses these tubes in continuity to double the length of the bowel. This procedure reduces the bowel diameter and improves absorption, but involves several anastomoses and has a risk of compromising the blood supply. This procedure, once done, cannot be repeated, unlike the STEP procedure. A large study over 20 years included 19 patients who underwent this procedure. Sixteen were weaned off TPN, but only eight responded to LILT, (Fig. 42.5) and the other eight still needed SBT.

Spiral Intestinal Lengthening and Tailoring (SILT)

SILT is a relatively new technique described in 2011, but only a few papers have been published showing the use of this technique. In SILT, the mesentery is carefully incised without damaging the vessels and then the intestine is spirally cut, stretched over a tube, and closed increasing its length and reducing its luminal diameter.

Advantages of SILT:

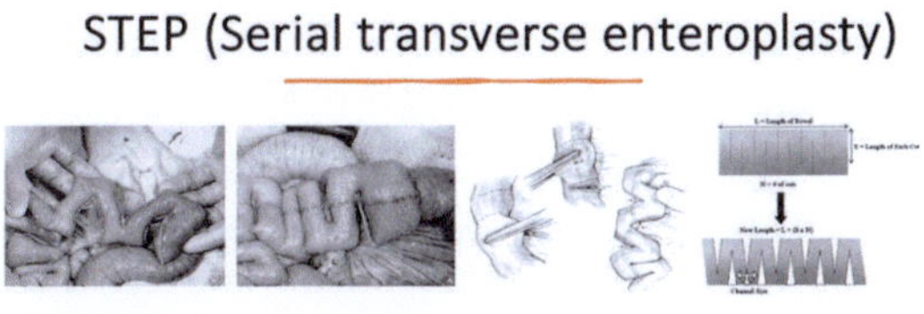

Fig. 42.4a STEP Technique

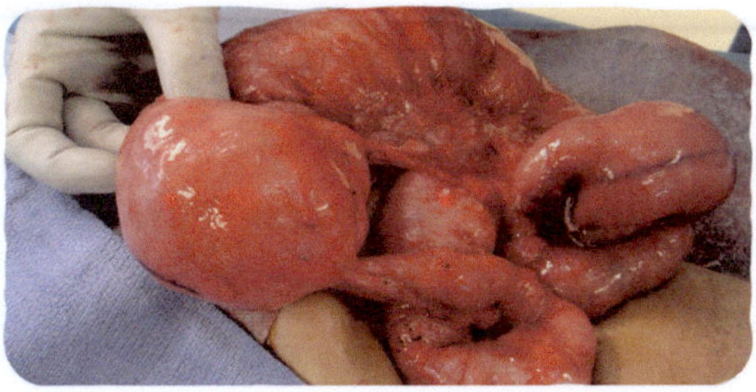

Fig. 42.4b Dilated bowel before STEP

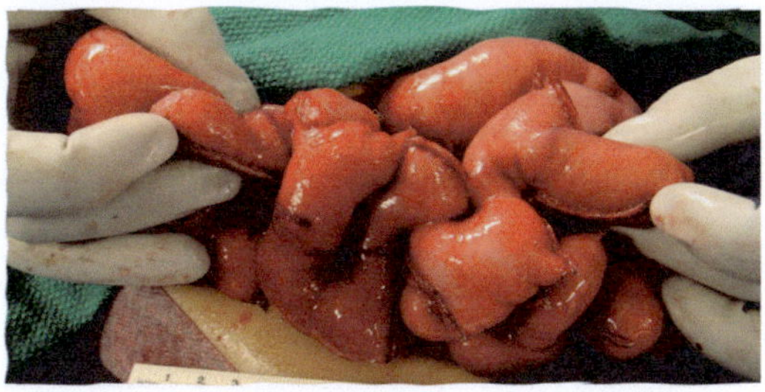

Fig. 42.4c Completed STEP

It can be performed even if the bowel is less dilated (<4 cm).

It does not alter the orientation of the muscle fibers. This prevents re-dilation of the bowel.

Mesenteric damage is minimal.

Disadvantage:

Bowel must be opened, increasing the risk of contamination and sepsis.

In a clinical study of five children who were operated on 5 years ago, reported by Coletta et al. The median increase in small bowel length with SILT was 56%, with a 50% decrease in diameter. In two of their patients, SILT was combined with duodenal was tailored with antimesenteric stapling, and in one other patient, SILT of a less dilated distal jejunum was combined with STEP of the proximally more dilated jejunum. There were no major complications like leakage, necrosis, fistula, obstruction, or intra-abdominal abscess. Median TPN requirement decreased from seven nights per week to four nights. Liver function was not much altered, and the weight increased in all.

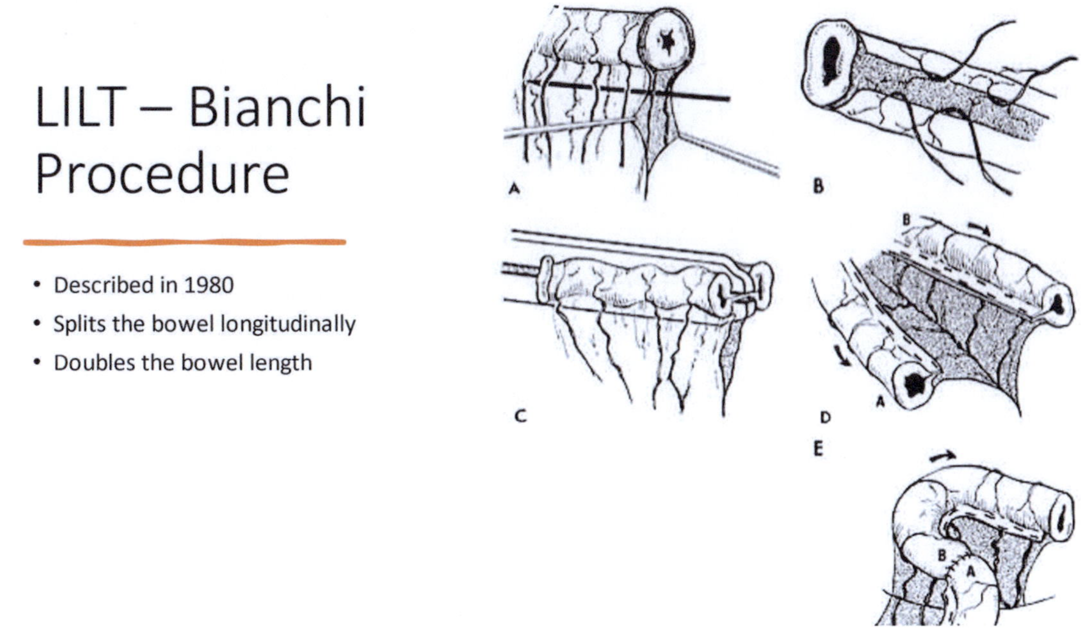

Fig. 42.5 Bianchi procedure

SILT is a good alternative for bowel lengthening in children with SBS and can be combined with other techniques to provide maximal benefits.

- **Experimental Techniques**
  - Distraction enterogenesis (Fig. 42.6 a, b)
    Distraction device is used for the elongation of isolated bowel segments. Significant increase in length, mucosal mass, and epithelial proliferation was achieved using these techniques, but they are still in experimental stages.
  - Tissue Engineering
    The primary role of tissue engineering in SBS is to develop strategies to restore or replace the damaged or missing intestinal tissue.

    Intestinal *Tissue Regeneration* aims to create functional intestinal tissue to replace or supplement the insufficient or damaged portion of the small intestine. This can involve the use of various approaches, such as scaffolds, cells, and growth factors, to encourage the growth and differentiation of intestinal tissue. Engineers design biocompatible *scaffolds* that mimic the structure and mechanical properties of the native small intestine. These scaffolds can provide structural support for cell growth, guide tissue regeneration, and facilitate nutrient absorption. *Stem cells* or other appropriate cell sources are used to populate the scaffolds. These cells can be differentiated into various cell types found in the small intestine, including enterocytes, goblet cells, and Paneth cells, to promote functional tissue formation. *Adequate blood supply (vascularization)* is crucial for tissue survival and function. Tissue engineering approaches also focus on promoting the formation of blood vessels within the regenerated tissue to ensure proper oxygen and nutrient delivery. Once ready, these constructs are *rigorously tested* to ensure they exhibit normal intestinal functions, including peristalsis, nutrient absorption, and barrier function. In vitro and in vivo studies are conducted to assess their efficacy. Once tissue-engineered constructs are successfully developed and validated, they can be *transplanted* into

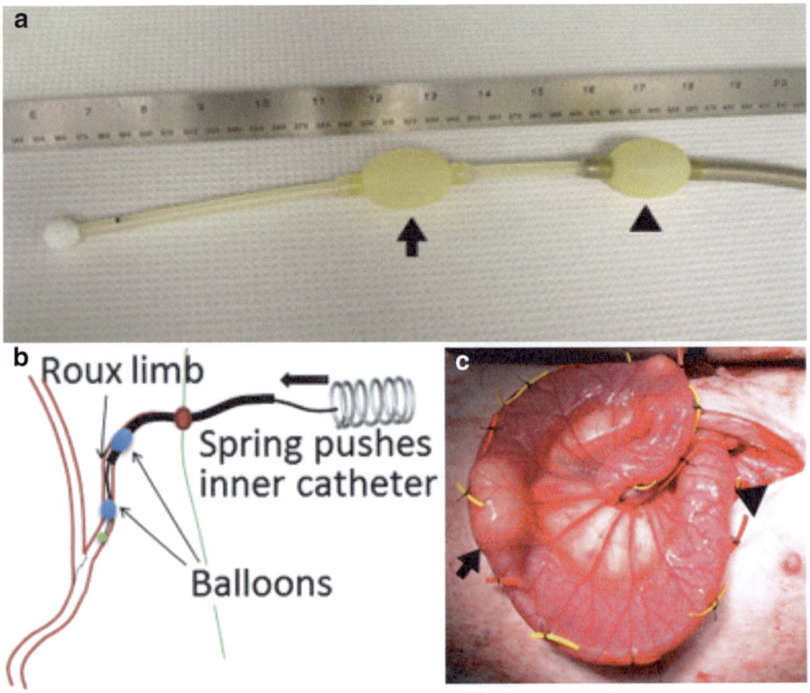

Fig. 42.6a Distraction using balloon and springs

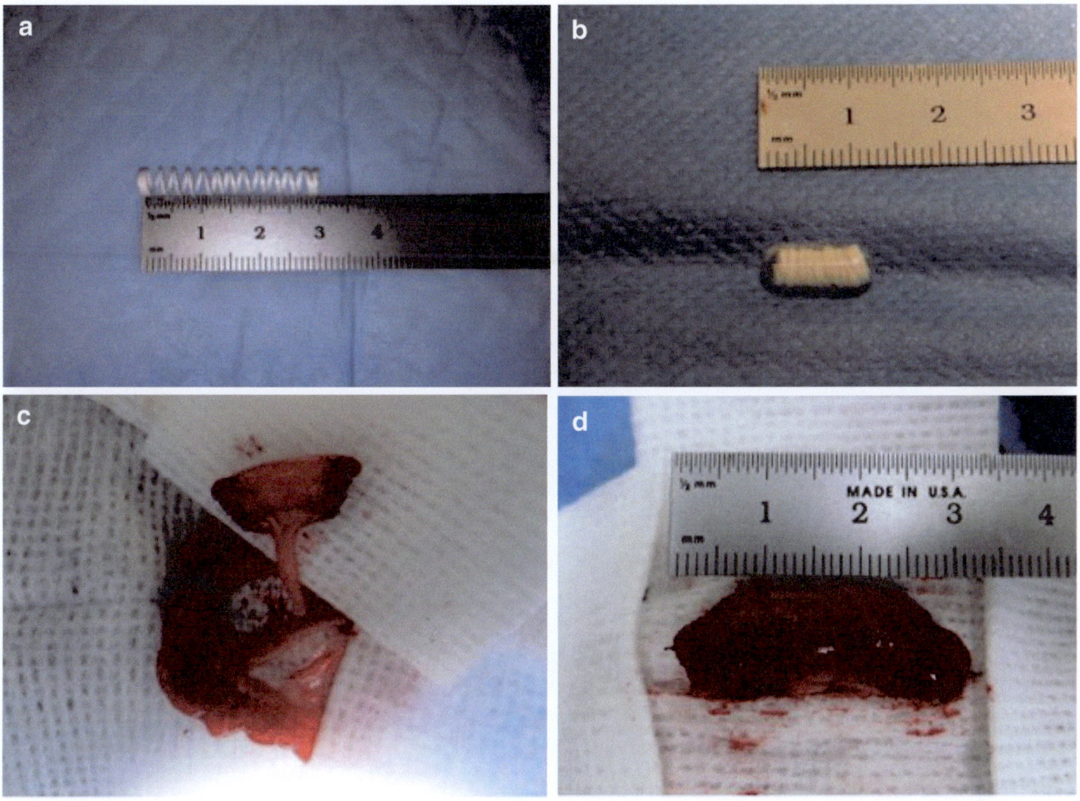

Fig. 42.6b Capsule has the spring, and the spring gets deployed within the bowel segment, causing distraction pressure and elongation

patients with SBS to augment their intestinal function.

Patient-specific tissue engineering strategies to the specific needs of individual patients may involve using the patient's own cells to minimize the risk of rejection. Small Intestinal organoids (Fig. 42.7) isolated from the host intestine are loaded onto scaffolds and are implanted in the host omentum. Tissue-engineered small intestine (TESI), three times the implanted size, can be obtained using human organoids. This is a major advance for kids with SBS.

It's important to note that while tissue engineering holds promise for treating SBS, there are still many challenges to overcome. These include ensuring the long-term functionality and safety of tissue-engineered constructs, addressing immune rejection issues, and optimizing the scalability and cost-effectiveness of these treatments. Research in tissue engineering for SBS is ongoing, and its clinical application is evolving.

42.14 Small Bowel Transplant

The number of children with SBS needing SBT has gone down significantly. Improvement of care due to specialized multidisciplinary programs which bring together a diverse team of experts within a dedicated center that focuses on SBS, aiming to optimize the administration of enteral feeding, gradual transition away from parenteral nutrition (PN), and the judicious application of pharmacotherapy and surgical interventions have significantly reduced the need for SBT. Indications for transplantation include children with severe IFALD, no available central venous access, and central venous line associated

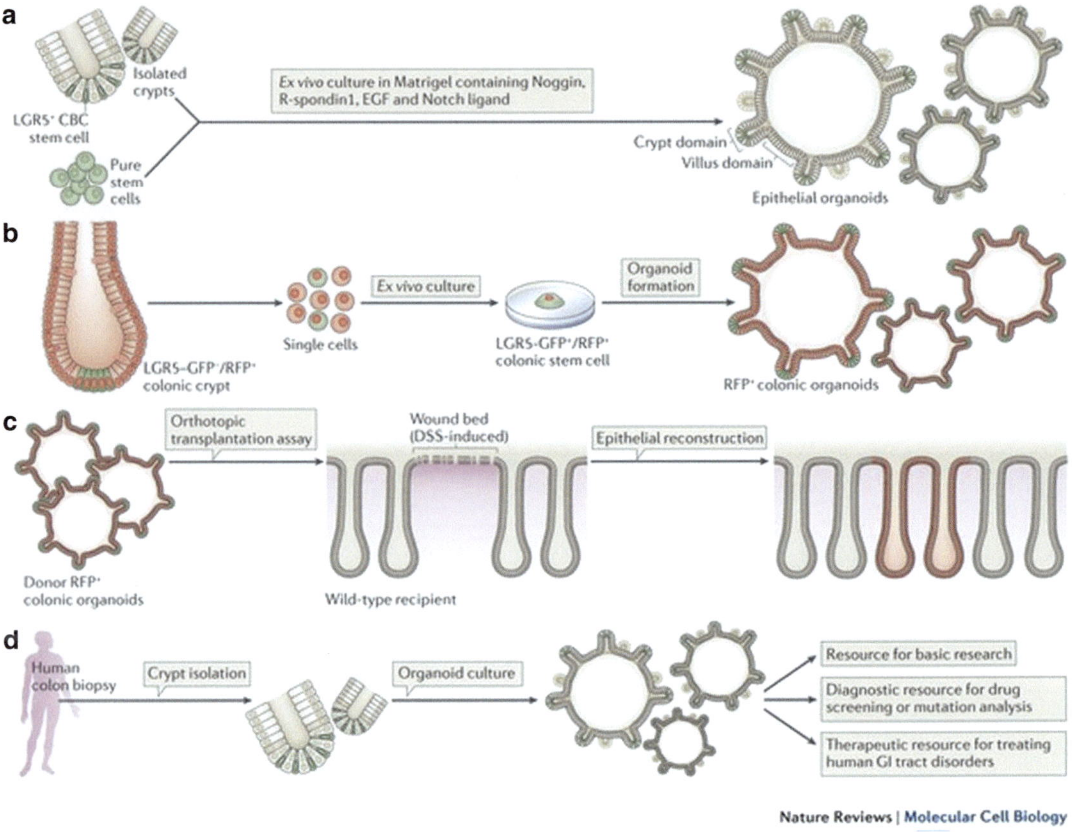

Fig. 42.7 Human organoids on scaffolds for TESI

with multiple life-threatening blood stream infections. Children who do not wish to lead a life dependent on TPN are also candidates for liver and small bowel transplant.

Summary

1. **Short Bowel Syndrome Overview:**
   - SBS is a condition resulting from the loss of gut tissue, either mechanically or functionally, leading to altered functions and nutritional deficiencies.
   - The length of the remaining gut, although crucial, is not the sole determinant of outcomes. Functional considerations include the amount of absorptive surface and nutrient absorption efficiency.
2. **Multidisciplinary Management:**
   - A collaborative, multidisciplinary approach is essential for the effective management of SBS.
   - Advances in medical and surgical interventions, including new drugs and parenteral nutrition options, have significantly improved treatment outcomes.

   - Surgical criteria for timing and type have been refined, reducing referrals for small bowel transplants.
3. **Etiology and Clinical Presentation:**
   - Common causes of SBS include necrotizing enterocolitis, gastroschisis, intestinal atresias, volvulus, and Hirschsprung disease.

- Clinical presentation includes severe diarrhea, malabsorption leading to failure to thrive, abdominal pain/distension, dehydration, electrolyte imbalance, nutritional deficiencies, delayed development, and intestinal failure-associated liver disease (IFALD).

4. **Bowel Length and Portion:**
    - The normal bowel length varies with age, and less than 75 cm remaining bowel poses a risk for SBS.
    - The likelihood of SBS increases with less than 38 cm remaining bowel, and less than 15 cm dramatically reduces the chance of independence from parenteral nutrition.
5. **Bowel Portion and Adaptation:**
    - Different portions of the bowel have distinct functions and adaptation capabilities.
    - Nutrient administration, including citrulline/arginine, long-chain triglycerides, and fish oils, stimulates adaptation.
    - Gut hormones like GLP2 and PYY play a role in adaptation, with GLP2 analogs showing promise in reducing PN requirements.
    - Small intestinal bacterial overgrowth (SIBO) is common in SBS, contributing to malabsorption, altered microbiome, and dysbiosis.
6. **Medical Management:**
    - **Central Venous Line:** Immediate use for fluid, electrolyte, and nutrition after gut loss.
    - **Total Parenteral Nutrition (TPN):** Balanced TPN with monitoring; consider fish oil-based lipids to prevent IFALD.
    - **Fluid Management:** Address significant fluid depletion with robust fluid and electrolyte replenishment; consider oral rehydration solutions.
    - **Treatment of Gastric Hypersecretion:** Addressed with H2 receptor blockers and proton pump inhibitors; wean off after surgery.
    - **Enteral Nutrition:** Gradual introduction, starting with trophic feeds; consider human milk for infants; advance gradually while monitoring fluid balance.
7. **Medications Useful in SBS:**
    - **Supplements:** Needed due to unpredictable absorption; routine administration in TPN; monitor and replace after weaning.
    - **Acid Suppression:** Needed initially; manage gastric hypersecretion.
    - **Reduction of Transit Time:** Use medications like loperamide, cholestyramine, and octreotide; cautious use in preventing bacterial stasis.
    - **Adaptation Stimulants:** GLP2 analogs like teduglutide are used for stimulation of adaptation.
8. **Multidisciplinary Bowel Rehabilitation Program:**
    - Specialized programs for SBS management enhance survival, optimize enteral feeding, and transition from parenteral nutrition with a comprehensive approach.
    - Collaboration among experts in nutrition, gastroenterology, and surgery contributes to improved patient outcomes.
9. **Indications for Bowel Lengthening (BL):**
    - Patient-specific criteria for pursuing BL, considering factors like enteral autonomy, TPN-associated risks, and recurrent SIBO.
    - BL may be indicated when TPN poses risks, and the bowel diameter exceeds 4 cm.
10. **Autologous Intestinal Reconstructive Surgery (AIRS):**
    - **Surgical Bowel Lengthening:** Procedures like serial transverse enteroplasty (STEP), Bianchi procedure/LILT, and spiral intestinal lengthening and tailoring (SILT) increase bowel length.
    - **Experimental Techniques:** Distraction enterogenesis and tissue engineering explore novel approaches.
    - **Challenges in Tissue Engineering:** Despite promising results, challenges include long-term functionality, immune rejection, and scalability.

11. **Small Bowel Transplant:**
    - **Reduced Need:** Specialized programs and multidisciplinary care have significantly reduced the need for small bowel transplant.
    - **Indications:** Severe IFALD, no central venous access, multiple life-threatening infections, and patient preference for independence from TPN.

Suggested Reading

Chan CF, Wu TC. Recent advances in the management of pediatric intestinal failure. Pediatr Neonatol. 2014;55:426.

Gura KM, Calkins KL, Puder M. Use of fish oil intravenous lipid emulsions as monotherapy in the pediatric intestinal failure patient: beyond the package insert. Nutr Clin Pract. 2020;35:108.

Lacaille F, Gupte G, Colomb V, et al. Intestinal failure-associated liver disease: a position paper of the ESPGHAN Working Group of Intestinal Failure and Intestinal Transplantation. J Pediatr Gastroenterol Nutr. 2015;60:272.

Merritt RJ, Cohran V, Raphael BP, et al. Intestinal rehabilitation programs in the management of pediatric intestinal failure and short bowel syndrome. J Pediatr Gastroenterol Nutr. 2017;65:588.

Modi BP, Langer M, Duggan C, Kim HB, Jaksic T. Serial transverse enteroplasty for management of refractory D-lactic acidosis in short-bowel syndrome. J Pediatr Gastroenterol Nutr. 2006;43:395–7. https://doi.org/10.1097/01.mpg.0000228116.52229.7b.

Pierret ACS, Wilkinson JT, Zilbauer M, Mann JP. Clinical outcomes in pediatric intestinal failure: a meta-analysis and meta-regression. Am J Clin Nutr. 2019;110:430.

Ramos Boluda E, Redecillas Ferreiro S, Manrique Moral O, et al. Experience With teduglutide in pediatric short bowel syndrome: first real-life data. J Pediatr Gastroenterol Nutr. 2020;71:734.

Stanger JD, Oliveira C, Blackmore C, et al. The impact of multi-disciplinary intestinal rehabilitation programs on the outcome of pediatric patients with intestinal failure: a systematic review and meta-analysis. J Pediatr Surg. 2013;48:983.

Meckel Diverticulum, Duplications, and Mesenteric Cysts

43

T. K. Jayakumar, Revathy Menon, and Rahul Saxena

43.1 Meckel Diverticulum

43.1.1 Introduction

Meckel diverticulum is a true diverticulum, i.e., it contains all three layers of the bowel wall and is usually present in the ileum. It was first reported by Hildanus (1598), and the embryology and pathology were described by Johann Frederick Meckel (1809) and Daniels (2000).

43.1.2 Embryology

During embryonic life, the terminal small bowel is connected to the yolk sac via the vitello-intestinal duct also called the omphalo-mesenteric duct, for nutrition. This duct is obliterated by five to nine weeks of gestation, and the placenta provides the nutrition. Meckel diverticulum is the commonest (90%) remnant structure of the vitello-intestinal duct. Other types of remnants like patent vitello-intestinal duct with umbilico-ileal fistula, cyst, and fibrous cord/band are rarer (see Chap. 31).

43.1.3 Epidemiology

The classical teaching about the rule of twos only gives a smaller picture: affects 2% of the population (up to 4% are symptomatic), is 2 inches long, age of presentation at 2 years (about 50% are operated under 4 years of age), 2 times more common in boys (reported range is two to five times), 2 types of heterotopic mucosa (gastric and pancreatic), and are situated 2 feet from the ileocecal valve (location varies with age; mean distance 34 cm at 2 years, compared to 67 cm at 21 years).

43.1.4 Pathology

The diverticulum sometimes has a blood supply of its own. The morphology can vary from long to short length and narrow to broad base (Fig. 43.1a–c). The diverticulum contains normal ileal mucosa in most cases, while heterotopic mucosa is seen in up to 60% of the cases (Fig. 43.2). The gastric mucosa is the most common one among symptomatic cases. Other het-

T. K. Jayakumar · R. Menon · R. Saxena (✉)
Department of Pediatric Surgery, All India Institute of Medical Sciences, Jodhpur, India

© The Author(s), under exclusive license to Springer Nature Singapore Pte Ltd. 2025

S. Roy Choudhury (ed.), *Pediatric Surgery*, https://doi.org/10.1007/978-981-96-1257-4_43

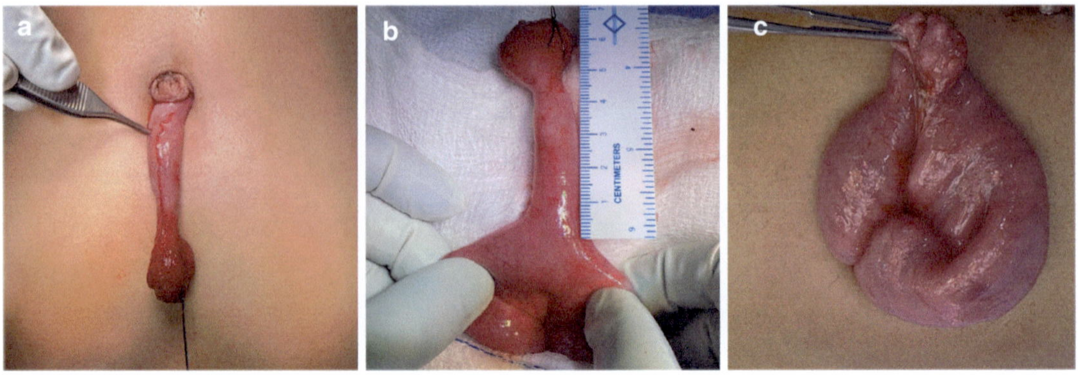

Fig. 43.1 (**a**) Meckel diverticulum (with its blood supply) delivered via the supraumbilical port incision during laparoscopy. (**b**, **c**) Different morphologies of the diverticulum (long and narrow base, short and broad base)

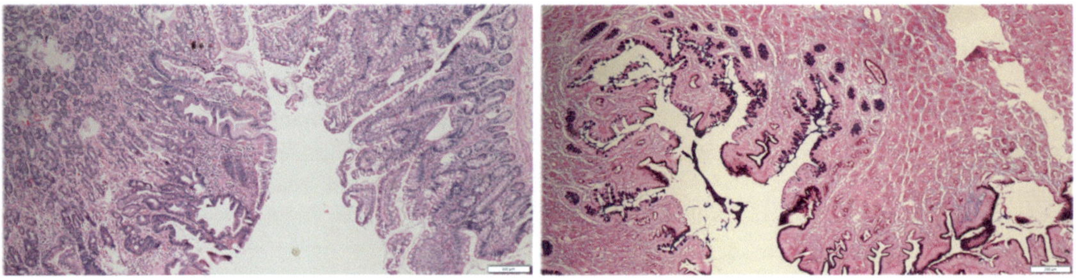

Fig. 43.2 Meckel diverticulum with gastric metaplasia [H&E 4x]. The Alcian blue–PAS stain highlights neutral mucin in gastric glands (pink) and acidic mucin in intestinal epithelium (blue). [ABPAS 4x]. (Courtesy Dr. Lavleen Singh, AIIMS, New Delhi)

erotopic tissues like pancreatic, duodenal, colonic, and endometrial are rare. It is difficult to rule out the heterotopic tissue from gross features like short or thickened diverticulum.

43.1.5 Presentation

Meckel diverticulum remains asymptomatic in most cases with a 4–6% lifetime risk of becoming symptomatic. It may be discovered incidentally at laparotomy or laparoscopy or present with symptoms of intestinal bleeding, abdominal pain, intestinal obstruction, or perforation. Children with symptomatic Meckel's present with lower gastrointestinal bleeding (40%), intestinal obstruction (30%), diverticulitis (20%), and umbilical discharge (6%). The literature from India reports intestinal obstruction as the commoner symptom compared to other Asian or Western countries where lower gastrointestinal bleeding is the commonest symptom.

- Bleeding: About 50% of children with lower gastrointestinal bleeding have Meckel diverticulum. Of those, 80% have gastric heterotopic tissue which may extend beyond the limits of the diverticulum into the adjacent ileum as well. The heterotopic gastric mucosal secretions cause ulceration and subsequently bleeding. The bleeding is usually painless, with a bright red (in severe bleeding) or maroon-colored or dark tarry blood in stools. Chronic anemia and a history of blood transfusions are frequently encountered. The risk of bleeding reduces with age as heterotopic gastric mucosa atrophies in most cases after 30 years of age.

- Intestinal obstruction: Mechanisms of obstruction are intussusception, volvulus, internal hernia, incarcerated Littre hernia, and rarely in late presentation of Meckel diverticulitis. Meckel diverticulum acts as a lead point and can cause ileo-ileal/ileocolic intussusception. When the intussusception is reduced, one may encounter an "inverted diverticulum" (Fig. 43.3a,b). Meckel diverticulum with a band connected to the umbilicus can act as an axis for the bowel to twist and cause volvulus (Fig. 43.4). Small bowel loops often herniate between the ileal mesentery and diverticular vessels causing internal herniation. Incarceration of Littre hernia (inguinal/femoral/umbilical) with Meckel diverticulum as content has been reported, though it does not cause obstruction. Rarely, the inflamed diverticulum can perforate and become gangrenous (Figs. 43.5 and 43.6).
- Inflammation: Patients present with features like that of acute appendicitis, like abdomen pain initially felt around the umbilicus, migrating to the right lower quadrant, nausea, vomiting, and fever. Inflammation can be attributed to heterotopic tissue or luminal obstruction due to fecal stasis, enteroliths, parasites, and foreign bodies. Finding of a normal appendix during an intended operation for appendicitis should prompt for the examination to look for the presence of a Meckel diverticulum

43.1.6 Diagnosis

Patients presenting with lower gastrointestinal bleeding must be resuscitated and investigated for the causes. Upper or lower gastrointestinal endoscopy may not identify the Meckel diverticulum but rule out other causes. Capsule endoscopy is reported to have been used for diagnosis. Meckel scan (Technetium 99m-pertechnate) is the preferred investigation, with Pentagastrin/Histamine-2 blockers for enhancement. It identifies the Meckel diverticulum only when heterotopic gastric mucosa is present (Fig. 43.7). It has high specificity but less sensitivity. Investigations like CT angiography and tagged RBC scans require active bleeding to be present for diagnosis. SPECT/CT is an upcoming investigation.

In children with no history of abdominal operations presenting with small bowel obstruction, Meckel diverticulum should be suspected. In patients presenting with abdomen pain, Meckel diverticulitis may or may not be identified on ultrasonography or CT scan. In all these scenarios, diagnostic laparoscopy has become the favored diagnostic and treatment modality. For patients undergoing laparoscopy for suspected appendicitis who are found to have a normal appendix, the small bowel must be inspected for Meckel diverticulum.

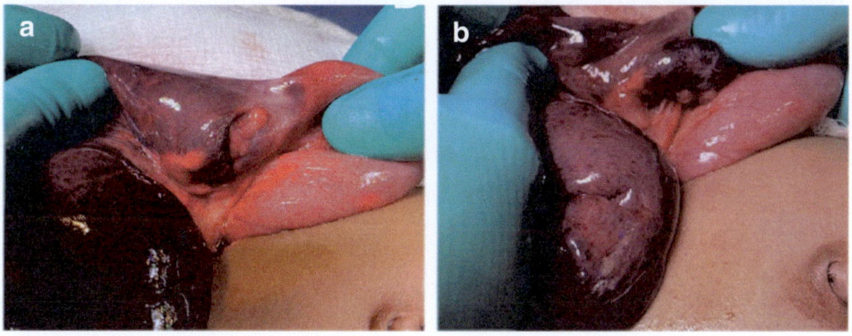

Fig. 43.3 (**a**, **b**) Before and after images of inverted Meckel diverticulum in a case of intussusception

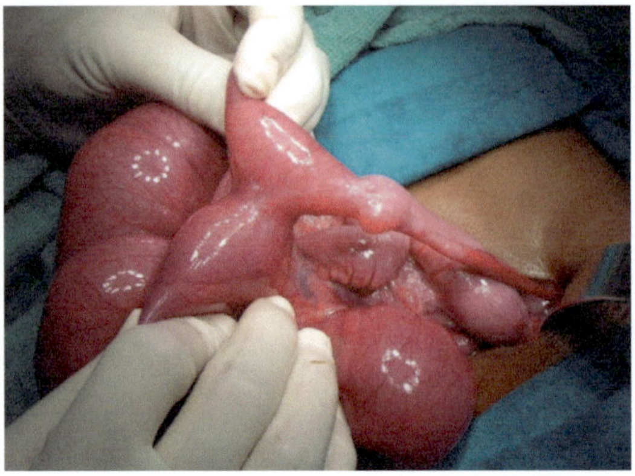

Fig. 43.4 Meckel diverticulum with band to umbilicus resulting in intestinal obstruction due to volvulus

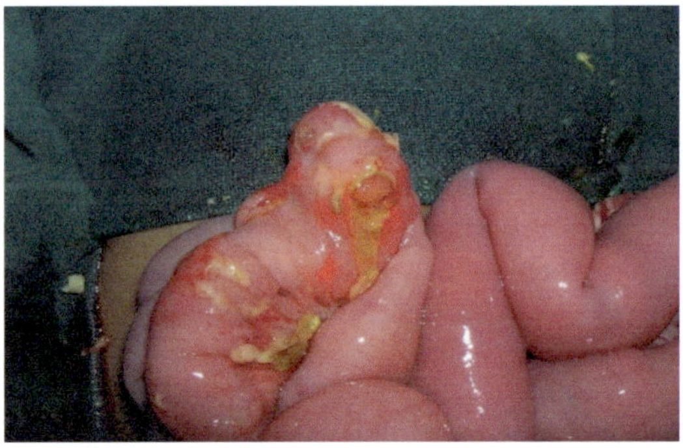

Fig. 43.5 Perforated Meckel diverticulum at open surgery

43.1.7 Treatment

Symptomatic Meckel diverticulum warrants removal. Laparoscopy followed by exteriorization of the ileal segment with Meckel diverticulum via the umbilical port incision is preferred

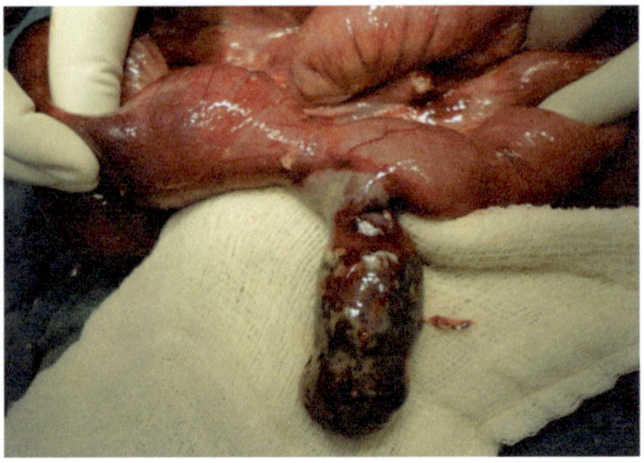

Fig. 43.6 Gangrenous Meckel diverticulum

(Figs. 43.1a–c and 43.8). Resection of the ileal segment (with Meckel diverticulum) is the safest and most definitive treatment. Alternative approaches like stapler resection of the diverticulum and wedge resection of the diverticulum are also done, but they risk leaving heterotopic tissue behind. Hence, they are best avoided when inflammation or bleeding is present. It is difficult to rule out heterotopic tissue by gross examination and requires histopathological examination.

There is no clear consensus on the treatment of incidentally detected Meckel diverticulum. Reasons for removal are the potential for the patient to become symptomatic in the future and rarely malignancy within the diverticulum. Some surgeons don't perform the resection to avoid surgical complications. Resection should be considered especially when the diverticulum is narrow mouth, thickened or connected to the umbilicus by a band, or a mesodiverticular band is present.

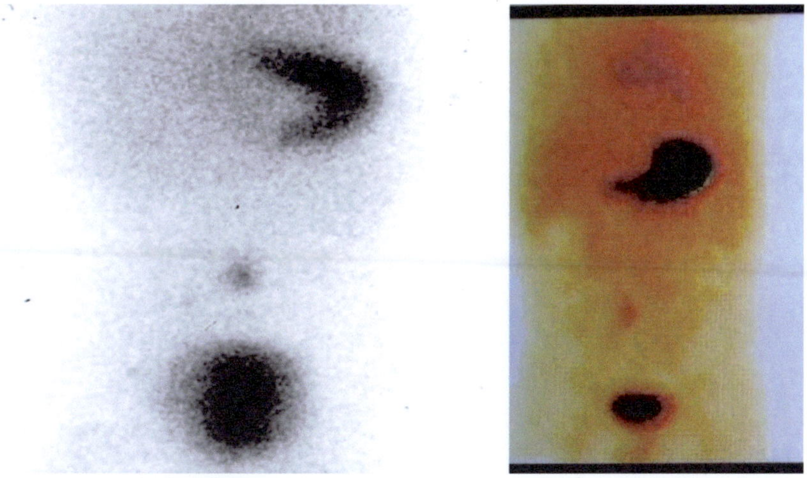

Fig. 43.7 Hot spot in nuclear scan suggestive of Meckel diverticulum

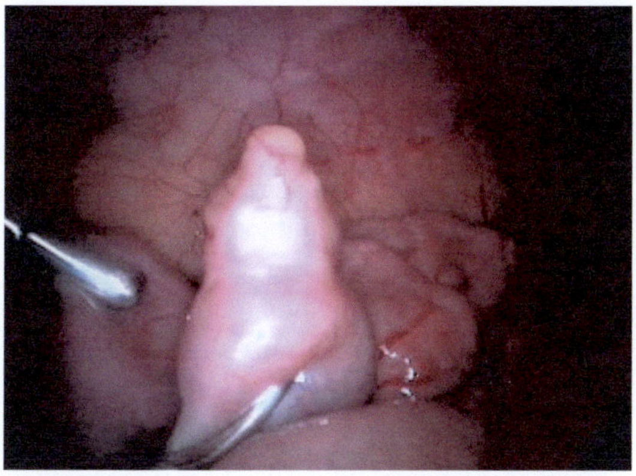

Fig. 43.8 Laparoscopic view of Meckel diverticulum

43.2 Duplications of Intestine

43.2.1 Introduction

The term duplication of the alimentary tract was first coined by William Ladd in 1937. Three common findings as described by him include (a) a well-developed smooth muscle coat, (b) an epithelial lining representing gastrointestinal mucosa, and (c) attachment to the alimentary tract. They usually present before the age of 2 years, the incidence being 1 in 4500 live births.

43.2.2 Embryology

They are associated with vertebral, spinal, and genitourinary anomalies in 20% of patients and this suggests a multifactorial process in their development.

43.2.3 Theories of Etiology

- Persistence of neuro-enteric canal
- Split notochord (gap in the notochord allows endoderm of the gut to herniate and form diverticula)
- Partial or abortive twinning
- Diverticula of the embryonic intestine and recanalization defects (all gastrointestinal organs begin as solid tubes slowly vacuolating and failure to do so results in duplications)
- Environmental factors (hypoxia, vascular accidents, trauma)

43.2.4 Pathophysiology

The distinct characteristics of duplication cysts are well-developed smooth muscle coats, epithelial lining, and attachment to the alimentary tract.

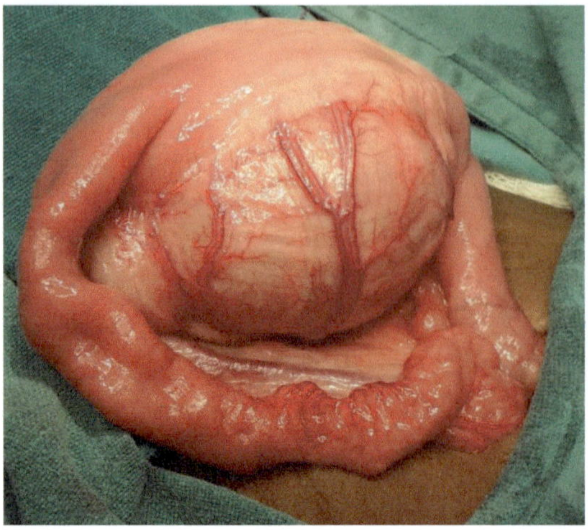

Fig. 43.9 Cystic duplication of the intestine

These duplication cysts may be found anywhere in the gastrointestinal tract from mouth to the anus, but the most common site is the ileum, jejunum, followed by the esophagus. There are two types of duplications, *cystic or tubular* (Figs. 43.9 and 43.10), of which cystic is the more common type. Cystic variants do not communicate with the gut lumen whereas tubular communicate with the gut lumen.

43.2.5 Clinical Presentation

They may be detected incidentally or manifest with symptoms such as abdominal pain, distension, obstruction, intussusception, bleeding, perforation, respiratory compromise, and painless mass. These symptoms are related to the location of the duplication, size, presence, or absence of heterotopic tissue. One-third of all duplications is seen to contain heterotopic gastric mucosa. This heterotopic tissue leads to ulceration, and bleeding, with subsequent anemia. They may even undergo malignant transformation. Those presenting with abdominal pain may be misdiagnosed with appendicitis or intestinal obstruction. Thus, duplication cysts must be considered an important differential while dealing with patients presenting with an obstruction or an abdominal lump.

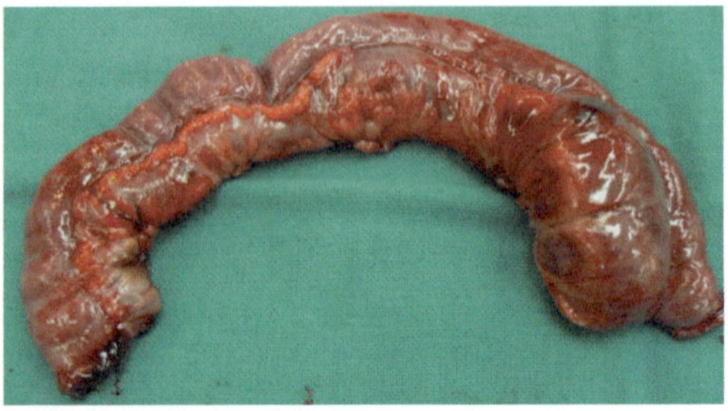

Fig. 43.10 Tubular duplication of the intestine (note double bowel with two lumens)

43.2.6 Diagnosis

- Ultrasonography may show an outer and inner tube with different echogenicity called *gut signature or double wall sign* which is useful in the diagnosis of duplication cysts.
- CECT scans and MRI scans are also very helpful in terms of preoperative planning.
- In cases of a vertebral anomaly with a duplication, an MRI is essential to rule out communication with the spinal cord.
- Contrast studies may demonstrate mass effect or communication with the alimentary tract.
- Tc-99m pertechnetate scan can detect ectopic gastric mucosa. A small bowel duplication may be mistaken for a Meckel diverticulum on Technetium Pertechnate scan.

43.2.7 Treatment

Surgical removal is the treatment of choice for duplication cysts to ensure the elimination of symptoms and avoidance of recurrence. Duplication cysts are usually benign but there is always preponderance for malignant transformation. This also necessitates surgical resection.

Since these cysts share a common blood supply with the native intestine, resection of the associated normal intestine is also usually required. Small cysts may be enucleated provided the native blood supply is left intact. For tubular duplications where resection of a large length of the bowel is anticipated, mucosal stripping through multiple enterotomies can preserve bowel length and decrease ulceration from ectopic mucosa if present.

43.2.8 Esophageal Duplication Cyst

They are the most common foregut duplication cysts and the second most common location of gastrointestinal duplication cysts after small bowel with an estimated prevalence of approximately 0.1–0.2% in the general population. Two-thirds of these lesions are found in the lower third of the esophagus and one-third is found in the upper or middle third of the esophagus. Patients may present with features of mass effect such as nonproductive cough, chest pain, and dysphagia. They are managed with thoracotomy or thoracoscopy and cyst excision.

43.2.9 Gastric Duplication Cyst

Gastric duplication cysts comprise around 4–9% of all enteric duplication cysts. These are usually solitary and do not communicate with the gastric lumen, and most are related to the greater curvature of the stomach. Patients are usually symptomatic owing to the secretory mucosal component. Management includes excision of the cyst or mucosal stripping leaving the muscular wall.

43.2.10 Small Bowel Duplication Cyst

Duodenal duplication cysts make up 2–12%, Ileal duplication cysts make up about 44%, and Jejunal duplication cysts make up about 50% of GI tract duplications. They arise from the mesenteric side. Small bowel duplications may manifest with a variety of abdominal symptoms such as pain, vomiting, and bleeding and this often leads to misdiagnosis if not evaluated properly. Laparotomy with excision of the cyst can be done but resection with end-to-end anastomosis may be required in tubular duplications or those closely associated with the bowel wall.

43.2.11 Colonic Duplication Cyst

It has an incidence of about 13%. Patients with colonic duplications can present at any age but up to 80% of patients do so within 2 years of age (Fig. 43.11a–d). Long tubular colonic duplications can be managed by connecting to the normal colon both proximally and distally.

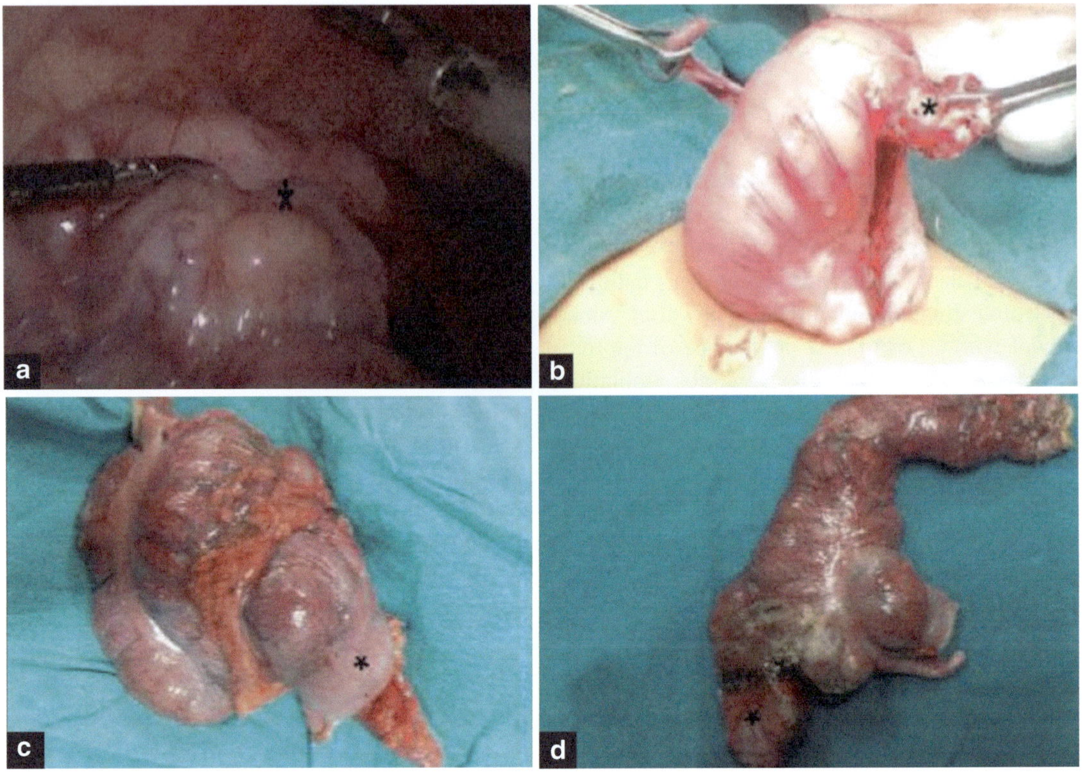

Fig. 43.11 (**a**–**d**) Cecal duplication cyst

43.3 Mesenteric Cyst

Incidence: they are rare lesions and account for 1 in 20000 admissions to a pediatric hospital. Any cyst seen to arise from a mesenteric location is usually grouped under the broad terminology of mesenteric cyst. The most common presentation is a palpable abdominal lump. Other symptoms include pain, vomiting, distension, features of obstruction, bleeding, perforation.

43.3.1 Classification

- Lymphatic origin (chylous or chylolymphatic cyst)
- Mesothelial cyst
- Enteric cyst
- Pseudocyst
- Dermoid cyst
- Cyst of urogenital origin

43.3.2 Embryology

There are several proposed theories to account for the development of mesenteric cysts which include failure of mesenteric leaves to fold, failure of lymphatic system space to join with venous system, occult trauma, neoplasia, and lymph nodal degeneration. The theory of benign lymphatic proliferation is the most accepted.

43.3.3 Pathophysiology

Mesenteric cysts may be single or multiple, unilocular or multilocular, and may contain serous, chylous, or hemorrhagic fluid (Figs. 43.12 and 43.13). They may be lined with cuboidal or columnar epithelium. They have no mucin-producing cells which is in contrast to duplication cysts. These cysts are usually chylous when involving proximal bowel

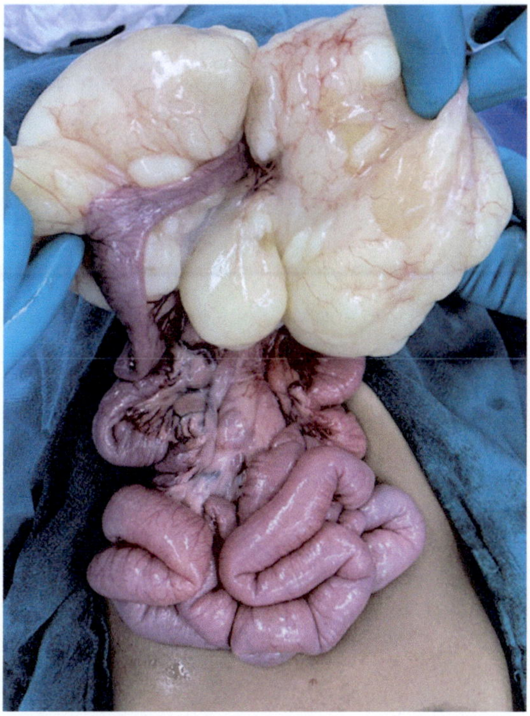

Fig. 43.12 Lymphatic cyst of the intestine

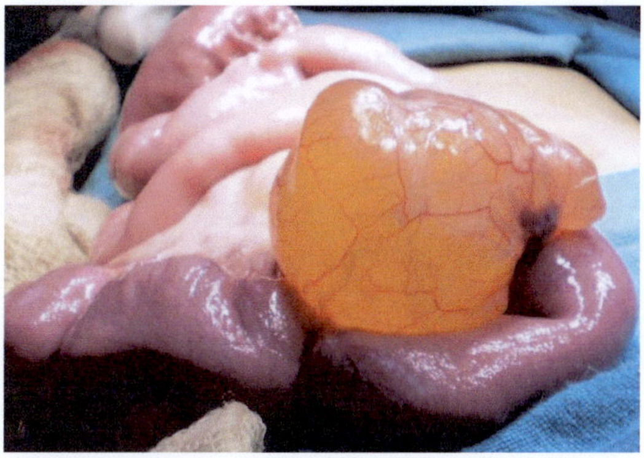

Fig. 43.13 Chylous cyst of the intestine

mesentery and serous when involving distal bowel mesentery. They may be present anywhere from the duodenum to the rectum. They extend from the base of the mesentery to the retroperitoneum. The most common location is the mesentery of the ileum.

43.3.4 Clinical Presentation

The most common presentation is a palpable abdominal lump. The differential diagnosis for a mesenteric cyst presenting as a palpable lump includes duplication cyst, ovarian cyst, choledochal cyst, pancreatic, splenic or renal cyst, hydronephrosis, teratoma, or a hydatid cyst. The mesenteric cyst is noted to be palpable and freely mobile in the transverse plane on examination. They may also present with other symptoms including pain, vomiting, distension, features of obstruction (the most common acute presentation in children), bleeding, and perforation (Tillaux).

43.3.5 Diagnosis

The diagnosis of a mesenteric cyst is made on ultrasound and CT scan. On ultrasound, it appears as a well-circumscribed thin-walled fluid-filled structure.

43.3.6 Treatment

Total removal of the cyst is the treatment of choice. Enucleation is generally unsuccessful and 50–60% of children seem to require concomitant bowel resection. Another available option is partial excision and marsupialization for an extensive cyst which precludes complete excision.

43.3.7 Lymphangioma

Lymphangiomas represent 90% of mesenteric cysts encountered. They are mostly seen in the mesentery of the small bowel followed by the omentum, mesocolon, and retroperitoneum. They have a thin endothelial lining. Extensive lymphangioma of the intestine is extremely rare (Fig. 43.14). Asymptomatic lymphatic lesions require follow-up, whereas symptomatic lesions undergo surgical excision.

43.3.8 Mesothelial Cysts

They are the majority of the non-lymphangiomatous cysts encountered in the omentum or mesentery (Fig. 43.15). They are serous-containing cysts lined by mesothelium. They are thought to arise from incomplete fusion of mesothelium of omentum or mesentery.

Management options include enucleation and surgical excision. If a plane of dissection can be achieved between the cyst and the adjacent bowel wall, the cyst is enucleated, and the mesenteric defect is closed. Surgical resection with the involved bowel and anastomosis results in a complete cure. In about 10% of cases, the lesion is very extensive which precludes complete excision. In these cases, partial excision with marsupialization of the remaining intestine is performed. The cyst lining in these cases should be destroyed by electrocautery, tincture of iodine, or hypertonic saline. Recurrence is reported in up to 14% requiring redo surgery.

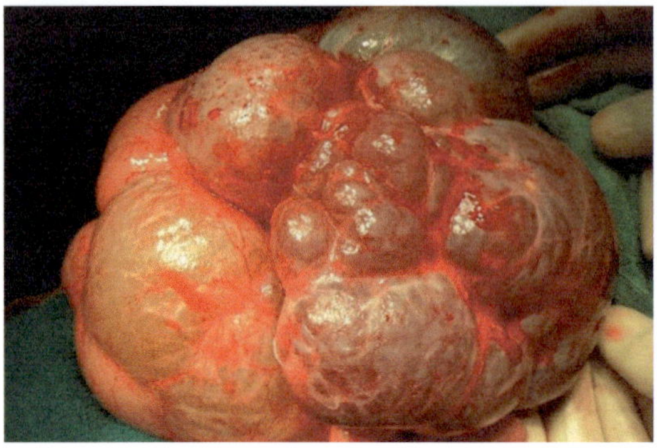

Fig. 43.14 Lymphangioma of the intestine

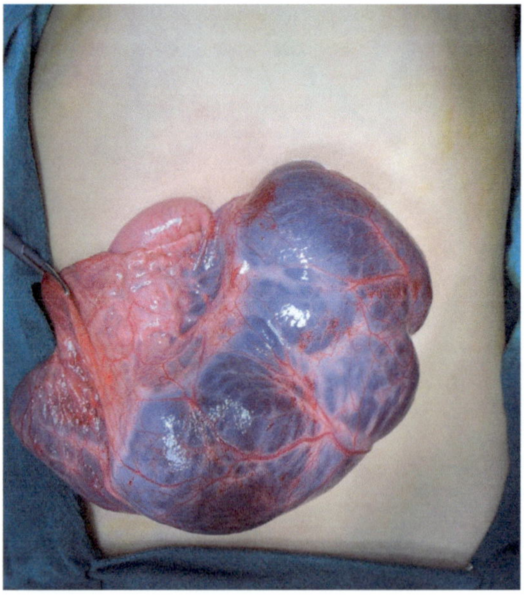

Fig. 43.15 Omental mesothelial cyst

Summary

Meckel diverticulum usually presents with lower gastrointestinal bleeding due to heterotopic gastric mucosa, intestinal obstruction, and an incidental finding during abdominal operations.

Definitive treatment is resection of the Meckel diverticulum including its base.

Duplication cysts are rare congenital anomalies of the alimentary tract and can involve anywhere from mouth to anus.

They have diverse clinical presentations and may contain heterotopic mucosa.

Complete surgical excision is usually the treatment of choice.

Suggested Reading

Meckel Diverticulum

Chen Q, Gao Z, Zhang L, Zhang Y, Pan T, Cai D, Xiong Q, Shu Q, Qian Y. Multifaceted behavior of Meckel's diverticulum in children. J Pediatr Surg. 2018;53:676–81. https://doi.org/10.1016/j.jpedsurg.2017.11.059.

Daniels IR. Historical perspectives on health: Johann Friedrich Meckel the younger and his diverticulum. J R Soc Promot Health. 2000;120:125–6. https://doi.org/10.1177/146642400012000211.

Karaman A, Karaman Í, Çavuşoğlu YH, Erdoğan D, Aslan MK. Management of asymptomatic or incidental Meckel's diverticulum. Indian Pediatr. 2010;47:1055–7. https://doi.org/10.1007/s13312-010-0176-1.

Keese D, Rolle U, Gfroerer S, Fiegel H. Symptomatic Meckel's diverticulum in pediatric patients—case reports and systematic review of the literature. Front Pediatr. 2019;7:267. https://doi.org/10.3389/fped.2019.00267.

Rattan KN, Singh J, Dalal P, Rattan A. Meckel's diverticulum in children: our 12-year experience. Afr J Paediatr Surg. 2016;13:170–4. https://doi.org/10.4103/0189-6725.194671.

Varcoe RL, Wong SW, Taylor CF, Newstead GL. Diverticulectomy is inadequate treatment for short Meckel's diverticulum with heterotopic mucosa. ANZ J Surg. 2004;74:869–72. https://doi.org/10.1111/j.1445-1433.2004.03191.x.

Yahchouchy EK, Marano AF, Etienne J-CF, Fingerhut AL. Meckel's diverticulum. J Am Coll Surg. 2001;192:658–62. https://doi.org/10.1016/S1072-7515(01)00817-1.

Mesenteric Cysts

Anand S, Aleem A. Duplication cyst. In: StatPearls. Treasure Island (FL): StatPearls Publishing; 2023.

Coran AG, Caldamone A, Scott Adzich N, Krummel TM, Laberge JM, editors. Pediatric surgery. 7th ed. Oxford: Elsevier Limited; 2012.

Gandhi D, Garg T, Shah J, Sawhney H, Crowder BJ, Nagar A. Gastrointestinal duplication cysts: what a radiologist needs to know. Abdom Radiol. 2022;47:13–27. https://doi.org/10.1007/s00261-021-03239-w.

Liu R, Adler DG. Duplication cysts: diagnosis, management, and the role of endoscopic ultrasound. Endosc Ultrasound. 2014;3:152. https://doi.org/10.4103/2303-9027.138783.

Puri P, Hollwarth ME, editors. Pediatric surgery. 2nd ed. Heidelberg: Springer; 2019.

Saxena R, Pathak M, Sinha A. Caecal duplication cyst: a rare disease with variable presentation and its management in the era of laparoscopy. J Minimal Access Surg. 2020;16:71. https://doi.org/10.4103/jmas.JMAS_220_18.

44 Intussusception

Y. N. V. S. Siva Kamesh, Rahul Saxena, and Subhasis Roy Choudhury

44.1 Introduction

First described in 1674 by Paul Barbette, intussusception is defined as the telescoping of a proximal segment of the bowel—the *intussusceptum* into the distal bowel—the *intussuscipiens*. The cause is that the majority of them remain idiopathic, while 10–25% of them have a definite lead point. Very rarely, retrograde intussusception can occur, e.g., through gastrojejunostomy.

44.2 Demographics

Male to female ratio is 2:1 to 3:2.

Age of presentation: Most common between 6 and 9 months, associated with weaning,

Nearly 75% of cases present within the first 2 years of life,

90% of cases present within 3 years of age.

Perinatal intussusception (0.3% of all intussusceptions) is rare.

44.3 Etiology

1. Idiopathic variety is common, often associated with preceding viral illness in 20–30% of cases.
2. Gastroenteritis often precipitates it. A probable explanation is that the change in diet causes alteration in gut flora, leading to inflammation of Peyer's patches within the submucosa of the small intestine, which swells up and acts as a leading point.
3. Seasonal occurrences of upper respiratory infection, adenovirus, and rotavirus infection are also seen.
4. Pathological lead point (PLP) is frequently present in older children and adults. The most common PLPs are an inverted Meckel diverticulum, followed by intestinal polyps (inflammatory fibroid polyp, hamartomatous polyp of Peutz-Jhegers syndrome). Rare lead points could be lipoma, fibroma, adenoma, etc. Postoperative intussusception can occur following any surgical procedure in children.

44.4 Pathology

Three cylinders of intestine are involved (Fig. 44.1).

Intussuscipiens: outer (covering) cylinder

Intussusceptum: Inner (entering) and middle cylinders

Apex: Tip of the inner tube (lead point)

Neck: entry point (Fig. 44.2)

Y. N. V. S. Siva Kamesh · R. Saxena (✉)
Department of Pediatric Surgery, All India Institute of Medical Sciences, Jodhpur, India

S. Roy Choudhury
Pediatric Surgery, Lady Hardinge Medical College and Associated Kalawati Saran Children's Hospital, New Delhi, Delhi, India

© The Author(s), under exclusive license to Springer Nature Singapore Pte Ltd. 2025

S. Roy Choudhury (ed.), *Pediatric Surgery*, https://doi.org/10.1007/978-981-96-1257-4_44

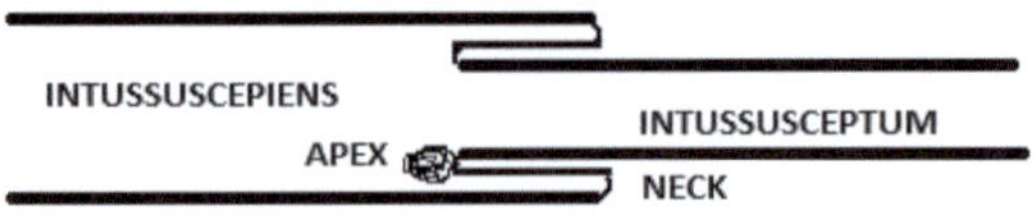

Fig. 44.1 Intussusception. (Courtesy: Dr. Rahul Saxena)

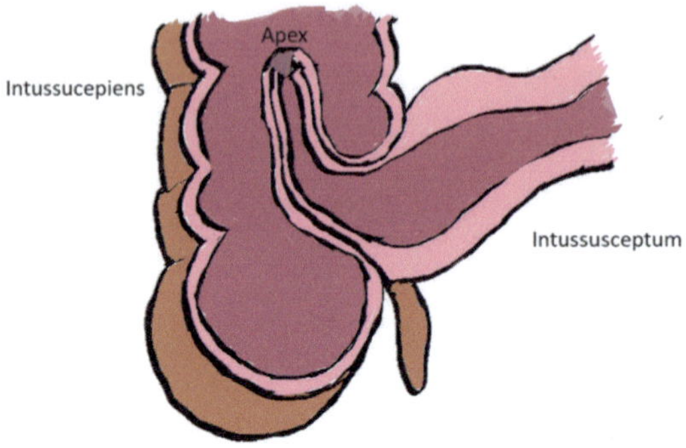

Fig. 44.2 Pathology of intussusception

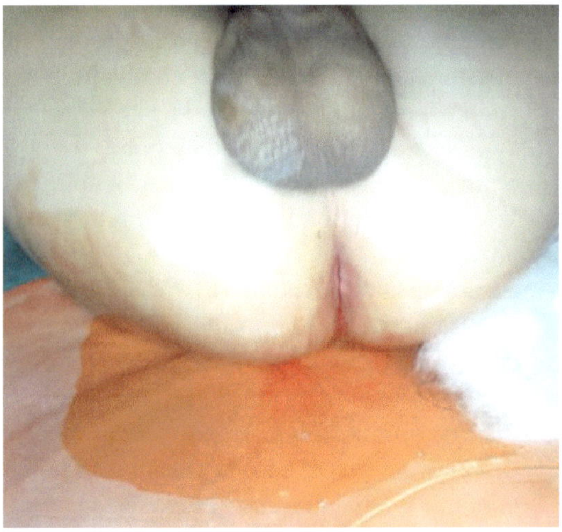

Fig. 44.3 Red currant jelly stools

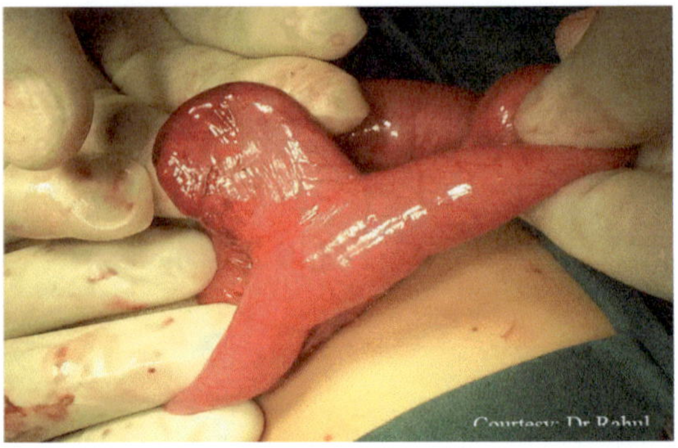

Fig. 44.4 Meckel diverticulum causing intussusception

Intussusception generally occurs in the last 50 cm of small bowel, where maximum aggregation of Peyer's patches is present. Mechanical bowel obstruction results from obstruction of the lumen. The mesenteric vessels get strangulated, which results in local edema and venous congestion. The venous congestion causes the oozing of blood and mucus from the intussusceptum, resulting in characteristic red currant jelly stools (Fig. 44.3). Finally, ischemia sets in, which results in bowel necrosis in cases with late presentation. Apex is the most vulnerable site for gangrene (Fig. 44.4).

44.5 Types of Intussusceptions

Ileo-ileal—5%, ileocolic—77%, ileo-ileocolic—12%, colocolic—2%, multiple—1%, retrograde—0.2%, others—2.8%.

44.6 Clinical Features

Usually, a lusty male child aged between 6 and 9 months presents with a sudden onset of paroxysmal abdominal pain, screaming, drawing up legs, vomiting, and facial pallor. In between attacks, the child becomes listless and drawn. This gradually becomes normal till the next bout of pain. Initially, the baby passes a normal stool, and then the character changes to blood and mucus, termed *red currant jelly*.

Examination in a quiet environment with a warm hand will help to detect a sausage-shaped lump with concavity toward the umbilicus and emptiness of the right iliac fossa, called *sign-de-dance*.

On rectal examination, the apex of the intussusception may be rarely felt, and red currant jelly staining on the finger can be seen. Features of intestinal obstruction with vomiting, abdominal distension, and visible bowel loops develop with the progression over time.

44.7 Diagnosis

(a) Abdominal X-ray findings include increased bowel gas shadow, absence of cecal gas, and multiple air-fluid levels. The presence of a normal gas-filled colon nearly rules out intussusception.
(b) Ultrasonography: Characteristic '*target sign*' (loop of bowel within another loop, Fig. 44.5a). Pathological lead point can also be seen.
(c) Contrast enema with air or barium can demonstrate the head as a filling defect called '*claw sign*' (not seen in ileo-ileal intussusception).

44.8 Differential Diagnosis

(a) Acute enterocolitis: Generally associated with the passage of fecal matter with blood (in contrast with only blood and mucous in cases with intussusception)
(b) Henoch-Schonlein purpura: Intussusception may be precipitated
(c) Prolapse of the rectum: Examination of the finger insinuated between the mass and the rectal wall will halt at the vault.

44.9 Treatment

1. Initial treatment starts with keeping the patient nil by mouth and hydration with intravenous fluids. A nasogastric tube needs to be inserted if a child is vomiting or the abdomen is distended.
2. Radiological reduction can be done with or without sedation. There is a slightly higher rate of perforation if done with sedation.

Two methods:
  (i) Hydrostatic reduction
  (ii) Pneumatic reduction

44.9.1 Hydrostatic Reduction

This was first described in a series by Hirschsprung in 1876. It can be done:

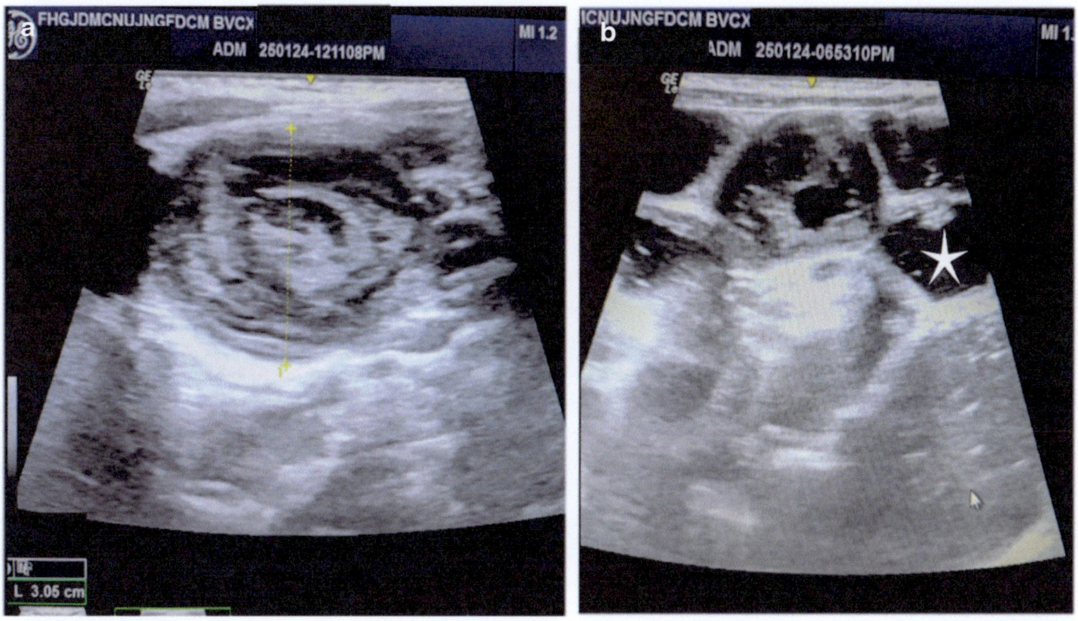

Fig. 44.5 Ileo-colic intussusception: (**a**) target sign and (**b**) shows disappearance of target sign and efflux of fluid into the rectum after successful reduction

- With water-soluble contrast under fluoroscopic guidance
  - Under fluoroscopy, the appearance of intussusceptum is that of a filling defect within the bowel.
  - Sometimes, a spring coil pattern is seen when contrast coats the intussuscipiens.
  - Sometimes, a thickened and edematous IC valve appears as a filling defect within the caecum.
- With saline under ultrasonographic guidance

Patient is made to lie supine on the bed in the ultrasound suite. The procedure can be done with or without sedation as per institutional protocol and based on the cooperation of the child. The diagnosis of intussusception is confirmed by *target sign* (Fig. 44.5a) on the transverse view and the *pseudo-kidney* sign on the longitudinal view. A large-bore Foley catheter is inserted per rectally after adequate lubrication. The bulb is instilled with saline, and the catheter is made to tug above the anal canal. Adequate saline must be instilled into the bulb so as to prevent a leak during reduction. Normal saline is infused through the Foley with an IV infusion set and placed on standby at the table. Reduction can be monitored with ultrasound (Fig. 44.5b).

44.10 Rule of 3

1. Fluid at a height of 3 feet,
2. For 3 minutes and
3. Three attempts.

Signs of success for enema reduction are passage of flatus and feces and contrast seen in small bowel loops during the procedure.

44.10.1 Pneumatic (Air-Enema) Reduction

It is done by introducing air through a rectal tube under fluoroscopic guidance, which was first described by Fiorito in 1959.

Applying air pressure up to 80–100 mm of Hg, with the help of a three-way Foley catheter inserted rectally and attached to an air insufflation/pressure gauze device under fluoroscopic control.

Absolute contraindications for enema reduction are features of peritonitis, suspected perforation, and shock. The success rate is close to 80–90%, even higher in cases with early diagnosis. In cases with prolonged obstruction, the chance of success is poor.

Operative reduction by laparotomy or laparoscopy may be required when radiological reduction is contraindicated, as mentioned above. Operative steps are identification of the sausage-shaped mass, starting squeezing from the apex, avoiding pulling as it can cause rupture, and compression with a warm saline pack, which reduces edema and thus helps in reduction.

In difficult cases, pressure squeezes to reduce edema of the ileocecal valve (Copes method) may be attempted. Bowel resection is required for irreducible and gangrenous intussusception. If a lead point is found like Meckel diverticulum (Figs. 44.6a,b and 44.7a,b), polyp, or any others, then resection is recommended. The recurrence rate is between 2% and 3%.

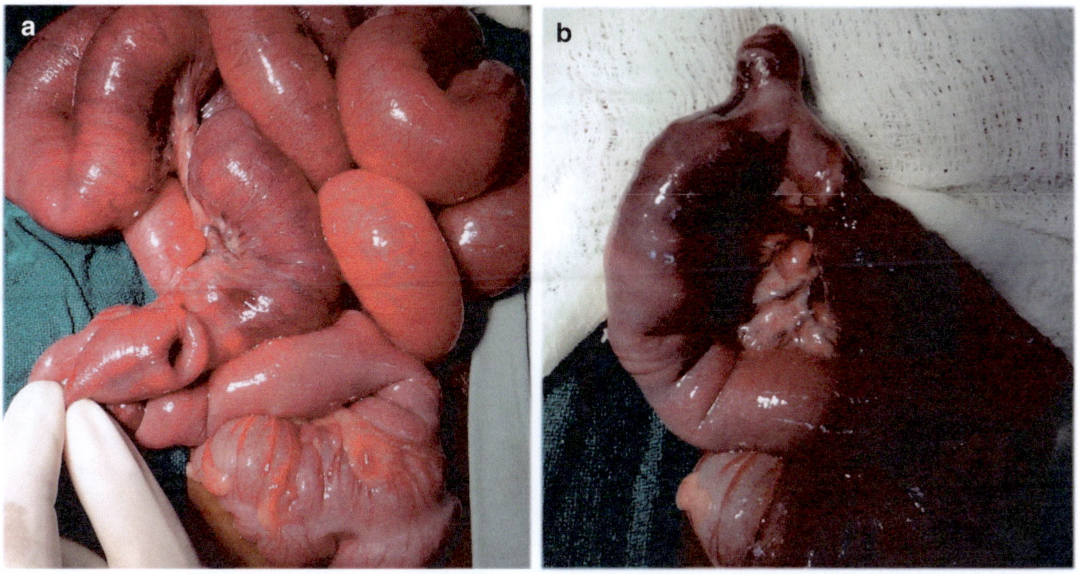

Fig. 44.6 (**a**, **b**) Inverted Meckel diverticulum causing intussusception

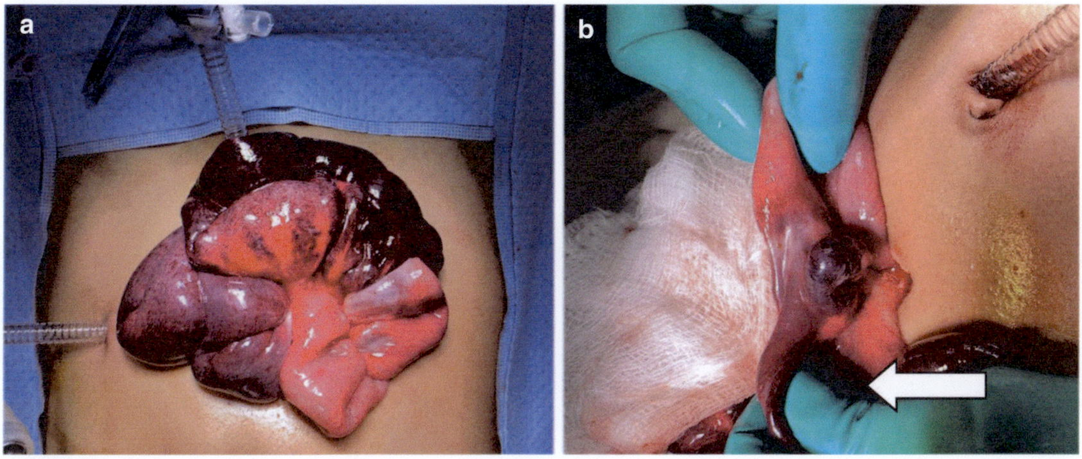

Fig. 44.7 (**a**, **b**) Ileo-ileal intussusception due to Meckel diverticulum (arrow)

Summary

1. Intussusception is the telescoping of a portion of gut into an adjacent segment from proximal to distal.
2. It is most commonly seen in children at the age of 6–9 months.
3. Commonly presents with pain in the abdomen, vomiting, irritability, excessive crying, blood in stools, and abdominal lump/distension.
4. Abdominal examination reveals a palpable lump, and on digital rectal examination, one may find *red-currant jelly* stools.
5. Diagnosis is usually confirmed by identifying the *target sign* and *pseudo-kidney* sign on ultrasonography.
6. Treatment consists of adequate hydration and non-operative reduction by either pneumatic or hydrostatic methods under fluoroscopic or ultrasound guidance.
7. Operative reduction is warranted in selected cases.

Suggested Reading

Coran AG, Caldamone A, Scott Adzich N, Krummel TM, Laberge JM, editors. Pediatric Surgery. 7th ed. Oxford: Elsevier Limited; 2012.

Vo NJ, et al "Intussusception in children"; UpToDate, Jan 20, 2023.

Part VII

Tropical Diseases in Pediatric Surgery

45 Abdominal Tuberculosis in Children

Niyaz Ahmed Khan and Subhasis Roy Choudhury

45.1 Introduction

As per the World Health Organization (WHO), children below 15 years constitute 11% of all tuberculosis patients worldwide. About 1.1 million children fall ill due to tuberculosis every year, and a large number of them lose their lives. Abdominal tuberculosis (ATB) remains common in developing countries, accounting for 0.9% to 1.95% of pediatric hospital admissions. Diagnosis of ATB in children is difficult due to the lack of specific clinical symptoms or tests and often requires invasive procedures like laparotomy or laparoscopy for a definitive diagnosis. The condition is primarily caused by *Mycobacterium tuberculosis*, though it can also result from *Mycobacterium bovis* or other atypical mycobacteria. ATB may occur alone or alongside extra-intestinal tuberculosis. The infection typically spreads through ingestion of tubercle bacilli or through hematogenous or local spread from other infected areas. Tissue damage occurs due to a type IV hypersensitivity reaction, where the bacilli trigger the immune system, leading to the formation of epithelioid granulomas and caseous necrosis. The most commonly affected areas in order are the ileum, ileocecal region, colon, jejunum, rectum, duodenum, stomach, and esophagus.

45.2 Types of Abdominal Tuberculosis in Children

1. Tuberculosis of mesenteric lymph nodes
2. Peritoneal tuberculosis
   (a) Wet- Ascitic
   (b) Dry- Plastic, adhesive type, cocoon formation (Fig. 45.1)
   (c) Miliary tuberculosis: granular peritoneal surface (Fig. 45.2)
   (d) Omental: mass, cake, miliary nodules (Fig. 45.3)
3. Intestinal tuberculosis
   (a) Ulcerative
   (b) Hypertrophic
   (c) Ulcerohypertrophic
   (d) Miliary
4. Tuberculosis of solid organs like liver, spleen etc.

The symptoms of abdominal tuberculosis are often vague and may include abdominal pain, loss of appetite, fever, diarrhea, vomiting, constipation, and cough. A common feature is weight loss of more than 5% over the past 3 months or an inability to gain weight during the same period despite proper nutrition, with no other obvious explanation. The clinical signs can vary and may

N. A. Khan (✉)
Department of Pediatric Surgery, Madhukar Rainbow Children's Hospital, New Delhi, Delhi, India

S. Roy Choudhury
Pediatric Surgery, Lady Hardinge Medical College and Associated Kalawati Saran Children's Hospital, New Delhi, Delhi, India

© The Author(s), under exclusive license to Springer Nature Singapore Pte Ltd. 2025
S. Roy Choudhury (ed.), *Pediatric Surgery*, https://doi.org/10.1007/978-981-96-1257-4_45

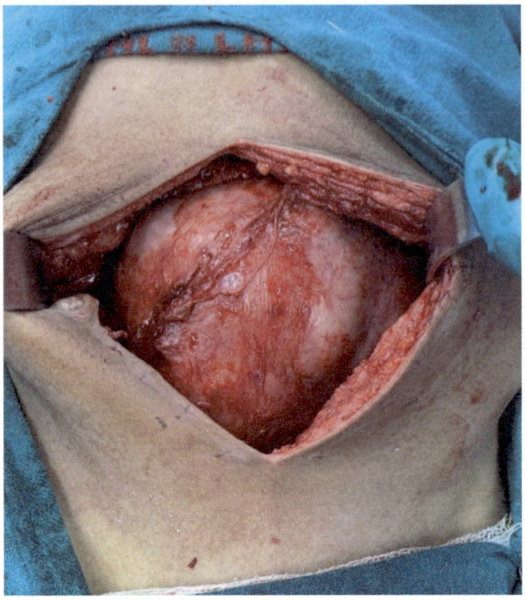

Fig. 45.1 Abdominal cocoon formation in a case of tuberculosis

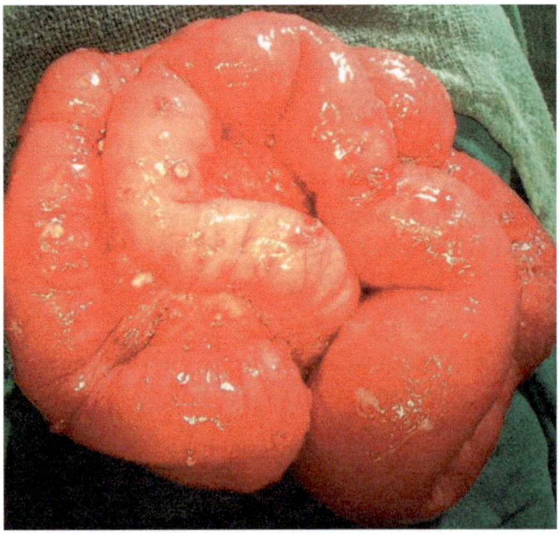

Fig. 45.2 Miliary tuberculosis on the bowel

include abdominal bloating, visible intestinal movements, a palpable mass, a soft or doughy abdomen, ascites, umbilical changes, liver and spleen enlargement, enterocutaneous fistulas, and swollen lymph nodes. Umbilical involvement in intraabdominal tuberculosis may present as puckering, inflammation, or a fecal fistula. Patients may also show signs of peritonitis.

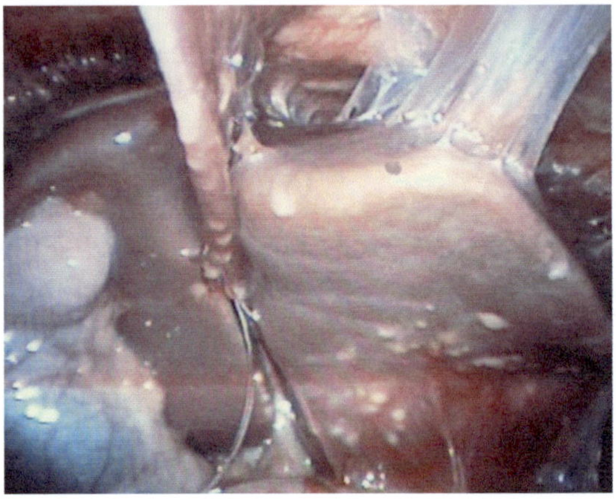

Fig. 45.3 Disseminated tuberculosis on the peritoneal surface and liver (laparoscopic view)

45.3 Diagnosis

When children present with subacute intestinal obstruction, tuberculosis should be considered in the differential diagnosis, particularly if there is a history of tuberculosis in the child or their family. The diagnosis primarily depends on the microscopic identification of acid-fast bacilli (AFB) in body fluids or tissue samples. However, since abdominal tuberculosis tends to be paucibacillary, AFB may not be detectable in the tissue or sputum. The presence of caseating granulomas with epithelioid giant cells in tissue specimens from patients suspected of having tuberculosis can be considered a diagnostic finding. With the advent of image-guided biopsy and laparoscopy, a concerted effort should be made to obtain a histopathological diagnosis of tuberculosis before starting antitubercular treatment.

45.4 Investigations

Hematologic findings in children with abdominal tuberculosis may be nonspecific but often show anemia and an elevated erythrocyte sedimentation rate (ESR). The ELISA test, which detects antitubercular antibodies, is nonspecific and therefore not recommended for diagnosing tuberculosis. A positive tuberculin (Mantoux) test can indicate previous exposure but does not distinguish between active or inactive infection.

The World Health Organization (WHO) now recommends Interferon-Gamma Release Assays (IGRAs), which assess a patient's blood for M. tuberculosis-specific hypersensitivity. Infected individuals' leukocytes release interferon-gamma (INF-γ) when exposed to M. tuberculosis-derived antigens. Unlike the Mantoux test, IGRAs do not require a follow-up visit for reading and do not cross-react with the BCG vaccine. However, a key limitation is that IGRAs cannot differentiate between latent and active tuberculosis, and the blood sample must be promptly transported to the laboratory, making the test more costly.

In abdominal tuberculosis, examination of abdominal fluid typically reveals an exudative fluid with increased lymphocytes, and the serum-ascites albumin gradient (SAAG) is usually less than 1.1 g/dL. Acid-fast bacilli (AFB) are rarely detected on a smear, but ascitic fluid cultures may yield the bacteria. A significant increase in the level of adenosine deaminase (ADA) in ascitic fluid, above 33 U/L, has shown high sensitivity and specificity for diagnosing tuberculosis, though this test is not widely available.

Recent advances in the diagnosis of abdominal tuberculosis in children include the use of the Gene Xpert MTB/RIF assay, a nucleic acid amplification test that detects M. tuberculosis by DNA sequencing (CBNAAT). While it has been widely applied for diagnosing pulmonary tuberculosis with high sensitivity and specificity, its application in abdominal tuberculosis is less established. The test is rapid, delivering results in about 2 hours, and can also detect rifampicin resistance, which is crucial for effective treatment. However, the yield of tubercular bacilli from ascitic fluid is generally low, so the test's diagnostic sensitivity for abdominal tuberculosis remains poor.

45.5 Radiological Imaging

A chest radiograph may reveal signs of either previous or active tubercular infection. In cases of intestinal obstruction due to stricture or adhesions, an abdominal radiograph may show multiple air-fluid levels. In ascitic forms of abdominal tuberculosis, the radiograph might show a gasless abdomen with diffuse haziness from ascitic fluid, and occasionally, calcifications may be observed.

Abdominal ultrasound is valuable in diagnosing abdominal tuberculosis and can reveal the following features:

- Echogenic or septate fluid in the abdomen
- Thickening and nodularity of the peritoneum
- Thickening of the mesentery with increased echogenicity (greater than 15mm)
- Enlarged mesenteric or retroperitoneal lymph nodes (larger than 1 cm) with central necrosis, conglomeration, and peripheral enhancement
- Thickened and dilated bowel loops
- Matted thickened bowel loops, especially in the ileocecal region

Barium meal follow-through (BMFT) is seldom necessary for diagnosis but may show:

- Ileal stricture with proximal bowel loop dilation
- Pulled-up or deformed cecum
- Abnormalities in the ileocecal valve area
- Irregular mucosal folds with ulcerations
- Loss of the normal ileocecal angle

A contrast-enhanced computed tomography (CECT) scan is a useful adjunct for identifying intraabdominal abnormalities such as:

- Thickened, dilated bowel loops
- Ileocecal thickening
- Dense peritoneal fluid
- Thickened omentum, mesentery, and peritoneum
- Hypodense lesions in solid organs that suggest miliary tuberculosis

45.6 Histopathology

For histopathological diagnosis, if an enlarged peripheral lymph node is present, fine needle aspiration or biopsy can be performed. Image-guided biopsy or laparoscopy may also be done

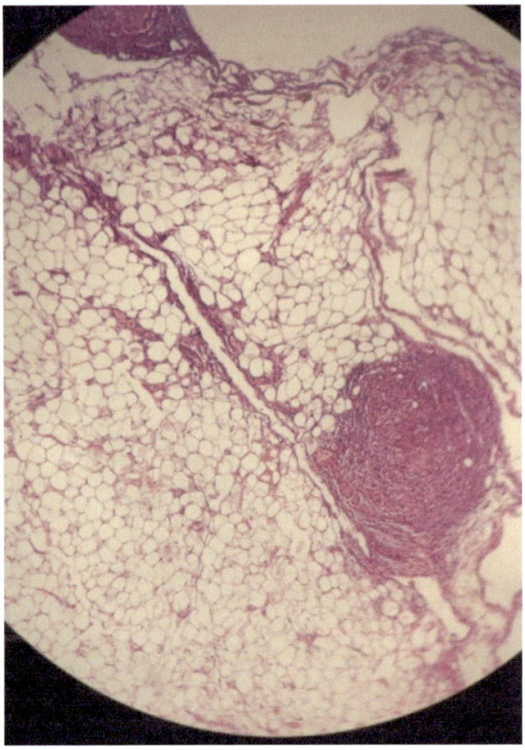

Fig. 45.4 Photomicrograph of epithelioid cell granuloma suggestive of tuberculosis

to obtain tissue samples from abdominal lymph nodes, omentum, or tubercles on the peritoneal surface for histological or cytological examination. The hallmark features for diagnosing tuberculosis include caseating epithelioid cell granulomas, Langhans giant cells, and the presence of acid-fast bacilli (Fig. 45.4).

In some cases, a strong indirect indication of the disease may come from the patient's response to antituberculous therapy, which can support the diagnosis.

45.7 Complications

The complication of abdominal tuberculosis includes intestinal obstruction from adhesion or stricture formation (Figs. 45.5 and 45.6), intestinal perforation, intra-peritoneal abscess, cocoon formation (Fig. 45.1), fistulization, hemorrhage, malabsorption, and malnutrition.

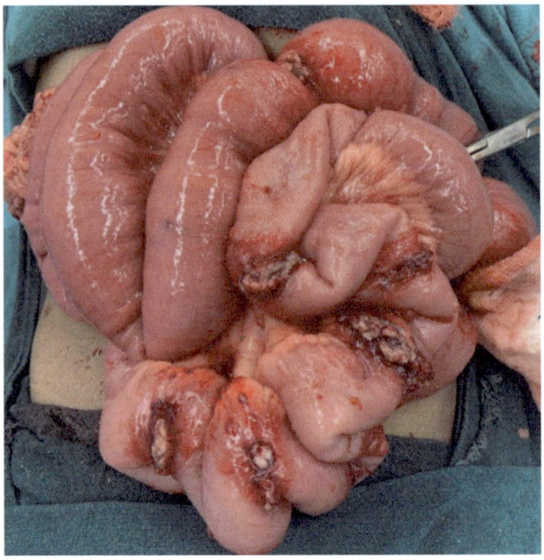

Fig. 45.5 Multiple intestinal strictures due to tuberculosis

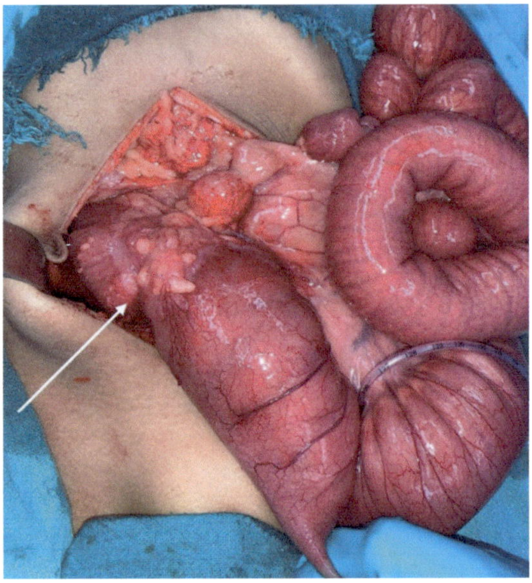

Fig. 45.6 Ileocaecal tubercular stricture (white arrow) with enlarged lymph nodes

45.8 Treatment

Medical treatment for abdominal tuberculosis involves antituberculous chemotherapy. Under India's National Tuberculosis Elimination Program (NTEP), patients are no longer categorized as new or previously treated. Instead, they are classified as either Rifampicin-resistant tuberculosis (RR-TB) or Rifampicin-sensitive tuberculosis (RS-TB). For all microbiologically confirmed cases of abdominal tuberculosis, as well as new clinically diagnosed (probable RS-TB) cases, the prescribed regimen consists of 2HRZE+ 4HRE drugs. The average dosages for this regimen are as follows: isoniazid (10 mg/kg/day), rifampicin (15 mg/kg/day), ethambutol (20 mg/kg/day), pyrazinamide (35 mg/kg/day), and streptomycin (20 mg/kg/day).

The NTEP has transitioned from using combi-packs and patient-specific drug boxes to fixed dose combinations (FDCs) for multi-drug tuberculosis therapy. FDCs minimize the risk of missing one or more drugs, thus reducing the potential for drug-resistant strains to emerge. There are two types of pediatric FDCs available under NTEP:

- *Intensive Phase (IP)*: Three-drug FDC dispersible tablets (H 50 mg, R 75 mg, Z 150 mg) in a 10:15:30 ratio
- *Continuation Phase (CP)*: Two-drug FDC dispersible tablets (H 50 mg, R 75 mg) in a 10:15 ratio

Since ethambutol is not available in a dispersible tablet form, a separate 100 mg non-dispersible ethambutol tablet is given alongside the FDC for both the intensive and continuation phases. Additionally, every patient receiving Isoniazid should be given a daily pyridoxine supplement (10 mg) to prevent neuropathy.

Monitoring: Clinical assessment should be done monthly during the treatment and then every 3 months. Ultrasound of the abdomen should be done at the end of treatment or if there is worsening or non-response to treatment.

45.9 Surgical Considerations

Indications: (a) Tissue biopsy for diagnosis by open or laparoscopic approach. (b) Complications arising out of tuberculosis like bowel stricture, intestinal perforation, obstruction, or massive uncontrolled hemorrhage.

Due to malnutrition and prolonged symptoms in these patients, it is important for surgeons to optimize the patient and improve nutritional status with parenteral nutrition. During surgery, the presence of disseminated tuberculosis on the bowel and peritoneal surfaces with adhesions is best left undisturbed, with only a peritoneal/ omental/ lymph node biopsy taken for confirmation of the diagnosis. Extensive bowel manipulation and adhesiolysis should be avoided in these situations, as they carry a high risk of bowel injury and subsequent fecal fistula, which could lead to prolonged recovery and morbidity. Postoperative antituberculous therapy should be started promptly. For patients receiving intravenous fluids, injectable streptomycin, and ciprofloxacin/levofloxacin can be administered before transitioning to oral antituberculous drugs.

For a short intestinal stricture, a stricturoplasty can be performed, which involves opening the stricture longitudinally and then closing it transversely. More extensive strictures may require bowel resection followed by end-to-end anastomosis. In cases of localized intestinal perforation, closure or resection with anastomosis is possible if the bowel edges are healthy. However, there is a high risk of postoperative leaks and fecal fistulas. Therefore, for severely diseased bowel with peritonitis, an initial bowel ostomy (such as an ileostomy) may serve as an effective temporary solution. The ostomy can be closed electively later, after a 3–6 months course of antituberculous therapy. It may be wise to perform a distal bowel contrast study to ensure a healthy bowel prior to the stoma closure.

45.10 Summary

Diagnosis of ATB in children is difficult due to the lack of specific clinical symptoms or tests and often requires invasive procedures like laparotomy or laparoscopy for a definitive diagnosis. The condition is primarily caused by Mycobacterium tuberculosis an acid-fast bacillus (AFB). The most commonly affected areas in order are the ileum, ileocecal region, colon, jejunum, rectum, duodenum, stomach, and esophagus. Diagnosis is suspected on clinical findings, imaging studies and supported by serological tests or tests for identification of the AFB or its genetic material (CBNAAT). The hallmark of tissue histological diagnosis is caseating epithelioid cell granuloma, Langhans type of giant cells and identification of AFB. Medical treatment with antituberculous chemotherapy is the cornerstone of treatment. Surgical interventions are required for diagnostic purpose like a tissue biopsy or for management of intestinal complications like perforation, obstruction or haemorrhage.

Suggested Reading

Pant N, Choudhury SR, Gupta A, et al. Umbilical signs of peritoneal tuberculosis in children. Indian J Pediatr. 2012;79:1192.

WHO operational handbook on tuberculosis: module 5: management of tuberculosis in children and adolescents. WHO consolidated guidelines on tuberculosis: module 5: management of tuberculosis in children and adolescents, 2022.

Splenic and Liver Abscess

46

Ankur Mandelia, Niyaz Ahmed Khan,
and Subhasis Roy Choudhury

46.1 Splenic Abscess

Splenic abscesses (SA) are rare in children, but their incidence has risen in recent years with advancements in diagnostic imaging.

46.1.1 Etiology

SA can result from hematogenous infection, immunocompromised states, malnutrition, hematologic disorders, malignancy, trauma, or diabetes. In developing countries, common etiological factors include enteric fever (salmonella and its subtypes), tuberculosis, and parasitic diseases.

46.1.2 Clinical Presentation

Patients typically present with fever, anorexia, and left upper quadrant pain. Occasionally, referred pain to the left shoulder may occur due to phrenic nerve irritation. On examination, tenderness in the left upper quadrant is often observed, with or without splenomegaly. Leukocytosis with a left shift is common but may be absent in immunocompromised individuals.

A. Mandelia (✉)
Department of Pediatric Surgery, Sanjay Gandhi Post Graduate Institute of Medical Sciences (SGPGIMS), Lucknow, India

N. A. Khan (✉)
Department of Pediatric Surgery, Madhukar Rainbow Children's Hospital, New Delhi, India

S. Roy Choudhury
Pediatric Surgery, Lady Hardinge Medical College and Associated Kalawati Saran Children's Hospital, New Delhi, Delhi, India

46.1.3 Imaging Studies

Modern imaging techniques have improved the diagnosis of SA.

- *Ultrasonography (US)* shows hypoechoic lesions with irregular margins and echogenic contents in the spleen.
- *CT scan* displays hypodense areas in the spleen and is considered the gold standard for diagnosis due to its high sensitivity and superior anatomical definition, albeit with higher radiation exposure (Fig. 46.1a, b).

CT scans are particularly useful for evaluating complex cases and multiple abscesses. US is valuable for guiding abscess aspiration and monitoring recovery.

46.1.4 Management

Treatment approaches for SA include antibiotics, percutaneous drainage, open drainage, and splenectomy (partial or total), used either independently or in combination.

© The Author(s), under exclusive license to Springer Nature Singapore Pte Ltd. 2025
S. Roy Choudhury (ed.), *Pediatric Surgery*, https://doi.org/10.1007/978-981-96-1257-4_46

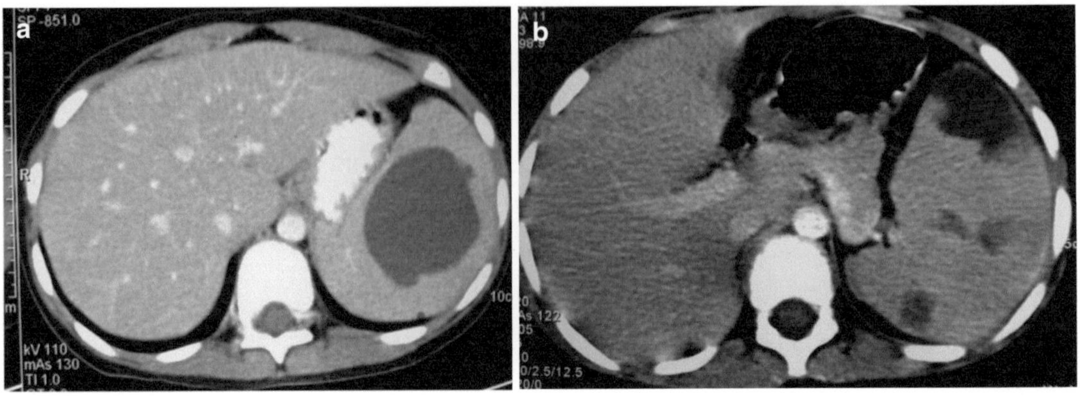

Fig. 46.1 (**a**) CT scan showing solitary splenic abscess. (**b**) Multiple splenic abscesses. (Reprinted with permission from Prof. S Roy Choudhury, Choudhury, S.R. (2018). Pyloric Stenosis. In: Pediatric Surgery. Springer, Singapore. https://doi.org/10.1007/978-981-10-6304-6_31)

- *Antibiotic Therapy*: Effective for abscesses smaller than 3 cm and is considered the first-line treatment.
- *Percutaneous Aspiration or Drainage*: Recommended for abscesses larger than 3 cm. US-guided needle aspiration is generally safe and effective, but percutaneous drainage (PCD) with a pigtail catheter is often preferred for larger or multilocular abscesses due to its higher success rate and cost-effectiveness. PCD is also more effective in abscesses with ill-defined cavities, necrotic debris, and thick, viscous fluid. However, catheter use may lead to complications such as slippage, blockage, or infection.
- *Splenectomy*: Reserved for cases where aspiration or drainage fails or when abscess rupture occurs.

Preserving the spleen is crucial in children to maintain its immunological functions, making conservative approaches the preferred initial strategy.

46.2 Liver Abscess

Liver abscesses (LA) in pediatric patients are predominantly observed in developing nations, particularly in tropical and subtropical regions.

46.2.1 Incidence

In developing countries, the prevalence of LA ranges between 4 and 7 cases per 1000 pediatric hospital admissions. Among these, pyogenic liver abscesses (PLA) account for the majority (80%), whereas amoebic liver abscesses (ALA) are comparatively less common. Tubercular and fungal liver abscesses are exceedingly rare. ALA demonstrates endemicity in regions such as Southeast Asia, Egypt, and South Africa.

46.2.2 Etiopathogenesis

46.2.2.1 Predisposing Factors

In previous years, perforated appendicitis was frequently associated with pediatric LA. In high-income countries, these abscesses are commonly linked to severe underlying illnesses, granulocyte dysfunction, sickle cell disease, parasitic infections, or immunosuppression. Conversely, in endemic regions, malnutrition, unhygienic living conditions, and parasitic infections like helminthiasis act as predisposing factors.

Various congenital anomalies and biliary tract obstructions may also facilitate bacterial growth and lead to multiple abscesses. Liver trauma represents another risk factor. A significant number of LAs are categorized as cryptogenic, often due to prior antibiotic therapy or challenges in culturing anaerobic organisms.

46.2.3 Pathophysiology

Bacteria and other pathogens typically reach the liver via the biliary system, the portal vein, or the hepatic artery. PLA frequently presents as a solitary lesion in the liver's right lobe (75%) due to preferential portal blood flow to this region. Left lobe abscesses are clinically significant as they are prone to severe complications like rupture into the peritoneal or pericardial cavities. Although multiple abscesses involving both lobes are less common (25%), ruptured liver abscesses can occur in either lobe.

ALA results from the hematogenous dissemination of trophozoites that penetrate the colonic mucosa and travel through the portal vein to infect the liver. It is the most prevalent extraintestinal manifestation of amebiasis and usually affects the right lobe. These abscesses contain thick, reddish-brown pus, often described as resembling chocolate or anchovy sauce. Secondary bacterial infections can change the pus to a yellow or green hue. Amoebae are typically identified in the abscess wall. Differentiating between PLA and ALA can be clinically and radiologically challenging, with mixed infections being common, especially in India.

46.2.4 Causative Organisms

ALA is predominantly caused by *Entamoeba histolytica*. In PLA, *Staphylococcus aureus* is the most frequently isolated organism, followed by Gram-negative bacteria (*E. coli, Klebsiella, Enterobacter*, and *Salmonella typhi*) and anaerobes. Tubercular abscesses are rare, and fungal microabscesses are usually seen in patients with leukemia.

46.2.5 Clinical Presentation

Children with LA typically present with fever, abdominal pain (commonly in the right upper quadrant), and tender hepatomegaly. Nonspecific symptoms such as fatigue, weight loss, and anemia may also occur. Jaundice, though uncommon, may arise due to sepsis, hepatic dysfunction, intrahepatic biliary obstruction, or bilio-vascular fistulas.

Subdiaphragmatic irritation or pleuropulmonary involvement can cause right shoulder pain or a dry cough. Pleural effusion or empyema may also be observed due to contiguous spread. While some cases exhibit a gradual onset, others may present acutely with severe sepsis or peritonitis due to rupture.

46.2.6 Investigations (Fig. 46.2)

Hematologic studies may reveal anemia, leukocytosis, and elevated ESR. Liver enzyme levels (e.g., alkaline phosphatase, SGOT, and SGPT) are elevated in approximately half of the cases. Coagulation profile may be deranged. Blood cultures often yield negative results due to prior antibiotic use. Serological tests such as indirect hemagglutination antibody titres (IHA) and ELISA are useful for diagnosing amebiasis but have limited specificity in endemic areas.

Ultrasonography is the initial imaging modality of choice, often showing hypoechoic, rounded lesions with defined walls. Contrast-enhanced CT is more sensitive for identifying small lesions and aids in planning interventions (Fig. 46.3a, b). On MRI, abscesses appear hypointense on T1-weighted images and hyperintense on T2-weighted sequences.

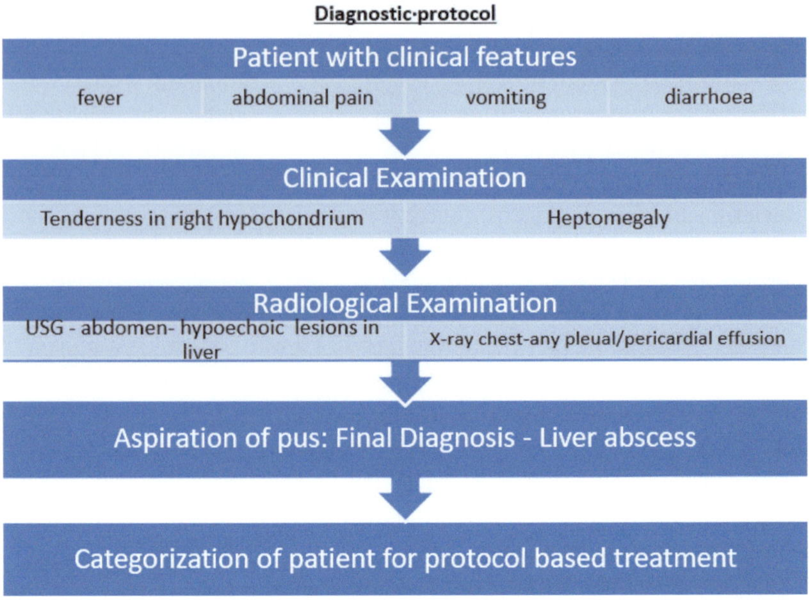

Fig. 46.2 Diagnostic protocol for liver abscess. (Reprinted with permission from Prof. S Roy Choudhury, Choudhury, S.R. (2018). Pyloric Stenosis. In: Pediatric Surgery. Springer, Singapore. https://doi.org/10.1007/978-981-10-6304-6_31)

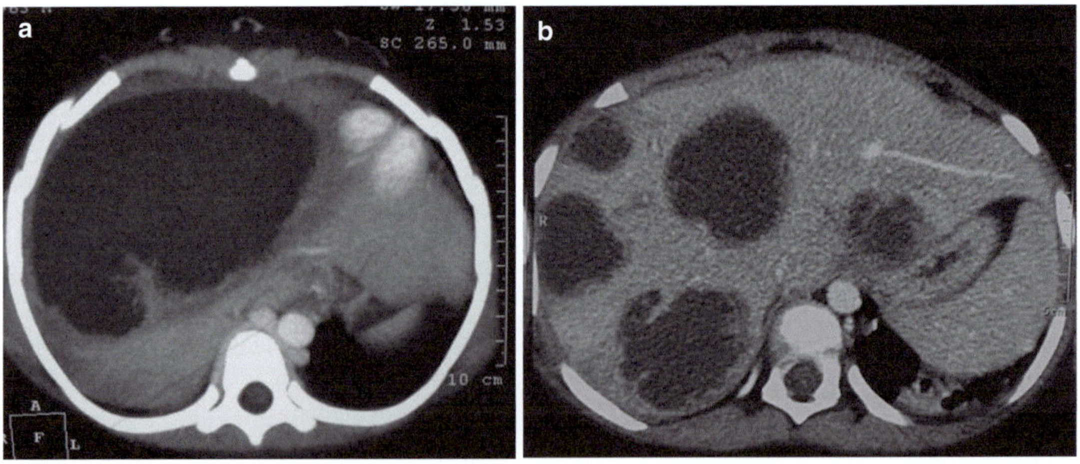

Fig. 46.3 CT Scan showing (**a**) single liver abscess; (**b**) multiple liver abscess. (Reprinted with permission from Prof. S Roy Choudhury, Choudhury, S.R. (2018). Pyloric Stenosis. In: Pediatric Surgery. Springer, Singapore. https://doi.org/10.1007/978-981-10-6304-6_31)

46.2.7 Treatment (Table 46.1, Fig. 46.4)

46.2.7.1 Medical Management

In some cases, antimicrobial therapy alone can successfully manage liver abscesses. However, the standard approach often involves combining it with percutaneous or surgical drainage. Conservative treatment is typically suitable for smaller abscesses (<5 cm), while larger ones usually necessitate pus drainage. For uncomplicated larger abscesses (>5 cm), percutaneous needle aspiration (PNA) under ultrasound guidance is considered the most effective technique, provided coagulopathy is corrected beforehand.

Antimicrobial regimens should cover the spectrum of pathogens commonly associated with liver abscesses. An initial combination therapy comprising an anti-staphylococcal agent, an anti-anaerobic drug, an anti-amoebic agent, and

Table 46.1 Treatment protocol for liver abscess

Patient selection	Type of treatment
All uncomplicated cases Abscess cavity <5 cm. Abscess with solid appearance on USG. Multiple small lesions	Medical management only (combination of higher-generation cephalosporin, aminoglycoside, and metronidazole)
Febrile even after 48–72 hours of adequate medical treatment with liquefied abscess. Abscess cavity >5 cm	Percutaneous needle aspiration with medical management (Repeated aspirations at certain interval may be required)
Large abscess with Impending rupture or pointing to the parietal wall	Percutaneous continuous catheter drainage with medical management
Abscess ruptured into peritoneal cavity. Abscess cavity not accessible by percutaneous drainage. Ongoing sepsis even after antibiotic therapy and percutaneous drainage	Surgical open drainage/laparoscopic drainage

Reprinted with permission from Prof. S Roy Choudhury, Choudhury, S.R. (2018). Pyloric Stenosis. In: Pediatric Surgery. Springer, Singapore. https://doi.org/10.1007/978-981-10-6304-6_31

either an aminoglycoside or cephalosporin for Gram-negative bacteria is recommended. This broad-spectrum approach is particularly effective given the frequent occurrence of mixed microbial infections. The final choice of antibiotics should be tailored based on the culture results and sensitivity patterns of isolated organisms.

Currently, a 4- to 6-week course of antimicrobial therapy is advised for adequately drained solitary abscesses. For multiple liver abscesses, the treatment duration may extend to 12 weeks. Ongoing clinical evaluations and imaging studies should determine the appropriate length of treatment.

46.2.7.2 Surgical Management

With advancements in image-guided procedures, percutaneous aspiration or drainage has become the preferred approach for managing liver abscesses (LA). Open surgical drainage is now primarily reserved for cases involving ruptured abscesses or unsuccessful percutaneous interventions.

46.2.7.3 Percutaneous Techniques

Percutaneous needle aspiration (PNA), combined with antimicrobial therapy, is highly effective for managing uncomplicated LA and should be considered the first-line treatment. Repeat aspirations of liquefied abscess contents under ultrasonographic guidance may be necessary in some cases.

46.2.7.4 Percutaneous Drainage (PD)

PD is indicated in specific scenarios, including:

(a) Large abscesses at risk of rupturing or those that have already ruptured into the parietal wall.
(b) Abscesses containing thick pus that cannot be adequately aspirated with a wide-bore needle.

A wide-bore catheter (>10 Fr) is preferred for PD, as it provides superior drainage compared to pigtail catheters. PD is associated with several advantages, including a lower risk of complications compared to open surgical drainage, avoidance of general anesthesia, shorter hospital stays, and better patient acceptance. However, PD is not without challenges, as complications such as catheter blockage, infection, and dislodgement can occur. Failure rates for PD range from 5% to 30%, according to published literature.

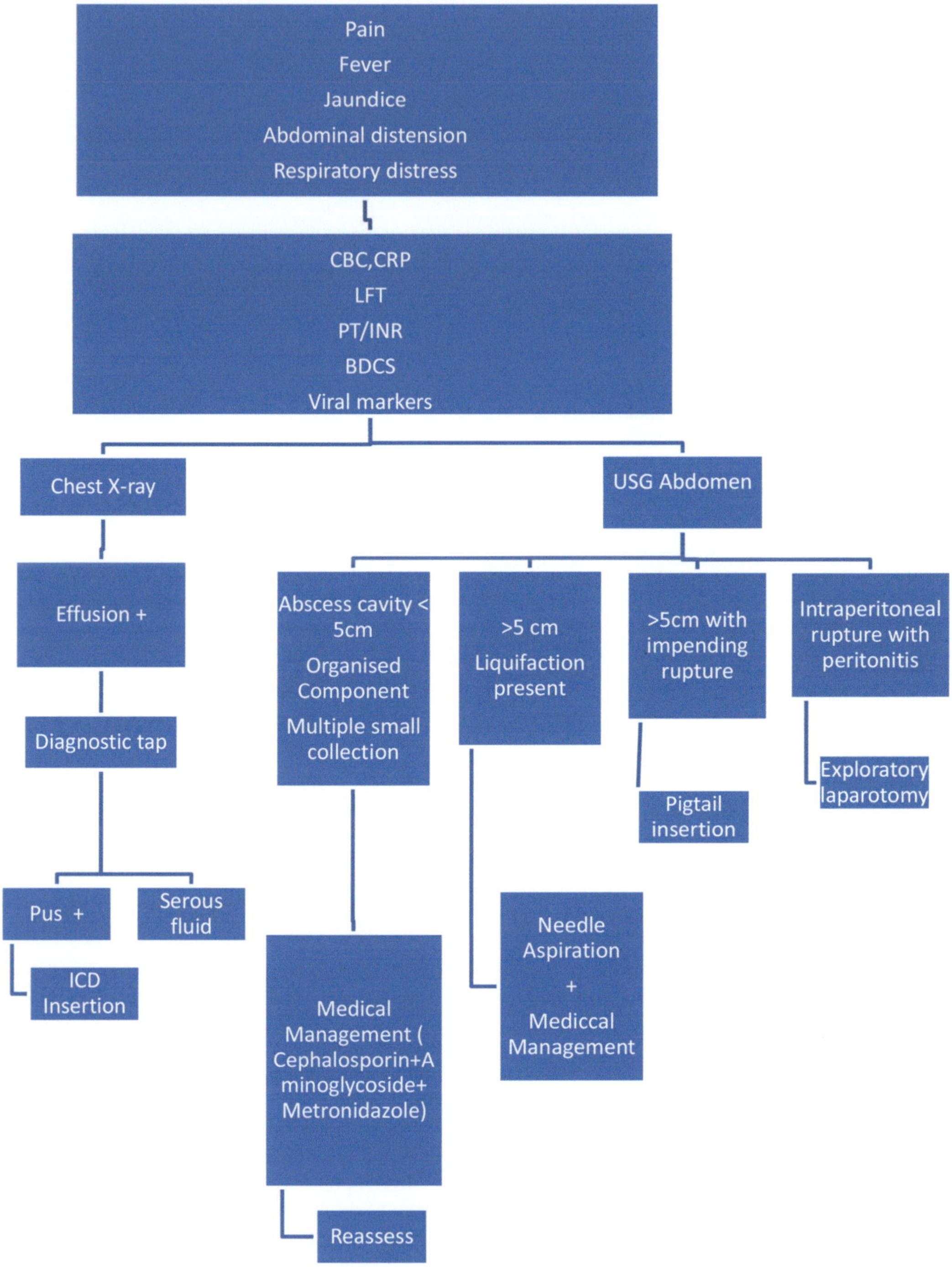

Fig. 46.4 Management algorithm for liver abscess. (Reprinted with permission from Prof. S Roy Choudhury, Choudhury, S.R. (2018). Pyloric Stenosis. In: Pediatric Surgery. Springer, Singapore. https://doi.org/10.1007/978-981-10-6304-6_31)

46.2.7.5 Open Surgical Drainage

Open surgical drainage remains essential in certain cases, including:

(a) Ruptured abscesses with associated peritonitis.
(b) Persistent abscesses following failed percutaneous drainage, especially in critically ill patients with ongoing sepsis.
(c) Abscesses located in regions inaccessible to image-guided techniques.

Laparoscopic drainage offers a minimally invasive alternative to open surgery and can be effective in selected cases.

In our clinical experience, distinguishing between different types of LA often lacks significant clinical relevance, as mixed microbial infections are common. A combined antimicrobial approach targeting both pyogenic and amoebic pathogens generally yields favorable outcomes.

For fungal abscesses, systemic antifungal therapy should be initiated following abscess drainage, either percutaneously or surgically. Amphotericin B and fluconazole are currently the first-line treatments for fungal LA.

46.2.8 Complications and Prognosis

The presence of jaundice, liver failure, acute abdomen, sepsis, coagulopathy, encephalopathy, and hypoalbuminemia (<2 g/dL) is recognized as a poor prognosticator. Complications such as pleural effusion and empyema are common but typically respond well to aspiration or tube drainage of the pleural fluid. A mortality rate of approximately 3% has been documented in a large study conducted in India. However, survivors generally do not experience any significant long-term morbidities.

46.3 Summary

Primary splenic abscess (SA) is an uncommon condition in children, often linked to immunosuppression and secondary to bacteremia. A good number of cases are related to infection with Salmonella or its subtypes. Treatment options include antibiotic therapy, percutaneous aspiration and drainage. Liver abscesses (LA) in children are now rare in developed nations but remain prevalent in the developing countries. Pyogenic liver abscesses account for most cases, followed by amoebic and fungal types. Diagnostic imaging modalities include ultrasonography (US) and computed tomography (CT). Treatment typically involves a combination of percutaneous drainage and appropriate antimicrobial therapy. However, open or laparoscopic surgical drainage may still be required in selected cases.

Suggested Reading

Roy Choudhury S, Debnath PR, Jain P, Kushwa AK, Puri A, Chadha R, Sonkar P. Conservative management of isolated splennic abscess in children. J Pediatr Surg. 2010;45:372–5.

Roy Choudhury S, Khan NA, Saxena R, et al. Protocol based management of 154 cases of Pediatric liver abscess. Pediatr Surg Int. https://doi.org/10.1007/s00383-016-4009-8. Published online 8th Nov. 2016. Pediatr Surg Int (2017) 33:165–172.

Zinner MJ, Ashley SW. Maingot's Abdominnal operation. 12th ed. McGraw Hill USA; 2013.

Hydatid Disease in Children

47

Hiramani Pathak and Subhasis Roy Choudhury

47.1 Introduction

Hydatid disease or echinococcosis is caused by the tapeworm *Echinococcus*. Four species of echinococcus produce clinical manifestations in humans; *E. granulosus* (dog tapeworm) is the most common and produces cystic echinococcosis. Alveolar echinococcosis is caused by *E. multilocularis* and it is infrequent. *E. vogeli* and *E. oligarthus* rarely manifest in humans (Oral et al. 2012).

Hydatid disease is endemic in many developing countries; however, global migration of people warrants that every healthcare professional be well aware of this disease.

Definitive hosts are the canids, especially dogs; cattles (goats, horses, and cows) are the intermediate hosts, and humans are the incidental hosts with no role in the transmission cycle. Adult tapeworms inhabit the small intestine of the definitive hosts and lay thousands of eggs per day that are expelled in feces. Intermediate or the incidental hosts ingest the eggs. Oncospheres hatch from the eggs and penetrate the intestinal mucosa, enter the blood and lymphatic system, and further migrate to the liver or other distant organs. Echinococcosis does not transmit from one human to another, as two mammalian species are required for the completion of echinococcal life cycle.

Hydatid disease usually occurs in adults (19–64 years) and is uncommon in children, comparatively. Prevalence of Liver and lung hydatidosis continues to increase with increasing age. Liver (70%) is the most commonly affected organ, followed by lungs (20%), and rarely other sites like muscles, bones, kidneys, heart, pancreas, central nervous system, and spleen are involved in much lesser frequencies. Barring hair, nail, and teeth, no other sites in the human body are spared (Gupta et al. 2014).

Cysts of E. Granulosus—Unilocular, expansile. Consists of three layers, the inner endocyst, which is a germinative layer; the mid exocyst, which is the parasite-derived acellular laminated layer, and the outer pericyst, which is a host-derived adventitial layer. Cysts of E. multilocularis are multilocular and lack pericysts, enabling tissue invasion.

Infections are mostly acquired in childhood but manifested in adults with a latency of three to four decades. Many are diagnosed incidentally, and many more are found at autopsy or are undiagnosed. Symptoms depend on the site and size of the cysts. Cysts grow at the rate of 1–5 cms in diameter per year.

H. Pathak (✉)
Birat Medical College Teaching Hospital, Tankisinuwari, Nepal

S. Roy Choudhury
Pediatric Surgery, Lady Hardinge Medical College and Associated Kalawati Saran Children's Hospital, New Delhi, Delhi, India

© The Author(s), under exclusive license to Springer Nature Singapore Pte Ltd. 2025

S. Roy Choudhury (ed.), *Pediatric Surgery*, https://doi.org/10.1007/978-981-96-1257-4_47

47.2 Liver

Two-thirds of hydatid cysts are found in liver. Right lobe is more frequently affected than the left. The pathology of the layers of the cyst is shown in Fig. 47.1. Large cysts in liver produce hepatomegaly with or without pain. Nausea, vomiting, and anorexia are other symptoms of liver hydatidosis. High index of suspicion is required for timely diagnosis and treatment. Complications of liver hydatid cysts include rupture into the biliary tree, causing obstructive jaundice, biliary colic, and cholangitis. They can also rupture into the peritoneal cavity, causing peritonitis, anaphylaxis, and multi-organ failure. Some rupture trans-diaphragmatically, causing pulmonary hydatidosis and inciting respiratory symptoms. Cysts may have pressure effects on the bile ducts resulting in cholestasis, on portal veins causing portal hypertension, and on the hepatic veins/IVC causing hepatic venous obstruction or Budd-Chiari syndrome.

Diagnosis is usually made by ultrasonography. For complicated cysts, computed tomography (CT) and/or magnetic resonance imaging (MRI) may be required. CT has the advantage of avoiding observer bias of ultrasonography and aids in planning management (Fig. 47.2a).

USG—USG has a sensitivity of 90–95% for the detection of echinococcal cyst. US appearance has been classified by Gharbi et al. into five types and by WHO into five types as shown in table below (Gharbi et al. 1981) (Table 47.1).

Classification of the cyst type dictates management of cystic hydatid disease of the liver.

Type I and II Gharbi lesions (types CE1 and CE3 WHO lesions) are routinely managed with percutaneous treatment(PAIR). More than 95% of these cysts are treated successfully with this technique. Few of the type III Gharbi lesions may be treated with percutaneous technique, while others require percutaneous evacuation (drainage) or modified catheterization. It should be noted that the success of the percutaneous tech-

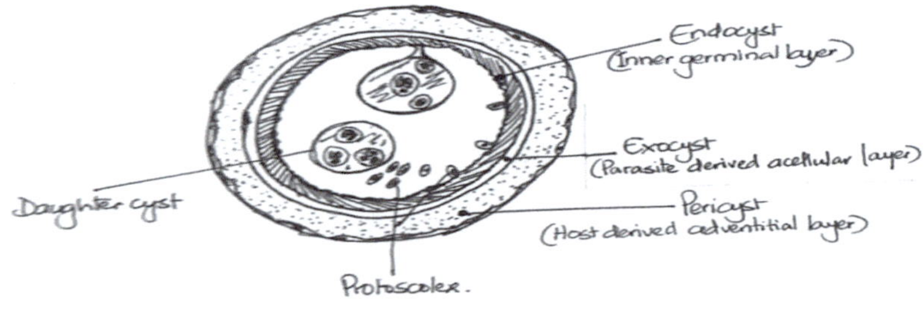

Fig. 47.1 Schematic diagram of a hydatid cyst

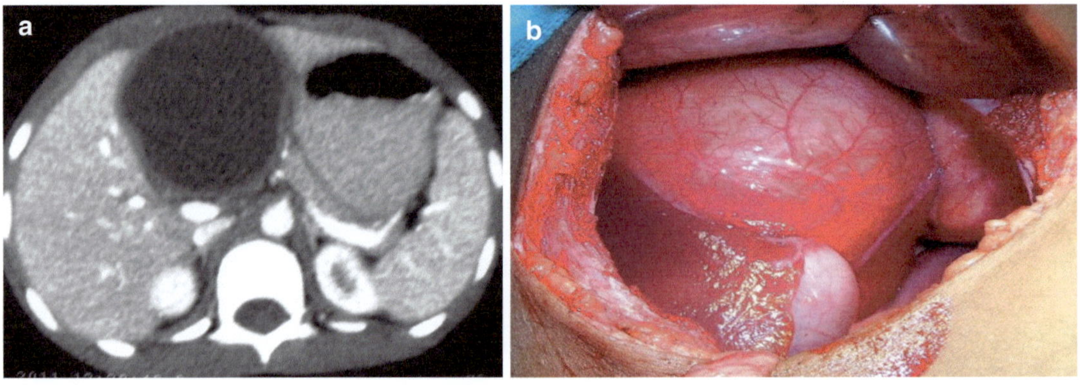

Fig. 47.2 (**a**) CT abdomen showing a large solitary hydatid cyst of the liver. (**b**) Intraoperative image of the same patient

Table 47.1 Gharbi et al. and WHO Classification of cystic echinococcosis based on ultrasonography

Gharbi (1981) type	Description	WHO type	Stage
Type I	Univesicular anechoic cystic lesion with double line sign	CE1	Active
Type II	Cyst with detached membranes, "waterlily sign"	CE3a	Transitional
	Cysts with daughter cysts in solid matrix	CE3b	
Type III	Multiseptated "honeycomb" cysts	CE2	Active
Type IV	Cyst with heterogeneous content, no daughter vesicles	CE4	Inactive
Type V	Solid plus calcified wall	CE5	inactive

nique depends on the amount of drainable content present within the cyst. Type IV and V cysts are inactive and do not require prompt treatment, and they can be safely managed with a wait-and-watch policy.

47.3 PEARLS of Management

1. Albendazole chemotherapy—Usually albendazole 10 mg/kg/dose twice daily regimen for 3 to 6 months with regular follow-up for cysts less than 5 cms in size. Albendazole is ovicidal, larvicidal and vermicidal. Some add Praziquantel to increase the protoscolicidal effect of Albendazole. Younger patients have a better response to chemotherapy. Although relapse after chemotherapy is high (up to 30%), >90% of relapses are sensitive to retreatment with chemotherapy.
2. For cysts located at the liver surface with the threat of rupture, surgery is recommended (Fig. 47.2b). Care should be taken not to spill during surgery. We use 10% povidone-iodine-soaked pads to contain inadvertent peritoneal contamination. An anesthetist should have an intravenous steroid and adrenaline injection ready in the event of any anaphylactic reaction following handling or spillage of the cyst fluid. Choice of surgery depends on the site, size, number, and complexity. Cyst decompression with removal of cyst wall, leaving part or entire pericyst in situ, may be done for most lesions. Endocysts are easily peeled in uncomplicated cysts. Cysts are decompressed using wide bore plastic suckers. Thick sediments with daughter cysts may be evacuated using tablespoons. While some complex cysts may require more radical procedures like pericystectomy or anatomic/non-anatomic liver resections.

   Residual cystic cavity may be left open or covered with an omental flap. Small, non-calcified, non-infected cavities may be closed with simple running absorbable sutures. Capitonnage, which involves spiral suture closure of the cavity from the bottom upwards, can be performed for cavity closure.

   Cystobiliary communication has to be looked for and treated with an intraoperative cholangiography and drainage procedure.

   Laparoscopic management of hepatic hydatid cysts follows the same principles as open surgical management. A disadvantage of the laparoscopic procedure is poor maneuverability and limited experience of surgeons if complex procedures need to be performed.
3. For cysts that are deep in liver parenchyma and multiple (Fig. 47.3a, b), the percutaneous drainage technique is utilized, as open surgery risks damage to vessels and intrahepatic ducts. Most hepatic hydatid cysts can be managed with PAIR (sequential steps of Puncture, Aspiration, Instillation, and Reaspiration).

   Cyst is punctured with a wide-bore needle through a non-dependent wall to avoid sediment. Daughter cysts, if present, are punctured. Around half of the cyst volume is aspirated, scolicidal agent is instilled, and completely reaspirated after 15–20 minutes. Scolicidal agents used for instillation are hypertonic saline 20%, ethanol 95%, cetrimide 0.1%, or povidone-iodine 10%. Cyst obliteration occurs 9–12 months after PAIR.

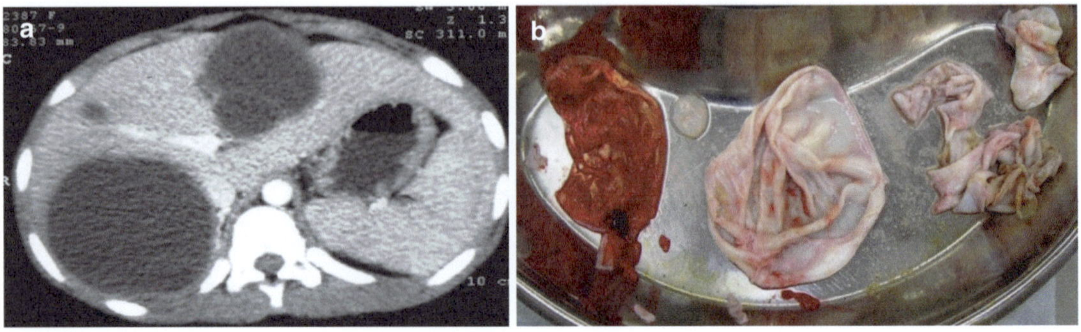

Fig. 47.3 (**a**) Multiple hydatid cysts of the liver. (**b**) Postoperative specimen of multiple liver cysts of the same patient

47.3.1 Indications for PAIR (Khuroo 2021)

- Cyst size >4cms
- Gharbi I and II cysts (WHO CE1 and CE3)
- Cysts in deep locations or inaccessible for surgery
- Cysts in high-risk patients, relapse after surgery, failed drug therapy, and refusal for surgery

Cysts of pancreas, spleen, kidney, lung, and brain are contraindicated for PAIR. Other contraindications are—difficult access, cysts with multiple septa, cysts with hyperechogenic solid patterns, calcified cysts, cysts with biliary communication.

47.4 Indications for Surgery

- Complicated cysts (hemorrhage, rupture, cysts with biliary fistulae)
- Cysts with multiple daughter cysts
- Cyst diameter >10cms
- Superficial cysts (as they pose a risk for rupture)
- Extrahepatic disease—kidney, brain, bone, lungs
- Unavailability of the percutaneous facility

47.5 Thorax

Thoracic involvement in hydatidosis is common and more so in children. In fact, the lung is the commonest site of involvement in children. Chest pain, cough with mucopurulent sputum, and hemoptysis are the commonest symptoms. Cysts attain large sizes before symptoms appear due to the compressible nature of lung tissue. Therefore, presentation is usually delayed in cases of lung hydatidosis, and a high index of suspicion is often required for early diagnosis. Sudden onset of cough, chest pain, hemoptysis, and anaphylaxis may suggest rupture of the cyst.

Cysts may be complicated by infection or rupture. Cyst rupture can be contained or complete. Contained rupture denotes detachment of pericyst from endocyst, and hence the contents are contained and do not produce anaphylaxis/ hemoptysis. On the other hand, complete ones rupture into bronchus and produce hemoptysis, chest pain, cough, and rarely expectoration of membrane, and they may rupture into pleural cavity, producing hydrothorax/hydropneumothorax.

Plain chest radiography antero-posterior and lateral views are sufficient for diagnosis in most cases, but for evaluation of complications and spread, higher imaging modalities like computed tomography (CT) and/or magnetic resonance imaging (MRI) are required. CT and MRI also aid in planning management. Primary lung cysts are usually single, unilateral, and present in the lower lobes. Lower lobe involvement is seen in 55–70%, multiple cysts (30%), and bilateral roughly 20%.

Well-circumscribed round radio-opacity is usually seen radiologically, Cannon ball in AP view and a Rugby ball in lateral view. Crescent sign, air fluid levels are noted in ruptured cysts, and air bubbles, rim enhancements are seen in infected cysts (Fig. 47.4).

Hydatid cysts of diameter >10cms are considered giant hydatid cysts and pose a therapeutic challenge. Treatment of lung hydatid cysts include chemotherapy, cystectomy, capitonnage, wedge resection, and sometimes even lobectomy (Figs. 47.5a–c and 47.6). Pleural disease may require decortication or pleurectomy. The usual precautions for any anaphylactic reaction and prevention of spillage of cyst contents should be followed. One should be prepared to find multiple airways and even bronchial communication leading to technical challenges in controlling airleak following the cyst removal. All airway communications should be meticulously closed with preferably non-absorbable suture.

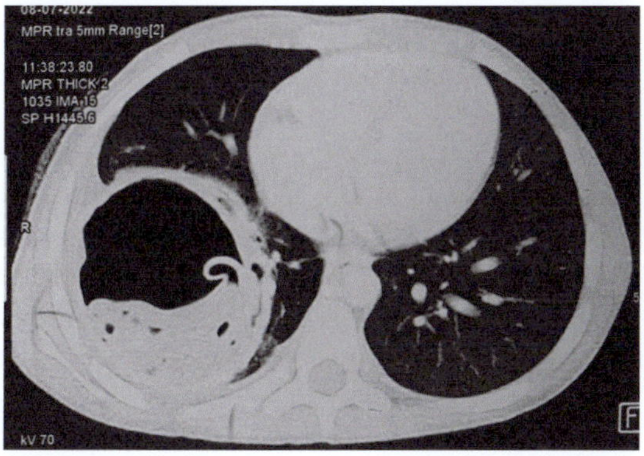

Fig. 47.4 Hydatid cyst right lung showing floating membranes

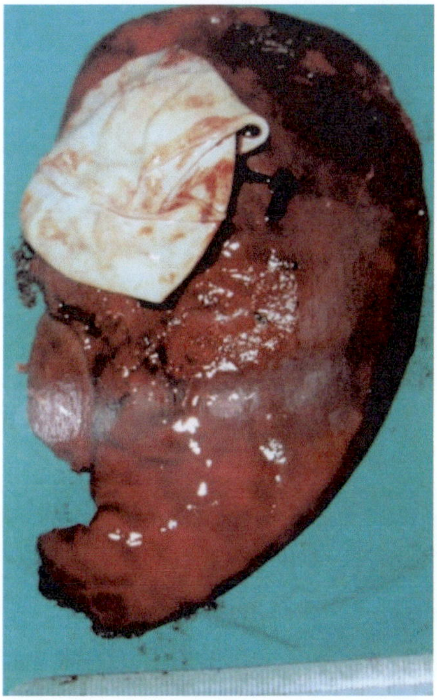

Fig. 47.6 Lobectomy specimen, hydatid cyst lung

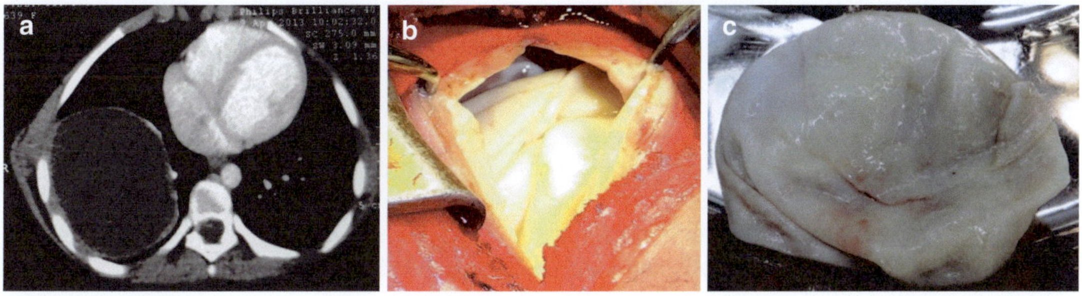

Fig. 47.5 (**a**) Right lung hydatid cyst, (**b**) cyst at thoracotomy, and (**c**) specimen of cyst cavity after cystectomy

47.6 Management of Combined Liver and Lung Hydatid Disease

Combined lung and liver lesions are rare and pose a significant management challenge. Lung lesions may be treated as stated in the thoracic section mentioned above, and liver lesions may be managed with PAIR or percutaneous drainage or cystectomy. When the liver lesion is located subhepatically and an ipsilateral lung lesion is present, both can be managed via thoracotomy followed by cystectomy through the diaphragmatic incision.

47.7 Brain

Cerebral hydatid disease is rarely encountered and affects children. They are usually single and have a thin capsule, involving mostly regions supplied by the middle cerebral artery; they may rupture into ventricles and cause diffuse spread. They are differentiated from abscesses by the absence of rim enhancement and surrounding edema. Other differential diagnoses of cerebral cystic lesions have to be borne in mind for appropriate management.

Cerebral hydatid cysts present with features of raised intracranial pressure and focal neurological deficits. Diagnosis is made by CT or MRI.

Treatment is mostly surgical excision and chemotherapy.

Reports of involvement of kidneys, pancreas, spleen, heart, peritoneum, soft tissues, orbits, spine, and bone are available in the literature. A case-based approach for management is required for the optimum treatment of hydatidosis.

47.8 Kidneys

Renal hydatid cysts are extremely rare. Computed tomography is required for diagnosis and surgical planning (Fig. 47.7). Cystectomy is the treatment of choice.

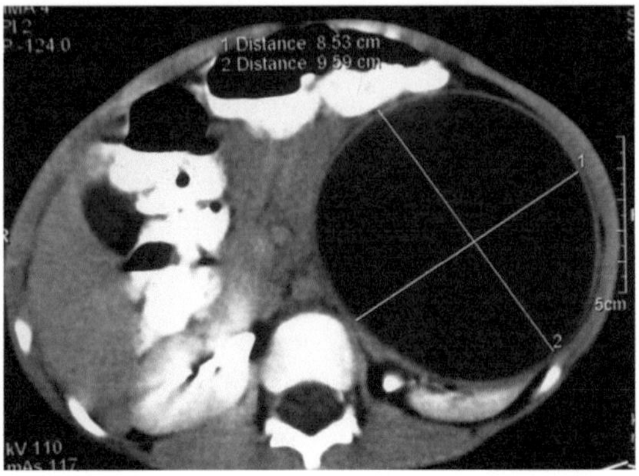

Fig. 47.7 CT showing left renal hydatid cyst

47.9 Postoperative Care and Outcome

Albendazole (10 mg/kg) is initiated 1 week prior to surgery and continued postoperatively for 4 weeks. This reduces the risk of secondary echinococcosis.

Intra-abdominal abscesses, secondary infection of the cyst cavity, secondary echinococcosis due to spillage, and anaphylaxis are complications that have to be watched for after treatment. Complication rates are low (<1%); however, recurrence stands at 2–25%.

Summary

- Hydatidosis is initially asymptomatic.
- Liver and lungs are the most commonly affected organs.
- Diagnosis is established by ultrasound imaging.
- Treatment depends on the type, site, size of lesion, and amount of drainable fluids in the cyst cavity.
- PAIR, percutaneous drainage and surgery along with adjunctive Albendazole are the mainstays of treatment in liver hydatidosis while cysts in other areas require surgery.
- Complications are low and can be further minimized with immaculate surgical handling

Suggested Reading

Gharbi HA, Hassine W, Brauner MW, Dupuch K. Ultrasound examination of the hydatic liver. Radiology. 1981;139(2):459–63.

Gupta R, Sharma SB, Prabhakar G, Mathur P. Hydatid disease in children: our experience. Formos J Surg. 2014;47(6):211–20.

Khuroo MS. Percutaneous drainage in hepatic hydatidosis-the PAIR technique: concept, technique, and results. J Clin Exp Hepatol. 2021;11(5):592–602.

Oral A, Yigiter M, Yildiz A, Yalcin O, Dikmen T, Eren S, Kantarci M, Salman AB. Diagnosis and management of hydatid liver disease in children: a report of 156 patients with hydatid disease. J Pediatr Surg. 2012;47(3):528–34.

Intestinal Complications of Worm Infestation in Children

48

Ankur Mandelia and Subhasis Roy Choudhury

48.1 Ascariasis

Ascaris lumbricoides is a common intestinal nematode affecting children worldwide, leading to major morbidity and mortality in endemic areas. The estimated prevalence of ascariasis is over 1 billion cases worldwide. Although most cases are asymptomatic, heavy infestation can cause various intestinal and biliary complications.

48.1.1 Lifecycle

Ascaris are very large (adult females: 20–35 cm; adult males: 15–30 cm) nematodes (roundworms) that parasitize the human intestine and are endemic in tropical and subtropical regions with poor sanitation (Fig. 48.1). Infection occurs through the faeco-oral route by ingestion of fertilized eggs. The eggs hatch in the small intestine and release larvae, which invade the intestinal mucosa and are carried via the portal, then systemic circulation to the lungs. They are excreted into the pulmonary secretions and are either coughed up or swallowed, thereby gaining entry back into the gut. In the gut, they have a predilection for the jejunum and the ileum, where they develop into adult worms. Adult worms can live up to 1 to 2 years.

48.1.2 Clinical Presentation

Adult worms usually do not cause acute symptoms; however, heavy infestation in children may cause stunted growth via malnutrition. High worm burden (> 60 worms) is likely to cause a wide spectrum of acute abdominal complications:

(a) Intestinal complications:
- Intestinal luminal occlusion:
  - This is the most common intestinal complication, accounting for 50–65% of ascariasis-related complications.
  - Multiple worms get entangled with each other, forming a large bolus (Fig. 48.2). This ascaris worm bolus mechanical obstruction of the bowel lumen, especially near the ileo-caecal valve, and aggravates spasticity of the distal ileum by the combined action of endo-toxins of worms and host inflammatory reactions.
- Intussusception or volvulus:
  - The bolus of worms can also serve as a lead point for intussusception or as a pivot for small bowel volvulus.
  - Incidence of volvulus and intussusception has been reported to be 24–36% and 2%, respectively.

A. Mandelia (✉)
Department of Pediatric Surgery, Sanjay Gandhi Post Graduate Institute of Medical Sciences (SGPGIMS), Lucknow, India

S. Roy Choudhury
Pediatric Surgery, Lady Hardinge Medical College and Associated Kalawati Saran Children's Hospital, New Delhi, Delhi, India

© The Author(s), under exclusive license to Springer Nature Singapore Pte Ltd. 2025

S. Roy Choudhury (ed.), *Pediatric Surgery*, https://doi.org/10.1007/978-981-96-1257-4_48

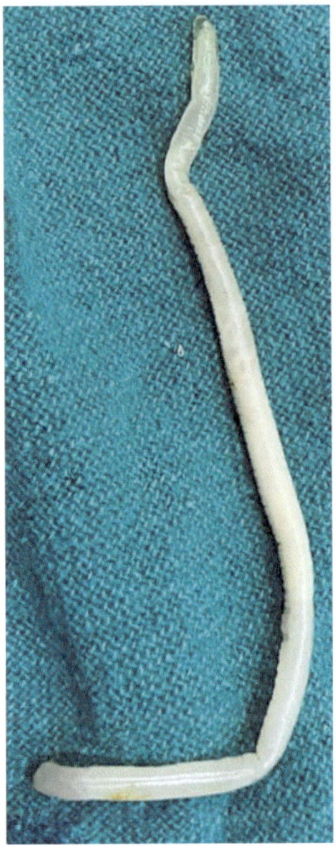

Fig. 48.1 Adult worm of Ascaris lumbricoides

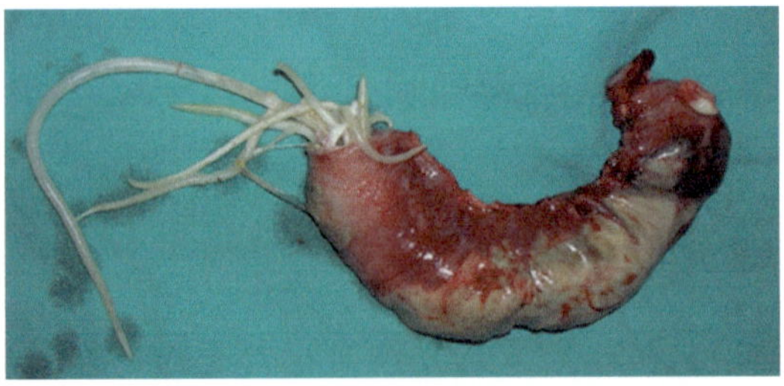

Fig. 48.2 Worm bolus obstruction with gangrene of intestine

- Intestinal perforation: Ascaris does not have teeth and stays in the bowel lumen. It can, however, still penetrate normal or pathologic bowel by the following mechanisms:
  - Worm bolus may obstruct the lumen of blind—ending structures, such as the Appendix or Meckel diverticulum, and cause perforation.
  - Perforation can also result from ischemic necrosis following volvulus.
  - Worms may exit from primary bowel pathologies such as tubercular, typhoid, amoebic, or other intestinal ulcers, following trauma, and through anastomotic suture lines.

(b) Biliary complications: In India, biliary ascariasis has been reported to be endemic in the Kashmir valley and Tamil Nadu. It accounts for 10–19% of ascariasis-related complications. Prior sphincterotomy, bilio-enteric anastomosis, and female sex are predisposing factors for bilio-pancreatic ascariasis. The migration of A. lumbricoides through the ampulla of Vater causes various hepatobiliary and pancreatic complications:

- Biliary colic
- Cholecystitis: *Ascaris* infection can induce acalculous cholecystitis
- Cholangitis
- CBD stricture
- Calculi: *Ascaris* eggs can also serve as a nidus for stone formation
- Hepatic abscess: persistent cholangitis can lead to portal pyaemia, predisposing to the formation of hepatic abscesses
- Pancreatitis: the worm may gain entry into the pancreatic ducts causing irritation and precipitating an attack of acute pancreatitis

48.1.2.1 Diagnosis

History taking is an extremely important component of diagnosing roundworm infestation. Children will usually present with typical features of intestinal obstruction, but parents may also give a history of vomiting of worms or passage of worms in stools. Peripheral eosinophilia, due to larval invasion of the blood, is common. Stool examination may show Ascaris eggs in the stool.

Plain radiographs of abdomen show multiple air fluid levels in case of intestinal obstruction, pneumoperitoneum in case of perforation, radiolucent areas, cigar bundle appearance and "whirlpool" sign (ball of worms) (Fig. 48.3). The sensitivity of ultrasonography (USG) in diagnosis of ascariasis ranges between 85% and 90%. USG findings suggestive of ascariasis include:

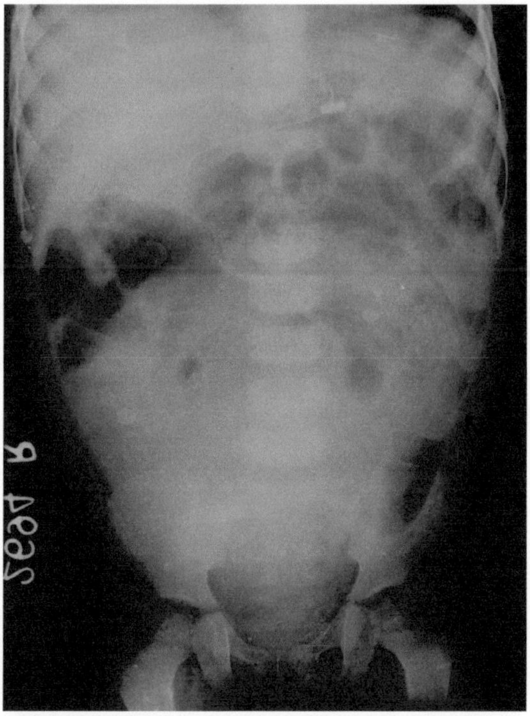

Fig. 48.3 Plain X-ray abdomen showing "cigar bundle" appearance (arrow)

(a) hypoechoic tubular structure with well-defined echogenic walls (adult worm) with or without characteristic movements; (b) multiple long, linear, parallel echogenic strips without acoustic shadowing in longitudinal (railway track) and transverse (bull's eye) views; (c) overlapping longitudinal interfaces in the main bile duct due to coiling of a single worm or several worms in the CBD (helmenthinoma). Endoscopic retrograde cholangio-pancreatography (ERCP) is both diagnostic and therapeutic for biliary ascariasis and usually shows the worm as a long filling defect.

48.1.2.2 Treatment

The management of uncomplicated ascariasis is usually conservative and consists of anti-helminthic chemotherapy with mebendazole, albendazole, levamisole, or pyrantel palmoate. If medical treatment fails, endoscopic retrograde cholangiopancreatography can be used to extract worms from the biliary tree, and surgical enterotomy can accomplish worm removal from the intestinal tract (Fig. 48.4). In cases of gangrene or perforation, resection anastomosis of the involved segment may become necessary.

The morbidity associated with surgical intervention for ascariasis complications is extremely high, as there is a high chance of leakage of suture lines or sutured enterotomies. A high index of suspicion, early diagnosis, and prompt intervention can prevent bowel ischemia or gangrene and significantly reduce morbidity and mortality associated with such cases. Primary prevention of ascariasis involves maintaining proper hygiene and sanitation practices, and periodic deworming on detection of ova/cysts on microscopic stool analysis.

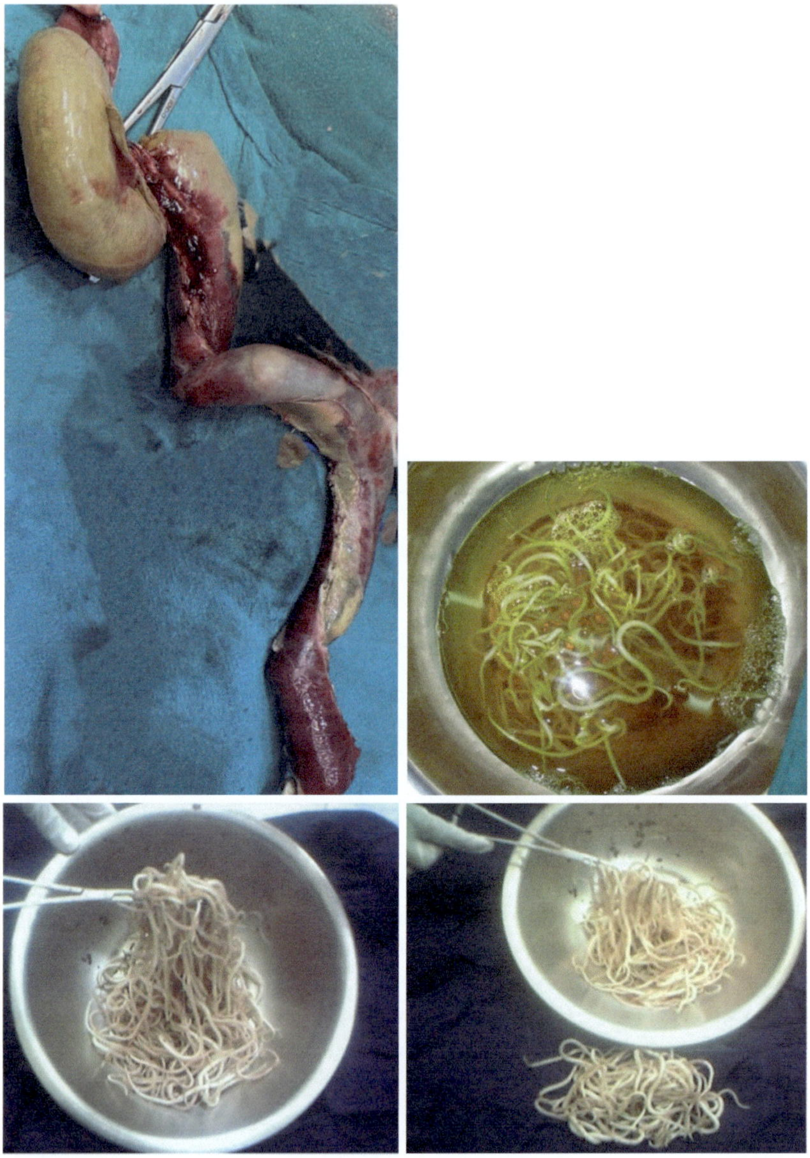

Fig. 48.4 Intestinal gangrene due to worm bolus needing enterotomy and extraction of worms

Suggested Reading

Ramareddy RS, Alladi A, Siddapa OS, Deepti V, Akthar T, Mamata B. Surgical complications of Ascaris lumbricoides in children. J Indian Assoc Pediatr Surg. 2012;17:116–9.

Vagholkar K, Pawanarkar A, Vagholkar S, Jawanjal A, Subudhi S, Chauhan P, et al. Surgical complications of round worm infestation. Int J Res Med Sci. 2016;4:1838–40.

Part VIII

Anorectal Disorders in Children

49 Anorectal Malformations

Subhasis Roy Choudhury and Rajiv Chadha

49.1 Introduction

The abnormal structural anatomy in anorectal malformations (ARM), commonly termed as "imperforate anus," has been well studied in recent times and is now better understood; however, although a broad consensus exists, the optimal surgical management of ARM is still evolving.

49.2 Embryology

At the tail-end of the embryo, the cloaca receives the hindgut, tailgut, and the allantois. Descent of the urorectal septum (URS) and its fusion with the cloacal membrane results in a urogenital sinus anteriorly and post-allantotic gut posteriorly. Rupture of the cloacal membrane opens the anus to the exterior. Any interference with the formation, growth, and descent of the URS or with the growth of mesenchymal tissue around the cloaca results in ARM.

Incidence is 1 in 4500–5000 live births with a slight male preponderance.

S. Roy Choudhury
Pediatric Surgery, Lady Hardinge Medical College and Associated Kalawati Saran Children's Hospital, New Delhi, Delhi, India

R. Chadha (✉)
Department of Pediatric Surgery, Lady Hardinge Medical College and Kalawati Saran Children's Hospital, New Delhi, Delhi, India

49.3 Associated Abnormalities

ARM is a part of the VACTERL (vertebral, anorectal, cardiac, trachea-esophageal, renal, and limb defects) and associated anomalies may be present in 50–70% of cases. Lumbosacral spinal malformations, urologic, and cardiac abnormalities are common. Thus, mandatory evaluation of a child with ARM includes renal and spinal ultrasound (US) and echocardiography. A nasogastric tube should be passed to rule out associated esophageal atresia with/ without tracheaesophageal fistula [TEF] (approximately 10% of cases).

49.4 Types

Traditionally, the three types are h*igh*, i*ntermediate,* and *low,* depending on the termination of the gut (Wingspread 1984): above, within the craniocaudal limits of the pelvic floor musculature, or caudal to the pelvic floor. Broadly, they are in relation to the levator muscle, hence called *supralevator* or *infralevator* anomaly (Fig. 49.1).

Males with ARM most frequently (90%) have a high anomaly with the lower end of the rectum ending in a fistulous communication with the urethra or, less commonly, the bladder neck. In female patients, a low anomaly with the terminal fistula of the rectum opening to the exterior is very common (90%). Imperforate anus without a terminal fistula (blind-ending rectum) is rare in

© The Author(s), under exclusive license to Springer Nature Singapore Pte Ltd. 2025
S. Roy Choudhury (ed.), *Pediatric Surgery*, https://doi.org/10.1007/978-981-96-1257-4_49

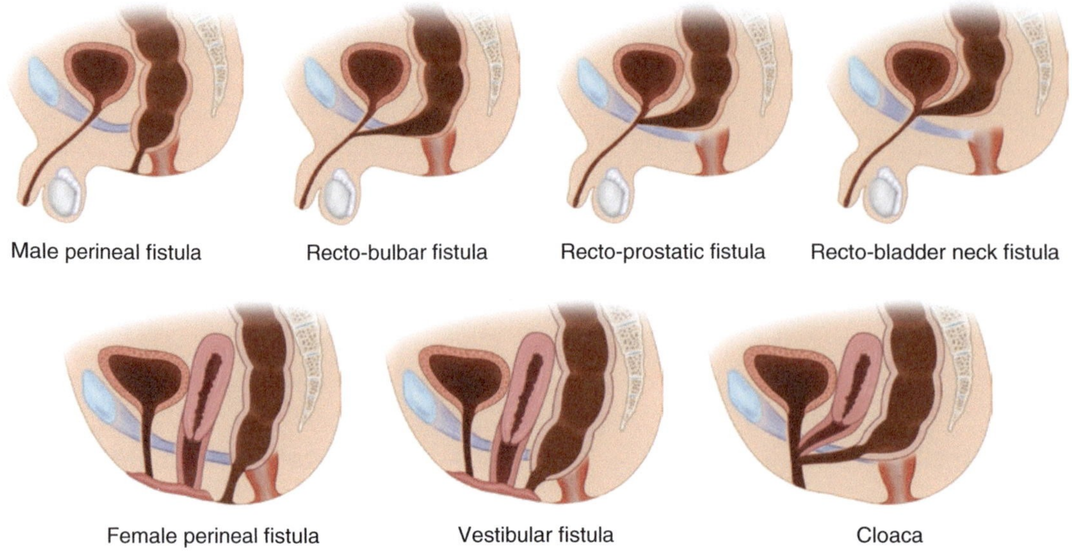

Fig. 49.1 Anatomical types of the common Male (above) and Female (below) ARM. (please check the 1st edition for this picture)

both sexes (5%) and frequently occurs in association with Down's syndrome. Rectal atresia/ stenosis, in which the anal canal and a small length of distal-most rectum are patent, is rare in both sexes (1–2%).

49.4.1 Usual Characteristics of High/Intermediate Anorectal Malformations (HARM)

Anorectum ends in fistula with the urinary tract in males and in a persistent cloaca, the vagina (uncommon) or vestibule in females.

Deficient pelvic and sphincteric musculature.

Sacral defects common.

Higher incidence of associated other organ system anomalies.

Relatively poor outcome regarding postoperative fecal continence.

Treatment is more challenging.

49.4.2 Usual Characteristics of Low Anorectal Malformations (LARM)

Anorectum ends in fistulous connection to the exterior.

Good sphincteric and pelvic musculature.

Normal sacrum.

Better chance of achieving satisfactory fecal continence.

Simpler treatment.

49.5 Classification

The most accepted current classification was derived in the international conference on ARM in the year 2005 in *Krickenbeck*. This classification is based on the anatomical fistula site with added rare and regional variants. It also addresses the follow-up and results post-surgery.

49.5.1 Major Clinical Groups

Perineal (cutaneous) fistula
Rectourthral fistula
- Bulbar
- Prostatic

Rectovesical fistula
Vestibular fistula
Cloaca
No fistula
Anal stenosis

49.5.2 Rare/Regional Variants

Pouch Colon
Rectal atresia/stenosis
Rectovaginal fistula
H-Type fistula
Others

49.6 Clinical Presentation

49.6.1 In Newborns

1. LARM: A meconium-filled tract along the median raphé and a meconium discharging perineal fistula are diagnostic of LARM in males (Fig. 49.2a). Anal stenosis, covered anus, anal membrane and bucket-handle deformity (Fig. 49.2b) are other variants of male LARM
2. Late presentation in girls with vestibular or perineal fistula may occur as they often decompress well through the fistula (Figs. 49.3 and 49.4). A perineal canal or H-type recto-vestibular/vaginal fistula (Fig. 49.5a, b) presents with passage of meconium or feces via the vestibule/ vagina in addition to the normal anal canal.
3. Signs suggestive of HARM: Meconium in urine (recto-urinary fistula) in males, a flat-bottom perineum (Figs. 49.6 and 49.7), and a single perineal opening (cloaca) in females (Fig. 49.8) are diagnostic of HARM.
4. Children with Down syndrome and ARM almost always (95%) have HARM without an associated fistula (Fig. 49.9).
5. Presence of associated malformations (described earlier).

49.6.2 Investigations

In cases where the type of ARM is not clearly evident by the clinical findings, an invertogram may be performed 18–24 hours after birth (exception-associated TEF because of risk of

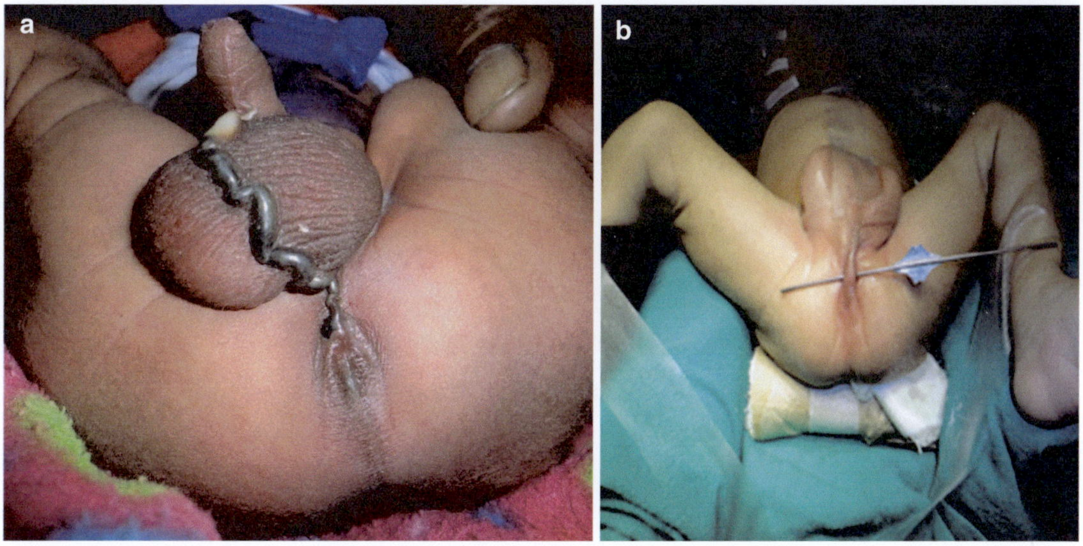

Fig. 49.2 Low ARM in male. Note meconium filled tract along median raphé (**a**); median skin tag called a bucket handle deformity (**b**)

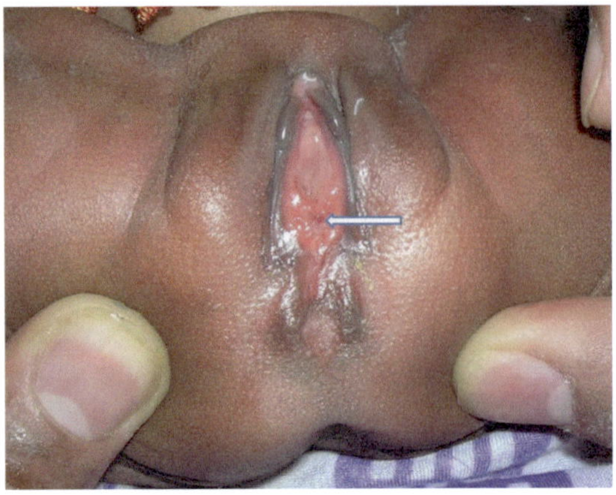

Fig. 49.3 Vestibular fistula (arrow)

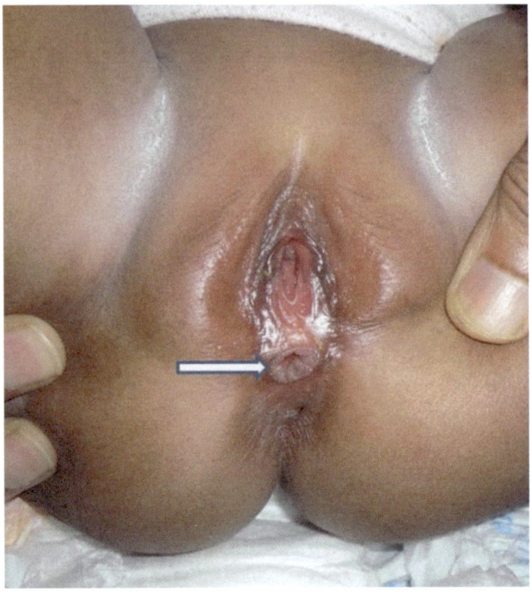

Fig. 49.4 Perineal fistula (Anterior perineal ectopic anus) [arrow]

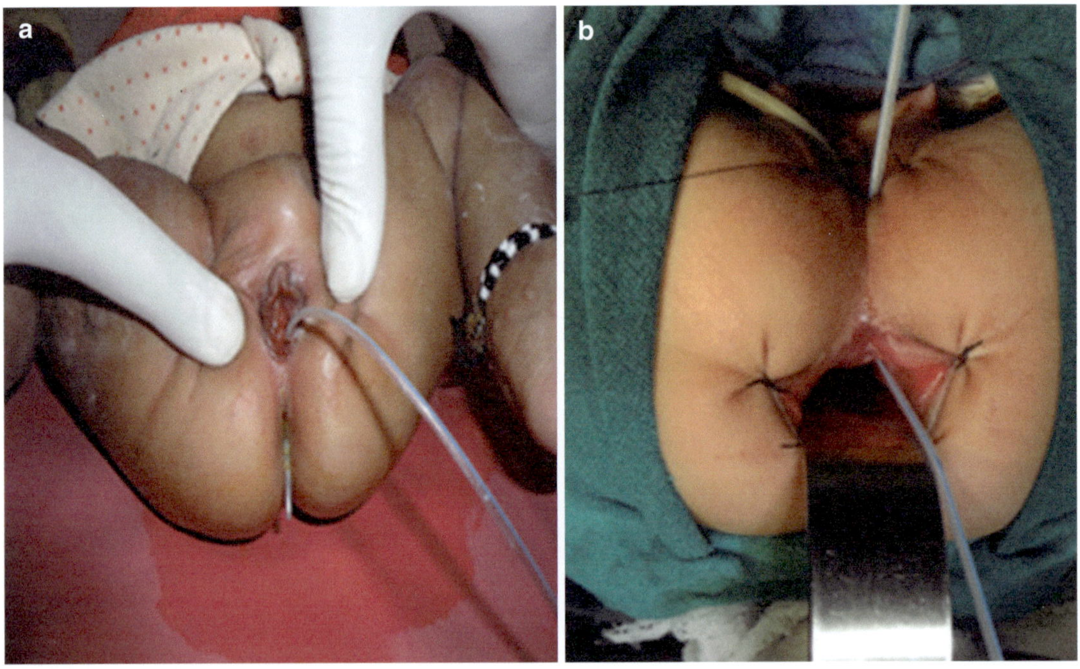

Fig. 49.5 H-type fistula (perineal canal). (**a**) opening in vagina (arrow); (**b**) anal opening (arrow)

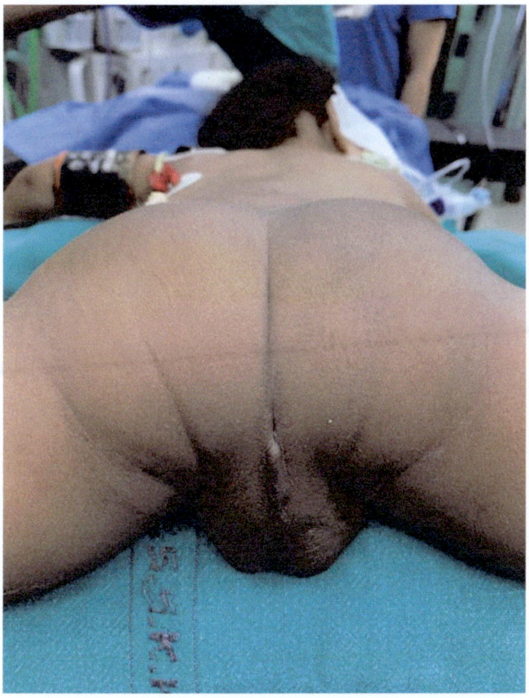

Fig. 49.6 HARM in male, no anal opening; note flat perineum

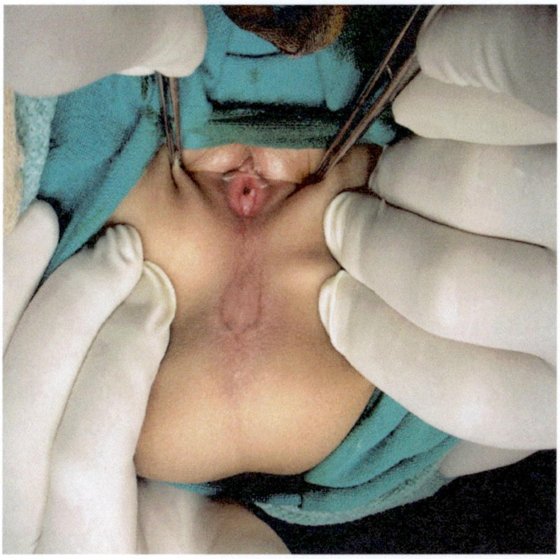

Fig. 49.7 Absence of anal opening, female HARM, flat perineum

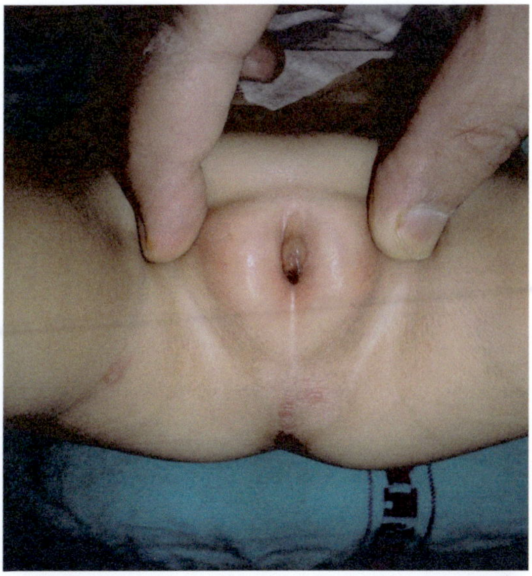

Fig. 49.8 Persistent cloaca with small-looking external genitalia. Note flat perineum

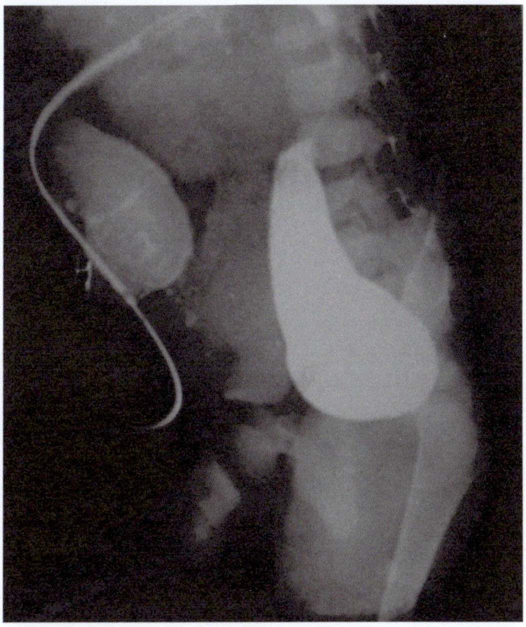

Fig. 49.9 Distal dye-study in child with Down syndrome and ARM without fistula. Note the blind-ending rectum

aspiration). A radio-opaque marker is placed at the anal dimple, the child is held upside down for a few minutes with slight flexion at hip joint and alignment of the greater trochanters. On the invertogram film, the lower limit of the rectal gas shadow is noted, and any obvious associated abnormalities like sacral agenesis are identified (Figs. 49.10 and 49.11). The level of ending of the rectal gas shadow is interpreted in relation to

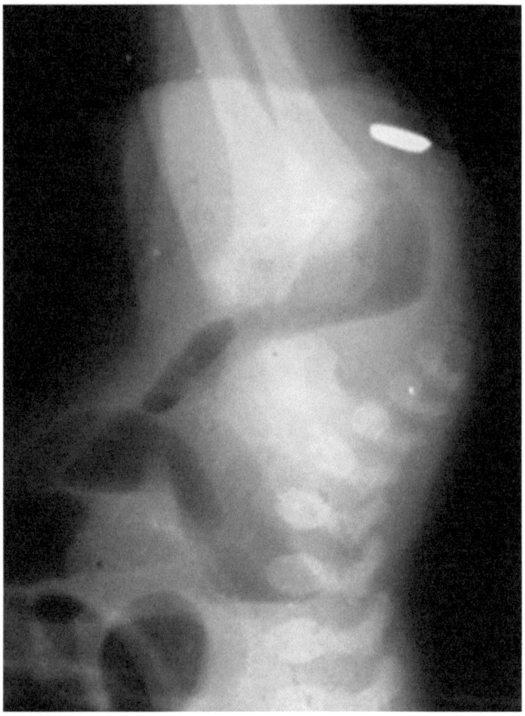

Fig. 49.10 Invertogram: Low ARM

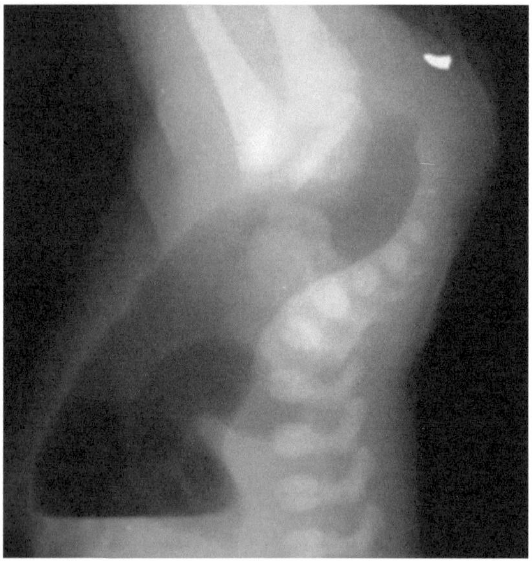

Fig. 49.11 Invertogram: High ARM

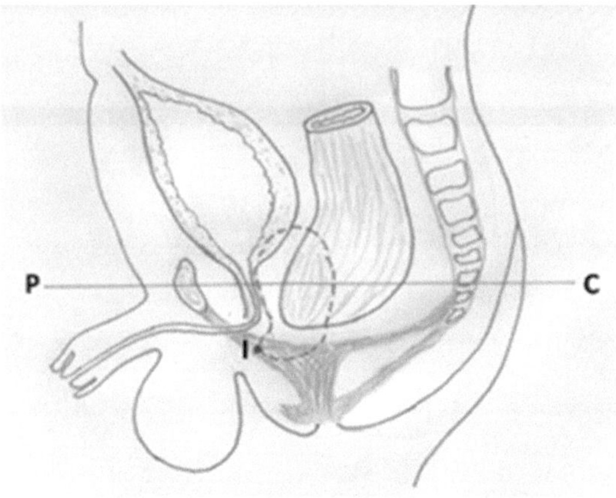

Fig. 49.12 Diagrammatic representation of P-C line and I-point in an invertogram

defined bony pelvic landmarks like the pubococcygeal line (PC line) and the I-line. The PC line joins the center of the pubis to the coccyx, while the I-line is parallel to PC line but passing through the lower border of the ischial tuberosity [I-point] (Fig. 49.12). Termination above PC line is HARM and below is intermediate (between PC and I-lines) or LARM.

At present, a cross-table prone X-ray with buttocks of the baby elevated is preferred over an invertogram (Fig. 49.13a, b). Relation of rectal gas to coccyx is given paramount importance in deciding management. If rectal gas is ending proximal to the coccyx, a preliminary colostomy is preferable but if it is extending beyond the coccyx, then anoplasty/ primary repair is feasible. Distance of bowel gas shadow more than 1 cm from the perineum is taken as intermediate or high anomaly. US may also be applied to determine the level of termination of the rectum. In centers where congenital pouch colon (CPC) is common, meconuria in males with a large air-fluid shadow occupying more than 50% width of abdomen on an erect abdominal X-ray suggests CPC (Figs. 49.14 and 49.15a, b).

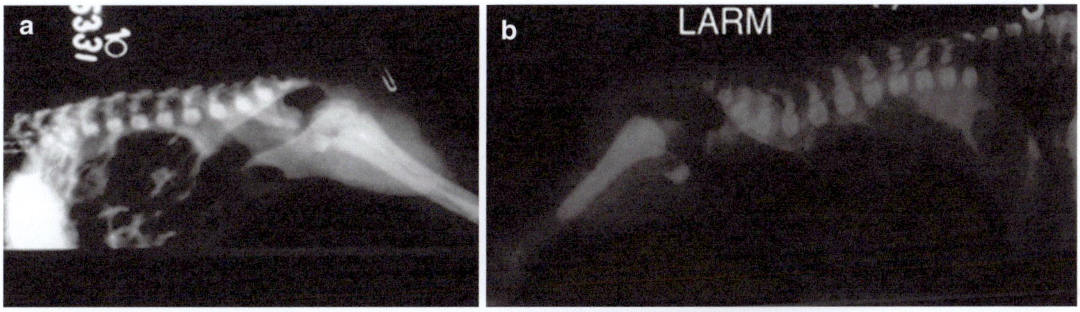

Fig. 49.13 Cross-table prone lateral view: (**a**) HARM, (**b**) LARM

Fig. 49.14 Erect abdominal X-Ray in newborn with CPC; air-fluid level occupying more than 50% of abdominal width

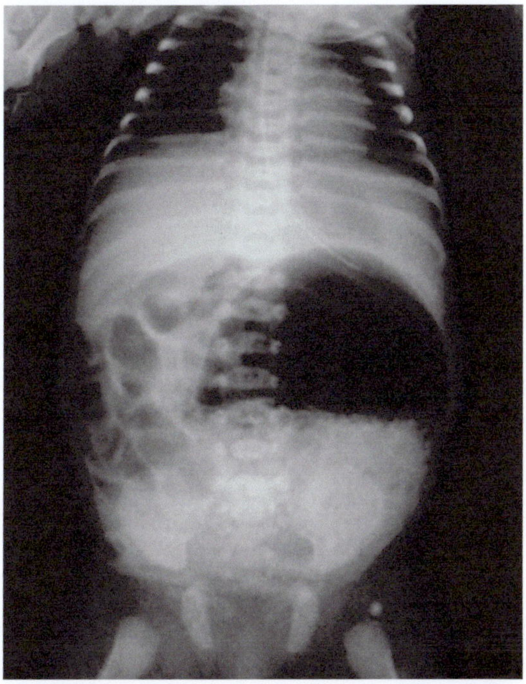

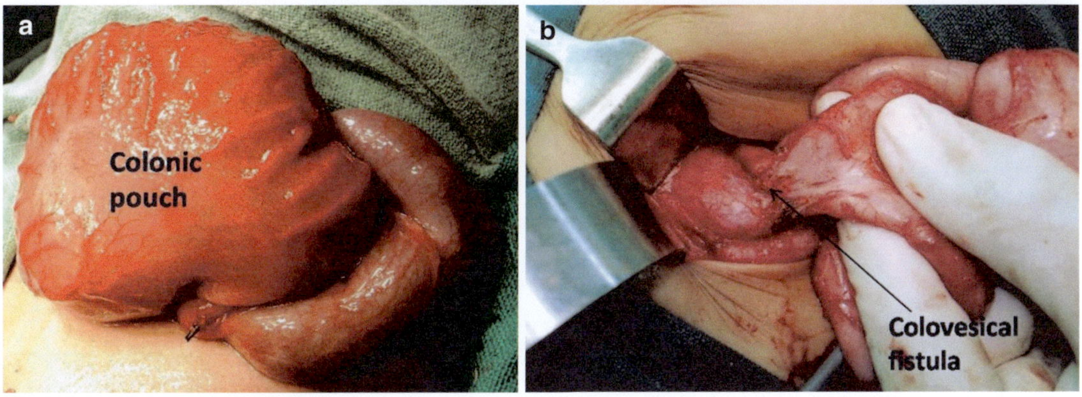

Fig. 49.15 (**a**) Congenital pouch colon, (**b**) colon terminating in high urinary fistula

49.7 Management

Suggested management algorithms for ARM are depicted in Figs. 49.16 and 49.17.

Initially, the baby is kept nil per oral on intravenous fluids with nasogastric aspiration, thermoregulation is ensured, and injection of vitamin K is administered, and the baby is stabilized. As soon as feasible, additional essential investigations to assess for associated abnormalities including USG spine, US abdomen for genitourinary anomalies, and a 2-D echogram to assess any associated cardiac anomaly, should be performed in all patients.

49.7.1 Low ARM

In these children, often an early corrective surgery is possible in a stable baby without significant associated abnormalities**.** Surgical options include:

Males

- Cut-back perineal anoplasty (laying open fistula posteriorly to the anal canal).
- Anal dilation for anal stenosis.
- Minimal Posterior Sagittal Ano-rectoplasty (MPSARP).

Females **(patients with perineal or vestibular fistula)**

- Anal transposition
- Anterior or limited posterior sagittal anorectoplasty (ASARP/ Limited PSARP)

49.7.2 High Anomalies

The preferred management is a preliminary colostomy followed by definitive staged correction. The different definitive surgical procedures for the correction of high ARM are:

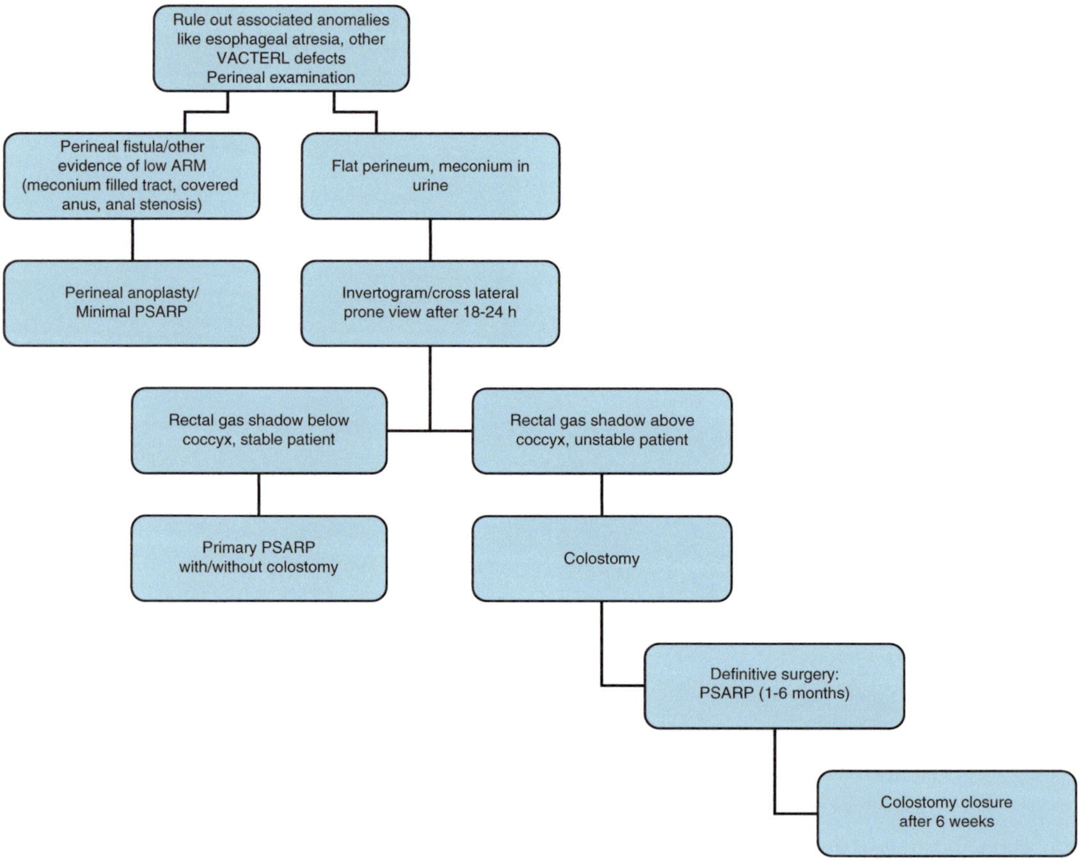

Fig. 49.16 Algorithm of management for male anorectal malformations

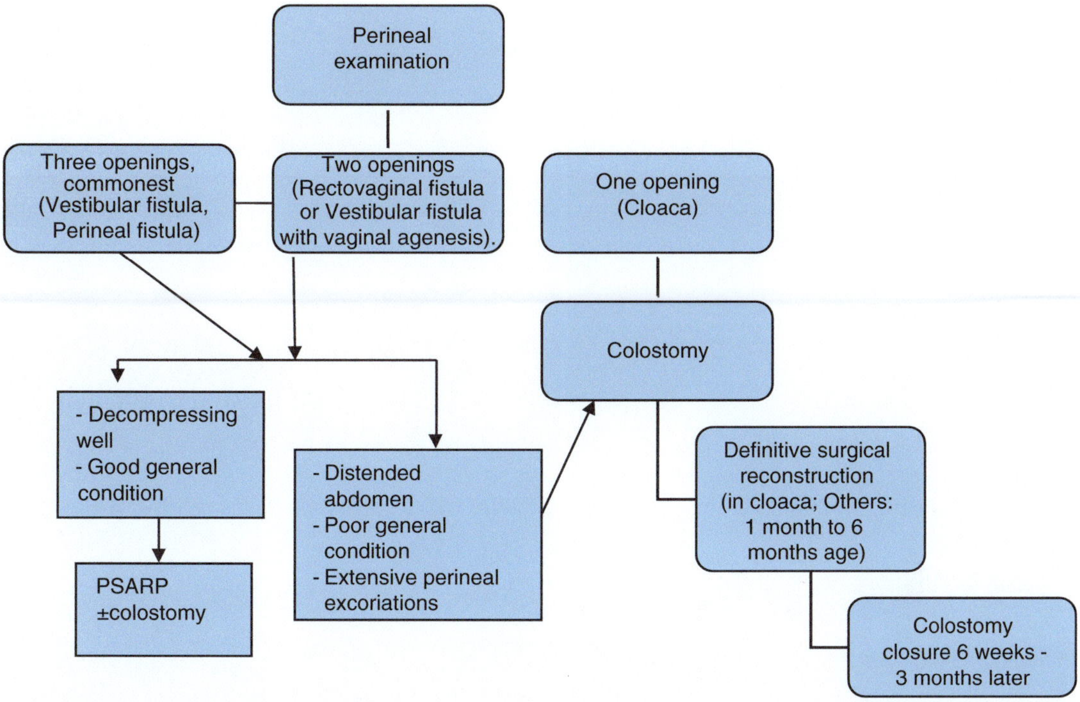

Fig. 49.17 Algorithm of management for female anorectal malformations

Posterior sagittal anorectoplasty (PSARP), abdomino-perineal, abdomino-sacroperineal, or a laparoscopic-assisted pull-through. Currently, PSARP, as described by Peña is the most commonly performed operation.

Prior to definitive reconstruction, a pressure-augmented distal colostogram, using water-soluble contrast, is invaluable in determining the level of ending of the distal rectum and the presence and level of opening of the terminal urinary fistula of the rectal pouch. A pressure-augmented distal cologram often fills up the bladder and urethra through the fistula thus eliminating the need for an MCU (Fig. 49.18a, b). A blind-ending rectum without fistulous communication (Fig. 49.9) is often seen in cases with Down syndrome.

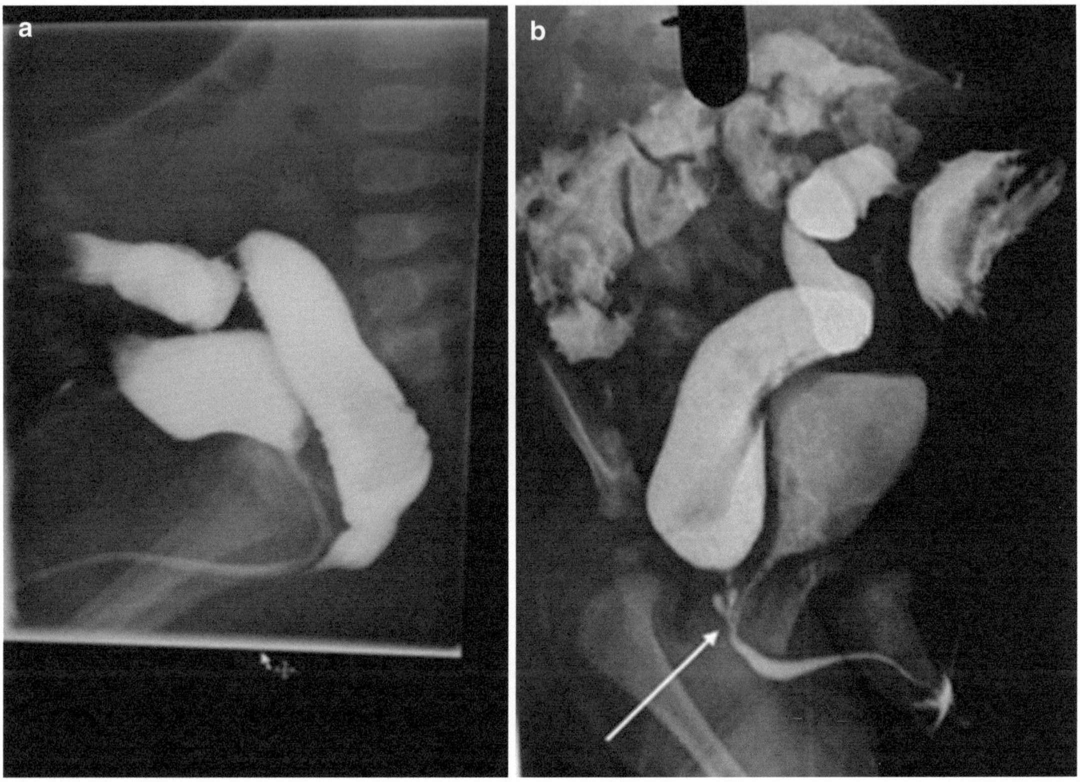

Fig. 49.18 (**a**) Distal cologram, recto-bulbar urethral fistula (long tract), (**b**) recto-prostatic-urethral fistula (arrow), short tract, note the dye in seminal vesicles

49.8 Steps of PSARP Operation For Male Patients (Fig. 49.19a, b).

- Catheterization of the bladder.
- Posterior midline (sagittal) incision extending from the mid-sacrum to the perineum.
- Division of the parasagittal fibers, muscle complex and levator ani muscles in the midline with splitting of the coccyx (if necessary).
- Identification of the rectum and securing the lower end with stay sutures.
- Opening the rectum in the midline, identifying the rectourethral fistula from inside.
- Separation of the rectourethral fistula with an initial anterior submucosal dissection followed by full-thickness separation of the rectum from the urethra (Fig. 49.20).
- Closure of the urethral fistula.
- Adequate mobilization of the rectum for bringing it to the perineum.
- The rectum is placed within the muscle complex, and the levator muscle approximated in the midline posterior to the rectum; anoplasty performed.

For recto-bladder neck fistula cases (very high anomaly), abdominal and/or laparoscopic approach for division of the fistula and pull-through of the anorectum is recommended (Fig. 49.21). Laparoscopic-assisted PSARP (LAARP) is also an option in some cases of HARM with a high prostatic-urethral fistula.

Rectal atresia In both sexes, rectal atresia is managed by a colostomy in the neonatal period followed later by anastomosis of the rectal pouch with the anal canal by the posterior sagittal route.

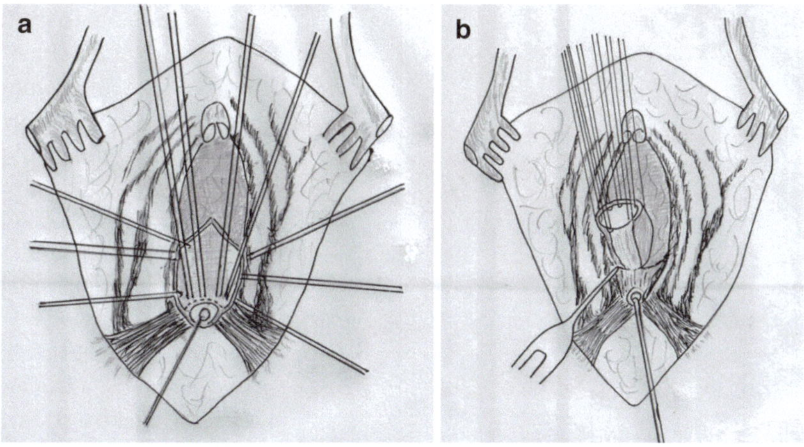

Fig. 49.19 Operative steps of PSARP for male HARM with rectourethral fistula; (**a**) fistula dissection, (**b**) rectal mobilization

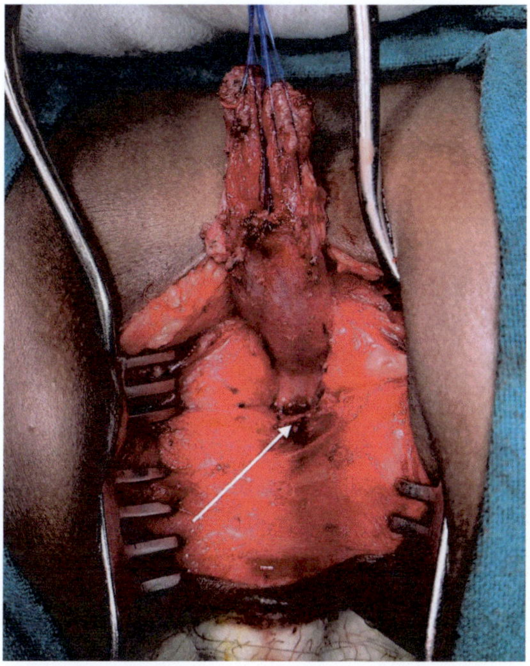

Fig. 49.20 Male PSARP with the rectum mobilized and disconnected from the recto-bulbar-urethral fistula (arrow)

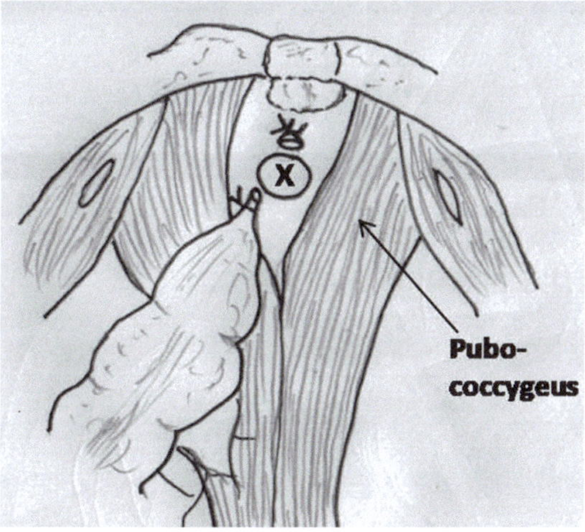

Fig. 49.21 Pelvic floor anatomy at LAARP for male HARM with bladder neck fistula after ligation of the fistula. X marks site for pull-through of rectum

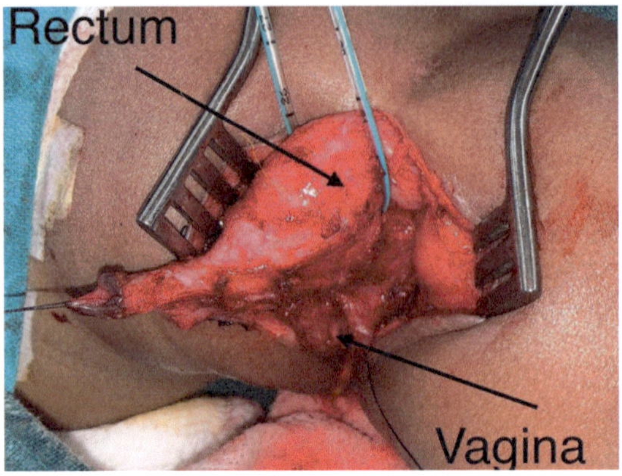

Fig. 49.22 Rectum mobilized off vagina during limited PSARP for vestibular fistula

49.9 Steps of Limited PSARP Operation for Female Patients

- Catheterization of the bladder.
- Posterior sagittal incision with division of the muscles in the midline as above.
- Complete separation of the rectum from the vagina with meticulous dissection (Fig. 49.22).
- Reconstruction of the perineal body.
- Rectum is placed within the muscle complex and anoplasty completed.

The management of persistent cloaca is covered in chapter 50.

Anal dilation is started 2 weeks after the definite repair and colostomy can be closed after 6 weeks if adequate healing has taken place.

49.10 Congenital Pouch Colon (CPC)

Congenital pouch colon (CPC) is an unusual malformation in which a pouch-like dilatation of a shortened colon is associated with an anorectal malformation (ARM). CPC is much more common in India than in the rest of the world, with about 90% of cases being reported from India, especially northern India, where it comprises around 15% of ARM. CPC is categorized into four subtypes based on the length of the normal colon proximal to the colonic pouch. In the more severe subtypes, either the normal colon is absent with the ileum opening directly into the colonic pouch (type I) or the ileum opens into a short segment of cecum, which then opens into the pouch (type II). The less severe subtypes have a longer length of normal colon proximal to the colonic pouch (types III and IV CPC) (Fig. 49.23). CPC has also been classified into '*Incomplete*' (types III–IV) or '*Complete*' CPC (types I–II), depending upon whether the length of the normal proximal colon is adequate or not for pull-through surgery after excision of the pouch. In males with CPC, the colonic pouch usually ends in a colovesical fistula (CVF) opening just proximal to the bladder neck. The opening of the terminal fistula in girls is more variable but correlates with the 'high' (more cranial) opening of the fistula in males. There is a high incidence of associated Meckel diverticulum and other anomalies of the distal limb of the midgut and the hindgut and, in males, a high incidence of vesico-ureteric reflux (VUR).

In patients with the more severe subtypes of CPC (types I–II), initial management usually consists of either an ileostomy/ colostomy proximal to the pouch or a window colostomy of the pouch, preferably after divison-ligation of the CVF (in males). In experienced hands and optimal conditions, division-ligation of the CVF, tubularization of the pouch and an end colostomy of the tubularized colon can be performed. Definitive surgery, 6 months to 18 months later, involves abdomino-perineal pull-through of the tubularized colon. In types III–IV CPC, initial surgery consists of a proximal colostomy with definitive surgery consisting, preferably, of ligation-division of the CVF and pull-through of the colonic pouch after its tubularization. Less commonly, the relatively small colonic pouch is excised and the proximal colon brought down to the perineum. Long-term results regarding fecal continence in patients with CPC are usually poor, especially in the more severe types I–II CPC. Post pull-through surgery, there is also a possibility of redilatation of the tubularized colon, often with recurrent enterocolitis.

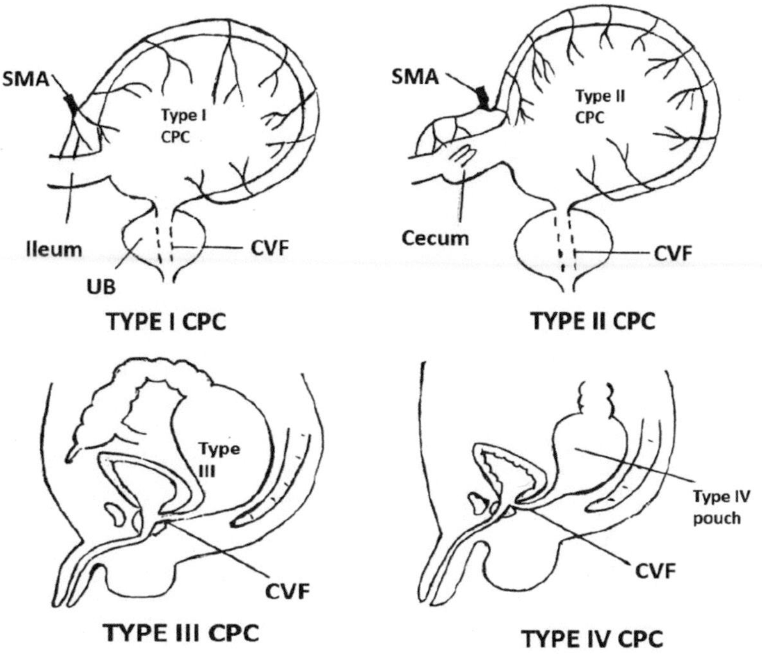

Fig. 49.23 Diagrammatic representation of subtypes of CPC. UB urinary bladder, SMA superior mesenteric artery, CVF colovesical fistula. (Note: Picture publication; permission granted by author Rajiv Chadha)

In recent years, primary PSARP and LAARP are increasingly becoming part of the management protocol for ARM.

Primary PSARP **for ARM can be performed in the presence of**

- Experienced surgeon, safe neonatal anesthesia facilities
- Babies with good birth weight
- No associated major organ system anomalies
- Bowel gas shadow extending below coccyx on prone, cross-table X-ray

Advantages of Primary PSARP

- Multiple surgeries and anesthesia exposure are avoided
- No colostomy related complications
- Recurrent UTI due to presence of recto-urinary fistula avoided
- Avoids multiple scars
- Early development of ano-cerebro-cortical reflux (role in post-repair continence)

Advantages of *Laparoscopic-Assisted Anorectal Pull Through (LAARP)*

- Major division and weakening of the striated sphincteric complex avoided
- Diminished perirectal and perineal scarring
- Optimal visualization of terminal recto-urinary fistula
- Allows precise placement of rectum within the external sphincter complex

49.11 Assessment of Fecal Continence After Definitive Repair of ARM

The following functions are assessed:

(a) Voluntary bowel movement
(b) Soiling
(c) Constipation

Several scoring systems (Kelly, Krickenbeck) for continence assessment are available for children above 3 years. Management of fecal incontinence includes a detailed bowel management program as discussed in Chap. 54.

Summary

Initial evaluation of ARM includes history-taking with a thorough perineal examination to assess the type of ARM and evaluation for the presence of any associated major organ malformations (VACTERL).

In males, the commonest ARM is recto-urethral fistula, and in females, a vestibular fistula. A meconium-filled tract and meconium discharging perineal fistula are definite signs of LARM in males and are usually managed easily by a perineal cut-back anoplasty.

ARM with a flat bottom, poorly developed anal dimple, meconium in urine (recto-urinary fistula) in males are diagnostic of HARM, usually managed with an initial colostomy. Findings on a prone cross-table lateral radiograph after 18–24 h of birth (rectal gas below/above the coccyx) can decide initial management of primary PSARP versus a preliminary divided colostomy.

In girls, three perineal openings suggest a vestibular fistula (commonest) or a perineal fistula; two openings suggest a recto-vaginal fistula or rectovestibular fistula with vaginal agenesis; and one opening suggest a persistent cloaca. Apart from persistent cloaca, girls who comply with the defined criteria (Fig. 49.17) can undergo primary anorectoplasty while an initial colostomy is needed otherwise.

A persistent cloaca, needs urgent genitourinary evaluation by US. The baby requires a 'high' colostomy. If present, a hydrocolopos needs drainage by a vaginostomy and occasionally urinary diversion by a vesicostomy.

Almost 95% of patients with Down syndrome and ARM have ano-rectal atresia without fistula. Rectal atresia or stenosis is rare in both sexes (1–2% cases). Congenital pouch colon presents with a distended abdomen and a large air-fluid level on an abdominal X-ray and is managed by an initial colostomy or a proximal ileostomy.

Suggested Reading

Coran AG, Caldamone A, Scott Adzich N, Krummel TM, Laberge JM, editors. Pediatric surgery. 7th ed. Oxford: Elsevier; 2012.

Stephens FD, Durham Smith E. Classification, identification, and assessment of surgical treatment of anorectal anomalies. Pediatr Surg Int 1986;1:200–5.

Holschneider AM, Hutson JM, editors. Anorectal malformations in children embryology, diagnosis, surgical treatment, follow-up. Heidelberg: Springer; 2006.

Pena A, Bischoff A, editors. Surgical treatment of colorectal problems in children. 1st ed. Springer; 2015.

50 Cloacal Anomalies and Congenital Pouch Colon (CPC) in Girls

Rajiv Chadha and Subhasis Roy Choudhury

Cloacal anomalies represent the most severe form of anorectal malformation (ARM) in females, constituting around 20% of female ARM. There is a single perineal opening, usually with "small-looking" genitalia (Fig. 50.1). The rectum, vagina and urinary tract open into a "single, common channel" which can be 1–10 cm long. Uterine septation and duplication are common, especially with a long common channel (Fig. 50.2), and the vagina(s) may be distended and full of secretions leading to hydrocolpos. The hydrocolpos can compress the trigone leading to hydroureteronephrosis. "Low" cloacal malformations (<3 cm common channel) (Fig. 50.2) usually have a well-developed sacrum, a normal appearing perineum, adequate pelvic nerves and musculature, and a good functional prognosis. Cloacal malformations with a common channel >3 cm have more complex defects.

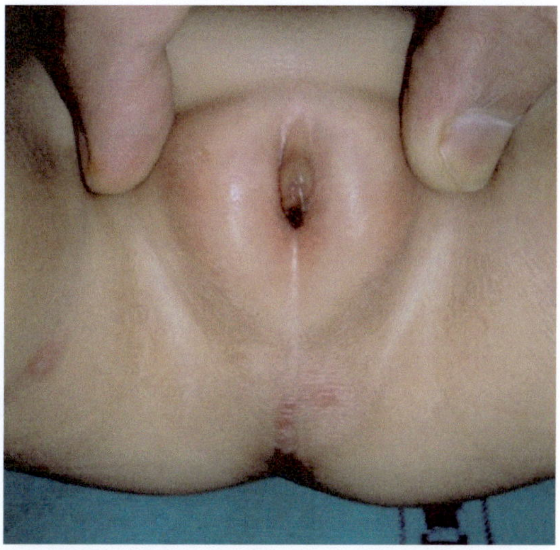

Fig. 50.1 "Small-looking external genitalia" in a girl with cloacal malformation. Note the flat perineum

Preliminary assessment of newborn girls with persistent cloaca includes an emergency genitourinary (GU) evaluation. In addition to a diverting colostomy, in the presence of hydrocolpos, a tube vaginostomy is usually adequate, although occasionally, urinary diversion in the form of a tube cystostomy or vesicostomy may be necessary.

R. Chadha (✉) · S. Roy Choudhury
Pediatric Surgery, Lady Hardinge Medical College and Associated Kalawati Saran Children's Hospital, New Delhi, Delhi, India

© The Author(s), under exclusive license to Springer Nature Singapore Pte Ltd. 2025
S. Roy Choudhury (ed.), *Pediatric Surgery*, https://doi.org/10.1007/978-981-96-1257-4_50

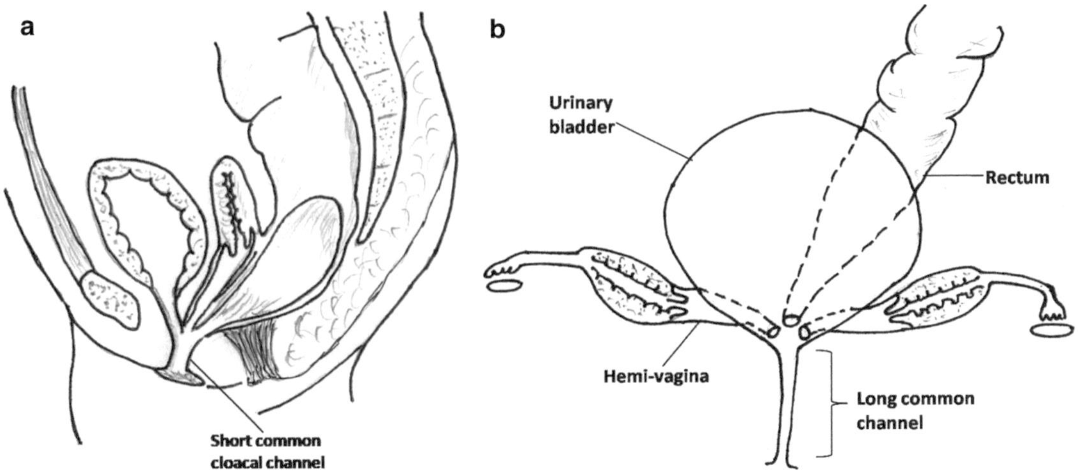

Fig. 50.2 (**a**) Cloaca with a short common channel (<3 cm), and (**b**) long common channel with uterovaginal duplication

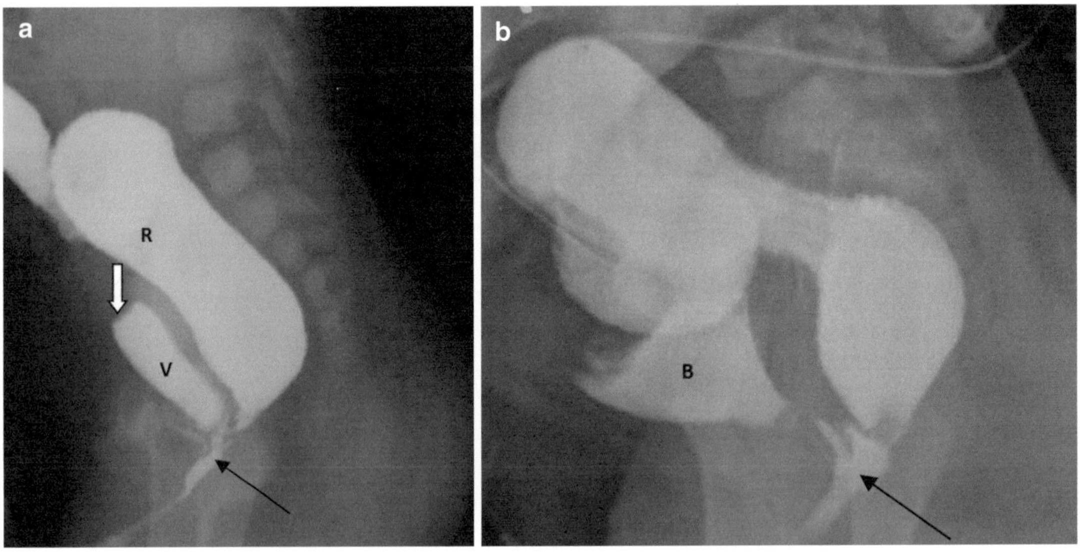

Fig. 50.3 (**a**, **b**) Distal cologram, cloaca (black arrow showing common channel). Note cervical impression above vagina (white arrow) (R rectum, V vagina, B bladder)

50.1 Management of Cloaca

Definitive repair of cloacal malformations is usually performed at 6 months to 1 year of age by the posterior sagittal route (PSARVUP). Preoperative assessment of the length and width of the common channel, the length of urethra and integrity of the bladder neck, the length of the vagina, any uterovaginal duplication, and the level of termination of the rectum are essential. This requires a dye-study via the common channel or colostomy (Fig. 50.3), detailed endoscopy, and 3D cloacogram or magnetic resonance imaging (MRI).

Patients with a common channel length less than 3 cm are >50% of all cases and can usually be managed by the posterior sagittal approach (PSARVUP) alone. The rectum is separated from the urogenital sinus and mobilized for perform-

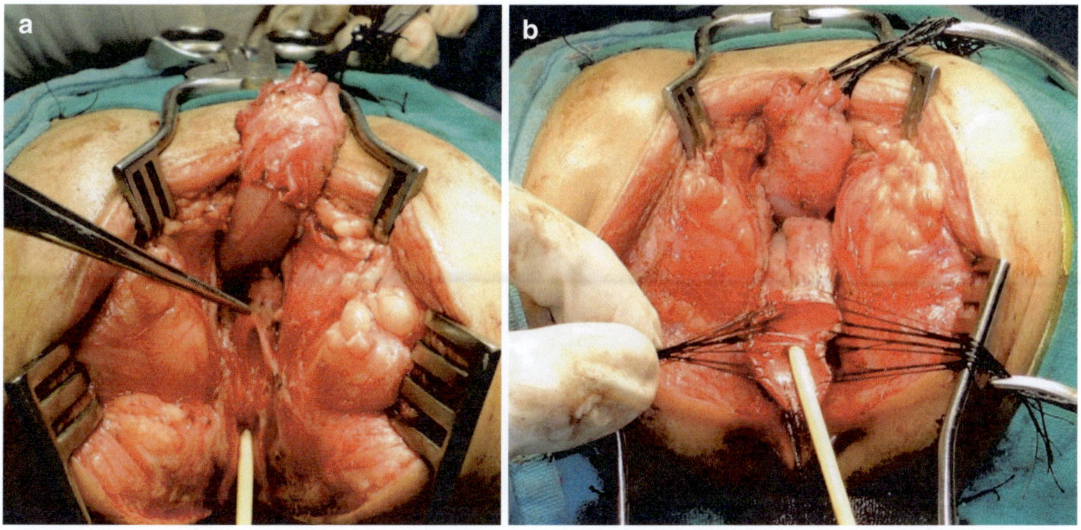

Fig. 50.4 (**a**) "TUM" showing mobilized rectum, forceps holding the posterior edge of urogenital (UG) sinus and (**b**) completion of TUM

ing an anoplasty. A total or partial urogenital sinus mobilization (TUM/PUM) can aid in bringing the urethra and vagina to the perineum (Fig. 50.4).

Patients with the common channel length 3–5 cm constitute 20% of all cases and may be managed by TUM or an "extended transabdominal TUM." Often, these patients, as well as those with common channel >5 cm long require a more extensive procedure including a laparotomy. In these, a "vaginal switch procedure" may be applicable for patients with separated hemiuteri, vaginal septum, and two large hemicolpi. Most patients, however, require vaginal replacement with a segment of bowel (sigmoid colon/small bowel), the common channel being preserved as the urethra for spontaneous voiding/clean intermittent catheterization (CIC). Patients with repaired cloacal malformations, especially with a long common channel, need long-term evaluation of functional outcomes, e.g., fecal and urinary continence, need for further urological reconstruction, the ability to pass menses without pain or obstruction, and successful sexual outcomes. These functional outcomes do not occur at the same time, stressing the need for commitment to a well-defined long-term care pathway.

50.2 Congenital Pouch Colon (CPC) in Girls

CPC in girls is usually of the more severe types I–III subtypes, and is associated with distinct genitourinary (GU) abnormalities. In contrast to "persistent cloaca," the external genitalia appear essentially normal with a wide posterior margin of the vestibule (Fig. 50.5). All girls have a hemiuterus and vagina on each side in the pelvis flanking the terminal fistula of the colonic pouch (Fig. 50.6). In newborns, there is often an appearance of folds radiating inwards and upwards from the margins of the vestibule, a "clover-leaf" appearance (Fig. 50.7). In outpatient examination in older girls or on examination under anesthesia (EUA), the position of the urethral opening and, thus, the meeting point (confluence) of the urethral and vaginal openings in the vestibule can be "low" or near normal (<1.5 cm from the base of the clitoris) (Fig. 50.8) or "high" (>1.5 cm from the base of the clitoris) (Fig. 50.9). The terminal fistula of the colonic pouch opens either into in the urethra distal to the bladder neck; high in the vestibule, almost "distal urethral" (Fig. 50.5); or in the vestibule, closer to the perineum in an intervaginal position just posterior to the urethral meatus (Fig. 50.8). The urethral opening is usually wider

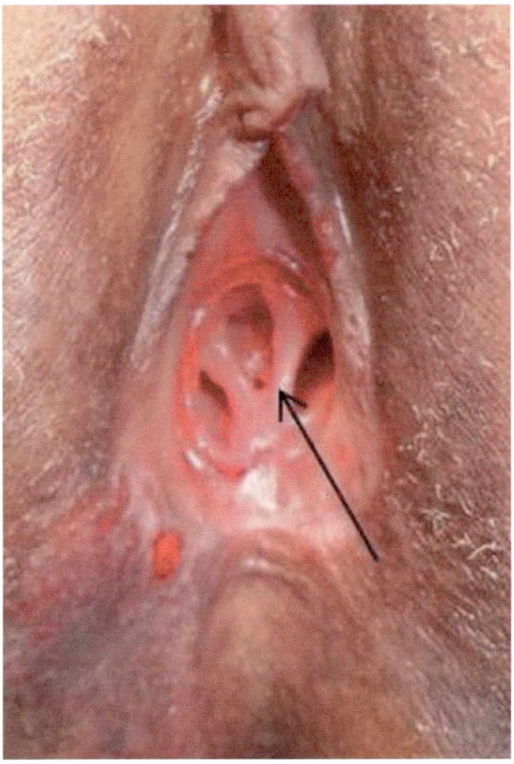

Fig. 50.5 External genitalia in girl with type II CPC, wide posterior margin vestibule, and perineal excoriations. Arrow points to the opening of terminal fistula of pouch in "distal urethral" position

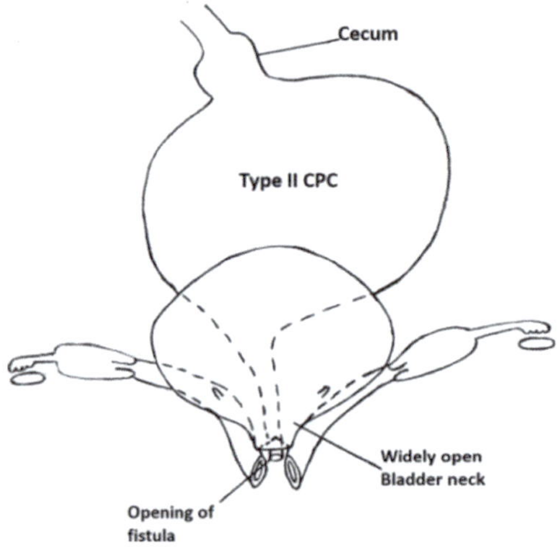

Fig. 50.6 Diagrammatic representation of pelvic anatomy in girls with CPC

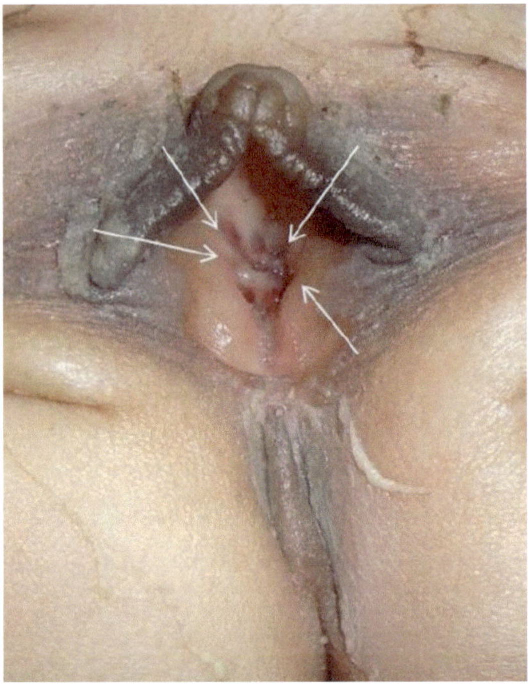

Fig. 50.7 "Clover-leaf" appearance in newborn girl with CPC. Arrows point to folds radiating inwards from margins of vestibule

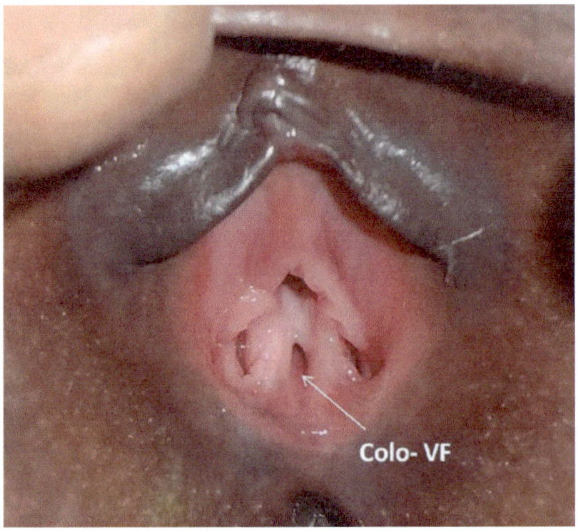

Fig. 50.8 "Low" confluence of four perineal openings. Colo vestibular fistula (VF), colo-vestibular fistula

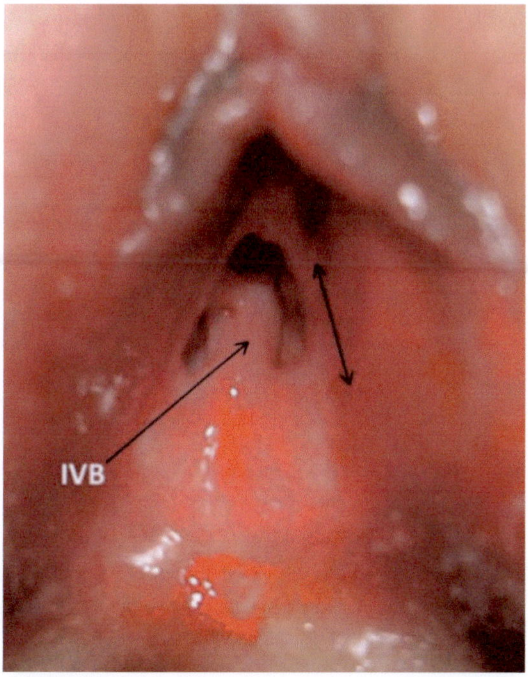

Fig. 50.9 "High" confluence of perineal opening with tilted vaginas (double-headed arrow). IVB wide intervaginal bridge

than normal, there is a wide intervaginal bridge and the vaginas often appear tilted and. Urinary incontinence (UI) ranges from 75% to 81%, and extensive peri-vulval and perineal excoriations may be present (Fig. 50.5). UI may be partial (PUI), the girls passing urine at intervals but with diurnal and nocturnal dribbling, or else complete (CUI). The UI is due to a varying severity of a structural abnormality of the lower urinary tract (LUT), the main anatomical features responsible being a short, wide urethra leading to a partially or widely open bladder neck, often with a V-shaped posterior defect, reduced bladder capacity, poorly developed trigone, and laterally placed ureteric orifices close to the bladder outlet.

Most patients present with gross abdominal distension, as in males, unless adequate decompression occurs through the associated fistula. Some girls present during infancy or later, with moderate abdominal distension, poorly managed constipation, perineal rashes, and often a doughy feeling over the abdomen due to retained feces. UI may be apparent or elicited on detailed history-taking. Abdominal X-rays in older girls may show a large soft-tissue shadow of retained fecal matter.

The principles of management are similar to those in males. An important consideration is that the clinical findings as well as micturating cystourethrogram (MCU) and cystourethrogenitoscopy(CUS) examination show a spectrum both as regards urinary continence as well as the anatomy of the LUT and external genitalia. Due to the anatomical features described earlier, UI is difficult to manage and may need bladder neck repair (BNR). If procedures to provide effective bladder outlet resistance with or without bladder augmentation do not achieve satisfactory results, an option may be surgical bladder neck closure (BNC), augmentation cystoplasty, usually ileocystoplasty, and creation of a catheterizable channel for emptying the urinary bladder or reservoir, usually a Monti's channel. The segment of bowel available for use for bladder augmentation in girls with CPC is limited by the fact that in the more common types I–II CPC, normal proximal colon is either absent (type I CPC) or very short (type II CPC) and a segment of the colonic pouch is usually preserved by tubularization for increasing the colonic absorptive area. Thus, using a substantially long length of terminal ileum for augmentation does aggravate the risk of short-bowel syndrome with its attendant metabolic and nutritional complications. One useful feature in types I–III CPC is that during tubularization of the colonic pouch, a segment of the pouch can be preserved with a leash of vessels for bladder augmentation if required later. This can avoid the risk of short-bowel syndrome due to ileocystoplasty in these patients who already have a shortened overall bowel length.

Girls with CPC do not have a "persistent cloaca" in the accepted sense of the term. Extensive surgeries for the urogenital sinus (UGS) component of the abnormality such as TUM are not required as there is a wide vestibule and a wide introitus. Division of the intervaginal septum and vagino-pouch remnant fistula on either side (if colo-vestibular fistula present) can produce a single capacious cavity with a relatively normal/hypospadic urethral opening. Monitoring for the obstetric implications of the uterovaginal abnormalities in these patients is a long-term requirement. It should be remembered, however, that a few cases of type IV CPC with a vestibular fistula and without the features described above have also been reported.

50.3 Summary

In cloaca the rectum, vagina and urinary tract open into a "single, common channel" which can be 1–10 cm long. Uterine septation and duplication are common and the vagina(s) may be distended and full of secretions leading to hydrocolpos which can compress the trigone leading to hydroureteronephrosis. Cloacal malformations with a common channel >3 cm have more complex defects. Management involves a diversion colostomy followed by a reconstructive operation at a later stage. A combination of posterior sagittal approach (PSARVUP) along with total urogenital sinus mobilization (TUM) is the operative procedure for reconstruction. CPC in girls pose a significant challenge for ano-rectal and genito-urinary reconstruction.

Suggested Reading

Chadha R, Roy Choudhury S, Pant N, et al. The anomalous clinical anatomy of congenital pouch colon in girls. J Pediatr Surg. 2011;46:1593–602.

Coran AG, Caldamone A, Scott Adzich N, Krummel TM, Laberge JM, editors. Pediatric surgery. 7th ed. Oxford: Elsevier Limited; 2012.

Holschneider AM, Hutson JM, editors. Anorectal malformations in children embryology, diagnosis, surgical treatment, follow-up. Heidelberg, Germany: Springer; 2006.

Yadav PS, Kapoor K, Khanna V. Pant N, Roy Choudhury S, Chadha R. Management of urinary incontinence in girls with congenital pouch colon. Pediatr Surg Int. 2024;40:168

51 Hirschsprung Disease

Kanishka Das and Subhasis Roy Choudhury

51.1 Introduction

Hirschsprung disease (HD) is a functional bowel obstruction due to the absence of ganglion cells in the distal colorectum commonly or involving more proximal bowel to varying extents less often.

51.2 History

Harald Hirschsprung, a Danish pediatrician, presented the first autopsy description of two patients who had died from constipation and abdominal distension (1886). The actual pathology of aganglionosis as the cause of constipation was realized by a Swedish pediatric surgeon who had recommended recto-sigmoidectomy as the surgical treatment. Considerable progress in the understanding and management of the disease has been made over the last several decades; currently, early diagnosis and single-stage surgical treatment is the standard of care in the common rectosigmoid form of the disease with excellent outcomes in the majority.

The incidence is 1 in 4500–7000 live births worldwide. There is a male preponderance with a male to female ratio of 4:1. In long segment disease, there is a relative female preponderance, and the male to female ratio approaches 1:1.

K. Das (✉)
Pediatric Surgery, AIIMS - Bhubaneswar, Bhubaneswar, Odisha, India

S. Roy Choudhury
Pediatric Surgery, Lady Hardinge Medical College and Associated Kalawati Saran Children's Hospital, New Delhi, Delhi, India

51.3 Etiopathogenesis and Pathology

The following are proposed in the etiopathogenesis

- Failure of the normal embryonic cranio-caudal neural crest cell migration.
- Absence of neurotrophic factors or cellular adhesion molecules in the developing gut leads to poor 'homing' of ganglion cells therein despite normal migration.
- Deficient nitric oxide synthetase (NOS), and hence NO production in the gut.
- Pacemaker cells (intestinal cells of Cajal) that mediate gut peristalsis have also been implicated.
- Genetic studies—Though most cases are sporadic, several genetic mutations have been identified in some cases of Hirschsprung disease, especially in long segment disease and familial variants. These include mutations of the RET proto-oncogene (familial variety has association with MEN 2B) and various other genes (GDNF, GFRa1, EDNRB, NRTN, ZFHX1B, ET3, PHOX2B, SOX10, and SHH). The chances of family members having the disease increases with the extent of agangli-

© The Author(s), under exclusive license to Springer Nature Singapore Pte Ltd. 2025

S. Roy Choudhury (ed.), *Pediatric Surgery*, https://doi.org/10.1007/978-981-96-1257-4_51

onosis - 3–7% in rectosigmoid aganglionosis and up to 20% in total colonic aganglionosis. Association of other congenital and genetic anomalies is seen in 10–25%, Trisomy 21 being the commonest. In Waardenburg-Shah syndrome, HD is associated with sensory neural deafness, hypopigmentation of the iris and hair. Neurocristopathy syndromes, multiple endocrine neoplasia type 2b, piebaldism, and congenital central hypoventilation syndrome with HD (Haddad syndrome) are other known associations.

51.3.1 Pathophysiology

The enteric nervous system consists of 'extrinsic' and 'intrinsic' pathways.

The 'extrinsic' system is a cholinergic system with acetylcholine (ACh) as the neurotransmitter, resulting in excitatory/contractile state of bowel. The adrenergic system has adrenaline/noradrenaline as neurotransmitters, they are mainly inhibitory and some excitatory. The 'intrinsic' system comprises the nonadrenergic/noncholinergic (NANC) system with nitric oxide (NO) as an inhibitory neurotransmitter, resulting in bowel relaxation. In HD, a decrease in NO (inhibitory) and increase in cholinergic and adrenergic excitatory function (all excitatory) tilts the balance to a persistent contractile state of the aganglionic segment and hence a functional mechanical obstruction.

Extent of the disease Rectosigmoid disease is the common (80%) form. Long segment colonic HD (aganglionosis extending to the descending colon and more proximal colon) is rare (10–15%). Total colonic aganglionosis (TCA) and total bowel/intestinal aganglionosis (TBA/TIA) and ultrashort segment HD (USSHD) are now considered biologically distinct from HD and are discussed later.

51.3.2 Pathology

Grossly, the aganglionic segment (collapsed, spastic) is generally distal to the ganglionic segment (dilated, hypertrophied) with an intervening transition zone that assumes a funnel shape with progressive tapering distally, all three segments being contiguous. Skip segments of aganglionosis with intervening ganglionic segments are anecdotal.

A histological diagnosis is crucial, and the following features establish the diagnosis.

- Absence of ganglion cells in the Auerbach (myenteric), Meissner (submucosal), and mucosal plexus.
- Hypertrophied nerve fibers extending into the submucosa are seen in hematoxylin and eosin staining, but are conspicuous and exhibit typical diagnostic patterns with acetylcholinesterase staining.

51.4 Clinical Features

They can present across childhood and adulthood, most present in the neonatal period or in infancy, yet late presentations are common in developing countries.

Neonates and early infants present with

- History of delayed passage of meconium (beyond 48 hours after birth) in term-born children with attendant abdominal distension & non-bilious vomiting. Bilious vomits occur with longer segment disease and mimic distal small bowel obstruction. Neonatal enterocolitis can present with generalized sepsis.
- Older infants may manifest later, often at weaning, with progressively worsening constipation, abdominal distension, poor feeding, and non-bilious vomits.
- Enterocolitis, at whatever age, is a gut-associated toxic presentation with lethargy, gross abdominal distension, bloody stool, bilious vomit, and features of peritonism/bowel perforation and peritonitis. An alternate constipation with diarrhea cycle is also described.

Physical signs—general and abdominal, vary with presentation and chronicity. Besides abdominal distension, palpable colon with/without fecalomas are common. A rectal examination reveals a tight anus that grips the finger with explosive passage of flatus and feces after withdrawing the finger in the typical rectosigmoid HD child. Longer segment afflictions would not manifest this sign. Enterocolitis is accompanied by fever or hypothermia, systemic sepsis and shock, and evolving peritoneal signs.

51.5 Investigations

- An erect, plain abdominal X-ray that includes the pelvis shows colonic distension with sigmoid colonic "cut off" and lack of bowel gas in the pelvis. Longer segment colonic disease will show correspondingly proximal cut-offs.
- *Contrast enema*—This is an important screening test that selects cases for the invasive rectal biopsy. The diagnostic features are narrow distal bowel (aganglionic), variable length of conical transition zone (ganglionic-aganglionic interface), and dilated proximal bowel (ganglionic). The common rectosigmoid form shows a transition zone at the sigmoid (Fig. 51.1) while longer colonic involvement have transition zones more proximally (Fig. 51.2). Generally, a bowel wash or rectal examination is avoided prior to the study as they may interfere with imaging the transition zone; however, established transition zones do not disappear with these maneuvers. The contrast is instilled by gravity flow through a rectal catheter, thereby avoiding overdistension. The study is terminated once the transition zone and proximal dilated bowel are demonstrated. Oblique and lateral films help in unfolding the convoluted sigmoid colon and imaging the transition zone. Where inconclusive, a delayed 24-hour film may help evaluate for significant contrast retention.
- A typical 'transition zone' may be absent in the following scenarios:
  - Neonates, occasionally
  - USSHD or TCA
  - Rectal examination or wash performed prior to the contrast enema.

  The normal maximal diameter of rectum is greater than that of the sigmoid colon, i.e., the *rectosigmoid ratio* is >1. This ratio is reversed in the classical rectosigmoid HD.
- *Anorectal manometry.* Normally, distension of rectum is associated with relaxation of the internal anal sphincter leading to loss of anal canal pressure termed as recto-anal inhibitory reflex (RAIR), an important physiology that ensures rectal ampullary storage, anorectal continence and coordinated evacuation of feces. Loss of RAIR suggests Hirschsprung disease.
- The status of manometry in the diagnosis of HD is as follows:
  - It is a screening test for the exclusion of HD, especially in habitual constipation and in the older child.
  - Because of technical expertise required, inconsistent results and operator variabil-

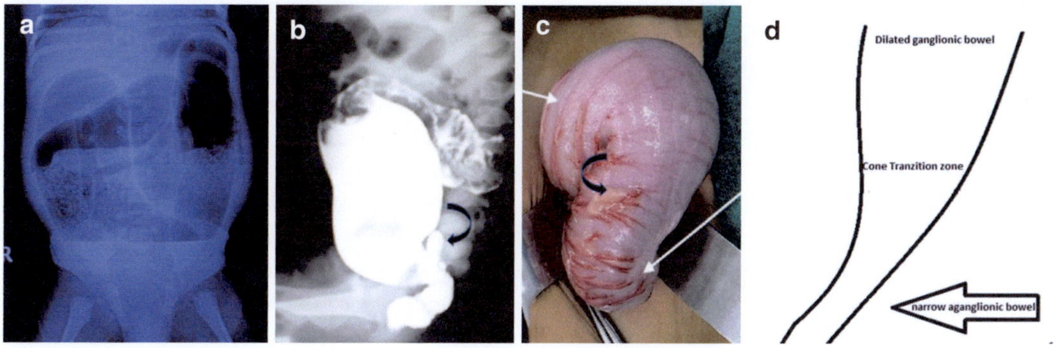

Fig. 51.1 Erect abdominal X-ray (**a**) showing distended colon with distal "cut off"/gasless pelvis. Note the typical rectosigmoid transition zone (curved arrow) between the dilated sigmoid and the narrow rectum (straight arrows) in the contrast enema (**b**) and at surgery (**c**). Corresponding diagrammatic representation in (**d**)

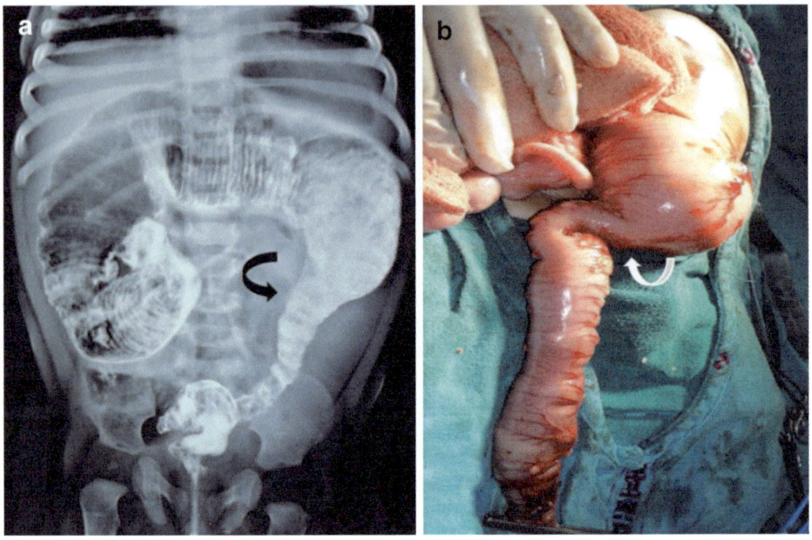

Fig. 51.2 Long segment colonic HD with mid-descending colon transition zone (curved arrow) in the contrast enema (**a**) and at surgery (**b**)

ity, a diagnosis of HD needs further histologic confirmation.

- Diagnosis of ultrashort segment HD/internal anal sphincter achalasia where transition zone is absent on contrast enema and routine histology of rectal biopsy is unremarkable.

- *Rectal biopsy*—An invasive investigation, this is the gold standard for establishing the diagnosis. It may be a suction rectal biopsy/ punch biopsy or open biopsy; the former is feasible on an outpatient basis. The biopsy should be taken from at least 2 cm above the *dentate line* as there is a physiological paucity of ganglion cells below this level. In suction/punch rectal biopsy, 2 or 3-minute specimens are generally taken between 2 and 5 cm above the dentate line. In the OR, a single larger specimen is adequate and may be full thickness or mucosubmucosal, depending on the staining procedures employed. A full thickness biopsy is preferred with routine hematoxylin & eosin staining while a mucosubmucosal biopsy with adequate submucosa suffices where frozen section with acetylcholinesterase (AChE) staining is used. Once aganglionosis is established with a rectal biopsy, leveling biopsies are obtained at 5–6 cm intervals proximally till the transition cone and into the dilated zone to map the innervation (leveling). At the 'distal most ganglionic level' of these one-point biopsies, a doughnut (ring of full-thickness bowel) biopsy is recommended for confirming normal circumferential innervation.

In USSHD/IASA, a strip of full-thickness longitudinal rectal biopsy beginning at the dentate line and coursing cranially for 2–4 cm, containing the muscle layers, may simultaneously serve as an internal sphincteric myectomy for the treatment of the pathology itself.

Histological findings of aganglionosis along with hypertrophied nerve bundles by staining with hematoxylin and eosin (Fig. 51.3) or calretinin stained paraffin sections confirm the diagnosis. Calretinin, a calcium-binding protein, is positive in thin nerve fibrils normally distributed in the lamina propria, muscularis mucosae, and submucosa. In HD, this calretinin expression is absent in the nerve trunks of the aganglionic bowel. Thus, biopsy, intraoperative frozen-aided or on routine paraffin sections postoperatively, confirms the aganglionosis and levels the extent for the purpose of a diverting stoma or pull-through surgery.

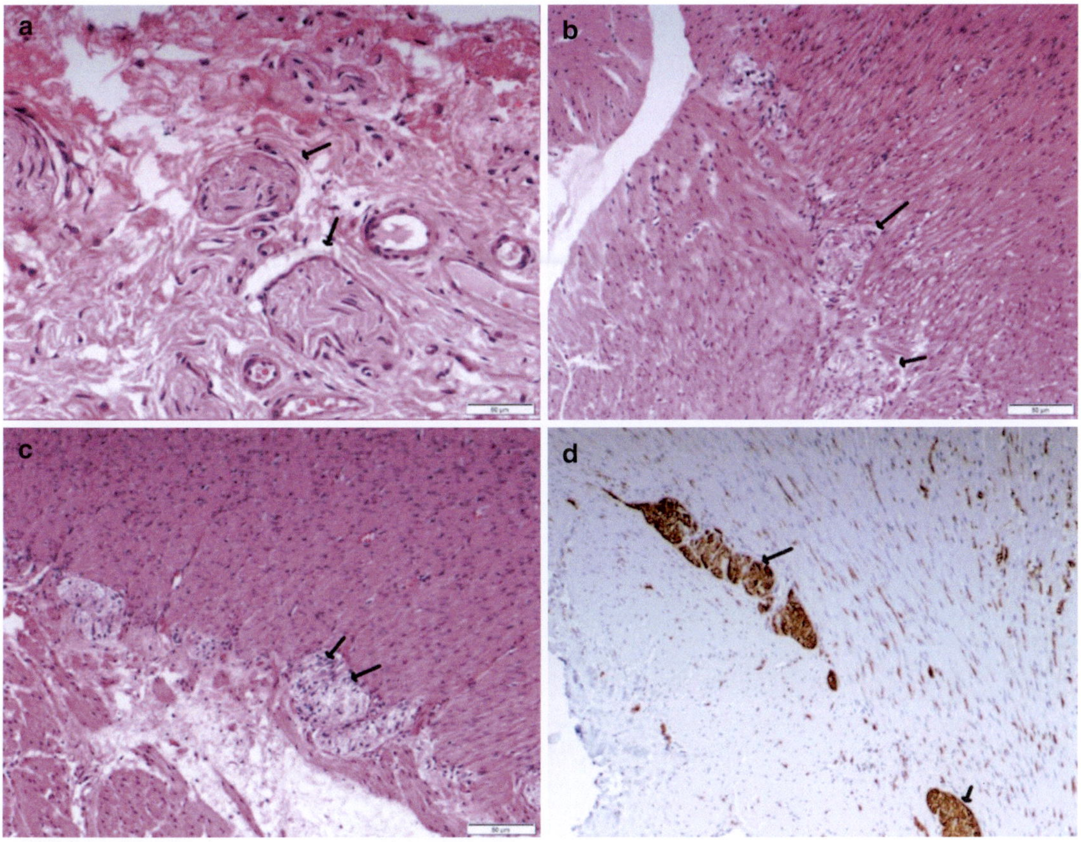

Fig. 51.3 Rectal biopsy showing absence of ganglion cells in the submucosal (**a**, arrows) and myenteric plexuses (**b**, arrows) with hypertrophied nerve bundles suggestive of Hirschsprung disease. [H & E, ×200] The hypertrophied nerve bundles are highlighted in **d** [PGP 9.5 stain, ×100]. In **c**, the rectal biopsy from another patient shows mature ganglion cells (arrows), excluding the diagnosis of Hirschsprung disease. [H&E, ×200]. (Courtesy Dr. Prasenjit Das, AIIMS, New Delhi)

51.6 Differential Diagnosis

- Neonatal period: Meconium ileus, distal ileal atresia, colonic atresia, low anorectal malformation, small left colon syndrome in infants of diabetic mothers.

  Other causes of delayed passage of meconium: prematurity, meconium plug, sepsis & dystelectrolytemia, hypothyroidism, variant HD including intestinal neuronal dysplasia, hypo/hyper/dysganglionosis, and intestinal motility disorders.
- Infant and older children: Improper weaning, functional/habitual constipation, and encopresis (fecal retention with liquid soiling) are common differential diagnoses (Table 51.1, Fig. 51.4).

Table 51.1 Clinical difference between idiopathic constipation and Hirschsprung disease

	Idiopathic constipation	Hirschsprung disease
Meconium history	Normal	Delayed
Diet	Poor, low in fiber	Relatively normal
Voiding issues	Often, as a part of bowel bladder dysfunction	Rare
Perianal fecal soiling (encopresis)	Common	Rare
Stool retentive behavior	Common	Rare
Obstructive symptoms, abdominal distension, dilated bowel loops	Rare	Common
Per rectal examination	Dilated rectal ampulla	Narrow, spastic rectum that grips the finger
Stool in rectal ampulla	Common, fecalomas	Rare, usually empty
Enterocolitis	Never	Possible

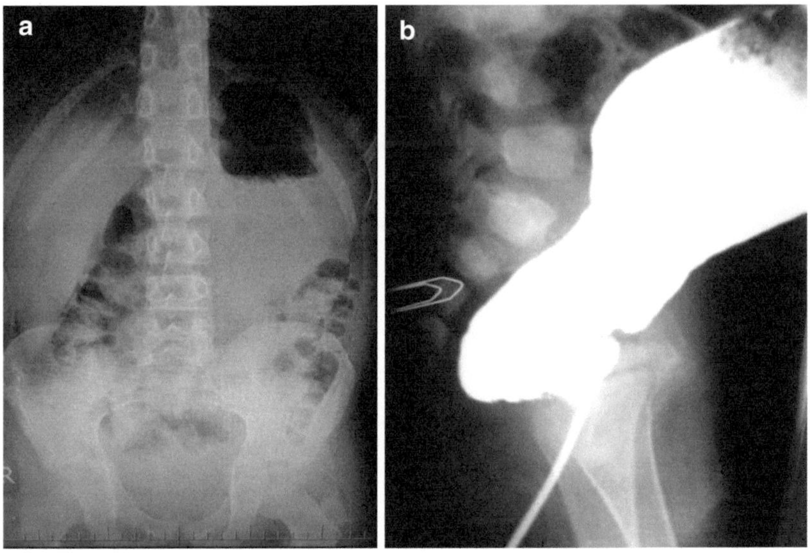

Fig. 51.4 Idiopathic constipation—The abdominal X-ray (**a**) shows extensive colonic fecal shadows, the contrast enema (**b**) delineates a dilated rectal ampulla up to the anal verge with a posterior shelf

51.7 Allied Disorders

Total colonic aganglionosis ***(TCA)*** In this form of long segment aganglionosis (3–12%), the whole colon and often part of the terminal ileum, up to 50 cm proximal to the ileocolic valve, is aganglionic. Rarely does aganglionosis extend further proximally to involve the proximal small bowel or even the total bowel (total intestinal aganglionosis – TIA). TCA presents with features of distal small bowel obstruction; the presentation is sometimes not classic and diagnosis is delayed by a few months. There is a higher chance of familial involvement in TCA. The contrast enema may show a narrow caliber and foreshortened colon with loss of splenic flexure and hence a "question mark" like appearance (Fig. 51.5). Rectal biopsy confirms the diagnosis of aganglionosis; however, the extent can only be determined by more proximal biopsies, usually at laparotomy or laparoscopy. The biopsy of the appendix is unreliable for identification of ganglion cells, especially intraoperatively on frozen sections; hence, colonic and small bowel biopsies are taken for leveling /mapping. Generally, a stoma is constructed at the distal-most site of the ganglionic ileum based on frozen section histopathological confirmation, and a pull-through surgery is scheduled later. The principle of pull-through surgeries is like the classical HD as described below, with the addition of a longitudinal colonic patch to provide a larger absorptive surface. The colonic patch may be drawn from the right side (Kimura) or the left side (Martin) or by creating a J pouch. The Martin modification of Duhamel pull-through with a long side-to-side colorectal anastomosis is preferred. Of late, some have waited for a year with a stoma for bowel adaptation and formation of a semi-solid effluent and proceeded with an ileal Duhamel procedure/straight ileoanal pull through with comparable results. Frequent bowel movements in the initial post-operative period settle down over a period; supplementation of nutrients absorbed in the terminal ileum is essential.

TIA is extremely difficult to manage. Sitting a stoma at the ganglionic bowel and total parenteral nutrition (TPN) with some enteral feeding is the initial management. Later, bowel lengthening procedures like Bianchi or STEP (serial transverse enteroplasty) may be attempted if significant bowel dilatation occurs. Zeigler suggested small bowel myectomy-myotomy of aganglionic bowel with limited success for TCA/TIA. Small bowel transplantation may be needed for long-term survival in some of these patients.

Internal anal sphincter achalasia Earlier termed USSHD—ultrashort segment HD, it has been renamed as internal anal sphincter achalasia. The clinical presentation is indistinguishable from HD, with no demonstrable narrowing or transition zone in contrast study. Routine rectal biopsy is unremarkable, but acetylcholinesterase staining on the strip biopsy/multiple anorectal biopsies special biopsy has typical findings. Diagnosis is established by demonstrating the absence of recto-anal inhibitory reflex (RAIR) on anorectal manometry. It is treated by anorectal myectomy or internal sphincterotomy and intra-sphincteric injection of botulinum toxin.

Variants of Hirschsprung disease This is a heterogeneous group of disorders that overlap in clinicopathological features with Hirschsprung disease but are distinct by themselves. They require an adequate full thickness rectal biopsy and specific histopathological evaluations including histochemistry, immunohistochemistry, and electron microscopy for a criterion-based diagnosis are briefly discussed.

- *Immature ganglia* are encountered in premature neonates and mature with advancing gestational age to term. They may account for

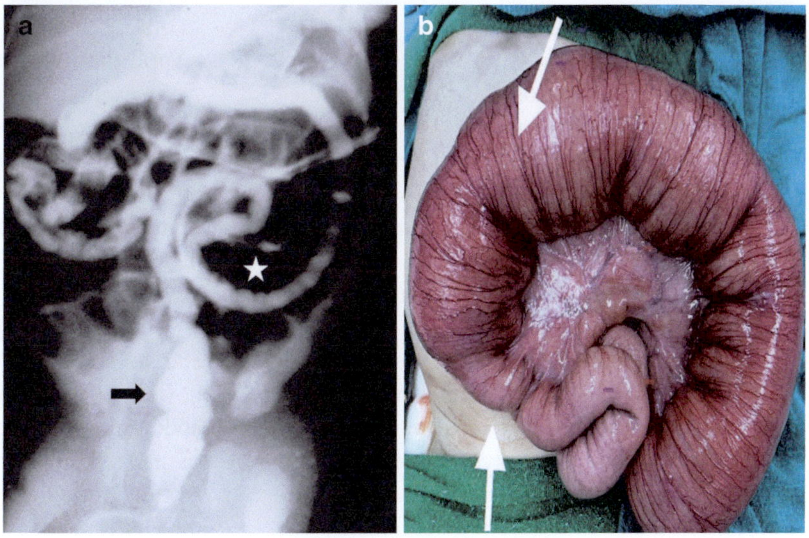

Fig. 51.5 Total colonic aganglionosis—The contrast enema (**a**) shows a question mark microcolon, also note dilated small bowel (star) and preserved rectosigmoid ratio (arrow). Intraoperative photograph (**b**) showing dilated and thickened proximal ganglionic ileum (oblique arrow), transition zone, and narrow distal aganglionic ileum (vertical arrow)

obstructive symptoms that gradually resolve with maturity.

- *Intestinal neuronal dysplasia*—Type A is a rare, primary sympathetic neural disorder that presents as an acute infantile form and is frequently fatal. Type B, a malformation of the parasympathetic myenteric plexus, is commoner and may coexist with Hirschsprung disease in the proximal ganglionic bowel. The diagnosis may be missed and lead to persistent obstructive symptoms after pull-throughs. A full-thickness biopsy that demonstrates specific features (hyperganglionosis, ectopic ganglia, and giant ganglia) clinches the diagnosis.
- *Isolated hypoganglionosis* is rarely encountered in evaluation for large bowel dysmotility and shows sparse and small myenteric ganglia; in contrast, a transition zone hypoganglionosis of HD is common encountered during leveling biopsies *Smooth muscle cell disorder and holovisceral myopathies* are primary smooth muscle intestinal disorders that involve other hollow viscera too (e.g. bladder and uterus), are rare, unresponsive to any form of management and generally fatal. MMIS-megacystic microcolon intestinal hypoperistalsis syndrome is the common form involving the bladder.

51.8 Management

The choice of investigation and treatment is dictated by the clinical presentation (Fig. 51.6). The child is resuscitated and stabilized first with one or more of the following measures

(a) Breast feeds/clear liquids/intravenous hydration.

(b) Gentle rectal washout, with/without liquefying agents and retention enemas (e.g., glycerine) to lyse the fecalomas.

Intravenous antibiotics/other medications for sepsis/enterocolitis are administered. Sick children unresponsive to rectal washout and antibiotics may need emergency diversion stoma—blind/leveling colostomy or ileostomy as appropriate, as a lifesaving procedure.

51.8.1 Surgical Treatment

(a) Staged operation

Staged operations consist of an initial siting of a stoma followed by a definitive pull-through operation after several months. The stomal siting is best done at the distal level of circumferentially ganglionic bowel determined by intraoperative doughnut frozen section histopathology or a 'leveling' stoma. In the absence of a reliable intraoperative leveling facility, a 'blind' stoma is sited 5–10 cm proximal to the gross transition zone. Where such a zone is not visible, the siting is difficult. A definitive pull-through procedure is scheduled after a period of diversion varying from several weeks to months to allow the hypertrophied dilated bowel to return to near normal dimensions and interim nutritional rehabilitation of the child.

(b) *Pull-through procedures* (Fig. 51.7) include the following standard ones.
- Duhamel (modified Martin)—aretrorectal pull-through procedure,
- Swenson procedure—an abdominal and trans anal pull through and
- Soave (modified Scott-Boley) procedure: An abdominal or transanal endorectal pull-through.

In each, most or all of the aganglionic bowel is excised, and part/whole of the circumference of the distal most ganglionic bowel is surgically placed within a cm or so of the dentate line by various technical modifications. The results of the three operations are comparable.

The Swenson operation creates a circular end to end anastomosis of the ganglionic bowel above the anal sphincter. It involves abdomino-pelvic circumferential dissection of the rectum followed by eversion of the rectum through the anal canal to complete the anastomosis from the perineal end.

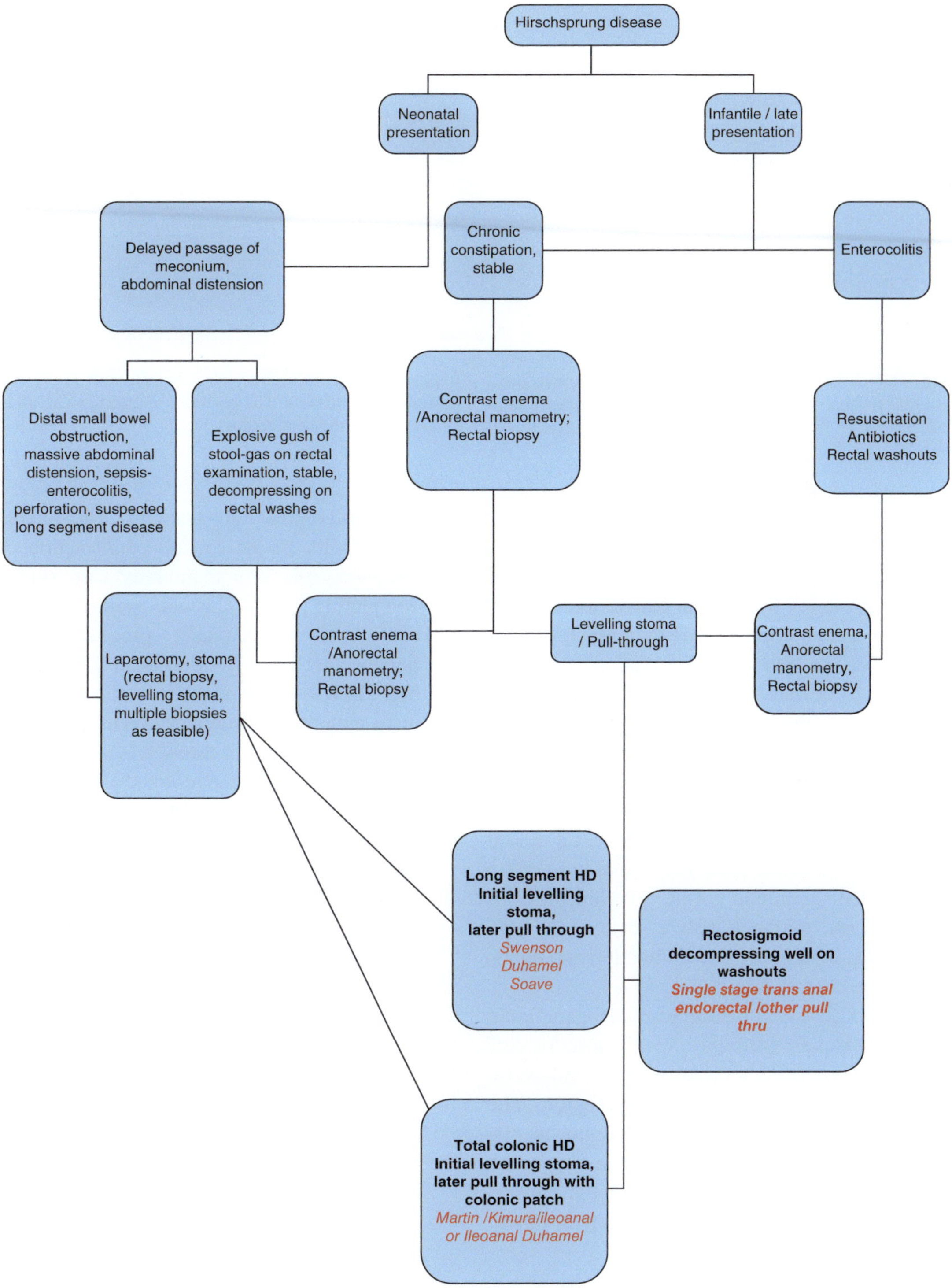

Fig. 51.6 Algorithmic management of Hirschsprung disease and total colonic aganglionosis

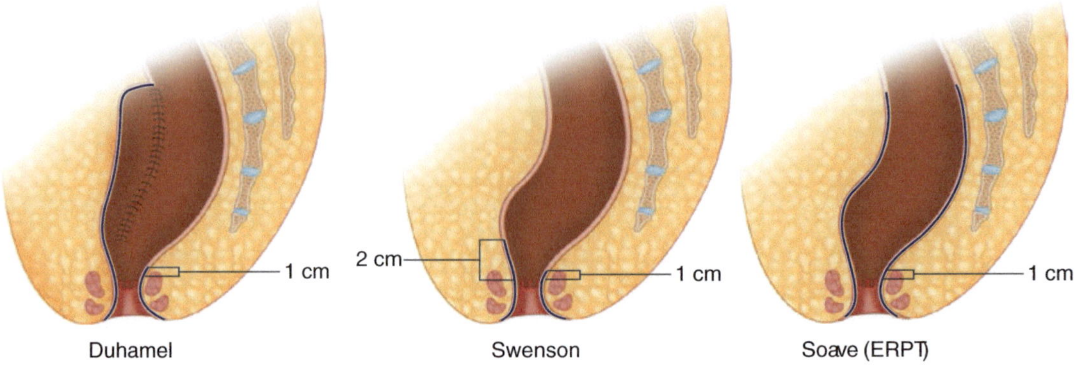

Fig. 51.7 Schematic diagram of the three common surgical pull-through procedures in the definitive management of HD. Note the varying lengths of the native bowel retained in each (blue line). The muscle cuff is divided posteriorly in Soave's. The posterior anastomosis in all is at a cm above the dentate line

In the Duhamel procedure, the proximal ganglionic colon is routed caudally through the retrorectal space. The common wall between the posterior wall of the native, narrow rectum and anterior wall of the pulled-through bowel is divided with various devices, clamps or linear cutter stapler, thereby leaving an anterior smaller circumference of aganglionic bowel and a relatively larger posterior circumference of ganglionic bowel. The Martin modification includes an end-to-side anastomosis between the rectal stump and the pulled colon at the cranial limit of the divided common wall. Technically, it involves minimal pelvic dissection, and results in terms of bowel function and continence are satisfactory.

In the Soave operation, the proximal ganglionic colon is pulled through a rectal muscular cuff that is retained after a submucosal endorectal dissection of the aganglionic anorectum. The pulled-through bowel is anastomosed circumferentially above the dentate line in the Scott–Boley modification and the muscle cuff is partially divided posteriorly to render it non obstructive.

A circumferential all-quadrant (doughnut) biopsy with frozen section confirmation of ganglion cells is a mandatory step before completing the pull-through operation, especially in single-stage procedures. A laparoscopy-assisted transanal endorectal pull (TERP) with frozen section biopsy and histo-pathological confirmation of the transition zone before pull-through is more appropriate for long segment colonic HD.

Neonates with rectosigmoid HD who are stable are now initially managed with rectal saline irrigation and stimulation for bowel movement. Those decompressing effectively can be managed with a home enema regimen and electively operated in the neonatal period or early infancy with a one stage procedure, provided the distal ganglionic bowel is not too dilated for the small pelvis. Though any of the procedures described above can be done primarily, a one-stage transanal endorectal pull-through (TERP) with or without laparoscopy assistance for leveling biopsy and mobilization has gained popularity in the management of classical rectosigmoid HD (Fig. 51.8).

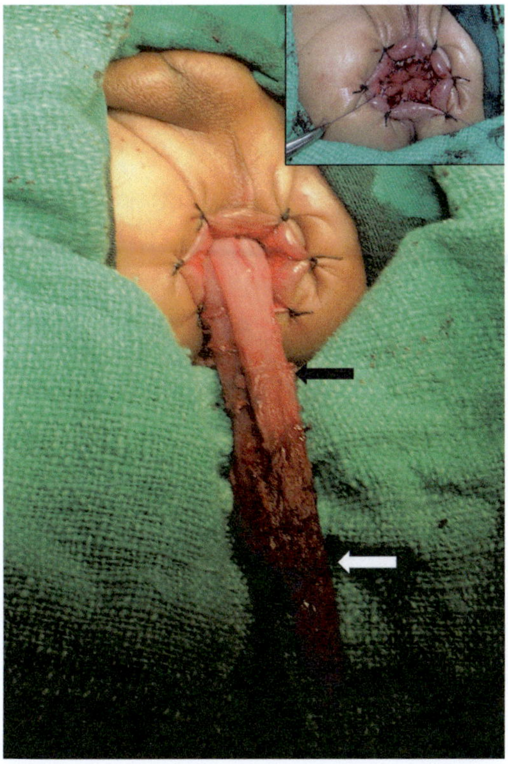

Fig. 51.8 Transanal endorectal pull-through (Soave) procedure in rectosigmoid HD. Note the transition zone (white arrow) between the proximal dilated bowel (black arrow) and the distal narrow rectum. A circumferential full-thickness biopsy confirms normal innervation at the dilated bowel 5–7 cm above the transition zone before the final anastomosis (inset)

51.9 Complications and Outcome

- Post-operative: anastomotic leak, stricture, intestinal obstruction, pelvic abscess, wound infection, and perineal excoriation.
- Chronic obstructive symptoms/constipation/ persistent aganglionosis/hypoganglionosis/ transition zone pull-through.
- Enterocolitis.
- Incontinence/diarrhea.
- Voiding dysfunction.

Constipation is commoner following the Duhamel operation. Enterocolitis is more commonly reported following the Swenson operation. Incontinence and diarrhea are complications associated with Soave and endorectal pull-through. Cuff-related problems following the Soave operation can be avoided by splitting the muscular cuff.

Enterocolitis can occur in up to 30% of patients with HD. This occurs due to obstruction leading to bacterial stasis and inflammation of the bowel wall and can progress to perforation. It can occur before or after surgery/removal of the aganglionic segment and is more commonly associated with long segment HD. The presentation and management have been discussed above.

Long-term functional outcome, bowel continence, and quality of life in optimally managed patients of rectosigmoid HD are generally excellent. A minority with fecal incontinence is managed with a bowel management program. The outcomes with long segment colonic HD are equally favorable, with an initial bowel frequency that settles over the years. The outcome in TCA is comparatively modest and quality of life improves over years. TIA is incompatible with life.

Patients with persistent obstructive symptoms after surgery are systematically reviewed for technical errors and histopathological errors in diagnosis and leveling. The treatment options are varied, ranging from botulinum injection to redo stomas/pull-through operations depending on the complication.

51.10 Summary

Hirschsprung disease (HD) / aganglionosis coli is a common cause of congenital large gut obstruction and must be differentiated from the commoner habitual constipation. Classical rectosigmoid HD (85%) is common in term males; long segment disease is preponderant in females and associated with familial, syndromic and genetic forms. Plain x rays are suggestive and the contrast enema / anorectal manometry are reliable screening tests. Rectal biopsy confirms the diagnosis while levelling biopsies map the proximal contiguous extent of abnormal innervation. Surgical treatment is individualized – single staged pull-through or staged (stoma followed by pull-through). Duhamel procedure and transanal endorectal pull through are the commonest definitive procedures for HD worldwide. Long term outcomes are excellent in rectosigmoid HD and comparatively modest with long segment disease. Rare forms of bowel aganglionosis (TCA/TIA, USSHD/IASA, skip lesions) are biological entities distinct from classical rectosigmoid HD.

Suggested Reading

Coran AG, Caldamone A, Scott Adzich N, Krummel TM, Laberge JM, editors. Pediatric surgery. 7th ed. Oxford: Elsevier Limited; 2012.

Holschneider AM, Hutson JM, editors. Hirschprung's disease and allied disorder. Heidelberg: Springer; 2006.

de Lorijn F, Boeckxstaens GE, Benninga MA. Symptomatology, pathophysiology, diagnostic work-up, and treatment of Hirschsprung disease in infancy and childhood. Curr Gastroenterol Rep. 2007;9:245–53.

Losty PD, Flake AW, Rintala RJ, Hutson JM, Iwai N. Rickham's neonatal surgery. London: Springer; 2018.

Puri P. Hirschsprung disease and allied disorders. 4th ed. Springer; 2019.

Teitelbaum DH. Hirschsprung's disease & related conditions. Semin Pediatr Surg. 2012;21:281–370.

52 Acquired Anorectal Disorders

Subhasis Roy Choudhury and Govind V. S. Murthi

The common acquired anorectal disorders in children are:

- Perianal abscess and fistula in ano
- Anal fissure and anal skin tag
- Hemorrhoids
- Rectal prolapse

52.1 Perianal Abscess and Fistula in Ano

Perianal or perirectal abscesses almost always occur during infancy. They are commoner in males as it is proposed that imbalance in androgen causes production of abnormal anal glands that are prone to infection. If perianal abscesses occur later in childhood, Crohn's disease should be considered.

The abscess typically presents as a firm, tender mass in the perianal region, often with discharging pus (Fig. 52.1). If detected in the early stages, conservative treatment with antibiotics is effective; a third of these will recur. If the abscess is fluctuant or recurrent, it is best incised and drained under GA. During this procedure, it is advisable to have the patient in lithotomy position, open the anus with a self-retaining retractor and search for the inner opening by gentle pressure on the abscess and this is revealed by pus. Then, a curved lacrimal probe can be placed into the abscess and the whole tract is laid open with diathermy. In this way, the incidence of fistula formation is reduced, as opposed to simple incision and drainage.

About a third of perianal abscesses progress to a fistula-in-ano. The child is usually seen after two or more flareups of a perianal abscess that

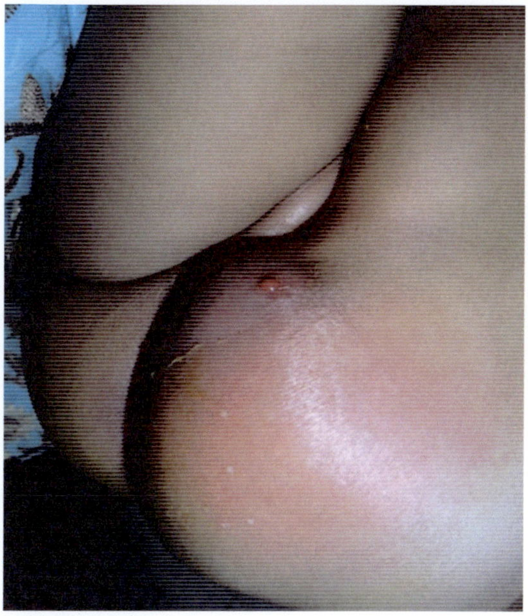

Fig. 52.1 Ruptured perianal abscess

S. Roy Choudhury
Pediatric Surgery, Lady Hardinge Medical College and Associated Kalawati Saran Children's Hospital, New Delhi, Delhi, India

G. V. S. Murthi (✉)
Paediatric Surgical Unit, Sheffield Children's Hospital, Sheffield, UK

© The Author(s), under exclusive license to Springer Nature Singapore Pte Ltd. 2025

S. Roy Choudhury (ed.), *Pediatric Surgery*, https://doi.org/10.1007/978-981-96-1257-4_52

either continues to drain or forms a small pustule that ruptures, heals, and forms again. The fistula is commonly located off the midline (Fig. 52.2). The preferred surgical procedure for fistula in ano is fistulotomy. With the patient under general anesthesia, the anus is gently opened with a retractor. A fine malleable probe is inserted through the fistula and gently advanced until it appears at the base of the involved crypt. An incision is made along the probe and is deepened until the whole fistula track is laid open over the probe. The base of the exposed fistula is denuded of granulation tissue with a curette. The wound is left open to heal by secondary intention with satisfactory results (Fig. 52.3). The fistula tract is superficial, below the sphincter complex, and radial. There are no long-term consequences following fistulotomy.

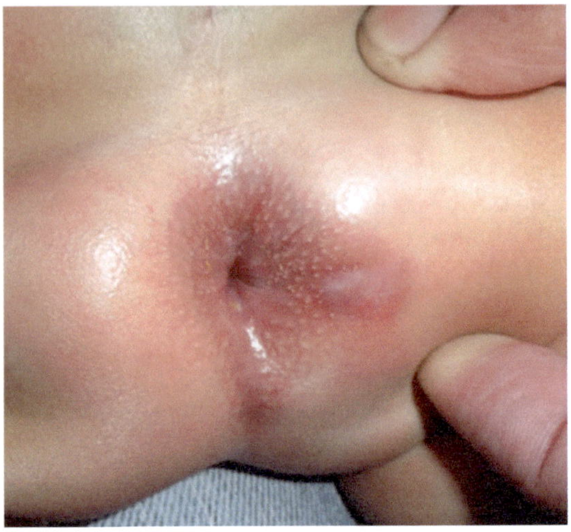

Fig. 52.2 Fistula in ano, note the lateral site

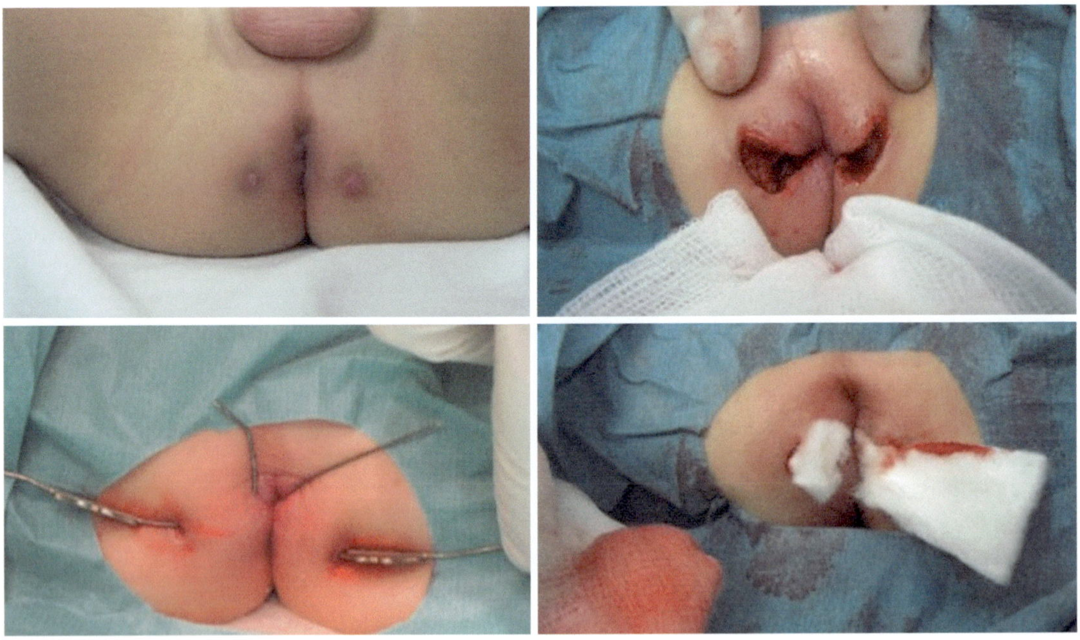

Fig. 52.3 Fistula in ano, probe in situ, and tract laid open

52.2 Anal Fissure

Anal fissure is a longitudinal tear or a ulcer in the distal anal canal. The cause in children is a period of constipation followed by hard, bulky stool that results in a posterior midline tear in the anoderm below the mucocutaneous junction. The discomfort in having a bowel movement associated with the fissure often leads to further constipation, which, in turn, aggravates the fissure with each stool and prevents healing. This theory now is considered an oversimplification of the pathology. Alternate theory proposes that raised anal sphincter pressure results in ischemia in the posterior midline anal canal—which ulcerates—leading to anal fissure. The diagnosis is made by the history of blood streaking on the stool, the child's crying during bowel movements and the recognition of a tear in the distal anal canal on examination.

Management of these patients includes a stool softener such as lactulose, and a local analgesic (2–5% lignocaine jelly). Most anal fissures will heal by these measures. In symptomatic or non-responding cases, chemical sphincterotomy can be performed by topical application of glyceryl trinitrate ointment or local injection of botulinum toxin.

Rarely, lateral sphincterotomy may be used in the older child. There is no role for fissurectomy and anal stretching is best avoided as it can lead to sphincter damage.

An anal fissure in an older child or a teenager may be associated with chronic inflammatory bowel disease, usually Crohn's disease.

A perianal skin tag may result from a healed fissure (Fig. 52.4). It is generally of no consequence and can be managed conservatively. A large tag can be bothersome and can affect adequate perianal hygiene. In these cases, local excision is reasonable.

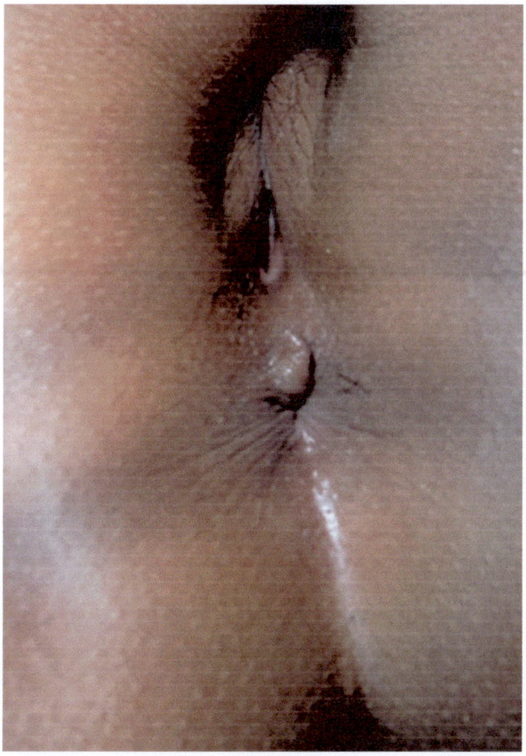

Fig. 52.4 Anal skin tag secondary to a fissure

52.3 Hemorrhoids

Hemorrhoids are extremely uncommon in the pediatric population. Children with portal hypertension are likely to develop hemorrhoids but are usually asymptomatic. The usual presentation is of bleeding, pain, prolapse, and itching (Fig. 52.5). Most children respond to conservative measures like management of constipation. If symptomatic (pain, bleeding, and irreducible), surgical intervention in the form of bipolar cautery excision is helpful. Often at examination under GA the hemorrhoids may not be prominent or clearly demarcated and hence care must be

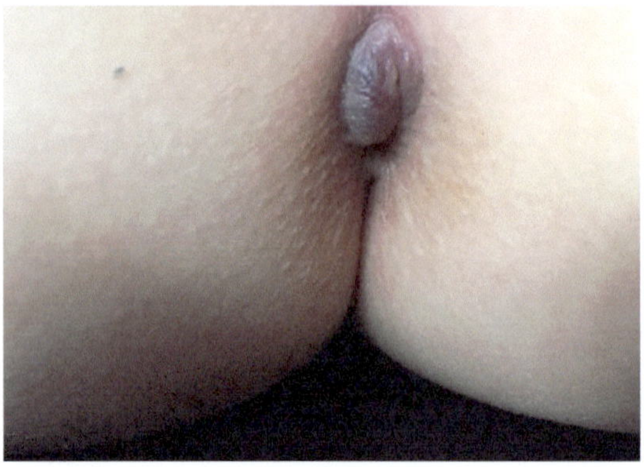

Fig. 52.5 Hemorrhoids (Photo taken by parent enabling diagnosis)

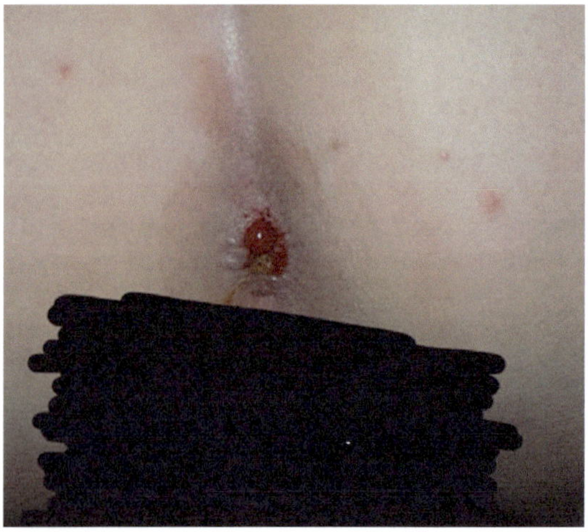

Fig. 52.6 Rectal polyp (Photo taken by parent enabling diagnosis)

taken to not remove too much of the mucosa around the circumference of the anus.

Rarely, a persistent, prominent hemorrhoid can be indicative of a rectal cavernous hemangioma; endoscopy of the rectum and sigmoid, and MRI to assess its extent may be useful. Such lesions are best treated conservatively, as surgical excision can be damaging.

52.4 Rectal Polyp

Occasionally, a low-lying rectal polyp may present as a protuberant mass (Fig. 52.6). This would warrant an endoscopy and excision. They are usually juvenile hamartomatous polyps and need no further intervention. Familial adenomatous polyp (FAP) in childhood is a congenital condition and the polyps are usually sessile and do not present as a prolapsing polyp.

52.5 Rectal Prolapse

Rectal prolapse is a relatively common problem in young children and causes distress to the child and the parents. Prolapse can range from the commoner mucosal prolapse that occurs during toilet training to full-thickness prolapse of the rectum, which usually occurs in the older child and is usually secondary to dysfunctional defecation. Non-accidental injury (sexual abuse) should be considered in the differential diagnosis of rectal prolapse.

Rectal prolapse in children is likely precipitated by:

- Weakness of the pelvic supporting musculature (levator mechanism).
- Loosely attached rectal submucosa to the underlying muscularis.
- Straining during stooling is caused by protracted diarrhea or constipation.
- Parasitic infection may also promote prolapse.
- Decreased anal tone due to previous surgery.
- Behavioral issues.

Rectal prolapse can be classified as follows:

- Partial: only the mucosa protrudes for 1–3 cm. Radial folds are seen (Fig. 52.7a). This usually occurs during the potty training period and is self-resolving.
- Full thickness: whole thickness of the rectal wall prolapses. Concentric mucosal folds are often seen (Fig. 52.7b).

The prolapse either reduces spontaneously as the child gets off the toilet or the parent pushes it back in. Many children very quickly learn to reduce their own prolapse. It generally does not recur until the next stool. It is uncommon for the child to be able to produce the prolapse in the examining room, and such attempts are not recommended; a photo taken by parents on their mobile phone helps

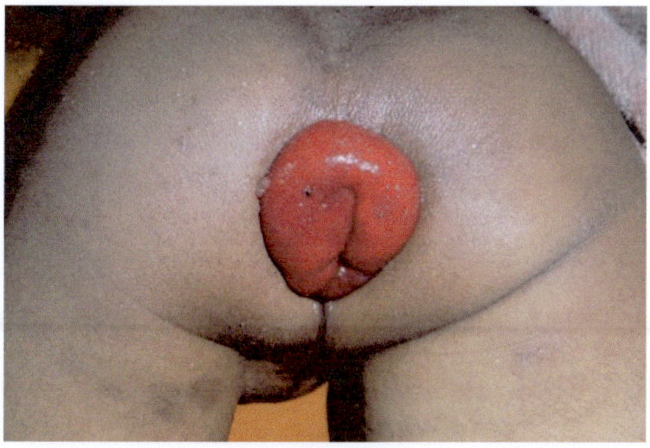

Fig. 52.7a Mucosal rectal prolapse with radial folds

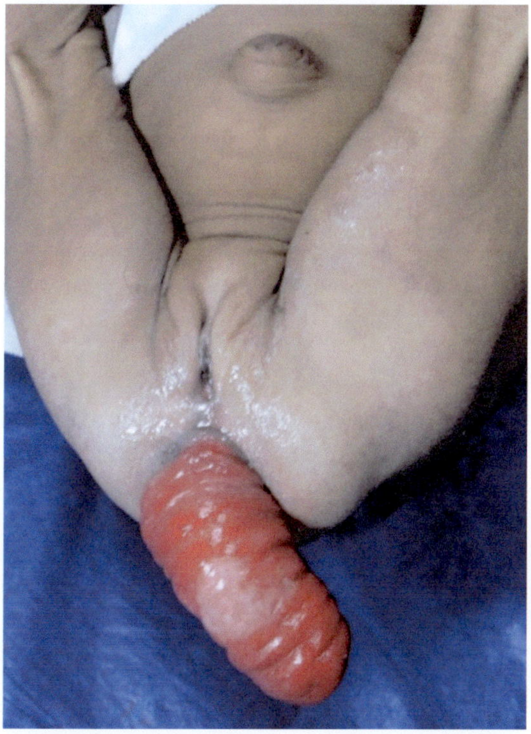

Fig. 52.7b Full-thickness rectal prolapse with concentric folds in a malnourished child

make the diagnosis these days. The typical prolapse is a rosette of mucosa, sometimes slightly longer posteriorly than anteriorly (Fig. 52.4a, b). One should be able to slip a finger alongside the prolapse and feel the sulcus 1 to 2 cm up inside the anusto differentiate it from intussusception. A deeper sulcus suggests intussusception rather than rectal prolapse (see Chap. 44).

52.5.1 Management

Most cases can be treated with conservative measures. Children who have failed conservative therapy or sclerotherapy, and in patients with full-thickness prolapse, operative fixation techniques are generally needed.

For mucosal rectal prolapse:

- Parental reassurance
- Treat underlying constipation and behavioral issues
- Encourage digital repositioning for mucosal prolapse
- Treat associated conditions
  - Bowel infections
  - Poor nutritional status
- Most resolve with the above measures
- If persistent and constipation is treated, and if associated with pain, bleeding, or irreducibility, surgical intervention in the form of sclerotherapy is undertaken. Hypertonic saline, 25% glucose, 5% sodium tetradecylsulfate, or 5% phenol in almond oil may be used. The agent is injected into the submucosal plane above the dentate line (1 mL in each quadrant); it produces an inflammatory response and scar that prevents the rectal mucosa from sliding downward. The injection procedure sometimes requires to be repeated.

For full-thickness rectal prolapse:

This requires surgical intervention. Approaches can be perineal or transabdominal (open or laparoscopic).

Perineal approaches include:

- Delorme's procedure (mucosal sleeve resection and folding in of prolapse).
- Altmeier's procedure (full-thickness excision and anastomosis).
- Thiersch procedure—(concentric suture to hold prolapse in); this is mentioned here only to state that it is best avoided as it does not address the underlying cause and severely impairs the quality of life of the patient by creating a fixed ring with constant leakage of feces.

Other approaches include:

- Open posterior rectopexy (fixing the rectum with the presacral pelvic fascia).
- Laparoscopic rectopexy.

There is an increasing recognition that rectal prolapse, particularly full-thickness and in the older child, is associated with bowel dysfunction. Hence, where available, investigative and treatment adjuncts such as anorectal manometry, biofeedback, and treatment of behavioral issues should be considered.

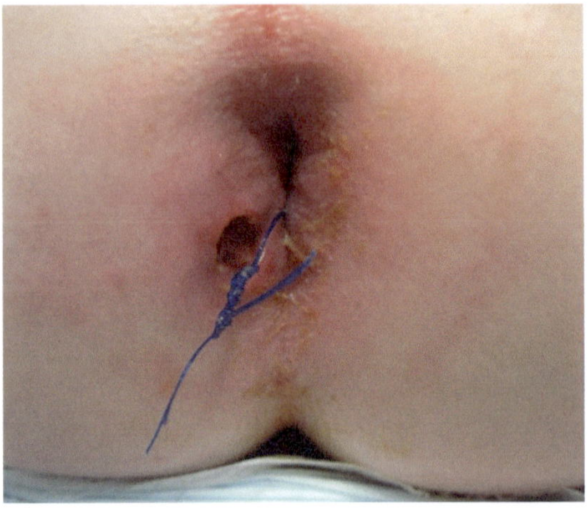

Fig. 52.8 Perianal Crohn's disease—seton inserted into fistula

52.6 Rectal Prolapse in Anorectal Malformations

Following PSARP repair for anorectal malformations, mucosal and full-thickness rectal prolapse can occur. The underlying causes include associated spinal pathology, poor pelvic floor musculature and tone, and dysfunctional defecation. Correction includes local resection and redo anoplasty.

52.7 Perianal Crohn's Disease

Crohn's disease may present as a perianal lesion—abscess, fissure, or fistula—in isolation or as part of other manifestations of bowel and extra-intestinal involvement (Fig. 52.8). In either case, treatment would involve medical management as directed by the gastroenterologists. Surgical intervention for perianal Crohn's disease would depend on the severity of involvement. While established abscesses have to be drained, I&D is best avoided, and the use of a seton is recommended to facilitate prolonged drainage. Severe perianal Crohn's disease may necessitate a defunctioning colostomy, and the patient and parents should be counseled about the potential for this being a long-term intervention. Defunctioning stomas usually enable healing of the perianal disease; however, reversal of the stoma can result in recurrence of perianal disease in ~30% of patients. Fistulas can complicate stomas in Crohn's disease and would usually necessitate bowel resection rather than simple revision of the stoma because of associated inflammation (a note of caution).

Severe perianal excoriation due to infective diarrhea and neutropenia in malnourished patients may need treatment with a diverting colostomy, allowing the ulcer to heal (Fig. 52.9a, b).

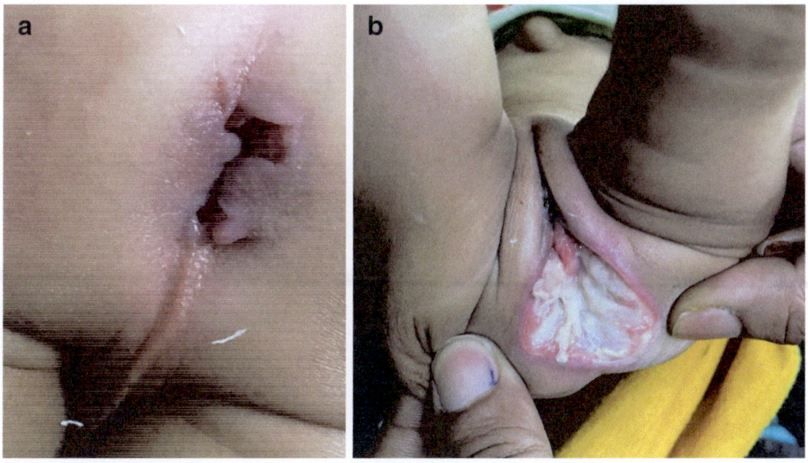

Fig. 52.9 (**a**, **b**) Severe perianal ulceration due to infective diarrhea with leukopenia

Summary

- Acquired anorectal disorders are largely treatable by simple conservative measures, such as treating the underlying constipation and behavioural issues.
- We should avoid performing a per rectal examination as it causes distress to the awake child and is usually uninformative.
- EUA—this should be used where conservative methods have failed and serves as both a diagnostic and treatment method.
- Local, limited interventions (sclerotherapy, excision of lesion, seton) are sufficient in majority of cases.

Suggested Reading

Wexner SD, Duthie GS, editors. Constipation—etiology, evaluation and management. 2nd ed. Heidelberg: Springer; 2006.

53 Lower Gastrointestinal Bleeding

Govind V. S. Murthi and Subhasis Roy Choudhury

53.1 Introduction

Lower gastrointestinal tract bleeding (LGIB) in children manifests as "bleeding per rectum." Clinically, this can manifest as fresh red blood, altered blood, or melaena. It can be mild, moderate (multiple drops/clots of blood) (Fig. 53.1), or severe (profuse bleeding), and the former is commoner than the latter presentation. The possible underlying causes for LGIB in children are shown in Table 53.1. A perusal of the causes shows that the causes are myriad and, to some extent, age-related. Bleeding episodes can be multiple, and severity can be variable too. Therefore, in modern practice, different diagnostic and treatment modalities have to be adopted in order to deal with the problem of "bleeding per rectum."

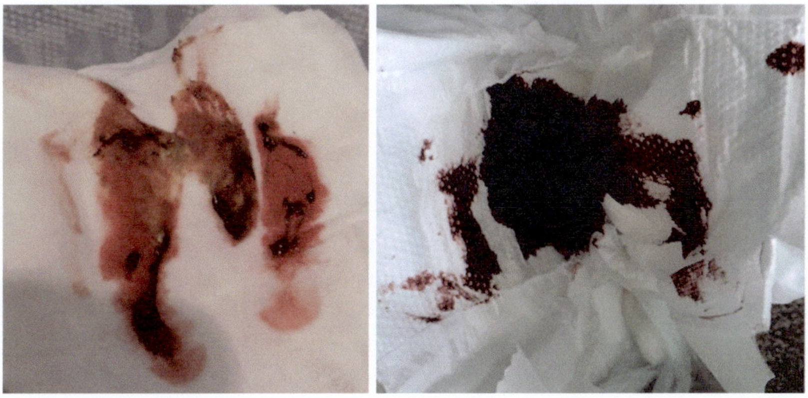

Fig. 53.1 Per rectal bleeding

G. V. S. Murthi (✉)
Paediatric Surgical Unit, Sheffield Children's Hospital, Sheffield, UK

S. Roy Choudhury
Pediatric Surgery, Lady Hardinge Medical College and Associated Kalawati Saran Children's Hospital, New Delhi, Delhi, India

© The Author(s), under exclusive license to Springer Nature Singapore Pte Ltd. 2025
S. Roy Choudhury (ed.), *Pediatric Surgery*, https://doi.org/10.1007/978-981-96-1257-4_53

Table 53.1 Possible causes of "bleeding per rectum" in children

Severity	Infant	Child	Adolescent
Mild bleeding	Anal fissure	Anal fissure	Infective colitis
	Dietary protein allergy	Infective colitis	Polyp
	Vitamin K deficiency	Polyp	IBD
		IBD	Solitary rectal ulcer
		Solitary rectal ulcer	Hemorrhoids
Moderate to severe rectal bleeding	Necrotizing enterocolitis	Intussusception	NSAID enteropathy
	Hirschsprung enterocolitis	Meckel diverticulum	IBD
	Duplication cyst	Typhlitis	Vascular malformation
	Vascular malformation	Henoch-Schonlein purpura	Meckel diverticulum
		Duplication cyst	

Abbreviations: *IBD* inflammatory bowel disease, *NSAID* non-steroidal anti-inflammatory drug

53.2 Approach to a Child with Rectal Bleeding

The treatment of gastrointestinal bleeding is threefold:

- Resuscitation and stabilization of the patient
- Careful history of the bleeding and associated features, and physical examination
- Assess for intervention
  - Is intervention needed to diagnose, locate, and treat the cause
  - Is intervention needed urgently, or can it be done electively
  - Type of intervention needed—endoscopic, surgical (including laparoscopic), or both

Depending on the clinical presentation, severity, and frequency of bleeding, and the findings of clinical examination, the timing and modality of intervention are determined. In modern clinical practice, endoscopy is often the primary modality of intervention, both as a diagnostic and therapeutic measure, and surgical intervention is reserved for select situations. Hence, pediatric surgeons and gastroenterologists should work together from the very beginning in cases of "bleeding per rectum," where the diagnosis and treatment are not evident.

Resuscitation will require prompt insertion of an intravenous line and fluid resuscitation of a child with shock. Blood transfusion and platelet transfusion may be required.

History taking should focus on family history, drug intake, underlying medical conditions, previous episodes, and interventions including previous operations. The colour of the blood should be ascertained in order to differentiate between fresh bleeding (bright red) and altered blood (dark, black, tarry). Clinical examination should include inspection of the blood (including photos/videos taken by parents on their mobile phones), lesions on the skin (oral pigmentation, vascular lesions) and perineal examination including a look for anal fissure, fistulae, skin tags. Per rectal examination is best avoided as it does not yield much information and distresses the awake child.

In modern practice, depending on the resources and skill mix available, there exists a wide range of intervention (both diagnostic and therapeutic) modalities that can be used for managing the child with "bleeding per rectum." These different options are shown in Table 53.2.

Constipation associated anal fissure and cow's milk protein allergy are common causes of mild bleeding per rectum in infancy and early childhood. In India, gastrointestinal infections are the leading cause of bleeding per rectum in children. Hence, in a stable patient without any obvious cause of bleeding, a course of combination antibacterial and antiparasitic drug therapy often settles the issue.

Table 53.2 The various diagnostic and therapeutic options available for the management of lower gastrointestinal (GI) bleeding in children

Endoscopy	Endoscopic hemostatic options
Gastroscope	Injection—adrenaline/sclerosant/adhesives/ethanol
Colonoscope	Argon Plasma Coagulation (APC)
Video capsule	Polypectomy snare
Small bowel enteroscope	Bipolar/multipolar probe
	Clips—through the scope (TTS), over the scope (OTS)
Surgery	Hemospray
Perineal examination	
Laparoscopy	*Others*
Laparotomy	Radionuclide scan—RBC scan, technetium pertechnetate
	Angiography
	Cross-sectional imaging—CT, MRI

Conditions that may require urgent surgical intervention are primarily those that lead to bowel necrosis. These children are sick at presentation with a tense, distended abdomen. The cause of intestinal gangrene can be internal herniation, volvulus, band obstruction with a fixed loop, or necrotizing enterocolitis.

Bleeding Meckel diverticulum, vascular malformations, typhoid ulcer, and duplications can present as an emergency. The management of suspected bleeding Meckel diverticulum has moved away from the technetium scan due to the low sensitivity (60%) and specificity (76%) of the test. Such patients are best approached with a laparoscopy initially, and if a Meckel is not found, upper and lower GI endoscopy is undertaken under the same anesthetic by the gastroenterologists.

Intussusception can present with bleeding per rectum and is detailed in a separate chapter. Anal fissure is the most common cause of rectal bleeding in the first 2 years of life. The condition has been discussed in detail in the chapter "acquired rectal disorders."

The most common cause of lower gastrointestinal bleed in school-going children is rectal polyps. The characteristic of bleeding from rectal polyps is painless, and fresh blood is passed in drops both before and after defecation. Juvenile polyps are the most common cause, which comprise 80% of childhood polyps. This is a mucous retention polyp and histologically features a cluster of mucoid lobes surrounded by flattened mucus-secreting glandular cells. There is no malignant potential. These polyps are most commonly seen in children between 3 and 10 years, with a peak at age between 5 and 6 years. The majority (85%) of children have a solitary polyp. The most common complaint is rectal bleeding, and occasionally, the polyps may prolapse out of the rectum. Diagnosis is by rectal examination and/or endoscopy. Removal by endoscopy snare or single ligation of the stalk is the treatment of choice.

Lymphoid polyps make up about 15% of childhood polyps. They begin to appear during the first year of life, peak at about the third year of life, and diminish in number by 5 years of age. These are multiple and may present with mild chronic blood loss. Diagnosis is made by contrast enema, endoscopy, and biopsy. No treatment is necessary since they will regress spontaneously.

Presence of multiple rectal polyps or rectal polyp in a child with family history of polyps suggests the diagnosis of familial adenomatous polyposis (FAP). FAP has an autosomal dominant inheritance. Hundreds of adenomatous colonic polyps may be present in childhood (rare), with virtually all developing adenocarcinoma of colon by the third decade of life. The most common and best recognized variant is patients with Gardner's syndrome, which combines the premalignant adenomatous colonic polyps with soft and hard tissue tumors. Diagnosis is by family history, and contrast studies are followed by biopsy. This condition requires monitoring in childhood under the guidance of a geneticist. Surveillance endoscopy is commenced after 10 years of age and is undertaken every 2 years till adulthood. Though the eventual management is surgery, it is aimed to manage the child conservatively till adulthood, and this is possible in the majority of children. Indications for colectomy in childhood would include genetics indicating a phenotype with high potential for malignancy and/or large polyp load. Surgery in childhood is usually sub-total colectomy and ileo-rectal anastomosis followed by endoscopic surveillance and APC coagulation of polyps in the rectal stump.

In Peutz–Jeghers syndrome, polyps are associated with melanin hyperpigmentation of the lips and oral mucosa. The polyps are usually multiple and hamartomas. They will appear anywhere, but the majority are limited to the jejunum and ileum. Chronic blood loss and anemia in a child with repeated bouts of colicky abdominal pain secondary to actual or incipient intussusception are typical. Diagnosis is by contrast studies. GI malignancy has been reported in 2–3% of patients. Females with Peutz-Jeghers syndrome seem predisposed to develop ovarian tumors, usually in adolescence. Treatments depend on the severity of symptoms and the extent of involvement. Rarely, in children who have had previous bowel resection and anastomosis, in particular between the ileum and colon, bleeding per rectum can occur from the anastomotic site. Endoscopy usually leads to the diagnosis and limited surgical resection, and re-anastomosis may be required in selected cases.

53.3 Summary

The management of "bleeding per rectum" or LGIB is variable depending on the presentation and findings. Most children can be managed in an elective manner, and severe life-threatening bleeding requiring emergency intervention is not common. A joint approach along with gastroenterologists is recommended as endoscopy forms an integral part of the management algorithm

Suggested Reading

Kliegman R, Stanton B, Geme JS, Nelson SN. Textbook of pediatrics. 20th ed. Philadelphia: Saunders, Elsevier; 2015.

54 Constipation and Fecal Incontinence

Joshua Rae, Govind V. S. Murthi, and Subhasis Roy Choudhury

54.1 Constipation

Constipation is a common problem in childhood with a prevalence of about 3–4%. The most widely accepted definition is as per Rome IV criteria:

- Two or fewer defecations per week
- At least one episode of incontinence per week
- History of excessive stool retention or retentive posturing
- History of painful or hard bowel movements
- Large fecal mass in the rectum
- History of large-diameter stools that may obstruct the toilet

Presence of 2 or more of these symptoms for more than 1 month in a child <4 years or for more than 2 months in a child >4 years is considered diagnostic for constipation.

54.2 Causes of Constipation

Functional constipation (Idiopathic) (commonest)

- Organic

Anorectal malformations
Pelvic mass
Neurogenic bladder secondary to spinal cord trauma or spinal cord pathology

Intestinal neural disorders

- Hirschsprung disease
- Visceral myopathies or neuropathies

Metabolic or hormonal conditions

- Hypothyroidism
- Hypercalcemia

Drugs

- Opiates
- Phenobarbiturates
- Antacids

Since the most common cause of constipation is functional, it needs to be differentiated from other causes which may require surgical intervention. The following are the signs and symptoms which alert the physician that the constipation is not idiopathic:

J. Rae · G. V. S. Murthi (✉)
Paediatric Surgical Unit, Sheffield Children's Hospital, Sheffield, UK

S. Roy Choudhury
Pediatric Surgery, Lady Hardinge Medical College and Associated Kalawati Saran Children's Hospital, New Delhi, Delhi, India

© The Author(s), under exclusive license to Springer Nature Singapore Pte Ltd. 2025
S. Roy Choudhury (ed.), *Pediatric Surgery*, https://doi.org/10.1007/978-981-96-1257-4_54

- Constipation in a neonate
- Delayed passage of meconium after 48 hours
- Family history of Hirschsprung disease
- Blood in stools (anal fissure ruled out)
- Failure to thrive
- Bilious vomiting
- Marked abdominal distension
- Anal abnormality (abnormal location, stenosis)
- Findings suggestive of a neurogenic cause
  - Absent anal or cremasteric reflex
  - Decreased lower limb power/tone/reflex
  - Spina bifida (hair/swelling in lumbosacral spine)
- Delayed milestones (suggestive of hypothyroidism/developmental causes)

54.3 Management of Functional Constipation

Treatment can either be medical, surgical, or a combination of both.

A bowel management program should be tailored toward the child and family. Children should be encouraged to consume a varied diet with appropriate fiber and water intake. Correct posturing on the toilet and encouragement from carers are required.

First line treatment includes oral laxatives—either osmotic (e.g. polyethylene glycol (PEG)) and/or stimulant (e.g. senna) or per rectal medications including enemas or suppositories (e.g. bisacodyl).

If a fecal mass is present this requires disimpaction with large doses of laxatives or, if this fails enema and/or manual evacuation. Once the patient is disimpacted, a maintenance dose of laxatives can be given. This is continued for a period of at least 2 months, and then the dose can be tapered off as tolerated.

The treatment of constipation is in three phases

- Fecal disimpaction: If a large fecal mass is obstructing the rectum, it needs to be removed by polyethylene glycol (PEG, 1–1.5 g/kg/day). In case PEG is unavailable, rectal enemas or even manual fecal disimpaction may be necessary. Rectal glycerin suppository at regular intervals is very helpful.
- Maintenance therapy: PEG at the dose of 0.4–0.8 g/kg/day is preferred; otherwise, lactulose at the dose of 1–2 mL/kg/day can also be given. The maintenance therapy is continued for at least 2 months, provided that the child is free from constipation for at least 1 month.
- Tapering off: The medications are gradually tapered.

For patients with longstanding functional constipation who have not responded to treatment, it is important to ensure compliance with medication first. If this is not a concern, patients should be considered for possible underlying Hirschsprung disease or anal achalasia with anorectal manometry +/− rectal biopsy +/− botulinum toxin injection to the anal sphincter (if high resting pressures are noted). Anorectal manometry is a useful tool as a positive recto-anal inhibitory reflex (RAIR) rules out a diagnosis of Hirschsprung disease. If pelvic floor dyssynergia is present, the patient may benefit from physiotherapy.

For patients with a normal RAIR and low anal resting pressures consideration should be for contrast enema and manometric studies.

54.4 Fecal Incontinence

54.4.1 Causes of Fecal Incontinence in Children

1. Anorectal malformations
2. Hirschsprung disease
3. Spina bifida
4. Pelvic and sacrococcygeal tumor
5. Trauma

54.4.2 True Fecal Incontinence Versus Fecal Pseudo-incontinence (Encopresis)

True fecal incontinence patients are those who lack the ability to make voluntary bowel movements. Fecal pseudo-incontinence or encopresis is generally due to fecal impaction with overflow, and once effectively treated, these patients may be able to have voluntary bowel movements.

Bowel management program for patients with tendency toward constipation and *dilated colon* includes:

(a) Dietary modification: avoid a constipating diet, a high-fiber diet (fruits, vegetables, juices, cereals, pulses, and honey) that acts as a laxative.
(b) Laxatives.
(c) Large volume enemas.

Bowel management program for patients with tendency toward diarrhea with *nondilated or narrow colon* includes:

(a) Constipating diet (avoidance of diarrhea-promoting food).
(b) Small volume enemas.
(c) Oral drugs: Loperamide, pectin (slowing the bowel).

54.4.2.1 High-Volume Enemas

Transanal irrigation consists of either saline or water with salt and either phosphate, glycerin, or soap added (Fig. 54.1a). The volume is determined by the age and size of the patient. The enema is administered over 15 minutes and held for a period of at least 10 minutes, and the patient then sits on the toilet until empty. The aim of these washouts is for the colon to be empty and the patient to be clean for 24 hours. This whole process is on a trial-and-error basis and requires considerable investment from the child and carer.

Most patients with functional constipation who have failed medical management or who cannot tolerate transanal irrigation will be successfully managed with ACE (Antegrade Continence Enema) washouts (Fig. 54.1b, c). The appendix is used to form a catheterizable channel for the administration of antegrade washouts to clear the colon (either in the RIF or at the umbilicus). This can be achieved with either open or laparoscopic surgery. If the patient is also undergoing simultaneous bladder augmentation with Mitrofanoff, the appendix can be split, or if the appendix is absent, a 'neo appendix' can be fashioned from the cecum, or a direct cecostomy can be used.

Patients can be managed with washouts as long as required, and some manage to transition back to oral laxative therapy.

For patients who do not respond to ACE washouts, care should be taken to ensure that there is

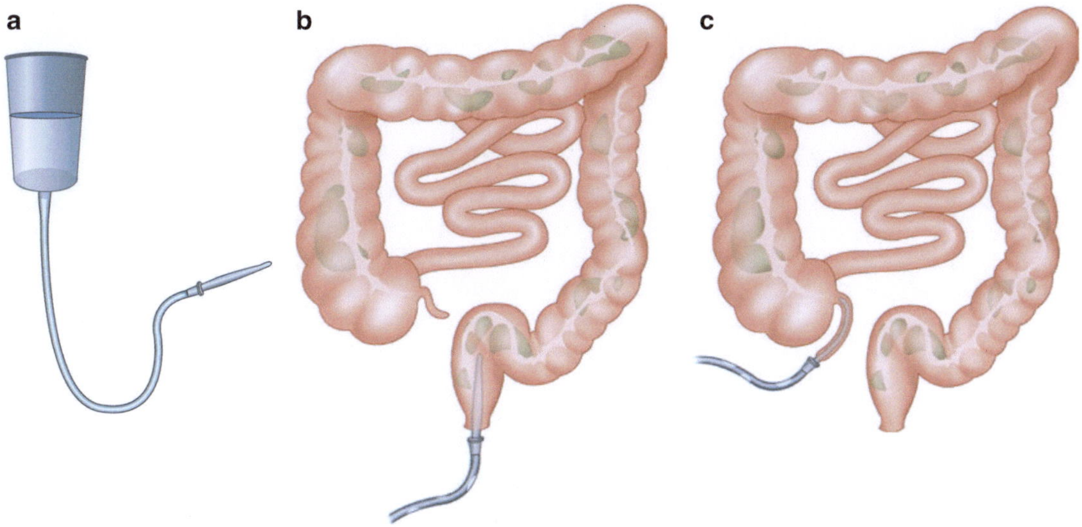

Fig. 54.1 (**a**) Home enema application with a can. (**b**) Patient education for enema therapy. (**c**) Antegrade continence enema (ACE) through an appendix stoma

no retrograde passage of the washout into the ileum—this can be confirmed by a contrast study.

If these treatments fail, then the options depend on the findings of contrast and manometry studies. Options include segmental or extended resection, or total colectomy with stoma or reconstruction.

Suggested Reading

Holschneider AM, Hutson JM, editors. Anorectal malformations in children embryology, diagnosis, surgical treatment, follow-up. Heidelberg: Springer; 2006.

Kliegman R, Stanton B, Geme JS, Schor N. Nelson textbook of pediatrics. 20th ed. Philadelphia: Saunders, Elsevier; 2015.

Levitt MA. Pediatric colorectal surgery: tips & tricks. 1st ed. CRC Press; 2022. https://doi.org/10.1201/9781003150015.

Wexner SD, Duthie GS, editors. Constipation—etiology, evaluation and management. 2nd ed. Heidelberg: Springer; 2006.

Stoma Care

55

Elizabeth Scudamore, Govind V. S. Murthi, and Subhasis Roy Choudhury

55.1 Introduction

Stomas are an essential component of pediatric surgical practice. Given that a stoma is an opening of a hollow viscus onto the body surface, stomas in pediatric practice are created either along the intestinal tract (esophagostomy, gastrostomy, jejunostomy, ileostomy, appendicostomy, and colostomy) or the urinary tract (vesicostomy, suprapubic cystostomy, Mitrofanoff stoma (appendix), Monti (small bowel), ureterostomy or rarely, urethrostomy, pyelostomy, or nephrostomy) (Fig. 55.1). They may be either temporary or permanent in nature.

Neonates and children undergo the formation of a stoma for many reasons. Stoma creation may be both lifesaving and a means of improving the quality of life of a child.

Common pathologies and indications for a stoma in neonates and children can be congenital such as anorectal malformation, Hirschsprung disease, intestinal atresia, or acquired such as necrotizing enterocolitis, meconium Ileus, malrotation, inflammatory bowel disease, or tumors.

Around 80% of stomas are formed within the first 6 weeks of life, and the majority are reversed before the child is 1–2 years old.

In modern clinical practice, the role of the specialist stoma nurse is pivotal to the planning and management of stomas.

Clinical issues related to stoma formation, management, and long-term care relate to its location, number, the volume and nature of its output, type (end, loop, and tube), duration (temporary, long-term, or permanent), and the associated complications that can occur.

For the purposes of discussion of stoma care, a broad division could be as follows:

- Intestinal stomas
- Urinary stomas

E. Scudamore · G. V. S. Murthi (✉)
Paediatric Surgical Unit, Sheffield Children's Hospital, Sheffield, UK

S. Roy Choudhury
Pediatric Surgery, Lady Hardinge Medical College and Associated Kalawati Saran Children's Hospital, New Delhi, Delhi, India

© The Author(s), under exclusive license to Springer Nature Singapore Pte Ltd. 2025
S. Roy Choudhury (ed.), *Pediatric Surgery*, https://doi.org/10.1007/978-981-96-1257-4_55

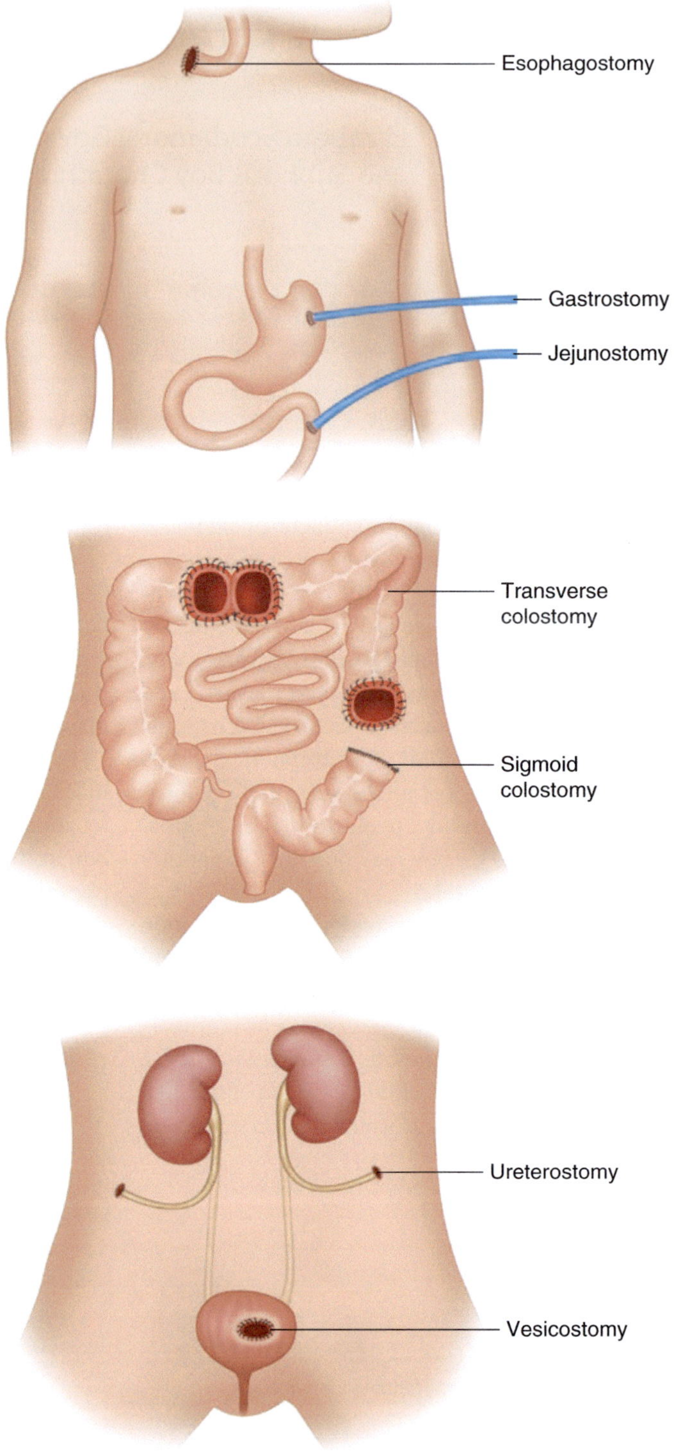

Fig. 55.1 Different sites of stomas in pediatric patients

55.2 Intestinal Stomas

Esophagostomy (Figs. 55.2a, 55.2b) is usually performed for managing esophageal atresia. Since there is a lot of saliva and hence sodium depletion can be a problem, it should be monitored.

Gastrostomy (Figs. 55.3 and 55.4)—these are usually a tube stoma, and a variety of tubes and buttons are available to secure these stomas. In resource-poor settings, because of the prohibitive cost of gastrostomy buttons and limited availability, either a Malecot or a Foley catheter can be used as effective alternatives. The common problem faced by gastrostomy is enlargement of the stoma with peri-catheter leakage of feeds. This can be prevented by the use of a Malekot catheter rather than a Foley catheter. The triangular shape of the bulb of Malecot (rather than the spherical shape in Foleys) prevents enlargement of the site. Also, a feeding nipple can be placed over the stoma and the catheter passed through it. The nipple limits the movement of the catheter and enlargement of the stoma. Some side holes are made in the nipple to allow air to pass through and keep the area dry.

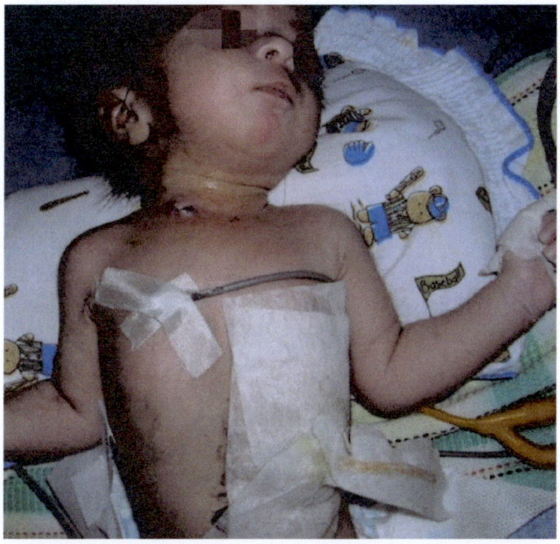

Fig. 55.2a Esophagostomy and gastrostomy (tube)

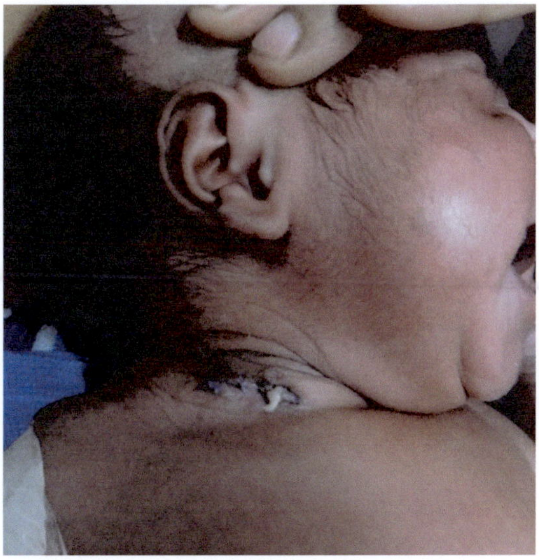

Fig. 55.2b Esophagostomy

Jejunostomy (tube) is usually used for feeding purposes. This is best created as a tube stoma, as

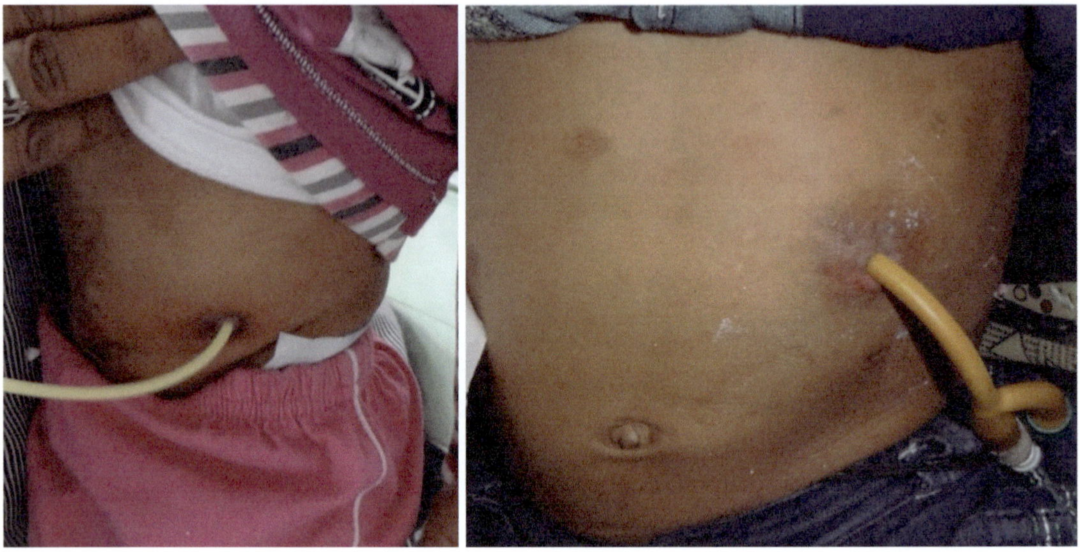

Fig. 55.3 Well-managed gastrostomy tube for feeding

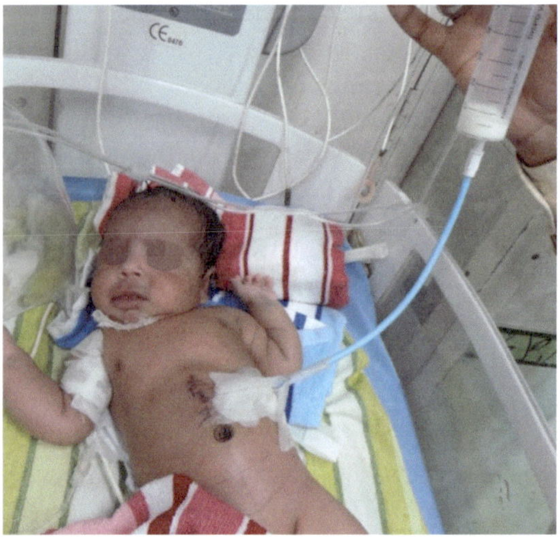

Fig. 55.4 Gastrostomy feeding in new born

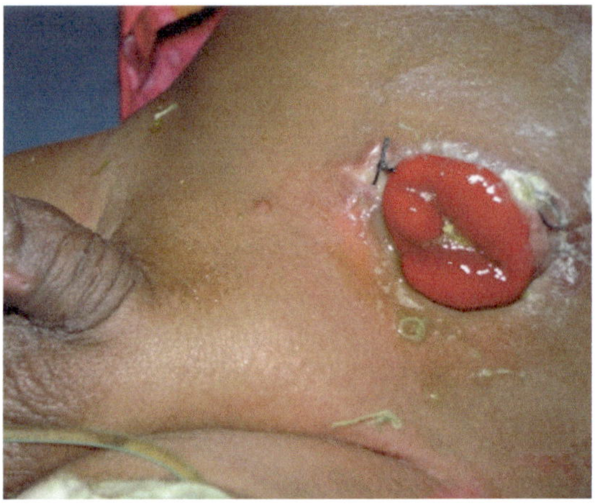

Fig. 55.5 Ileostomy (single end stoma)

the high volume of effluent and its enzymatic contents can cause problems due to dehydration and skin excoriation.

55.2.1 Fecal Stomas (Ileostomy, Colostomy)

Ileostomy (Fig. 55.5) and colostomy (Figs. 55.6, 55.7 and 55.8) are frequently performed in children for fecal diversion. The stoma effluent may vary from liquid to semisolid to solid, depending on the level and duration, with distal stomas having a more solid effluent.

Appendicostomy—an indwelling catheter (Foley) or a gastrostomy button can be left in situ as this stoma is usually for long-term management of bowel dysfunction and administration of antegrade enemas.

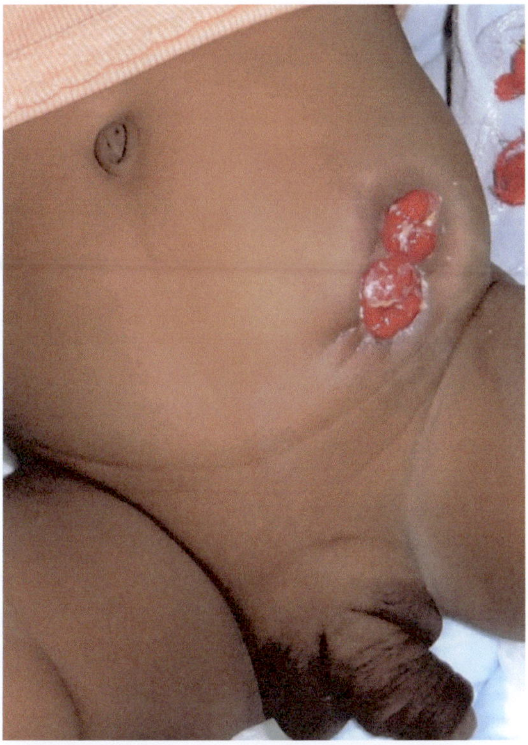

Fig. 55.6 Divided sigmoid colostomy (double stoma)

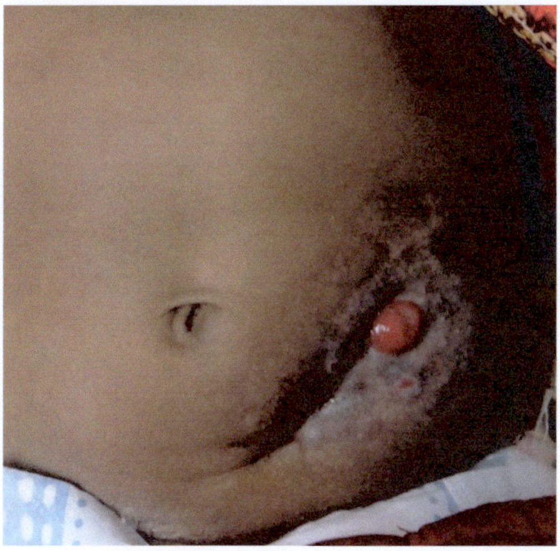

Fig. 55.7 Sigmoid end colostomy, note stoma site skin excoriation

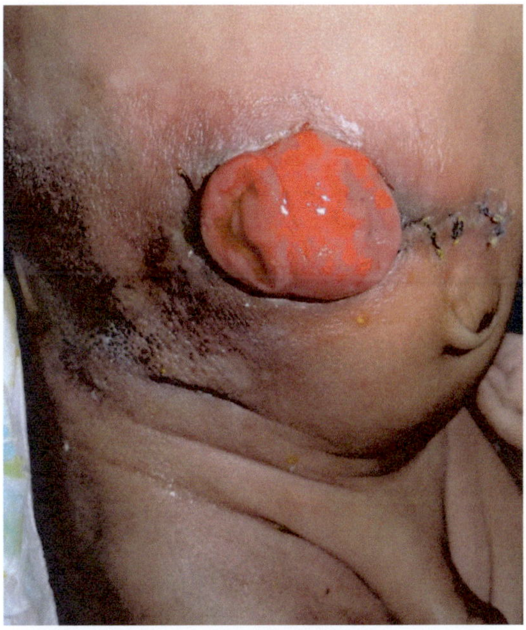

Fig. 55.8 Transverse loop colostomy

55.3 Urinary Stomas

Suprapubic cystostomy—this can be a tube stoma with a Foley catheter, or, if for long-term use, a gastrostomy button can be inserted.

Vesicostomy/ureterostomy (Fig. 55.9)—a small urostomy bag may be applied, or in neonates and infants, the urine can be allowed to leak into nappies.

Mitrofanoff/Monti—a catheter or button can be left in situ as these stomas are usually for long-term use.

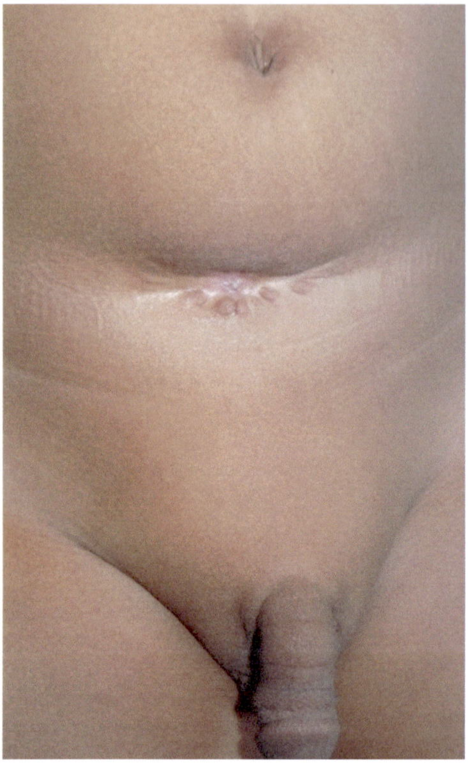

Fig. 55.9 Vesicostomy

55.4 Stoma-Related Complications

The common stoma-related problems are bleeding from the muco-cutaneous junction leading to anemia, skin excoriation, prolapse, retraction, stenosis, dehydration, and electrolyte imbalance due to high output (Figs. 55.10, 55.11, 55.12, 55.13 and 55.14).

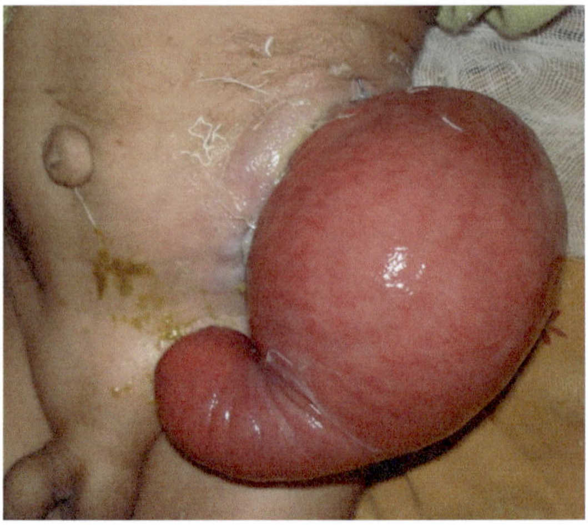

Fig. 55.10 Colostomy prolapse (pouch colon)

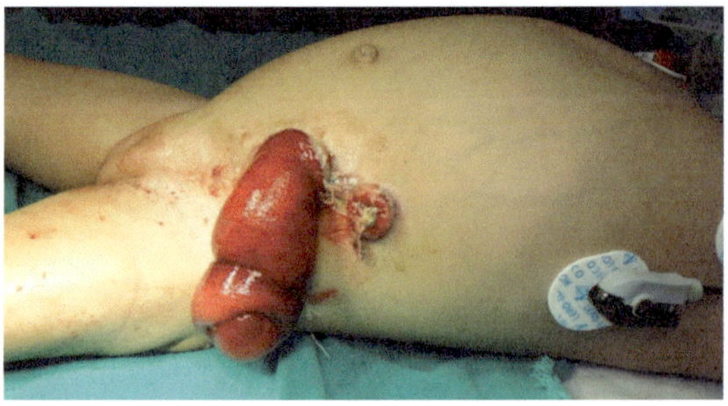

Fig. 55.11 Colostomy prolapse (distal stoma), a common complication

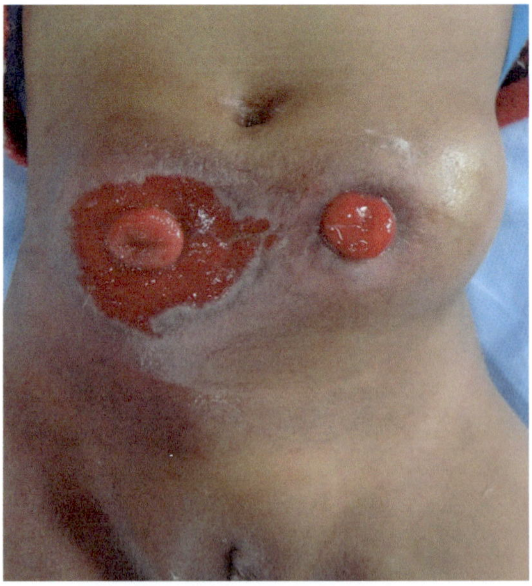

Fig. 55.12 Divided stoma (ileostomy and mucous fistula), with skin excoriation

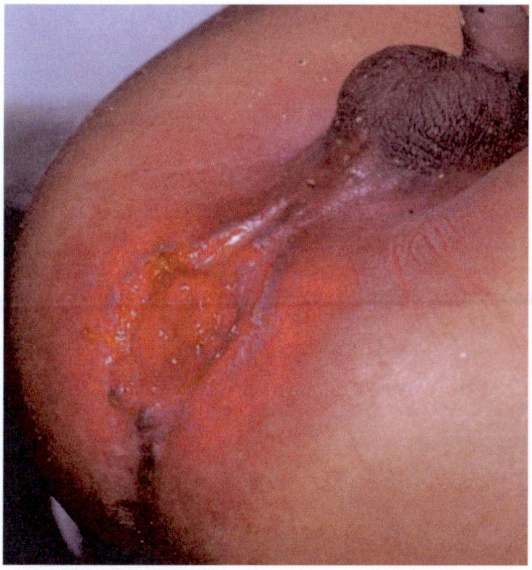

Fig. 55.13 Perianal excoriation following ileal pull-through

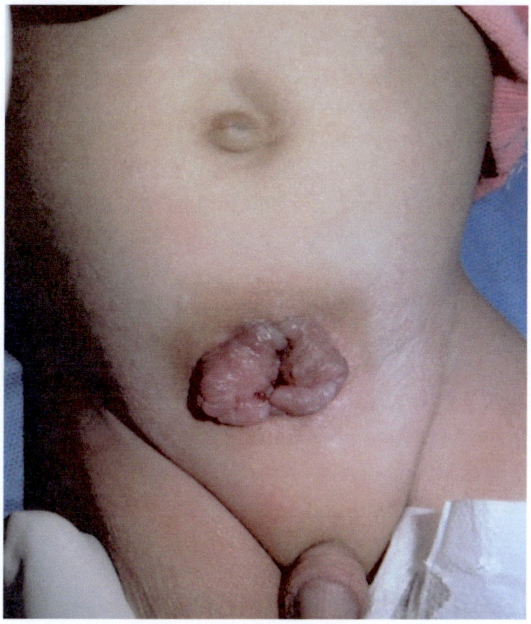

Fig. 55.14 Prolapsed vesicostomy

55.5 Stoma Care

Pediatric stoma care presents many challenges. Skin characteristics and the body profile of neonates and children need to be considered when caring for the stoma and selecting the appropriate appliance. In a poorly neonate, there will often be other things to consider when choosing a stoma bag on an already small abdomen, for example, the stoma being close to the umbilicus, central IV lines, or additional stomas. It is often necessary to be creative with the products selected to ensure a secure fit and minimize the risk of leaking stoma bags (Coloplast 2018). Several types of stoma collection bags are available for the collection of the effluent (Fig. 55.15a, b). They can be simply tied around the abdomen or fixed with stoma adhesive paste and powder.

When carrying out post-operative stoma care, the stoma should be observed for signs of edema or ischemia. An assessment of the stoma appearance, condition of peristomal skin, and the consistency of effluent should be documented. On return from the operation theater, the stoma will be covered by soft paraffin (Jelonet) gauze to keep the stoma moist. Once the stoma starts to function, an appropriately sized stoma bag should be applied.

55.5.1 In Resource-Poor Settings

Simple application of cotton cloth with frequent changing and gently cleaning the site appears to be effective in majority of our patients as they are generally small and their parents handle it very effectively. It is necessary that cotton should not be kept directly on the stoma as it will become adherent to it and may cause bleeding during removal. To prevent trauma, it is necessary to keep a paraffin gauge or a cotton cloth dipped in oil over the stoma and then cover it with a pad or other cloth. The surrounding skin can be protected with application of coconut oil or any emollient cream and a paste of zinc oxide with calamine (siloderm) or a stoma adhesive paste (karaya gum, adept). Weak steroid (betamethazone) and antifungal (co-trimazole) creams are effective in managing troublesome peristomal skin excoriation. While cleaning the stoma, a non-abrasive moist cloth should be used to minimize the damage to the stoma. It is necessary to keep the peristomal area dry by frequent cleaning and application of powder/paste. Excessive stoma

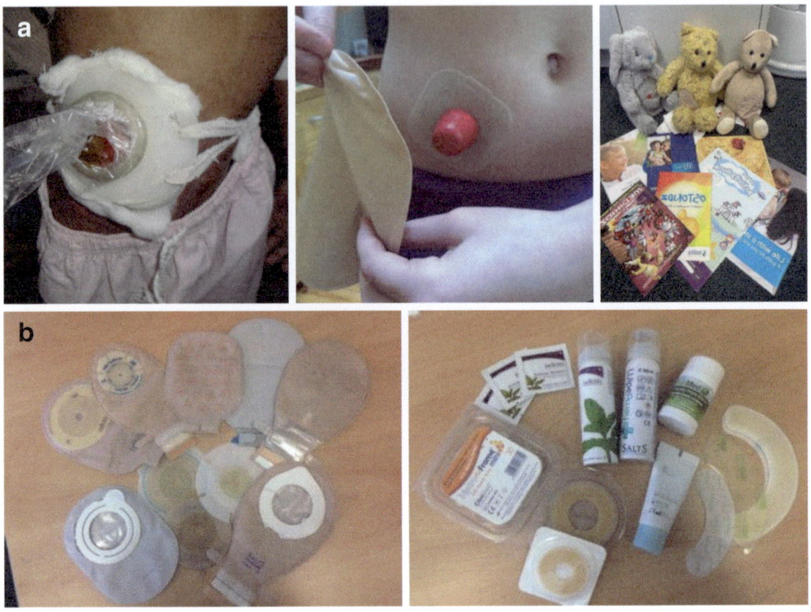

Fig. 55.15 (**a**) simple stoma bag with strapping and (**b**) stoma adhesive stoma bags and accessories

output with dehydration needs medical attention with adequate fluid and electrolyte replacement. Minor prolapse can be managed by simple reduction; however, stoma retraction or stenosis may require surgical revision.

The opening in the stoma appliance baseplate should be no more than 1–2 mm in diameter, larger than the stoma diameter at skin level. This will minimize the skins exposure to stool. If the mucous fistula (distal end) is close to the proximal stoma, the opening should be cut to accommodate both stomas in a figure of eight shape. Any exposed skin can be covered with protective paste/seal.

Once a template has been cut, it can be saved for future sizing. The size of stoma should be checked at each bag change for the first few weeks following surgery, as the size and shape of the stoma may change as edema subsides. The goal is to have a stoma product in place for a minimum of 24 hours. If the barrier is still functional, the wear time can be prolonged up to 4 days in an infant with an average wear time of 2–3 days. In premature infants, acceptable wear time decreases. This may be 12–24 hours initially (Coloplast 2018). The stoma bag should be emptied regularly when no more than a third full, and the stoma bag should be changed if leakage is observed from the baseplate of the bag.

When changing the stoma bag, the peristomal skin should be assessed for any signs of skin redness or skin breakdown. In the initial postoperative period, if the neonate/child has an ileostomy, the amount of effluent, its color, and consistency should be recorded to ensure the output is within normal limits and the child is not at risk of dehydration. As a rule of thumb, any effluent >20 ml/kg of body weight should be replaced by oral or IV routes.

It is advisable to initiate child/parental teaching of stoma care as soon as possible in preparation for discharge.

55.6 Role of Pediatric Stoma Nurse Specialist

The role of a pediatric stoma nurse specialist is to provide care, support, and education to children with a stoma and their families. It is a multifaceted role with the main aim being to help the child adjust to living with a stoma, improving their quality of life, and empowering them to manage the stoma with confidence and live a healthy, active life.

Formation of a stoma can result in physiological, psychological, and emotional problems for the child, young person, and their family (Coloplast 2018); therefore, the stoma nurse's role in stoma counseling is paramount. Children who are properly informed and prepared for surgery are less anxious and experience a shorter and less psychologically traumatic recovery. Parental worries or fears are also lessened. Education, and the way it is delivered, should take into account the developmental age, physical, emotional, and religious needs of the child and their family.

There are many resources available to help prepare a child and their family for stoma surgery. These range from parent and children's information booklets, online information, coloring booklets, to the use of stoma teddy bears for play therapy or demonstration. Pre-operative kits are available, which aim to simulate what it is like to wear a stoma bag and can help alleviate concerns regarding visibility and security. Photo albums can be used to show the journey of a child while in the hospital, showing places, equipment, or people who the child may encounter. Some children and families find it beneficial to make contact with others who have been through a similar experience.

If the surgery is planned, the stoma nurse specialist is able to meet with the child and family prior to admission. The number of times this happens is dependent on the needs of the child/family. For babies/children who have had a stoma formed as a result of emergency surgery, information/teaching is given post-surgery.

Stoma site marking is recommended for school-aged children and teenagers having elective surgery. Selection criteria of the site follow the same criteria as those of an adult. The stoma nurse specialist will assess the child in various positions taking into consideration the child's sporting activities, hobbies, and clothing habits (Coloplast 2018). In children with additional special needs, consideration when selecting a stoma site needs to take into account wheelchair use or other additional medical devices. It's recommended that both the child and parent are involved in these discussions.

Following surgery, the stoma nurse specialist, alongside ward staff, will educate the child/family on how to care for the stoma, including how to change a stoma bag, care for the peristomal skin, and discuss potential complications and what action to take. Teaching is ongoing, but the aim is to support the child and family so they feel competent at caring for their stoma by the time of discharge home.

Stoma nurse specialists will collaborate with other members of the multi-disciplinary team (MDT) to ensure a smooth discharge. Referrals are made to local pediatric community teams to ensure support is available in the community and that stoma supplies are arranged for discharge and ongoing supplies.

All children and young people with health needs should enjoy the same rights and opportunities as other pupils within an educational environment to enable them to reach their full potential. For a child who has had a stoma, returning to school can be a worrying and distressing time for both the child and their parents. A stoma nurse specialist is able to support this transition by ensuring the child is well supported in school, any concerns or worries have been addressed prior to their return, appropriate staff training has been delivered to nursery/school staff, and support given with writing an Educational Health Care plan if needed.

Following discharge, a stoma nurse specialist remains an advocate for the child, family, and other healthcare professionals involved. They act as a resource, troubleshooting any potential problems to ensure the child lives a full and active life. Regular follow-up and support are offered through clinic appointments and/or home visits if needed.

Children with stomas are supported by their pediatric nurse specialist and local pediatric community teams until they reach 16 years of age, or, if the child has additional complex needs, they may remain under the care of a pediatric team until they reach 18 years old. At this point, they will be transitioned over to the adult service. Transition of a patient aims to be a purposeful, planned process that addresses the medical, psychosocial, educational, and vocational needs of a young person (DfES and DH 2006). The stoma nurse specialist will assist in ensuring this process is as smooth as possible for the patient.

References

Coloplast. Paediatric Stoma care: Global best practice guidelines for neonates, children, and teenagers. 2018.
DfES and DH. Transition: getting it right for young people. 2006.

Part IX

Pediatric Oncology

Principles of Cancer Chemotherapy in Children

56

Madhavi Redkar

56.1 Introduction

Improved survival for childhood cancer has been one of the successes of modern medicine. In 1970, the 5-year overall survival from all types of childhood cancer was only 28%; now it is 75%. For acute lymphoblastic leukemia, the survival has improved from 9% in 1960 to 85% today. This dramatic improvement in survival is due to chemotherapy, sometimes as the only treatment modality, especially, for leukemia and lymphoma, but more often in combination with surgery and radiotherapy for solid tumors.

56.2 Critical Differences Between Pediatric and Adult Cancers

Cancer has a very diverse and intricate pathophysiology involving genetic, epigenetic, and environmental factors. Understanding the critical differences between pediatric and adult cancers is very important. This helps investigate the underlying pathophysiologic and molecular mechanisms for developing new diagnostic/therapeutic approaches.

First, types of cancers are different between children and adults. Childhood cancers are not triggered by lifestyle as in adults, and very few are inherited from parents.

For example, while brain and bone cancers are rare in adults, they have much higher rates in children. Similarly, leukemia is also more prevalent in children.

Second, even though cancers in children tend to respond better to therapy, children and adults differ in genitourinary pH and transit, intestinal motility and conjugation, and transport of bile salts. All of these factors affect the metabolism of chemotherapeutic drugs. Pediatric tissues and organs are very fragile and immature and have higher metabolic rates because children rapidly develop. Treatment dosages that are safe to administer to adults are often severely toxic to a child's developing organs, which absorb, distribute, and eliminate substances more rapidly than the same type of organ in an adult.

Finally, genetic stability in children and adults also differs, affecting cancer mutation rates.

The majority of malignancies occurring in childhood are sensitive to cytotoxic chemotherapy. This chemosensitivity is generally attributed to the high proliferation rate of childhood malignancies and the capacity of the malignant cells to become apoptotic.

M. Redkar (✉)
Department of Pharmacology, BKL Walawalakar Rural Medical College and Hospital, Kasarwadi, At Post Sawarde, Chiplun, Maharashtrav, India

© The Author(s), under exclusive license to Springer Nature Singapore Pte Ltd. 2025
S. Roy Choudhury (ed.), *Pediatric Surgery*, https://doi.org/10.1007/978-981-96-1257-4_56

Therefore, chemotherapy plays a major role in treating pediatric malignancies and improves outcomes for most of them.

The management of patients with cancer is complex and requires contribution from a range of healthcare professionals working alongside specialist oncology consultants to address patients' needs and optimize outcomes.

Among various disciplines actively involved in cancer management include pediatricians, pediatric surgeons, pediatric oncologists, pathologists, and radiologists, along with specialized nursing staff and technicians. The recent advances in cancer management also require an expert geneticist, nutritionist, and psychologist/counselor.

56.3 Commonly Occurring Childhood Malignancies (American Academy of Pediatrics, 2020)

I. Head Face Neck:
- Retinoblastoma
- Neuroblastoma
- Rhabdomyosarcoma
- Nasopharyngeal carcinoma

II. Thoracic:
- Neuroblastoma
- Teratoma

III. Abdominal:
- Neuroblastoma
- Hepatoblastoma
- Wilm's tumor
- Rhabdomyosarcoma
- Mesoblastic nephroma

IV. Extremity:
- Fibrosarcoma
- Rhabdomyosarcoma
- Ewing's sarcoma
- Soft tissue sarcoma
- Osteosarcoma

V. Genitourinary:
- Teratoma
- Germ cell tumors

Hemopoietic malignancies may present with lymph node enlargements or a mass.

56.4 Chemotherapy

Chemotherapy is an aggressive form of chemical drug therapy meant to destroy rapidly growing cells in the body. It's usually used to treat cancer, as cancer cells grow and divide faster than other cells.

Knowledge of the cell cycle determines the development of various protocols and regimes, while protocols are a combination of chemotherapeutic agents with the idea of destroying cancer cells while protecting normal cells.

Cellular growth, development, and differentiation are exceptionally well controlled by a conserved biological mechanism: the cell cycle. The cell cycle represents a series of tightly integrated events that allow the cell to grow and proliferate.

The cell cycle is a set of coordinated events that culminate in the formation of two cells from one mother cell. It's composed of four major phases: G1 (growth phase 1), S (DNA synthesis phase), G2 (growth phase 2), and M (mitosis), which function to integrate environment-sensing signaling pathways with cell growth and proliferation. This process is classically described as four sequential phases that progress from quiescence (G0 phase) to proliferation (G1, S, G2, and M phases), and then back to the G0 phase (Diagram 56.1).

Cell cycle progression is primarily controlled by two regulatory processes: phosphorylation of specific proteins by cyclin-dependent kinases

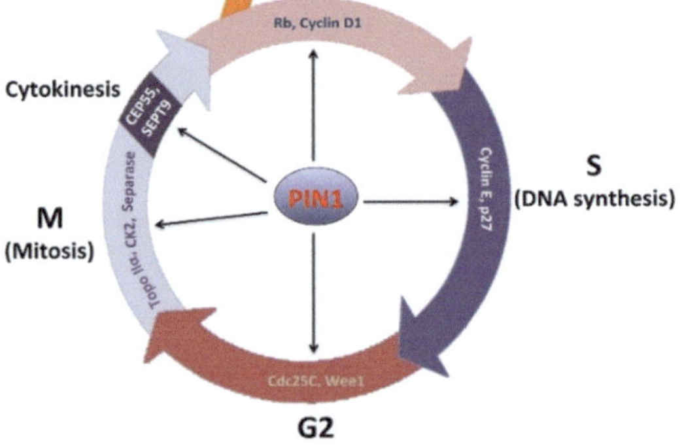

Diagram 56.1 Representation of a cell cycle

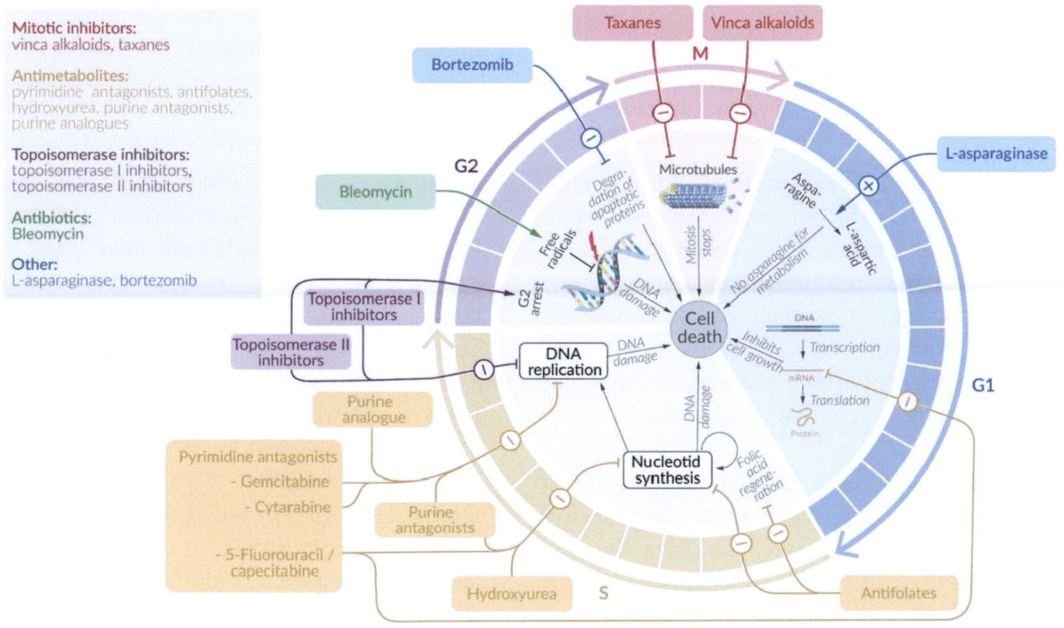

Diagram 56.2 Mechanisms of action of various chemotherapeutic agents on different cell stages of cell cycle

(CDKs) and their dephosphorylation by phosphatases, and specific proteolytic degradation by the ubiquitin-proteasome system.

Knowledge about the cell cycle is critical to understanding how best to clinically develop these agents, both as single agents and in combination with chemotherapy.

Cell cycle inhibition represents an opportunity for therapeutic intervention in treating proliferative diseases like cancer. Most anti-cancer drugs perturb the proliferation cycle of tumor cells by inhibiting/damaging cell cycle events, which activate checkpoints arrest cells and induce apoptosis (Diagram 56.2).

Most regimes involve the use of acronyms for agents used. Some commonly used protocols are as follows:

56.4.1 Hodgkin's Lymphoma

COPP Protocol: Cyclophosphamide, Oncovin(Vincristine), Prednisolone, and Procarbazine.

ABVD Protocol: Adriamycin, Bleomycin, Vinblastine, and Dacarbazine.

56.4.2 Non-Hodgkin's Lymphoma

COMP Protocol: Cyclophosphamide, Oncovin, Methotrexate, and Prednisolone.

CHOP Protocol: Cyclophosphamide, Hydroxydaunorubicin (Doxorubicin), Oncovin, and Prednisolone.

Cycle/schedules on the other hand use the knowledge of cell cycle to decide the timing of various regimes. A cycle is the block of time in which a regimen is given. Each regimen can have a different cycle time.

For example, a cycle of CHOP is usually 21 days. This is how the cycle breaks down:

- Cytoxan, adriamycin, and oncovin (Vincristine) are given on day 1.
- Prednisone is given on days 1-5.
- 16 days "off" without chemotherapy. This totals 21 days, completing one cycle.
- Another new cycle starts.

56.5 Classification of Chemotherapeutic Agents Used in Pediatric Oncology (Table 56.1)

Chemotherapy Fundamentals Combined chemotherapy accounts for most chemotherapy treatments for cancer. There are many reasons why this is done. In combination chemotherapy, agents with distinct mechanisms of action are administered concurrently, whereby their cumulative or synergistic effects facilitate a more rapid and effective destruction of cancer cells.

The drugs used have different mechanisms to develop resistance and hence the combination prolongs the effectiveness of the chemotherapy. The drugs used in combination may reduce or ameliorate the side effects of other drugs or modalities used.

However, when combination chemotherapy is used, it is important to be aware of drug–drug interactions and exacerbation of toxicity while using multiple drugs.

Terms Associated with Chemotherapy Chemotherapy encompasses a wide variety of therapy treatments. Following are some examples:

Neo-adjuvant Chemotherapy (Preoperative): This chemotherapy is given before the patient is taken up for surgery. Neoadjuvant chemotherapy may be given to attempt to shrink cancer, so the surgical procedure may not need to be as extensive. It may help in organ preservation. Neoadjuvant chemotherapy may help achieve sensitivity for particular receptors or biomarkers.

Adjuvant Chemotherapy (Postoperative): This chemotherapy is given after the surgery. The idea behind the usage is to kill micrometastatic disease and increase disease-free survival.

Induction chemotherapy: This chemotherapy is given to induce remission. This term is commonly used in the treatment of acute leukemias.

Consolidation chemotherapy: This chemotherapy is given once remission is achieved. The goal of this therapy is to sustain remission. Consolidation chemotherapy may also be called intensification therapy. This term is commonly used in the treatment of acute leukemias.

Maintenance chemotherapy: This chemotherapy is given in lower doses to assist in prolonging remission. Maintenance chemotherapy is used only for certain types of cancer, most commonly acute lymphocytic leukemias and acute promyelocytic leukemias.

First-line chemotherapy: This chemotherapy has, through research studies and clinical trials, been determined to have the best probability of treating a given cancer. This may also be called standard therapy.

Second-line chemotherapy: This chemotherapy is given if a disease has not responded or reoccurred after first-line chemotherapy. Second-line chemotherapy has, through research studies and clinical trials, been determined to be effective in treating a given cancer that has not responded or reoccurred after standard chemotherapy. In some cases, this may also be referred to as salvage therapy.

Palliative chemotherapy is given specifically to address symptom management without expecting to reduce cancer significantly.

Chemoradiation: Integration of chemotherapy with radiotherapy. This modality results in the enhancement of tumor response to radiation. Some drugs known to sensitize cancerous cells include 5-flurouracil and cisplatin. The use of these drugs helps protect the normal tissue from adverse effects of radiation.

Table 56.1 Classification of chemotherapeutic agents according to their main mechanisms of action

S No	Class of drugs	Mechanism of action	Examples of drugs
1.	Anti- metabolites	Interferes with precursors of DNA /RNA of the rapidly multiplying cancer cells	Pyrimidine antimetabolites: Cytarabine Gemcytabine 5-Flurouracil Purine antimetabolites: 6-Thioguanine 6-Mercaptopurine Fludarabine Cladribine
2.	Anti-folates Distinct group of antimetabolites	Inhibit diydrofolate reductase which in turn inhibits synthesis of purines and pyramidines. Also inhibit the synthesis of thymidates, a precursor of DNA strands	Aminopterin Methotrexate Trimethrexate
3.	Anti-microtubule compounds Include many of Vinca alkaloids	Interfere with the formation of microtubules which are essential for maintaining the cellular architecture	Vincristine Vinblastine Vinorelbine
4.	Alkylating agents One of the older classes of chemotherapeutic agents. Also have a broad spectrum of action	Form covalent bond between alkyl group and cellular molecules like deoxyribose in DNA. This in turn alters the DNA and subsequent replication. This group of agents also cause a lot of toxicity due to the nonspecific alkylation within the cells	Mechlorethanamine Cyclophosphamaide Ifcophosphamide Melphalan Busulfan Nitrosoureas-like Carmustine
5.	Platinum Compounds	Forms complex with DNA/RNA proteins and the platinum atom thereby damaging the cell and causing apoptosis	Cisplatinium Carbaplatinum
6.	Topoisomerase II inhibitors: Includes several classes of drugs which may have additional mechanisms of action	Inhibits topoisomerase II enzymes interferes in DNA replication, transcription and repair. Some drugs do cause oxidative damage to the cells in addition to TPII inhibition. Mitoxantone additionally causes intercalation of DNA strands	Epipodophyllotoxins: Etoposide Teniposide Anthracyclines: Doxorubicin Epirubicin Daunorubicin Mitoxantone
7.	Topoisomerse I inhibitors These show great promise in treatment of some solid tumors in pediatric age group	Interfere in DNA replication	Topotecan Irinotecan
8.	Anti-tumor antibiotics	Oxidative damage of DNA of cancerous cells	Bleomycin Dactinomycin
9.	L-Aspariginase Forms mainstay of ALL management	Depletes an essential amino acid aspartame which is essential for the cell to survive	
10.	Miscellaneous agents	At higher doses, they are known to induce apoptosis of malignant cells by binding to steroid receptors of the cell membrane	Retinoic acid: (very high doses of retinoic acid are used in The treatment of neuroblastomas and retinoblastomas Corticosteroids

The main mechanisms of action are mentioned here. Many drugs/classes of drugs do have many different modes of action contributing to their therapeutic efficacy. These drugs are elsewhere in the book along with the respective tumor management

56.6 Recent Advances

Pediatric cancers pose unique challenges when compared to adult malignancies. Pediatric malignancies tend to have a lower mutational burden and are often driven by specific genetic alterations rather than the accumulation of multiple mutations over time.

Pediatric tumors are typically characterized by high genetic heterogeneity, meaning that different cells within the same tumor may harbor distinct genetic abnormalities. This complexity can make it difficult for traditional chemotherapy to effectively target and eliminate cancer cells, underscoring the need for more precise, targeted treatment strategies.

Although pediatric chemotherapy is a proven and effective treatment for various childhood cancers, a wide range of short-term and long-term toxicities associated with chemotherapy can significantly impact the quality of life of young patients.

Hence, one finds precision medicine and personalized modalities to be fast emerging in pediatric oncology.

At the heart of precision medicine in pediatric oncology is the concept of genomic profiling, which involves the comprehensive analysis of a patient's tumor genetic makeup to identify specific genetic alterations driving cancer growth and progression.

This information can then pinpoint potential therapeutic targets, enabling clinicians to select treatments targeting these molecular abnormalities.

56.7 Pharmacogenomics

Pharmacogenomics studies how an individual's genetic makeup influences their response to drugs. Understanding the genetic factors that affect drug metabolism makes it possible to personalize chemotherapy regimens for each patient, optimizing drug doses to maximize efficacy and minimize toxicity.

For example, genetic variations in the *TPMT* gene can influence the metabolism of the chemotherapy drug 6-mercaptopurine (6-MP), which is used to treat acute lymphoblastic leukemia (ALL). Patients with certain TPMT variants are at higher risk of experiencing severe side effects, and therefore may benefit from a reduced 6-MP dose.

56.8 Tumor Profiling

Tumor profiling involves analyzing the molecular characteristics of cancer cells to identify potential therapeutic targets or prognostic markers. This information can help guide the selection of more effective and less toxic treatments for individual patients.

For example, in neuroblastoma, a common pediatric cancer, the presence of the MYCN oncogene amplification is associated with more aggressive disease and poorer prognosis. Patients with MYCN-amplified neuroblastoma may benefit from more intensive chemotherapy regimens or the addition of targeted therapies, such as ALK inhibitors.

Various technologies like next-generation sequencing technologies and identifying actionable targets are under study to help the development of newer therapeutic agents.

Stem Cell Therapy Hematopoietic stem cell transplantation (HSCT) involves the intravenous infusion of hematopoietic stem cells to reestablish blood cell production in patients whose bone marrow or immune system is damaged or defective. Over the past half-century, this technique has been used increasingly frequently to treat numerous malignant and nonmalignant diseases.

AutologousBoneMarrowTransplantation The bone marrow products are collected from the patient and are reinfused after purification methods. The advantages include no graft versus host disease (GVHD.) The disadvantage is that the bone marrow products may contain abnormal cells that can cause relapse in the case of malignancy; hence, theoretically, this method cannot be used in all cases of abnormal bone marrow diseases.

Cord Cell Transplants Whenever possible use of stem cells from umbilical cords is preferred.

Allogenic Transplantation The donor is an HLA-matched family member, unrelated matched donor, or mismatched family donors (haploidentical).

Hematopoietic stem cell transplantation (HSCT) is indicated in diverse malignant conditions like multiple myeloma, various types of leukemia, lymphomas, myelofibrosis, and many other conditions. Many non-malignant conditions like aplastic anemia, severe combined immune deficiency disorder also benefit from HSCT.

HSCT plays a vital role in the management of solid tumors. Hematopoietic stem cell transplantation (HSCT) has also been investigated in medulloblastoma, metastatic breast cancer, and other solid tumors that are refractory to conventional chemotherapy.

Angiogenesis inhibitors are unique cancer-fighting agents because they block the growth of blood vessels that support tumor growth rather than blocking the growth of tumor cells themselves. Angiogenesis inhibitors interfere in several ways with various steps in blood vessel growth.

Angiogenesis, the formation of new blood vessels from preexisting ones, is required for the growth and metastases of solid tumors. Angiogenesis is mediated by the stabilization of the master transcription factor (hypoxia-inducible factor-α), leading to the transcription of several pro-tumorigenic factors, including VEGF. Inhibiting this pathway has emerged as an important target for antineoplastic therapy, and over the past several years, it has been the focus of extensive research and drug development. VEGF signaling pathway (VSP) inhibitors have been approved for the treatment of a broad spectrum of malignancies

Angiogenesis inhibitors battle cancer in a unique way. They don't attack cancer cells directly. Instead, they strike a tumor's blood supply. They block the growth of new blood vessels, so the tumor doesn't get the oxygen and nourishment it needs to grow. In some cases, the tumors may shrink.

Some of these drugs target the signals that help the tumor get blood. They usually don't harm normal cells in your body. These novel agents also aren't as likely to cause your body to start resisting the drug.

In some cases, these medicines work best with other cancer-fighting treatments. They only work in cancers with solid tumors. They don't work for blood cancers like leukemia.

Angiogenesis inhibitors interfere with the creation of blood vessels in three main ways (Table 56.2).

- *By blocking blood vessel growth factors.* The main growth factor in angiogenesis is vascular endothelial growth factor (VEGF). It binds to receptors on the cells of blood vessels and jump-starts the creation of new blood vessels. Some angiogenesis inhibitors find VEGF or other growth factors, then bind to them, so they can't do their job.
- *By interfering with VEGF receptors.* This stops them from sending signals to blood vessel cells. Without these signals, angiogenesis won't start. Example: tyrosine kinase inhibitors.
- *By interfering with the cellular signals.* This can block their activities and keep blood vessels from growing.

Although this modality of therapy holds a great promise in the management of several solid

Table 56.2 Mechanisms of action of novel angioneogenesis inhibitors with examples

By blocking blood vessels growth factors	By interfering with VEGF receptors	By interfering with the cellular signals
Bevacizumab	Axitinib	Everolimus
Ramucirumab	Cabozantinib	Lenalidomide
Ziv-aflibercepts	Lenvatinib mesylate	Thalidomide
	Pazopanib	
	Sorafenib	
	Sunitib	
	Vandetanib	

tumors, they have been extensively tried in adults. They are used in children in being studied or in various phases of clinical trials. The side effects associated with these agents are many and serious in nature.

56.9 Targeted Therapies

56.9.1 Monoclonal Antibodies

Monoclonal antibodies are laboratory-produced molecules that can specifically recognize and bind to target proteins on the surface of cancer cells. By doing so, they can either directly inhibit the target protein's function or recruit the immune system to attack and destroy the cancer cells.

Some examples of monoclonal antibodies used in pediatric chemotherapy are:

Rituximab for non-Hodgkin lymphoma CD20-positive lymphomas
Trastuzumab for certain types of pediatric solid tumors
Dinutuximab for neuroblastoma
Brentuximab vedotin for CD30-positive lymphomas

Monoclonal antibodies are associated with fewer side effects compared to traditional chemotherapy drugs, as they do not affect healthy cells. The biggest disadvantage of this class is the fast development of resistance.

56.9.2 Small Molecule Inhibitors

Small molecule inhibitors are designed to specifically target and inhibit the function of proteins or enzymes that play a crucial role in cancer cell growth and survival. Many small molecule inhibitors target kinases, which are enzymes that regulate various cellular processes, including cell proliferation, differentiation, and apoptosis.

Tyrosine kinase inhibitors (TKIs) are another class of targeted therapies that work by inhibiting the function of specific enzymes (tyrosine kinases) involved in cancer cell growth and survival. TKIs are promising in treating various pediatric cancers, including chronic myeloid leukemia (CML) and certain types of solid tumors.

Examples include the following:

Imatinib, which has been tried and tested in CML as well as Philadelphia chromosome-positive acute lymphoblastic leukemia and some pediatric solid tumors
Crizotinib for ALK-positive neuroblastoma

This modality offers improved survival rates and reduced toxicity compared to conventional chemotherapy.

56.10 Immunotherapies

Immunotherapies harness the power of the patient's immune system to fight cancer. Examples of immunotherapies used in pediatric oncology include:

- Immune checkpoint inhibitors block proteins that prevent the immune system from attacking cancer cells. Several such molecules are being studied .One such drug acts against a checkpoint protein called CTLA-4. Other immune checkpoint inhibitors act against a checkpoint protein called PD-1 or its partner protein PD-L1.
- Chimeric antigen receptor (CAR) T-cell therapy, in which a patient's T cells are genetically engineered to recognize and attack cancer cells expressing a specific antigen. CAR T-cell therapy targeting CD19 has shown promising results in treating pediatric patients with relapsed or refractory B-cell acute lymphoblastic leukemia.

56.11 Innovative Drug Delivery Systems

Advancements in drug delivery systems, such as nanoparticle-based carriers, can help improve the therapeutic index of chemotherapy drugs and reduce toxicity by selectively targeting cancer cells and minimizing exposure to healthy tissues. These include dendrimers, liposomes, micelles, and quantum dots. Several clinical trials are currently underway to study the efficacy of these drug delivery systems.

Use of newer drug infusion systems like Portacath, Chemports, Hickman lines, Broviac lines, and peripherally inserted central catheters (PICC) go a long way in improving the quality of life for pediatric patients.

56.12 Conclusion

To ensure the best possible outcomes for patients and minimize the long-term consequences of treatment, it is mandatory to reduce toxicity in pediatric chemotherapy.

By exploring and implementing various modalities and strategies, such as risk-adapted therapy, dose modifications, targeted therapies, and supportive care, physicians can provide effective treatment while minimizing toxicity and enhancing the quality of life for pediatric cancer patients.

As the field of pediatric oncology continues to evolve, further advancements in precision medicine, drug development, and drug delivery systems will undoubtedly lead to even more effective and less toxic treatment options for children with cancer.

Summary

Pediatric chemotherapy continues to be the mainstay of cancer management in children. A short overview of the chemotherapeutic management of pediatric malignancies is provided, including a brief mention of mechanisms of action. Recent advances and newer treatment modalities like precision medicine, pharmacogenomics, and targeted delivery are discussed. Newer molecules like small molecules inhibitors (tyrosine kinase inhibitors), monoclonal antibodies, and agents used in immunotherapy will have a significant role in cancer chemotherapy in future. Many of these molecules are being studied in different phases of clinical trials.

Suggested Reading

Childhood Cancer Genomics (PDQ®)–Health Professional Version published by the National Cancer Institute. Updated: April 14, 2023. https://www.cancer.gov/types/childhood-cancers/pediatric-genomics-

Kanakia S. Chemotherapy. In: Redkar R, editor. IAPS textbook of pediatric surgery. 1st ed. Jaypee Brothers Medical Publishers; 2020. p. 583–92.

Krasin MJ, Davidoff AM. Principles of pediatric oncology, genetics of cancer and radiation therapy. In: Conran AG, editor. Pediatric surgery, vol. 1. Elsevier Saunders; 2012. p. 397–416.

Nazer B, Humphreys BD, Moslehi J. Effects of novel angiogenesis inhibitors for the treatment of cancer on the cardiovascular system: focus on hypertension. Circulation. 2011;124(15):1687–91.

Roychoudhary S. Pediatric surgery: a quick guide to decision making. In: Pediatric oncology. 1st ed. Springer; 2018. p. 253–87.

57 Principles of Radiation Oncology in Children

Shikha Halder

57.1 Introduction

Most pediatric cancers are curable with proper treatment, and survival rates are around 70–80%. Improved cure rates add 50–60 years to the child's life. Hence, there is a concern for treatment-related late effects, quality of life, and their integration into society, which are as important as the cure.

Treatment of malignant tumors in children is multimodality, and Radiotherapy is an important modality. In 1988, Donaldson, reviewing the role of radiotherapy in modern pediatric oncology, stated that an estimated 70–80% of children with cancer would need and receive radiotherapy at some time in their course of treatment.

In the last decade, with the concern about the late effects of radiotherapy, such as the neuropsychological effects of irradiation of the central nervous system (CNS), orthopedic effects, and the fertility effect, chemotherapy regimens have become more intensive, consequently reducing the proportion of children receiving radiotherapy has been reduced to approximately 40–50%.

Pediatric radiation oncology has evolved as an essential sub-specialty. In the last two decades, national and international working groups, such as the Children's Cancer and Leukemia Group and the International Society of Pediatric Oncology, have supported standard radiotherapy treatment protocols.

57.2 Principles of Radiation Therapy

Pediatric Radiation Oncologists must provide the highest possible standard of radiotherapy. Careful planning involving multiple steps is required to achieve local tumor control with minimum irradiation to normal tissues and minimal late effects.

Radiation therapy, unlike chemotherapy, affects only the site where it is delivered. Hence, targeting tumors in specific locations and delivering radiation to the tumor's exact location is important.

Radiation damages the DNA of rapidly growing malignant cells but may also affect the normal tissue or cells surrounding the target area of radiation. However, normal cells have a better capability of repair than malignant cells, which translates into tumor control without an acceptable loss of normal tissue function.

S. Halder (✉)
Department of Radiation Oncology, Sir Gangaram Hospital, New Delhi, India

© The Author(s), under exclusive license to Springer Nature Singapore Pte Ltd. 2025
S. Roy Choudhury (ed.), *Pediatric Surgery*, https://doi.org/10.1007/978-981-96-1257-4_57

57.3 Interaction of Ionizing Rays with Tissue

Absorption of energy from ionizing radiation incident upon a cell damages the DNA. Radiation therapy acts on the tissues in two ways: -

Direct action: The incident photon (ionizing radiation) directly hits the DNA molecule and disrupts molecular structure. Such structural change leads to cell damage or even cell death.

Indirect action: The incident photon hits the water molecules, the principal constituent of the cell, and other organic molecules in the cell, thereby producing free radicals such as hydroxyl (HO•) and alkoxy (RO2•), Free radicals are characterized by an unpaired electron in the structure, which is very reactive, it reacts with DNA molecules and causes molecular structural damage. Hydrogen peroxide, H_2O_2, is also toxic to DNA molecules. The result of the indirect action of radiation on DNA molecules is the impairment of function or death of the cell (Fig. 57.1).

The role of the six typical radiobiological phenomena determining the response of both malignant and normal tissues are the 6Rs:

Reoxygenation—In the process of radiation damage, as described above, oxygen is essential to produce lethal damage. The fractionated radiation allows the hypoxic tumor center of a growing tumor to be re-oxygenated during intervals between fractions, leading to increased tumor cell killing by free radical formation.

Repopulation—During the radiation treatment, both normal stem cells and malignant cells can repopulate; normal cell repopulation leads to decreased radiation side effects, whereas malignant cell repopulation results in disease recurrence.

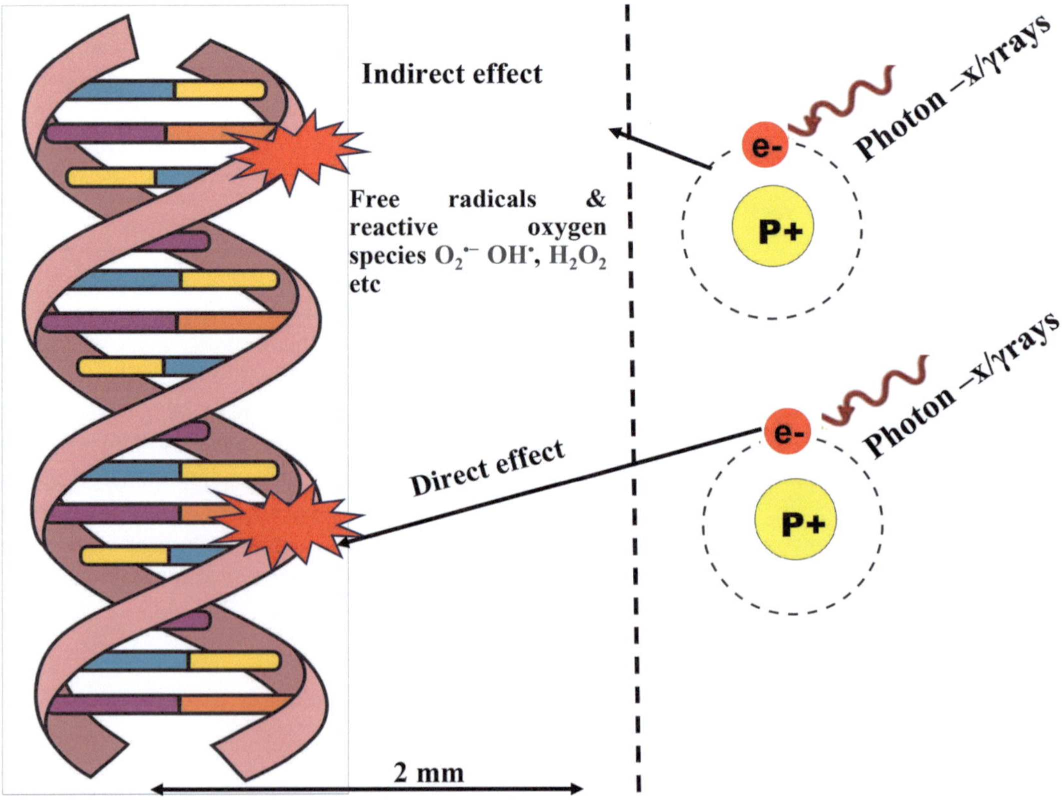

Fig. 57.1 Direct & indirect Radiation affect on cell. (Acknowledgement the DNA structure: Ramchandra Pokale, Chief Artist, CCM, AIIMS, Delhi)

Repair—Damage can be lethal or sublethal. Fractionation allows normal cells to repair radiation-induced sublethal damage much better than malignant cells.

Redistribution—cells are more sensitive to radiation in the G2 and M phases of the cell cycle and resistant in the late S phase. Fast-multiplying neoplastic cells are more prone to radiation damage as cells get redistributed to a more sensitive phase than normal tissues, which proliferate sluggishly depending on the tissue type.

Radiosensitivity—the response to radiation varies by tumor intrinsic and individual radiosensitivity.

Reactivation of the immune system—Recent Advances in radiobiology have revealed that Radiotherapy can modify the tumor microenvironment and induce a local and systemic immune response. Conversely, Radiotherapy (RT) can increase some immunosuppressive barriers, leading to tumor radio-resistance.

57.4 Types of Ionizing Radiation for Therapy

Ionizing radiation takes a few forms: Alpha, beta, and neutron particles, and gamma and X-rays (photons). All types are caused by unstable atoms, which have either an excess of energy or mass (or both). They must release that extra energy or mass through radiation to reach a stable state.

Commonly used ionizing radiation for therapy are:

Photons (X-rays and gamma rays): Photons can penetrate deep into your tissue, killing cancer cells. Nearly all radiotherapy treatments use photons.

Electrons: Electrons are produced by a linear accelerator. Because of their defined track length within the tissue, it can be used to irradiate superficial tumor volumes, with relative sparing of deeper tissues.

Protons: Protons produced by a high-energy cyclotron have the advantage of depositing their energy within the Bragg peak, a short track length at a depth within tissue. It has potential advantages over photon therapy because Proton beam therapy lacks an "exit dose" due to the Bragg peak. It enables one to deliver highly conformal doses to the tumor volume and nearly completely spares normal healthy tissue (Fig. 57.2a, b).

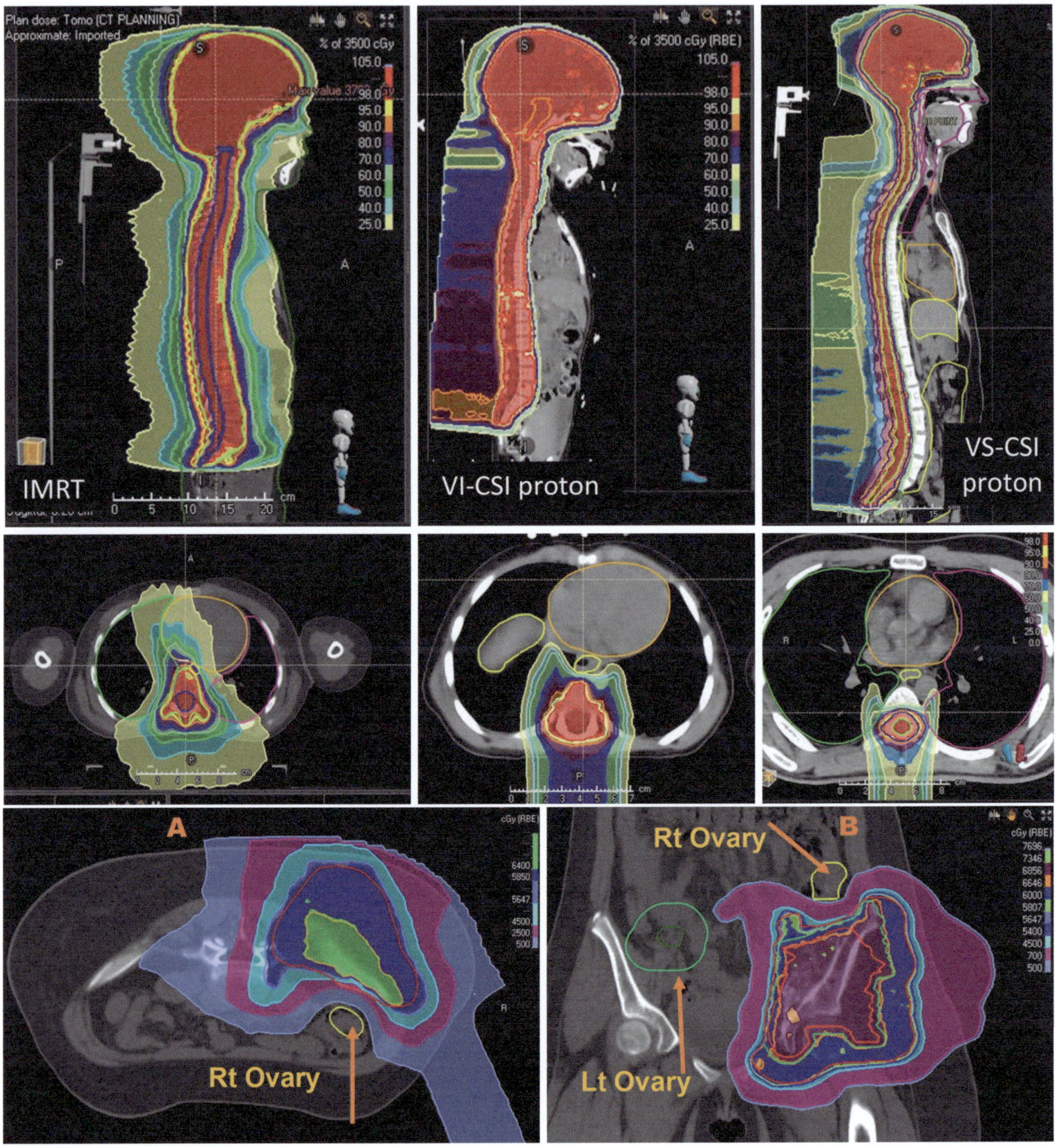

Fig. 57.2 (**a**) Dose colour wash between treatment plans with IMRT, vertebral-inclusive CSI (VI-CSI, opted in prepubertal patients), and vertebra-sparing CSI (VS-CSI, opted in a post-pubertal patient, i.e., who have attained skeletal maturity Proton therapy plans allow superior sparing of anterior and lateral OARs, including esophagus, DARS, midline mucosa, thyroid, heart, lungs, kidneys, liver, and bowel bag- demonstrated in the sagittal section. Representative axial section through the heart shows sparing of anterior OARs in VS-CSI ≫ VI-CSI ≫ IMRT plan. (Acknowledgement: Dr. Jalali, Apollo Proton Center). (**b**) 15 year young girl with unresectable osteosarcoma. Dose prescription to CTV 74Gy equivalent with sparing of bilateral ovary Rt ovary receiving 3.6 Gy and Lt ovary 2.8Gy (Acknowledgement: Dr Srinivas Chikuri, Apollo Proton Centre)

57.5 Delivery of Radiation Therapy

Radiation therapy can be delivered in two ways: Teletherapy or external beam radiotherapy and Brachytherapy (Fig. 57.3a, b).

External beam radiation therapy (EBRT) is a type of radiation therapy that directs a radiation beam from outside the body toward the malignant tumor inside the body.

Most external beam radiation therapy types are done by a linear accelerator (LINAC) or Cobalt machine. Most Cobalt machines are being replaced by linear accelerators from the radiation safety point of view, and linear accelerators are doing more accurate treatment.

The majority of pediatric cancers are treated with external radiation.

Brachytherapy—Gamma rays produced by radioactive decay of radioactive sources such as *Co-60* and *Ir-192* are used for brachytherapy. Brachytherapy means placing the source in the vicinity of the malignant tumor either placing hollow needles into the tumor tissue, also called interstitial brachytherapy, or special applicators can insert into the body cavity like the esophagus, vagina, and uterine cavity, which is called intracavitary brachytherapy.

Brachytherapy has an established role in the treatment of localized retinoblastoma, rhabdomyosarcoma, especially vaginal rhabdomyosarcoma, but other sites such as head and neck & bladder may be suitable.

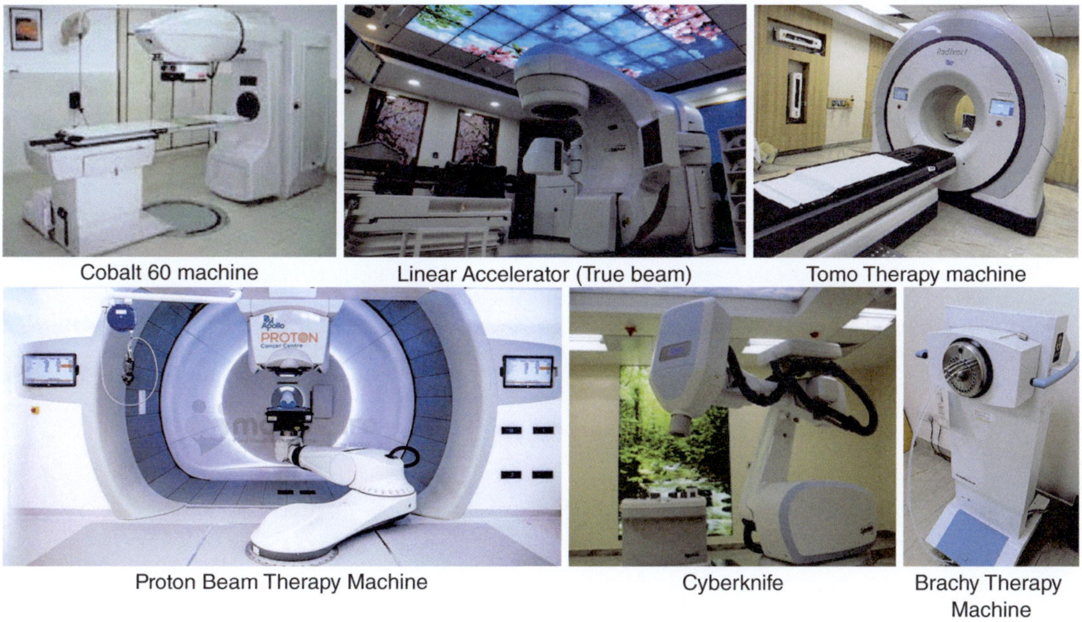

Fig. 57.3 (**a**) Radiation Therapy delivery machines. (Acknowledgement: BLK Max Super-speciality Hospital, Delhi and Dr. Piyusha Kulshrestha, Metro Hospital & Cancer Institute, Delhi). (**b**) Radiation delivery machines. (Acknowledgement: BLK Max Super-speciality Hospital, Delhi and Dr. Sapna Nangia, Apollo Proton Centre, Chennai)

57.6 Radiation Therapy Planning

57.6.1 Immobilization and Simulation

Patients must be immobilized during both simulation and treatment, and the setup must be reproducible throughout the treatment period to avoid geographically missing the tumor bed and irradiating the normal tissue. Some children require general anesthesia for simulation, probably in part or throughout the treatment.

With advances in technology and the various equipment capable of delivering radiation, it is essential to maintain proper immobilization (Fig. 57.4) and accurately to ensure proper treatment.

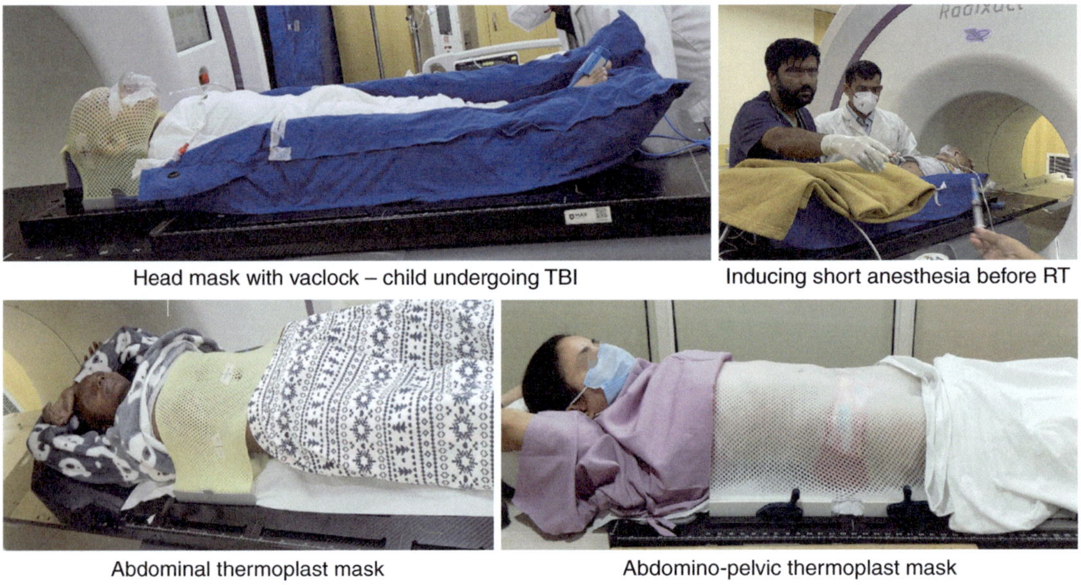

Fig. 57.4 Radiation delivery mask, immobilization, etc. (Acknowledgement: BLK Max Super-speciality Hospital, Delhi and Dr. Piyusha Kulshrestha, Metro Hospital & Cancer Institute, Delhi)

57.7 Target Delineation

Definition of target volume for radiotherapy planning.

The target volumes are defined as follows:

1. *The gross tumor volume (GTV)* is the gross tumor that is clinically palpable or visible and demonstrable on imaging such as CT, MRI, and positron emission tomography (PET) scans (Figs. 57.5 and 57.6).
2. *The clinical target volume (CTV)* is the tissue volume that contains the GTV + subclinical tumor.
3. *The planning target volume (PTV)* is defined to select the area to cover patient movements, errors of patient setup on the machine, and beam inaccuracies to ensure that the prescribed dose is delivered to the whole of the CTV (Fig. 57.7) and avoiding critical organs (Fig. 57.8).

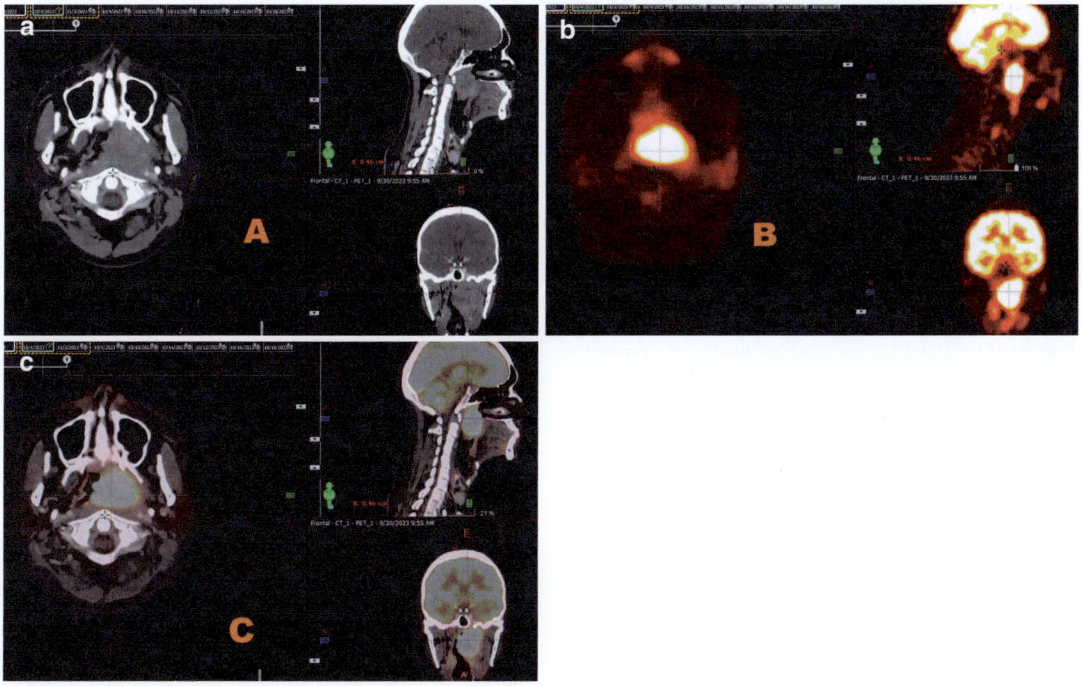

Fig. 57.5 Different imaging modalities for identifying disease area. A 19-year-old boy with Nasopharynx cancer. (**a**) Acquired CT simulation images. (**b**) Diagnostic PET images. (**c**) PET fused with CT simulated image. (Acknowledgment—BLK Max Super-specialty Hospital, Delhi

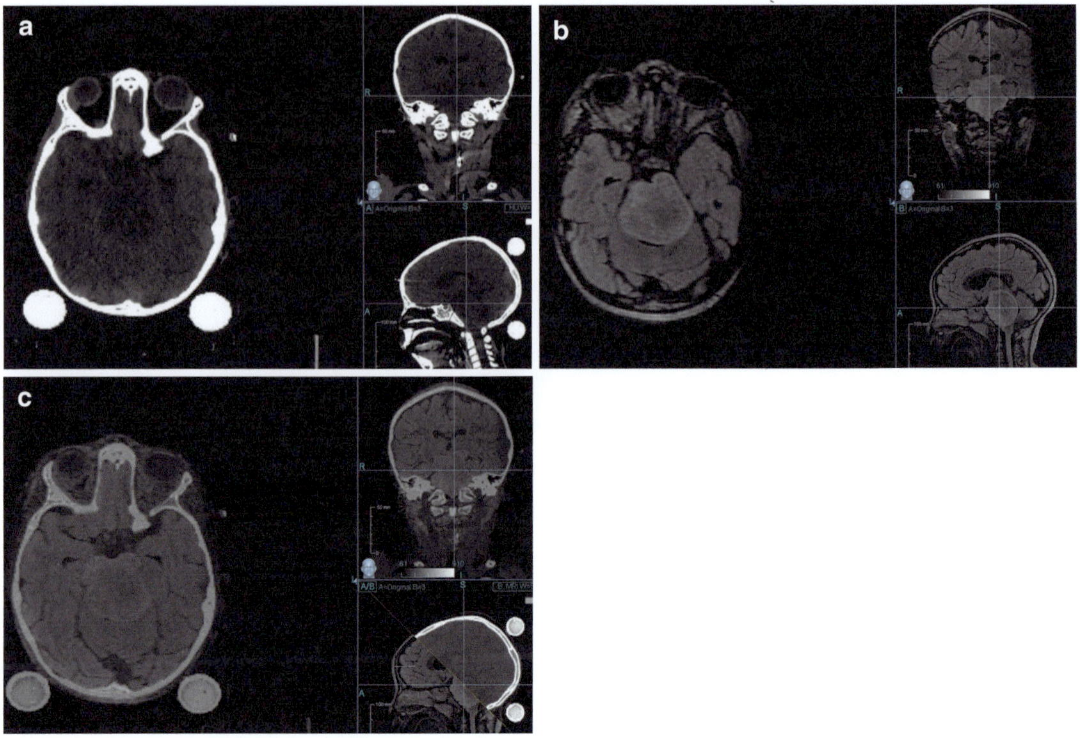

Fig. 57.6 Different imaging modalities for identifying disease area. A 7-year-old boy with brain stem glioma. (**a**) Acquired CT simulation images. (**b**) Diagnostic MRI image. (**c**) MRI fused with CT simulated image. (Acknowledgment—BLK Max Super-specialty Hospital, Delhi

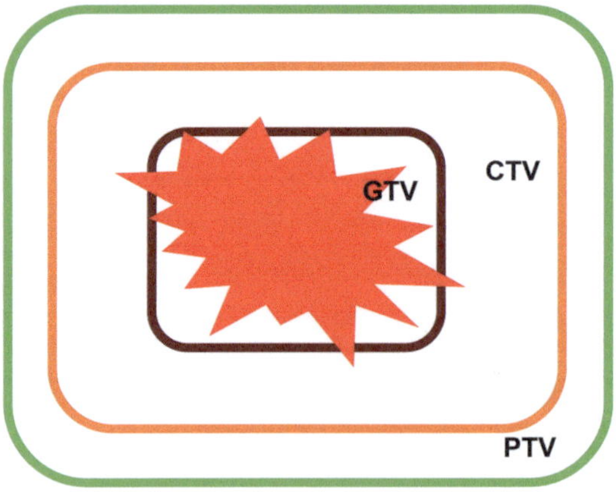

Fig. 57.7 Concept of Tumour/ Target volume. Gross target volume (GTV), Clinical target volume (CTV), Planning target volume (PTV)

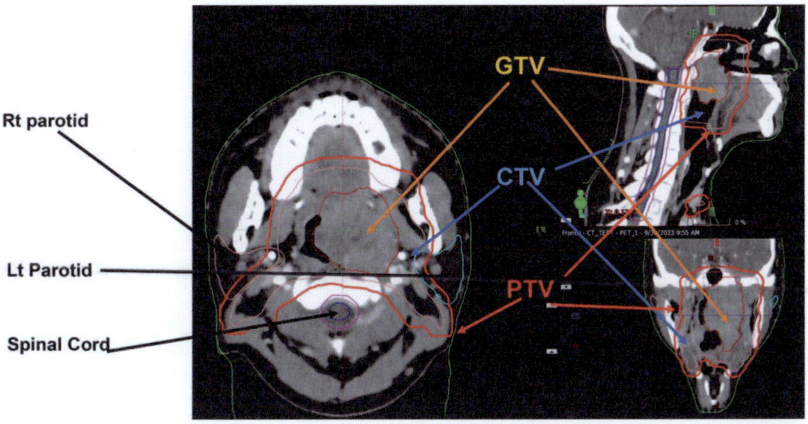

Fig. 57.8 Delineation of GTV, CTV, PTV & Critical structure on a CT scan planned for Radiation therapy

57.8 Radiation Technique

Radiation therapy has come a long way from treatment planning based on orthogonal radiographs with large margins around tumors. A quest to improve the survival rates and adverse effect profile of 2DRT led to widespread adoption and application of 3D imaging (CT scan) based methods for definitive/curative treatment

1. 3 Dimensional radiotherapy—3DCRT
2. Intensity-modulated radiotherapy—IMRT
3. Image-guided radiotherapy—IGRT
4. Stereotactic ablative RT (SBRT)

Advances in radiation planning software have also led to further three-dimensional conformal radiotherapy (3DCRT) to intensity-modulated radiotherapy (IMRT). IMRT permits the sparing of normal tissues and hence dose-escalation to tumors, exquisitely sculpted dose distributions with IMRT (Figs. 57.9 and 57.10).

Image-guided radiotherapy (IGRT) is onboard imaging before and during radiation delivery that can reduce Patient setup errors, tumor motion, and anatomical changes such as tumor regression and weight loss during radiotherapy, an essential part of modern radiation delivery (Figs. 57.11 and 57.12).

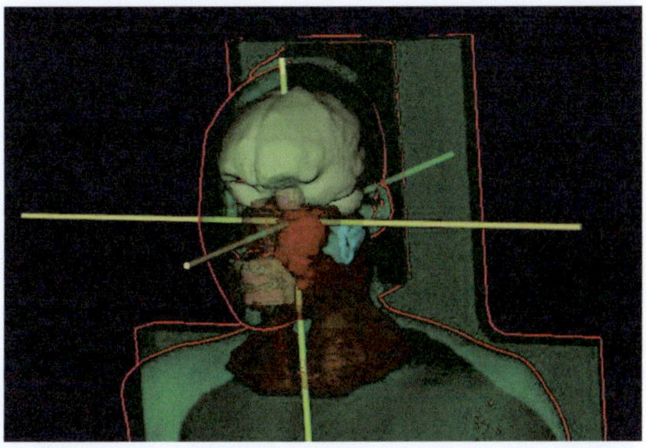

Fig. 57.9 3D Reconstruction

Registration of cone beam CT obtained in treatment position on treatment machine to plan CT scan for abdominal RT in three dimensions: (**a**) coronal, (**b**) axial, and (**c**) sagittal slices each illustrate the registration between the CT scans used on the treatment machine to ensure alignment.

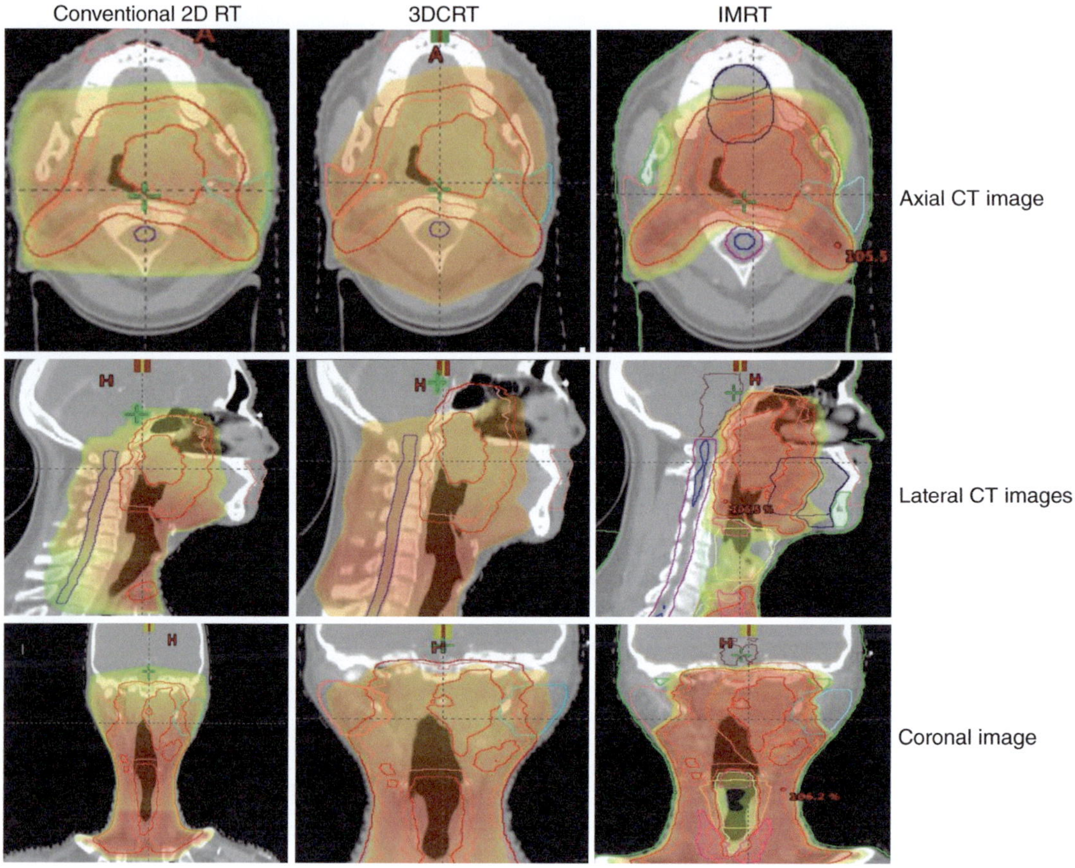

Fig. 57.10 Sculpting of dose & sparing of normal tissue with IMRT compared to 2DRT & 3DCRT. (Acknowledgment: BLK Max Super-specialty Hospital, Delhi)

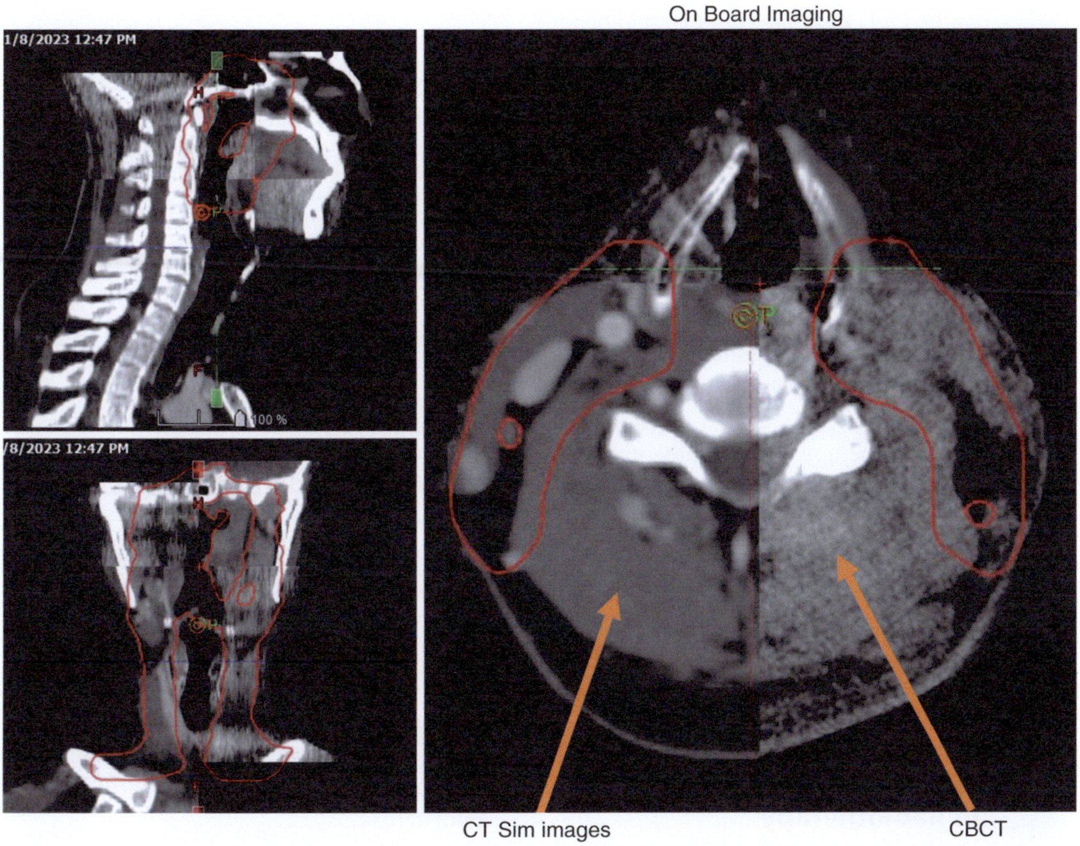

Fig. 57.11 Fusion of CT Sim with Cone beam CT (CBCT) acquired before RT -complete match with CT sim images

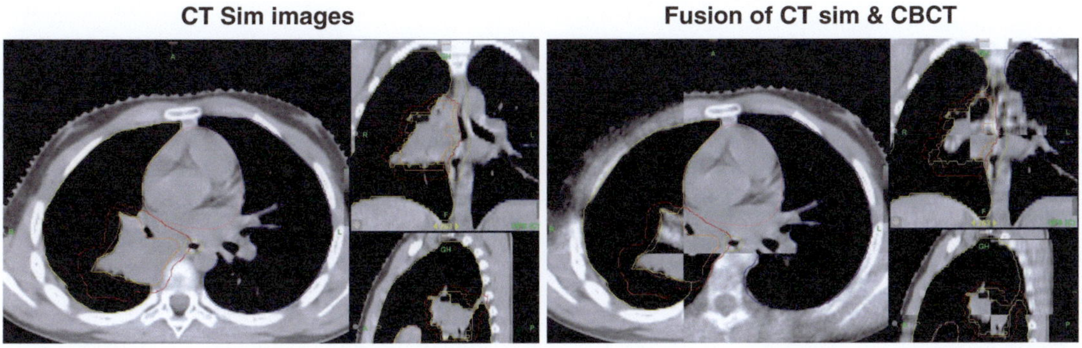

Fig. 57.12 A case of Rhabdomyosarcoma of mediastinum—Appreciable tumor regression after few fractions of RT. (Acknowledgment: BLK Max Super-specialty Hospital, Delhi)

Stereotactic body radiotherapy-external beam radiotherapy (EBRT) that accurately delivers a high irradiation dose to an extracranial or extracranial target in one or few treatment fractions.

57.9 Fractionation of Radiotherapy

Fractionation of radiotherapy is defined as radiation dose over time that is considered one of the essential factors that control the outcome of radiotherapy.

Standard radiotherapy is generally given in 1.8–2 Gray (Gy) per fraction; in specific situations like large areas of irradiation or age below 3 years, the dose is reduced to 1.5 Gy per fraction, and the dose is delivered over 5 days per week.

The total dose ranges from 10 Gy (Wilms tumor) to 60 Gy (gliomas) to improve local control and reduce toxicity.

57.10 Summary of the Current Role of Radiotherapy in the Treatment of Cancer in Children

Tumors treated by radiotherapy	Dose required for local control (Gy)
Radiotherapy alone for control of primary	
Retinoblastoma	40–45 Gy
Stage 1A Hodgkin disease	36 Gy
Intracranial Germinoma	45 Gy
Brain stem glioma	54–60 Gy
Post-operative RT adjuvant for residual/ microscopic disease	
Ewings sarcoma	45–54 Gy
Stage lll Wilms' tumor	10.8 Gy
Rhabdomyosarcoma	45–50.4 Gy
Medulloblastoma	Craniospinal RT –36 Gy + boost to the primary tumor to a total dose of 54 Gy
Glioma (astrocytoma's ependymoma)	54–60 Gy (depending on histology and grade)
Stage III neuroblastoma	21–36 Gy
Radiotherapy for sanctuary site's	
CNS prophylaxis in ALL	12–18 Gy
Total body irradiation as part bone marrow transplant to reduce incidence of graft vs host & ablation of bone marrow	2 Gy single fraction, 12–14 Gy/ 6–8 fraction in bis in die (BID) doses
Palliative	
Bone metastasis	8–30 Gy/single or fractionated RT

57.11 Acute Radiation Effects

These result from the depletion of rapidly dividing stem cells. They are generally related to dose and treatment time but have little relation to fraction size. Even when severe, they are self-limiting, and recovery occurs if the tolerance dose has not been exceeded.

Nausea/vomiting: usually controlled by antiemetics.

Erythema: Moisturizing cream can provide beneficial symptomatic relief from soreness or itching.

Mucositis: This is frequent when the head and neck area are treated. Regular use of benzydamine or soda bicarbonate and salt mouthwash is advisable. NSAID and local anesthetics are used for painful sores.

Myelosuppression: It occurs following wide-field radiotherapy to areas including significant amounts of marrow. The use of granulocyte colony-stimulating factor (GCSF) has been shown to reduce the tendency to neutropenia in patients undergoing craniospinal.

Alopecia: This will be complete following 24 Gy prophylactic cranial irradiation, but regrowth occurs. The choice of radiation technique can be an essential determinant of the extent and/or severity of alopecia.

57.12 Late Effects

The incidence of late effects is related to the total radiation dose, particularly the fraction size. In this respect, there is a dissociation between acute and late effects risk.

Bone growth: Impairment of bone growth is one of the distressing late effects. The proliferative cells' epiphysial growth plate is sensitive to radiation. Meticulous radiotherapy planning is vital to minimize the late orthopedic effects of radiation. Epiphyses should be excluded from the radiation field, if possible.

Central nervous system: Radionecrosis is rare below 60 Gy, and generally occurs with a latency of 6 months to 2 years. It results from a direct effect on glial tissue.

Neuropsychological effects: an IQ reduction of approximately 13 points is seen in children given 24 Gy prophylactic cranial irradiation (PCI) compared with siblings. Hence, the present protocol for PCI is reduced to 12 Gy and therapeutic cranial irradiation (cerebrospinal fluid (CSF) ve for leukemic cells) to 18 Gy. Following higher doses for brain tumors, an increased risk of learning and behavior difficulties is seen. An important risk factor for neuropsychological late effects is the age at diagnosis.

Lung: Late effects include radiation pneumonitis, which may lead to lung fibrosis.

Kidney: Late effects on renal function are usually seen 2–3 years following radiotherapy. Signs and symptoms ranging from hypertension to renal failure.

Endocrine: Endocrine deficiencies following radiotherapy are common. Pituitary irradiation is a matter of concern for growth hormone deficiency. Radiotherapy to the head and neck area, which includes the thyroid gland to a dose 25–40 Gy leads to hypothyroidism requiring thyroid hormone replacement therapy.

Reproductive: The germinal epithelium is susceptible to the effects of low-dose irradiation.

Testicular radiation of 2–3 Gy in adult males often results in transient oligospermia. Slow recovery is usually observed after 3–5 Gy, and beyond 5 Gy, recovery is unlikely.

In females, the oocytes are less sensitive to radiation, and 10–12 Gy radiation is required to cause infertility.

Tolerance of critical organs to radiotherapy frequently limits the dose of radiation. The critical organs and their 'tolerance doses' are given in Table 57.1 The incidence of late effects is related to the total radiation dose, particularly the fraction size. In this respect, there is a dissociation between acute and late effects risk.

Bone growth: Impairment of bone growth is one of the distressing late effects. The proliferative cells' epiphysial growth plate is sensitive to radiation. Meticulous radiotherapy planning is vital to minimize the late orthopedic effects of radiation. Epiphyses should be excluded from the radiation field, if possible.

Central nervous system: Radionecrosis is rare below 60 Gy, and generally occurs with a latency of 6 months to 2 years. It results from a direct effect on glial tissue.

Neuropsychological effects: an IQ reduction of approximately 13 points is seen in children given 24 Gy prophylactic cranial irradiation (PCI) compared with siblings. Hence, the present protocol for PCI is reduced to 12 Gy and therapeutic cranial irradiation (CSF + ve for leukemic cells) to 18 Gy. Following higher doses for brain tumors, an increased risk of learning and behavior difficulties is seen. An important risk factor for neuropsychological late effects is the age at diagnosis.

Lung: Late effects include radiation pneumonitis, which may lead to lung fibrosis.

Kidney: Late effects on renal function are usually seen 2–3 years following radiotherapy. Signs

Table 57.1 Normal tissue Tolerance Doses

Tissue	Tolerance in Gy
Whole lung	20 Gy
Kidney	<18 Gy
Mean liver dose	23 Gy
Spinal cord	10 cm–45 Gy

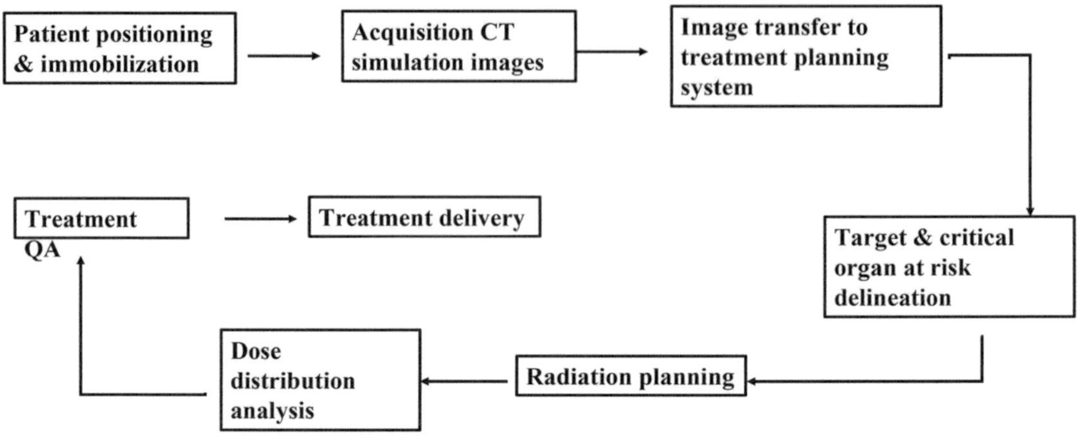

Flowchart 57.1 Workflow in an advanced radiation therapy setup

and symptoms ranging from hypertension to renal failure.

Endocrine: Endocrine deficiencies following radiotherapy are common. Pituitary irradiation is a matter of concern for growth hormone deficiency. Radiotherapy to the head and neck area, which includes the thyroid gland to a dose 25–40 Gy leads to hypothyroidism requiring thyroid hormone replacement therapy.

Reproductive: The germinal epithelium is susceptible to the effects of low-dose irradiation.

Testicular radiation of 2–3 Gy in adult males often results in transient oligospermia. Slow recovery is usually observed after 3–5 Gy, and beyond 5 Gy, recovery is unlikely.

In females, the oocytes are less sensitive to radiation, and 10–12 Gy radiation is required to cause infertility.

Tolerance of critical organs to radiotherapy frequently limits the dose of radiation. The critical organs and their 'tolerance doses' are given in Table 57.1.

A typical workflow in an advanced radiation therapy setup is given in Flowchart 57.1.

Suggested Readings

Donaldson SS. The place of radiotherapy in modern paediatric oncology. Br J Radiol. 1988;Suppl. 22:54–65.

Mandeville HC. Chapter 21: Principles of paediatric radiation oncology. In: Hoskin P, editor. Radiotherapy in practice: external beam therapy. 3rd ed. Oxford University Press; 2019.

Sánchez LM. Pediatric radiation oncology: overview and summary note. J Cancer Prev Curr Res. 2015;3(3):119–22.

Taylor RE. Cancer in children: radiotherapeutic approaches. Br Med Bull. 1996;52(4):873–86.

Taylor RE. Paediatric clinical oncology. Clin Oncol. 2013;25:1–2.

Pediatric Renal Tumors

58

Basant Kumar and Subhasis Roy Choudhury

Incidence and mortality rates of childhood cancers vary worldwide. Incidence of renal tumors ranges from 3.2% to 11.1% of all pediatric tumors worldwide and it has significant ethnic and pathological variations. The Wilms' tumor (WT; Nephroblastoma) is the most common kidney tumor, and it is the fourth most common childhood cancer overall. WT is usually occurs in children less than 5 years of age. The exact cause is unknown, but hypothesized that it occurs due to genetic alterations affecting the normal embryological development of the genitourinary system. *WT1*, *CTNNB1*, and *WTX* gene alterations have been associated with Wilms tumor and are found in about 1/3 cases of WT patients. Current overall survival of WT patients in developed countries after successful treatment is above 90%. Multimodal treatment includes surgery, chemotherapy and radiotherapy. Radiotherapy has made a significant improvement in overall survival compared to surgery alone. To prevent the drug toxicity associated with combined chemotherapy and radiotherapy is the primary research issue. The SIOP–RTSG 2016 (UMBRELLA) program seeks to further enhance overall outcome in high-risk patients by validating novel prognostic indicators, such as blastemal tumor volume and molecular markers like 1q gain. Most WT patients survive rather well, particularly those with "favorable" histology that do not have anaplasia and who are detected early and receive the right care. For the majority of patients, one working kidney is enough to lead a normal life. Vigilant approach, early detection and prompt referral to the oncologist are the key for improved outcome.

B. Kumar (✉)
Department of Pediatric Surgical Superspecialties, Sanjay Gandhi Post Graduate Institute of Medical Sciences, Lucknow, India

S. Roy Choudhury
Pediatric Surgery, Lady Hardinge Medical College and Associated Kalawati Saran Children's Hospital, New Delhi, Delhi, India

Worldwide the incidence of kidney tumors comprises 3.2–11.1% of all pediatric cancers and has significant racial and pathological variations. The highest reported incidence is in sub-Saharan Africa, while the lowest proportions occur in East Asia. The overall incidence and survival vary according to the age of diagnosis, sex, race, and geography. The most prevalent malignant juvenile kidney tumor in the world is Wilms tumor (WT; nephroblastoma); other kidney masses that can be diagnosed include renal rhabdoid tumors, renal cell carcinomas (RCC), renal sarcomas, and other uncommon cancers (Tables 58.1 and 58.2).

© The Author(s), under exclusive license to Springer Nature Singapore Pte Ltd. 2025

S. Roy Choudhury (ed.), *Pediatric Surgery*, https://doi.org/10.1007/978-981-96-1257-4_58

Table 58.1 Pathological classification of pediatric kidney tumors

Nephroblastoma (Wilms' tumor; WT) (~85%)	Histology Favorable (~90%) Unfavorable Focal anaplasia Diffuse anaplasia
Congenital mesoblastic nephroma	3–4%; mesenchymal tumor with low malignant potential
Cystic renal tumors	Cystic nephroma Cystic partially differentiated nephroblastoma (CPDN)
Clear cell sarcoma of kidney	3–4%
Malignant rhabdoid tumor of the kidney	Rare, highly malignant
Renal cell carcinoma	Rare, young adolescents
Metanephric stromal tumor	Rare, benign, purely mesenchymal neoplasia
Ossifying renal tumor of infancy	Extremely rare benign tumor
Others	Renal cell sarcoma Renal adenocarcinoma Renal angiomyolipoma Renal neurogenic tumors Renal teratoma, etc.

Table 58.2 Revised SIOP-working-classification of kidney tumors and its risk categories based upon pre-chemo and post-chemotherapy histopathology

Risk category	With preoperative chemotherapy	Without preoperative chemotherapy (primary surgery/nephrectomy)
Low-risk tumors	Mesoblastic nephroma Cystic partially differentiated nephroblastoma (CPDN) Complete necrotic nephroblastoma	*Mesoblastic nephroma* *Cystic partially differentiated nephroblastoma (CPDN)*
Intermediate-risk tumor	Nephroblastoma- Epithelial type/stromal type/mixed type/regressive type, and nephroblastoma with Focal Anaplasia	*Non-anaplastic nephroblastoma and its variants* *Nephroblastoma with focal anaplasia*
High-risk tumor	Nephroblastoma Blastemal type/Diffuse anaplasia Clear cell sarcoma of the kidney Rhabdoid tumor of the kidney	*Nephroblastoma with diffuse anaplasia* *Clear cell sarcoma of the kidney* *Rhabdoid tumor of the kidney*

58.1 Wilms' Tumor

Wilms' tumor (WT; nephroblastoma); the most common childhood renal tumor, was first described by a German physician, Dr. Max Wilms, in 1899. Overall, it is the fourth most common childhood malignancy. It originates from nephrogenic blastemal cells. Also, it is the second most common solid tumor in children after neuroblastoma, excluding tumors arising from the central nervous system. About 7% of all pediatric malignancies and the majority (about 90%) of kidney tumors are WT. Globally, the reported incidence is roughly 1 in 10,000 children under the age of 15.

58.1.1 Epidemiology

Pediatric kidney cancers occur in roughly 8 per million children under the age of 15 years. Wilms' tumor accounts for approximately 90% of pediatric kidney cancers. Wilms tumor is more common in blacks than in whites, and it is uncommon among East Asians. The average age of diagnosis is 3 years, with the majority of children diagnosed between the ages of 1 and 4 years. Bilateral WTs occur in 4–13% of patients. A positive family history is present in 1–2% of instances.

58.1.2 Etiopathogenesis

The exact cause of WT is unknown. It is believed to be brought on by changes in the genes that govern healthy genitourinary development. Wilms' tumors are caused by a sequence of events that are still poorly understood. Nephrogenic rests, which can occasionally be found in normal kidneys in intralobular or perilobular locations, are clusters of primitive metanephric cells generated from renal stem cells. Patients with unilateral Wilms' tumors (30–40%) and all patients with bilateral Wilms' tumors are more likely to experience these nephrogenic rests. Consequently, these early nephrogenic rests are thought to be a forerunner to Wilms' tumor.

Despite being taken into consideration, environmental exposures do not appear to be a major factor in the etiopathogenesis of Wilms tumors. Children with Wilms' tumor have been found to have several foci of genetic abnormalities, which may make them more susceptible to developing Wilms' tumor.

58.1.3 Molecular Genetics

Knudson and *Strong* put up a genetic model for Wilms tumor growth at the beginning of the 1970s. Wilms' tumor (WT) gene heterozygosity and a number of chromosomal locations have been mapped. The tumor suppressor gene WT-1 (11p13) is mutated in children with Denys–Drash syndrome and deleted in those with WAGR. A specific loss of maternal allele is linked to the familial form of Beckwith-Wiedemann syndrome (BWS) and loss of heterozygosity (LOH) of the WT-2 gene (11p15). According to the National Wilms tumor study (NWTS-5), LOH at the 16q and 1p loci is linked to a worse prognosis and a higher risk of relapse. Seventy-five percent of patients with anaplastic histology have been discovered to have the p53 tumor suppressor gene.

58.1.4 Associated Anomalies and Syndromes

WAGR syndrome (Wilms' tumor, aniridia, genitor-urinary anomalies, mental retardation), Beckwith–Wiedemann syndrome (macroglossia, hemihypertrophy, visceromegaly, hypoglycemia, and abdominal wall defects), and Denys-Drash syndrome (male pseudohermaphroditism, Wilms' tumor, and progressive renal disease) are all linked to Wilms' tumors. Septal deficiency, microcephalus, von-Willebrand's disease, hyperinsulinism, Frasier syndrome, and other related anomalies are also associated with WTs.

58.1.5 Clinical Presentation

About 80% of Wilms tumors show as a smooth, non-tender, asymptomatic abdomen or flank mass (Fig. 58.1a). The traditional trio of flank bulk, hematuria, and loin discomfort may be present in late instances (25%). Varicocele and urinary tract infections are less frequent, but 5–30% of individuals have fever, hypertension, and extensive hematuria. Less frequently, intratumor bleeding causes fever, anemia, and hypotension. It is uncommon for advanced illnesses to present with respiratory symptoms associated with lung metastases. Weight loss, malaise, dysuria, abdominal crisis due to intraperitoneal tumor rupture, tumor thrombus involving IVC with dilated abdominal veins, and heart thrombus are possible side effects.

Syndromic associations were observed in up to 10% of children with WT, and approximately 5–7% of patients with WT may have bilateral disease. Familial occurrence has been recognized. The role of heredity is under study.

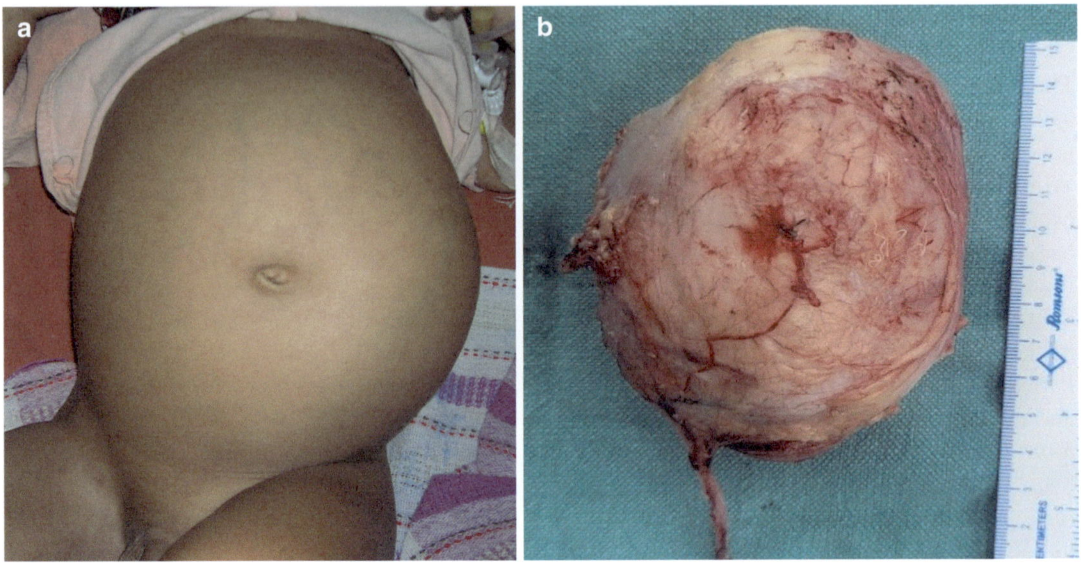

Fig. 58.1 (**a**) Left flank mass (Wilms' tumor) (**b**) Gross appearance of nephroureterectomy specimen (WT)

58.1.6 Examination

A palpable, painless abdominal tumor was frequently observed during physical examination. Aniridia, genitourinary abnormalities, and indications of overgrowth are characteristics of related diseases such as WAGR syndrome and Beckwith–Wiedemann syndrome (BWS) that require attention.

58.1.7 Differential Diagnosis

The primary differential is neuroblastoma (Table 58.3). Congenital mesoblastic nephroma, cystic nephroma, CPDN, cystic Wilms' tumor, teratoid WT, renal cell carcinoma, kidney clear cell sarcoma, kidney rhabdoid tumor, nonmalignant mass, hydronephrosis, multicystic kidney disease, renal cyst, kidney dysplasia, etc., are examples of additional differential diagnoses.

Table 58.3 Differences in the presentation of Wilms' tumor and neuroblastoma

	Neuroblastoma	Wilms' tumor
Age of presentation	Younger age (<2 years of age)	Older age: Peak 3–5 years of age
Calcification	Common: 90%	Uncommon: 10–15%
Encasement and invasion	Encases vascular structures but does not invade them Elevates the aorta from the vertebral column	Displaces adjacent structures without invading IVC/renal vein/atrium tumor thrombus
Nature of mass	Poorly marginated and surface nodular	Well circumscribed
Midline crossing	Common	Uncommon, except for very large tumors
Displacement of kidney	Displaced and common	Kidney parenchyma involved (claw sign)

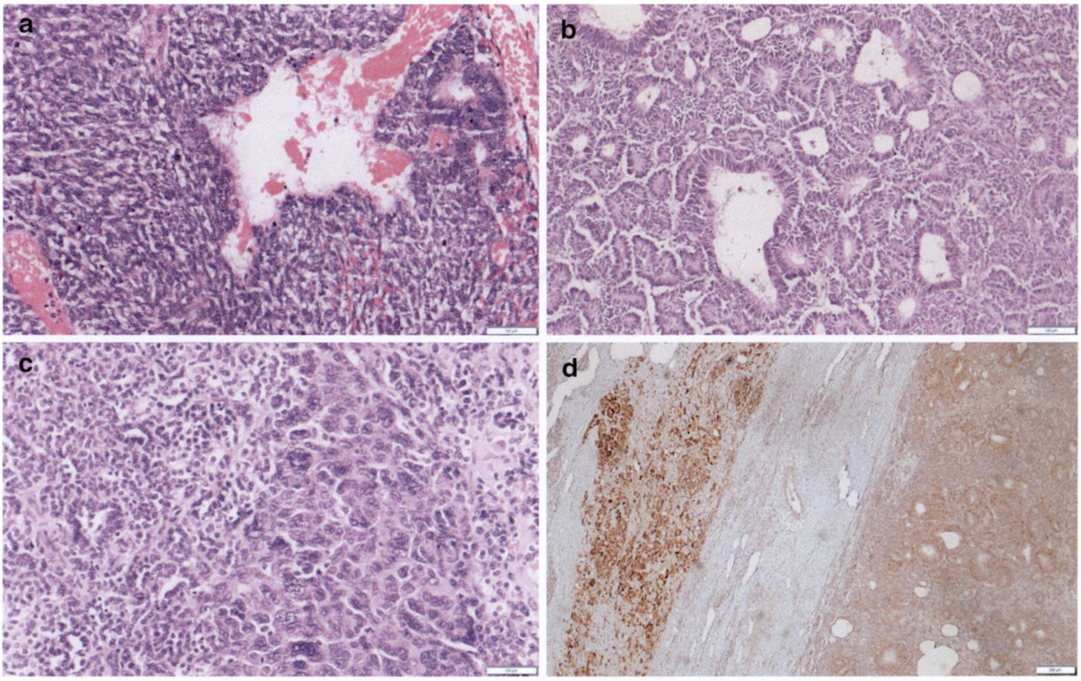

Fig. 58.2 (**a**) Blastemal predominant nephroblastoma. The blastemal component comprises small blue round cells showing brisk mitotic activity, and the epithelial component is noted in the upper right corner (H&E 10X). (**b**) Epithelial predominant nephroblastoma composed of the epithelial component only ("monophasic") (H&E, 10X). (**c**) Nephroblastoma showing focal anaplasia (H&E, 10X) (**d**) Anaplastic focus showing p53 positivity (IHC 4X). (Courtesy Dr. Lavleen Singh, AIIMS, New Delhi)

58.1.8 Pathology

Grossly, the WT appears grayish white, with a fleshy cut surface that has bleeding, necrosis, and cystic areas (Fig. 58.1b). Perhaps the only characteristic that separates WT from hyperplastic nephrogenic rests is the fibrous pseudocapsule.

Abnormal glomeruli and heterogeneous tissue, including bone, cartilage, muscle, and adipose tissue, are visible under *a microscope* (Fig. 58.2a–d). Three components (triphasic) are characteristic of Wilms' tumor histopathology: (a) blastemal elements, which are characterized by spherical, blue cells; (b) stromal elements; and (c) epithelial elements, which include abnormal glomeruli and tubules. A favorable WT may be: monophasic or triphasic while. Anaplastic (diffuse or focal) denotes unfavorable pathology.

- *Rhabdoid tumor of kidney (a tumor that spreads to the brain) and clear cell sarcoma of kidney (a tumor that spreads to the bone) are now categorized as distinct diseases and are no longer regarded as Wilms' tumor.*

58.1.8.1 Spread and Metastasis

- Locally—adjacent organs, renal sinuses, ureter, renal vein, IVC (4%–10%), right atrium.
- Lymphatics—locoregional lymph nodes (15–20%).
- Hematogenous—lung (80%), liver (15%), bone, brain, etc.

58.1.9 Prognostic Factors

Numerous factors, including histology, stage, age at diagnosis, response to chemotherapy, and—above all—molecular/genetic indicators, influence the prognosis of Wilms tumor.

58.1.10 Investigations and Approach in Wilms' Tumor

- Physical examinations for nutritional status, side and size of tumor, liver span, BP measurement, suspected lymph nodal or other masses, and examination for other congenital anomalies or syndromic features, if any
- Complete hemogram and biochemistry: LFT, KFT, and coagulation profile
- Urinalysis
- Abdominal ultrasonography with Doppler
- Chest X-ray
- CECT of abdomen and chest (Figs. 58.3a–c and 58.4)
- +/− MRI/cytogenetic studies

58.1.11 Features to Search for in Imaging

- Size/site of mass and its nature
- Laterality/extension- function of the other kidney
- Involvement +/− of tumor in one/both kidneys
- +/− of IVC/renal vein/cardiac thrombus

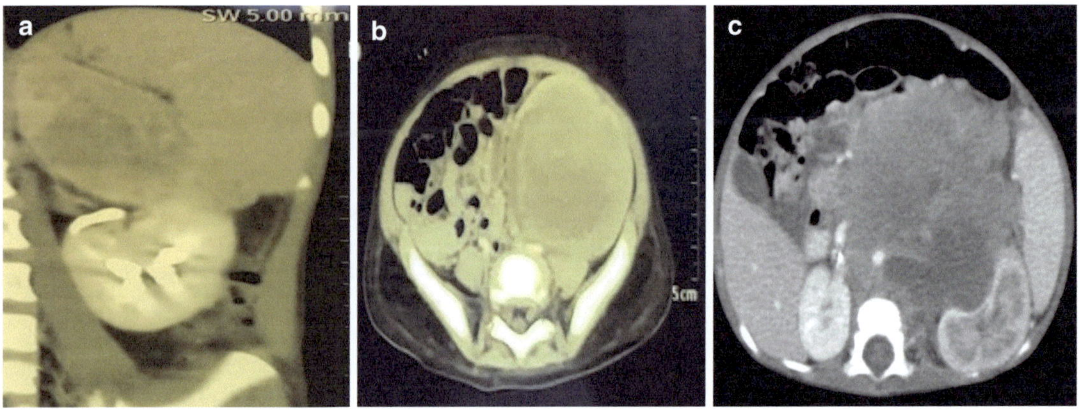

Fig. 58.3 (**a** and **b**) CT scan showing left Wilms' tumor. (**c**) CT scan showing neuroblastoma for comparison (see Chap. 59)

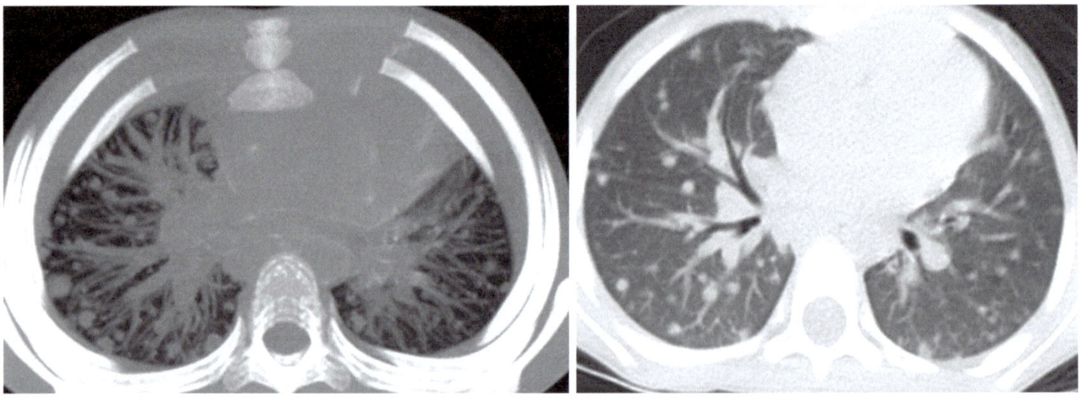

Fig. 58.4 CT showing pulmonary metastasis

- Metastasis
- LN status and relation of mass with major vessels and adjacent vital organs

58.1.12 Diagnosis: *Clinical/Radiological/Histological*

According to the *COG protocol*; before starting neoadjuvant chemotherapy, histological confirmation is necessary for all patients, while in the *SIOP protocol*, the diagnosis is entirely based on radiology.

Biopsy

- FNAC, open or Tru-cut biopsy.
- Open/Tru-cut biopsy will upstage the tumor stage (COG-NWTS) while a FNAC does not upstage.

58.1.13 Staging of WT

According to *Children's Oncology Group (COG-NWTS)*

- *Stage I*: The tumor is confined within the kidney tissue and is fully excised without spilling. No prior effort at biopsy was made. There is no breach in the renal capsule.
- *Stage II*: The tumor is fully excised with distinct margins, but it has breached the renal capsule or renal sinus. Before resection, a biopsy is performed.
- *Stage III*: Gross or microscopic residual tumor in abdomen. No haematogenous spread. Abdominal lymph nodes involvement. Tumor rupture, transacted tumor thrombus, and positive resection margins. Inoperable tumors.
- *Stage IV*: Haematogenous metastases to lung, liver, bone, brain, or lymph node metastases outside the abdomen.
- *Stage-V*: Bilateral WT.

58.1.14 Management

Multimodal therapy is the gold standard of care, utilizing radiotherapy, surgery, and chemotherapy.

- Children with unilateral Wilms tumors should have *surgery first* for staging and treatment, according to the *Children Oncology Group (COG-NWTS)*. Treatment is then risk-based on tumor stage histology and risk group.
- *International Society of Pediatric Oncology (SIOP)* advises *preoperative chemotherapy* in the first place for all children without a preoperative histological or cytological diagnosis.
- *When a child presents with a big or incurable tumor, the Modified COG approach is used. FNAC/Tru-cut/open biopsy is used to obtain a cytological or histological diagnosis in these children, and chemotherapy is administered prior to surgery. The standard COG regimen is used to manage patients with smaller tumors.*

58.1.15 Surgical Treatment

- Surgery objectives for Wilms tumor (Fig. 58.5)
- For unilateral Wilms' tumor, the entire tumor must be removed *"en-bloc"* as part of a nephrouretecomy; for bilateral tumors or

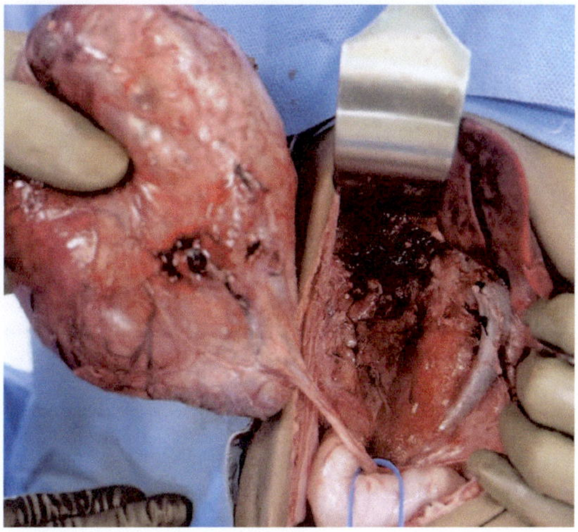

Fig. 58.5 Intraoperative picture of left nephrectomy

tumors in a single kidney, a partial nephrectomy or wedge resection of the tumor with distinct margins is necessary.

- Tumor rupture and spilling must be prevented.
- Sufficient LN sampling (minimum six).
- Tumor staging.
- Renal tumor bed clip-marking.

The Following Are the Key Steps in the Procedure

- Sufficient supra-umbilical transverse incision and accurate tumor extent evaluation. Contralateral kidney examination is not advised if CECT reveals a normal contralateral kidney.
- Over the Gerotas fascia, it medially mobilizes the colon, preventing damage to the renal capsule. Before moving the kidney, vascular management of the renal arteries is advised to stop the tumor's vascular spread. To prevent spills, tumors should be handled carefully.
- It is important to thoroughly inspect the ureter, renal vein, and IVC for any signs of tumor extension or thrombosis. It is necessary to split and ligate the ureter as low as feasible. It is best to remove the tumor *"en-bloc,"* meaning that it should not be cut.
- If not implicated, removal of the adrenal glands can be avoided; however, in cases with upper polar lesions, adrenal gland removal may be necessary.
- It is necessary to sample lymph nodes and remove any palpable or visible lymph nodes from the iliac, para-aortic, and celiac regions.
- Finally, clips are used to indicate the tumor bed in order to facilitate future treatment.

58.1.16 Tumor Thrombus in Inferior Vena Caval/Right Atrial Thrombus (Fig. 58.6a–c)

For the surgical excision of tumor thrombus involving the supra-hepatic vena cava and atrium, cardiopulmonary bypass is necessary. Preoperative chemotherapy can be used to control extension into the right atrium or above the level of the hepatic veins. It makes it easier for the intravascular thrombus to decrease in its extent, which eliminates the need for cardiopulmonary bypass surgery to remove the tumor thrombus. Cardiopulmonary bypass is not necessary for tumor removal with thrombus if the tumor can be localized and controlled below the atrium.

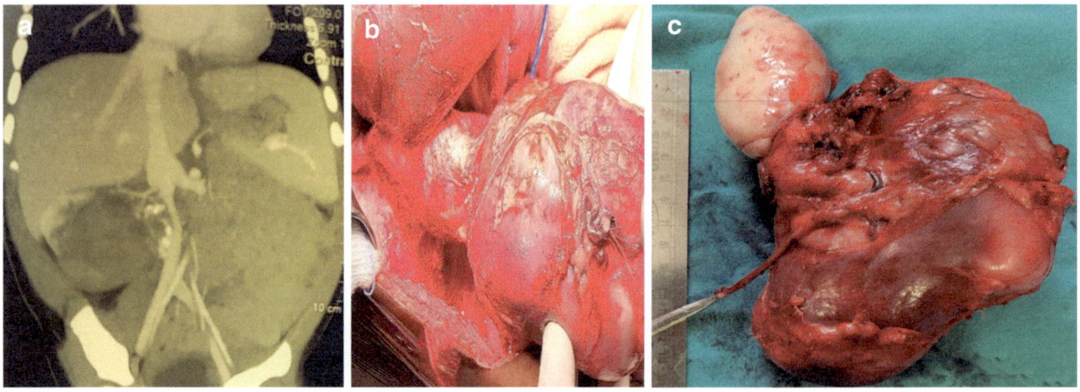

Fig. 58.6 (**a**) CT showing IVC thrombus (**b** and **c**) Intraop and excised IVC thrombus with tumor

58.1.17 Bilateral Wilms' Tumor (Fig. 58.7a, b)

Compared to children with unilateral lesions, children with bilateral tumors are typically younger. The average age of presentation is 25 months. For these kids, maintaining sufficient renal parenchyma is crucial to preventing post-operative renal failure. If imaging indicates a Wilms' tumor, the COG does not advise biopsy for bilateral tumors. To improve the likelihood of renal salvage, these patients are placed on neoadjuvant chemotherapy for 6 weeks before being reviewed. Partial nephrectomy may be performed on individuals with polar tumors that involve one-third or less of the renal parenchyma. For tiny hilar tumors, a tumorectomy or wedge resection with a margin can be carried out.

- *Nephron sparing surgery* (Fig. 58.8): Patients with bilateral Wilms' tumor and those with unilateral WT who are at high risk of renal failure, such as those with Denis Drash syndrome and WAGR association, should have nephron sparing surgery. There should be a clear tumor-free margin available with complete tumor removal confirmed by *frozen-section* histology. In patients with a unilateral tumor, those with solitary kidney, tumor in a horseshoe kidney, or very small tumor as defined by imaging are ideal candidates for partial nephrectomy or nephron sparing surgery. Complete nephrectomy is the recommended course of treatment for patients with high-risk histology, such as anaplasia or prominent blastemal components.

58.1.18 Rhabdoid Tumors of Kidney (RTK)

Of all pediatric kidney tumors, RTK is the rarest, fastest-growing type and has proven to be the most difficult to cure. They occur at a younger age

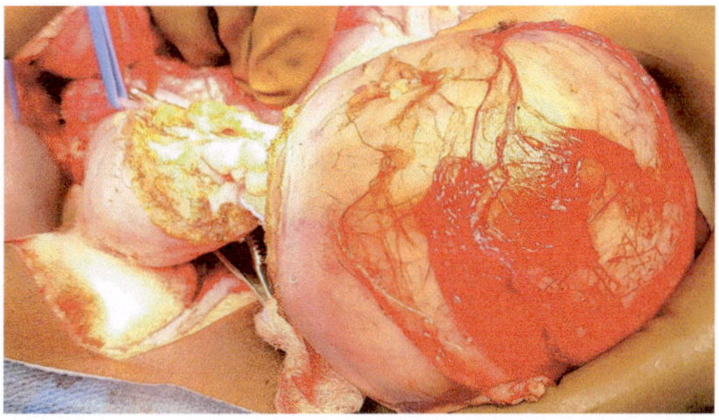

Fig. 58.8 Intraoperative picture of Nephron sparing surgery

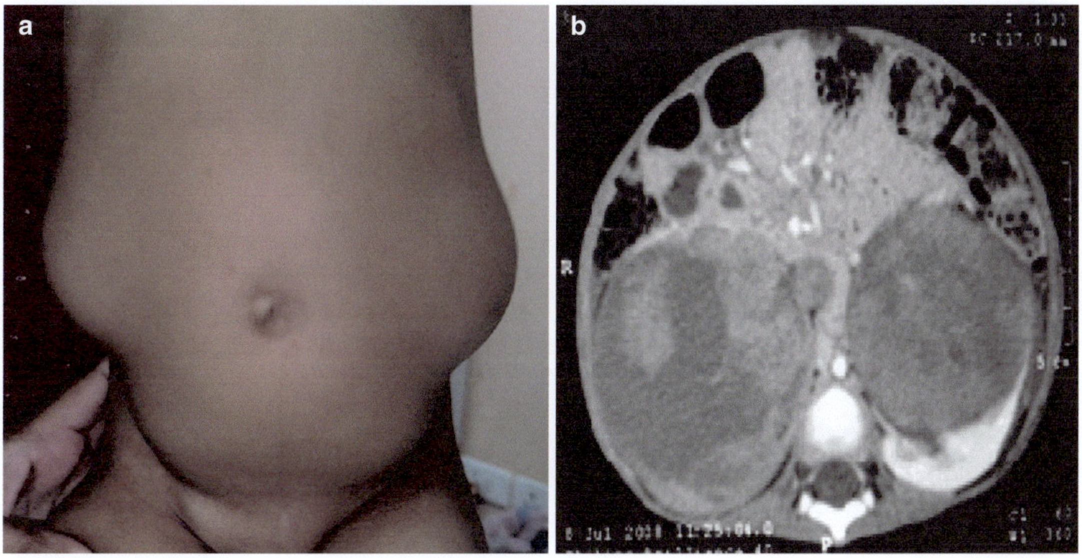

Fig. 58.7 (**a**) Bilateral flank mass [WT] (**b**) CT picture showing bilateral WT

(infancy or early childhood), and 85% of cases present within 2 years of life. RTKs are usually bulky masses centered in the renal hilum with a grossly indistinct tumor border reflecting aggressive invasion. It has prominent acidophilic cytoplasm resembling rhabdomyoblasts. A genetic mutation in the *SMARCB1* gene, which controls cell growth, is the cause of it in most of the cases. The tumor is widely metastatic at presentation and has a very aggressive nature, known for its potential to metastasize in the brain. Metastasis occurs most frequently in the lung (70%). NWTS-5 employed cyclophosphamide, carboplatin, and etoposide as part of an aggressive treatment. Sadly, there was no increase in survival.

58.1.19 Clear Cell Sarcoma of Kidney (CCSK)

CCSK is a rare (3–5% of all pediatric renal tumors), aggressive renal tumor that can spread to other organs. It is another malignant variant of pediatric renal tumor, histologically characterized by predominantly clear cytoplasm of the malignant cells. A notably high rate of recurrence and death is linked to CCSK, which primarily metastasizes in the bone (bone-metastasizing tumor of infancy) and occasionally in the brain. The chemotherapy regimen, which includes vincristine, doxorubicin, etoposide, and cyclophosphamide, is comparable to that for Wilms' tumor. The survival of this high-risk group of tumors depends on the stage and is similar to Wilms' tumor. Both CCSK and RTK can be renal and extra-renal in origin.

Neoadjuvant Chemotherapy: Preoperative chemotherapy for Wilms' tumor is generally recommended in certain clinical situations like

(a) Solitary functioning kidney.
(b) Unresectable/locally advanced tumors.
(c) Bilateral kidney tumors.
(d) Tumor in a horseshoe kidney.
(e) Intravascular/intracardiac extension of the tumor.
(f) Metastatic tumor.
- Prior to receiving neoadjuvant chemotherapy, histopathology is necessary. A follow-up CT scan is often performed 6 weeks following treatment to review operability. If necessary, a re-evaluation for resectability in bilateral Wilms is typically conducted 6 or 12 weeks following chemotherapy.

COG-NWTS Protocol for the Treatment of Wilms' Tumor

Treatment of favorable tumors				
Risk group	Criteria	Surgery	Chemotherapy	Radiotherapy
Very low risk	<2 years of age, <550 g, Stage I, No loss of heterozygosity (LOH)	Surgery only	No	No
Low risk:	Stage I/II, No LOH at 1p or 16q	Yes	Yes EE 4A regimen	No
Standard risk	Stage I/II with LOH or Stage III/IV without LOH at 1p or 16q	Yes	Yes DD4A regimen	Yes
High risk	**Stage III and IV with loss of heterozygosity at 1p or 16q**			
(a) Stage III	–	Yes	Chemotherapy DD4A After 6 weeks—M regimen	Yes
(b) Stage IV	CR to the metastatic lesion by 6 weeks	+/–	DD4A regimen	No chest RT (abdominal as per local stage)
(c) Stage IV.	IR Of metastatic lesion by 6	+/–	DD4A regimen for 6 weeks followed by regimen M	Chest RT and abdominal as per local stage

Treatment of Unfavorable Tumor/Anaplastic Tumors

Stage I	Focal	DD4A	***Flank irradiation to all patients**
	Diffuse	DD4A	
Stage II	Focal	DD4A	
	Diffuse	UH-1	
Stage III	Focal	DD4A	
	Diffuse	UH-1	
Stage IV	Focal or diffuse	UH-1 UH-2 (poor responders)	***Lung irradiation with flank/abdomen**

Regimens

- *EE4A*: Vincristine and dactinomycin X 18 weeks
- *DD4A*: Vincristine, daactinomycin, and adriamycin X 24 weeks
- *M*: Vincristine, dactinomycin, driamycin cyclophosphamide, and etoposide X 24 weeks
- *UH-1*: Vincristine, adriamycin, cyclophosphamide, carboplatin, and etoposide X 24 week
- *UH-2*: UH-1 with additional vincristine and irinotecan

SIOP Protocol for Treatment of Wilms' Tumor

Preoperative management		
Clinical staging	Chemotherapy	
Localized tumor	DAM/VCR × 4 weeks	**Surgical staging**
Metastatic tumor	DAM/VCR/EPI × 6 weeks	**Histological diagnosis**

DAM dactinomycin/actinomycin-D, *VCR* vincristine, *EPI* epirubicin/etoposide

Post-surgery management	
Clinical staging	Management
Localized Stage I, low-grade tumor	None
Stage I, intermediate grade tumor + anaplasia	DAM/VCR/EPI × 6 weeks
Stage II—(LN negative)	DAM/VCR × 18 weeks
Stage II + and III	DAM/VCR/EPI × 28 weeks + Tumor bed irradiation
High-grade tumor	EPI/IF/VP16/CARBO × 34 weeks + irradiation
Metastatic Stage IV	As per the local stage of tumor + metastases Mx—RT and/or excision of mets

DAM dactinomycin, *VCR* vincristine, *EPI* epirubicin, *IF* ifosfamide, *VP-16* etoposide, *CARBO* carboplatin, *RT* radiotherapy

58.1.20 Prognosis and Outcome

Stage, tumor histology, and LOH at 1p and 16q all affect the prognosis. Age and tumor weight are also significant factors in Stage I favorable histology. Since LOH-positive individuals are known to be a poor prognostic factor, the COG has begun treating these patients with more aggressive chemotherapy. In Stages I and II, the current 5-year survival rate is greater than 90%, but in Stages III and IV, it is roughly 73%.

58.1.21 UMBRELLA Protocol (Fig. 58.9)

Based on the findings of earlier national and international trials and studies, the International Society of Paediatric Oncology's (SIOP–RTSG) Renal Tumor Study Group has created a new study protocol for pediatric renal tumors called the UMBRELLA SIOP-RTSG 2016 protocol (the UMBRELLA protocol). In order to further enhance outcomes for high-risk patients, the UMBRELLA protocol seeks to evaluate novel prognostic indicators, such as blastemal tumor volume and molecular markers like 1q gain. The SIOP-RTSG pathology panel has reached a consensus to establish the updated SIOP-RTSG pathology and molecular biology procedure for Wilms tumors in order to facilitate widespread adoption of the UMBRELLA methodology. Although Wilms tumor patients currently have great overall outcomes, there are still subgroups with poor prognoses and higher relapse rates. Finding these subgroups is crucial for better treatment stratification, which may lessen the immediate and long-term consequences of chemotherapy.

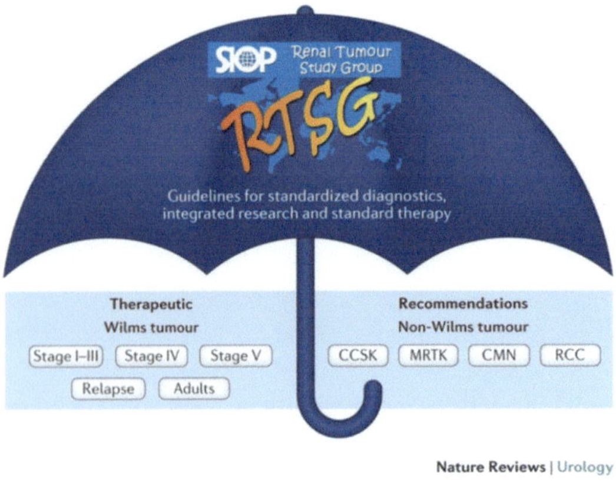

Fig. 58.9 Pictorial dipiction of umbrella protocol

58.1.22 Renal Cell Carcinoma (RCC)

RCC rarely manifests in childhood, in contrast to Wilms tumor. It typically manifests as hematuria and abdominal bulk in the second decade of life. Weight loss, fever, anemia, malaise, flank discomfort, and urine retention are some of the symptoms. RCC makes up about 6% of pediatric and adolescent malignant kidney tumors. The translocation morphology type is the most prevalent among a number of histologic subtypes. About 40% of pediatric RCCs are translocation-type, or clear cell neoplasms, which are identified by chromosomal translocations involving the Xp11.2 TFE3 gene. Papillary tumor, renal medullary carcinoma, chromophobe RCC, and RCC "not otherwise specified" are further forms of RCC that have been seen in children. Since they are not susceptible to chemotherapy or radiation, the mainstay of treatment consists of complete tumor excision and lymph node dissection. The stage of the tumor is the most important prognostic factor.

58.1.23 Renal Angiomyolipoma

Renal angiomyolipoma is a benign hamartomatous lesion typically associated with tuberous sclerosis and made up of varying amounts of blood vessels, smooth muscle cells, and fat. They can be bilateral with characteristic CT scan findings suggestive of fatty elements. Larger than 4 cm size of lesions are associated with a higher incidence of bleeding. Symptoms include flank pain, blood in urine, anemia, fever, kidney pain, palpable mass, and hypertension. Flank pain or acute abdomen due to bleeding is the most common presentation and indication of surgery. Angio-embolization can be effective in the management of bleeding from such tumors; otherwise, partial nephrectomy/nephron sparing surgery is recommended. Mechanistic targets of rapamycin (mTOR) inhibitors have been found to be promising in reducing the size of this tumor.

58.1.24 Cystic Renal Tumors

Cystic nephroma (CN), also known as multilocular cystic nephroma (MCN) (Fig. 58.10a, b), cystic Wilms' tumor (CWT), and cystic partially differentiated nephroblastoma (CPDN) are kidney cystic tumors that are radiologically identical. They are a spectrum of tumors, with CPDN in the intermediate zone, CN at the benign end, and CWT at the malignant end. The lining of the cysts and septa distinguishes them histologically. While CWT has more solid tissue in between the cysts with typical Wilms' tumor blastemal, stromal, and epithelial components, CPDN is represented by poorly differentiated tissue or blastemal cells observed in the septa. The cornerstone of treatment for CN and stage 1 CPDN is complete surgical excision, which is curative. CWT and higher stage CPDN requires additional chemotherapy.

58.1.25 Congenital Mesoblastic Nephroma (CMN)

A rare benign kidney tumor, CMN, is typically discovered in the first year of life. In neonates and infants (those under 6 months old), it is the most prevalent kidney tumor. It frequently shows up as an abdominal mass in newborns and babies and is discovered during prenatal ultrasounds. It differs from Wilms' tumor and has unique histological features. The classic type (24%), cellular type (66%), and mixed type (10%) are the three histologic subtypes that are described. Uniform spindle-shaped cells grouped in bundles with sporadic foci of entrapped normal glomeruli and tubules are the hallmarks of the classic variation. The cellular variety tends to penetrate, recur locally, and manifests late. Chemotherapy and radiation are ineffective, and total surgical excision is curative. Excellent results are obtained without adjuvant therapy with an OS rate of approximately 95%.

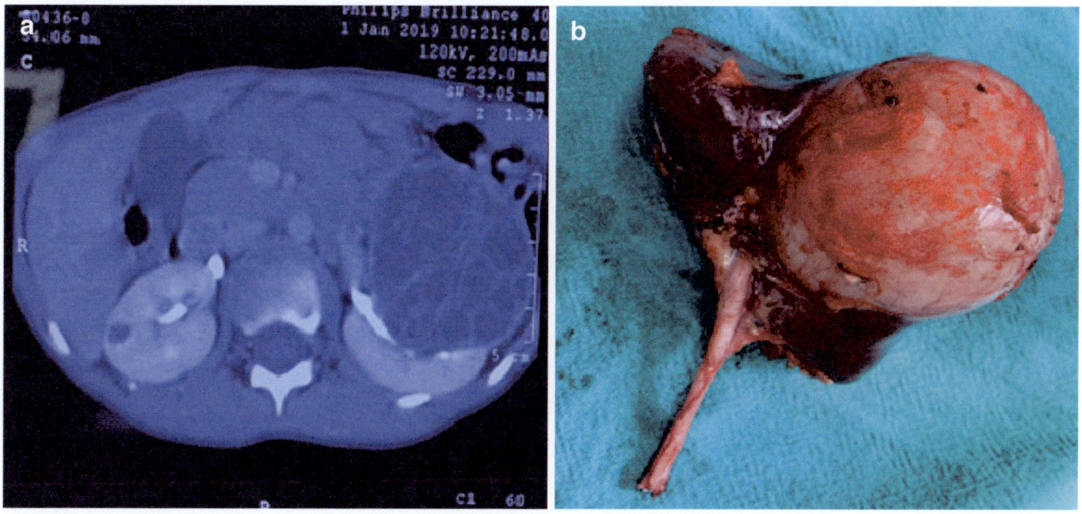

Fig. 58.10 Multilocular cystic nephroma (MCN) (**a**) CT picture, (**b**) Nephrectomy specimen

58.1.26 Summary

Wilms' tumor (Nephroblastoma) is the 2nd most common solid tumor in children after Neuroblastoma. It has significant racial and pathological variations. The overall incidence and survival vary according to the age of diagnosis, sex, race, and geography. Other kidney masses include congenital mesoblastic nephroma common in infants, renal rhabdoid tumors, renal cell carcinomas (RCC), renal sarcomas, and other uncommon cancers. Current multimodal treatment including surgery, chemotherapy and radiotherapy results overall survival above 90% in developed countries. The SIOP–RTSG 2016 (UMBRELLA) program seeks to further enhance overall outcome in high-risk patients by validating novel prognostic indicators. Vigilant approach, early detection and prompt referral to the oncologist are the key for improved outcome.

Suggested Reading

Carachi R, Grosfeld JL, Azmy AF. The surgery of childhood Tumours. 2nd ed. Heidelberg: Springer-Verlag; 2008.

Coran AG, Caldamone A, Scott Adzich N, Krummel TM, Laberge JM, editors. Pediatric surgery. 7th ed. Oxford: Elsevier Limited; 2012.

De Kraker J, Graf N, Pritchard-Jones K, Pein F. Nephroblastoma clinical trial and study SIOP 2001, protocol. SIOP RTSG; 2001.

Gupta DK, Carachi R. Pediatric oncology- surgical and medical aspects. 1st ed. JAYPEE BROTHERS Medical Publishers (P) Ltd.; 2007.

Poplak DG, Pizzo PA. Principles and practice of pediatric oncology. Wolters Kluwer; 2016.

Sarin YK. Wilms' tumor. Springer; 2022. https://doi.org/10.1007/978-981-19-3428-5.

Vujanić GM, Gessler M, et al. The UMBRELLA SIOP–RTSG 2016 Wilms tumour pathology and molecular biology protocol. Nat Rev Urol. 2018;(15):693–701.

Neuroblastoma

59

Nitin J. Peters, Saswati Behera, and Subhasis Roy Choudhury

59.1 Introduction

Neuroblastoma is the most common extracranial solid tumor in children, worldwide accounting for about 8–10% of cancers. The overall incidence is 1 per 10,000 children. The incidence is highest in the first year of life. Neuroblastomas arise from primordial neural crest cells and occur in the adrenal medulla or anywhere along the sympathetic ganglia, most notably in the retroperitoneum and posterior mediastinum.

59.2 Pathology

The exact etiology behind such tumors is still unknown, however, studies suggest a role of genetic factors and gene-environment interactions in the perinatal period. Neuroblastoma can also occur as part of genetic syndromes like Hirschsprung disease and Neurofibromatosis, etc.

Neuroblastomas are made up of immature neuroblasts; they are small, uniform cells with dense, hyperchromatic nuclei and scant cytoplasm. Differentiated cells have a more mature ganglion cell appearance with well-defined nucleoli and eosinophilic cytoplasm. Characteristic features of neuroblastoma include the presence of neuropil and arrangement in rosettes. Immunohistochemistry with specific markers (Neuron-specific enolase, chromogranin) can help in the diagnosis of doubtful cases (Fig. 59.1). The Shimada classification, modified later as the International Neuroblastoma Pathology Classification, is based on the biological behavior and prognosis of tumors.

Neuroblastoma typically represents a poorly differentiated tumor, whereas *ganglioneuroma* is its well-differentiated, benign counterpart. *Ganglioneuroblastoma* represents both, having features of immature, poorly differentiated neuroblasts and mature ganglion cells. Based on the type of tumor, degree of differentiation, age, and percentage of mitotic/ karyorrhectic cells, the tumor is classified as *favorable or unfavorable histology.*

N. J. Peters (✉)
Department of Pediatric Surgery, Post Graduate Institute of Medical Education and Research, Chandigarh, India

S. Behera
Department of Pediatric Surgery, All India Institute of Medical Sciences, Bhatinda, Punjab, India

S. Roy Choudhury
Pediatric Surgery, Lady Hardinge Medical College and Associated Kalawati Saran Children's Hospital, New Delhi, Delhi, India

© The Author(s), under exclusive license to Springer Nature Singapore Pte Ltd. 2025

S. Roy Choudhury (ed.), *Pediatric Surgery*, https://doi.org/10.1007/978-981-96-1257-4_59

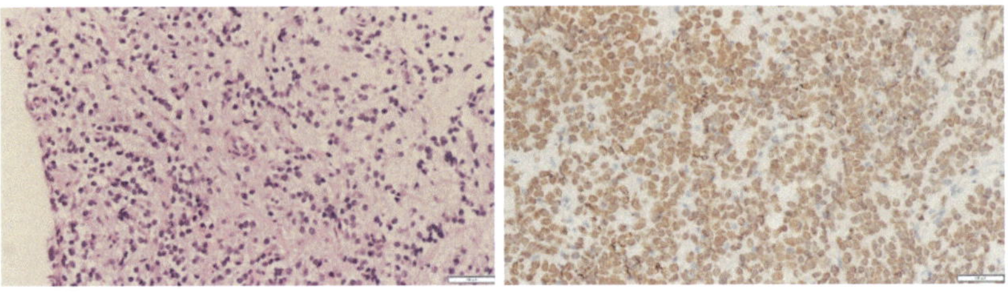

Fig. 59.1 Poorly differentiated neuroblastoma: The tumor shows neuroblasts embedded in neuropil. [H&E 10x]. The tumor cells are immuno-positive for PHOX2B[IHC 10x] (Courtesy Dr. Lavleen Singh, AIIMS, New Delhi)

Table 59.1 Current prognostic factors for neuroblastoma

	Favorable	Poor
Clinical		
Age	<18 months	>18 months
Site	Non adrenal Thoracic, pelvic	Adrenal
Stage	L1, MS	L2,M
Histological	Differentiation, Low mitosis-Karyorrhexis index (defined as fewer than 100 mitotic or karyorrhectic cells per 5000 cells) Stroma-rich tumors	Poorly differentiated High MKI Stroma poor
Biological		
N-Myc	Non-amplification	Amplification (> 10 copies)
DNA content	Hyper-diploid	Diploid, tetraploid
1p Del	–	Present
LOH 1p 36	–	Present
Trk A	Present	–
Trk B	–	Present
NGF	Present	–
CD 44	Elevated	Lack
Ferritin	–	Elevated
NS enolase	–	Elevated
LDH	–	Elevated (>1500 U/ml)
17 q gain	–	Present
MDR-1	–	Present
P-glycoprotein	–	Elevated
NM 23	–	Present
Bcl 2	–	Present
Caspase	Elevated	–

59.3 Prognostic Factors

Age and tumor biology play an important role in the prognosis of these children. In recent times, several molecular markers of prognosis in neuroblastoma have been mentioned, however, they may not be easily available in all centers, especially in the LMICs (Table 59.1).

59.4 Clinical Presentation

The presentation can be in several ways:

- Due to a large primary tumor: Cervical, thoracic, abdominal, or pelvic mass. Cervical masses are apparent at an early stage. *The most common site is the adrenal* (approx. 50% of cases, Fig. 59.2).

- Due to local extension or compression by the primary tumor (Fig. 59.3):
  - Cervical: Horner syndrome due to involvement or origin from the stellate ganglion
  - Intraspinal extension: Motor and sensory deficits
  - Compression of the bladder/ rectum by pelvic tumor: Difficulty in passing urine and stool
- Due to metastases:
  - Skin nodules, especially in Stage MS (Blueberry muffin-like spots)
  - Proptosis/periorbital ecchymosis (raccoon eyes, Fig. 59.4)
  - Pancytopenia—Involvement of the bone marrow
  - Hepatomegaly—Liver metastases
  - Bone pains, pathological fractures—Bone metastases
- Paraneoplastic syndrome:
  - Secretory diarrhea: Caused by the secretion of vasoactive intestinal peptide (VIP) by tumor cells
  - Opsoclonus myoclonus syndrome "*dancing eyes, dancing feet*": Caused by presence of anti-neuronal antibody.

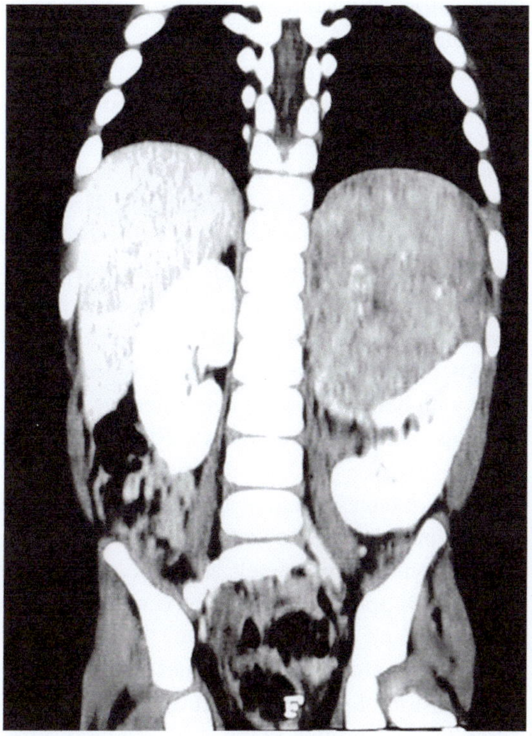

Fig. 59.2 Left adrenal neuroblastoma

The progression of neuroblastoma is variable, which may range from spontaneous regression as in neonatal tumors to widespread metastasis on presentation. In some rare cases, paraneoplastic symptoms like opsoclonus-myoclonus-ataxia could be the only presenting symptoms. Other nonspecific symptoms include loss of appetite, fever, fatigue, and weight loss.

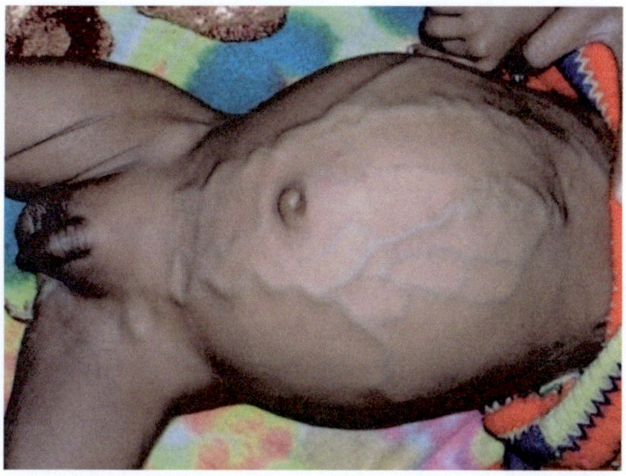

Fig. 59.3 Dilated veins due to IVC obstruction from abdominal neuroblastoma

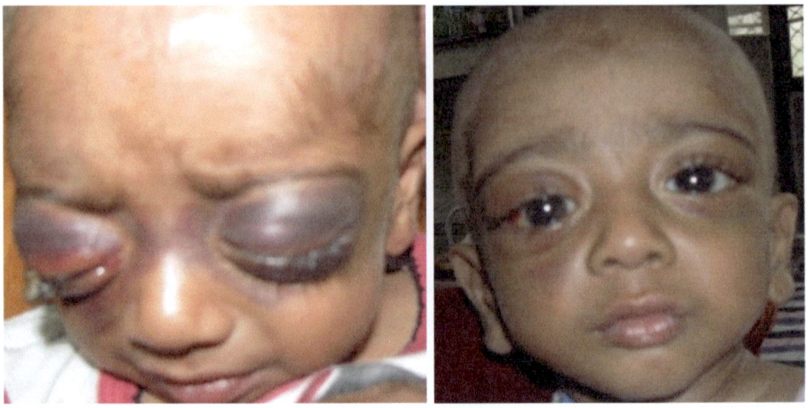

Fig. 59.4 "Raccoon eye" neuroblastoma (pre- and post-chemotherapy).

59.5 Screening

Screening is done by 24-h urinary VMA (vanillylmandelic acid) and HVA (homovanillic acid) levels. Neonatal screening which was performed in Japan, Germany, etc., has been stopped because of overdiagnosis of neuroblastoma and unnecessary treatment and no benefit in outcomes.

59.6 Diagnosis

59.6.1 Radiological Investigations

- X-ray, ultrasound, contrast CT, and MRI.
- Nuclear medicine investigations.

Cervical and thoracic neuroblastomas present as a posterior mediastinal mass which could be appreciated as mediastinal opacities in the posterior-anterior view and lateral views. Additional mediastinal shifting, cardiomegaly, enlarged lymph nodes, pulmonary infiltrates, and even minute stippled calcifications can be appreciated in some cases. Intraspinal neuroblastoma sometimes presents as erosions of vertebral bodies or pedicles. Due to limited assessment, clinicians usually plan ultrasonography and cross-sectional imaging. Ultrasonography (USG) is noninvasive, widely available, and devoid of non-ionizing radiation with the advantage of real-time imaging. It is highly effective to detect tumor mass in cervical, abdominal, and pelvic neuroblastoma. USG can also be used for biopsy when required. USG provides information like an organ of origin, size, and consistency (solid or cystic), heterogeneity like necrosis and stippled calcification, abnormal vascularity, tumor wall and its relationship with adjoining organs, enlarged lymph nodes, and signs of metastasis like malignant ascites or pleural effusion, etc. In cervical NB, USG can assess many surgery-related risk factors like the relationship with major vessels (carotid artery and internal jugular vein), enlarged cervical lymph nodes, and intraspinal extension. In the abdomen, NB is seen as a retroperitoneal tumor mass with homogenous or heterogenous content. Margins, calcifications, mass effect, and tumor necrosis can be well appreciated. More often, vessels are encased rather than just compressed in such patients. Tumor vascularity and its relationship with major vessels are more apparent in the USG Doppler study. Inferior vena cava (IVC) thrombus and residual patency can be well assessed by Doppler. Suprarenal mass causing compression of renal vasculature is another condition to be identified in the case of a large adrenal NB.

Very often, the findings of USG are confirmed and correlated with cross-sectional imaging like computed tomography (CT) and magnetic resonance imaging (MRI).

The availability of fast acquisition, with modern multi-slice CT imaging, makes it possible to scan, within a few minutes without the need for anesthesia or pre-procedure preparation, which is a boon in children. In addition to the USG findings, CT can detect features like a degree of vascular encasement, tumor thrombus, enlarged lymph nodes, loss of fat planes, and the presence of calcification (Fig. 59.5).

MRI is the investigation of choice when there is spinal cord involvement, especially in cases with paraplegia or other neurological deficits.

59.6.2 Image-Defined Risk Factors (IDRF)

International Neuroblastoma Risk Group Staging System (INRGSS) has employed image-defined risk factors (IDRFs) comprised of *twenty specific radiologic features* (Table 59.2) like vascular encasement, involvement of adjacent structures, and intraspinal extension which could add to the complexity of intraoperative tumor resection and further outcome. CT images are ideal for preoperative evaluation of such IDRFs and planning before surgery. The presence of IDRFs denotes advanced locoregional disease which demands a critical assessment of these patients before surgery.

59.6.3 Nuclear Medicine Scan

Radiolabeled metaiodobenzylguanidine (MIBG) scan is highly specific and sensitive for evaluating bone and bone marrow disease. Over 90% of

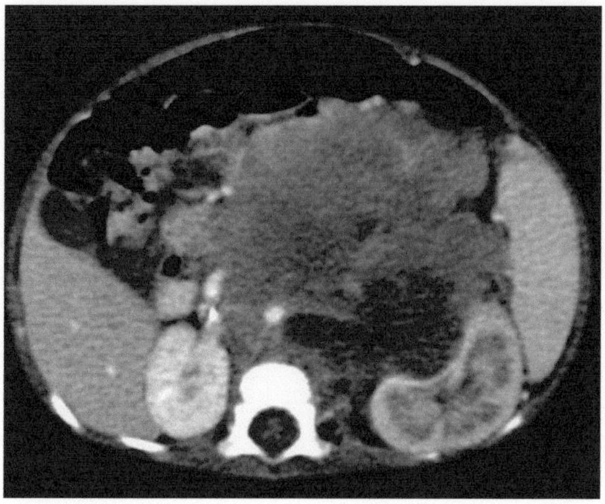

Fig. 59.5 CT scan, abdominal neuroblastoma; note tumor crossing the midline, encasing and lifting the aorta with fine calcifications

Table 59.2 Image-defined risk factors (IDRFs)

Anatomical regions	Descriptions
Multiple body compartments	Ipsilateral tumor extension within two body compartments (e.g., neck and chest, chest and abdomen or abdomen and pelvis)
Neck	Tumor encasing carotid artery, vertebral artery and/or internal jugular vein Tumor extending to base of skull Tumor compressing trachea
Cervicothoracic junction	Tumor encasing brachial plexus roots Tumor encasing subclavian vessels, vertebral artery and/or carotid artery Tumor compressing trachea
Thorax	Tumor encasing aorta and/or major branches Tumor compressing trachea and/or principal bronchi Lower mediastinal tumor infiltrating costovertebral junction between T9 and T12 vertebral levels
Thoracoabdominal junction	Tumor encasing aorta and/or vena cava
Abdomen and pelvis	Tumor encasing porta hepatis and/or hepatoduodenal ligament Tumor encasing branches of superior mesenteric at mesenteric root Tumor encasing origin of celiac axis and/or origin of superior mesenteric artery Tumor encasing one or both renal pedicles Tumor encasing aorta and/or vena cava Tumor encasing iliac vessels Pelvic tumor crossing sciatic notch
Intraspinal tumor extension	Intraspinal tumor extension (above L2) provided that (any of the following): More than one third of spinal canal in axial plane is invaded Perimedullary leptomeningeal spaces are not visible Spinal cord signal intensity is abnormal
Infiltration of adjacent organs and structures	Pericardium Diaphragm Kidney Liver Duodenopancreatic block Mesentery

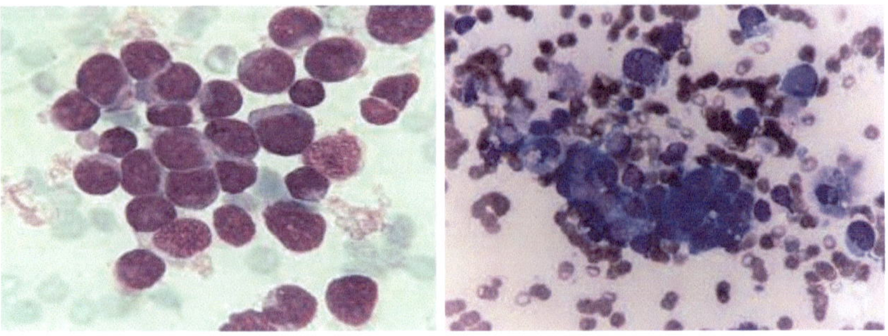

Fig. 59.6 Bone marrow infiltration of neuroblastoma cells (H and E stain)

NB masses are metaiodobenzylguanidine (MIBG) sensitive, however, rest of them can be picked up by ^{99}Tc diphosphonate scintigraphy, especially bony disease. FDG-PET (positron emission tomography) scan can help in the localization of metastasis or viable tumor after therapy. In 10% of cases of neuroblastomas that are not MIBG avid with I $^{131 \text{ or } 123}$, PET/CT with DOTA conjugated peptides such as ^{68}Ga-DOTATATE could be extremely helpful. The role of bone scan when MIBG is being performed is controversial. It is still included in the workup of a patient with neuroblastoma.

59.6.4 Histopathological Investigation

- FNAC/biopsy of the primary or secondary mass for histopathological diagnosis and genetic testing for prognostication
- Bone marrow aspiration and biopsy from bilateral posterior iliac spines (Fig. 59.6)

59.6.5 Other Tests

Catecholamines and their metabolites like HVA (homovanillic acid) and VMA (vanillylmandelic acid) produced from adrenal medulla are useful tumor markers of neuroblastoma. Twenty-four-hour urinary HVA and VMA are also used to monitor the response to treatment (chemotherapy and surgical excision). However, around 5–10% of neuroblastoma do not cause elevation in their levels.

Immunohistochemistry It is useful to differentiate neuroblastoma from other small round cell tumors like Ewing's sarcoma (CD99 positive), Lymphoma (CD45 positive), and Rhabdomyosarcoma (desmin and myogenin positive) (Fig. 59.1).

59.7 Staging

There has been a significant evolution in the staging systems of NBL, over the decades. As far as histopathology is concerned, the traditional Shimada classification has been replaced by the International Pathological Classification System (INPC). This system divides tumors into favorable and unfavorable categories based on factors like age, degree of neuroblastic differentiation, Schwannian stroma, and Mitosis-Karyorrhexis Index. The first three categories are considered maturational sequences, viz.: Neuroblastoma, Ganglioneuroblastoma, Intermixed, and Ganglioneuroma. The fourth category is Ganglioneuroblastoma (nodular variety), which is a multi-clonal tumor.

The *International Neuroblastoma Staging System (INSS)*, which was based on surgical findings, is no longer used in clinical protocols of NBL. The current system in use is the *International Neuroblastoma Risk Group Staging System (INRG)*. This system is based on radiological findings guided by the image-defined risk factors (IDRFs) (Table 59.3).

Table 59.3 International Neuroblastoma Risk Group Staging System (INRG)

Stage	Description
L1	Localized tumor not involving vital structures as defined by the list of image-defined risk factors (IDRF) and confined to one body compartment
L2	Locoregional tumor with the presence of one or more image-defined risk factors
M	Distant metastatic disease (except stage MS)
MS	Metastatic disease in children younger than 18 months with metastases confined to skin, liver, and/or bone marrow

59.8 Risk Stratification

Factors utilized for risk stratification are age, stage of disease, histopathological grading, DNA ploidy, MYCN gene amplification status, segmental chromosomal aberrations, serum lactate dehydrogenase, and serum ferritin. Risk stratification has facilitated intensity-adjusted neuroblastoma therapy and resultant outcomes. INPC has been helpful in guiding stratification in the hands of trained pathologists. The status of MYCN gene amplification is essential for children with stage 4 tumor who are <18 months of age and children with stage 3 tumors. Presence of DNA ploidy in infants with stage 4 or 4S disease without MYCN amplification has significantly worse survival and might warrant for more intensive therapy (Tables 59.4a, 59.4b and 59.4c).

Table 59.4a Treatment of low-risk neuroblastoma

Criteria	Management
Antenatal or perinatal (age < 3–6 months) small adrenal mass	Close observation
Stage L1, any age, absence of MYCN amplification	Close observation/ surgery
Unresectable stage L2, age < 18 months, absence of MYCN amplification	Close observation with 3-monthly imaging
Stage MS, age < 12 months, absence of MYCN amplification	If life-threatening symptoms/chromosomal aberrations present chemotherapy 2–4 cycles 2–4 cycles of chemotherapy and follow-up

Table 59.4b Treatment of intermediate-risk neuroblastoma

Criteria	Management
Stage L2, age > 18 months, absence of MYCN amplification or low serum ferritin/ LDH (when MYCN status is unknown)	INPC—Differentiated—4 cycles of chemotherapy INPC—Undifferentiated/poorly differentiated—6 cycles of chemotherapy, surgery, radiotherapy, and cis retinoic acid followed by tumor response assessment
Stage L1 with MYCN amplification, age < 10 years	If no tumor response and IDRF persists—Surgery followed by chemotherapy If only IDRF—Chemotherapy alone 6 cycles of chemotherapy followed by surgery Postop radiotherapy and 6 cycles of 13-cis-retinoic acid
Stage M with age < 12 months, absence of MYCN amplification or low serum ferritin and LDH (when MYCN status is unknown)	Chemotherapy to achieve metastatic remission followed by surgical resection

Table 59.4c Treatment of high-risk neuroblastoma

Criteria	Management
Stage L2 with MYCN amplified or high serum ferritin/LDH (when MYCN status is unknown) Stage M with age < 18 months and MYCN amplified or high serum ferritin/LDH (when MYCN status is unknown) Stage MS with MYCN amplified Stage M, age 12–18 months, MYCN non-amplified with segmental chromosomal aberrations	High-risk protocol (induction chemo, surgery, autologous hematopoietic stem cell transplant, radiotherapy)
Stage M, age > 18 months Stage M, age 12–18 months, MYCN non-amplified with numerical chromosomal aberrations	High-risk protocol (only induction chemotherapy and surgery)

LR low risk, *IR* intermediate risk, *HR* high risk
In low-risk disease, residual tumor (<50%) is acceptable, as the outcome remains excellent
b-IR therapy entails chemotherapy + surgery to achieve>CR/VGPR/PR. IR will entail a minimum of 4 cycles and up to 8 cycles of intermediate risk therapy
if MYCN is unavailable for low-risk patients, we would assume that they are low risk. Unavailability of MYCN with LDH > =750 units and/or ferritin > = 120 ng/microliter in stage 3 and 4 disease would upstage to high-risk approach
Stage 4S symptomatic patients, inability to obtain biology, consider treatment until symptom resolution with up to 8 cycles

59.9 Treatment

59.9.1 Principles of Treatment

Based on these prognostic factors, the tumor is classified as low-, intermediate-, and high-risk groups (Tables 59.4a, 59.4b and 59.4c).

A combined modality of surgery, chemotherapy, and radiotherapy based on disease stage and risk group is applied in the treatment of neuroblastoma.

Low-Risk Tumors

In low-risk disease, post-surgery residual tumor (<50%) is acceptable, as the outcome remains excellent. Chemotherapy is not needed. Stage MS may require no treatment at all if it is low risk. Follow-up remains in the form of USG /CT every 4 months in the first year followed by semi-annually in the second year.

Prenatally detected neuroblastomas are known to regress, therefore, an adrenal mass in a child less than 3 months of age and a localized tumor less than 5 cm within the adrenal gland without any vascular invasion can be closely observed. Six to eight weekly monitoring with clinical examination and USG is warranted till resolution. Any increase in size or change in behavior with increased NSE value would warrant surgical excision.

Intermediate-Risk Tumors

This group comprises heterogeneous patients like infants with metastasis and large unresectable nonmetastatic tumors at diagnosis. A chemotherapy regimen comprising cyclophosphamide, doxorubicin, carboplatin, and etoposide is recommended. A reapeat bone scan should be done in case of bone marrow infilteration in the pre chemotherapy assessment.

Radiotherapy is reserved for progressive disease and unresectable primary tumors.

Surgery: The most complete tumor resection is performed while preserving full organ and neurological function even if it necessitates leaving minimal residual disease over vital structures. Follow-up using clinical examination, radiology (USG), and urinary catecholamines is recommended quarterly in the first year followed by semi-annually second and third years, and annually thereafter (Parikh et al. 2015).

High-Risk Tumors

They require intensive induction chemotherapy, myeloablative consolidation, and chemotherapy with autologous stem cell rescue. 13-Cis-retinoic acid is administered for promoting the differentiation of tumor cells. Targeted treatment for minimal residual disease like MIBG therapy and targeted immunotherapy is also used wherever indicated. Surgical resection of the residual tumor (90–95% safe resection) is recommended and has shown better EFS and OS in various series.

59.9.2 Chemotherapy

Various chemotherapy regimens are known for neuroblastoma. The chemotherapy dose and schedule will depend on the risk stratification. The regimens mentioned here are simplified, and in-depth reading will be required, especially for detailed doses and complications.

Very Low Risk/Low Risk
Chemotherapy may be indicated sparingly in cases where surgical excision/observation may not be feasible. In case of life-threatening symptoms (LTS), VP/Carbo 2–4 cycles may be administered (Etoposide/Carboplatin). In the event of resolution of LTS, surgery is to be considered if IDRF is negative; otherwise, 4 cycles of CADO may be administered (Cyclophosphamide/Adriamycin/Vincristine).

Intermediate Risk
In this subset, the same philosophy of low risk is applied. VP/Carbo ×4 weeks should be followed by reassessment and surgery planned if IDRF is negative. In case of poor or no response, CADO is to be administered.

High Risk
The treatment is extensively spread over a period of 1 year and requires a multimodality approach. The components of care include chemotherapy, surgery, autologous stem cell transplant, radiotherapy, and differentiating therapy.

There are several regimens, and however, the most commonly used regimen is Rapid COJEC used for induction [Cisplatin (C), Vincristine (O), Carboplatin (J), Etoposide (E), Cyclophosphamide (C)]. For inadequate metastatic response, 2 courses of TVD [Topotecan, Doxorubicin, Vincristine] are indicated.

59.9.3 Surgical Excision

59.9.3.1 Preoperative Preparations

Blood work like hemogram and coagulation values should be overlooked and optimized with a proper preoperative stock of blood products. Consultation and discussion of difficult cases, e.g., mediastinal involvement, vascular encasement, etc., should be done with surgical super specialties like a cardiothoracic and vascular team. Pediatric intensive care beds with vital monitoring facilities and mechanical ventilation should be available for perioperative optimization.

Written informed consent is always an integral part and should never be missed. Parents should be informed about possible postoperative sequelae in special cases like Horner syndrome and intraspinal extension.

The anesthesia team with expertise in difficult cases should be available. The need for single lung ventilation, intraoperative blood product transfusion, and the risk of both hypotension and hypertension crisis due to catecholamine release should be kept in mind.

59.9.3.2 Cervical Neuroblastoma

Cervical NB is generally picked up early and has favorable tumor biology. The intraspinal and intrathoracic extension should be anticipated.

The patient is laid supine with the neck extended and the head rotated to the contralateral side to improve exposure. A shoulder roll and head ring are secured to maintain stability. The entire neck and upper chest are exposed as per the requirement. A transverse incision is given along Langer's line. One should be careful to avoid injury to the greater auricular nerve along the anterior border of the sternocleidomastoid muscle (SCM) and spinal accessory nerve. Large lesions might require the division of SCM for better exposure. Vascular encasement of the internal jugular vein (IJV) and the carotid artery should be dissected out carefully by taking prior vascular controls and hemostatic clamps with careful handling of the vagus nerve lying in the carotid sheath.

In the case of gross cervical lymphadenopathy, a formal neck dissection is performed involving lymphadenectomy.

59.9.3.3 Cervicothoracic Neuroblastoma

Due to the presence of complex neurovascular structures of the thoracic inlet and mediastinal components, operating in this area is a surgical challenge. Generally, approaches like trans-manubrial and trapdoor thoracotomy (anterior thoracotomy) are used to access most of the tumor mass.

These incisions and approaches are often modified according to the site and extent of the tumor mass. Larger lesions occupying most of the mediastinum and reaching both thoracic cavities might require bilateral anterior thoracotomy (clamshell thoracotomy). Newer approaches like cervical-parasternal thoracotomy incisions are also explained to access tumors reaching posterior costovertebral spaces (Martucciello et al. 2021).

Lesions with intraspinal extensions might require laminectomy or foraminectomy to achieve complete resection but the risks outweigh the benefits. Gross resections have better outcomes even in the case of intermediate-risk diseases. Strong adherence of the tumor to the neural foramina should not be disrupted in order to attempt complete resection at the cost of serious neurological deficits afterward. Nerve damage and resulting *Horner's syndrome* should always be explained to parents beforehand in case of high cervical lesions.

59.9.3.4 Thoracic-Abdominal Neuroblastoma

The majority of abdominal NB arise from the adrenal gland or sympathetic ganglia in the upper abdomen covering the retroperitoneum. In such cases, thoracoabdominal approaches are favorable and provide excellent visualization of encased vessels and involved lymph nodes. Surgeons should not risk extensive resection and loss of vital organs or major vessels in case of tumors with *favorable biology*.

A right-sided incision along with kocherization helps in the dissection of tumors from encased vena cava and right renal vessels. Reflecting hepatic flexure, ascending colon, and right lobe of the liver medially, the retroperitoneum is exposed completely.

Similarly, left-sided tumors are dissected carefully from the left renal hilum, aorta, and its branches like the celiac axis, superior mesenteric artery, etc. Splenic flexure of the colon, stomach, tail of pancreas, and spleen is mobilized after dividing splenorenal and splenophrenic ligaments to expose the retroperitoneal space.

59.9.3.5 Pelvic Neuroblastoma

Neuroblastomas arising in the pelvis are difficult to handle due to encasement of iliac vessels, lumbosacral trunk, and variable degrees of bowel and bladder involvement. However, primary pelvic tumors present early without metastasis and usually have favorable biology and respond well even after gross macroscopic resection.

Preoperative MRI is extremely crucial to determine the extent of the tumor and surgical planning. Wherever required, procedures like cystoscopy, urodynamics, and rectal manometry are useful. Mechanical bowel preparation should be strictly followed preoperatively. Vascular controls should be ensured beforehand to prevent injury to major vessels like the aortic bifurcation and iliac complex. Nerve stimulation is useful intraoperatively to delineate the lumbosacral trunk and pelvic complex. At times, preoperative stenting of the ureters may be required for ease of dissection of the tumor from the lateral pelvic walls.

Postoperative morbidity like foot drop, due to injury of pelvic nerves should be explained beforehand. Other complications due to neurologic impairment include neuropathic bladder, partial cauda equina syndrome, and variable degrees of fecal and urinary incontinence.

Alternative approaches to the pelvis such as retropubic, trans perineal, and other approaches used for common pelvic tumors like rhabdomyosarcomas and congenital anomalies like anorectal malformations. However, outcomes are comparable in all the above-described approaches and should be planned according to the scenario (Fati et al. 2021).

59.9.3.6 Minimal Invasive Approach

Operative strategies of minimal invasive surgery (MIS) must consider individual case profiles. There are no strict guidelines on MIS, and however, some studies have preferred well-confined smaller tumors without IDRFs or involvement of major vessels (Galazka et al. 2019). However, the horizon of MIS has increased nowadays and with the feasibility to operate on more difficult cases.

Surgical steps should not be compromised in order to complete the procedure in a minimally invasive approach. Factors like pneumatic pressure, tissue handling, hemostasis, and extent of resection should be anticipated. Conversion to open surgery is always a safer alternative in certain situations.

The extent of lymph node sampling using MIS is variable as per the surgical expertise and often the most common deviation from principles of oncological surgery. The impact of lymph node sampling on survival and disease outcome is still debatable in the literature, and however, various reports emphasize poor lymph node retrieval with the MIS approach. Thus, MIS in neuroblastoma is developing with each passing day.

59.9.3.7 Thoracic Neuroblastoma

MIS used for diagnostic purposes is extremely beneficial in preventing the comorbidities of open thoracotomy.

Keeping in mind the presence of IDRFs, resection of thoracic NB arising as a posterior mediastinal mass is widely performed. Special cases like NB arising from the lower mediastinum are considered IDRF even in the absence of bronchial or vascular affection. Similarly, patients suffering from opsoclonus myoclonus syndrome usually have thoracic NB which need not be resected always for good oncologic outcomes. However, failure of conservative management and pressure effect may mandate resection where MIS could provide less trauma.

Intraspinal extensions or proximity to neural foramina require neurosurgical backup intraoperatively. Extensive tumor resection jeopardizing neurological function is not advisable, and thus, preoperative stratification is extremely important in such cases taking into consideration the tumor biology and markers.

The size, nature, and site of thoracic NB have to be critically assessed by the operative team as per their expertise and resources for minimally invasive interventions. The thoracic cavity is space-limited as compared to the abdominal cavity and may require special situations like single lung ventilation to improve exposure.

Horner's syndrome is one of the most commonly encountered complications faced postoperatively.

59.9.4 Special Considerations

59.9.4.1 Vascular Dissection

Major vessels like the aorta and its branches are often found encased while attempting resection of tumors arising in the abdominopelvic region. It is vital to trace the course and origin of these vessels which is followed by finding an appropriate plane between the tumor mass and the adventitia of the vessel. This maneuver is carefully done using the "*bivalving technique*" with a gently curved dissector after taking prior vascular control. Energy sources like bipolar cautery or harmonic scalpel are utilized to dissect the tumor parenchyma from the vessel in toto or in piecemeal. In cases where the periadventitial plane is obliterated, the sub-adventitial vascular plane is accessed. This approach can weaken the vessel under dissection and make it vulnerable to rupture or avulse due to traction during surgery. It is advisable to leave a small portion of the adhered tumor tissue rather than jeopardize major vessels.

Special care should be taken while dissecting veins like the vena cava and its tributaries which are thin-walled and fragile as compared to the aorta and can bleed profusely if avulsed during surgery.

59.10 Radiotherapy

Radiotherapy is administered following ASCT and prior to therapy with 13-cis-retinoic acid (RA). SIOP-PODC recommends the administration of 21.6 Gy radiation to the primary tumor bed and to residual bone metastases (< 6 sites). Radiotherapy is typically administered 60 day after Bu to avoid Bu-enhanced radiotoxicity.

59.11 Differentiating Therapy and Newer Modalities

13-Cis-retinoic acid (RA), a differentiation-promoting biological agent, has been shown to enhance EFS in high-risk NBL. It is not useful for gross residual disease. Dose: 160 mg/m^2/day (5.33 mg/kg/d in ≤12 kg) orally in 2 divided doses for 14 day a month, for a total of 6 months.

Anti-ganglioside (GD2) monoclonal antibody ch14.18 immunotherapy, consisting of ch14.18 with granulocyte–macrophage colony-stimulating factor (GM-CSF) and IL2, significantly improves outcomes for high-risk NBL patients by acting on minimal residual disease. An improvement in 2 year EFS of up to 20% has been demonstrated. It is expensive and is not commercially available in India currently.

59.12 Summary

In summary, for low-risk patients, surgical excision of the tumor is usually curative and avoids the risks associated with chemotherapy. Intermediate-risk patients are usually treated with surgery and standard chemotherapy. The poor prognosis in high-risk patients justifies a much more intense treatment regimen, including combination chemotherapy followed by complete surgical excision (if possible), radiation therapy to achieve local control, myeloablative treatments, and autologous stem cell transplant.

Suggested Reading

Brignole C, Pastorino F, Perri P, et al. Bone marrow environment in metastatic Neuroblastoma. Cancers (Basel). 2021;13(10):2467.

Chen AM, Trout AT, Towbin AJ. A review of neuroblastoma image-defined risk factors on magnetic resonance imaging. Pediatr Radiol. 2018;48(9):1337–47.

Dumba M, Jawad N, McHugh K. Neuroblastoma and nephroblastoma: a radiological review. Cancer Imaging. 2015;15:5.

Fati F, Pulvirenti R, Paraboschi I, Martucciello G. Surgical approaches to Neuroblastoma: review of the operative techniques. Children. 2021;8(6):446.

Galazka P, Czyzewski K, Marjanska A, Daniluk-Matras I, Styczynski J. Minimally invasive surgery in pediatric oncology: proposal of guidelines. Anticancer Res. 2019;39(11):5853–9.

Matthay KK, Maris JM, Schleiermacher G, et al. Neuroblastoma. Nat Rev Dis Primers. 2016;2:16078. Published 2016 Nov 10

Li J, Liu X, Chen M, Wang J, Wang X. Values of serum CA125, NSE and 24-hour urine VMA in diagnosis and prediction of treatment of paediatric neuroblastoma. Int J Clin Pract. 2021;75(12):e14932.

Lonergan GJ, Schwab CM, Suarez ES, Carlson CL. Neuroblastoma, ganglioneuroblastoma, and ganglioneuroma: radiologic-pathologic correlation. Radiographics. 2002;22(4):911–34.

Maris JM, Hogarty MD, Bagatell R, Cohn SL. Neuroblastoma. Lancet. 2007;369(9579):2106–20.

Martucciello G, Fati F, Avanzini S, Senes FM, Paraboschi I. The Cervico-parasternal thoracotomy (CPT): a new surgical approach for the resection of Cervicothoracic Neuroblastomas. Children. 2021;8(3):229.

McHugh K. Renal and adrenal tumours in children. Cancer Imaging. 2007;7(1):41–51.

Parikh NS, Howard SC, Chantada G, et al. SIOP-PODC adapted risk stratification and treatment guidelines: recommendations for neuroblastoma in low- and middle-income settings. Pediatr Blood Cancer. 2015;62(8):1305–16.

Sebire NJ, Gibson S, Rampling D, Williams S, Malone M, Ramsay AD. Immunohistochemical findings in embryonal small round cell tumors with molecular diagnostic confirmation. Appl Immunohistochem Mol Morphol. 2005;13(1):1–5.

Shimada H, Umehara S, Monobe Y, et al. International neuroblastoma pathology classification for prognostic evaluation of patients with peripheral neuroblastic tumors: a report from the Children's Cancer Group. Cancer. 2001;92(9):2451–61.

Taggart DR, London WB, Schmidt ML, et al. Prognostic value of the stage 4S metastatic pattern and tumor biology in patients with metastatic neuroblastoma diagnosed between birth and 18 months of age. J Clin Oncol. 2011;29(33):4358–64.

60 Liver Masses in Children

Anjan Kumar Dhua and Subhasis Roy Choudhury

Liver masses in children can stem from a variety of benign and malignant causes (refer to Fig. 60.1). Hepatoblastoma is the most frequent primary malignant liver tumour in infants and young children. In neonates, infantile hepatic hemangioma is the most common liver mass. Hepatoblastoma typically occurs between 4 months and 4 years of age, whereas hepatocellular carcinoma is more prevalent in older children. Among benign tumours, mesenchymal hamartoma and focal nodular hyperplasia are often observed in young infants and children.

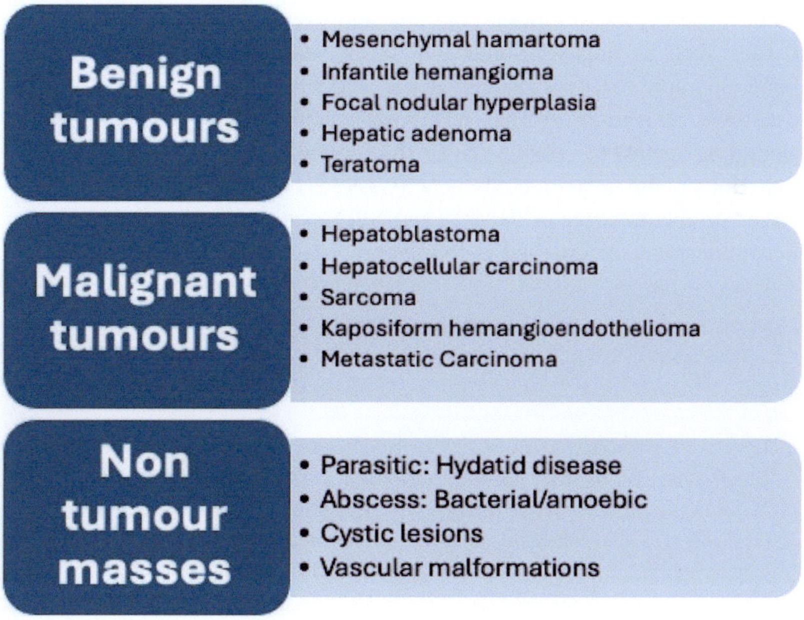

Fig. 60.1 Differential diagnosis of liver masses in children

A. K. Dhua (✉)
Mother and Child Block, AIIMS, New Delhi, India

S. Roy Choudhury
Pediatric Surgery, Lady Hardinge Medical College and Associated Kalawati Saran Children's Hospital, New Delhi, Delhi, India

© The Author(s), under exclusive license to Springer Nature Singapore Pte Ltd. 2025
S. Roy Choudhury (ed.), *Pediatric Surgery*, https://doi.org/10.1007/978-981-96-1257-4_60

60.1 Hepatoblastoma

The incidence of hepatoblastoma in the United States is reported to be 1.2 cases per million population, with a male-to-female ratio of 1.7:1. While most cases are sporadic, there are associations with conditions such as Beckwith-Wiedemann syndrome, prematurity, Gardner's syndrome, trisomy 18, trisomy 21, Aicardi syndrome, Li-Fraumeni syndrome, Goldenhar syndrome, type 1a glycogen storage disease (von Gierke disease), and familial polyposis coli. The tumour predominantly affects the right lobe in 50% of cases, the left lobe in 15%, and is centrally located in 27% of cases. Although rare, the global incidence of hepatoblastoma is on the rise.

60.2 Pathology

Hepatoblastoma is a tumour characterised by diverse patterns of differentiation, ranging from foetal hepatocytes to embryonal cells and even tissues such as muscle, connective tissue, and bone. Sporadic cases are strongly associated with excessive activation of the WNT/beta-catenin signalling pathway, often driven by somatic mutations in the beta-1 catenin gene (CTNNB1). Based on the presence of these varied cell types, hepatoblastoma is classified as follows:

60.3 Pathological Types

Hepatoblastomas are classified into two types (Fig. 60.2) based on their pathological features: epithelial and mixed epithelial-mesenchymal.

The pure foetal type (Fig. 60.3a, b) has the best prognosis, whereas the small cell undifferentiated (SCUD) type has the worst prognosis.

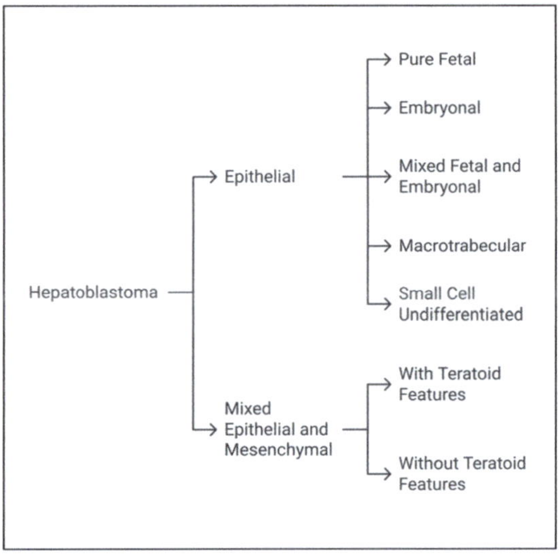

Fig. 60.2 Classification of hepatoblastoma based on the pathological features

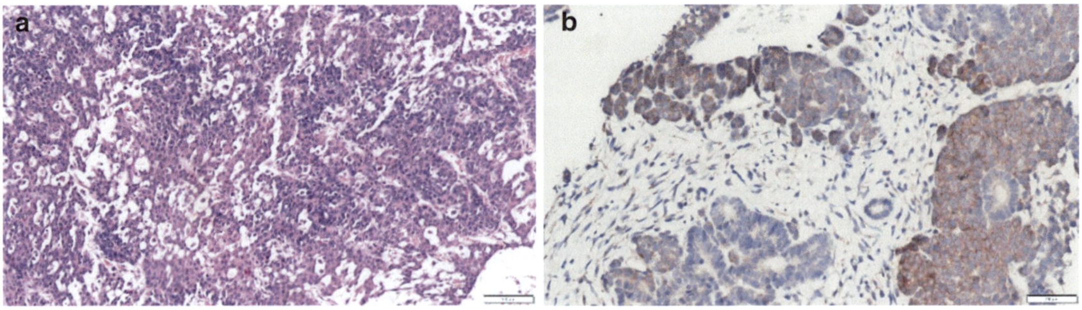

Fig 60.3 (**a**, **b**) Hepatoblastoma Fetal type- (**a**) The neoplastic cells are arranged in cords and resemble adult liver. There is minimal mitosis or pleomorphism. [H&E 10x]. (**b**) The tumor cells are immuno-positive for arginase. [IHC 10x] (courtesy Dr. Lavleen Singh, AIIMS, New Delhi)

60.4 Presentation

In infants, the typical presentation is an asymptomatic abdominal mass located in the right upper quadrant (Fig. 60.4). Nonspecific symptoms may include low-grade fever, anorexia, and poor weight gain or failure to thrive. In rare cases, large tumours can lead to complications such as portal hypertension due to portal vein obstruction, ascites resulting from obstruction of the portal and hepatic veins, and obstructive jaundice caused by bile duct compression. Additionally, large tumours at the time of diagnosis may sometimes rupture, resulting in hemoperitoneum.

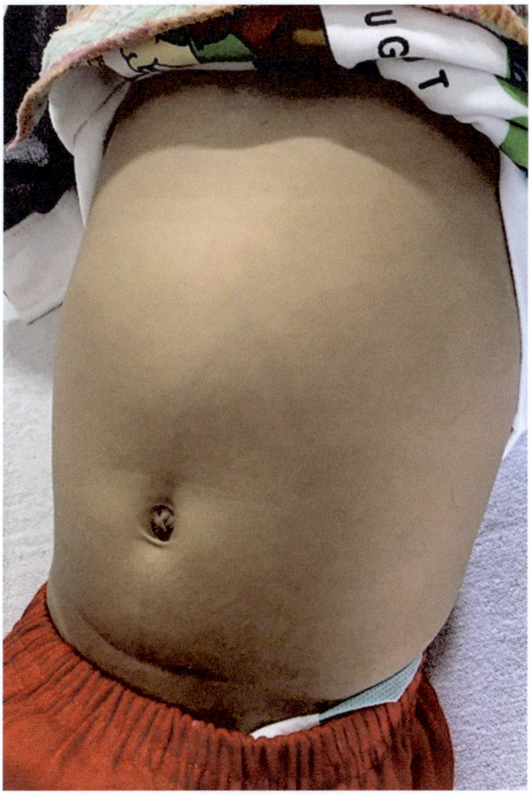

Fig. 60.4 Upper abdominal mass in an infant due to hepatoblastoma

Uncommon presentations of hepatoblastoma include "sexual precocity", which can result from ectopic synthesis of beta-human chorionic gonadotropin. In some cases, children may experience osteopenia and pathological fractures due to disrupted calcium metabolism. Additionally, ectopic production of adrenocorticotropic hormone (ACTH) or parathyroid hormone-related protein (PTHrP) may lead to Cushing's syndrome and hypercalcemia, respectively.

60.5 Diagnosis

Tumour Marker

Alpha-fetoprotein (AFP) is elevated in the majority of hepatoblastoma cases and serves as an essential marker for both diagnosis and treatment monitoring. AFP levels typically normalise after complete tumour resection within 4–6 weeks. It is important to note that neonates naturally have high AFP levels at birth, which decrease to adult levels by 6–8 months. Normal AFP levels range from approximately 40,000 ng/mL in full-term newborns to over 100,000 ng/mL in premature infants. AFP also provides prognostic value, as hepatoblastomas with AFP levels below 100 ng/mL are generally poorly differentiated and associated with a worse prognosis. Such tumours often exhibit aggressive behaviour, extensive disease at presentation, resistance to chemotherapy, and a two-year survival rate of only 24%. Consequently, patients with localised disease and AFP levels below 100 ng/mL at diagnosis are categorised into high-risk groups in most major hepatoblastoma risk stratification models.

Additionally, hepatoblastoma is frequently associated with elevated platelet counts due to tumour cell secretion of thrombopoietin. This thrombocytosis may aid in supporting the diagnosis of hepatoblastoma in uncertain cases.

60.6 Imaging Studies

- Ultrasonography (USG) is the preferred initial imaging modality to determine the origin of the mass. It typically reveals a hyperechoic, solid intrahepatic mass of varying size and location.
- Contrast-enhanced computed tomography (CECT) or MRI of the abdomen (Fig. 60.5a, b) is used to assess the extent of tumour involvement. A triphasic CT scan can highlight the vascular anatomy of the liver in relation to the tumour. Additionally, chest CT evaluation is essential since the lungs are the most common site for metastases. MRI is often favoured over CT as it provides more precise details regarding tumour dimensions, margins, involvement of adjacent organs, and multifocality.
- Hepatoblastomas are usually FDG-PET positive, making PET scans useful for evaluating disease extent and chemotherapy response. However, routine use of PET scans is not recommended. FDG-PET may, however, be explored in certain situations during the post-resection surveillance when a recurrent mass cannot be palpated or picked up by CECT despite rising tumour markers.

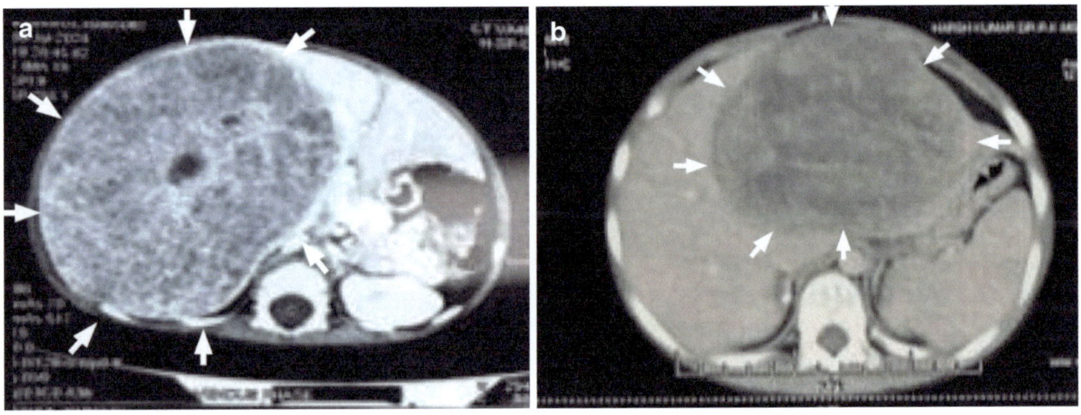

Fig. 60.5 (**a**) CT scan, right lobe hepatoblastoma. (**b**) CT scan, left lobe hepatoblastoma

60.7 Histopathology/Cytology

Fine-needle aspiration cytology or percutaneous needle biopsy is required to confirm the diagnosis in children scheduled for upfront chemotherapy. However, due to the potential risks associated with percutaneous biopsy, some groups suggest that children aged 6 months to 3 years with serum α-fetoprotein (AFP) levels exceeding 1000 ng/mL or more than three times the normal age-specific level may be presumed to have hepatoblastoma, eliminating the need for a biopsy in these cases.

60.8 Staging and Risk Stratification

Management of hepatoblastoma is currently guided by the PRETEXT (pretreatment extent of disease) staging system developed by the International Society of Pediatric Oncology Liver Tumor Group (Fig. 60.6).

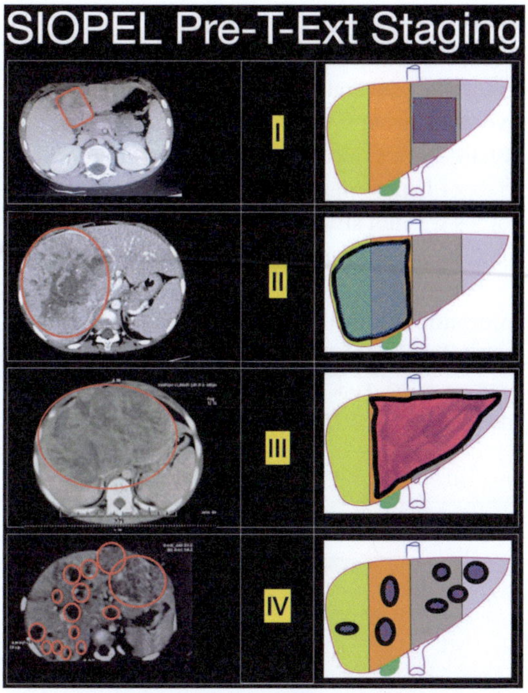

Fig. 60.6 SIOPEL staging of hepatoblastoma

- *PRETEXT 1*: Tumour confined to one sector, with three adjoining sectors unaffected.
- *PRETEXT 2*: Tumour involving two sectors, with two adjoining sectors unaffected.
- *PRETEXT 3*: Tumour involving two or three sectors, with only one sector or two non-adjoining sectors unaffected.
- *PRETEXT 4*: Tumour involving all four sectors, with no sector unaffected.

Additional tumour extensions or characteristics are denoted using the following "Annotation Factors":

- *V*: Involvement of the inferior vena cava or all three hepatic veins.
- *P*: Involvement of the porta hepatis.
- *E*: Extrahepatic spread.
- *F*: Multifocal tumours.
- *R*: Tumour rupture at diagnosis.
- *C*: Involvement of the caudate lobe.
- *M*: Presence of metastases.

Advanced hepatoblastoma, defined as PRETEXT stage III or higher, involving more than two liver sectors, presents a considerable challenge for surgical resection.

60.9 Risk Stratification

In the past several decades, four major cooperative trial groups—COG, SIOPEL, GPOH, and JPLT—have undertaken prospective randomised trials of hepatoblastoma. The comparison of outcomes was not straightforward as their risk stratification system varied (Fig. 60.7).

The Children's Hepatic Tumours International Collaboration (CHIC) was conceptualised to develop a common global approach to risk stratification in hepatoblastoma. A "risk stratification tree" referred to as the Children's Hepatic tumours International Collaboration–Hepatoblastoma Stratification (CHIC-HS) has been developed based on the PRETEXT status, metastasis, age, AFP ≤100 ng/mL, PRETEXT annotation factors, and surgical resectability at diagnosis into four risk levels: very low, low, intermediate, and high (Fig. 60.8).

The new risk stratification system is essential as it will allow a comparison of treatment outcomes of past and future studies. Also, it may provide a platform for global collaborative trials in paediatric hepatoblastoma.

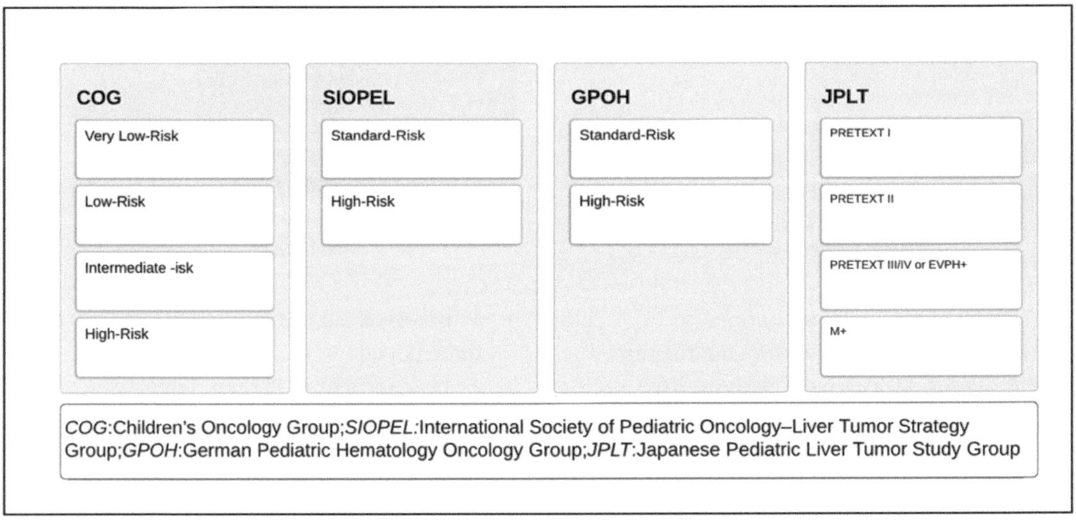

Fig. 60.7 Schema showing the variations in risk stratification existing in various pediatric oncology collaborative study groups worldwide

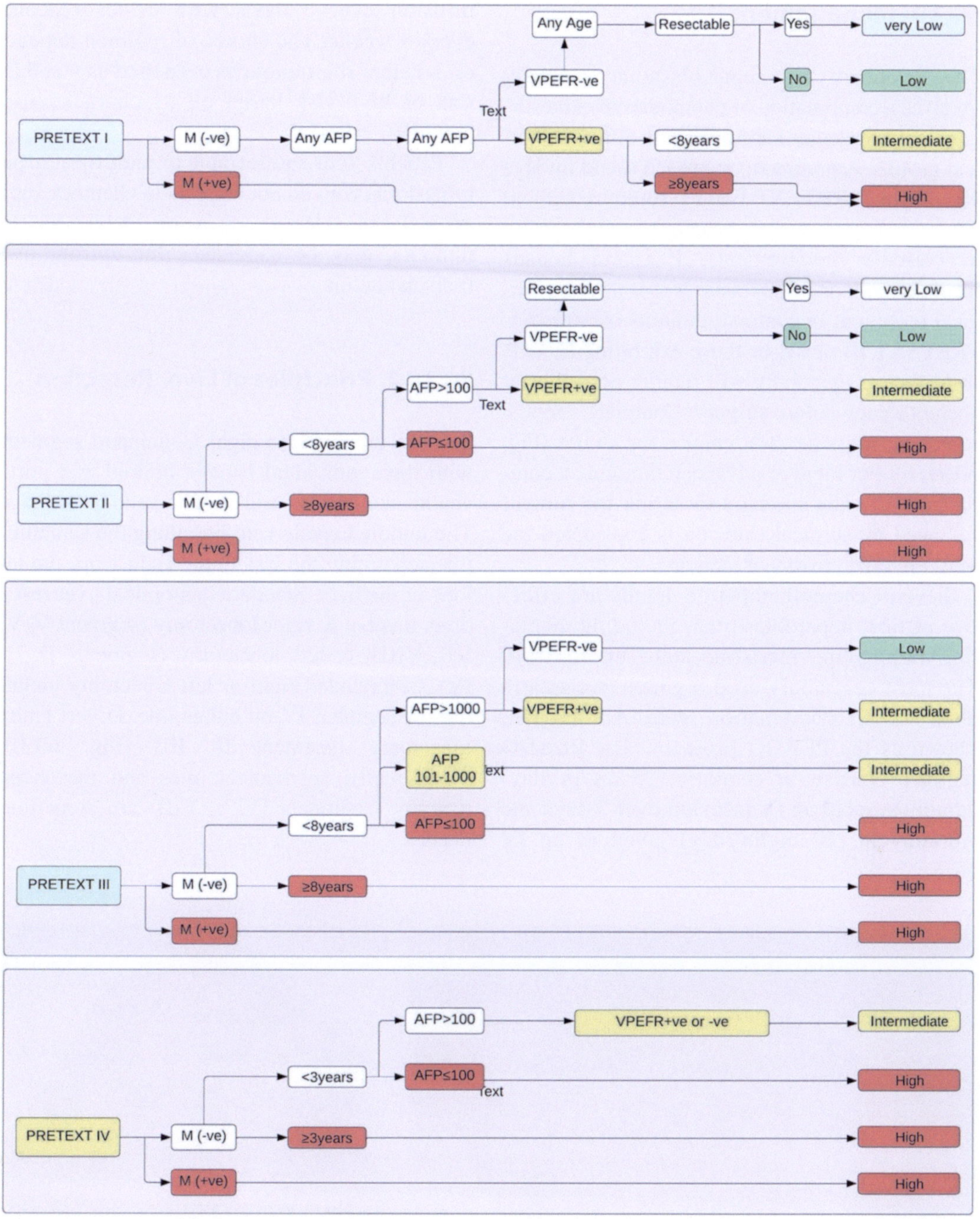

Fig. 60.8 Risk stratification trees for the Children's Hepatic Tumours International Collaboration–Hepatoblastoma Stratification (CHICHS). PRETEXT PRETreatment EXTent of disease, AFP Alfa-fetoprotein levels in ng/ml, M Metastasis, VPEFR PRETEXT annotation factors

60.10 Management

The treatment of hepatoblastoma typically involves a combination of chemotherapy and surgery, with strategies varying across different clinical groups. A pragmatic approach could involve considering PRETEXT I and II tumours without extension factors such as E (extrahepatic spread), V (vascular involvement), P (porta hepatis involvement), or M (metastases) for primary surgical resection. In contrast, tumours classified as PRETEXT III or IV, or those exhibiting E, V, P, or M factors, generally will require neoadjuvant chemotherapy before surgery. Complete surgical resection offers the best chance for a cure (Fig. 60.9a, b). For large or advanced tumours, a combination of chemotherapy to shrink the tumour followed by surgical excision is considered the most effective treatment strategy.

Several chemotherapeutic agents are effective against hepatoblastoma, including cisplatin, Adriamycin, vincristine, and 5-fluorouracil. The most commonly used regimen is cisplatin alone or in combination with Adriamycin, known as the PLADO protocol. The PLADO regimen consists of cisplatin (25 $mg/m^2/day$) administered as an IV infusion over 3 days and Adriamycin (20 $mg/m^2/day$) given as an IV infusion over 3 days, with cycles repeated every 3 weeks. The choice of regimen depends on whether the tumour is classified as standard risk or high risk based on its characteristics (SIOPEL criteria).

Patients with unresectable or multifocal hepatoblastoma who do not respond to chemotherapy, as well as selected cases of PRETEXT IV tumours, may be candidates for upfront liver transplantation.

60.10.1 Principles of Liver Resection

Liver is divided into eight Couninaud segments with their individual hepatic arterial and portal venous connection and hepatic venous drainage. The middle hepatic vein lies along the Cantalie's line separating the functional right from the left lobe of the liver. Standard anatomical liver resections involve a. right lobectomy (segment V, VI, VII, VIII), b. left lobectomy (segments II, III, IV), C. extended right or left lobectomy including the segment IV on either side. D. left lateral lobectomy (segment II, III) (Fig. 60.10). Additionally, segmentectomies and mesohepatectomy (segments IV, V, VIII) are sometimes needed.

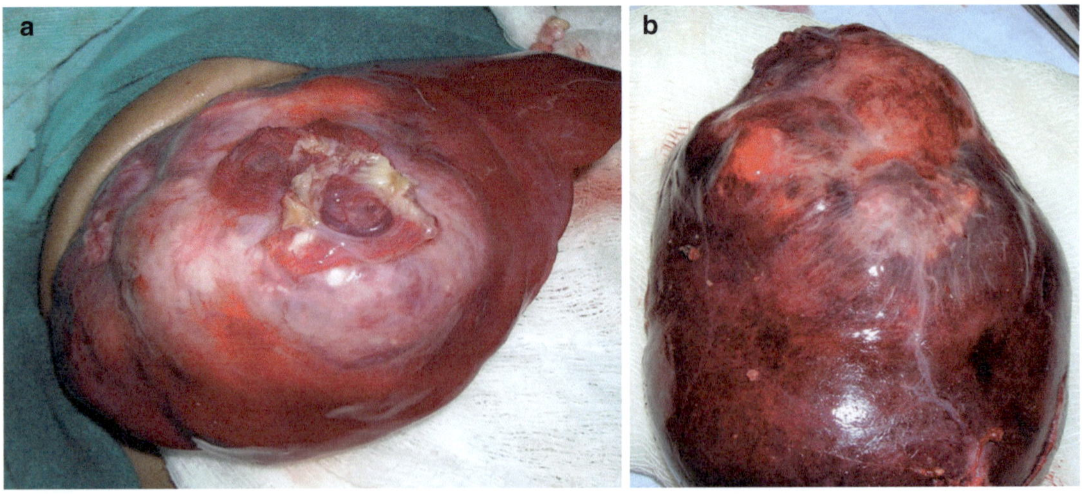

Fig. 60.9 (**a**) Right lobe hepatoblastoma at surgery (**b**) Resected specimen of hepatoblastoma (right hepatectomy)

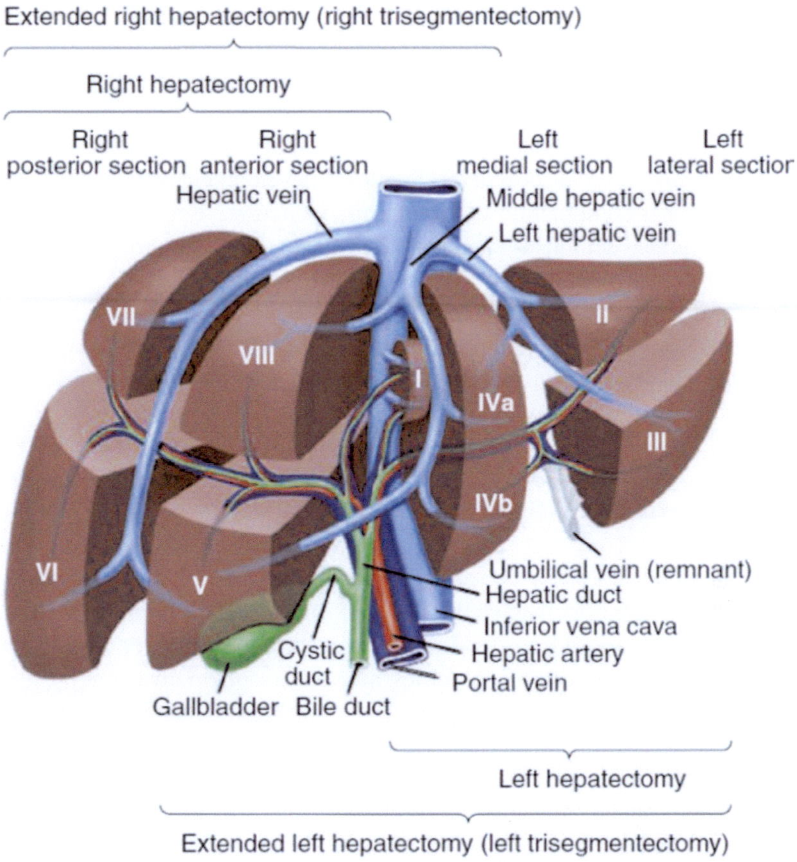

Fig. 60.10 Segments of liver in relation to liver resection

60.11 Role of Orthotopic Liver Transplant

As mentioned earlier, patients who are not eligible for liver tumour resection but have achieved complete resolution of lung metastases (through chemotherapy, surgical resection, or both) may be considered candidates for liver transplantation. In such cases, liver transplantation serves as the sole means of achieving local control. The effectiveness of liver transplantation in treating hepatoblastoma is now well established. Consequently, it is strongly recommended to refer all newly diagnosed unresectable cases to a liver transplant centre for evaluation at the earliest opportunity rather than delaying until after initial chemotherapy to decide on transplantation.

60.12 Treatment of Relapsed Disease

Patients with recurrent disease may present with isolated lung relapse, isolated local/liver relapse, a combination of local and lung relapse, or distant metastases in non-pulmonary sites. These cases pose significant challenges in terms of oncological management and outcomes. While the overall prognosis in relapse cases is generally poor, a subset of patients may achieve long-term survival through a combination of chemotherapy and surgical intervention. The integration of both modalities is critical for achieving sustained remission.

There is no standardised chemotherapy protocol for relapsed cases. For patients who have not previously received doxorubicin, a regimen including doxorubicin (e.g. ifosfamide/doxorubicin or carboplatin/doxorubicin) is often considered. Alternative options for those who have already been treated with doxorubicin include the ICE regimen (ifosfamide/carboplatin/etoposide), carboplatin with etoposide, or docetaxel. Single-agent irinotecan or a combination of irinotecan and vincristine has also demonstrated potential in managing recurrent disease.

In select cases, such as those with isolated pulmonary metastases, surgical removal through pulmonary metastasectomy alone may be an effective treatment approach.

60.13 Long-Term Toxicities

As the outcome of hepatoblastoma has improved over time, the long-term effects of chemotherapy in the survivors also warrant the attention of clinicians. The two most prominent toxicities are cardiotoxicity and ototoxicity.

For cardiotoxicity, dexrazoxane is the only US Food and Drug Administration (FDA) approved drug specifically aimed towards preventing anthracycline-mediated cardiotoxicity. Trials that had included doxorubicin being administered as a continuous infusion for as long as 96 h were less cardiotoxic than bolus dosing but were more cumbersome to administer and required longer inpatient treatment. Current hepatoblastoma trials utilise bolus doxorubicin dosing, where dexrazoxane co-administration is advisable for cardioprotection. The suggested dosage ratio of dexrazoxane to doxorubicin is 10 to 1 (e.g. 500 mg/m^2 dexrazoxane to 50 mg/m^2 doxorubicin). It is advisable to give dexrazoxane before doxorubicin. A diluted solution of dexrazoxane in lactated Ringer's intravenously is administered over 15 min before doxorubicin.

Hearing loss is one of the most concerning long-term toxicities associated with platinum agents (predominantly cisplatin) for hepatoblastoma therapy. Severe grades of hearing impairment can hinder subsequent speech and language development and impair overall neurocognitive function. Several strategies include the early detection of ototoxicity in children receiving platinum agents. This would minimise the risk of severe impairment in the frequencies required for speech recognition by providing an opportunity for treatment alterations before auditory damage becomes severe. Primarily based on two studies (COG ACCL0431 and SIOPEL- 6), the FDA has approved sodium thiosulfate to decrease the risk of cisplatin-related ototoxicity in paediatric patients aged 1 month or older who have a diagnosis of localised, nonmetastatic solid malignancy. It is used as a single dose of 20 g/m^2 administered over 15 min, 6 h after each of the six cisplatin doses.

Hepatocellular carcinoma, undifferentiated embryonal sarcoma, and rhabdomyosarcoma of the biliary tree are other rare malignant conditions affecting children.

60.14 Other Liver Tumours

Infantile hepatic hemangioma (IHH) is the most common benign solid liver tumour in children seen in the first year of life. They can be small focal lesions or large diffuse lesions. A triad of hepatomegaly, congestive heart failure, and anaemia, cutaneous hemangiomas has been found in 80% of the cases. Thrombocytopenia, consumptive coagulopathy (Kasabach-Merritt syndrome), and congenital hypothyroidism are other features of this lesion. Syndromes such as Osler-Weber-Rendu, Klippel-Trénaunay-Weber, Ehlers-

Danlos, Beckwith-Wiedemann syndromes, diaphragmatic hernia, trisomy 21, transposition of the great arteries, and extra numeric digits have been associated with infantile hepatic hemangioendothelioma. Computed tomography (CT) with intravenous contrast classically shows diffusely enhancing lesions (Fig. 60.11). MRI with intravenous gadolinium improves the accuracy of diagnosis. There are distinct histological characteristics of hepatic hemangioendothelioma as shown in (Fig. 60.12a, b).

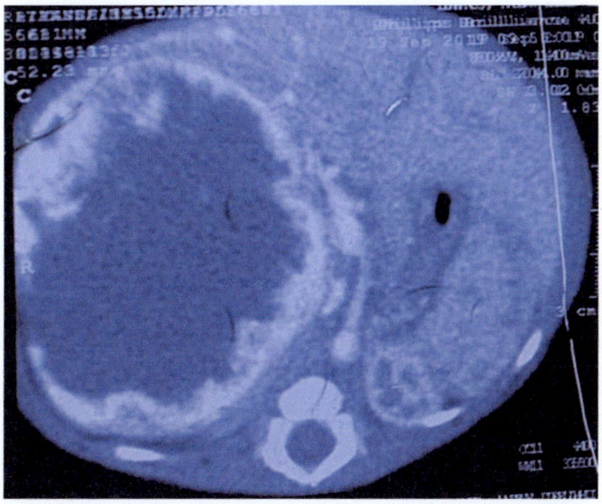

Fig. 60.11 CT scan showing hemangioendothelioma of the liver, note diffuse vascular lesion with peripheral enhancement

60.14.1 Management

These lesions tend to grow in the first year of life and then begin to regress spontaneously. Asymptomatic lesions should be observed. Patients with features of congestive cardiac failure, coagulopathy, or respiratory distress need intervention. Digitalis and diuretics are used for heart failure. Steroids in the form of prednisolone 2–3 mg/kg/day and vincristine have been successfully used. Interferon alpha has fallen in disrepute due to complications like spastic diplegia. Propranolol is a new addition to drugs effective in this disease. Embolisation for large lesions is often successful. Localised lesions can be resected with a good outcome. Any residual lesion after successful conservative treatment should be resected as malignant transformation to angiosarcoma is a possibility.

60.15 Mesenchymal Hamartoma of the Liver

This is the third most common solid tumour and the second most common benign tumour of the liver. It presents with an abdominal mass, respiratory distress, and congestive cardiac failure. Antenatal diagnosis by ultrasonography is sometimes possible.

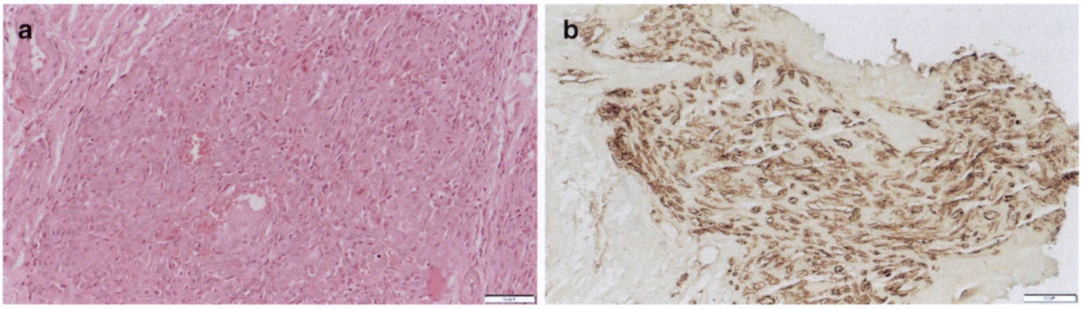

Fig. 60.12 (**a**, **b**). Hemangioendothelioma. (**a**) Nodular aggregates of plump endothelial cells. Neoplastic endothelial have abundant eosinophillic cytoplasm, distinct nucleoli and presence of intracytoplasmic lumina. [H&E x10] (**b**). Tumor cells are immune positive for CD31. [IHC 10x] (courtesy Dr. Lavleen Singh, AIIMS, New Delhi)

Pathologically, these are large, well-circumscribed lesions with cystic and solid areas mainly involving the right lobe of the liver. CT, USG, and MRI are all helpful in the diagnosis (Fig. 60.13), and serum alpha-fetoprotein level is often raised. Complete surgical excision is the treatment of choice as transformation to an undifferentiated embryonal sarcoma is possible; for large lesions, temporary marsupialisation (Fig. 60.14a, b) may be done, followed by close follow-up and complete surgical excision in the future. The characteristic histopathological feature is shown in (Fig. 60.15).

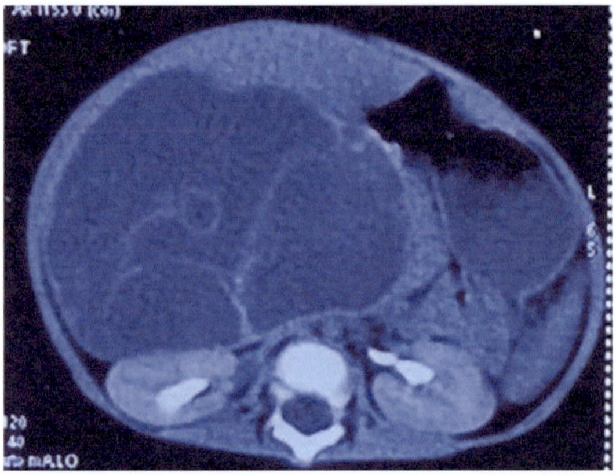

Fig. 60.13 CT scan, mesenchymal hamartoma of liver, Multiple cystic and solid areas with septations

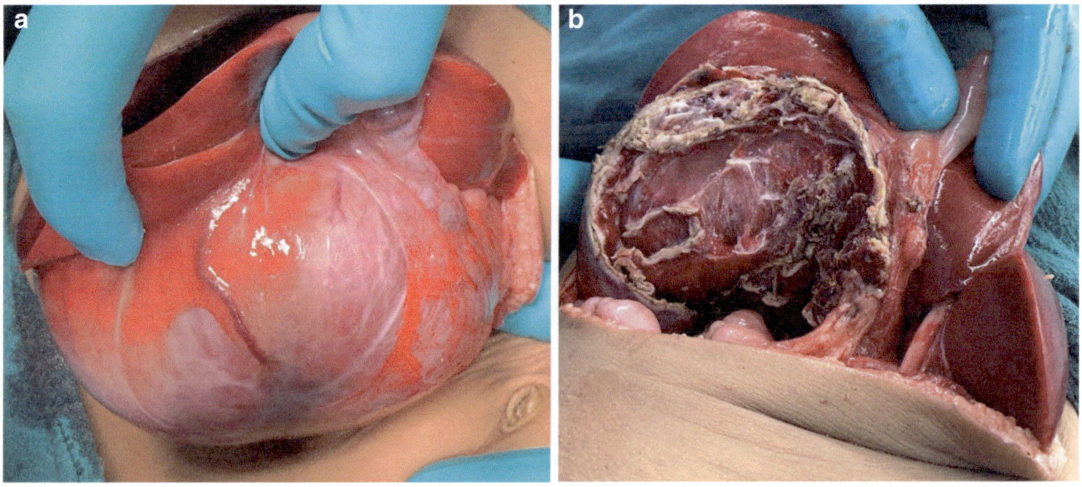

Fig. 60.14 (**a**) Mesenchymal hamartoma of the liver. (**b**) Near complete surgical excision of mesenchymal hamartoma of the liver

Fig. 60.15 Mesenchymal hamartoma. MH shows disorganized arrangement of primitive mesenchymal and epithelial elements. Note the dilated bile ducts surrounded by myxoid stroma and peripherally located benign hepatocytes. [H&E 2x] (courtesy Dr. Lavleen Singh, AIIMS, New Delhi)

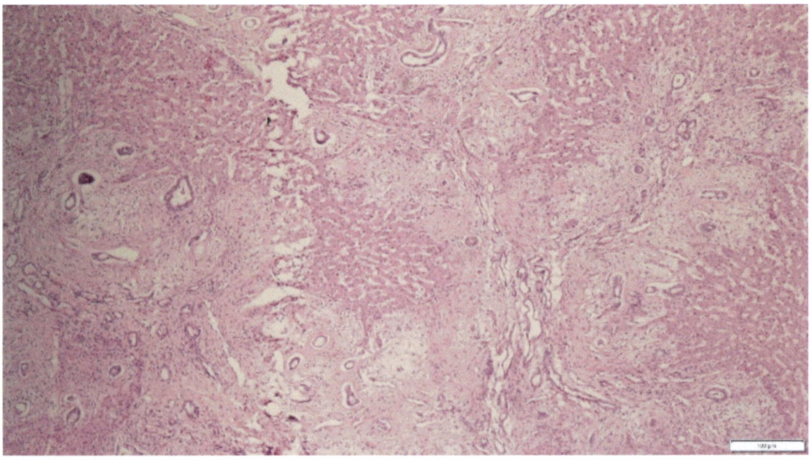

60.16 Focal Nodular Hyperplasia

This tumour occurs relatively late, with a mean age of 7 years and female preponderance. Association with oral contraceptives has been documented in adults. Paediatric focal nodular hyperplasia often shows regression; hence, an expectant treatment may be offered. Symptomatic cases and those with persistent lesions and doubtful diagnosis are better removed surgically (Fig. 60.16).

Congenital giant liver cyst (Fig. 60.17a, b) is rare in children. It can be managed with simple cyst excision.

60.17 Summary Points

1. Hepatoblastoma is a rare tumour but the most common primary paediatric malignant hepatic neoplasm.
2. Complete evaluation (high-quality cross-sectional imaging, biopsy, and serum AFP) and multimodality treatment (cisplatin-based chemotherapy, response evaluation, and complete tumour resection) as per risk stratification form the backbone for managing all newly diagnosed cases of hepatoblastoma.
3. Early referral to a liver transplant centre for management is recommended for all newly

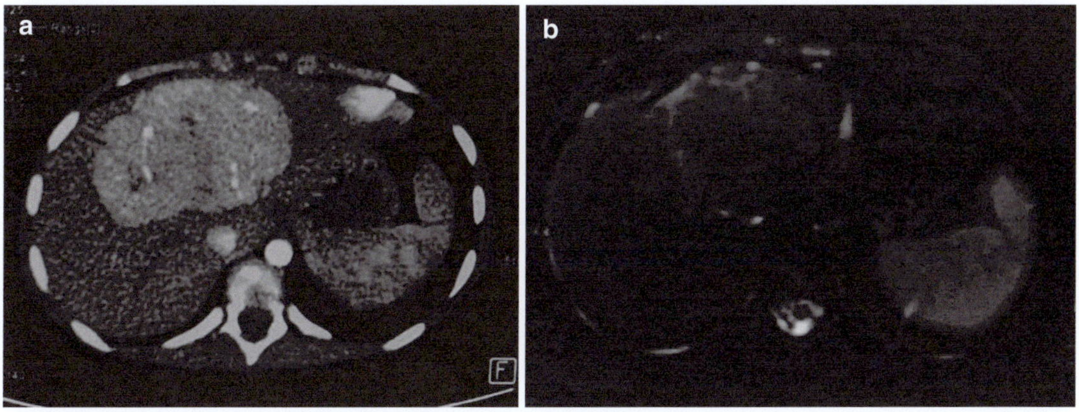

Fig. 60.16 (**a**) CT Scan (**b**) MRI showing focal nodular hyperplasia of liver

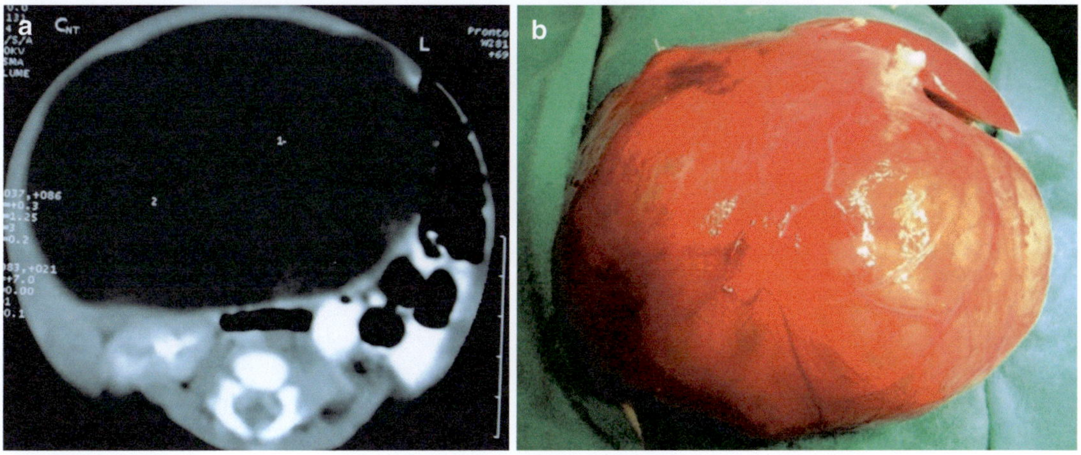

Fig. 60.17 (**a**) CT scan Giant Liver cyst in newborn (**b**) Gross appearance at surgery

diagnosed unresectable patients rather than referring after checking the response of initial chemotherapy.
4. Clinico-radiological follow-up with biomarkers should identify early relapses.
5. Survivors should be screened for ototoxicity and cardiotoxicity depending on the prior chemotherapy.
6. Hepatic hemangiomas need a tailored approach for management depending on the patient's clinical profile.
7. Mesenchymal hamartoma is managed by complete surgical resection as far as possible for a cure.

Suggested Reading

Agarwala S, Gupta A, Bansal D, Vora T, Prasad M, Arora B, Kapoor G, Chinnaswamy G, Radhakrishnan V, Laskar S, Kaur T, Dhaliwal RS, Rath GK, Bakhshi S. Management of Hepatoblastoma: ICMR consensus document. Indian J Pediatr. 2017;84(6):456–64.

Coran AG, Caldamone A, Scott Adzich N, Krummel TM, Laberge JM, editors. Pediatric surgery. 7th ed. Oxford: Elsevier Limited; 2012.

Meyers RL, Maibach R, Hiyama E, Häberle B, Krailo M, Rangaswami A, et al. Risk-stratified staging in paediatric hepatoblastoma: a unified analysis from the children's hepatic tumors international collaboration. Lancet Oncol. 2017;18(1):122–31.

Poplak DG, Pizzo PA. Principles and practice of pediatric oncology. Wolters Kluwer; 2016.

Germ Cell Tumors

61

Sandeep Agarwala and Subhasis Roy Choudhury

61.1 Extracranial Germ Cell Tumors

61.2 Introduction

Germ cell tumors (GCT) originate from the primordial germ cells that migrate from the allantois to the various gonadal sites. During this migration, they can get arrested at various extra-gonadal sites, and so GCT can be gonadal or extra-gonadal in origin. The overall incidence of GCT is about 1 in 100,000 children less than 15 years of age. There are two peaks of occurrence. In the neonates and infancy, it is usually the extra-gonadal and testicular sites, while in the adolescents, it is the ovarian and mediastinal sites. The distribution of germ cell tumors is shown in Table 61.1.

The following are the common features of germ cell tumors in children:

- Extra-gonadal sites predominate compared with gonadal locations and account for about 60% of cases. Of the extra-gonadal sites, the sacrococcygeal site is the commonest, the other sites being mediastinum, retroperitoneum, the head and neck and brain.
- Ovarian germ tumors account for 30%, and testicular germ cell tumors account for the remaining less than 5% cases of GCT.
- Overall, 80% of GCTs are benign.
- The most common benign tumors are teratomas.
- The most common malignant histology is yolk sac tumor (endodermal sinus tumor), which has alpha-fetoprotein (αFP) as a sensitive marker. The other malignant components are choriocarcinoma and embryonal carcinoma.

Table 61.1 Distribution of primary sites of pediatric GCT

SITE	%	SITE	%
Ovary	27	Chest	5.1
Sacrococcygeal	47	Cervical	4.5
CNS	3.6	Pelvic	0.8
Pharynx	2.2	Retroperitoneal	4.0
Testis	4.5	Others	1.0

61.3 Pathology

GCTs can be mature teratoma, immature teratoma, or malignant GCT (MGCT). Most childhood germ cell tumors are benign, comprising mature and immature teratomas (Figs. 61.1a, b and 61.2). Immature teratomas contain primitive neuroepithelium, and based on that, they are

S. Agarwala (✉)
Department of Pediatric Surgery, AIIMS, New Delhi, India

S. Roy Choudhury
Pediatric Surgery, Lady Hardinge Medical College and Associated Kalawati Saran Children's Hospital, New Delhi, Delhi, India

© The Author(s), under exclusive license to Springer Nature Singapore Pte Ltd. 2025
S. Roy Choudhury (ed.), *Pediatric Surgery*, https://doi.org/10.1007/978-981-96-1257-4_61

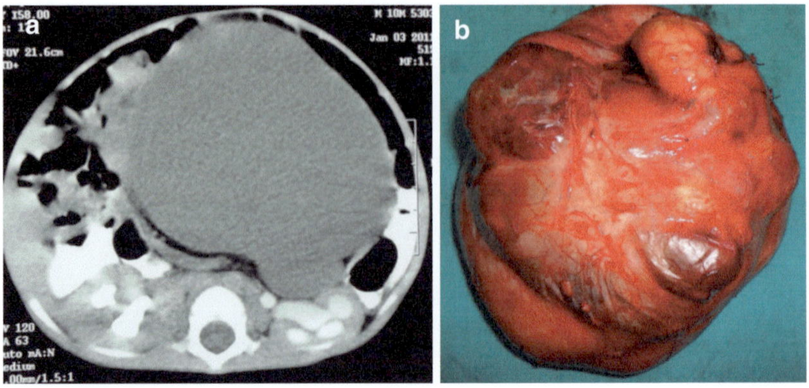

Fig. 61.1 (**a**) CT scan showing intra-abdominal mass, (**b**) surgically removed, mature teratoma

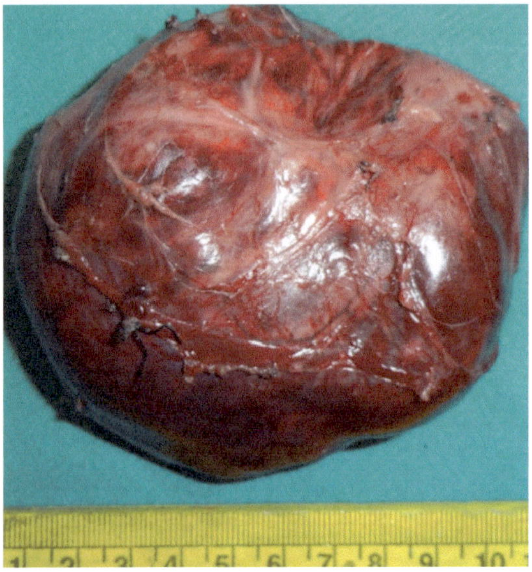

Fig. 61.2 Large pelvic teratoma resected from a newborn

graded between I and III (Norris grading). The pathological types of malignant GCT are yolk sac (endodermal sinus) tumor, dysgerminoma (or seminoma), choriocarcinoma, embryonal carcinoma, polyembryoma, teratocarcinoma and mixed GCT. Yolk sac tumor, also called endodermal sinus tumor (EST), is the most common malignant histologic variant in infancy and childhood.

The most important predictor of tumor recurrence in pediatric immature teratomas is the presence of microscopic foci of yolk sac tumor. Because of their small size, they may be missed by the pathological sampling process.

61.4 Clinical Presentation

The presentation of GCT is either as an asymptomatic mass or due to the mass effect on the surrounding organs.

Ovarian tumors: These are usually seen in adolescent girls. They present with a painless mass in the lower abdomen. Some may present as an acute abdomen due to rupture, hemorrhage, or torsion of the ovary. Torsion is seen invariably in benign ovarian tumors. Occasionally, large pelvic masses can present with urinary obstruction and/or constipation (Fig. 61.3).

Testicular tumors: Testicular GCTs are usually seen in 3–5 year age group. They usually present with a painless mass in the scrotum (Fig. 61.4). Occasionally, pain and inflammatory signs may be present, and differentiation from benign conditions like torsion testis, epididymo-orchitis or traumatic hematoma becomes necessary.

Sacrococcygeal teratoma (SCT): Is the most common neoplasm of the fetus and newborn with an incidence of 1 in 20,000–40,000 live births and has a female predominance. Most SCTs in neonates are histologically benign, and however, at older ages increasing proportions are malignant.

A mass is the usual presentation (Fig. 61.5a, b). Large masses may present with symptoms of mass effect like urinary retention or constipation. Rarely in older children, they may present as a discharging sinus in the gluteal region.

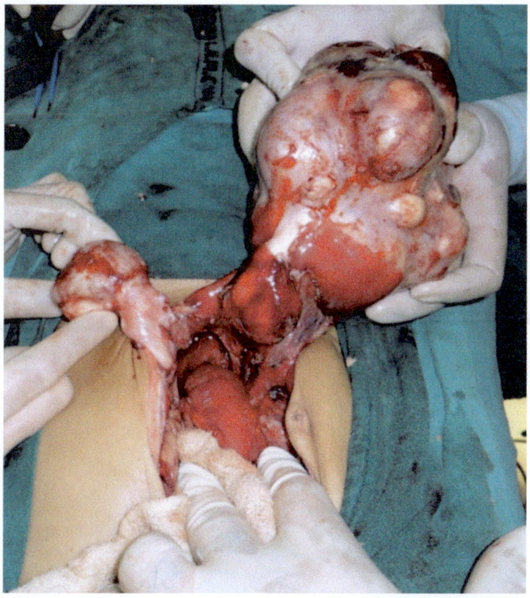

Fig. 61.3 Bilateral ovarian germ cell tumor (left larger than right)

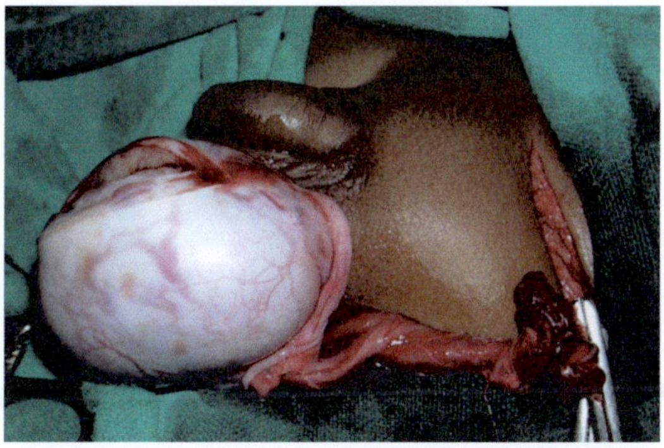

Fig. 61.4 Testicular germ cell tumor; note inguinal approach for orchidectomy

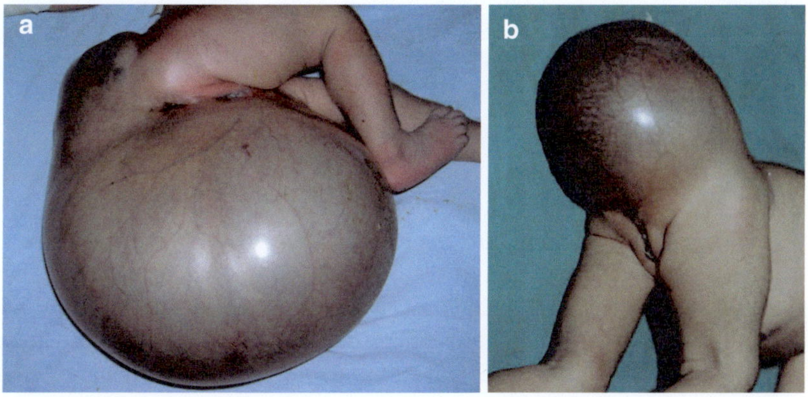

Fig. 61.5 (**a**, **b**) Sacrococcygeal teratoma in a neonate (**a**: Lateral and **b**: Posterior views)

Antenatal diagnosis is also frequently made with the increasing use of antenatal ultrasound scans. The tumor is retrorectal and so can easily be diagnosed with the digital rectal examination. The tumor is present in relation to the coccyx and usually protrudes externally and may extend across the pelvis into the abdomen.

Altman classification has been described based on its local extent. (Fig. 61.6)

Type I lesion has only an external component.

Type II lesion has primarily external but also has pelvic extension.

Type III lesion has little external component and has significant abdomino-pelvic extension.

Type IV lesion does not have an external component.

Risk of malignancy is highest in type IV lesions, probably because they present late.

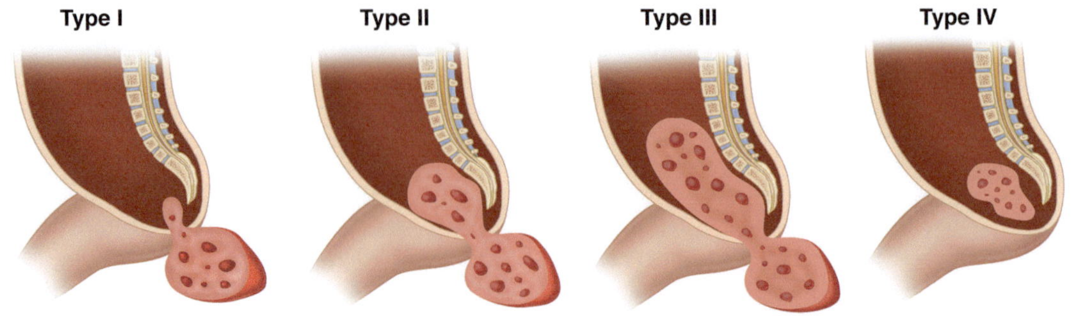

Fig. 61.6 Altman classification of fore types of sacrococcygeal teratoma (kindly reproduce)

Table 61.2 Normal ranges of serum αFP in infants

Age	Mean ± SD (ηg/mL)
Premature	134,734 ± 41,444
Newborn	48,406 ± 34,718
0–2 weeks	33,113 ± 32,503
2 week–1month	9452 ± 12,610
2 month	323 ± 278
3 month	88 ± 87
4 month	74 ± 56
5 month	46.5 ± 19
6 month	12.5 ± 9.8
7 month	9.7 ± 7.1
8 month	8.5 ± 5.5

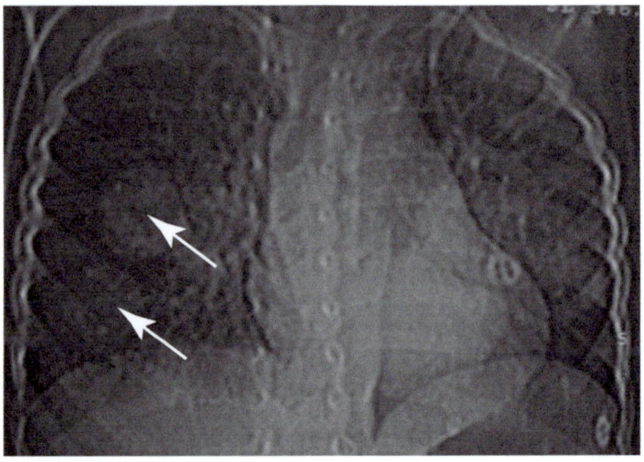

Fig. 61.7 Chest X-ray showing metastatic germ cell tumor

61.5 Investigations

Radiological examinations are done for ascertaining the diagnosis and to look for local extent and for metastases. In infants of less than 2 months of age with sacrococcygeal teratoma, and with a normal aFP value (according to the age-related values—Table 61.2), metastatic workup can be avoided, as the chances of malignancy are very less. A contrast-enhanced CT scan (CECT) is the preferred cross-sectional imaging both for the local extent and the metastatic extent. The benign GCTs have a heterogeneous appearance with areas containing fat, cystic areas and calcification. Calcification is often seen as chunky radio-opaque shadows in plain radiographs and CECT scans. Metastatic workup is done by CECT of the thorax and the abdomen to detect retroperitoneal lymph node metastases or lung metastases. The commonest site of metastasis is the lungs (Figs. 61.7 and 61.8a, b). Bone and bone marrow metastases are extremely rare, and so these sites are not evaluated routinely in GCTs.

Biochemical markers: Serum alpha-fetoprotein (αFP) and beta human chorionic gonadotrophin (βhCG) are markers for EST and choriocarcinoma, respectively. These biomarkers are used for diagnosis, assessment of response and detection of residual disease and recurrence. However, it must be remembered that αFP is normally high in neonates and comes to adult values at approximately 8 months of age. The half-life of αFP is 5 days, and that for βhCG is about 2.5 days. The decline of these serum markers after surgical resection is a log fall, and so it may take some time for these to return to normal levels depending on the initial levels.

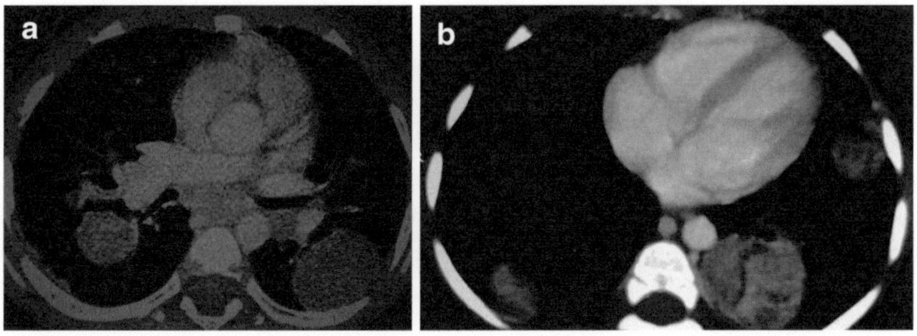

Fig. 61.8 (a, b) CT scan chest, metastatic germ cell tumor

Table 61.3 Staging of malignant germ cell tumors

Testicular	
I	Limited to testis, completely resected by high inguinal orchiectomy; no clinical, radiographic, or histologic evidence of disease beyond the testis; tumor markers normal after appropriate half-life decline; patients with normal or unknown markers at diagnosis must have negative ipsilateral retroperitoneal lymph node sampling to confirm stage 1 disease
II	Transcrotal orchiectomy; microscopic disease in scrotum or high in spermatic cord (<5 cm from proximal end); retroperitoneal lymph node involvement (<2 cm) and/or increased tumor markers after appropriate half-life decline
III	Tumor-positive retroperitoneal lymph node(s) >2 cm diameter: no visceral or extra abdominal involvement
IV	Distant metastases that may include liver
Ovarian	
I	Limited to ovary, peritoneal washings negative for malignant cells; no clinical, radiologic, or histiologic evidence of disease beyond the ovaries (gliomatosis peritonei did not result in upstaging); tumor markers negative after appropriate half-life decline
II	Microscopic residual or positive lymph nodes (<2 cm); peritoneal washings negative for malignant cells (gliomatosis peritonei did not result in upstaging); tumor markers positive or negative
III	Gross residual or biopsy only, tumor-positive lymph node(s) >2 cm diameter; contiguous visceral involvement (omentum, intestine, bladder): peritoneal washings positive for malignant cells
IV	Distant metastases that may include liver
Extragonadal	
I	Complete resection at any site, coccygectomy included as management for sacrococcygeal site, negative tumor margins
II	Microscopic residual; lymph nodes negative
III	Gross residual or biopsy only; regional lymph nodes negative or positive
IV	Distant metastases that may include liver

61.6 Staging

The basic format of staging is stage I being local tumor completely resected, stage II being locally extensive tumor, stage III with lymph nodal metastases and stage IV with distant metastases. Staging is done differently for testicular, ovarian and extra-gonadal tumors, the details of which is given in Table 61.3.

61.7 Treatment

Benign GCT

Excision of the tumor is the primary treatment for all benign GCTs. There is no role of chemotherapy for benign GCTs, and these need to be resected at presentation. In benign GCTs of the testis and ovaries, organ preservation should be the aim by performing tumor enucleation and preserving the affected testis or ovary.

Immature Teratomas

Immature teratoma, in children regardless of histological grade, is treated with surgical resection without any adjuvant chemotherapy. However, for immature teratoma grade III in adolescents, some advocate adjuvant chemotherapy due to the high risk of recurrence and malignant transformation.

Malignant GCT

The treatment of malignant GCT is multi-modal and risk-based. The risk categorization and the treatment are basically based on the location and the stage of the tumor (Table 61.4). Low-risk tumors are treated with surgery alone, and these include stage I testicular EST and stage I ovarian tumors. However, later study results (AGCT0132) showed that stage I ovarian tumors treated with surgery alone had an unacceptably low 3-year EFS, and therefore, stage I ovarian tumors are now considered as intermediate risk and given adjuvant chemotherapy. All malignant GCTs require chemotherapy (adjuvant or neoadjuvant + adjuvant) except stage I EST of the testis.

Malignant GCTs are extremely chemosensitive tumors and respond very well to cisplatin-based chemotherapy like PEB regime (cisplatin, etoposide and bleomycin). Therefore, in large malignant GCTs where upfront extensive surgery may result in incomplete resection, tumor spill or cause significant surgical morbidity or lead to significant deformity, upfront resection should not be attempted. Neoadjuvant chemotherapy is advocated in such cases to achieve tumor reduction, thereby making the resection complete without tumor spill and also less morbid and less deforming.

The current importance of radiotherapy is mainly in the treatment of the seminoma and the ovarian dysgerminoma. The other subtypes are not as responsive. This too has been diminished after the emergence of platinum-based chemotherapy. Recurrent germ cell tumors (unresectable tumor following salvage chemotherapy) may also be treated with radiotherapy. Therefore, radiotherapy is not routinely advocated in the management of most malignant germ cell tumors.

61.8 Surgical Principles for Germ Cell Tumors

Upfront surgery is the treatment of choice for all benign tumors like teratomas and also for malignant germ cell tumors, if feasible. In cases of malignant tumors, the resection should not involve any vital structures as effective chemotherapy is available which can substantially reduce the bulk of the tumor and make resection less morbid.

Ovarian tumors: Operative management is the mainstay of treatment of pediatric germ cell tumors but it is imperative to use reproductive sparing techniques for benign tumors. Ovarian sparing surgery should not be attempted in malignant ovarian GCT. The basic steps are as follows: laparotomy and collection of ascitic fluid of peritoneal washings for cytology; examination of the entire peritoneal surface and liver and biopsy of any suspicious lesions; unilateral oophorectomy. Salpingo-oophorectomy should be done only if the salpinx is involved with the tumor, otherwise attempt should be made to salvage the salpinx. Wedge biopsy of any suspicious lesions of the contralateral ovary. Bilateral involvement is present in 10–15% of dysgerminoma, but is extremely rare with other histological types of GCT (Fig. 61.3). Omentectomy of only the portions adherent to the tumor.

Testicular tumors: The surgical approach mandates an inguinal incision with occlusion of the cord structures by a vascular clamp (Fig. 61.4). The testis is then mobilized into the operative field, and a radical orchiectomy is performed with ligation of all cord structures at the level of the internal ring (high inguinal orchidectomy). Exploration through a scrotal approach should be avoided whenever a

Table 61.4 Risk categorization and treatment for malignant germ cell tumors

Risk	Testicular	Ovarian	Extra-Gonadal	Treatment
Low	Stage I	–	–	Surgery alone
Intermediate	Stage II/II/IV	Stage I/II/III	Stage I	Surgery + PEBx4 cycles
High	–	Stage IV	Stage II/III/IV	Surgery + PEBx4 cycles (6 courses for SCT)

testicular tumor is suspected as it contaminates another lymphatic area and can lead to recurrence.

Testicular endodermal sinus tumors (EST): These tumors are localized (stage I) in up to 85% of the cases. For stage I tumors, only surgery is recommended with a prolonged follow-up. While for stage II or III disease, surgery should include high ligation and orchiectomy followed by chemotherapy with platinum-based regime, namely PEB or JEB. Retroperitoneal lymph node (RPLN) sampling is rarely indicated. RPLN, that is >5 cm on CECT, is taken as involved and the patient is accordingly staged. All RPLN <5 cm are considered not involved to begin with. In these cases, if the αFP shows a log fall after high inguinal orchidectomy and achieves normal range, then these patients are stage I and are risk categorized and treated accordingly. In case the αFP does not decline or declines initially but then starts to rise again, then these nodes are considered involved and the patient is staged as stage III and treated accordingly. In a small proportion of case where the αFP is not elevated at presentation (5% of testicular EST), and the RPLN is < than 5 cm in size, RPLN biopsy must be carried out for accurate staging and appropriate treatment. *Testicular teratomas*: These consist of 10% of all testicular neoplasms in children and occur mostly before the age of 4 years. If the preoperative evaluation has revealed that the mass is occupying a part of the testis and/or is cystic in nature, it is likely to be a testicular teratoma. A testicular teratoma can be safely enucleated and sent for frozen section. If the frozen confirms a teratoma, the cord's blood supply is restored and the testis is repositioned back into the scrotum. Testicular teratomas are mostly mature and benign lesions accounting for 10–40% of the pediatric germ cell tumors (67) and can be safely treated by enucleation alone.

Extra-gonadal germ cell tumors: A benign sacrococcygeal teratoma needs to be excised completely and at diagnosed. The excision should always be combined with coccygectomy, or else there is a very high risk of recurrence rate to the tune of 37–40%. An inverted "V" incision is the one commonly employed but for tumors extending cranially beyond the bony pelvis an abdominal mobilization may first be required. In older infants and children who present with large malignant sacrococcygeal teratoma, preoperative cytoreduction with 2 courses of PEB regimen is recommended which is then followed by surgery and adjuvant chemotherapy. As most neonatal sacrococcygeal teratomas are mature or immature teratomas, they are treated with surgery alone with postoperative follow-up with serum αFP levels which should decline to normal levels (for age) within 3–4 weeks postoperatively. Any elevation in serum αFP levels after normal decline or a persistently elevated αFP should be evaluated for recurrent or residual disease, respectively. All malignant and recurrent teratomas need to be treated with chemotherapy. The survival rate for malignant sacrococcygeal teratoma has improved from 11% (before 1978) to 86% (after 1978) basically because of the institution of platinum-based regimens, namely PVB, PEB and JEB.

61.9 Fetus in Fetu

Fetus in fetu is nothing but a benign mature teratoma containing derivatives of all three germinal layers. This is characterized by organized musculoskeletal, vertebral and organ structures resembling a fetus (Fig. 61.9). The presence of

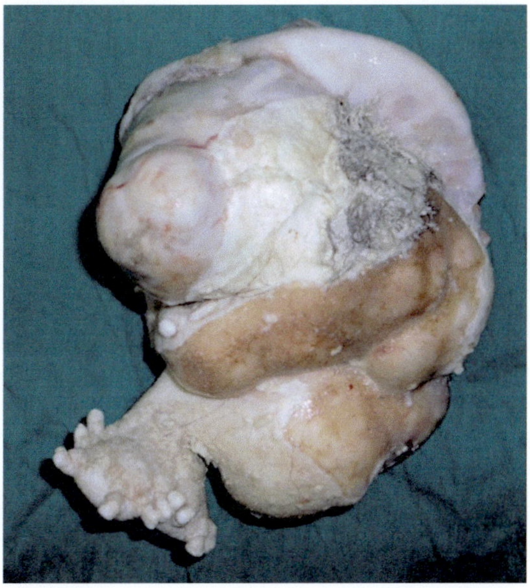

Fig. 61.9 Fetus in fetu specimen, showing hair and mature body parts

derivatives of the notochord (vertebral column) is essential to label a mature teratoma as a fetus in fetu. Complete surgcal removal is the treatment.

61.10 Summary

1. These tumors arise on the path of the migration of the germ cells from the yolk sac to the genital ridge.
2. 60% are extra-gonadal. Most GCT are benign and need to be excised at presentation.
3. The most common histological type of malignancy is Endodermal sinus tumor (Yolk sac tumor).
4. Raised serum αFP is a very sensitive biomarker for EST and serum βhCG for choriocarcinoma.
5. Malignant tumors are very chemo sensitive to Platinum based chemotherapy and so respond well.
6. All GCT's need to be excised. Malignant GCT's that are very large benefit from neoadjuvant chemotherapy prior to excision.
7. The malignant GCT's (MGCT) require additional adjuvant chemotherapy in nearly all cases.
8. Radiation therapy is not used in the treatment of MGCT.
9. The overall outcome is better for gonadal MGCT as compared to extra-gonadal MGCT's. The overall survival is at present greater than 90%.

Suggested Reading

Carachi R, Grosfeld JL, Azmy AF. The surgery of childhood tumours. 2nd ed. Heidelberg: Springer; 2008.

Coran AG, Caldamone A, Scott Adzich N, Krummel TM, Laberge JM, editors. Pediatric surgery. 7th ed. Oxford: Elsevier; 2012.

Poplak DG, Pizzo PA. Principles and practice of pediatric oncology. 7th ed. Philadelphia: Wolters Kluwer; 2016.

Soft Tissue Sarcomas

62

Sandeep Agarwala, Subhasis Roy Choudhury, and Lavleen Singh

62.1 Introduction

Soft tissue sarcomas (STSs) are a diverse group of malignant tumors that originate in the connective tissues, including lymphatics, vessels, smooth and striated muscles, fat, fascia, synovium, endothelium, and reticuloendothelium. These tumors are found to be more prevalent in males as compared to females. Among STS, rhabdomyosarcoma (RMS), which is committed to skeletal muscle lineage, is the third most common pediatric extracranial neoplasm after neuroblastoma and Wilms' tumor, comprising 15% of all solid tumors. The remaining cases comprise a diverse group of non-rhabdomyosarcomas (NRSTS), including synovial sarcoma, fibrosarcoma, and malignant peripheral nerve sheath tumors, among others. RMS exhibits a bimodal incidence pattern, with nearly two-thirds of cases diagnosed in children under 6 years of age, followed by a second peak in mid-adolescence. RMS can arise in various anatomical regions, with 35% occurring in head and neck, 22% in the genitourinary followed by trunk (27%) and extremities (14%) (Table 62.1). For localized rhabdomyosarcoma, the five-year overall survival rate reaches around 70% with local control being achieved in 80–90% of these cases.

S. Agarwala (✉)
Department of Pediatric Surgery, AIIMS, New Delhi, India

S. Roy Choudhury
Pediatric Surgery, Lady Hardinge Medical College and Associated Kalawati Saran Children's Hospital, New Delhi, Delhi, India

L. Singh
Department of Pathology, AIIMS, New Delhi, India

© The Author(s), under exclusive license to Springer Nature Singapore Pte Ltd. 2025

S. Roy Choudhury (ed.), *Pediatric Surgery*, https://doi.org/10.1007/978-981-96-1257-4_62

Table 62.1 Sites of RMS

Region (incidence)	Favorable sites	Unfavorable sites
Head and neck (35%)	Nonorbital non-parameningeal (30%-oral cavity, larynx, parotid region, cheek, scalp, and soft tissues of the neck)	Parameningeal (44%-ear, mastoid, nasal cavity, paranasal sinuses, infratemporal fossa, and pterygopalatine fossa)
	Orbital (25%)	
Genitourinary (22%)	Vulva, vagina, uterus, paratesticular	Bladder, prostate, kidney, and ureters
Extremities (14%)		All
Trunk (27%)		All
Others		Biliary, retroperitoneum, perineum and perianal

62.2 Diagnosis of RMS

62.2.1 Clinical Presentation

RMS of Head and Neck Region (Fig. 62.1): According to the site of origin, tumors involving nasopharynx, paranasal sinuses and middle ear present early with swelling or bleeding from nose or ear. Orbital RMS generally presents with symptoms like chemosis, proptosis or a conjunctival mass. Although regional lymph nodes are mostly not involved, these tumors behave in an aggressive manner with erosion of bony margins and infiltration in various head and neck spaces.

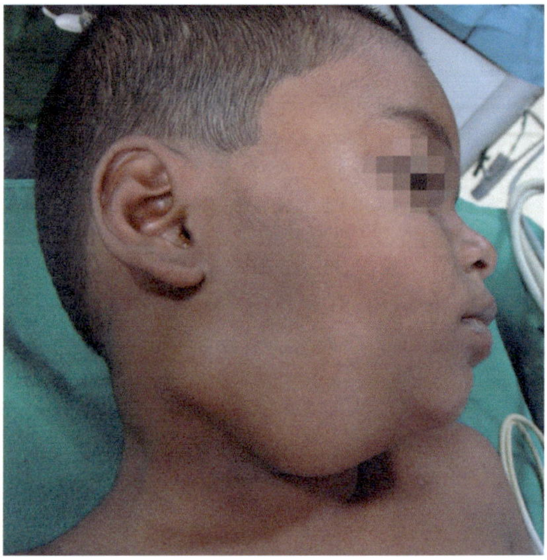

Fig. 62.1 RMS of the head and neck region

RMS of Trunk and Extremities (Fig. 62.2): RMS at these locations presents with a tender or non-tender swelling at the local site, which can be mistaken as a hematoma following a trivial trauma or an abscess. RMS of the extremities are more prevalent in the older age group and present more commonly in the lower limbs. Regional lymph nodes are positive in 30–50% cases but all may not be clinically palpable.

RMS of the Genitourinary System (Fig. 62.3): RMS of the bladder/prostate can present with varied lower urinary tract symptoms including storage symptoms such as urinary urgency, frequency; voiding symptoms like intermittency and retention and sometimes even with gross hematuria. Paratesticular tumors manifest as a painless, hard scrotal mass which can also indicate secondary symptoms due to a larger intra-abdominal mass. Vaginal RMS presents as fleshy polypoidal tissue protruding from the vaginal orifice or as bleeding per vaginum in a young child (Fig. 62.4).

Imaging Initial plain X-ray of the local site may demonstrate a soft tissue mass with calcifications. Sonography is the most useful investigation particularly in genitourinary RMS to locate the site of origin of the tumor and detect hydronephrosis or a large bladder indicating an obstructive lesion. For definitive histopathological diagnosis, USG- or CT-guided core needle biopsies can be performed. For detailed evaluation of the primary site and tumor extent, cross-sectional

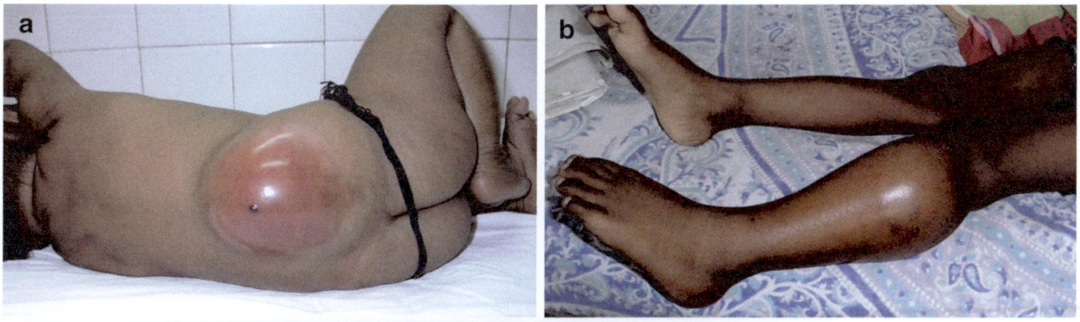

Fig. 62.2 (**a**) RMS trunk (**b**) RMS lower limb

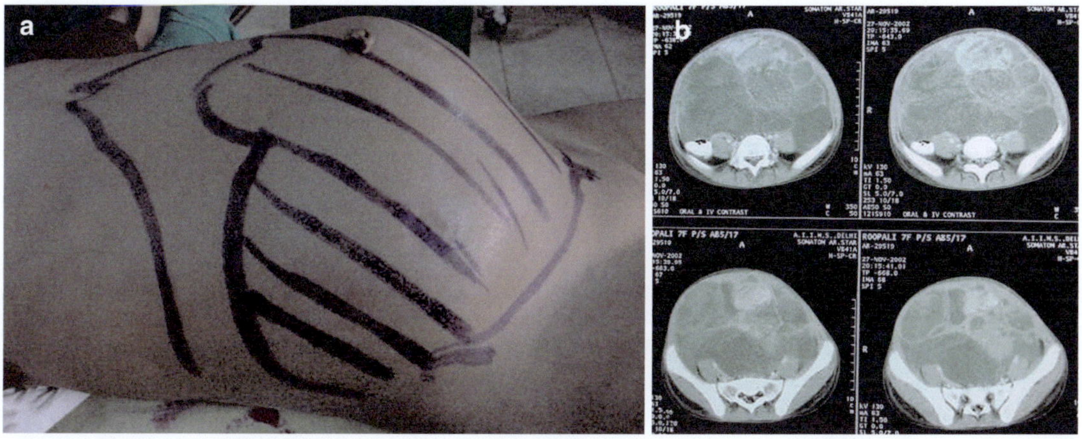

Fig. 62.3 (**a**) RMS bladder in a female child (**b**) Contrast-enhanced CT scan of the same patient showing a large heterogenous mass

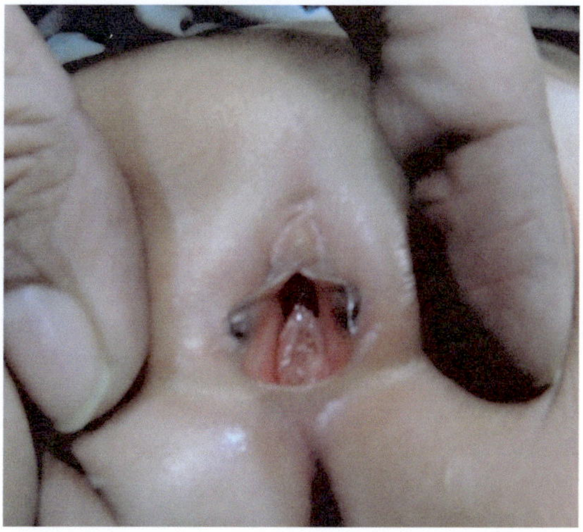

Fig. 62.4 Vaginal polyps in a girl child with RMS vagina

imaging like contrast-enhanced CT scan (CECT) and/or magnetic resonance imaging scans (MRI) of the affected region are required (Figs. 62.5, 62.6 and 62.7). CT scan of the chest is the most sensitive imaging modality to assess for pulmonary metastases, even more sensitive than FDG-PET for this purpose, and is required irrespective of the radiological study performed. Nuclear imaging modalities utilizing technetium 99 m diphosphonate are used for detecting bony metastases. In cases of extremity RMS, Tc-99 labeled radiocolloids injected in and around the primary tumor can map the sentinel draining lymph nodes. The utility of positron emission tomography (PET scans) in soft tissue sarcomas is still being investigated.

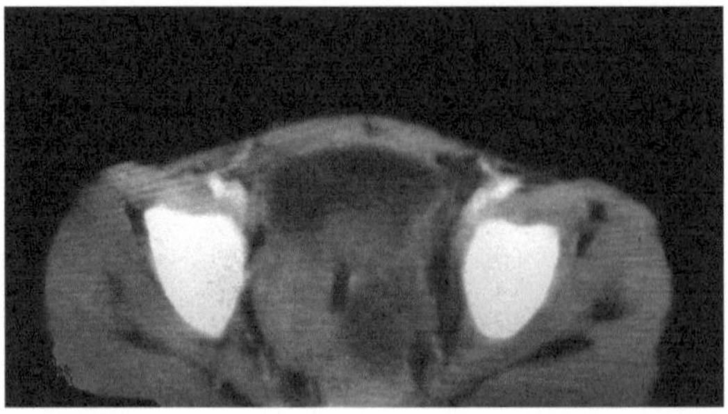

Fig. 62.5 Contrast-enhanced CT scan of a child with RMS Bladder/prostate showing involvement of the bladder base and the prostatic region with compression of the urethra

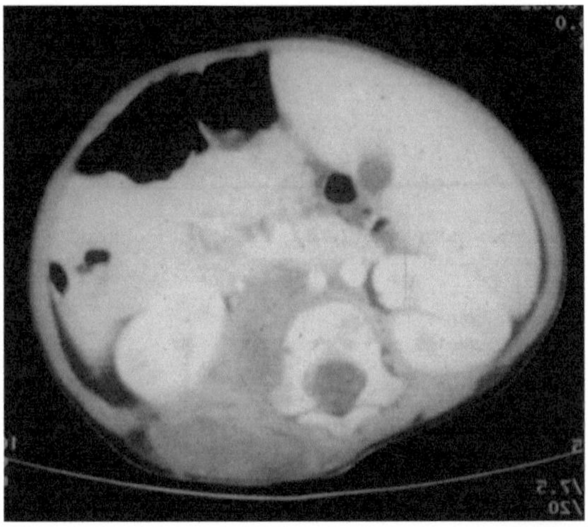

Fig. 62.6 CECT scan of a child with RMS of the trunk

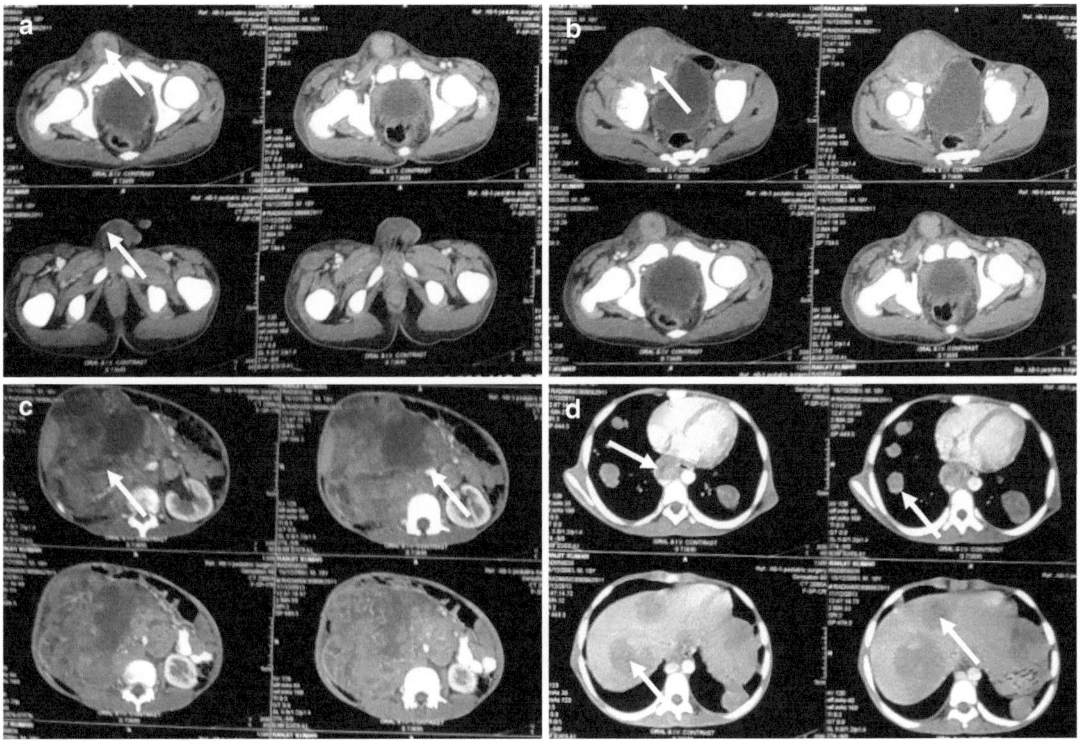

Fig. 62.7 (**a**) CECT scans of a boy with paratesticular RMS (**b**) Extension into the cord structures in the inguinal canal (**c**) Massive right retroperitoneal lymphadenopathy encasing the aorta and inferior vena cava (**d**) Multiple hepatic metastases, nodal involvement of the mediastinum, and multiple bilateral pulmonary metastases

Biopsy The biopsy of the affected region can be obtained either by an open incisional technique or USG or CT-guided core needle biopsy. Biopsies of the trunk and extremity RMS should be done along the long axis of the tumor, so as to include the biopsied site in the eventual formal resection. No attempt should be made at en bloc resection of the tumor at the initial presentation as there is a high risk of compromising adjacent vital tissues which may have been invaded by the primary tumor and also landing with positive margins on subsequent pathological evaluation.

Staging For subsequent management and prognostication of RMS, it is vital to properly stage every patient of RMS. Staging requires thorough clinical examination, laboratory, and radiological investigations. Size prior to treatment is assessed by clinical measurements or CT/MRI, depending upon the anatomical location. CT is utilized as a means of lymph nodal assessment in cases of less accessible primary sites. Metastatic workup involves some form of imaging (but not histologic confirmation, except for bone marrow examination). Biopsy is essential for histopathological diagnosis. Clinical grouping system used by the International Rhabdomyosarcoma Study Group (IRSG) is the most widely used staging system (Table 62.2).

Modified TNM pre-treatment staging classification for RMS is also used for risk categorization of RMS (Table 62.3).

Table 62.2 Clinical grouping (CG) system used by the International Rhabdomyosarcoma Study Group (IRSG)

Group I: Localized disease, completely resected
A confined to the organ or muscle of origin.
B infiltration outside organ or muscle of origin; regional nodes not involved.
Group II: Total gross resection with evidence of regional spread
A grossly resected tumors with "microscopic" residual tumor.
B regional disease completely resected with regional nodes involved, tumor extension into adjacent organs, or both.
Group III: Incomplete resection or biopsy with gross residual disease remaining.
A localized or locally extensive tumor, gross residual disease after biopsy only.
B localized or locally extensive tumor, gross residual disease after "major" resection (>50% debulking).
Group IV: Any size primary tumor, with or without regional lymph node involvement, with distant metastases, irrespective of surgical approach to the primary tumor.

Prognostic Factors, Risk Categorization and Outcome of Management of RMS The Prognostic analysis of patients with RMS takes into account multiple factors. The clinical grouping, TNM staging, primary tumor site and histology are used concurrently for risk categorization of the tumor and predicting the outcome for a patient (Table 62.4).

Table 62.3 TNM pre-treatment staging classification for RMS

Stage	Sites	T	Size	N	M
1	Favorable	T1 or T2	a or b	N0 or N1 or Nx	M0
2	Unfavorable	T1 or T2	a	N0 or Nx	M0
3	Unfavorable	T1 or T2	a	N1 M0	
		b	N0 or N1 or Nx	M0	
4	Either	T1 or T2	a or b	N0 or N1	M1

Definitions:

Site:

Favorable sites: Orbit, head and neck (excluding parameningeal), or genitourinary (excluding bladder/prostate)

Unfavorable sites: Bladder/prostate, parameningeal, extremities, trunk, and all others

Tumor: T1 = Tumor confined to anatomic site of origin

a) ≤5 cm in diameter

b) >5 cm in diameter

T2 = Extension and/or fixation to surrounding tissues

a) ≤5 cm in diameter

b) >5 cm in diameter

Regional nodes:

N0: Regional nodes not clinically involved

N1: Regional nodes clinically involved by tumor

Nx: Clinical status of regional nodes unknown (especially sites which preclude lymph node evaluation)

Metastasis:

M0: No distant metastases

MI: Metastases present

Table 62.4 Risk categorization for RMS

Risk group	TNM	CG	Site	Histology	Outcome (EFS)
Low subset A	1 or 2	I or II	FH or UFH	ERMS	Excellent (<85%)
	1	III	Orbit only	ERMS	
Low subset B	1	III	FH	ERMS	Very good (70–85%)
	3	I or II	UFH	ERMS	
Intermediate	2 or 3	III	UFH	ERMS	Good (50–70%)
	1–3	I–III	FH or UFH	ARMS	
High	4	IV	FH or UFH	ERMS or ARMS	Poor (<35%)

See Table on TNM for list of FH and UFH sites

FH Favorable site, *UFH* Unfavorable site, *ERMS* Embryonal RMS, *ARMS* Alveolar RMS

62.3 Pathology

Histology and Immunohistology Histologically, RMS depicts small round blue cell morphology which also comprises neuroblastoma, Ewing's sarcoma, small cell osteogenic sarcoma, and lymphomas. These tumors are histologically differentiated by H and E staining and molecular genetic analysis. The widely used international classification system for childhood RMS (Table 62.5) divides RMS into superior, intermediate, and poor prognosis based on histological types. Embryonal RMS (ERMS) which is the commonest type (70% of all RMS) has an intermediate prognosis. Spindle cell and botryoid subtypes of embryonal RMS have a superior prognosis. Alveolar RMS (ARMS) comprises 30% of RMS. The anaplastic variant of RMS is extremely rare in children (<1%) and is the same as pleomorphic in adults. On IHC staining, skeletal or smooth muscle-specific proteins such as anti-desmin, muscle-specific actin, and Myo D can be identified.

Table 62.5 International classification system for childhood rhabdomyosarcomas

I	Superior prognosis
	(a) Botryoid
	(b) Spindle cell
II	Intermediate prognosis
	(a) Embryonal
III	Poor prognosis
	(a) Alveolar
	(b) Undifferentiated sarcomas

Molecular Cytogenetics Distinct specific genetic alterations have been found in ERMS and ARMS. 80% of ERMS have an allelic loss of heterozygosity at 11p15.5. Similar percentage of ARMS have translocation between FKHR gene on chromosome 13 and either PAX3 gene on chromosome 2, t(2:3)(q35;q14) or PAX7 gene on chromosome 1, (t1:13)(p36;q14) resulting in PAX3/FOXO1 or PAX7/FOXO1 fusion gene, respectively, which results in formation of PAX3-FKHR and PAX7-FKHR fusion proteins, respectively. These fusion genes aid in the diagnosis of ARMS. Twenty percent of ARMS do not have these fusion proteins (Fusion negative ARMS), and this subset of ARMS behaves clinically as ERMS, with outcomes also being similar to the latter.

62.3.1 Treatment of RMS

Multimodality treatment comprising surgical resections, radiation therapy (RT), and systemic chemotherapy is utilized in RMS.

Principles of Chemotherapy All patients with RMS receive chemotherapy. The VAC regime (vincristine, actinomycin D, cyclophosphamide) is the gold standard chemotherapy protocol.

Principles of Radiation Therapy It is a vital prong for treatment in RMS as it improves local disease control and outcomes. In general, all patients receive RT, except for low-risk subset A(CG I). Those patients who on evaluation are found to have node-positive disease, the radiation protocol includes the involved lymph node site.

Resection of Primary Tumor The cornerstone in surgery for RMS is complete resection of the tumor along with a rim of normal tissue, also offering maximum possible functionality and good cosmetic outcomes. Complete oncological resection with no residual microscopic disease provides the best cure rates. Debulking surgery has no role in case of RMS. The surgical management depends on the primary site of origin, size of tumor, regional lymph nodal positivity, and distant metastases. At primary resection if there is a suspicion of positive margin, a biopsy of the margin should be obtained. Titanium clips should be placed in cases of gross residual disease or microscopic positivity which is unresectable so as to direct re-excision and later RT. Most tumors are either large or involve adjacent vital structures, hence being unresectable at presentation and so will require neo-adjuvant chemotherapy with or without RT for a safe and complete surgical resection.

Primary Re-Excision (PRE) PRE is done prior to the institution of any other adjuvant therapy. It comprises complete re-excision of the prior operative site which on histopathology shows negative margins. PRE is usually done in cases where only biopsy was performed initially but the primary tumor was resectable, or if a non-oncologic surgical excision was done, and if the margin status is not defined. PRE improves survival outcomes in localized RMS of the trunk and extremities.

Lymph Node (LN) Evaluation LN evaluation is required for deciding a treatment approach, lymph nodal positivity being considered as an important poor prognostic marker. Regional LN assessment includes clinical and radiological evaluations in conjunction with pathology for extremity RMS, where there is a high incidence of regional lymph nodal metastases (40–50%). The draining lymph nodes include the axillary nodes for upper extremity and inguinal nodes for lower extremity. Only about 3% of head and neck RMS have regional lymph nodal metastases, and hence, routine biopsy is not required. However, enlarged nodes should be biopsied. In the case of paratesticular RMS, if the retroperitoneal nodes (iliac and para-aortic/paracaval) are larger than 2 cm on CT evaluation, they are taken as positive and staged accordingly, with no need of being biopsied.

Second Look Operation (SLO) SLO consists of surgical exploration and resection of residual primary tumor being found on repeat imaging after completing the multiagent neoadjuvant chemotherapy with or without RT.

62.3.2 Surgical Principles for Various Sites

In the *head and neck RMS* at the orbital site, biopsy followed by chemoradiotherapy usually suffices.

Genitourinary RMS In the case of bladder prostate RMS, extensive resections may not be required after completion of chemotherapy and RT. Upfront surgical resection at these sites is only reserved for a small subset of patients who have a primary tumor involving the bladder dome. Resection through an inguinal incision is required in all paratesticular tumors along with the entire spermatic cord being excised, either upfront or following neoadjuvant chemotherapy. Attempt to biopsy or excision via scrotal approach should be avoided in view of alteration of lymphatic drainage which will then require hemiscrotectomy. RPLN biopsy and ipsilateral RP lymph node dissection are undertaken only for children aged more than 10 years. In case of vulval, vaginal, and uterine RMS, if radiological CR is not attained or those with early disease progression on induction chemotherapy and RT, surgical resection is needed.

Extremity RMS Most of the patients will require tumor resection following neoadjuvant chemotherapy. Upfront resection is only reserved for tumors which are smaller in size, which can be resected completely with negative margins, and will preserve the maximum possible functionality. All other lesions should only undergo an incisional biopsy. Sentinel draining lymph nodal sampling should always be performed during the initial biopsy, even if not clinically palpable and not enlarged on radiological evaluation.

62.3.3 Non-rhabdomyosarcoma Soft Tissue Sarcoma (NRSTS)

NRSTS are uncommon pediatric tumors, making up less than half of all pediatric soft tissue sarcomas, and can originate in any part of the body (Table 62.6, Fig. 62.8 a,b). The most frequent histologic types are synovial sarcoma, neurofibrosarcoma, and fibrosarcoma. Clinically, they manifest as painless masses at the site of origin, 15% being already metastatic at diagnosis. Lungs and brain remain the most common sites for metastases, while regional lymph node metastases and bone marrow involvement are extremely uncommon. Tumors involving the trunk comprise mainly malignant fibrous histiocytomas (MFH), malignant peripheral nerve sheath tumors, neurofibrosarcoma, and malignant schwannoma, latter three being neurogenic in origin.

Histology and Grading of NRSTS (Table 62.7): On histologic examination, most of the pediatric NRSTS are immature and show

Table 62.6 Some common and uncommon NRSTS seen in children

Common	Rare
Synovial sarcoma	Angiosarcoma
Fibrosarcoma	Hemangiopericytoma
Peripheral neuroectodermal tumor	Clear cell sarcoma
Malignant fibrous histiocytoma	Epitheloid cell sarcoma
Leiomyosarcoma	Intra-abdominal desmoplastic tumor
Neurogenic tumors	Malignant mesenchymoma
Malignant schwannoma	
Neurofibrosarcoma	
Malignant peripheral nerve sheath tumor	Extra-skeletal chondrosarcoma

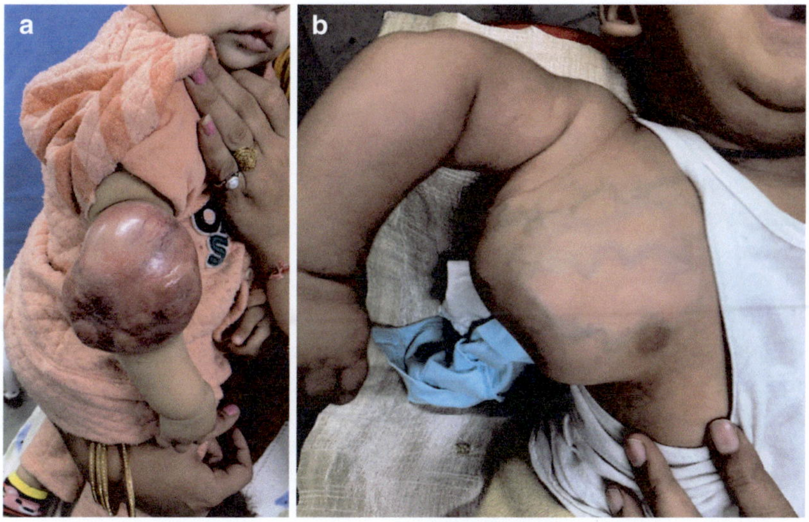

Fig. 62.8 (**a**, **b**) Non-rhabdomyomatous soft tissue sarcoma in infants

Table 62.7 Schema for grading of NRSTS in children

Grade 1
Myxoid well-differentiated liposarcoma
Deep-seated dermatofibrosarcoma protuberans
Well-differentiated or infantile (age < 5 years) fibrosarcoma.
Well-differentiated or infantile (age < 5 years) hemangiopericytoma
Well-differentiated malignant peripheral nerve sheath tumor.
Angiomatoid malignant fibrous histiocytoma
Grade 2
Sarcomas not specifically included in grade 1 or 3; <15% of tumor showing geographic necrosis or the mitotic index is <5 per 10 high-power fields.
Grade 3
Pleomorphic or round cell liposarcoma
Mesenchymal chondrosarcoma
Extra-skeletal osteosarcoma
Malignant triton tumor
Alveolar soft part sarcoma

poor differentiation with around half of these tumors having a histologic grade 3.

Prognostic Factors Depends upon: Extent of primary tumor (metastatic vs non-metastatic); histologic grade (low vs high); size of primary tumor (< 5 cm vs > 5 cm); extent of surgical resection (resectable vs unresectable).

62.3.4 Clinical Evaluation and Staging of NRSTS

The imaging investigation of choice is MRI for evaluation of the locoregional disease, irrespective of the tumor being located in the head and neck region, pelvis, or extremities. The modified TNM staging system used for RMS as described before is currently being employed for NRSTS as well. For histopathological subtyping, cytogenetic and molecular studies, core needle biopsy is essential. Excisional biopsy is only used when the primary tumor is small (<2.5 cm), otherwise should be rarely undertaken. Routine regional lymph node evaluation is not required as regional metastases are rare.

Treatment of NRSTS The treatment approach is multi-pronged, mostly similar to that in adults with only some differences. Cornerstone is the achievement of local control, and wide local excision (WLE) should be undertaken wherever feasible. According to the current COG guidelines, negative margins are defined as the presence of at least 0.5 cm of nonmalignant tissue around the resected specimen. In cases where periosteum or fascia lie in close relation and about the tumor, their removal in continuity with the tumor is taken as negative margins. Adjuvant RT is considered when the surgical reaction achieved is less than as described for WLE. Neoadjuvant chemotherapy and/or RT is used in unresectable NRSTS. No standard guidelines currently exist for RT in pediatric NRSTS, and external beam radiation therapy (EBRT) is considered the preferred modality. Pediatric NRSTS are not frequently chemosensitive, and guidelines for the same are not currently well defined. Indications for administration of chemotherapy include unresectable tumors and large, high-grade resected tumors which show a high propensity for metastatic recurrence. Doxorubicin and Ifosfamide are two chemotherapeutic drugs which show some response in NRSTS.

62.3.5 Ewing Sarcoma and Undifferentiated Small Round Cell Sarcomas of Bone and Soft Tissue

Ewing sarcoma (ES) represents an undifferentiated small round cell sarcoma (USRCS) characterized by the fusion of a member of the FET gene family (including FUS, EWSR1, and TAF15) with an ETS family transcription factor.

The USRCS classification has undergone a major shift in recent years, facilitated by the emergence of sophisticated high-throughput molecular methodologies that elucidate various underlying molecular phenomena. Within the fifth edition of the World Health Organization (WHO) classification of soft tissue and bone tumors, released in 2020, USRCS has been established as a distinct chapter that encompasses Ewing sarcoma alongside three additional sarcoma subsets: (1) round cell sarcoma exhibiting EWSR1::non-ETS fusions, (2) CIC-rearranged sarcomas, and (3) sarcomas harboring BCOR genetic alterations.

ES accounts for approximately 6–8% of all primary malignant bone neoplasms. In the pediatric age group, it ranks as the second most prevalent malignant bone tumor following osteosarcoma. The peak incidence of bone Ewing sarcoma is during the second decade of life, while soft tissue Ewing sarcoma presents at a slightly older age. There exists a notable male predominance, with a male-to-female ratio of 3:2. The remaining USRCS variants are exceedingly rare.

Clinical Presentation

Individuals afflicted with Ewing sarcoma and other undifferentiated round cell sarcomas (URCS) typically exhibit localized manifestations such as pain, stiffness, or swelling, persisting for several weeks to months. The emergence of systemic manifestations, including pyrexia and unexplained weight loss, frequently signifies the presence of metastatic disease.

Morphology and IHC

Ewing sarcoma is morphologically identified by sheets of uniform malignant small blue round cells, characterized by frequent mitotic activity and varying degrees of necrosis. The individual neoplastic cells exhibit stippled chromatin, subtle nucleoli, and a scant amount of clear to eosinophilic cytoplasm (Fig. 62.9a, b). These tumor cells are abundant in glycogen, which can be highlighted using Periodic acid–Schiff (PAS) staining in conjunction with diastase. The tumor cells demonstrate diffuse membranous positivity for the MIC-2 antigen; additionally, NKX2.2 (nuclear) is regarded as highly specific (Fig. 62.10a, b). Moreover, positivity for FLI-1 and ERG is contingent upon the specific translocation partner. The adamantinoma-like variant of Ewing sarcoma reveals diffuse positivity for epithelial markers, including cytokeratin and p40.

The EWSR1-non-ETS fusion sarcoma typically exhibits uniform round cells interspersed with a myxoid matrix. The neoplastic cells demonstrate diffuse expression of CD99 in approximately 50% of instances; expression of NKX2–2 may also be observed. Emerging biomarkers such as AGGRECAN and NKX3–1 could provide additional diagnostic value.

CIC-rearranged sarcomas reveal a diffuse or indistinctly lobular or nodular architectural pattern. The neoplastic cells present as small to medium-sized, exhibiting round to oval shapes with localized spindling. A moderate degree of

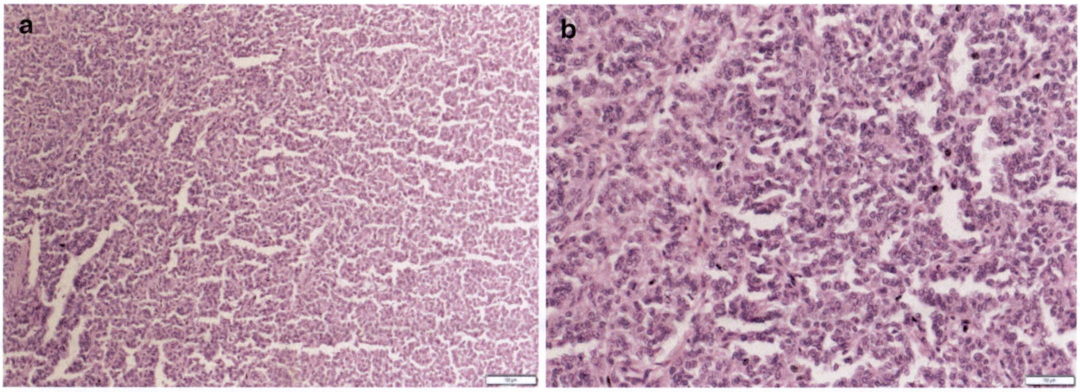

Fig. 62.9 Photomicrograph showing a case of Ewing sarcoma exhibiting a densely cellular tumor with a predominantly solid growth pattern [**a**; H&E x10]. The neoplastic cells showing round to oval nuclei with high nucleocytoplasmic ratio, hyperchromasia, stippled chromatin, indistinct nucleoli, and a scant amount of clear to eosinophilic cytoplasm [**b**; H&E x20]

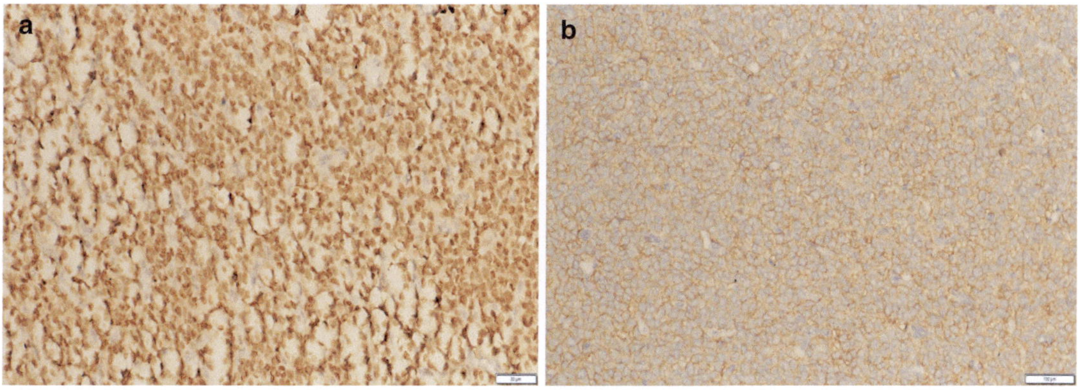

Fig. 62.10 Photomicrograph showing the immunohistochemical staining for NKX2.2(nuclear) [**a**, IHC NKX2.2] and MIC2 (membranous) [**b**, IHC MIC2] in a case of Ewing sarcoma

nuclear pleomorphism and intra-tumoral heterogeneity may be evident. The cytoplasmic composition ranges from pale eosinophilic to clear, with the nuclei predominantly displaying a vesicular form accompanied by prominent nucleoli, and mitotic figures are frequently encountered. The epithelioid or rhabdoid morphologies are commonly observed.

Upon immunohistochemical analysis, the tumor cells exhibit positivity for CD99 (which may be diffuse or patchy, membranous and/or cytoplasmic), WT-1 (nuclear with or without cytoplasmic expression in up to 95% of cases), and ETV-4.

Sarcomas characterized by BCOR genetic alterations encompass both BCOR rearranged sarcomas and those exhibiting BCOR internal tandem duplications. The histopathological features of BCOR rearranged sarcomas reveal a nesting architecture consisting of primitive, small, round to slightly elongated cells, which are enveloped by an abundant capillary network. Areas of hypocellularity interspersed with discohesive spindle cells in a conspicuous myxoid matrix are often noted. The nuclei show finely dispersed chromatin, with nucleoli generally remaining inconspicuous. The mitotic activity within these sarcomas presents variability.

BCOR-ITD soft tissue tumors, including infantile undifferentiated sarcoma and PMMTI, exhibit heterogeneous cellularity that ranges from solid aggregates of small primitive ovoid cells to hypocellular regions featuring dispersed stellate cells arranged within a myxoid matrix accompanied by delicate vascular structures. Tumors demonstrating a predominance of spindle cell morphology may closely resemble infantile fibrosarcoma. Furthermore, these tumors infiltrate adjacent tissues and exhibit a high frequency of mitotic figures.

On immunohistochemistry, all sarcomas harboring BCOR gene alterations manifest robust and diffuse nuclear BCOR positivity; additionally, in a majority of instances, there is expression of SATB2, TLE1, and cyclin D1. MIC-2 (CD99) positivity is observed in approximately 50% of cases. Moreover, BCOR:CCNB3 sarcoma exhibits reactivity to CCNB3, a feature not observed in other tumors associated with the BCOR family. BCOR-ITD soft tissue tumors demonstrate strong and diffuse positivity for EGFR.

62.3.6 Management

Ewing sarcoma (ES) patients are managed through a combination of systemic chemotherapy alongside surgical intervention and/or radiation therapy aimed at achieving local tumor control. Initially, patients are administered chemotherapy prior to the implementation of local-control strategies. The assessment of surgical margins and the histological response is critical factors influencing postoperative therapeutic decisions. Patients exhibiting metastatic disease frequently demonstrate a favorable response to preoperative chemotherapy. Effective local management of metastatic sites, particularly those involving bone metastases, is of paramount importance.

Utilizing this multimodal treatment strategy, the prognosis for ES has markedly improved, achieving a cure rate of 65–70% for localized cases. Conversely, the prognosis for metastatic and early relapsing tumors remains dismal, with a 5-year survival rate falling below 30%.

CIC-sarcomas are characterized by their high aggressiveness, exhibiting a 5-year event-free survival rate ranging from 17–43%, which is considerably inferior to that of stage-matched Ewing sarcoma or BCOR-altered sarcomas.

BCOR::CCNB3 sarcoma demonstrates a favorable response to treatment regimens designed for Ewing sarcoma, yielding comparable outcomes.

Information pertaining to EWSR-1::non-ETS sarcoma is scarce; however, responses to standard systemic chemotherapy regimens have been documented as minimal to modest.

62.4 Summary

1. RMS is the commonest sarcoma in children.
2. Though RMS can occur anywhere in the body, Head and neck region is the commonest site followed by genitourinary locations.
3. Contrast enhanced CT scans or MRI scans are used for radiological assessment of the extent of the primary lesion and metastatic evaluation.
4. Biopsy is necessary for confirmation of the diagnosis and ascertaining the histological type of RMS.
5. Tumors are then staged, risk categorized and treated according to the risk categorization.
6. The treatment is multimodal using surgery, chemotherapy and radiation therapy.

Suggested Reading

Carachi R, Grosfeld JL, Azmy AF. The surgery of childhood tumours. 2nd ed. Heidelberg: Springer; 2008.

Coran AG, Caldamone A, Scott Adzich N, Krummel TM, Laberge JM, editors. Pediatric surgery. 7th ed. Oxford: Elsevier; 2012.

Poplak DG, Pizzo PA. Principles and practice of pediatric oncology. Wolters Kluwer; 2016.

WHO Classification of Tumours Editorial Board. Paediatric tumours WHO classification of tumours, vol. 7. 5th ed. International Agency for Research on Cancer; 2023. ISBN: 978-92-832-4510-0.

63 Adrenal Tumors in Children

Devendra Kumar Yadav

63.1 Introduction

The adrenal glands are situated in suprarenal location and are continuously evolving gland. Cell proliferation in the fetal adrenal as a continuous process arises from outer zone and move to the center. Adrenal glands are much larger in fetus than in adults because of the existence of a prominent fetal cortex. In early post-natal life, remodeling of the adrenal cortex structure takes place which causes the gland shrinkage. The adrenal glands are suppressed in early life due to loss of fetal zone and gradual production of DHEA/DHEAS starts by the age of 8 years (*adrenarche*).

Adrenal tumors can be classified based on origin of mass from the glands and the functioning effect of the mass. They might arise from the medulla or cortex and are hyperfunctioning (approximately 90%) or nonfunctioning. Primary medullary tumors comprise of sympathetic neuroectodermal tumors, which are neuroblastoma, ganglioneuroblastoma, ganglioneuroma, and pheochromocytoma, all of which originate from the neural crest and may take place anywhere along the sympathetic chain aside from the adrenal gland itself. Tumors arising from the cortex part of adrenal glands are adrenocortical carcinoma, adenoma and lesions of uncertain malignant potential.

D. K. Yadav (✉)
Paediatric Surgery, All India Institute of Medical Sciences, New Delhi, India

63.2 Adrenocortical Tumor

Pediatric adrenocortical tumors (PACTs) are seen in less than 5 years old, with a high frequency up to the third year of life. The female–male ratio varies widely with age. Females predominated in the age groups 0–3 years (ratio 1.7:1). Worldwide annual incidence is thought to be 0.3–0.38 cases per million children less than age 15 years [International Pediatric Adrenocortical Tumors Registry (IPACTR), hosted by St. Jude Hospital].

Genetic counseling and testing are required in PACTs because of early onset, distinct biological activity, and syndromic association. The most involved pathways in the adrenal tumorigenesis are b-catenin, Insulin-like growth factor (IGF)-II/IGF-IR, p53/Rb signaling, and the chromatin remodeling process. Germline mutations associated with cancer predisposition syndrome contribute to childhood ACT, corresponding to approximately 50% of cases. Somatic genetic alterations are also common in PACTs. Tumor syndromes that show an increased incidence of pediatric ACT include the Li-Fraumeni syndrome (LFS), Beckwith–Wiedemann syndrome, CNC, Lynch syndrome, MAS, APC-associated polyposis conditions, and MEN1. TP53 mutation may contribute to the cause of most cases of ACT in children.

Pediatric ACT may present as abdominal mass (5%) or pain but usually present with various types of endocrinopathy (Fig. 63.1). Most of the

© The Author(s), under exclusive license to Springer Nature Singapore Pte Ltd. 2025

S. Roy Choudhury (ed.), *Pediatric Surgery*, https://doi.org/10.1007/978-981-96-1257-4_63

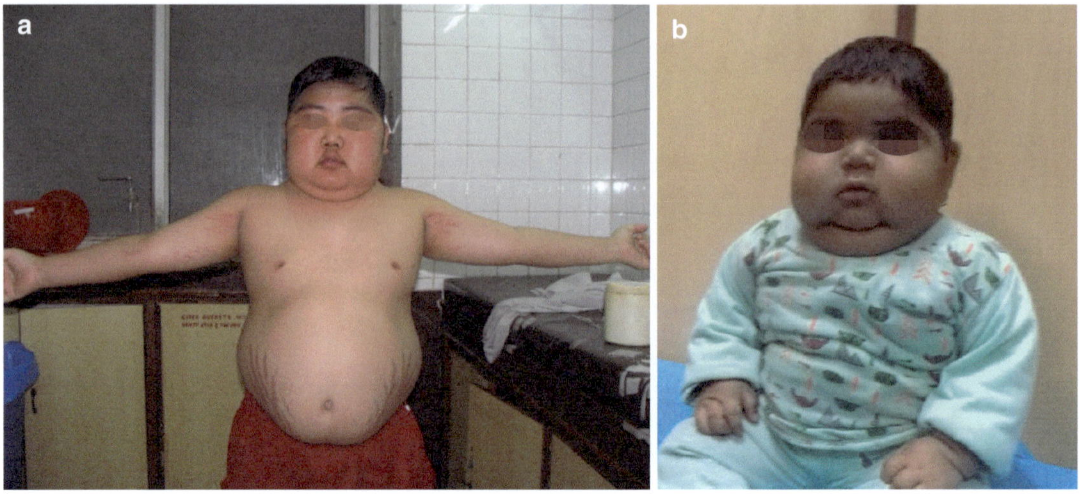

Fig. 63.1 (a) Cushingoid facies (b) Cushingoid features due to adrenal tumor

children present secondary to hormonal excess with isolated virilization (linear growth acceleration, advanced bone age, pubic hair, hirsutism, acne, deepening voice, muscle hypertrophy, clitoromegaly or increase in penis size) or combination of hypercortisolism and virilization (Fig. 63.2). The mixed secretion of androgen and glucocorticoids in PACTs ranges between 25% and 50% of cases, and rarely, they present isolated hypercortisolism and much more infrequent, isolated hyperaldosteronism or estrogen secretion. Less than 10% of cases presented with feminization or no clinical evidence of hormonal secretion. Pediatric ACT Registry shows that most patients [75.5% (192 of out 254 patients)] present with localized disease, and metastatic disease was found at diagnosis in less than 5% of cases.

Based on clinical features, comprehensive hormonal (adrenal and gonadal axis) and radiological evaluation is required for PACT evaluation. Hormonal evaluation is useful in the detection of persistent or recurrent disease. Level of testosterone, androstenedione, and particularly DHEA-S are often significantly increased. Estradiol, 17-hydroxyprogesterone, and 11-deoxycortisol levels may be increased. Cortisol secretion measurement may be abnormal, including lack of suppression in response to dexamethasone and increased 24-h urinary cortisol and midnight salivary cortisol levels.

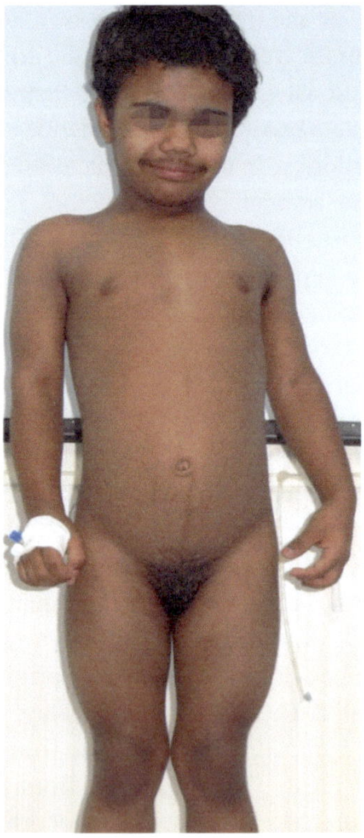

Fig. 63.2 Virilizing adrenal tumor (precocious puberty)

Imaging studies are helpful in establishing the extent of the disease, such as tumor location, tumor size, invasion of local structures, and the presence of tumor thrombus in the inferior vena cava and right atrium. The most common locations of distant metastases are the liver and lungs, so chest imaging is required in addition to abdominal imaging. CT scan is required for chest lesion and CT scan/MRI (preferably), if available, is required for evaluation of abdominal lesions (Fig. 63.3). COG ARAR0332 protocol recommends MRI abdomen + CECT chest + MDP Bone scan. Frequently, imaging studies cannot define the benignity of the lesion, and only the presence of metastases determines the malignancy. Other imaging studies, such as MRI of brain and bone scintigraphy, are required only under suspected metastasis.

It may be difficult to differentiate between a benign adrenocortical adenoma and adrenocortical carcinoma. Preoperative biopsy is not preferred. Weiss criteria correlate well with prognosis in adults but not in children. The Weineke system includes 11 items, and more weightage has been given to tumor size, and local invasion in addition to measures of cellular atypia. The scoring expressed three categories: (1) patients with up to 2 criteria had a benign long-term clinical outcome; (2) those with 3 criteria were indeterminate for malignancy; and (3) tumors meeting 4 or more criteria are characterized as malignant and those patients had poor outcomes.

Children's Oncology Group (IPACTR) has proposed a staging system which reveals Stage I: as Completely resected, small tumors (≤100 g and ≤200 cm3) with normal postoperative hormone levels, Stage II: Completely resected, small tumors (≥100 g or ≥200 cm3) with normal postoperative hormone levels, Stage III: Unresectable, gross or microscopic residual disease, tumor spillage, Stage I and II tumors with hormone levels that fail to normalize after surgery, retro-

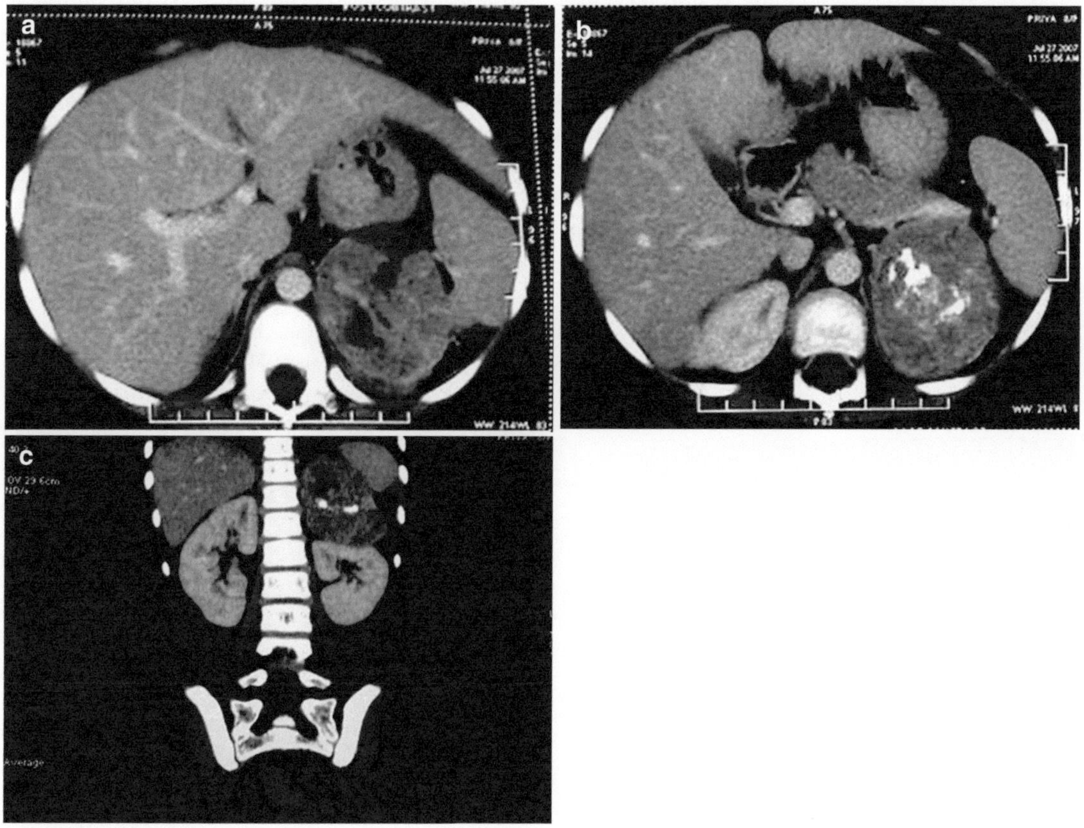

Fig. 63.3 (**a–c**) CECT of left adrenocortical tumor with calcification and few cystic areas

peritoneal lymph node involvement, Stage IV: distant metastasis.

The mainstay of treatment is complete surgical removal with microscopic clearance (Fig. 63.4). More invasion and surrounding adherence are features of malignant ACTs and en-bloc resection of involved organs like kidney, liver segments, or portions of the pancreas may be required (should only be tried if complete resection is possible; otherwise, biopsy only is preferable). As much as possible, rupture of the tumor should be avoided, whichever is the approach either laparoscopic or open. Adrenocortical tumors seem to have a thin capsule and are friable, so easy chance of rupture. Intraoperative tumor spillage worsens the long-term prognosis. Only COG ARAR 0332 protocol recommends lymph node sampling in stage I and retroperitoneal lymph node dissection (RPLND) for stage II–IV.

Because of the extreme rarity of ACTs in children, the role of chemotherapy is not very well standardized and may be given in cases of intraoperative tumor spillage, residual disease, or in those with local or distant metastases. Mitotane is the only recommended drug. The Children's Oncology Group trial (ARAR033, between 2003 and 2016) uses 8 cycles of cisplatin, etoposide, doxorubicin, and mitotane but shows significant toxicity. Adrenocortical tumors are radioresistant.

The overall 5-year survival for children with adrenocortical tumors depends on stage and the resectability. The poor prognostic factors are tumor weight (>200 gm), metastatic disease, age >4 years, microscopic tumor necrosis, para-aortic lymph node involvement, Incomplete resection or spillage during surgery, Low HLA class II antigen expression, and higher Ki-67 labeling index. The follow-up plan includes hormonal evaluation and radiography (CT Chest, MRI) every monthly for the first year, every 4 monthly for the 2nd year, every 6 monthly for 3rd year, once a year for 4th and 5th year. Six year and after that only hormone evaluation is required yearly.

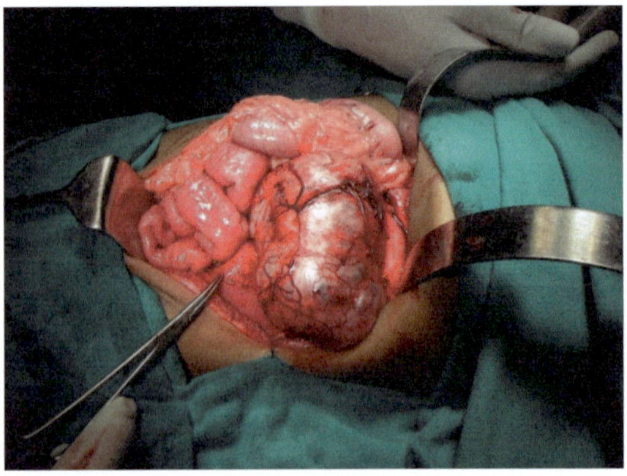

Fig. 63.4 Left adrenocortical tumor

63.3 Incidentaloma

Adrenal incidentaloma (AI) is an asymptomatic mass present in the adrenal gland and usually detected during diagnostic imaging performed because of other health issues than the suspected adrenal disease. AI is an extremely rare finding in the pediatric population and the prevalence is around 0.2% and it is increased with age. The differential diagnosis includes neuroblastoma, ganglioneuroblastoma, teratoma, adrenocortical tumor, hematoma, and simple cyst.

63.4 Pheochromocytoma/Paraganglioma

Pheochromocytomas (PHEOs) and paragangliomas (PGLs) are neuroendocrine tumors arising from chromaffin tissue of the adrenal medulla or extra-adrenal sympathetic ganglia in the thorax, abdomen, and pelvis. Depending upon the site of origin, tumors termed as pheochromocytomas when arising within the adrenal gland, and termed as paragangliomas when tumors arising from somewhere else.

PHEOs/PGLs represent <7% of tumor arising from the sympathetic nervous system and are rare findings in childhood and adolescent. The average age of diagnosis in childhood is 11 years, with slight predominance in boys. PHEOs represent most of the cases and are functional while PGLs represent less number of cases and may be functional (abdominal) and nonfunctional (head and neck, mediastinal).

PHEOs often occur as a sporadic tumor but can also develop as a part of various hereditary syndrome including VHL disease, MEN2A, MEN2B, Nf1, familial PGL syndrome. SDHB, SDHC, SDHD, VHL, RET, and NF1 mutations are prevalent. In the pediatric population, germline mutations seem to be even more common, with estimates ranging from 50% to 70%. The gene most mutated in PHEO is VHL, while in PGL it is SDHB. Comprehensive molecular profiling shows 3 types of clusters in nearly 70% of the cases of PHEO and PGL. Clusters 1A and 1B pseudohypoxia-related, cluster 2 kinase signaling-related, and cluster 3 Wnt signaling-related. Assignment to the cluster depend upon various clinical, biochemical, and imaging characteristics that may help guide the treatment and follow-up of patients.

Pediatric PHEO/PG can be identified by symptomatic catecholamine hypersecretion, as incidentaloma, tumor mass effect, and during screening of hereditary tumor syndrome. Headache, tachycardia, diaphoresis, and pallor are commoner symptoms than the weight loss, abdominal pain, fever, and seizures. Hypertension is seen in most patients.

The major diagnostic approach to PHEOs/PGL is measurement of plasma-free metanephrine levels or 24-h urinary metanephrine level, including both metanephrine and normetanephrine. Elevation of these metabolites greater than 4 times the upper limit of normal is associated with 100% of the possibilities of catecholamine-secreting tumor. Epinephrine-producing tumors are diagnosed later. Chromogranin A may be a useful tumor marker in these cases. It is recommended to confirm PHEO/PGL biochemically before moving to imaging studies.

Radiographic studies are required for proper localization in the form of CT or MRI of abdomen and pelvis, if unrevealing neck and chest should be involved (Fig. 63.5a). The other recommended functional test includes nuclear scintigraphy test, preferably Ga-DOTA-SSA PET/CT or scintigraphy for any PGL or for PHEO associated with SDHx mutations and 18F-FDOPA PET/CT or scintigraphy for PHEO not associated with SDHx mutations.

Malignancy in PHEO/PGL is defined by the presence of metastatic disease (at the site where the paraganglia are not located (i.e. lymph node, liver, lung) rather than by histologic examination. Although metastasis at presentation is uncommon in children (14% in a national French data-

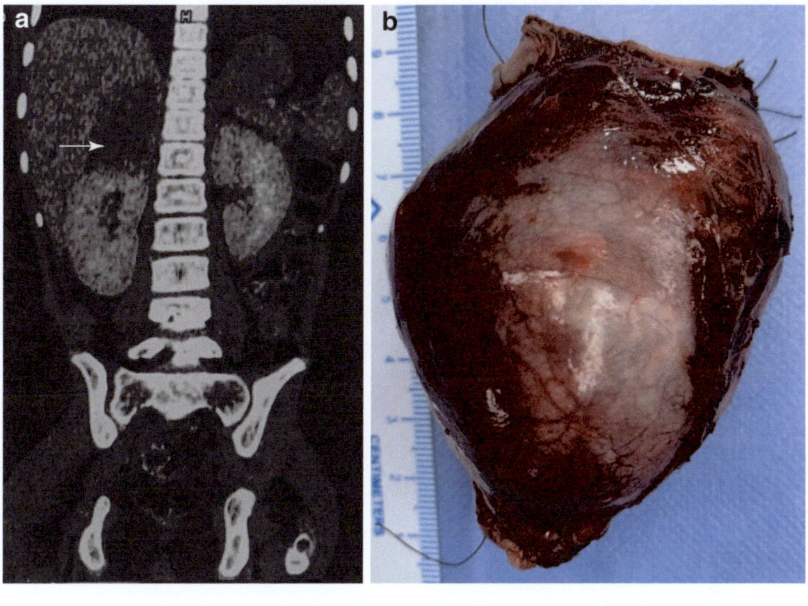

Fig. 63.5 (**a**) Right suprarenal pheochromocytoma, (**b**) completely excised specimen of pheochromocytoma

base), all PHEO/PGL should be considered as potentially malignant and evaluated accordingly. There is no clinical staging system for PHEO or PGL.

Surgery of localized tumors is the mainstay of the treatment (Fig. 63.5b). Complete resection is more likely in cases of PHEO than in PGL (>90% vs 50%–75%). Adequate preoperative preparation is necessary to avoid hypertensive crises, and mortality during operation. Current recommendations are to establish adrenergic blockade for 10–14 days at gradually increasing doses to control blood pressure. A laparoscopic surgical approach is preferable for small (<6 cm) and noninvasive PHEOs. Open procedures are appropriate for large PHEOs and PGLs to optimize tumor resection and to avoid tumor rupture. Cortical sparing partial adrenalectomy should be considered in cases of bilateral PHEO or if a PHEO develops in the contra-lateral gland after prior adrenalectomy, with the goal of preventing postoperative adrenal insufficiency. Radiation therapy can also be used in unresectable PGLs.

For patients with metastatic disease, responses have been documented to some chemotherapeutic regimens such as gemcitabine and docetaxel or different combinations of vincristine, cyclophosphamide, doxorubicin, and dacarbazine. Chemotherapy may help alleviate symptoms and facilitate surgery, although its impact on overall survival is less clear. Responses have also been obtained to high-dose 131I-MIBG and sunitinib. Alternative treatments for patients with non-resectable disease include radiofrequency ablation, tumor embolization, or peptide receptor radionuclide therapy with 131I-MIBG for those with uptake on scintigraphy or with Lu-DOTATATE (dodecanetetraacetic acid-tyr3-octreotate).

Repeat biochemical testing for PHEO/PGL is recommended 2–4 weeks after surgery to demonstrate a biochemical cure and should be repeated annually. Given the high rate of germline mutations, metachronous disease, recurrences, and metastases are common. The prognosis is good in PHEO/PGL with 5 years survival rate of 98%.

An algorithm for diagnosis and management of adrenal mass in children is given below (Fig. 63.6).

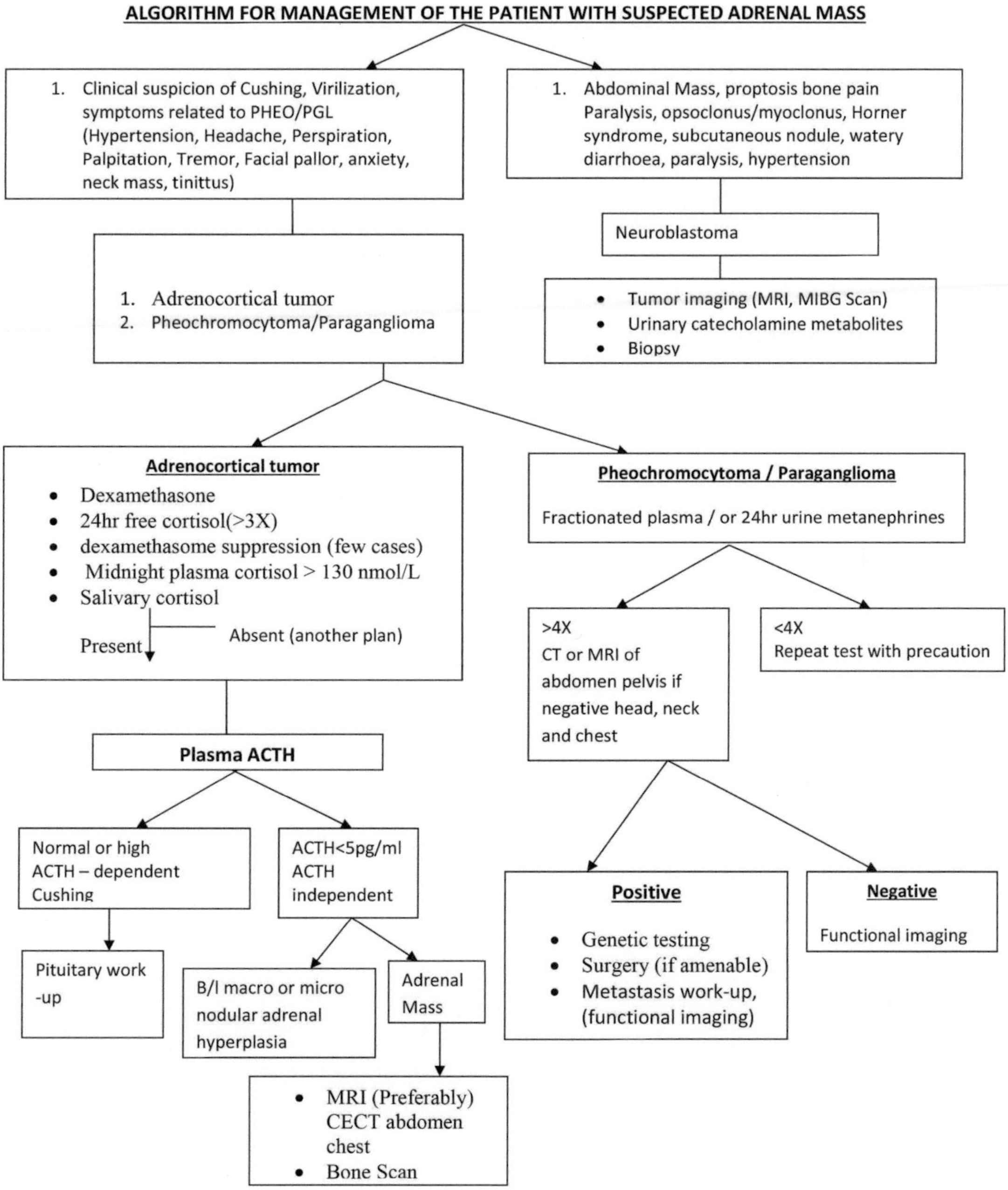

Fig. 63.6 Algorithm for management of the patient with suspected adrenal mass

Suggested Reading

Blaney SM, Adamson PC, Helman LJ. Principles and practice of pediatric oncology. 8th ed. Wolters Kluwer; 2016.

Part X

Pediatric Urology

64 Hydronephrosis and Other Cystic Diseases of Kidney

Prabudh Goel, Mehak Sehgal, Vishesh Jain, and Lavleen Singh

64.1 Introduction

Dilatation of the renal pelvis, with or without calyces is termed as hydronephrosis. It essentially implies an underlying abnormality in urinary flow dynamics, either due to an obstruction, due to reflux of urine back into the kidney, or due to production which is in excess of what can be handled by the kidney. Hence, the etiology of this dilatation can be due to congenital anomalies of kidney and urinary tract (CAKUT) including but not limited to pelvi-ureteric junction obstruction, vesico-ureteric junction obstruction and posterior urethral valves, vesico-ureteric reflux or transient hydronephrosis (Table 64.1).

Table 64.1 Causes of Renal dilatation

Isolated renal dilatation:	Physiological/transient hydronephrosis
	Pelvi-ureteric junction (PUJ) obstruction
Associated with dilatation of ureter:	
Ureteral pathology	Intrinsic lesion: Stricture, polyp, stone
	External compression: Pelvic tumors
	Ectopic ureter
Ureterovesical junction pathology	Vesico-ureteric reflux
	Ureterovesical junction obstruction
	Ureterocele
Obstructive pathology in the bladder or urethra usually result in bilateral hydroureteronephrosis	Bladder pathology: Bladder bowel dysfunction, neurogenic bladder, bladder diverticulum
	Urethral pathology: Posterior urethral valve (males only), urethral stricture, stone, polyp, meatal stenosis, anterior urethral valve/polyp

P. Goel (✉) · M. Sehgal · V. Jain
Department of Paediatric Surgery, All India Institute of Medical Sciences, New Delhi, India

L. Singh
Department of Pathology, AIIMS, New Delhi, India

© The Author(s), under exclusive license to Springer Nature Singapore Pte Ltd. 2025
S. Roy Choudhury (ed.), *Pediatric Surgery*, https://doi.org/10.1007/978-981-96-1257-4_64

64.2 Antenatal Hydronephrosis

Incidence of antenatal detection of hydronephrosis is around 0.5–4% of all pregnancies, with unilateral hydronephrosis being more common than bilateral. Most of these are physiological or transient hydronephrosis, often resolving by birth or in the early postnatal period. All cases diagnosed antenatally need to be under continued evaluation and monitoring.

Various grading systems have been developed to assess and characterize the severity of hydronephrosis in the fetus. Some of the commonly utilized ones are as follows:

64.2.1 Society of Fetal Urology (SFU) Hydronephrosis Grading System

The SFU grading system evaluates the degree of HDN based on the effect on the pelvi-calyceal system and renal parenchyma. This does not take into consideration the condition of the ureters or the bladder (Table 64.2).

64.2.2 Fetal Renal Pelvic Antero-Posterior Diameter

One of the most common methods of grading hydronephrosis in the second and third trimester is by the measure of renal pelvic antero-posterior diameter (RAPD). This is based on the effect of the HDN on the collecting system, and thus should not be used in isolation. Hydronephrosis is defined as a RAPD >4 mm in the second trimester or > 7 mm in the third trimester. Renal pelvic AP diameter > 10 mm in the second trimester and > 15 mm in the third trimester is significantly associated with a pathological cause. The following grades of hydronephrosis can be defined according to this system (Table 64.3):

Table 64.2 SFU hydronephrosis grading system

SFU grade	Pattern of renal sinus splitting
0	No splitting
1	Slight splitting of the central renal complex without calyceal involvement, normal parenchyma
2	Splitting of the central renal complex with extension to non-dilated calyces
3	Wide splitting of the renal pelvis, dilated outside the renal border, calyces uniformly dilated, normal parenchyma
4	Large, dilated calyces (may appear convex); thinning of the parenchyma to </=50% of the ipsilateral (normal) kidney

64.2.3 Urinary Tract Dilatation Classification System

This is a more extensive classification system which takes into account the following sonological (antenatal or postnatal) parameters: anterior and posterior RAPD, calyceal dilation, renal parenchymal thickness, renal parenchymal appearance, bladder abnormalities, and ureteral abnormalities. Based on these, a grading system has been devised as described in Table 64.4.

Other classification systems have also been described such as the Onen and Radiology grading systems. If hydronephrosis has been antenatally diagnosed and graded, it is important to also look for: laterality, renal parenchymal involvement, ureteric dilatation, urinary bladder, amniotic fluid, presence of any urinoma or urinary ascites, any other non-genitourinary anomalies. All cases need complete clinical examination and formal evaluation post-delivery. An ultrasound is performed usually 48 h of birth to tide over the initial period of dehydration, unless renal function is expected to be impaired, such as in cases of bilateral gross hydroureteronephrosis, solitary kidney, etc. An early ultrasound can then assist in the decision to rule out posterior urethral vales and other causes of obstructive uropathies, appropriately. These conditions should also be ruled out in children detected with bilateral hydrone-

Table 64.3 Grading of HDN based on RAPD

Degree of HDN	Second trimester	third trimester
Mild	4 to <7 mm	7 to <9 mm
Moderate	7 to <10 mm	9 to <15 mm
Severe	>10 mm	>15 mm

Table 64.4 Grading of HDN based on UTD system

Antenatal	Postnatal
UTD A1: RAPD <28 weeks: 4 mm to <7 mm (or) ≥28 weeks: 7 mm to <10 mm	*UTD P1*: Anteroposterior renal pelvic diameter 10 mm to <15 mm (or) Central calyceal dilatation
UTD A2,3: RAPD <28 weeks: ≥7 mm (or) ≥28 weeks: ≥10 mm (or) Any calyceal dilatation, with APRPD ≥4 mm or calyceal dilatation (or) Any ureteric dilatation, with APRPD ≥4 mm or calyceal dilatation (or) Parenchymal abnormality, bladder abnormality, or oligohydramnios	*UTD P2:* Anteroposterior renal pelvic diameter ≥ 15 mm (or) Peripheral calyceal dilatation (or) Ureteric dilatation ≥4 mm, with APRPD ≥10 mm or calyceal dilatation
	UTD P3: Parenchymal abnormality, bladder abnormality, or oligohydramnios, and any of the following: Anteroposterior renal pelvic diameter ≥ 15 mm (or) Any calyceal dilatation

phrosis, and in those where the ureter is also seen dilated. In a kidney demonstrating mild to moderate hydronephrosis, a repeat scan is generally performed after 4–6 weeks, and the child can be electively followed up in clinic.

In a unilateral hydronephrotic kidney, obstructive hydronephrosis secondary to pelvi-ureteric junction obstruction (PUJO) should be considered, as it is the most common pathological cause in this scenario. The natural history is variable and controversial, which is why multiple modalities of management have been described.

64.2.4 Pelvi-Ureteric Junction Obstruction

Pelvi-ureteric junction obstruction (PUJO or UPJO) is an important cause of hydronephrosis. Of the antenatally detected cases of fetal hydronephrosis, 30–44% are due to PUJO. The male to female ratio is 2:1, and 10–20% cases are bilateral.

Pathology

According to a classification by Koff, PUJO can be of the following types:

1. *"Intrinsic"*
   - Presence of an "adynamic segment" which interferes with ureteral peristalsis—Most common cause results in functional obstruction.
   - Morphologically it is narrower than the rest of the ureter and histology shows deficient and disorganized circular muscle fibers.
2. *"Extrinsic"*
   Due to mechanical factors such as
   - Crossing vessels
   - Ureteral folds (Ostling's folds)
   - Adhesive bands
   - Arteriovenous malformations

   These create extrinsic abrupt angulation/kinking of the PUJ and cause obstruction to the urinary outflow.

"Intraluminal" cause of obstruction could be due intraluminal pathology such as ureteral valves and fibroepithelial polyps.

Pathogenesis and Histology:

- *Kidneys with extrarenal pelvis* (Fig. 64.1a)—obstruction leads to initial pelvic dilatation later followed by pressure atrophy of the renal parenchyma (generally late damage of renal parenchyma).
- *Kidneys with intrarenal pelvis* (Fig. 64.1b)—obstruction leads to more parenchymal atrophy, resulting in a thin walled hydronephrotic sac (early damage of renal parenchyma).

Backpressure changes secondary to an increase in pelvic pressure causes increase in the hydrostatic pressure in the collecting and tubular system of the kidney. Subsequent to this, there is an effect on the intra-glomerular pressure which leads to decrease in glomerular filtration rate. Some of the reasons for this could be tubular ischemia, mechanical compression of tubular cells, and alteration in urinary shear stress. This results in hemodynamic, functional, and structural changes in the nephron. While compensatory mechanisms act to stabilize the pressure changes, significant obstruction causes irreversible damage

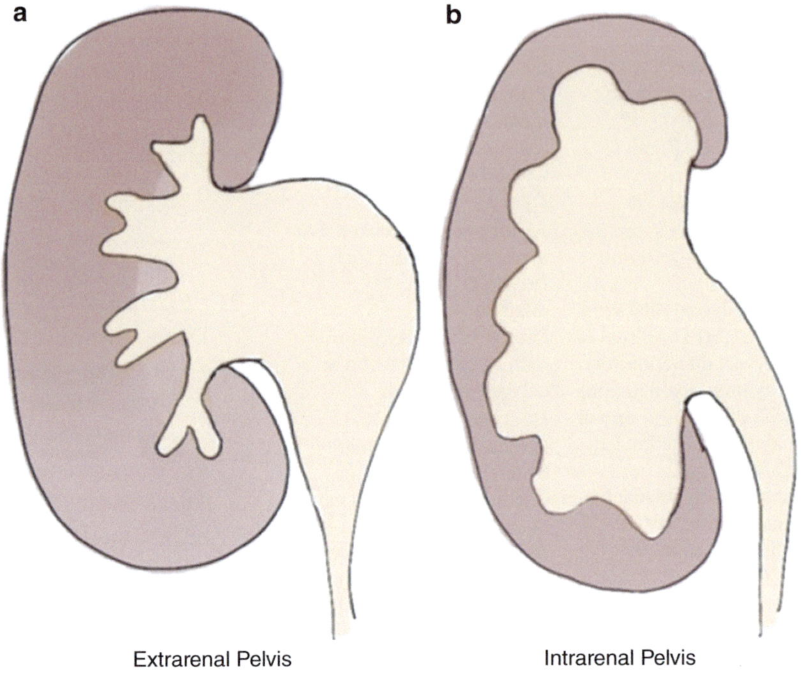

Fig. 64.1 Types of pelvis encountered in hydronephrosis, (**a**) extrarenal (**b**) intrarenal

to the kidney at later stages leading to tubular damage, glomerular damage, inflammation, and fibrosis. This may affect the concentrating ability of the kidney and sodium resorption.

Several chemical mediators of inflammation have been identified and activation of renin-angiotensin system appears to play a significant role in obstruction. The expressions of growth factor TGFβ up-regulation have been demonstrated in obstructed kidneys. This forms the basis of detection of urinary biomarkers, such as various proinflammatory cytokines and tubular enzymes, before conventional modalities detect renal damage.

Clinical Presentation:

- Antenatal
- Incidental
- Pain, usually dull aching
- Poor appetite or nausea, especially with left-sided involvement
- Palpable renal lump
- Acute colic followed by lump—then passage of large volume of urine—disappearance of pain and swelling: classically described as the *Dietl's crisis*
- Uncommon presentations: renal colic secondary to urolithiasis, UTI, Pyelonephritis, hypertension or detected after a history of renal trauma

Imaging:

- *USG*—To assess pelvic dilatation, calyceal cupping or clubbing, diameter of pelvis, thickness of renal parenchyma, any associated ureteric dilatation, contralateral kidney, or any associated pathology (Fig. 64.2).
- False-positive studies may be due to:
  - Extrarenal pelvis
  - Peri-pelvic cyst
  - Residual dilatation from previous obstruction
  - Dilatation following reflux
  - Pyelonephritis
  - Fetal and neonatal kidney: sonolucent appearance of the medulla and pyramids
  - MCDK: seen as multiple non-communicating cysts. In PUJO the largest cyst representing the renal pelvis is medial in location and the dilated calyces are seen as communicating cysts.
- False-negative studies may be due to:

- Acute obstruction
- Extrinsic compression from metastases and retroperitoneal fibrosis
- Oliguric states (such as in a healthy newborn)

• *Dynamic Isotope Renography* is the investigation of choice for functional assessment (Figs. 64.3, 64.4 and 64.5). The commonly used isotopes for renal function and drainage are: Tc 99 labeled Diethylene Triamine Pentacetic Acid (DTPA), Mercapto Acetyl Triglycine(MAG3),andL,L,ethylenedicysteine for scan (LLEC). MAG3 is, at present, the agent of choice for evaluation of renal function and drainage pattern, due to its higher renal extraction. It is especially preferred in infants and those with poor renal function. Diuretic is often given in the study to confirm the diagnosis of obstruction.

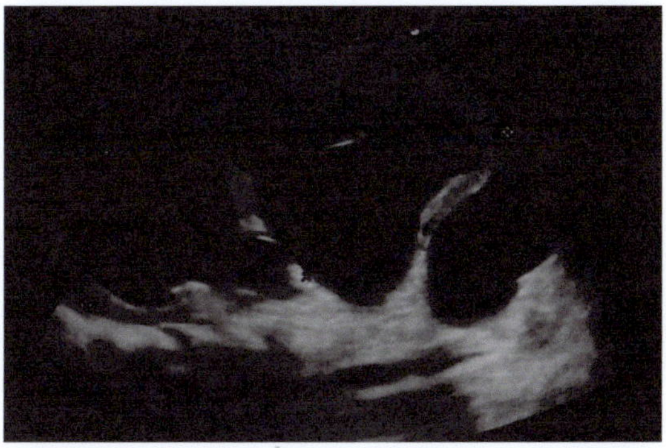

Fig. 64.2 Significant hydronephrosis with parenchymal thinning and calyceal clubbing as seen on ultrasound

Generally, the radionuclide is cleared from the renal pelvis within 10–15 min, defined as the "t1/2." The t1/2 is normal if <10 min, while a t½ >20 min indicates obstruction (post diuretic) (Fig. 64.3).

Some determinates that affect renal scintigraphy include: placement of the region of interest, time of measurement, state of hydration, bladder fullness, reservoir effect, type of protocol, renal response to furosemide, and the concept of supranormal function.

Supranormal function is defined as greater than 55% of differential renal function in the hydronephrotic kidney in children with unilateral hydronephrosis and is considered an indication for pyeloplasty by some clinicians.

Cortical transit time (normally <3 min) is said to be delayed if >3 mins, also helps in the diagnosis of PUJO.

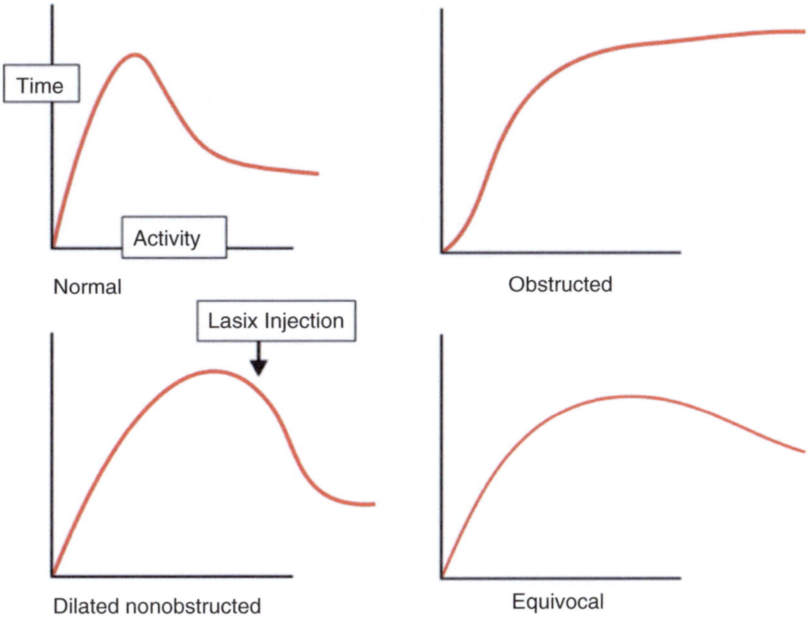

Fig. 64.3 Renogram patterns

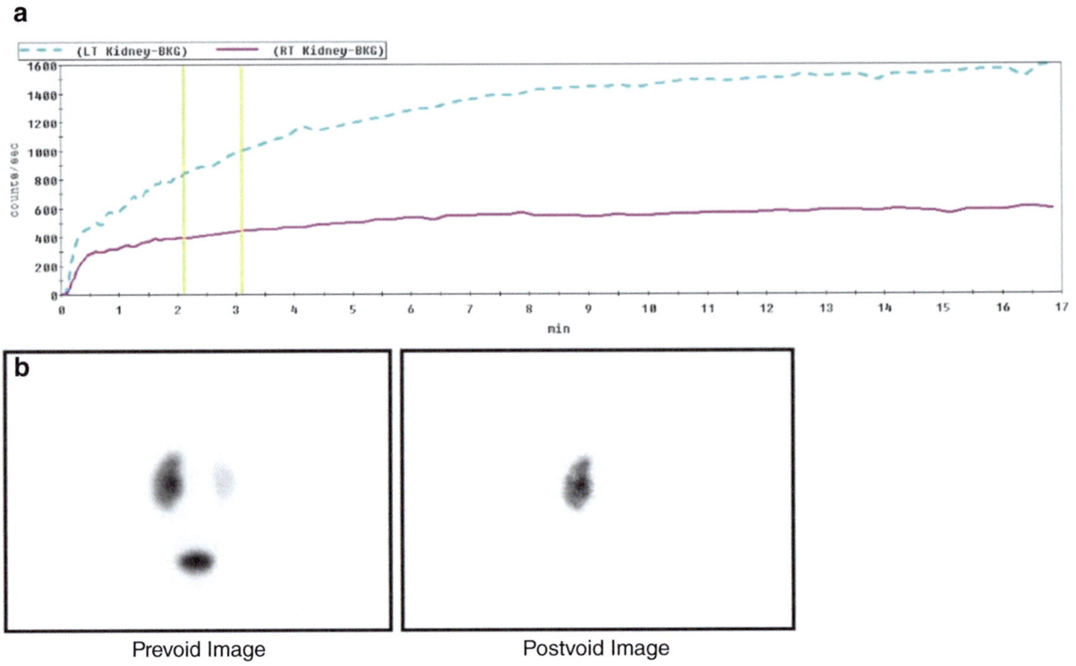

Fig. 64.4 (**a**) Renogram curve showing obstructed pattern in the left kidney. (**b**) Renogram showing retention of tracer in left kidney in delayed post void image

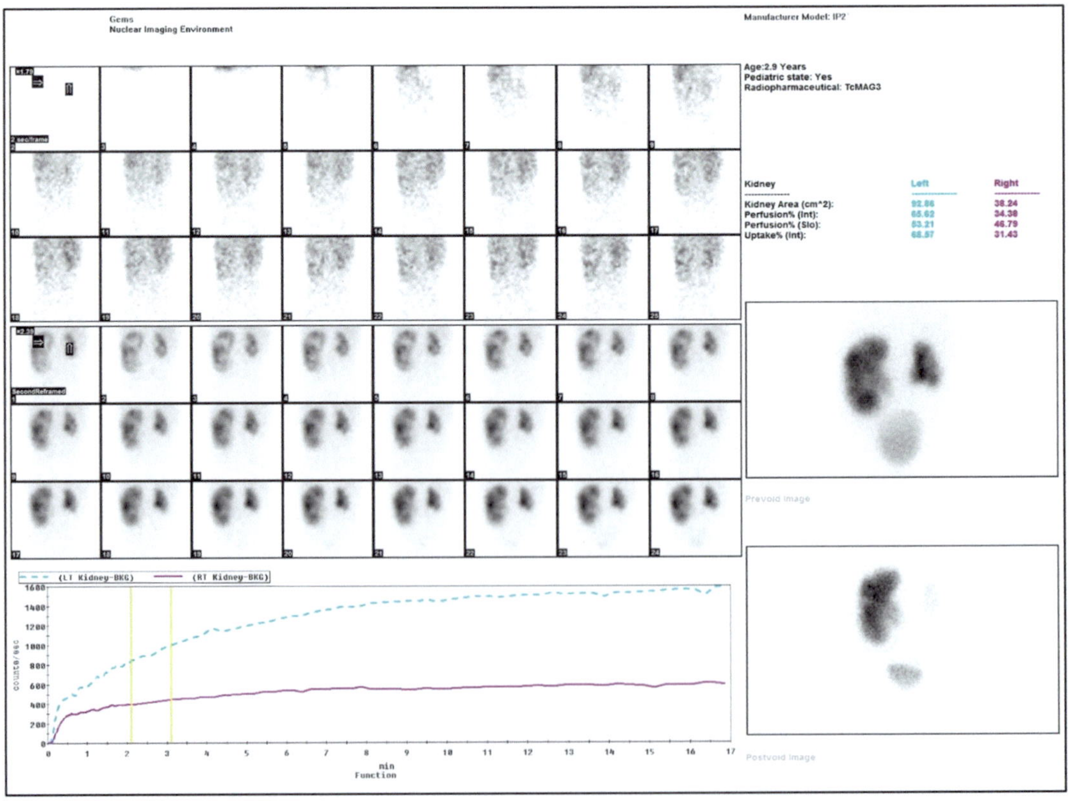

Fig. 64.5 MAG-3 Renogram showing obstructed left kidney (pelvi-ureteric junction)

- Intravenous Pyelography (IVP)- rarely performed, defines anatomy well if the renal function is good. Inaccurate in poor functioning kidneys.
- CT scan or CT Urography is rarely necessary (Fig. 64.6), high radiation exposure is a disadvantage. It helps to detect a rare crossing vessel and is the investigation of choice for its detection.
- Gadolinium Enhanced Magnetic Resonance Urography (CE-MRU) provides information on anatomy and function but is uncommonly used at present.
- Whitakar test (Pressure flow study)- Historically performed. Infusion of fluid via nephrostomy with measurement of pelvic pressure (rarely performed).
- Micturating cystourethrogram (MCUG) is recommended for bilateral hydronephrosis to rule out vesico-ureteric reflux or lower tract pathology. It is also done in cases of solitary kidney with contralateral MCDK and in those with dilated ureter on USG (Fig. 64.7).
- Biomarkers such as Plasma Renin Activity, Urinary NGAL, EGF, TGFβ1, MCP1, Kim1 are currently under evaluation for their role in the diagnosis of obstructive uropathy.

Management

The management algorithm of post-natal hydronephrosis is shown in Fig. 64.8.

1. *Conservative management*: Asymptomatic children with preserved renal function with stable hydronephrosis can be considered for observation. They can be monitored with serial USG and renal scintigraphy. Can be considered for antenatally diagnosed HDN, no symptoms, SRF > 40% and AP Pelvis <20 mm. Follow-up done with sequential USG and RDS.

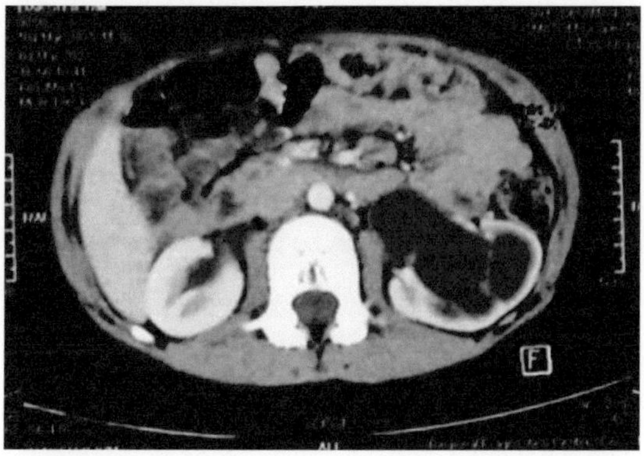

Fig. 64.6 Incidental detection of gross hydronephrosis on imaging an older child for pain abdomen of uncertain etiology

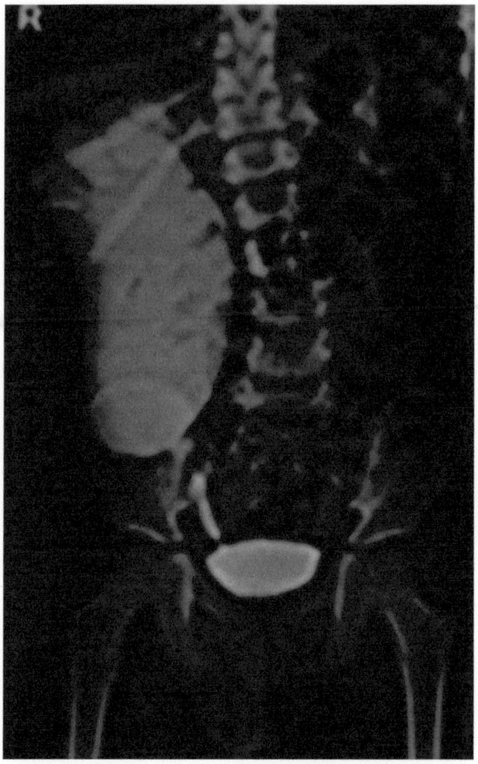

Fig. 64.7 MCU showing right PUJ obstruction with right vesico-ureteric reflux

2. *Percutaneous Nephrostomy*: It can be placed as a temporary diversion in large hydronephrotic kidneys, function <10%, and in cases of pyonephrosis. A repeat functioning imaging is done 4 weeks after placement to evaluate for renal recovery.
3. *Surgery*: The indications for surgery are as follows:
   - Increasing hydronephrosis on follow-up ultrasonography (increase in renal pelvic AP diameter 30 mm and above) with parenchymal thinning, calyceal clubbing.
   - Obstructive pattern on diuretic renogram.
   - Decreasing renal function (<40% differential renal function on diuretic renogram

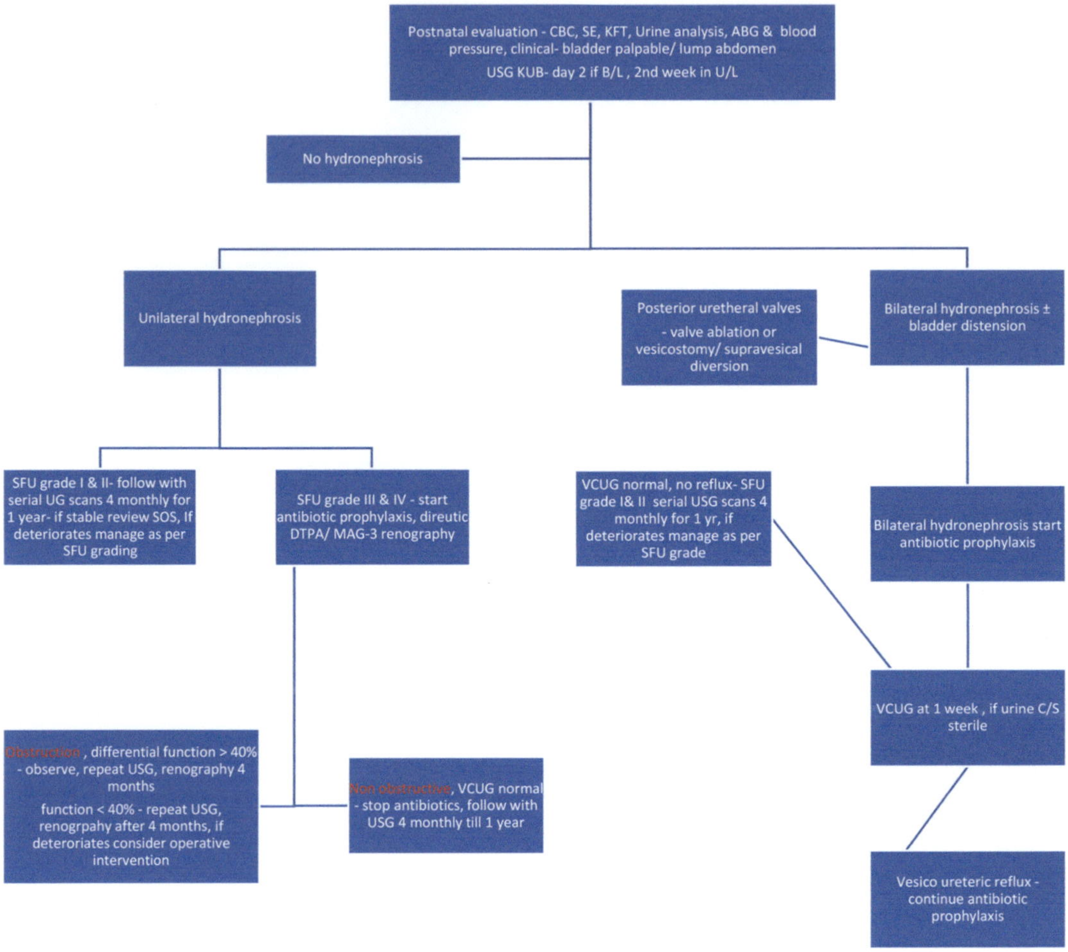

Fig. 64.8 Algorithm of management for post-natal hydronephrosis

and fall in function by 10% on sequential renograms).

- Clinical symptoms: Palpable lump, récurrent UTI, pain.

Anderson-Hynes Dismembered Pyeloplasty

This is the most commonly performed procedure and considered the gold standard for pelvi-ureteric junction obstruction (PUJO). Wide and dependent anastomosis of the spatulated ureter is done to a projection of the lower aspect of the pelvis after a redundant portion is excised (Fig. 64.9). The anastomosis can be performed over a trans-anastomotic stent (DJ or nephron-stent), stentless, or with a nephrostomy. The senior author prefers to use a nephron-stent that is a long stent fenestrated along its length. The tube is positioned inside the pelvis, across the neo-pelvi-ureteric junction and into the proximal half of ureter and exits by piercing the renal parenchyma. The tube serves as a trans-anastomotic stent and drains both the pelvis and the ureter. The stent can be removed from outside after 1 week ensuring satisfactory internal drainage.

Steps of Pyeloplasty

The operation can be done by open or laparoscopic or robotic technique with almost similar results in experienced hands. The minimally

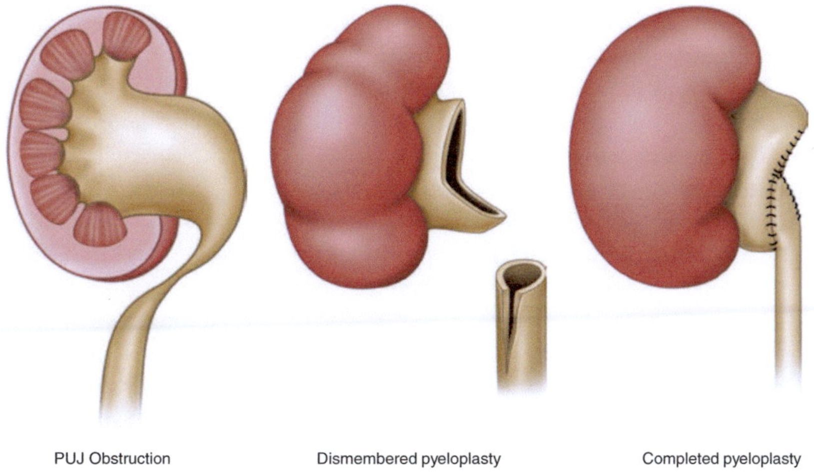

Fig. 64.9 Steps of Anderson-Hynes pyeloplasty

invasive surgery has the advantages of early recovery; however, the cost and available instrument size, especially for robotic surgery is currently under evaluation.

In the open method, the kidney can be approached anteriorly, laterally (flank approach) or posteriorly (lumbotomy approach) depending upon the preference and experience of the surgeon. The position of the patient can be semi lateral, lateral decubitus, or prone depending upon the approach. The steps involved are similar and as follows:

1. Division of the skin, subcutaneous and muscle layers while avoiding opening of the peritoneum.
2. Identification and opening of the Gerota's fascia.
3. Identification the PU junction and any crossing vessel.
4. Taking stay sutures at the ureter and the dependent part of the pelvis for orientation.
5. Dismembering of the pelvi-ureteric junction.
6. Lateral spatulation of the normal ureter.
7. Excising the redundant renal pelvis.
8. Anastomosis as described above over the desired stent (Fig. 64.9).
9. Peri-nephric drain insertion.
10. Closure in layers.

Non-dismembered Pyeloplasty

- *Culp flap/Spiral Flap/Culp-DeWeerd pyeloplasty*: Spiral flap is created from the renal pelvis, which is then used to repair the defect at the UPJ. Bridge the gap between the pelvis and healthy ureter over a distance of several centimeters (e.g. when UPJO and a relatively long segment of proximal ureteral narrowing or stricture occur in the same setting).
- *Scardino and Prince vertical flap*: Vertical flap designed in a situation of a dependent UPJ with a large, square-shaped extrarenal pelvis.
- *Foley's V-Y plasty*: performed in the situation of a high ureteral insertion.

Ureterocalicostomy: Performed in situations such as redo surgery, relatively long length of the obstructed ureteral segment, small intrarenal pelvis, etc. Proximal ureter distal to the obstruction is anastomosed to a dependent lower pole calyx instead of the renal pelvis.

Endopyelotomy and Balloon Dilatation: A full-thickness lateral incision through the obstructing proximal ureter performed using cold knife, electrocautery, or laser. Avoid in long segment narrowing, crossing vessel.

Laparoscopic (transperitoneal) and robotic pyeloplasty are the currently favored minimally invasive technique. Others include lumboscopic assisted and retroperitoneoscopic approaches.

Complications

Early complications following pyeloplasty can be bleeding, urinary tract infection including postoperative pyelonephritis, delayed opening of the ureteropelvic anastomosis due to clot or edema causing prolonged leak, urinoma formation.

Late complications include urolithiasis, restenosis, kinking or angulation/non-dependent anastomosis, fibrosis or stenosis.

Special Situations

1. Bilateral PUJO: Seen in 30%, appropriate to operate on a more severely dilated kidney and monitor the contralateral kidney for need for surgery later.
2. Crossing Vessel: A lower pole crossing vessel contributes to significant kinking at the PUJ and results in intermittent obstruction. Managed by a dismembered pyeloplasty or "vascular hitch" where the lower pole vessels are mobilized and moved to a more cranial position overlying the renal pelvis rather than the PUJ without dismembering the PUJ itself.
3. Very poorly functioning kidney: function <5% despite PCN—undergo nephrectomy.

64.3 Cystic Diseases of the Kidney

Cyst formation in the kidney is seen in many diseases. They may be genetically acquired, fetal malformations or acquired. Often, they may have associated extra-renal manifestations.

1. *Multi Cystic Dysplastic Kidney (MCDK)*: It is a severe variety of renal parenchymal malformation, characterized by replacement of the renal parenchyma with multiple small cysts giving a bunch of grapes appearance (Fig. 64.10a, b). MCKD is often associated with ureteral atresia on the same side. This condition usually affects one side (more commonly left) and needs to be differentiated from the PUJ obstruction (see above), and other forms of renal cystic diseases like polycystic renal disease. On histology, the kidney is seen to contain numerous non-communicating cysts separated by dysplastic tissue (Fig. 64.11).

   It is usually detected antenatally, post-natal symptomatology is infrequent, with most cases detected incidentally. Multicystic dys-

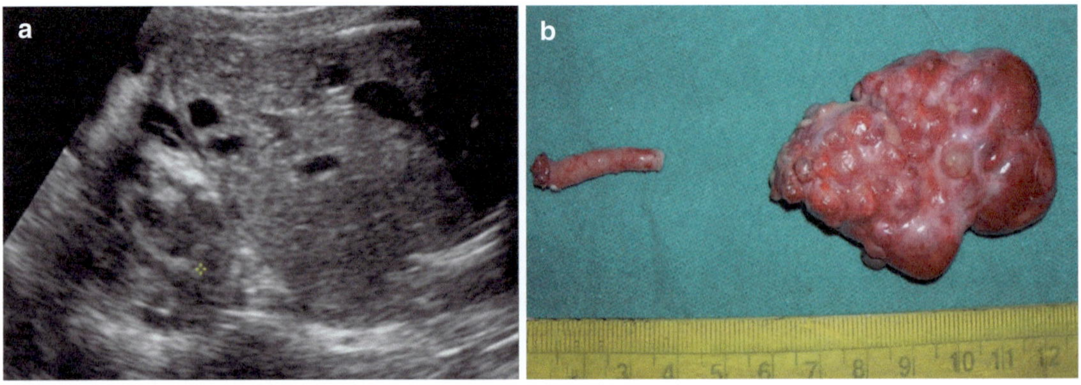

Fig. 64.10 (**a**) Multicystic dysplastic kidney on ultrasonography (**b**) MCKD specimen with atretic ureter

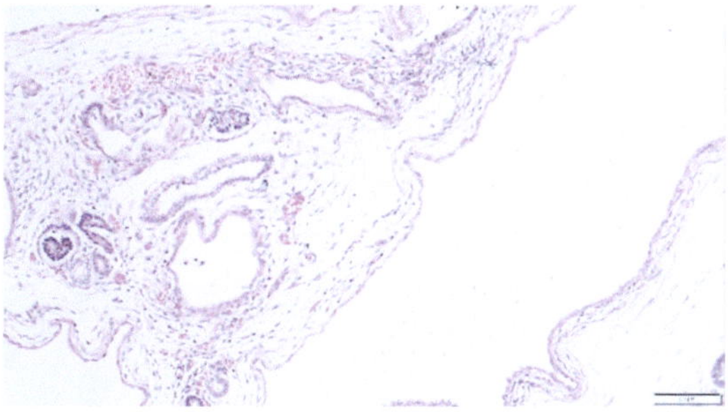

Fig. 64.11 Multiple Cysts lined by flattened epithelium with surrounding immature mesenchyme, primitive tubules and abortive glomeruli. [H&E 10x]. Diagnosis-Cystic Renal Dysplasia

plastic kidneys are poorly functional and bilateral cases are incompatible with life. Unilateral MCDK kidney usually undergoes atrophy, there could however be a small risk of future malignancy and hypertension.

Unilateral cases with normal opposite kidney are treated conservatively with serial ultrasound scans. Symptomatic cases with large lump, recurrent UTI, or hypertension may require surgical removal. Contralateral kidney needs screening for anomalies such as vesico-ureteric reflux, PUJO, rotation/position anomalies, etc. Further evaluation is based on sonographic findings.

2. *Genetically Acquired Cystic Renal Diseases*: These conditions present with a significant family history. They include polycystic kidney disease (Table 64.5, Fig. 64.12), glomerular renal cyst, and tubular renal cyst disorders. Other renal cystic disorders include Medullary sponge kidney, Medullary Cystic Kidney Disease.
3. *Isolated Renal Cysts*: They occur in children and adults, not associated with a genetic predisposition. The Bosniak renal cyst classification characterizes these cysts based on CT findings into 4 categories.

   Simple renal cysts present in children with infection, pain, or hypertension. They have a thin wall without septa, calcifications, or solid components. They done increase in size and usually arise from the upper pole. Primary conservative management is recommended but intervention can be considered symptomatic large compressive cysts, increase in cyst size on follow-up imaging, and when there is uncertainty about the underlying diagnosis. Percutaneous drainage has been tried. Laparoscopic marsupialization may also be considered.

   Complex cysts are rarely seen in children. Acquired renal cysts may be seen in children post liver transplantation and in those with end stage renal disease.
4. *Multilocular Cystic Nephroma (see Chap. 58)*

   It is a benign, cystic renal tumor that is made up of non-communicating cysts of differing size separated by thin septa. It usually occurs in children younger than 24 months of age and second peak incidence is at 30 years. This tumor is distinguished by the finding of only mature cell types within the septa of the cyst wall. It may present as an abdominal mass. The cut surfaces reveal a well-circumscribed multilocular tumor composed of cysts ranging from several millimeters to several centimeters in greatest diameter. It is a benign lesion which is cured by nephrectomy. If partial nephrectomy is considered, frozen section

Table 64.5 Description of common genetic associated renal cystic disorders

Type	Genetics	Pathology	Clinical Features	Investigations	Treatment
ARPKD (Autosomal recessive Polycystic Kidney Disease)	Recessively inherited PKHD1 gene mutation DZIP1L gene mutation	Bilateral enlarged, reniform shaped kidneys Spongy appearance with pinpoint dots on surface Cyst size increase over time Associated congenital hepatic fibrosis, Caroli syndrome' Histopathology	Antenatally detected Potters sequence Abdominal distension/lump Renal failure Hypertension Dyselectrolytemia Urinary tract infection Portal hypertension	USG: Enlarged kidney with raised echogenicity, poor corticomedullary differentiation; micro and macrocysts IVP: Radial streaks Molecular genetic testing	Respiratory stabilization Unilateral/bilateral nephrectomy Renal replacement therapy Management of hypertension, dyselectrolytemia, portal hypertension Genetic counseling
ADPKD (Autosomal dominant Polycystic Kidney Disease)	Dominantly inherited PKD1 and PKD2 gene mutations	Cystic dilatations in all parts of the nephron Initially normal architecture, later fibrosis and glomerulosclerosis Dysfunctional cilia Extrarenal manifestations: Cerebral vessel malformations, risk of mitral valve prolapse	Antenatally detected: Oligohydramnios, respiratory distress, large kidneys in neonates Asymptomatic, incidentally detected on screening Hypertension, pain, lump, distension, UTI, renal stones, proteinuria Aortic and intracranial aneurysms, mitral valve prolapse, extra-renal cysts	USG: Large cysts, heterogenous, increased echogenicity, asymmetry Genetic evaluation CT/MRI MRA brain	Management of renal failure, UTI, hypertension Tolavaptan: Slow the progression (trials) Rapamycin: Stabilizes cyst growth
Nephronophthisis	Autosomal recessive Gene mutations in NPHP1–NPHP11, AHI1, and CC2D2A	Severe tubular damage with thickened and split basement membrane Tubular atrophy, periglomerular fibrosis Cysts in tubules and collecting ducts Extrarenal: Mental retardation. Liver fibrosis, retinal degeneration, cardiac malformation	Renal concentration defect, glycosuria, proteinuria Growth retardation, fatigue, symptoms of renal osteodystrophy Hypertension	USG: Hyperechoic kidneys with loss of CMD; normal or decrease in size; medullary cysts	No specific treatment Symptomatic Treat for CKD

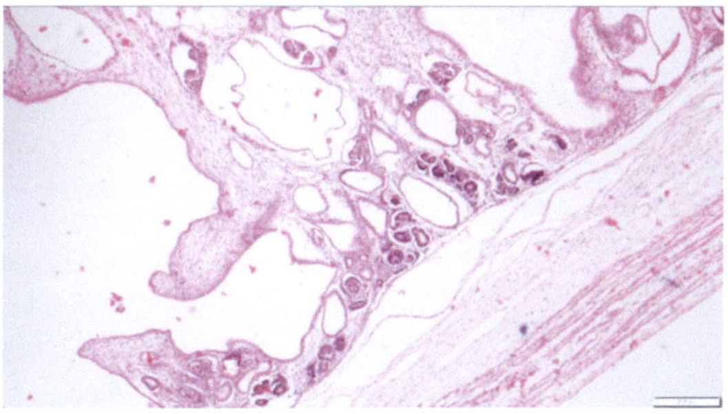

Fig. 64.12 Autosomal recessive polycystic kidney disease. Lesion shows Dilated radially arranged cysts in cortex and medulla lined by flattened/cuboidal epithelium. The intervening stroma shows few abortive glomeruli. [H&E 4x]

is indicated to exclude cystic, partially differentiated nephroblastoma.

64.4 Summary

1. Hydronephrosis and other cystic diseases of kidney are commonly diagnosed on antenatal scan.
2. Although the majority of them are physiological and resolve over time, it is important to identify the pathological and progressive obstruction.
3. Post natal renal imaging and diuretic functional renal scan are applied in combination for planning further management.
4. Surgical correction ranges from open to robotic restoration of the obstructive pathology with optimal preservation of renal function.
5. MCKD has characteristic imaging pattern to differentiate it from other form of obstructive hydronephrosis; they can be managed conservatively.
6. Several cystic diseases of kidney have genetic associations.

Suggested Reading

Docimo SG, Canning D, Khoury A, Salle JLP, editors. The Kelalis-King-Belman textbook of clinical pediatric urology. 6th ed. CRC Press; 2018.

Partin AW, Dmochowski RR, Kavoussi LR, Peters CA, Wein AJ, editors. Campbell-Walsh-Wein urology 2020. 12th ed. Elsevier.

Coran AG, Caldamone A, Scott Adzich N, Krummel TM, Laberge JM, editors. Pediatric surgery. 7th ed. Oxford: Elsevier Limited; 2012.

Herndon ACD, Cain MP. AUA update series lesson 3; 28 Prenatal diagnosis of urological disease; 2009.

Capolicchio JP, Braga LH, Szymanski KM. Canadian Urological Association/pediatric urologists of Canada guideline on the investigation and management of antenatally detected hydronephrosis. Can Urol Assoc J. 2018;12(4):85–92.

Nguyen HT, Benson CB, Bromley B, et al. Multidisciplinary consensus on the classification of prenatal and postnatal urinary tract dilation (UTD classification system). J Pediatr Urol. 2014;10:982–98.

Onen A. Grading of Hydronephrosis: an ongoing challenge. Front Pediatr. 2020;8:458.

Gordon I, Piepsz A, Sixt R. Guidelines for standard and diuretic renogram in children. Eur J Nucl Med Mol Imaging. 2011;38:1175–88.

Sinha A, Bagga A, Krishna A, Bajpai M, Srinivas M, Uppal R, Agarwal I. Revised guidelines on management of antenatal hydronephrosis. Indian J Nephrol. 2013;23(2):83–97.

Wilcox DT, Thomas DFM. Essentials of pediatric urology. 3rd ed; 2021.

Riedmiller H, Androulakakis P, Beurton D, Kocvara R, Gerharz E. European Association of Urology. EAU guidelines on paediatric urology. Eur Urol. 2001;40(5):589–99.

65 Urinary Stones in Children

Priyank Yadav and Sujit K Chowdhary

65.1 Introduction

Urolithiasis affects both adults and children worldwide, with an increasing incidence in the pediatric population. Managing urinary stones in children poses unique challenges due to anatomical and developmental differences. When conservative measures fail, surgical intervention becomes crucial. The surgical approaches employed aim to effectively remove or fragment stones, alleviate symptoms, prevent complications, and minimize long-term effects. Factors like stone characteristics, obstruction, patient age, and health status influence the choice of surgical intervention. This article examines various surgical management options for urinary stone disease in children, covering rationale, techniques, outcomes, and potential complications.

65.2 Types of Urinary Stones

- Calcium Stones:
  - Most common type of urinary stone
  - Composed primarily of calcium oxalate or calcium phosphate
  - Often associated with hypercalciuria, hyperoxaluria, hypocitraturia, and hypomagnesemia
- Struvite Stones:
  - Also known as infection stones
  - Composed of magnesium ammonium phosphate
  - Typically form in the presence of urinary tract infections, particularly with urease-producing bacteria
  - Alkaline urine environment promotes their formation
- Uric Acid Stones:
  - Formed due to elevated levels of uric acid in the urine
  - Associated with conditions such as gout, high-purine diet, or certain metabolic disorders
  - Radiolucent, requiring specialized imaging techniques like CT urography or ultrasound for detection
- Cystine Stones:
  - Formed due to cystinuria, a genetic disorder affecting renal tubular reabsorption of cystine
  - Cystine has poor solubility in urine, leading to stone formation
  - Can be accompanied by other metabolic conditions and may form mixed-composition stones.
  - One of the hardest stones
  - High recurrence rate and often require long-term management

P. Yadav
Sanjay Gandhi Post Graduate Institute of Medical Sciences, Lucknow, UP, India

S. K Chowdhary (✉)
Indraprastha Apollo Hospital, New Delhi, Delhi, India

© The Author(s), under exclusive license to Springer Nature Singapore Pte Ltd. 2025

S. Roy Choudhury (ed.), *Pediatric Surgery*, https://doi.org/10.1007/978-981-96-1257-4_65

- Mixed Stones:
  - Combinations of different stone types, such as calcium oxalate and uric acid
  - Can have variable characteristics and treatment approaches
  - Comprehensive stone analysis is essential to guide management decisions
- Matrix Stones:
  - Less common type of urinary stones characterized by a soft, gelatinous matrix material that holds together various mineral deposits
  - Consist of a mixture of organic and inorganic components, such as bacteria, proteins, and crystalline substances
  - Often associated with chronic urinary tract infections and occur in individuals with a history of recurrent urinary tract infections
  - The matrix material provides a favorable environment for the growth and aggregation of bacteria, leading to stone formation.

65.3 History and Examination

History and examination features may vary depending on the individual case, and additional investigations such as imaging studies and laboratory tests are usually required for a definitive diagnosis and to determine the characteristics of the urinary stones. History features in urinary stones include the following:

- Older children tend to present with hematuria and flank pain, while very young children may present with non-specific symptoms (e.g., irritability, vomiting).
- Children are less likely to suffer from hematuria, which may be visible or painless. It is more common to see non-visible hematuria in children as the only symptom.
- History of recurrent or previous episodes of renal colic, which is severe flank pain caused by the movement of stones in the urinary tract.
- History of urinary tract infections (UTIs).
- Previous history of urinary stones or family history of stone disease.
- Dietary habits, including fluid intake, high sodium intake, and consumption of foods high in oxalate (like spinach, rhubarb, beets, and chocolate) or purines (like organ meats, seafood, and certain legumes).
- Medical conditions that may increase the risk of stone formation, such as hyperparathyroidism, gout, or certain metabolic disorders.
- History of surgical interventions including previous surgeries for stone must be noted.

Examination features in urinary stones consist of the following:

- Physical examination may reveal tenderness or pain in the flank or lower back region.
- Abdominal examination may reveal a palpable mass or tenderness in the renal area.
- Examination of the genitals may be done to evaluate for any abnormalities or signs of infection.
- Blood pressure measurement may be performed to assess for hypertension, which can be associated with urinary stones due to shared risk factors like obesity and metabolic syndrome as well as medicines like diuretics.
- Neurological examination assesses underlying conditions, bladder dysfunction, and related symptoms in stone disease, guiding diagnosis, management, and prevention.

65.4 Diagnostic Work Up

The choice of diagnostic tests should be based on the individual patient's clinical presentation, available resources, and the healthcare provider's discretion. The goal is to balance diagnostic accuracy with minimizing radiation exposure in pediatric patients. Following tests are useful in the diagnostic work up:

- Urinalysis
  - Aids in detection of microscopic hematuria.

  - Assessment of Urine pH and identification of crystals such as calcium oxalate, uric acid, or struvite can help in determining the underlying stone type.
  - Evaluation of UTIs: Urinalysis can detect the presence of urinary tract infections, which are commonly associated with urinary stones, particularly struvite stones. The presence of bacteria, white blood cells, or nitrites in the urine may indicate an infection, prompting the need for appropriate treatment and further management.
- Renal Ultrasound (US):
  - Recommended as the initial imaging modality for urinary stone evaluation in children.
  - Highly effective in detecting stones within the kidneys, visualization of ureters is poor though.
  - Non-invasive and does not involve radiation exposure.
- Abdominal X-ray:
  - Limited application in routine evaluation of urolithiasis.
  - Useful for identifying radiopaque stones.
- Non-Contrast Helical CT Scanning:
  - Considered the most sensitive test for identifying stones, particularly ureteric stones.
  - Safe and rapid, with high diagnostic accuracy.
  - Offers 97% sensitivity and 96% specificity.
  - Reserved for cases when US and abdominal X-ray results are inconclusive.
  - Potential radiation hazards should be taken into account.
- Low-Dose CT Protocols:
  - Developed to reduce radiation dose while maintaining adequate image quality.
  - Used as an alternative to standard CT scanning in some cases.
- Intravenous Pyelography (IVP):
  - Rarely used in children for stone evaluation.
  - May be necessary to assess the caliceal anatomy before certain endoscopic management of stones.

65.5 Surgical Treatment of Renal and Ureteric Stones

65.5.1 Extracorporeal Shockwave Lithotripsy (ESWL)

ESWL is a non-invasive treatment modality that uses shockwaves to break down urinary stones into smaller fragments, allowing for their spontaneous passage through the urinary tract. ESWL has a significant role in the management of pediatric urolithiasis, providing a safe and effective treatment option for children. The principle behind ESWL involves the generation of high-energy shockwaves outside the body, which are focused on the stone using imaging guidance. These shockwaves create mechanical stress, leading to the fragmentation of the stone into smaller pieces. Indications for ESWL in pediatric urolithiasis include stones located in the kidney or upper ureter, with a size typically ranging from 4 mm to 20 mm.

Advantages:

- Non-invasive procedure
- Outpatient treatment, allowing for shorter hospital stays and reduced postoperative recovery time
- Well-tolerated by children, with anesthesia or sedation options
- High success rates, ranging from 70% to 90% for stone clearance

Disadvantages:

- Limited efficacy for certain stone compositions (e.g., cystine or hard calcium oxalate monohydrate stones)
- Larger stone sizes or presence of unfavorable anatomy (such as inferior calyx location, narrow infundibulopelvic angle, long infundibular length, narrow infundibular width) may require multiple sessions or alternative interventions
- Small risk of complications, such as bruising, bleeding, or injury to surrounding tissues
- Suitability may be affected by urinary tract obstruction, abnormal anatomy, or certain medical conditions such as coagulopathy

65.5.2 Percutaneous Nephrolithotomy (PCNL)

PCNL is a minimally invasive surgical procedure used in the management of pediatric urolithiasis, which involves the removal of kidney stones through a small incision in the back. It has a significant role in the treatment of complex or larger stones that cannot be effectively treated with other non-invasive methods. Under ultrasonographic or fluoroscopic guidance, a needle is placed percutaneously into the renal calyx having the stone or at a straight path to the stone. The percutaneous tract is subsequently dilated and a nephroscope is then used for direct visualization and removal of the stones. The stones may be fragmented prior to removal using lithotripter or laser. PCNL is indicated in pediatric patients with large renal stones (typically greater than 2 cm), complex stones, staghorn calculi, or stones that are resistant to other treatment modalities. It is commonly performed under general anesthesia, and the procedure can be modified depending on the location and characteristics of the stone. Miniaturized instruments and specialized techniques, such as mini-PCNL or ultramini-PCNL, are often used to ensure optimal outcomes and minimize complications in pediatric patients.

Advantages:

- Direct Visualization
- High Stone Clearance (86–98% after single session)
- Minimally Invasive when compared to open surgery resulting in less postoperative pain and shorter hospital stays
- Suitable for Complex Cases, including staghorn calculi and stones associated with anatomical abnormalities

Disadvantages:

- Potential Complications such as bleeding, infection, injury to surrounding structures like colon, and postoperative urinary leakage
- Longer Learning Curve
- Anesthesia and Hospital Stay

65.5.3 Ureterorenoscopy (URS)

URS is a minimally invasive endoscopic procedure that involves the use of a thin instrument called ureteroscope to visualize and treat stones located in the ureter and renal pelvis. The urinary tract is accessed through the natural urinary passage, without the need for external incisions. The procedure is typically performed under general anesthesia. The ureteroscope is inserted through the urethra and advanced through the bladder and ureter until it reaches the site of the stone. Once the stone is visualized, various techniques can be employed to remove or fragment it, such as laser lithotripsy or basket extraction. Indications for URS in pediatric urolithiasis include small to medium size stones located in the upper urinary tract (renal pelvis or upper ureter) and stones resistant to other treatment modalities like ESWL. URS can be classified into two types: flexible ureterorenoscopy and rigid ureterorenoscopy. Flexible ureterorenoscopy allows for easier navigation through tortuous anatomy and access to the entire upper urinary tract, including the kidney. On the other hand, rigid ureterorenoscopy is more commonly used for stones located in the ureter only.

Advantages:

- High success rate (90%)
- Precise stone targeting
- Minimal invasiveness (no incisions), resulting in reduced postoperative pain, shorter hospital stays, and faster recovery compared to open surgery

Disadvantages:

- Lower stone free rate for stones larger than 20 mm compared to PCNL
- Technical expertise and learning curve
- Risk of complications such as ureteral injury, bleeding, and urinary tract infection
- Need for anesthesia

65.5.4 Open and Minimally Invasive Stone Surgery

65.5.4.1 Open Nephrolithotomy/Pyelolithotomy/Ureterolithotomy

Open nephrolithotomy (also called anatrophic nephrolothotomy) was traditionally performed for stones in the renal calyces (including staghorn calculi). For this procedure, the kidney is exposed, the renal pedicle is dissected, and the posterior segmental artery is clamped. Methylene blue is given intravenously for visualization of the remaining parenchyma. The intersegmental plane is marked, and the main renal artery is occluded with ice slush for renal cooling. An incision is made along the marked lines, and the parenchyma is separated to access the stone. Open pyelolithotomy is performed by dissecting the renal pelvis and then making an incision on it to remove the stones in renal pelvis. An open ureterolithotomy is performed by dissecting the ureteric segment containing the stone and then making an incision on the ureter to remove the stone. For a stone that is impacted, the ureter is commonly inflamed and friable; the segment of the ureter just proximal to it is usually healthy and dilated allowing the stone to be removed easily from an incision in that segment. In the present era, open stone removal procedures are rarely performed, the main indications being:

- Very young children with large stones and/or congenital obstruction (simultaneous surgical correction for a congenitally obstructed system)
- Children with severe orthopedic deformities, limiting positioning for endoscopic procedures

Advantages:

- Provides direct access to the urinary tract, allowing complete stone removal.
- Suitable for large or complex stones that may require extensive reconstruction.

Disadvantages:

- Invasive procedure with longer recovery time.
- Increased risk of complications, such as bleeding, infection, and scarring.
- Potential for more pain and longer hospital stay compared to minimally invasive procedures.

65.5.4.2 Laparoscopic Pyelolithotomy/Ureterolithotomy

Laparoscopic pyelolithotomy and ureterolithotomy involve creating a pneumoperitoneum and inserting trocars for laparoscopic access. The affected kidney and ureter are identified and isolated. The kidney can be additionally dissected and mobilized to provide exposure. An incision is made in the renal pelvis for pyelolithotomy and the ureter for ureterolithotomy to remove the stone. The renal pelvis or the ureter are then closed over a double J stent. It is preferred to open surgery wherever the expertise is available. Following are the indications:

- History of previously failed endoscopic procedures
- Complex renal anatomy (ectopic or retrorenal colon)
- Concomitant UPJ obstruction or caliceal diverticula
- Mega-ureter
- Large, impacted stones

Advantages:

- Minimally invasive approach with smaller incisions and reduced postoperative pain.
- Provides excellent visualization of the surgical field.
- Allows precise stone removal and reconstruction if needed.

Disadvantages:

- Requires specialized training and expertise.
- Longer operative time compared to open surgery.

- Potential for complications associated with laparoscopic procedures (e.g., injury to surrounding structures, pneumoperitoneum-related issues).

65.5.4.3 Robotic Pyelolithotomy/Ureterolithotomy

The steps of robotic pyelolithotomy and ureterolithotomy are essentially similar to the laparoscopic procedures except that they are done using the surgical robot which offers more degrees of freedom, better instrument control, very precise suturing and elimination of hand tremors. The indications are the same as laparoscopic surgery.

Advantages:

- Enhanced dexterity and precise control offered by robotic-assisted technology.
- Improved visualization with a 3D camera system.
- Minimally invasive approach with smaller incisions and reduced postoperative pain.

Disadvantages:

- Requires specialized training and expertise in robotic surgery.
- Costly due to the need for robotic equipment and resources.

65.6 Surgical Management of Bladder Stones

65.6.1 Endoscopic Transurethral Cystolitholapaxy

This minimally invasive procedure involves inserting a cystoscope through the urethra and into the bladder to visualize and remove the stones. The stones are fragmented using laser or mechanical devices, and the fragments are then removed or flushed out.

65.6.2 Open Cystolithotomy

In certain cases, particularly when the bladder stones are large or there are complicating factors, open surgery may be performed. An incision is made in the lower abdomen, and the stones are directly accessed and removed from the bladder.

65.6.3 Percutaneous Suprapubic Cystolithotomy

This procedure involves making a small incision in the lower abdomen and inserting a scope directly into the bladder through the abdominal wall. The stones are then fragmented and removed.

65.6.4 Shock Wave Lithotripsy (SWL)

In SWL, high-energy shock waves are directed at the bladder stones externally, without the need for any incisions just like the ESWL for renal stones. The shock waves break the stones into smaller fragments, which are then passed out through urine (Fig. 65.1).

65.7 Metabolic Work Up

In general, for a first-time urinary stone former, there is 50% chance of forming another stone within the next 10 years. Children have a high tendency to form recurrent stones and frequently these stones arise due to metabolic abnormalities tipping the balance between stone promotors and

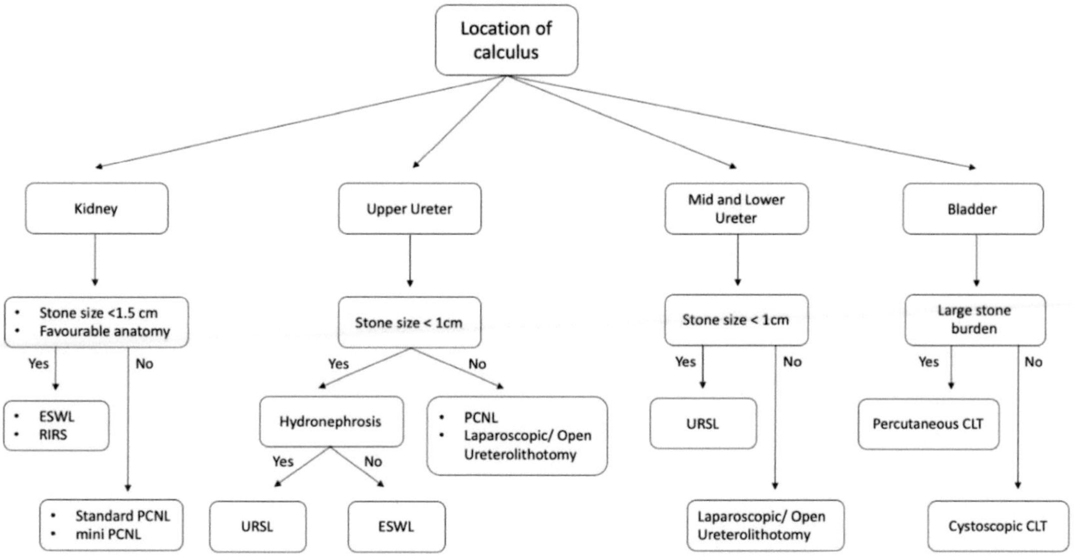

Fig. 65.1 Treatment options for pediatric urolithiasis. ESWL Extracorporeal Shockwave Lithotripsy, RIRS Retrograde Intrarenal Surgery, PCNL Percutaneous Nephrolithotomy, URSL Ureteroscopic Lithotripsy, CLT Cystolithotripsy. (*Yadav P, Madhavan K, Syal S, Farooq A, Srivastava A, Ansari MS. Technique, complications, and outcomes of pediatric urolithiasis management at a tertiary care hospital: evolving paradigms over the last 15 years. J Pediatr Urol. 2019;15(6):665.e1–665.e7.* https://doi.org/10.1016/j.jpurol.2019.09.011)

stone dissolvers in urine. The metabolic work up therefore must be done for every child who forms urinary stones. It is important to know the family and dietary history in detail. There are many blood and urinary tests that are listed below. Besides, any stone that is passed or removed must undergo analysis to determine its composition. This will impact subsequent medical management for stone prevention.

Blood investigations for metabolic work up		
CBC	Potassium	Albumin
Blood urea nitrogen	Phosphorous	Alkaline phosphatase
Creatinine	Bicarbonate	Parathyroid hormone
Calcium	Uric acid	
Sodium	Total protein	

Urine investigations for metabolic work up		
Urinalysis	24-hour Protein	24-hour Phosphorous
Urine culture	24-hour Uric acid	24-hour Magnesium
Spot urine calcium:creatinine	24-hour Oxalate	
24-hour Calcium	24-hour Citrate	

65.8 Medical Treatment

The metabolic workup for stones in children can identify various abnormalities, and the treatment depends on the specific condition. In general, increased fluid intake is recommended for all identified abnormalities to decrease the chance of urine supersaturation and stone formation. Here are some common abnormalities and their corresponding treatments:

- Hypercalciuria
  - Reducing sodium and animal protein
  - Increasing fruits and vegetables
  - Thiazide diuretics
- Hyperoxaluria
  - Avoiding high-oxalate foods such as spinach and nuts
  - Pyridoxine (vitamin B6) supplementation in certain cases
  - Reduced intake of vitamin C supplements
- Hyperuricosuria
  - Limiting purine-rich foods like organ meats and seafood
  - Allopurinol in certain cases

- Cystinuria
  - Limiting sodium and animal protein
  - Urine alkalinization
  - Chelating agents (such as tiopronin or D-penicillamine) to bind cystine in the urine
- Renal tubular acidosis (RTA)
  - Alkali supplementation for distal RTA
  - Treatment of underlying causes
- Hypocitraturia
  - Citrate-rich foods like lemonade
  - Potassium citrate supplementation

65.9 Summary

The management of urinary stones in children requires a comprehensive approach that considers various factors, including stone characteristics, obstruction, patient age, and health status. Conservative measures are the initial approach, but when they fail, surgical intervention becomes necessary. Different surgical options are available, such as ESWL, PCNL, and URS. ESWL is a non-invasive procedure that uses shockwaves to break down stones, while PCNL involves the removal of stones through a small incision in the back. URS is a minimally invasive endoscopic procedure used to visualize and treat stones in the ureter and renal pelvis. Open and laparoscopic/robotic procedures are reserved for specific cases. The choice of surgical intervention depends on several factors, including stone size, location, and patient characteristics. Successful surgical management aims to remove or fragment stones, alleviate symptoms, prevent complications, and minimize long-term effects. Close follow-up and long-term management are crucial to prevent recurrence and optimize outcomes.

Suggested Reading

EAU Guidelines. Edn. presented at the EAU Annual Congress Milan 2023. ISBN 978-94-92671-19-6.

Schneck FX, Ost MC. Surgical management of pediatric stone disease. In: Partin AW, Dmochowski RR, Kavoussi LR, Peters CA, Wein AJ, editors. Campbell-Walsh-Wein Urology. 12th ed. Elsevier; 2020.

Inguinal Hernia, Hydrocele Acute Scrotum, and Varicocele

66

Rohit Kapoor and Subhasis Roy Choudhury

66.1 Inguinal Hernia

66.1.1 Introduction

Inguinal hernia is one of the most common surgical ailments affecting children. It generally occurs when contents of the abdomen such as bowel, omentum, or preperitoneal fat protrude through a defect in the inguinal area. The incidence of inguinal hernia in children is estimated to be 8 to 50 every 1000 live births in various series. In premature babies however, the incidence is higher and reaches approximately 20%. Despite varying incidence and prevalence reported in the literature, the lifetime chance of a person being operated for inguinal hernia is quite high, 27% in men and 3% in women. Most cases present within first year of life and there is a clear mare preponderance with male to female ratio 3:1 to 10:1 in various series.

66.1.2 Embryology and Pathogenesis

(a) *In Males*- At the end of first trimester of pregnancy, processus vaginalis is formed in fetus from a diverticulum of peritoneum into the deep inguinal ring (DIR). In the canalicular phase (seventh to ninth months), testes descends through processus vaginalis into the scrotum. This processus vaginalis normally get obliterated spontaneously after testes descend but may persist till 2 years of age. The presence of this patent processus vaginalis (PPV) may lead to indirect inguinal hernia. Generally, if sac and the internal opening is large, then a hernia results and if they are small, then a hydrocele can occur. Indirect inguinal hernia, that occurs due to PPV, is the commonest type of hernia in children.

(b) *In Females*- In females, ovaries do not leave the abdominal cavity during descent. Diverticulum or canal of Nuck in females corresponds to the processus vaginalis in males. It is a pocket of peritoneum that extends from uterus to labia majora. Spontaneous closure of this diverticulum occurs at about 7 month's gestation. Failure of closure of this diverticulum may lead to the formation of indirect inguinal hernia in females.

66.1.3 Side

PPV (patent processus vaginalis) of left side closes earlier than right side and is responsible for increased incidence of inguinal hernia on the right side when compared to left (60% vs 30%, respectively).

R. Kapoor (✉)
Department of Paediatric Surgical Superspecialties, Sanjay Gandhi Postgraduate Institute of Medical Sciences, Lucknow, India

S. Roy Choudhury
Pediatric Surgery, Lady Hardinge Medical College and Associated Kalawati Saran Children's Hospital, New Delhi, Delhi, India

© The Author(s), under exclusive license to Springer Nature Singapore Pte Ltd. 2025

S. Roy Choudhury (ed.), *Pediatric Surgery*, https://doi.org/10.1007/978-981-96-1257-4_66

Incidence of bilateral hernia is 10% in full-term babies.

66.1.4 Risk Factors for Development of Inguinal Hernia

While most of the cases of inguinal hernia in children are isolated, the following conditions, if present, are associated with high risk of inguinal hernia:

1. Undescended testis,
2. Anterior abdominal wall defects such as Extropy bladder, Exomphalos, etc.
3. Eagle-Barret (prune belly) syndrome
4. Condition that increase intrabdominal pressure
   (a) Gross ascites
   (b) V.P. Shunt
   (c) Peritoneal Dialysis
   (d) Chronic respiratory disease like cystic fibrosis
5. Connective tissue disorders (e.g. Ehlers–Danlos syndrome)

Apart from this, as per a few recent studies, pediatric inguinal hernias may have a relationship with maternal inguinal hernias, but the underlying reason for this relationship is unknown and requires further investigation.

66.1.5 Classification

Types of inguinal hernia can be classified based on where and to what degree the processus vaginalis becomes obliterated, content of sac, and clinical presentation (Fig. 66.1).

I. *Indirect Inguinal Hernia*- This is the most common type of inguinal hernia in pediatric population and occurs due to PPV. It can be further classified on the basis of:
   (a) Extent of obliteration of PPV- Based on the extent of obliteration of processus vaginalis, Indirect inguinal hernias may be classified as:-
      (i) Vaginal(Complete)- Sac and its contents reach down completely in the scrotum
      (ii) Funicular- The sac and its content pass beyond the superficial inguinal ring but not up to the base of scrotum.
      (iii) Bubonocele- Sac and its content are limited to the inguinal canal and do not cross the superficial inguinal ring.
   (b) Content of sac- Contents of the hernia sac can be bowel, omentum, ovary and fallopian tube (only in females), appendix, caecum, etc. Based on content, Inguinal hernias can of the following types:
      (i) Sliding hernia- They have an organ such as caecum, urinary bladder, ovaries, and fallopian tube (in females) forming one wall of sac. It is important to identify them during surgery to prevent injury to the involved organ.
      (ii) Littre's hernia- They have Meckel's diverticulum as content.
      (iii) Richter's hernia- They have a portion of the circumference of the intestine as content.
      (iv) Amyand's hernia- Occurs when the appendix is trapped within an inguinal hernia.
   (c) Clinical presentation- Based on the clinical presentation, Inguinal Hernia can be classified into following types:
      (i) Reducible inguinal hernia- Contents get reduced either spontaneously or on applying gentle pressure.
      (ii) Incarcerated inguinal hernia- Content may not get reduced even on applying ample pressure but there are no signs of bowel obstruction or strangulation.
      (iii) Obstructed Inguinal hernia (Fig. 66.2a,b,c.)- incarcerated inguinal hernia presenting with signs of acute intestinal obstruction such as bilious vomiting, abdominal distension, inability to pass stool and flatus, etc.

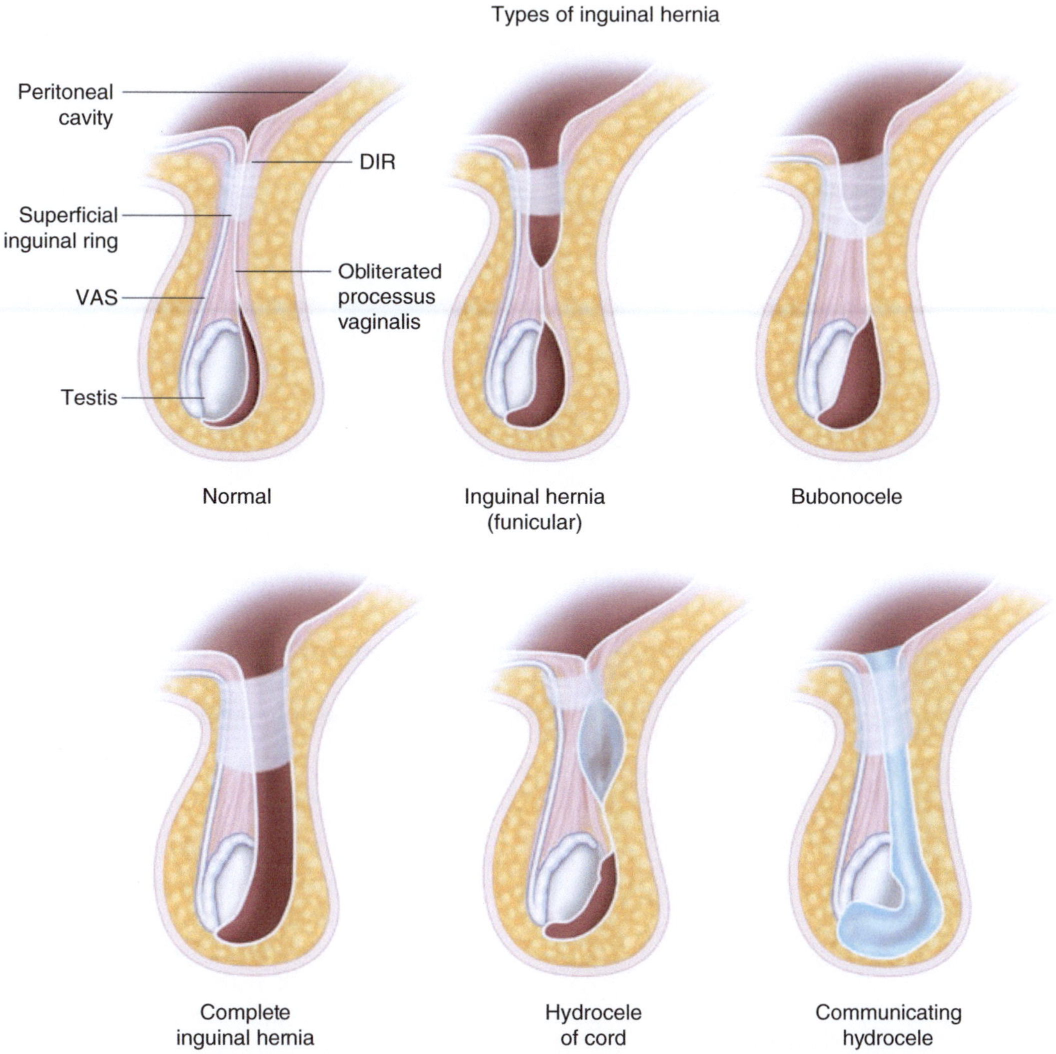

Fig. 66.1 Types of inguinal hernia and hydrocele (See previous edition for illustration)

(iv) Strangulated Inguinal hernia- incarcerated inguinal hernia presenting with signs of strangulation or bowel ischemia such as severe pain, blood in stool, sepsis, etc.

66.1.6 Clinical Features

Clinical presentation of these children is variable and may range from a painless reducible bulge in the inguinal region to a non-reducible incarcerated mass with or without features of obstruction or strangulation. Most commonly, they present as an asymptomatic groin swelling which typically appears when child is crying or straining disappears when the child is relaxed or is sleeping (Fig. 66.3). Additionally, reducibility with a gargling sound is characteristic of bowel in the hernia sac. The diagnosis of Inguinal hernia is essentially clinical and a proper history from the parents or referring physician, as well as a photograph, are often reliable in determining the diagnosis. Various maneuvers such as straining, crying, Valsalva maneuver, etc., can make the hernia visible. However, in some cases, the her-

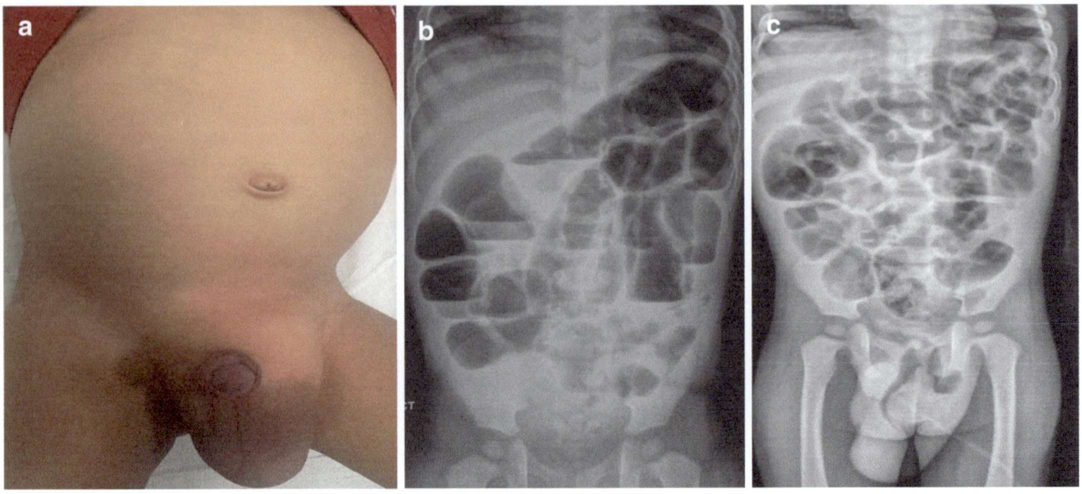

Fig. 66.2 (**a**) Obstructed Left inguinal hernia, male (Note the abdominal distension along with irreducible hernia); (**b**) Erect X ray abdomen of same patient showing multiple air fluid levels suggestive of acute intestinal obstruction; (**c**) Supine X ray abdomen of same patient showing bowel with air in scrotum along with dilated bowel loops

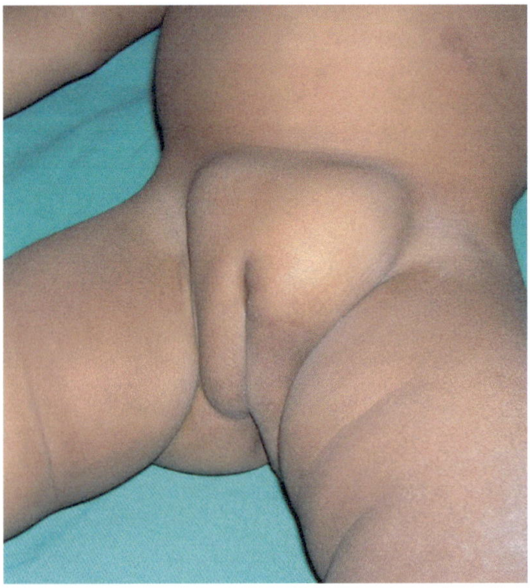

Fig. 66.3 Bilateral inguinal hernia, female

nia is not visible even on straining or crying. In such cases, a "Silk glove sign" in the spermatic cord on palpation indicates an indirect hernia sac. This sign is considered positive if the surgeon gets the feeling of two pieces of silk rubbing together when he rubs the spermatic cord side to side on the pubic tubercle. This sign has a positive predictive value of 86.73% which makes it an important sign to detect Inguinal hernia when inguinal bulge is not visible.

66.1.7 Differential Diagnosis

Differential diagnosis of inguinal hernia includes other causes of Inguinal swelling such as-

A. *In Males*
   1. *Hydrocele* (Fig. 66.4) *and encysted hydrocele of cord:* Hydrocele generally occur due to accumulation of fluid in the tunica of testis or spermatic cord in males and usually present with a scrotal swelling. Generally, swelling is firm in consistency, non-reducible, and it is possible to get above the swelling. Fluctuation and transillumination tests are positive. Although hydrocele is irreducible, it may reduce slowly during sleep in cases of communicating hydrocele.
   2. *Femoral Hernia:* Femoral hernias are a rare incidence in children (<1% of all pediatric groin hernias). Due to their rarity and close resemblance to inguinal hernias, they are often misdiagnosed especially if incarceration occurs and may lead to delay in treatment with disastrous complications. They can be differentiated from inguinal hernia on careful physical examination as the swelling is below and lateral to the pubis tubercle in these cases. However, in many cases, ultrasonography

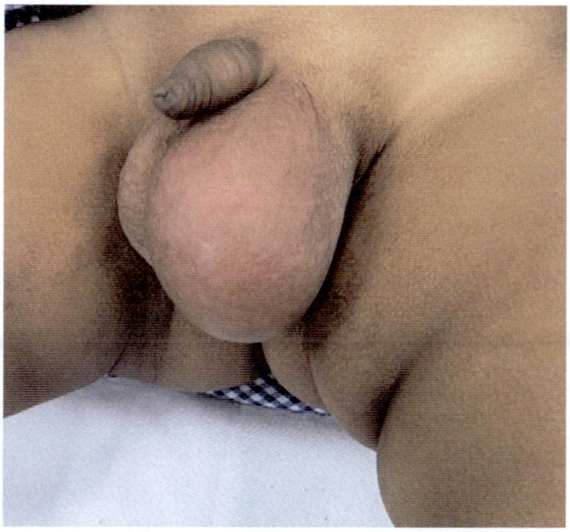

Fig. 66.4 Left hydrocele

or Laparoscopy is needed to correctly make a diagnosis.

3. *Varicocele:* They are commonly seen in adolescent age group with approximately 15% prevalence in pediatric age group. They are caused by dilated veins in the pampiniform plexus of the spermatic cord and usually manifest as a scrotal mass that grows in size with valsalva maneuver and has a distinctive "bag of worms" sensation on touch.
4. *Undescended/retractile Testis:* The Undescended or retractile testis in the inguinal canal may be felt as a firm mobile structure in the inguinal canal. However, pain and testicular sensation on pressure along with empty scrotum differentiates them from inguinal hernias.
5. *Lipoma of the cord-* Although lipoma of the spermatic cord is found in more than 20–70% of all operated cases of Inguinal hernia as per the literature, in approximately 8%, they can present as an inguinal bulge even without a hernia sac.

B. *In Females*

Hydrocele of the canal of Nuck- It is usually encountered in young girls less than 5 years old and occurs due to the accumulation of fluid in the canal of nuck. It generally presents as a firm, non-reducible swelling in inguino-labial region.

66.1.8 Role of Imaging

Although inguinal hernia is a clinical diagnosis, ultrasonography is often helpful in special circumstances such as the absence of any visible swelling on examination or equivocal clinical presentation, or to determine etiology of acute inguinoscrotal swelling.

66.1.9 Laboratory Evaluation

Laboratory workup in a case of inguinal hernia in children includes preoperative workup and is not helpful in diagnosis of these patients. However, all phenotypic females presenting with palpable bilateral inguinal mass infancy require additional workup such as Karyotyping and hormonal workup to rule out complete androgen insensitivity syndrome (CAIS) as it has an incidence of 1–2% in such patients.

66.1.10 Treatment

The Recommended treatment for Inguinal Hernia in children of any age is essentially Surgical. Although surgery is recommended as soon as feasible (Preferably within a month of diagnosis) in reducible hernia to avoid complications such as incarceration/obstruction or strangulation, it is not an emergency. For premature babies however, timing of surgery is controversial. In these patients, the increased risk of incarceration has to be balanced with postoperative respiratory and systemic complications of anesthesia in these babies while deciding the timing of surgery. However, most pediatric surgeons due to increased risk of complications, recommend surgical repair before their discharge from the hospital preferrably after attaining the weight of 2 kilogram.

In incarcerated hernia, however, reduction should be attempted immediately on presentation either manually or surgically, if manual reduction fails. Unless there are signs of obstruction or strangulation or child is very ill, manual reduction of an incarcerated hernia should always be attempted as it is successful in 95–100% of patients and has lower complication rate than emergency open surgical reduction. There are many techniques that one can use for manual reduction but preferred technique is the one in which thumb and index finger of one hand of examiner form a funnel where the mass exits the inguinal ring and steady circumferential pressure is exerted by the other hand on the inferomedial aspect of mass.

66.1.11 Surgical Procedure

The recommended surgical procedure in children for treatment of Inguinal Hernia is Herniotomy, which is defined as high ligation and division of the PPV. In Herniotomy, the hernial sac is isolated, ligated, and divided. In case of complete hernial sacs, it is advisable to lay open distal sac to prevent the formation of hydrocele in postoperative period. It is advisable to inspect the proximal hernial sac before ligation to detect any sliding hernia, especially in females. If the sliding hernia is present, then the sac can be ligated distal to the contents and the deep ring can be tightened (*Bevan repair*).

If the deep inguinal ring (DIR) has enlarged due to long-standing hernia, it is recommended to plicate the floor of inguinal canal (transversalis fascia) medial to the ring using a non-absorbable interrupted suture to narrow the ring and push the spermatic cord laterally (called *Lytle's repair*), in addition to herniotomy.

In case of very large hernias in small infants with very large deep inguinal ring defect and weakness of transversalis fascia, complete reconstruction of floor of inguinal canal is recommended by suturing conjoined tendon and transversalis fascia with inguinal ligament, thus strengthening the floor of inguinal canal (*Modified Bassini Repair*).

Additionally, laparoscopic hernia repair is gaining popularity so much so that the term "Inguinal hernia repair" is now slowly being used in place of "Herniotomy" to describe surgical procedure for inguinal hernia because in laparoscopy, sac is not divided, only the ring is closed using purse string suture (Fig. 66.5a,b). In girls, laparoscopy allows visualization of the internal genitalia. Another advantage is that asymptomatic Contralateral PPV can be diagnosed and managed in the same sitting. Laparoscopic hernia repair is also gaining popularity in incarcerated hernia because it allows for direct visualization of bowel after it is reduced in abdomen. Also, laparoscopic hernia repair in males have a distinct advantage as there is minimal handling of cord structures, therefore decreasing the risk of vas and vessel injury as compared to open (theoretical- yet to be proven).

The surgery can be done as a day care case except in premature babies (postconceptional

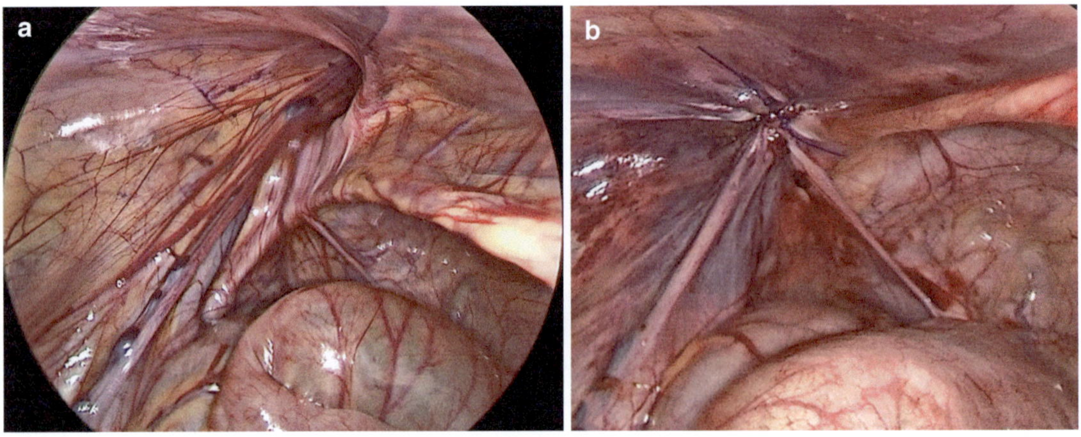

Fig. 66.5 (**a**) Laparoscopic view of Left Side inguinal hernia in a male with an open Deep Inguinal Ring (DIR); (**b**) Laparoscopic view of same patient after purse-string closure of DIR

age < 60 weeks) who should be observed overnight due to high risk of postoperative apnea.

Unilateral versus bilateral groin exploration is a controversial issue. The mean contention is that contralateral patent processus vaginalis (CPPV) is present in approximately 30–50% of children undergoing herniotomy. Of these children, 30–50% may develop a contralateral hernia, so routine contralateral inguinal exploration may benefit only 15–20% of cases. Hence contralateral exploration for clinical unilateral inguinal hernia is generally not recommended as in 75% cases it is unnecessary. With introduction of laparoscopy, this CPPV can be managed without any significant increase in operative time or cost. However, contralateral exploration is still recommended in children with ventriculo-peritoneal shunt who present with hernia as because of increased intra-abdominal fluid, it is very likely that the contralateral side will also become symptomatic.

In patients with associated inherited disorders of the connective tissue, herniorrhaphy is performed as recurrence rate of herniotomy alone is very high.

66.1.12 Postoperative Care and Complications

Most children have an uncomplicated postoperative course. Scrotal edema commonly occurs postoperatively especially after herniotomy of large inguinal hernia, but resolves spontaneously over a period of 1–3 weeks. Other postoperative complications include hematomas and hydroceles that can take many months to resolve and may rarely require surgical drainage. Postoperative infection in these cases is generally rare with incidence <1%, thus, routine use of postoperative antibiotics is generally not recommended in these cases. Recurrence after herniotomy is rare (<1%) when performed by expert pediatric surgeons. Vas deference and testicular vessel being part of spermatic cord are closely related to sac and may get injured during dissection especially in inexperienced hands. These injuries are fortunately very rare but catastrophic.

66.1.13 Direct Inguinal Hernias

Direct Inguinal hernia are rare in children and result from a defect resulting from weakness of muscles of floor of inguinal canal. Generally, the site of this defect is just medial to inferior epigastric vessel in the Hasselbach's triangle. It is very difficult to distinguish from indirect inguinal hernia clinically and diagnosis in most cases is made intraoperatively, especially in laparoscopy (Fig. 66.6). On the basis of etiology, it may be classified as primary direct inguinal hernia occurring due to inherent weakness of floor of inguinal canal or secondary direct inguinal hernia occurring due to weakness of floor of inguinal canal secondary to indirect hernia repair. In some cases, in which inguinal hernia repair had already been done previously, direct inguinal hernia may be misdiagnosed as recurrence especially if an associated direct inguinal hernia is missed during herniotomy for indirect inguinal hernia.

66.1.14 Adolescent Hernias

Adolescent patients (10 years to 18 years age) represent a "gray zone" between children and adults, and there is no consensus on the most appropriate surgery for inguinal hernias in these patients. Type of operation in these patients largely depends on the surgeon. Adult surgeons prefer to repair adolescent hernias with a mesh repair and pediatric surgeons tend to repair them with a high ligation of the sac. However, given

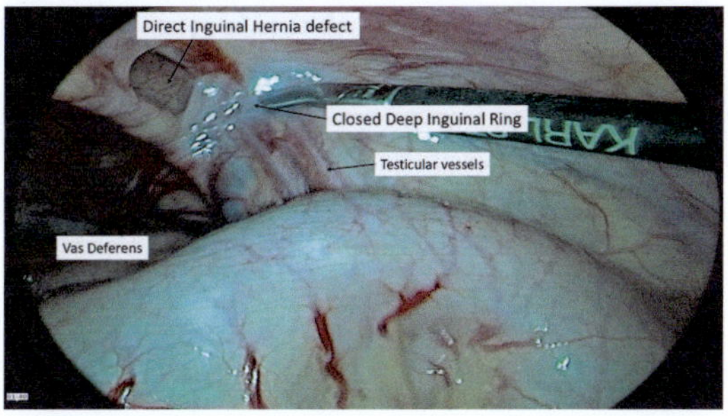

Fig. 66.6 Right side **Direct** inguinal hernia diagnosed intraoperatively during laparoscopy for Right **indirect** inguinal hernia (Misdiagnosed)

the complications involved with use of mesh in children, it is generally avoided and a tension-free tissue repair is considered prudent in most cases along with herniotomy.

66.2 Hydrocele

A hydrocele is defined as a collection of peritoneal fluid in the PPV or within the tunica vaginalis of testis.

66.2.1 Types of Hydrocele (Fig. 66.7)

66.2.2 Clinical Presentation and Diagnosis

Most cases of hydrocele in children are asymptomatic and present as painless, nonreducible, firm, fluctuant, transilluminate scrotal swelling (Fig. 66.4). If a history of reducibility or significant change in size is present, then communicating hydrocele can be suspected. Diagnosis of hydrocele is generally clinical; however, ultrasonography is useful in differentiating it from other causes of scrotal swelling in doubtful cases.

Hydrocele of the cord: When hydrocele is present above the testis, it is diagnosed as hydrocele of the cord. It can either be encysted (if it does not communicate with peritoneal cavity) or funicular (if it communicates with peritoneal cavity). Although it is mobile, traction test (which is elicited gently pulling the testis down), fixes it due to attachment to the cord thus decreasing its mobility.

66.2.3 Treatment of Hydrocele

Treatment involves watchful waiting till the age of 2 years as natural history suggest that the majority of congenital hydrocele resolve spontaneously by the age of 2 years. Beyond 2 years, the natural history of congenital hydrocele is poorly understood, However, surgery is indicated if the hydrocele persists beyond 2 years of age and in cases of communicating hydrocele with PPV. The surgery most commonly done is herniotomy (high ligation of processus vaginalis) with drainage of the distal hydrocele sac fluid.

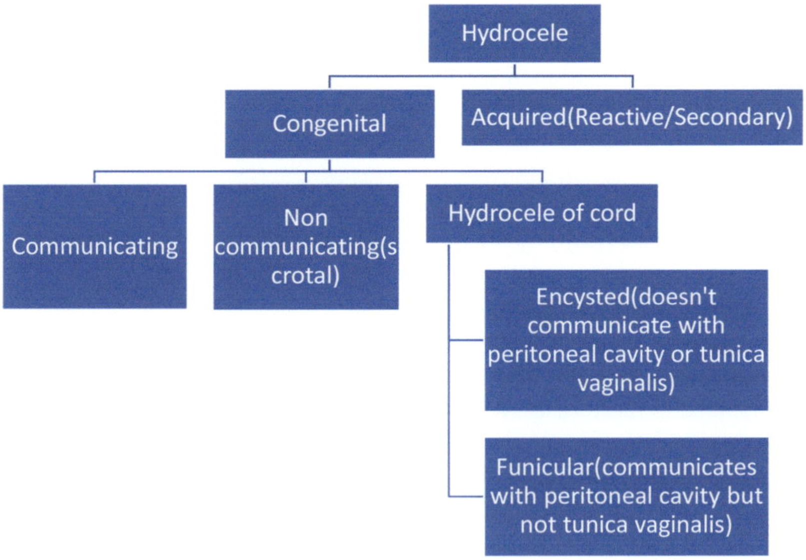

Fig. 66.7 Classification of hydrocele in children

66.2.4 Postoperative Complications

These include Scrotal swelling, iatrogenic undescended testis, recurrence, injury to vas deferens, testicular atrophy, and intestinal injury.

66.3 Acute Scrotum

66.3.1 Definition

Acute scrotum in children is a medical emergency that presents as acute pain or redness or swelling in the scrotum. The incidence is variable in various series however, testis is ischemic in approximately 20% of these cases. Thus, proper evaluation is needed in all cases of acute scrotum to find out its cause to prevent testicular loss due to ischemia.

66.3.2 Causes of Acute Scrotum in Children

The differential diagnosis of acute scrotum in children are varied and can be grouped as follows (14):

A. Torsion
   (a) Torsion of the appendix of testis
   (b) Torsion of the testis
B. Infection
   (a) Epididymitis
   (b) Epididymo-orchitis
C. Trauma
   (a) Hematoma
   (b) Hematocele
   (c) Testicular Rupture
D. Systemic Causes- Henoch–Schönlein purpura, Lymphoma/Leukemia
E. Incarcerated inguinal hernia
F. Acute hydrocele
G. Idiopathic Scrotal edema

66.3.3 Torsion of the Testis

Testicular torsion is a condition that occurs due to sudden rotation of testis on its axis thus causing twisting of the spermatic cord resulting in testicular ischemia. It is regarded as the most important and serious cause of acute scrotum that may result in testicular loss which may result from even 4 hours of testicular ischemia. They have a bimodal age distribution with peak occurrence in age groups, neonatal and pubertal. Their incidence is 1 in 4000 in males less than 25 years of age and approximately 65% of cases occur in males between 12 years to 18 years of age. This increased incidence during puberty results from increase in weight of testis during puberty.

Predisposing factors for torsion are:

(a) Inversion of the testis is the commonest. Lie of the testis transverse/horizontal or upside down.
(b) High investment of the tunica vaginalis "bell clapper" deformity: because of which the testis hangs free and can twist within the tunica vaginalis. Many children with this deformity have a transverse lie of testis in the scrotum.
(c) Rapid cremaster muscle contraction may also cause rotation of the testis.
(d) It is also proposed the pubertal testis with increased vascularity and weight is more prone to torsion.

66.3.4 Intravaginal and Extravaginal Torsion

Generally, neonatal torsion is generally extravaginal that occurs due to twist of the spermatic cord and pubertal torsion is intravaginal, due to "clapper bell" deformity. This is because in neonates the loose tissue around the testis allows the testis along with its tunica vaginalis to twist. Post neonatal age once the tunica vaginalis is fixed in the scrotum, extravaginal torsion cannot occur.

66.3.5 Clinical Features

Children with acute testicular torsion present with sudden onset excruciating pain in the groin and lower abdomen often associated with nausea and vomiting in nearly 90% of the patients. Symptoms of torsion are often precipitated by trauma, straining, or physical activity. On examination, scrotum may have reddish discoloration and may have abnormal lie on palpation with characteristically a thickened, tender, and twisted spermatic cord.

Acute epididymo-orchitis is clinically similar to testicular torsion, making it difficult to distinguish between the two. Elevation of the testis alleviates discomfort in epididymo-orchitis but exacerbates it in cases of torsion (Phren's sign). However, Phren's sign is not a valid diagnostic sign since it cannot distinguish between torsion and other causes of acute scrotum in children. Epididymo-orchitis is often accompanied by urethritis, a urinary tract infection (*E. coli*), and viral infections. In mumps orchitis, the chord is not thickened.

66.3.6 Diagnosis

Diagnosis of testicular torsion is generally made on clinical examination. Recently, TWIST score has been suggested in various prospective studies to diagnose testicular torsion clinically. The score consists evaluation and scoring based on 5 parameters as follows:

S No.	Parameter	Score
1	Nausea or vomiting	1
2	Testicular Swelling	2
3	Hard Testis on palpation	2
4	High riding testis	1
5	Absent cremasteric reflex	1

A score of ≥5 has a sensitivity of 76%, specificity 100% and positive predictive value 100% to diagnose testicular torsion.

66.3.7 Role of Imaging

When a clinical diagnosis of testicular torsion is unclear or uncertain, a *color doppler ultrasound of the scrotum* should be performed. Testicular torsion is characterized by a "whirlpool sign" on real-scale ultrasound images of the cord with reduced blood flow in color doppler. Doppler ultrasonography has been shown to have a sensitivity of 69–100% and a specificity of 77–100% in detecting testicular torsion.

Radionuclide study with technetium 99 can also show whether the testis is perfused or not with reported sensitivity and specificity of 100% and 97%, respectively. However, a nuclear scan takes several hours is not available everywhere promptly enough to permit timely operative decisions and orchidopexy. Thus, doppler ultrasound has supplanted nuclear scan as test of choice for testicular torsion. These investigations are of doubtful utility in children who are prepubertal, as the testis volume is small and accuracy of these tests is limited.

66.3.8 Management (Fig. 66.8)

In suspected cases, immediate surgical exploration is needed. Exploration is done through a midline scrotal incision. The involved testis is derotated and testis is covered with warm sponge. The involved testis is assessed for viability and managed as below.

- Necrotic testis- orchidectomy. A non-viable testis may be removed with prior consent (Fig. 66.9)
- Viable testis- orchidopexy
- Doubtful viability—age > 10 years—orchidectomy because of risk of alloimmunization secondary to damage to blood testis barrier
  age < 10 years- orchidopexy

Surgery should never be delayed on assumption of nonviability based upon a clinical estimate of duration of torsion.

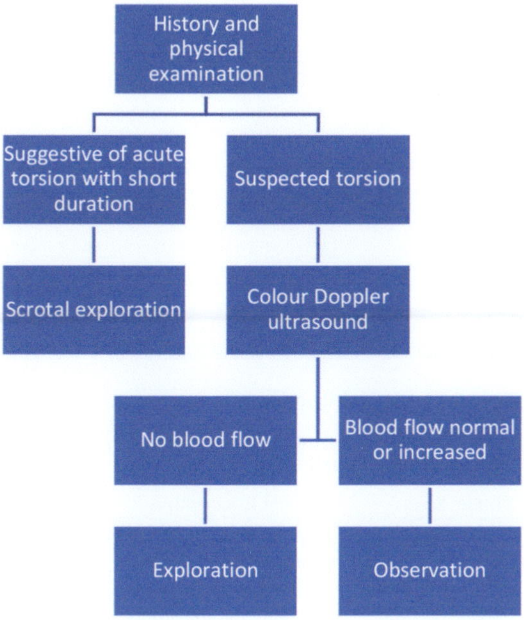

Fig. 66.8 Algorithm of evaluation and management of acute scrotum in children

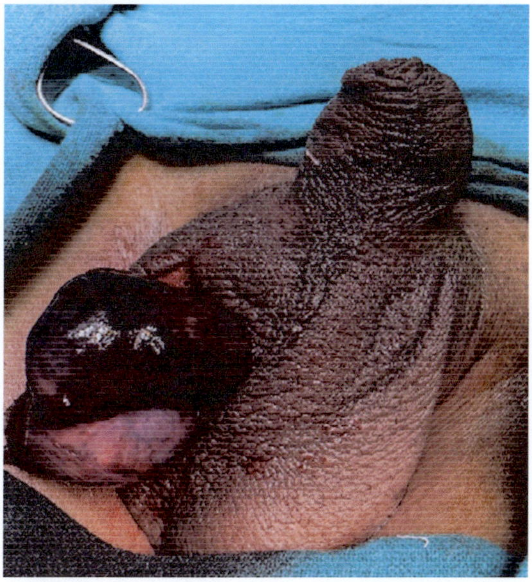

Fig. 66.9 Discolored/gangrenous testis due to torsion

The contralateral testis should always be fixed as the predisposing pathology is similar on both the sides (Fig. 66.10).

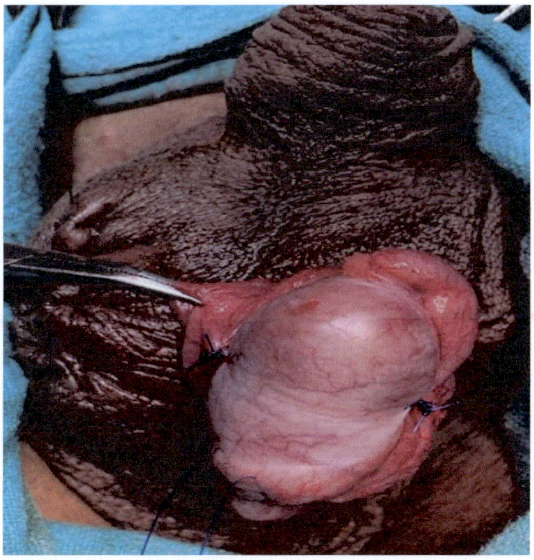

Fig. 66.10 Contralateral orchidopexy being done after orchidectomy for torsion testis

66.3.9 Torsion of the Appendix Testis (Hydatid of Morgagni)

This occurs due to sudden rotation of the appendix of testis and has incidence approximately 4 times more common than torsion of testis. It generally occurs in 7–10-year old boys and presents with gradual or sudden onset pain associated with nausea and vomiting and resembles symptoms of torsion testis. On examination, tenderness at the upper pole of the testis with the "blue dot" sign on transillumination is characteristic. Spontaneous involution due to ischemic necrosis of the appendix can happen. Treatment consists of supportive therapy with analgesics, limited mobility, and warm compresses. Surgery is only indicated if torsion of the testis cannot be ruled out. However, it may sometimes require scrotal exploration with excision of the twisted appendix.

Idiopathic scrotal edema presents at 4–12 years of age with red swollen scrotum without much pain or tenderness. The swelling may extend to the perineum, groin, and penis. It is probably due to allergic reaction and generally subsides in a day or two.

66.4 Varicocele

Varicocele is a condition affecting mainly adolescents that occurs due to abnormal dilatation of veins in the pampiniform plexus surrounding the spermatic cord. On the basis of etiology, varicocele can be classified into primary varicocele and secondary varicoceles. While the cause of primary or idiopathic varicocele is not clear and is proposed to be a result of increased venous pressure and incompetent valves, causes of secondary varicoceles include

1. IVC thrombus
2. Renal vein thrombosis especially on right side with clot propagation down the IVC
3. Abdominal mass (e.g. Retroperitoneal tumors, renal tumors, or lymphadenopathy)

Varicoceles can lead to decreased fertility and even testicular atrophy due to abnormally raised scrotal temperature. The left side is impacted in 95% of cases because the left spermatic vein joins the left renal vein at a 90-degree angle, while the right spermatic vein empties at a more obtuse angle directly into the inferior vena cava, allowing for more continuous flow.

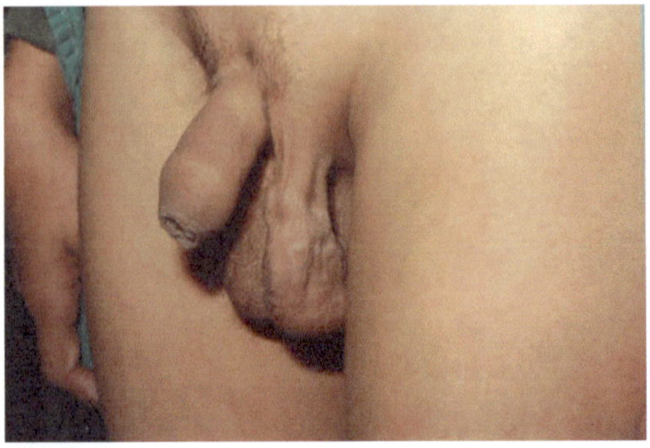

Fig. 66.11 Left varicocele

Table 66.1 Varicocele grading

Grade	Size	Clinical Description
1	Small	Palpable only on Valsalva maneuver
2	Moderate	Nonvisible on inspection but palpable upon standing
3	Large	Visible on gross inspection

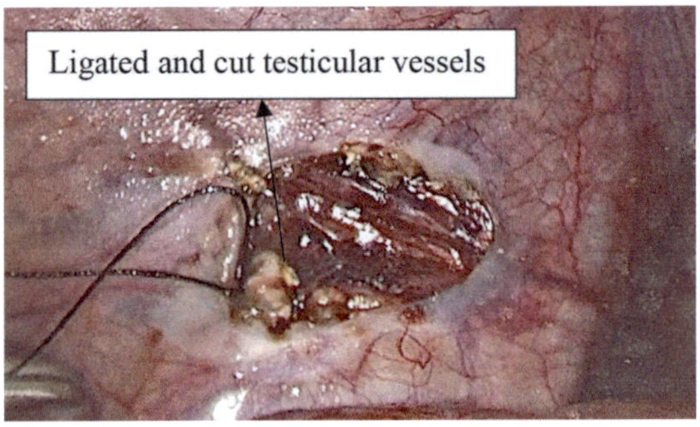

Fig. 66.12 Laparoscopic Palomo Procedure

66.4.1 Clinical Features

The scrotum on the affected side hangs lower than normal, and the dilated vessels feel like a "bag of worms" when palpated (Fig. 66.11). Based on the clinical description, it can be classified into three grades (Table 66.1).

Doppler ultrasound is often used to diagnose testis varicocele, but its accuracy may be limited in children due to the testis's smaller size. Peak Retrograde flow (PRF) during Valsalva maneuver can be used as a prognostic marker in adolescents and adults to predict testicular atrophy. As per the literature, PRF >38 cm/sec is generally associated with poor testicular growth and testicular asymmetry. Ultrasonography also helps to rule out causes of secondary varicocele.

When there is noticeable testicular atrophy or persistent pain or discomfort, surgery may be necessary. Surgery is also recommended for adolescents and young adults who exhibit related subfertility on semen analysis as correction has been linked to better semen analysis in these patients.

Operative procedure consists of ligating the testicular vein, ideally above the inguinal ligament. However, the most popular procedure is mass ligation of the testicular vessels above the inguinal ligament (*Palomo operation*; Fig. 66.12). Laparoscopy is a very efficient method for accomplishing this. This process guarantees that all of the veins are ligated. Collaterals help to keep the testis' circulatory supply intact. Embolization of the testicular vein under radiological control is an alternative therapy.

Postoperative complications include recurrence, reactive hydrocele, and testicular atrophy (rare). The recurrence rate after surgery is very high due to filling up of the collateral veins.

66.5 Summary

1. Inguinal hernia is very common in chlildren with the incidence of 1–5% in fullterm babies and 20% in preterm babies. Bilaterality incidence is 10%. Incarceration and obstruction are two common problems which warrents for an early surgical repair by herniotomy.
2. Hydrocele is a relatively benign condition in infants and can be observed till 2 yeras of age.
3. Testicular tortion is an emergency and requires immediate surgical exploration to avoid ischaemic injury to the testis.
4. Vericocele in adolescent boys can be corrected by laparoscopic ligation of retroperitoneal testicular veins (Palomo procedure).

Suggested Reading

Auger N, Del Giorgio F, Le-Nguyen A, Bilodeau-Bertrand M, Piché N. Maternal risk factors for paediatric inguinal hernia. Br J Surg. 2021;109(1):129–35.

Coran AG, Caldamone A, Scott Adzich N, Krummel TM, Laberge JM, editors. Pediatric Surgery. 7th ed. Oxford: Elsevier Limited; 2012.

De Los RT, Locke J, Afshar K. Varicoceles in the pediatric population: diagnosis, treatment, and outcomes. Can Urol Assoc J. 2017;11(1-2S):34.

Hall NJ, Ron O, Eaton S, Pierro A. Surgery for hydrocele in children—an avoidable excess? J Pediatr Surg. 2011;46(12):2401–5.

Morini F, Dreuning KMA, Janssen Lok MJH, Wester T, Derikx JPM, Friedmacher F, et al. Surgical management of pediatric inguinal hernia: a systematic review and guideline from the European Pediatric Surgeons' Association Evidence and Guideline Committee. Eur J Pediatr Surg. 2022;32(03):219–32.

Zhang K, Zhang Y, Chao M. Clinical characteristics and identification of risk factors of testicular torsion in children: a retrospective study in a single institution. Front Surg. 2023;9:1040487.

Undescended Testis

67

Ashitosh Pokharkar and Subhasis Roy Choudhury

67.1 Embryology

Cryptorchidism is the failure of testicular descent, which relies on the development and hormonal activity of the growing testis. The indifferent gonadal tissue located on the genital ridge of the embryo begins differentiating into a testis around 41 to 44 days after the expression of SRY (Sex determining region on Y chromosome) and SOX9 (SRY containing 9).

The hormonal function of the human fetal testis is crucial for the masculinization of the reproductive tract and testicular descent. Sertoli cells produce Mullerian inhibitory substance (MIS), which causes regression of the Mullerian duct structures. Leydig cells start producing testosterone by the ninth week, stimulating the development of Wolffian structures, including the epididymis and vas deferens. From the seventh to the ninth month, the testis descends through the inguinal canal into the scrotum.

67.2 Factors Influencing Testicular Descent

67.2.1 Gubernaculum

This is a mucofibrous structure attached to the testis and scrotum that guides the descent of the testis into the scrotum. The epididymis also plays a role in the descent.

There are two phases of testicular descent:

1. Transabdominal descent (5–28 weeks): During this phase, the testis descends from the retroperitoneum to the deep inguinal ring. This descent occurs due to the regression of the cranial suspensory ligament attached to the diaphragm and the thickening of the gubernaculum under the influence of androgens and ILGF3 (insulin-like growth factor 3) from the Leydig cells. Anti-Müllerian hormone (AMH/MIS) from Sertoli cells causes regression of the cranial suspensory ligament and thickening of the gubernaculum.
2. Inguinoscrotal migration (28–35 weeks): This phase is under androgenic control and may be due to the release of calcitonin gene-related peptide from the genitofemoral nerve. Other factors identified to influence gonadal descent are EGF, neonatal hormonal surge from the hypothalamo-pituitary-gonadal (HPA) axis, and inhibin B from Sertoli cells. Migration may be aided by the transmission of intra-abdominal pressure through the patent processus vaginalis (PPV).

A. Pokharkar (✉)
BJ Wadia Hospital for Children's, Mumbai, India

S. Roy Choudhury
Pediatric Surgery, Lady Hardinge Medical College and Associated Kalawati Saran Children's Hospital, New Delhi, Delhi, India

© The Author(s), under exclusive license to Springer Nature Singapore Pte Ltd. 2025

S. Roy Choudhury (ed.), *Pediatric Surgery*, https://doi.org/10.1007/978-981-96-1257-4_67

67.2.2 Incidence

Cryptorchidism is the most common congenital defect in boys, affecting 1–4% of full-term babies and 1–45% of premature babies. The descent of the testis can occur postnatally but is rare after the age of 6 months. UDT (undescended testis) is associated with 500 documented syndromes. The majority of cases are isolated, with a non-syndromic to syndromic UDT ratio of 6:1.

67.3 Epidemiology

1. Congenital: the most common variety.
2. Genetic susceptibility: The disease is heritable, but susceptibility is likely polygenic and multifactorial.
3. Environmental risk factors: Maternal alcohol consumption, maternal smoking, and increased consumption of analgesics increase the risk. Paternal horticulture-related professions also increase the risk.

67.4 Definitions

Normal scrotal position- Positioning of the midpoint of testis at or below the mid scrotum.

1. True UDT (cryptorchid): Absence of one or both testis in normal scrotal position. The sites could be intraabdominal, intracanalicular, or pre-scrotal in the superficial inguinal pouch (common).
2. Agenesis: Testis that was never present and hence is associated with ipsilateral mullerian duct persistence.
3. Acquired UDT: Testis documented scrotal at initial examination without intervening surgery.
4. Ascended UDT: Previously descended, then "ascends" spontaneously. It occurs because of failure of spermatic cord to lengthen adequately while the length of inguinal canal increase as the child is growing.
5. Secondary UDT: Suprascrotal location of testis after inguinal hernia repair and as a complication of orchidopexy surgery.
6. Retractile Testis: Testis in the upper part of scrotum which can be pulled down to the lower part of scrotum and remains there for more than 10 seconds. It is due to cremasteric reflex active in early childhood phase.
7. Ectopic UDT: Testis descends normally through inguinal canal but then moves into an abnormal position in the groin. The testis is usually fully developed however, main hazard is liability to injury. The most common sites are superficial inguinal pouch followed by femoral canal, suprapubic region, perineum, and contralateral scrotum (Fig. 67.1).
8. Peeping testis: This are non-palpable testis which can be moved into inguinal canal with application of intra-abdominal pressure.
9. Gliding testis: testis can be manipulated into upper scrotum but retracts when released.

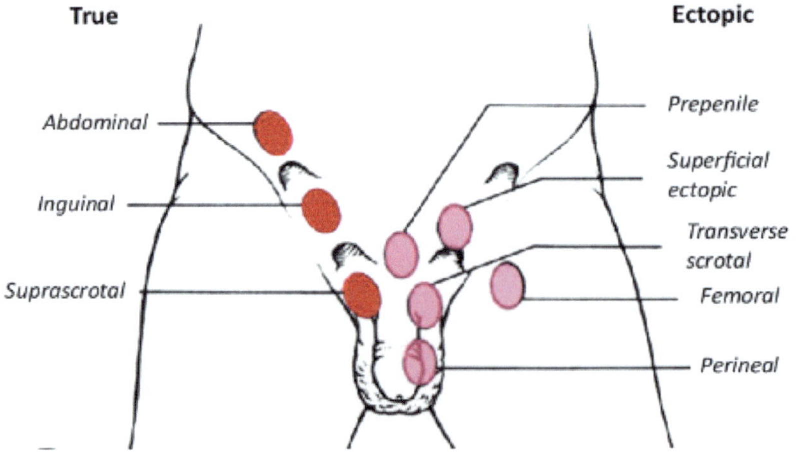

Fig. 67.1 Cryptorchid testis location

67.5 Clinical Features and Examination

The majority of undescended testes (UDTs) are palpable, with 75–80% being detectable through physical examination. About 60–70% of cases involve unilateral involvement, with the right side being more commonly affected due to delayed descent on that side (Figs. 67.2a, b and 67.3).

Careful history taking and a thorough physical examination are essential for diagnosis and planning the appropriate management. The examination should be conducted in a comfortable room, with the patient in a supine position, and ideally in a cross-legged or standing position. Abduction of the thighs helps inhibit the cremasteric reflex. The examination should document the palpability, position, mobility, size, and any possible associated findings such as hernia or hypospadias.

Gliding test: This involves rolling the fingers of one hand from the deep to the superficial inguinal ring and attempting to push the subcutaneous structures towards the scrotum using gel or powder. The fingers of the other hand are placed at the root of the scrotum, trying to grasp or roll the testis. In cases of micropenis with bilateral cryptorchidism, further evaluation, including an endocrine profile test with follicle-stimulating hormone (FSH), luteinizing hormone (LH), and testosterone levels, is necessary to assess for vanishing testes or hypogonadotrophic hypogonadism. Hypospadias may be present in 10–20% of cases, and if proximal penile hypospadias is observed in conjunction with UDT, chromosomal analysis is warranted due to the higher likelihood of associated abnormalities (32–47%).

Differentiating between a low undescended testis and a retractile testis is often challenging and may coexist in some cases. Both a retractile testis and a low undescended testis can be manipulated into the scrotum. However, the retractile testis remains in the scrotum temporarily without traction, while the low undescended testis does not remain in the scrotum. Pathological changes are observed in UDT but not in retractile testis. The ipsilateral hemiscrotum is poorly developed in cases of true undescended testis. Human Chorionic Gonadotropin (HCG) stimulation may facilitate the descent of a retractile testis, but a true undescended testis will not respond to this stimulation.

Distinguishing between anorchia (bilateral absence of testis) and intra-abdominal testis (cryptorchidism) can be done through the HCG stimulation test. Baseline testosterone, FSH, and LH levels are measured. Elevated baseline FSH levels indicate anorchia. If baseline FSH/LH lev-

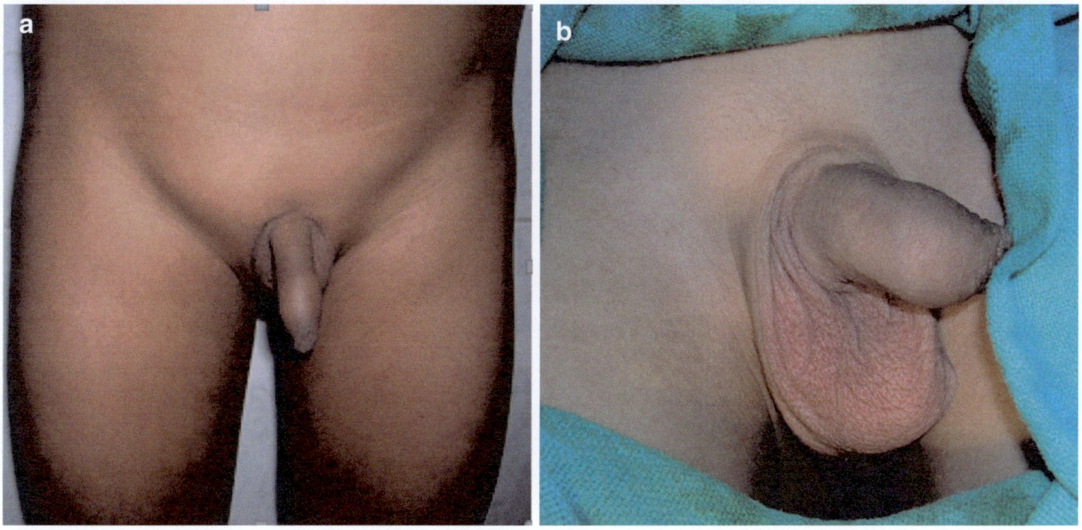

Fig. 67.2 a and b Right UDT, note the empty scrotum

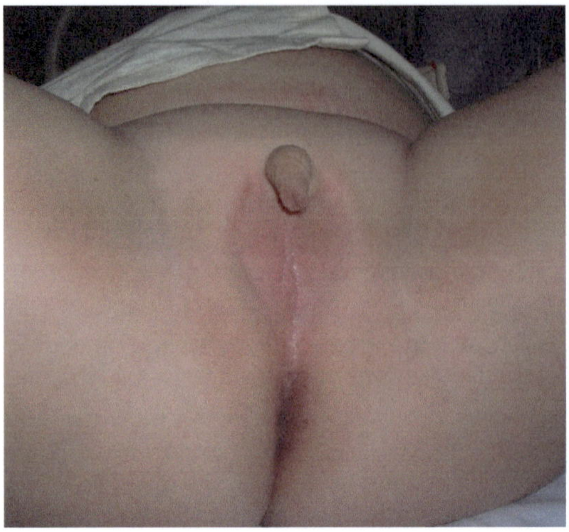

Fig. 67.3 Bilateral empty scrotum, UDT

els are normal, an elevation of serum testosterone following CG stimulation (2000 IU intramuscular daily for 3 days) indicates the presence of functioning testicular tissue. However, a negative response does not exclude the presence of a testis, and exploratory surgery is indicated in such cases. This test is currently not widely used due to non-standardization and potential for false results.

Radiological imaging, such as ultrasound scan, CT scan, or MRI, is generally unnecessary for localizing the testis. MRI is considered superior and may be useful in obese children, with gadolinium MR angiography offering high sensitivity for localization. For impalpable testes, imaging is not reliable in determining the need for definitive surgical intervention. Laparoscopy is the preferred procedure in such cases.

67.6 Associated Pathology

1. Testicular Maldevelopment: It involves abnormal germ cell development, along with a decreased number of Leydig cells (at the earliest stages), and degeneration of Sertoli cells.
2. Anomalies of Epididymis: The reported frequency of anomalies in the epididymis varies from 16% to 75%. Anatomic findings may include partial or complete non-fusion between the caput or cauda epididymis and the testis, elongated or looping epididymis, and atresia.
3. Other Pathologies: These include a patent processus vaginalis that can cause inguinal hernia, anomalies of the tunica that predispose to torsion, and abnormal attachment of gubernacular remnants, which are commonly observed.
4. Rare Associations: Polyorchisms (presence of more than two testes), splenogonadal fusion (fusion of the spleen with the gonad), and transverse testicular ectopia (abnormal position of the testis across the midline) are rare associations that have been reported.

67.7 Complications

Infertility: Despite histological abnormalities in UDT and the contralateral descended testis, as well as abnormal seminal analysis, the fertility rate of men with unilateral UDT is close to that of the normal population. However, bilateral UDT the sperm counts are low and is associated with a 50% chance of infertility.

Malignancy: The risk of developing malignancy in UDT cases is two to five folds higher than in the normal population. Early orchidopexy (surgical procedure to bring the testis into the scrotum) reduces the risk and facilitates testicular examination and cancer detection. The contralateral normally descended testis also carries a risk of developing malignancy. The highest risk is associated with an intra-abdominal testis. The most frequent malignant tumors associated with UDT are seminomatous and non-seminomatous germ cell tumors. Seminomas are the most common tumor associated with an intra-abdominal testis.

Other Complications: Other complications that can arise include pain, hernia, torsion (twisting of the testis), epididymo-orchitis (inflammation of the epididymis and testis), and atrophy (shrinkage of the testis).

To remember these complications, the acronym "TESTIS" can be used:

T—Torsion (Fig. 67.4a, b)

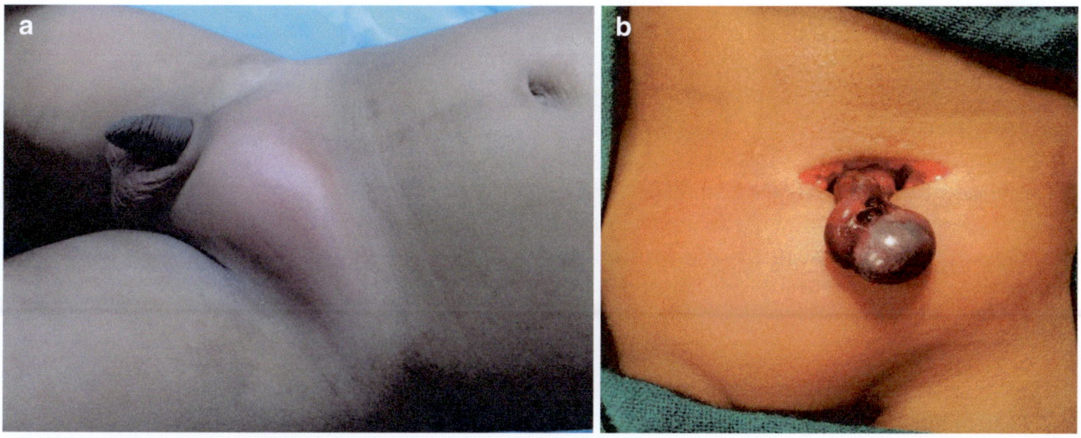

Fig. 67.4 (**a**) Testicular torsion in undescended testis. (**b**) Vascular insufficiency due to torsion

E—Epididymo-orchitis
S—Strangulation of Hernia
T—Trauma
I—Infertility
S—Seminoma (Tumor)

67.8 Treatment

67.8.1 Medical

In the past, hormonal therapy was attempted for certain forms of undescended testis (UDT) such as retractile testis or low UDT. However, the role of hormonal treatment, including low-dose human chorionic gonadotropin (HCG) and analogues of luteinizing hormone-releasing hormone (LHRH) like Buserelin, is not standardized and is currently not in use, except in some European countries.

67.8.2 Surgical

The American Urological Association recommends surgery for UDT after 6 months of birth and within 18 months. Early surgery is indicated for associated inguinal hernia. In infants, observation is recommended for up to 6 months after birth to allow for spontaneous descent. For premature babies, a waiting period of 6 months adjusted for the period of gestation is acceptable. After spontaneous descent, continued observation is necessary due to the risk of recurrent cryptorchidism.

In post-pubertal men with unilateral palpable UDT, orchidopexy (surgical fixation of the testis in the scrotum) should be performed if the testis appears normal. If the testis appears abnormal (soft, small, atrophic), orchidectomy (removal of the testis) is recommended. Orchidectomy is the preferred treatment for unilateral intra-abdominal testis in post-pubertal men due to the high risk of cancer. Prior consent for orchidectomy and post-removal histopathological examination is mandatory.

Retractile testes are more common than true undescended testis and do not require treatment. Reassurance should be provided to parents that the testis will likely descend and stay in the scrotum by puberty. The American Urological Association guidelines suggest yearly monitoring with physical examination for suspected retractile testis, as some cases may turn out to be true or ascended UDT.

67.8.3 Surgical Treatment

Surgical treatment is necessary to optimize testicular function, potentially reduce or facilitate the diagnosis of testicular malignancy, provide cosmetic benefits, and prevent complications such as clinical hernia or torsion.

The choice of operative treatment depends on the palpability of the testis:

(a) *For palpable testis: open orchidopexy is the standard treatment.*
(b) *For non-palpable testis: laparoscopy is currently the best procedure* (Fig. 67.9a, b).

Inguinal orchidopexy for a palpable testis is relatively easier. The following maneuvers may be employed to achieve adequate length of the vas and vessels so that the testis can reach the subdartos pouch in the scrotum:

1. Dissecting the processus vaginalis completely free from the cord (Fig. 67.5).
2. Incising the deep inguinal ring and mobilizing the cord structures retroperitoneally.
3. Dividing all retroperitoneal attachments.
4. Dividing the floor of the inguinal canal and fascia transversalis.
5. Dividing the deep epigastric vessels (Prentiss maneuver) to achieve a straighter route to the scrotum.

If the testis cannot be brought down during open orchidopexy, the following maneuvers can be performed:

- Staged orchidopexy: initial mobilization and fixation of the testis at the lowest possible site, followed by a second operation after a period of 6 months to bring the testis down to the scrotum, which is often successful.
- Fowler–Stephens (F-S) procedure.
- Microvascular anastomosis of testicular vessels to the deep inferior epigastric vessels.

There is no need for a biopsy in a normal-looking undescended testis (UDT). To retain the testis in the sub-dartos pouch, the neck or entry point can be narrowed, and care should be taken to avoid suturing through the tunica albuginea. Suturing through the tunica albuginea can disrupt the barrier and initiate an autoimmune reaction, potentially causing further damage to the testis. An atrophic testis should be removed and send for histopathological examination (Fig. 67.6).

*Scrotal orchidopexy (*Bianchi)*:* This option can be considered when the testis is palpable close to the scrotum and can be drawn easily into scrotum (Fig. 67.7).

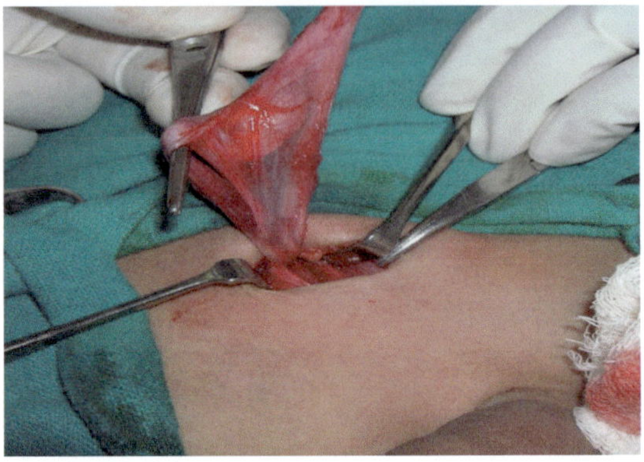

Fig. 67.5 Open orchidopexy, note separation of the intact sac from the spermatic cord structures

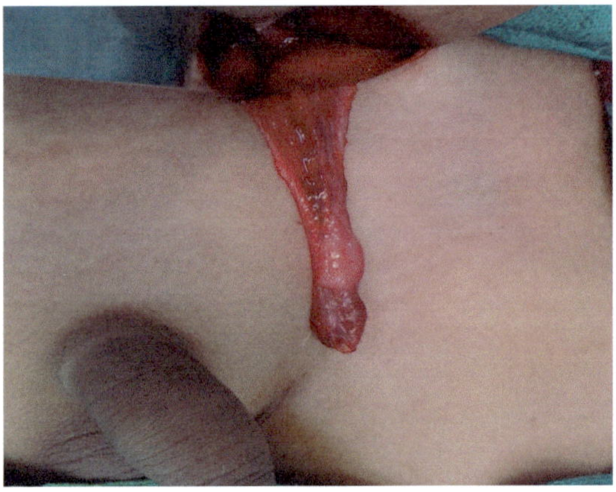

Fig. 67.6 Atrophic UDT in the inguinal canal

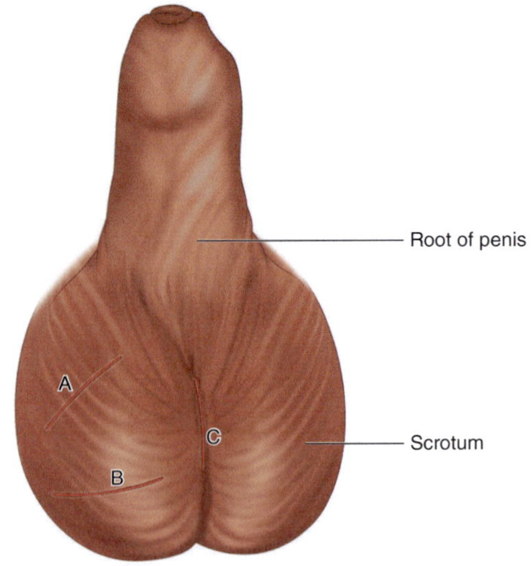

Fig. 67.7 Incisions for scrotal orchidopexy

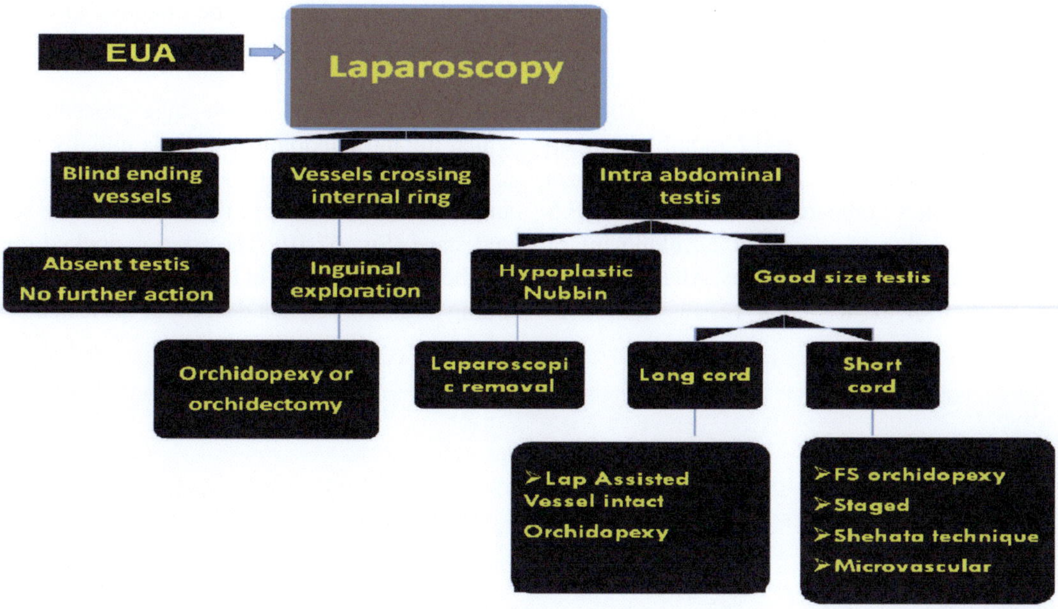

Fig. 67.8 Surgical management of impalpable testis

Laparoscopic orchidopexy is performed for non-palpable testis (Fig. 67.8). The procedure begins with an examination under anesthesia to palpate the testis. During laparoscopy, the testis may be atrophic, absent, or located in the abdomen or inguinal canal. Depending on its location, it can be peeping, canalicular, low intra-abdominal, or high intra-abdominal. The mobility of the testis, the length of the spermatic vessels, and the distance of the testis from the mid scrotum determine the appropriate operative procedure.

Based on the laparoscopic findings, the following scenarios and their corresponding management guidelines are outlined:

- Blind ending vas and vessels: This indicates an absent testis, and no intervention is required. Blind ending vessels are a definite indication of an absent testis.
- Atrophic intra-abdominal testis: Orchidectomy is performed.
- Low intra-abdominal testis with adequate mobility: Laparoscopy-assisted orchidopexy is performed (Fig. 67.9).
- Very high intra-abdominal testis: The Fowler–Stephens staged procedure is performed.
- Vas and vessels entering the inguinal ring: Inguinal exploration is performed. If the deep inguinal ring is open, then look for the testis through the open ring. If the deep inguinal ring is closed, then the presence of a sizable testis is practically negligible.

The main limiting factor in bringing an intra-abdominal testis to the scrotum is the length of the spermatic vessels. A low-lying intra-abdominal testis or a mobile testis that can be flipped to the opposite inguinal canal can be primarily brought down. On the other hand, a short length of the vessels requires a staged procedure. Caution should be exercised before initiating the mobilization of an intra-abdominal testis, as failure to bring it down may jeopardize the development of collateral circulation.

Fowler–Stephens (F-S) orchidopexy involves the high ligation and division of the testicular vessels to facilitate the lengthening of the cord and bring down an intra-abdominal testis. The vascular supply of the testis relies on collateral circulation from various sources, including the inferior vesical artery, the artery to the vas deferens, and the cremasteric artery surrounding the peritoneal covering of the testis. A two-stage operation with a gap of 6–12 months between stages as described by Dr Ransley, has shown better outcomes compared to a single-stage F-S orchidopexy due to improved development of collateral circulation to the testis. Alternatively, a low ligation of the testicular vessels (known as Koffs) has also proven to be effective in establishing adequate collateral circulation for the testis.

Shehata described a two-stage procedure in which the intra-abdominal testis is initially fixed to the opposite deep inguinal ring in the first stage, and then brought down to the scrotum in the second stage (Fig. 67.10). The traction applied during the first stage helps in lengthening the vessels, aiding in the subsequent descent of the testis.

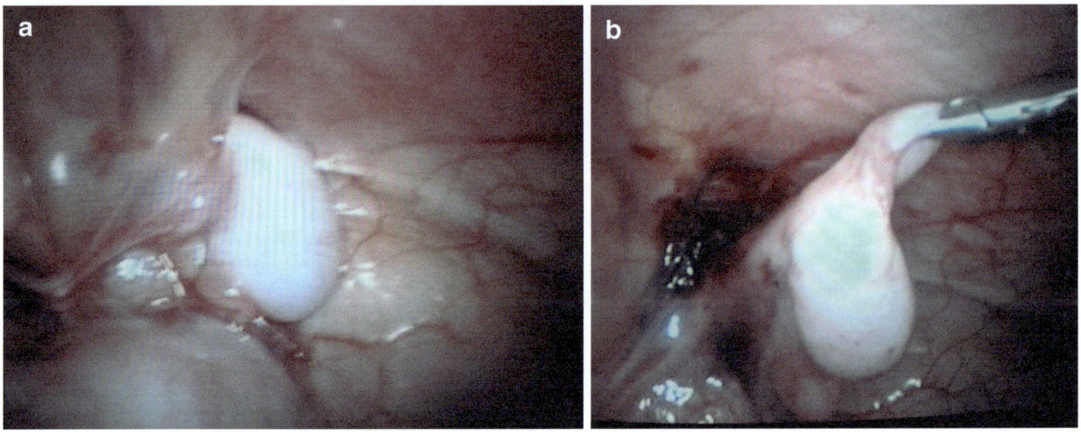

Fig. 67.9 Laparoscopic view of peeping testis

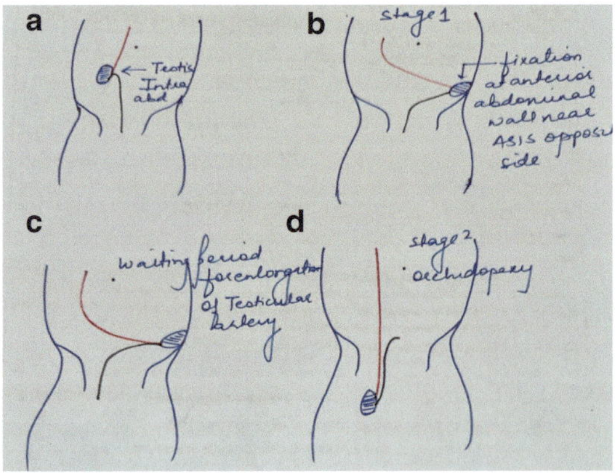

Fig. 67.10 (**a**–**d**) Hand drawn pictures may please be reproduced by artist

Summary

1. Development of human testis occurs under the influence of the SRY gene and SOX9 (SRY containing 9) as early as 5–9 weeks of gestation. The testis develops in the genital ridge in the retroperitoneum of the embryo and descends into the scrotum by seventh to ninth month during the fetal life under the guidance of gubernaculum. MIS from the Sertoli cells, testosterone and insulin-like growth factor 3 from the Leydig cells, EGF, hormones from the HPA axis, calcitonin gene-related peptide, inhibin B, genitofemoral nerve, PPV are all responsible for the testicular descend.
2. UDT is found in 30% preterm babies, 4% term babies, and 1% at 1 year of age. The chance of spontaneous descend is practically negligible after 6 m of age. Isolated UDT more common than syndromic variety.
3. Clinical examination of palpable versus impalpable UDT forms the foundation of planning treatment. Eighty percent are unilateral, 75% are palpable.
4. Palpable UDT is managed by open orchidopexy and currently laparoscopic approach is the best for the management of non-palpable testis.
5. Ideal age for orchidopexy is after 6 m and before 18 m.
6. Chance of fertility for men with unilateral UDT are close to normal population despite of reduced sperm count; however, in bilateral cases, both the sperm count and chances of fertility decreases.
7. The risk of developing malignancy (testicular germ cell tumor) in UDT cases is two to five folds higher than in the normal population. Intra-abdominal testis has higher malignant potential and early orchidopexy reduces the risk of developing malignancy.

Suggested Reading

Coran AG, Caldamone A, Scott Adzich N, Krummel TM, Laberge JM, editors. Pediatric surgery. 7th ed. Oxford: Elsevier Limited; 2012.

Docimo SG, Canning D, Khoury A, Salle JLP, editors. The Kelalis-King-Belman textbook of clinical pediatric urology. (6th ed.). ed. CRC Press; 2018.

Partin AW, Dmochowski RR, Kavoussi LR, Peters CA, editors. Campbell-Walsh -Wein urology. 12th ed. Philadelphia: Elsevier; 2020.

68 Hypospadias and Epispadias

Subhasis Roy Choudhury and Satish Aggarwal

68.1 Hypospadias

Hypospadias is a birth defect where the opening of the urethra is on the under surface (ventral surface) of the penis. It is essentially a ventral hypoplasia of penis wherein all the components on the ventral aspect ventral to the corporal bodies are hypoplastic to varying extent resulting in a triangular defect on the undersurface of penis with the base of triangle lying on the glans and apex lying where the corpus spongiosum starts deviating on either side of midline.

Urethral Plate It is the urothelial strip extending from the meatus to the tip of the glans. It may be wide and supple, producing a good groove in the glans, or it could be narrow, fibrotic, and projecting on the glans without a groove. The quality and width of the urethral plate have a good bearing on the surgical procedure. Wide and supple urethral plate with a good glans groove is suitable for tubularized incised plate (TIP) repair.

68.2 Development of the Penile Urethra

(a) This occurs between the 7th and 14th week of intrauterine development.
(b) *Genital tubercle* forms the body of the penis. Mesenchymal tissue forms the corporal bodies, Bucks fascia, dartos fascia, and corpus spongiosum.
(c) *Urethral folds* form on either side of the urethral groove on the ventral side of the genital tubercle to form the penile urethra. The urethral groove folds from proximal to distal to complete urethral tube formation. An arrest in the folding process results in abnormal opening. Glanular urethra is formed either by invagination of the ectodermal glanular tissue or by endodermal cellular differentiation.
(d) Two *Genital swellings* fuse to form the scrotum.

68.3 Components of Hypospadias

(a) Abnormal location of meatus
(b) Ventral triangular defect
(c) Ventral chordee (ventral curvature of penis)
(d) Hooded preputial skin on the dorsum
(e) Abnormal glans rotation: An inherent component of hypospadias. The glans rotation is outward, lateral, and downwards (OLD). This rotation gives rise to glanular tilt giving an appearance of false chordee, but it is cor-

S. Roy Choudhury
Pediatric Surgery, Lady Hardinge Medical College and Associated Kalawati Saran Children's Hospital, New Delhi, Delhi, India

S. Aggarwal (✉)
Sir Ganga Ram Hospital, New Delhi, Delhi, India

© The Author(s), under exclusive license to Springer Nature Singapore Pte Ltd. 2025

S. Roy Choudhury (ed.), *Pediatric Surgery*, https://doi.org/10.1007/978-981-96-1257-4_68

rected by glanuloplasty. The wider the glanular rotation, difficult is the repair and more is the need for raising wide glans wings during surgery. The glans anatomy is crucial in deciding the type of repair. There are four hillocks on the glans that define the meatal imprint (between the distal hillocks) and the line of glansplasty (the line between the distal and proximal hillocks on either side). Wider the lower hillocks, the more difficult is the glans repair. Modifications in the technique are often needed to circumvent difficult glans anatomy (see later).

(iii) Corporal disproportion: If the chordee persists after division of the urethral plate and excision of fibrosis underneath the plate, it is due to corporal disproportion, wherein the ventral corpora are shorter than the dorsal corpora. To correct this chordee, ventral Angle cuts or ventral corporotomy or ventral grafting (with de-epithelialized skin, or tunica vaginalis) is required.

(iv) False chordee can be due to glanular tilt which is caused by abnormal glans rotation (as described earlier). This is corrected by glansplasty.

68.4 Causes of Chordee

(i) Hypoplasia of ventral skin, dartos, and corpus spongiosum. This chordee can be corrected by degloving in most cases.

(ii) Fibrotic urethral plate and fibrosis underneath the urethral plate. If mild, it can be corrected by dorsal plication or Nesbit procedure. If severe, it should be corrected by division of the urethral plate.

68.5 Classification

Clinical classification is based on the location of the meatus (Fig. 68.1).

Anterior (50% cases)
- Glanular
- Coronal (Fig. 68.2)

Middle (30% cases)
- Distal Penile
- Mid penile (Fig. 68.3)
- Proximal penile (Fig. 68.4a, b)

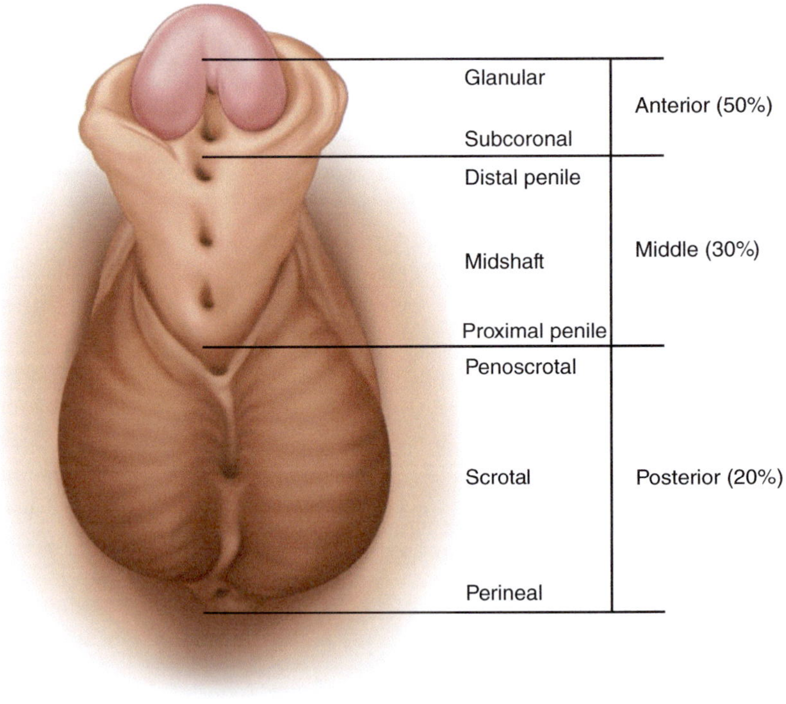

Fig. 68.1 Classification of hypospadias

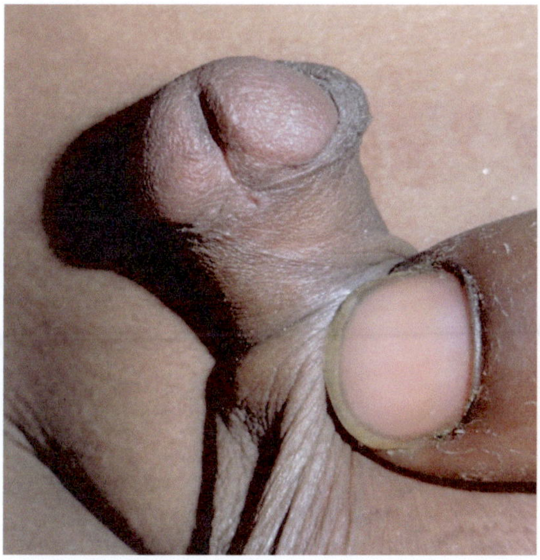

Fig. 68.2 Coronal hypospadias

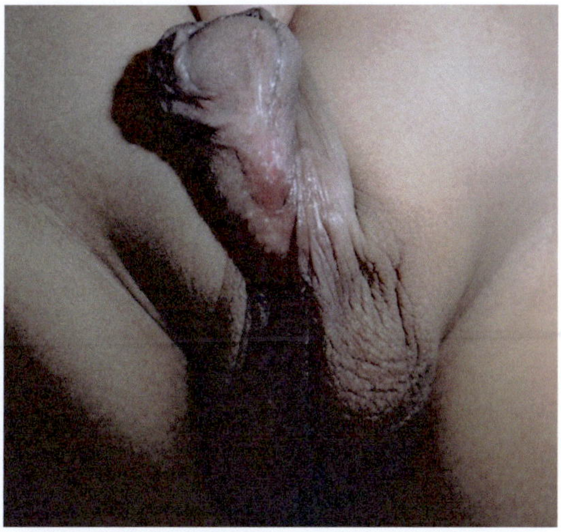

Fig. 68.3 Mid penile hypospadias

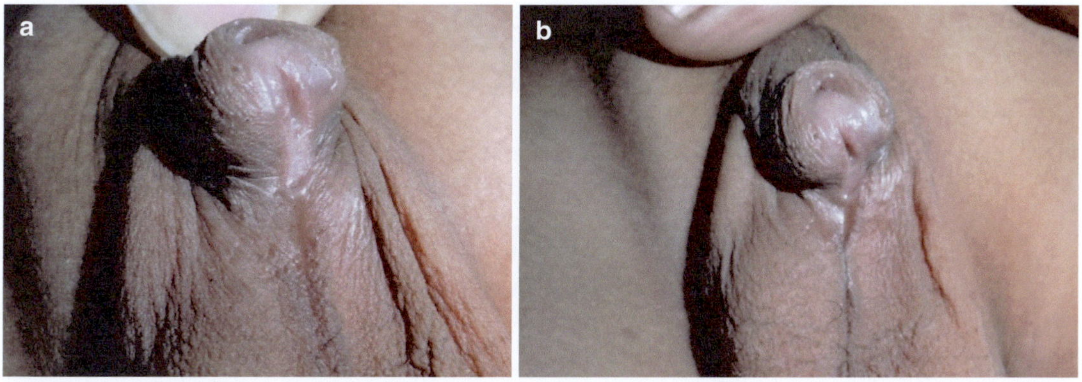

Fig. 68.4 (**a**, **b**) Proximal penile hypospadias with chordee

Posterior (20% cases)

- Penoscrotal (Fig. 68.5a, b)
- Scrotal
- Perineal

However, this classification is fallacious depiction of the true defect in hypospadias. Urethral meatus is a depiction of the level where the urethral plate is continuous with skin but hypoplasia of ventrum extends much more proximally. The true abnormality starts at a level where the corpus spongiosum surrounding the urethra starts deviating from midline to either side.

A more practical classification is Distal Hypospadias (glanular, coronal, and mid shaft) and Proximal Hypospadias (proximal penile, penoscrotal, scrotal, and perineal).

Hypospadias Sans Hypospadias (Chordee Without Hypospadias) The meatal location is on the glans but there is chordee. It is generally due to a congenital short urethra causing a bow and string effect.

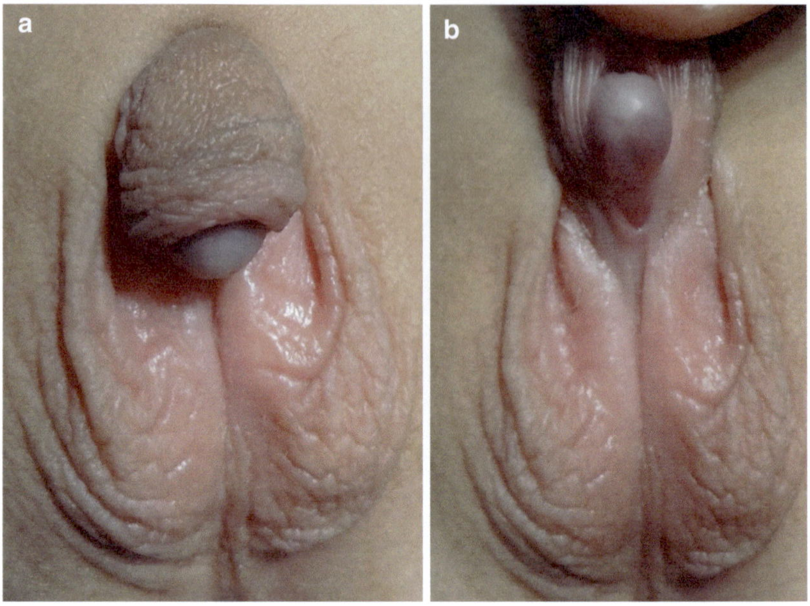

Fig. 68.5 (a, b) Penoscrotal hypospadias with chordee, hooded prepuce

68.6 Incidence

Incidence of hypospadias is 1 in 300 boys; it is one of the most common urinary anomalies in boys. Incidence is increasing day by day.

68.7 Etiology

Etiology is multifactorial. Increasing incidence is attributed to increasing genetic pool (boys operated for hypospadias becoming fathers and passing it on to the next generation and so on), increasing influence of androgen disruptors on the environment due to increasing use of oral contraceptives containing synthetic estrogens, use of chemical fertilizers and pesticides (evidenced by higher incidence in farming belts), and increased exposure to phytooestrogens through use of plastics in kitchen and water bottles. Defects in androgen stimulation during embryogenesis, enzymatic defects, and chromosomal anomalies also contribute.

68.8 Associated Anomalies

Anterior hypospadias are usually isolated defects.

Proximal and posterior hypospadias may have associated disorders of sexual differentiation (DSD). Undescended testis, inguinal hernia, enlarged prostatic utricle, pseudovaginal diverticulum, and upper urinary tract anomalies are frequent associations. A screening ultrasound should be done in such cases.

Cases of severe penoscrotal /Perineal hypospadias, asymmetry of gonads, hypospadias with undescended testis or micropenis, hypospadias with severe scrotal defects should be investigated with karyotyping and other tests to exclude DSD anomalies (see Chap. 79 on disorders of sexual differentiation, DSD).

68.9 Ideal Time of Repair

Between 6 and 18 months of age as, the child is less likely to have memory of genital manipulation later in life, will have less psychological disturbances, and the repair is complete before the child starts schooling.

Circumcision should not be done in cases of hypospadias, as the prepucial skin is often required for the repair.

68.10 Objectives of Repair

1. Straight penis (orthoplasty): This is the first objective. A straight penis with coronal meatus may still be ok for penetrative sex but a perfect meatus on glans but with curved penis will not be acceptable.
2. Vertically slit meatus of good caliber at the tip of glans with good firlit collar.
3. Hairless urethra of uniform and adequate caliber.
4. Symmetric conical glans (glansplasty).
5. Satisfactory configuration of the meatus (meatoplasty).
6. Satisfactory cosmetic skin cover.

Sequential steps in Chordee correction:

1. Degloving
2. Division of the urethral plate
3. Degloving + dorsal plication
4. Degloving + Nesbitt's procedure
5. Division of the urethral plate
6. Angle cuts on the ventrum
7. Ventral corporotomies
8. Ventral corporectomy and corporal grafting

68.11 Principles of Repair

The commonly used techniques are shown in Fig. 68.6.

68.11.1 Management of Distal Hypospadias

Most distal hypospadias can be corrected in a single stage using the native urethral plate with few exceptions. Most proximal hypospadias are better repaired in stages with few exceptions.

In Single-stage repair, prerequisite is that the chordee should be completely corrected. Native urethral plate is used for urethroplasty in the following ways:

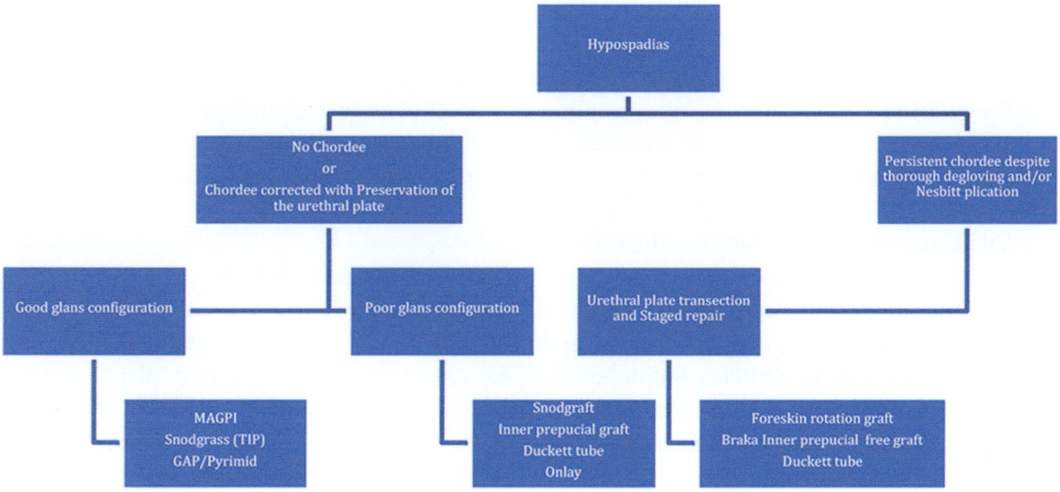

Fig. 68.6 Algorithm of surgical management of hypospadias. (MAGPI meatal advancement and glanuloplasty, GAP glans approximation procedure, TIP tubularized incised plate urethroplasty)

1. Most common is *Snodgrass's Tubularized Incised Plate (TIP) Repair*: Prerequisites for successful TIP Repair are no or minimal chordee (corrected by degloving), a supple and wide urethral plate projecting onto the glans which is well grooved. Incision is made around the corona, incision running parallel to the urethral plate on the ventrum. Degloving is performed in the plane between Buck's fascia and dartos. Correction of chordee is confirmed. The urethral plate is incised in midline, stopping short of the tip of the urethral plate. The thus widened urethral plate is then tubularized, glans wings are raised on both sides, and ventral glansplasty is performed ventral to the urethroplasty. Urethroplasty is covered by the soft tissue of the Dartos. Skin closure is performed in the midline using transposition of the dorsally hooded foreskin. According to Snodgrass, the midline incision in the urethral plate widens the plate and the raw area epithelializes within 72 hours. An important aspect of this operation is that the midline incision in the urethral plate does not extend for the entire length of the urethral plate and stops short of the tip of the glans.
2. Modifications in TIP Repair: (1) The raw area created by midline dorsal incision in the urethral plate can be grafted (inner foreskin) to create a circumferentially epithelialized urethra. Some surgeons refer to this as *"SnodGRAFT"* (2). Further, the midline incision on the urethral plate can be extended beyond in to the glans (hinging of the urethral plate on glans). This step enhances the urethra and helps in creating a better and wider meatus with good cosmesis at glansplasty. It is necessary if the urethral plate was not projecting on the glans adequately, and the meatal imprint on the glans was deficient. (3) Glans substitution and Frenuloplasty (Aggarwal): The operation starts as modified TIP repair with hinging of the urethral plate and grafting of the raw area with inner foreskin. After tubularization, the glans is approximated ventral to the meatus by a single stitch (to create a vertical meatus). Rest of the ventral glans is left open (otherwise, a tight closure would have caused ischemia, because of the difficult glans anatomy). An island of inner foreskin (approximately 1.5 × 1.5 cm) is mobilized on Dartos and swung on the ventrum using the Dartos as a Glans substitute and the overlying skin as the frenulum. Skin closure is then done. This procedure results in good and robust vascularized soft tissue at the glans and corona, thus preventing fistula, meatal stenosis, and meatal regression. Further, recurrent chordee becomes less likely as the hypoplastic ventrum has received a lot of normal tissue to support the urethra.
3. *Onlay Flap Procedures* (partial supplementation of urethral plate): When the urethral plate is not wide enough for TIP repair but the chordee gets corrected completely without urethral plate division, the Urethral plate is supplemented ventrally with inner preputial skin raised on a dartos flap. This could be done in Asopa style—a strip of inner skin brought ventrally with the outer skin without raising Dartos flap, or Duckett style—a strip of inner skin raised as an island on Dartos flap.
4. *Mathieu Procedure* (Peri-meatal skin flap from ventral skin): An essential requirement for the Mathieu procedure is a wide meatus with good peri-meatal skin and with good blood flow.
5. Primary Tubularization of Urethral Plate Without Dorsal Midline Incision: If the urethral plate is very wide and supple, it can be tubularized without the need for midline incision. Generally, it is not possible.

68.12 Complications

Fistula It is the most common complication. Acceptable rate of fistula in distal repair is 5–10%. The most common cause is a tight glans closure over the tube near the corona. It results from either inappropriate selection of the procedure for a given case or inadequate glans wings. If it occurs within the first 2 weeks, it may be treated with further urethral catheterization for 10 days to 2 weeks. Fifty percent of fistulas heal with this method. The rest require a formal surgical closure about 6 months later. If the fistula is very close to the glans, generally there is a very thin epithelial bridge between the meatus and the fistula; dividing the bridge generally suffices. More proximal fistula needs epithelial closure with support from Dartos-based skin flap. A diverticulum should be looked for and excised at the time of fistula closure. To define it better, cystourethroscopy is, at times, necessary to define diverticulae. As a general rule, distal obstruction (like meatal stenosis or distal stricture or additional distal fistulae) should be ruled out or addressed before fistula closure.

Meatal Regression and Stenosis It is a common complication after TIP repair specially if the case selection was not appropriate. Home calibration generally helps.

Urethral Stricture

Dehiscense Glans dehiscence is possible if the glans closure was tight or if the glans wings had become ischemic. At times, specially after Duckett repair, the skin becomes necrotic because the Dartos has been separated from it.

Recurrent Chordee Occurs late more commonly after TIP repair probably because of differential growth on a hypoplastic ventrum and a normal dorsum.

Complete dehiscence of repair happens if the wound became infected or the technique was not executed properly.

Late psychological and sexual dysfunction / erectile dysfunction.

68.12.1 Management of Proximal Hypospadias

They have higher incidence of associated upper tract anomalies, urethral diverticulum, pseudo-vaginal diverticulum, and prostatic utricle. Thus, cystoscopy should be done before correction of hypospadias for assessment of the posterior urethra. If required, on table, MCUG should be done. In narrow mouth prostatic utricle, obstructing membrane is ablated endoscopically. The catheter may have to be passed on a guide wire.

Most proximal hypospadias repairs have severe chordee, correction of which requires division of the urethral plate. Hence two-staged repair is a good alternative in these patients; In the first stage, chordee is corrected which generally requires division of the urethral plate. At times, more maneuvers are necessary to correct chordee such as ventral corporotomies. Ventral raw surface over the corpora is covered by either an inner prepucial foreskin graft or by Byar's flap transposition. Second stage (tubularization) is done 6 months later.

68.12.2 Single-Stage Repair in Proximal Hypospadias

Some surgeons prefer single-stage repair which can be achieved in the following way:

Asopa/Duckett Tubed Foreskin Repair Chordee is corrected by degloving and division of the urethral plate. The inner foreskin (when plenty available) is then rolled into a tube and transposed to the ventrum to reconstruct the entire length of the urethra from the hypospadiac meatus to the glans. The transposition could be in Asopa style (the inner skin and outer skin together come to the ventrum), or in Duckett style (the inner foreskin is raised as an island flap on Dartos separating the inner and outer foreskin). The difference is cosmetic. While the Asopa operation resulted in a degree of penile twist, the Duckett island tube was better cosmetically. Dr. Asopa, in his modifications, addressed this issue by making an oblique incision in the foreskin prior to ventral transposition. The use of inner preputial skin to form the urethral tube was originally described by Dr. H. S. Asopa (from Agra) in the early 1970s and later modified by Duckett in the 1980s.

A common problem with these techniques is the formation of urethral diverticulum, meatal stenosis, and skin dehiscence (more so in the Duckett operation). Also the meatus is not like a vertical slit.

Some surgeons also perform TIP-type of repair or hybrid procedures for less severe types of proximal hypospadias.

68.12.3 Management of Small Glans/Phallus in Hypospadias

If glans is very small or penis is very small, then preoperative stimulation is done with 12.5% DHT(Di-hydrotestosterone) cream. It is difficult to get commercially. It is the active form of testosterone and is more effective as compared to injection testosterone or testosterone gels. Stimulation is used for 4 weeks and surgery is performed after another 4 weeks.

68.12.4 Redo Hypospadias Repair and Hypospadias Cripples

Main issues are ventral scarring, persistent chordee, and nonavailability of foreskin which has already been used. These cases are best managed in stages (***Bracka***). First, a complete excision of fibrous tissue on the ventral aspect is done to the level of corporal bodies. Curvature is tested by Gitte's test. The glans is slit in the midline. The resultant raw surface of corporal body and the slit glans is then covered by a graft which can be sourced from buccal mucosa or other sources of hairless skin such as inner aspect of upper arm or postauricular skin. In desperate cases, even SSG (split skin graft) from the thigh can be taken. But it should be a thin graft so as to leave behind the hair follicles in the deeper half of the dermis. The graft is secured by a tie-over dressing for 7 to 10 days.

Once the graft has taken up the next step is the treatment of the graft with massage to prevent graft contracture. Six months later, the graft is tubularized.

68.13 Epispadias

The meatus is present on the dorsal surface of the penis and the penis is bent dorsally.

It occurs more commonly as a part of Bladder Exstrophy Epispadias Complex (BEEC), but isolated defects are also seen (Fig. 68.6).

When it is an isolated defect, it can be ***Continent Epispadias*** (bladder neck is normal and the defect is at the level of penile shaft), or ***Incontinent Epispadias*** (bladder neck is incompetent).

Types

- Glanular (Fig. 68.7)
- Penile
- Penopubic (Fig. 68.8)

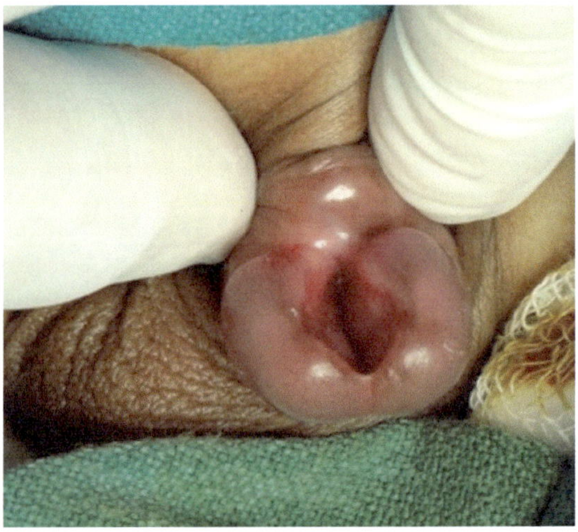

Fig. 68.7 Glanular epispadias

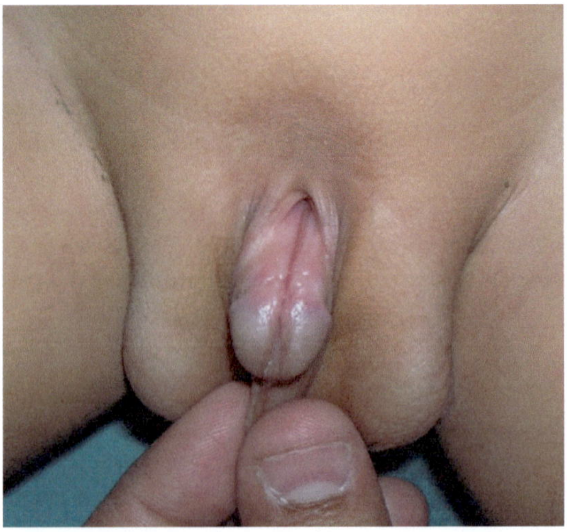

Fig. 68.8 Epispadias (peno pubic)

Incidence 1 in 120,000 in boys, and 1 in 500,000 in girls

The defect is characterized by pubic diastasis wherein the pubic bones do not fuse in the midline. This leads to deviation of the corporal bodies, which are attached to the inferior pubic rami which are also displaced and lie away from midline. This causes shortening of the visible length of the phallus as well as dorsal chordee.

68.14 Treatment

Principles of repair are similar to hypospadias repair (see above), which involves (a) correction of dorsal chordee, (b) urethral reconstruction, (c) glans reconstruction, and (d) approximation of penile skin.

The two techniques commonly applied are:

- Modified Cantwell-Ransley Repair (Preferred technique): This is a partial penile disassembly technique with placement of the urethra in a near-normal position. The IPGAM maneuver results in the placement of the urethral meatus more ventrally.
- Mitchell's Penile Disassembly Technique (See Chap. 70 on Exstrophy of Bladder): This technique uses complete penile disassembly, and occasionally leaves the meatus in the hypospadiac position for staged correction.

Suggested Reading

Hadidi AT, editor. Hypospadias surgery. 2st ed. Germany: Springer-Verlag Heidelberg; 2022.

Partin AW, Dmochowski RR, Kavoussi LR, Peters CA, Wein AJ, editors. Campbell-Walsh-Wein urology. 12th ed. Elsevier; 2020.

Prepuce and Circumcision

69

Rohit Kapoor and Subhasis Roy Choudhury

Prepuce can be defined as a double-layered covering over the glans of penis in males and its abnormality is often a cause of concern for the parents or the doctor.

69.1 Embryology, Anatomy, and Physiology of Prepuce

The development of penis starts from seventh week of gestation and continues till 17th week of intrauterine life. The prepuce (foreskin) is formed when the integument of the penis folds on itself. The frenulum, sometimes known as the “little bridle,” is an extremely sensitive tissue that attaches the prepuce to the undersurface of the glans. During birth and the first few years of life, the inner portion of the foreskin is attached to the glans and hence nonretractile (Fig. 69.1). It gets separated later in life, thus increasing retractability. Sometimes, this developmental nonretractability of the foreskin is often wrongly termed as phimosis by some clinicians. Preputial separation continues after birth, and males still exhibit some preputial adhesion at the age of five. When left alone, the majority of boys’ foreskin becomes completely and readily retractable at physical maturity. As a result, “ballooning” of the foreskin during micturition is a typical event in early childhood while the foreskin is still nonretractile. It requires no treatment because it is both temporary and self-limiting, resolving as the prepuce becomes more retractable. Pathological ballooning occurs after voiding and causes urinary blockage.

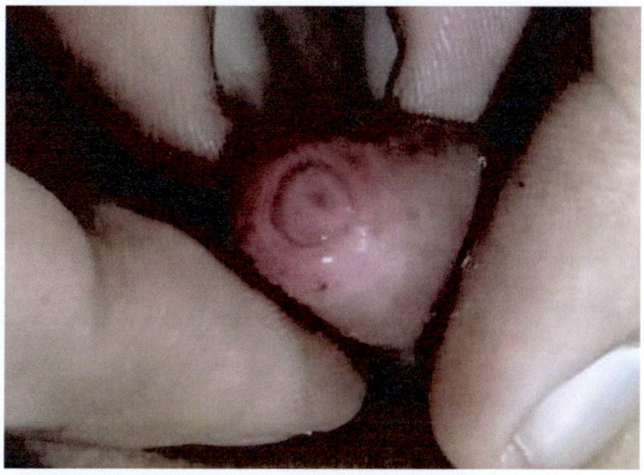

Fig. 69.1 Preputial adhesion

The foreskin typically protects the glans. The prepuce has a rich somatosensory innervation, forming a vital component of the penile erogenous tissue and thus sexual satisfaction. Thus prepuce has many roles that include protective, immunologic, and erogenous functions.

R. Kapoor (✉)
Department of Paediatric Surgical Superspecialties, Sanjay Gandhi Postgraduate Institute of Medical Sciences, Lucknow, India

S. Roy Choudhury
Pediatric Surgery, Lady Hardinge Medical College and Associated Kalawati Saran Children’s Hospital, New Delhi, Delhi, India

© The Author(s), under exclusive license to Springer Nature Singapore Pte Ltd. 2025

S. Roy Choudhury (ed.), *Pediatric Surgery*, https://doi.org/10.1007/978-981-96-1257-4_69

69.2 Management of Nonretractable Foreskin

Many patients are brought to the outpatient clinic by anxious parents due to nonretractile prepuce with or without ballooning while micturition. Majority of them are due to physiologic phimosis as described above, which is seen in almost all newborn males and is considered developmental. However, few patients may present with pathological phimosis, or distal scarring of the prepuce which is caused by fibrosis because of infection and inflammation and requires correction (Fig. 69.2a–d). Thus, management of phimosis depends upon identifying and differentiating physiological phimosis from pathological one. For Physiological phimosis, just reassurance with watchful waiting and local cleaning is advised. However, for Pathological phimosis with associated dysuria, balanitis, or scarring, intervention (medical or surgical) is required.

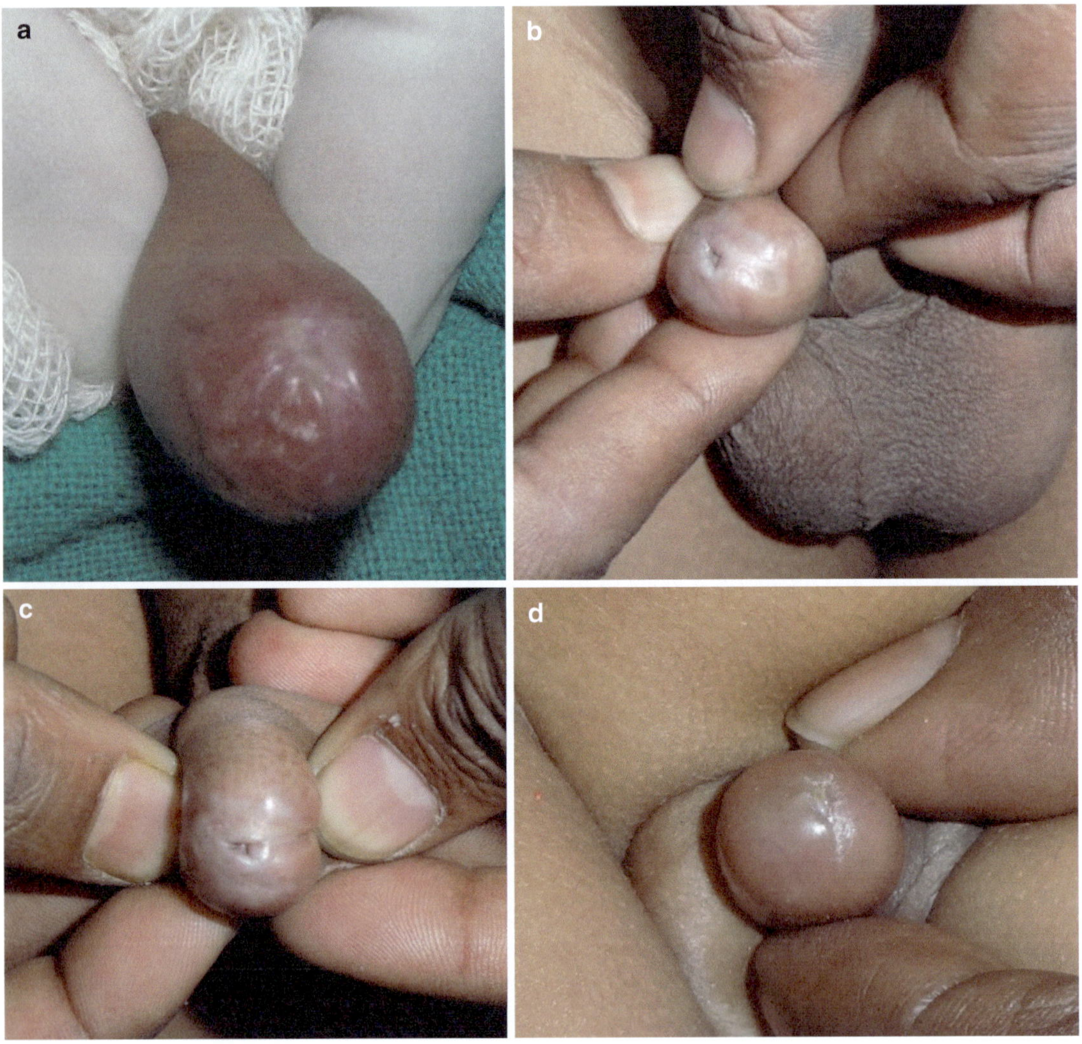

Fig. 69.2 (**a–d**) Pathological phimosis; note the scarred nonretractable foreskin

69.3 Medical Management of Phimosis

For almost two decades, *topical steroids* have been used to treat phimosis. Topical treatments have shown significant success in treating phimosis. Efficacy may vary from 65% to 95%, but they may be associated with side effects such as thinning of skin. Although their exact mechanism of action is unknown, it is thought to be due to their immunosuppressive or anti-inflammatory property. Most clinicians suggest Betamethasone 0.05% application twice a day over a 4-week period for best results. Due to side effects of using topical steroids, some authors have recommended the use of topical Nonsteroidal Anti-inflammatory creams with good results. Forceful retraction of the foreskin in young boys with restricted preputial opening should be avoided since it can cause further scarring and pathological phimosis.

69.4 Surgical Management for Phimosis

Surgical management is reserved for pathological recalcitrant phimosis that fails to respond to steroid therapy or has significant scarring. Recurrent balanoposthitis also forms an indication for surgical management. There are two surgical options available-

A. *Conventional Circumcision:* Circumcision involves complete excision of the prepuce and is one of the oldest procedures known to man. There are many techniques and devices of circumcision described in the literature such as sleeve circumcision (most common), Dorsal slit, Guillotine method (using bone cutter), Shield and clamp method (using Mogen clamp), use of other devices such as Plastibell, Smartklamp, Prepex, etc.
B. *Preputioplasty:* It is a plastic surgical procedure that allows for treatment of pathological phimosis without complete excision of the prepuce. There are many techniques described for preputioplasty but dorsal slit with transverse closure is most simple and has good results. Preputioplasty has an advantage over conventional circumcision because it has comparatively far less complication, but the recurrence of phimosis is more than conventional circumcision.

69.5 Contraindications of Circumcision

Circumcisions should not be performed until absolutely required, especially in males under the age of five. All parents of boys with hypospadias, as well as those with epispadias, ambiguous genitalia, and a buried penis, should avoid circumcision since the foreskin may be needed for reconstructive procedures. A family history of bleeding disorders is a relative contraindication for circumcision.

69.6 Complications of Circumcision

Circumcision is fraught to be associated with a plethoraofcomplications,someofwhichareasfollows-

- Bleeding
- Meatal stenosis
- Urethral injury
- Redundant skin and skin bridges
- Glanular injury

69.7 Balanitis Xerotica Obliterans (BXO)

Balanitis xerotica obliterans (BXO) is a chronic atopic dermatitis and an uncommon foreskin pathological disorder that occurs more commonly in males aged 9 to 11 years. The etiology of BXO is uncertain. It is a genital variant of lichen sclerosus et atrophicus, distinguished by white atrophic plaques on the glans penis and foreskin. Circumcision is the primary treatment option. For milder cases of BXO, a powerful topical steroid (e.g., 0.05% mometasone furoate, 0.05% clobetasol propionate, or 0.05% betamethasone cream) may alleviate local discomfort and improve the look of the foreskin.

69.8 Smegma Collection

This is a frequent issue, characterized by a white mass behind the foreskin (Fig. 69.3a–c). In most situations, the kid is asymptomatic, and parents may be comforted that retraction of the prepuce will clear the accumulation. Treatment consists of retracting the foreskin, cleaning the collection, and preserving local hygiene by frequent cleaning.

Acute Balanoposthitis: The inflammation of the prepuce is called posthitis, and that of the glans is called balanitis. This is treated with topical and or systemic antibiotics and maintaining local hygiene.

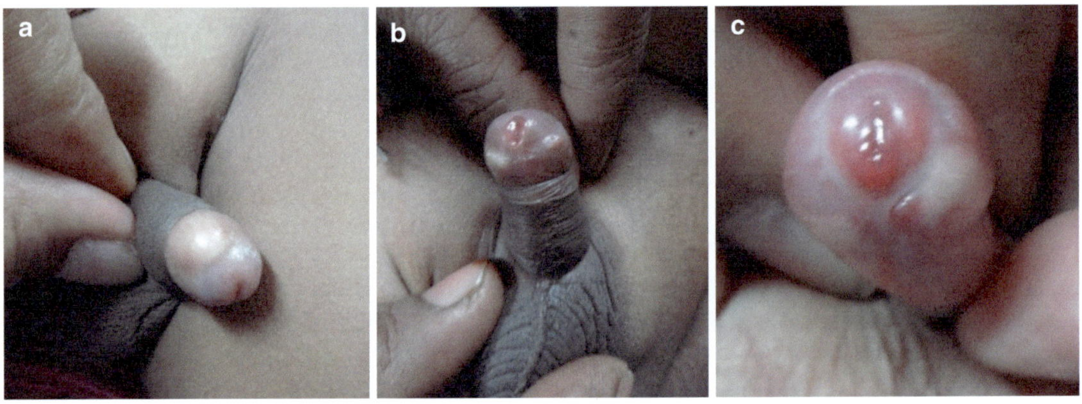

Fig. 69.3 (**a–c**) Smegma collection

69.9 Paraphimosis

Paraphimosis (Fig. 69.4) is caused by a tight foreskin that, following vigorous retraction over the glans, cannot be reduced. Venous and lymphatic blockage causes swelling of the foreskin and glans. This is a painful condition. Manual compression with ice helps to alleviate edema. The reduction of paraphimosis is uncomfortable and should be performed under local anaesthesia. In an emergency, if the prepuce is difficult to be repositioned, a dorsal slit may be needed.

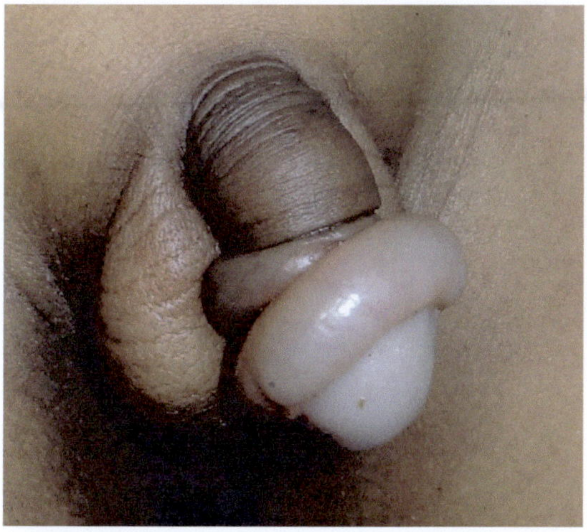

Fig. 69.4 Paraphimosis

References

Abdulwahab-Ahmed A, Mungadi I. Techniques of male circumcision. J Surg Tech Case Rep. 2013;5(1):1.

Atilla KM, Dundaroz R, Odabas O, Ozturk H, Akin R, Gokcay E. A nonsurgical approach to the treatment of phimosis: local nonsteroidal anti-inflammatory ointment application. J Urol. 1997;158(1):196–7.

Celis S, Reed F, Murphy F, Adams S, Gillick J, Abdelhafeez AH, et al. Balanitis xerotica obliterans in children and adolescents: a literature review and clinical series. J Pediatr Urol. 2014;10(1):34–9.

Choe JM. Paraphimosis: current treatment options. Am Fam Physician. 2000;62(12):2623–28. PMID: 11142469.

Shahid SK. Phimosis in children. ISRN Urol. 2012;2012:1–6.

Exstrophy of Bladder

70

Amit Gupta and Subhasis Roy Choudhury

70.1 Introduction

Exstrophy of the bladder is the commonest clinical presentation of a spectrum of anomalies clubbed together under the term Bladder-exstrophy-epispadias-complex (BEEC). Epispadias is a milder form and cloacal exstrophy is the most severe form in the spectrum. It is a developmental anomaly resulting from defective formation of lower abdominal wall, pelvis, and pelvic organs. The diagnosis is very much apparent on clinical examination and does not require any additional investigations.

Incidence is 1 in 50,000 live births, with a male/female ratio of 4:1.

70.2 Embryology

According to the most accepted theory by Marshall and Muecke, an abnormally large cloacal membrane prevents medial migration of mesenchymal tissue and development of underlying pelvic structures. Subsequent rupture of this cloacal membrane results in herniation of the incompletely developed underlying pelvic organs through the musculoskeletal defects consequent to incomplete mesenchymal growth. If the urorectal septum is incomplete at the time of rupture of the cloacal membrane, then cloacal exstrophy results. Usually, the urorectal septum is complete before the rupture of the membrane, resulting in the most common presentation of classic bladder exstrophy.

70.3 Antenatal Diagnosis

The following findings in the fetus indicate the diagnosis: (1) A solid mass bulging in the lower anterior fetal abdomen, (2) absence of bladder filling, (3) normal amniotic fluid volume, (4) low-set umbilical cord, (5) normal fetal kidneys, (6) splayed iliac bones, (7) umbilical arteries situated alongside the bulging mass, (8) scrotum anteriorly displaced with a small phallus in male fetuses.

70.4 Clinical Features

A constant feature across the spectrum is the musculoskeletal defect manifesting as pubic bone diastasis along with divergent recti and bony pelvic skeleton, clinically apparent as a lower abdominal wall defect and broad, stretched-out scrotum. The skeletal anomaly of the bony pelvis predisposes to *abnormal gait and hip dysplasia* in long term.

A. Gupta (✉)
Department of Pediatric Surgery, AIIMS Bhopal, Bhopal, Madhya Pradesh, India

S. Roy Choudhury
Pediatric Surgery, Lady Hardinge Medical College and Associated Kalawati Saran Children's Hospital, New Delhi, Delhi, India

© The Author(s), under exclusive license to Springer Nature Singapore Pte Ltd. 2025

S. Roy Choudhury (ed.), *Pediatric Surgery*, https://doi.org/10.1007/978-981-96-1257-4_70

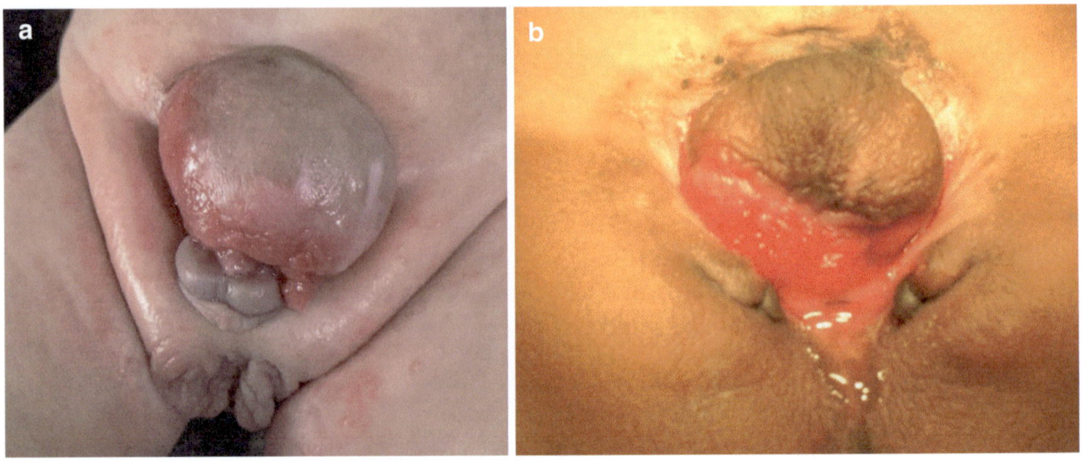

Fig. 70.1 Late presentation in (**a**) male, (**b**) female, note epithelialization of the bladder plate

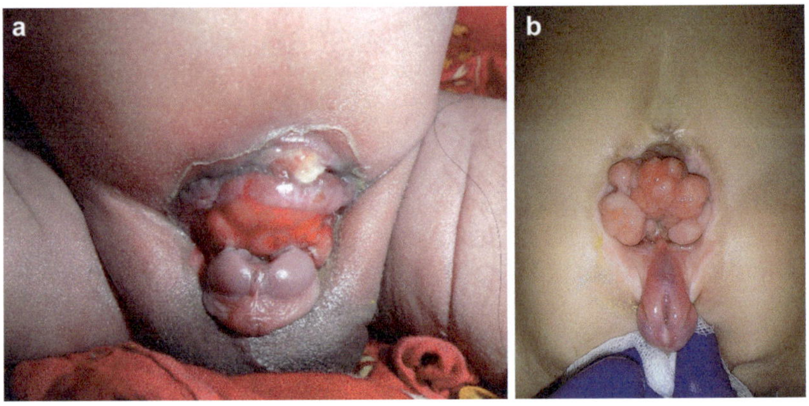

Fig. 70.2 Exstrophy bladder (**a**) new born male, (**b**) polypoidal bladder mucosa in a late presentation

Classic Bladder Exstrophy: This is the most common presenting form with the following typical features in addition to the musculoskeletal defect described above:

- Exposed bladder plate, the extent of bulge on straining or inversion with examining thumb indicates the bladder capacity achievable on reconstruction. Due to chronic inflammation, the exposed mucosa becomes polypoidal and squamous metaplasia may occur (Fig. 70.1) predisposing to recurrent stone formation and malignant change in the long term.
- Low-Set Umbilicus: malformed (with varying degree of exomphalos), located more caudal than normal at the uppermost extent of exposed bladder plate.
- Bilateral inguinal herniae are not unusual. The superficial and deep inguinal rings overlap without any obliquity in the inguinal canal.
- Anteriorly displaced anus. Anomalous weak pelvic floor muscle support associated with skeletal anomaly predisposes to rectal prolapse.
- Genital Anomalies:
  - *Males:* (Fig. 70.2): Epispadias with wide & short urethral plate exposed along its entire length, wide flattened glans, shorter length of anterior corporal bodies causing significant shortening in penile length, dorsal curvature of penile shaft (dorsal chordee), dorsally deficient prostate gland and prepuce, penoscrotal dissociation due to widely separated base of the penis and scrotum, testis are normally descended.
  - *Females*: (Fig. 70.3): Epispadias, bifid clitoris with small laterally displaced labia

minora and deficient mons pubis, the vaginal introitus is anteriorly displaced, the fallopian tubes and ovaries are normal, predisposition to uterine prolapse due to weak pelvic muscle support.

Exstrophy Variants: They account for 10% of cases and have muscular, fascial, and bony defect similar to classic exstrophy of the bladder.

1. Covered exstrophy
2. Duplicate exstrophy
3. Pseudoexstrophy
4. Superior vesical fissure (Fig. 70.4a,b)

70.5 Cloacal Exstrophy (Fig. 70.5)

Exstrophy of the cloaca with exposed and prolapsed intestine in the center of the defect (elephant trunk deformity), hemi-bladder on both sides, and varying degrees of exomphalos.

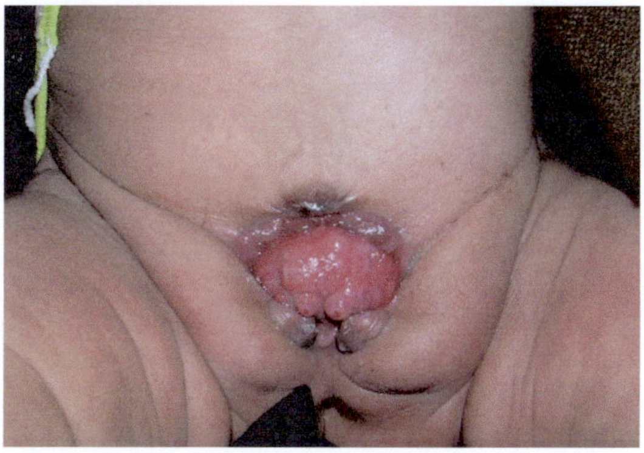

Fig. 70.3 Exstrophy bladder, female

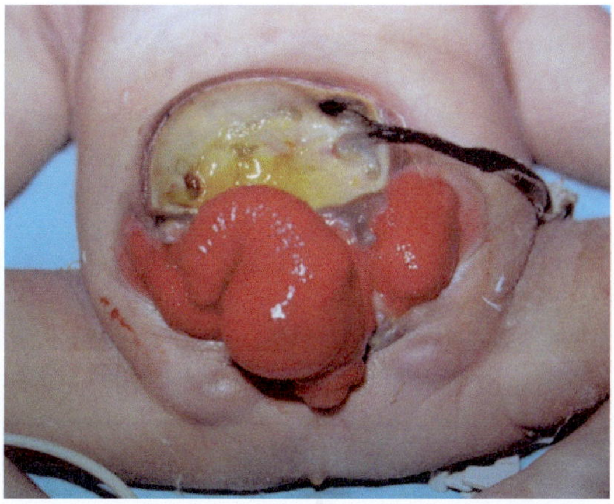

Fig. 70.5 Cloacal exstrophy

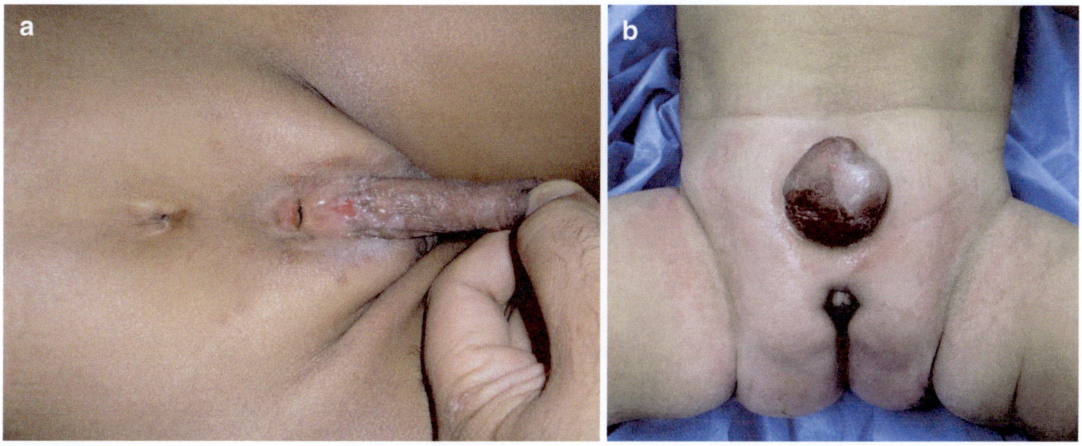

Fig. 70.4 Exstrophy variant (**a**) superior vesical fissure (male), (**b**) incomplete exstrophy (female)

70.6 Management

Staged repair is widely practiced as it shortens the duration of the anesthesia and surgical procedure in neonates and infants. It decreases the exposure of the bladder mucosa to prevent / restrict / reverse the deleterious effects of chronic inflammatory changes (poor bladder capacity and malignancy due to squamous meataplasia). The stages *of Modern Staged Repair (MSRE)* of bladder exstrophy are described below:

1. *Neonate*: Early surgical *closure of the bladder and abdominal wall defect*, and pubic bone approximation with or without osteotomy are recommended. Osteotomy may not be needed for pubic approximation if the child is operated on within 72 hours of life, as the ligaments are lax under the influence of maternal hormone relaxin. Osteotomy achieves the most anatomical repair with median pubic bone approximation and decreases the chances of postoperative dehiscence of the repair. Although theoretically, it should improve bowel-bladder continence, it has not shown a significant advantage in the long term and the pubic diastasis recurs as the patient grows older.
2. *6 Months to 1 Year of Age (in Males)*: *Epispadias repair*: salient steps are constructing a urethra from the open urethral plate to provide some bladder outlet resistance and stimulate growth in bladder capacity, correct the dorsal chordee, and increase the apparent length of penis. There are two surgical procedures described-
   (a) Modified Cantwell-Ransley Repair: Partial penile disassembly technique, more common and easy to learn & perform, achieves a urethral meatus at the tip, but this limits the increase in penile length.
   (b) Mitchell Complete Penile Disassembly Technique: Achieves better penile length, but urethral meatus remains hypospadiac which requires a late repair, and there is a risk of vascular compromise.
3. *4–5 Years Age*: *Bladder neck repair with or without bladder augmentation.* This is a reasonable time period to allow the urinary bladder to grow following the partial urinary continence achieved with the epispadias repair. Assessment of bladder volume is done to decide the appropriate procedure for achieving near normal (social) urinary continence before the child starts schooling. Also if bladder neck repair (BNR) is done, the child is old enough to physically and psychologically participate in a formal voiding or CISC program to become self-dependent while attending school.
   - Bladder Volume > 80 ml: Bladder neck repair (BNR). The popular technique is modified Young-Dees-Leadbetter (YDL) BNR.

OR

   - Bladder Volume Poor: Bladder augmentation with self-catheterizable stoma (Mitrofanoff).

One-stage combined primary exstrophy epispadias *repair (CPRE)* is regaining popularity with the advancement in anesthetic management to safely manage babies undergoing long-duration surgery. In these patients, bladder closure with / without bilateral ureteric reimplantation, epispadias repair, and bladder neck repair are performed in a single operation (Fig. 70.6). The Kelly tech-

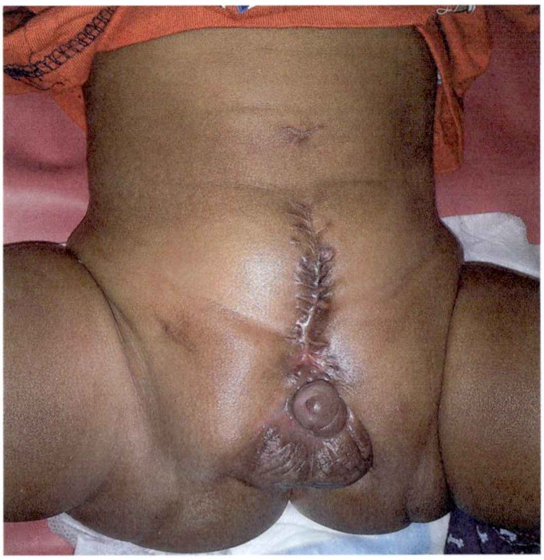

Fig. 70.6 Post-op Exstrophy Bladder Complete Primary Repair

nique of exstophy repair involves extensive soft tissue mobilization avoiding an osteotomy. It has been reported to be successful in achieving continence for exstrophy bladder patients.

Besides the repair of the urinary tract, it is also important to address the following anatomical and functional limitations due to the musculoskeletal anomaly—wound closure, short penis, anomalous weak pelvic muscle support to the pelvic organs, inguinal hernia(e), and urinary incontinence. The commonly practiced procedure to address these is osteotomy and approximation of pubic bone and divergent recti, but there is a morbidity related to external fixator pins used to achieve and maintain correction. *An alternative*, to avoid this morbidity as well as the needed assistance from an Orthopedic surgeon, is *Kelly's procedure* which achieves complete functional repair with radical soft tissue mobilization, leaving the bony defect as it is, but involves a risk of vascular compromise from injury to the pudendal vessels. Kelly's procedure has the potential to achieve better results than osteotomy. In case of nonavailability of expertise for both these procedures, *other options to bridge the gap without correcting the musculoskeletal anomaly and still achieve a secure closure are*: (1) Rectus muscle flap *or* (2) anterior rectus sheath flaps *and* Z-plasty during skin closure. It is important to note that *clinically manifesting inguinal hernia* has both direct and indirect component requiring herniotomy and herniorrhaphy to strengthen the lax posterior wall of inguinal canal in males or suture closure of deep inguinal ring in *females* respectively.

Umbilicoplasty also is an integral part of the surgical repair. It is performed mid-way between the line joining the xiphisternum to pubic symphysis.

Failed Repair or Small Fibrotic Bladder Plate: Continent urinary diversion is considered: (1) *Bladder augmentation* with a segment of bowel (ileum / sigmoid) with self-catheterizable channel (Mitrofanoff) is the commonly practiced option but requires regular long-term bladder wash to manage mucus secretion from bowel mucosa which predisposes to stone formation. The reservoir is insensate and self-catheterization at regular intervals is necessary to empty the urine. (2) *Ureterosigmoidostomy*, a less popular choice, offers the advantage of rectosigmoid as a sensate reservoir and voluntary continence due to anal sphincter without any need for self-catheterization to empty the urine, but at the cost of higher risk of sigmoid colon malignancy than bladder augmentation. Long-term complications of these procedures are stricture of reimplanted ureteric orifices, ascending UTI, hyperchloremic acidosis, and sigmoid malignancy (adenocarcinoma).

70.6.1 Cloacal Exstrophy

It requires multistage repair with bowel ostomy, bladder closure, bladder neck reconstruction, bladder augmentation, and anorectal reconstruction. The first stage is usually making a bowel stoma after separation and tubularization of the intestinal segment from the hemibladder which are joined in the midline to persist as exstrophy. The bladder closure follows subsequently in stages. Most children are reared as females as the size of phallus is very small. Most children survive with permanent stoma with clean intermittent catheterization of the urinary reservoir.

70.7 Complications and Follow-Up for Exstrophy Bladder

- *Wound dehiscence.*
- *Cutaneous fistula* anywhere along the suture line, most commonly in the penopubic and suprapubic regions.
- *Vesicoureteric reflux.*
- *Poor bladder capacity.*
- *Urinary incontinence* almost invariably occurs. However, with additional surgical procedures either bladder neck repair or bladder augmentation and clean intermittent catheterization before the schooling age, social urinary

continence (significant dry interval) can be achieved in up to 80% cases.

- *In males,* sexual dysfunction due to short penis and low fertility due to ejaculatory dysfunction.
- *In females,* successful pregnancies have been reported. Weakness due to divergent pelvic floor muscles predisposes to uterine prolapse.
- Psychosocial problems.
- Urinary stone formation.

Long-term follow-up and support is required to help them blend into the society of "normals".

Suggested Reading

Docimo SG, Canning D, Khoury A, Salle JLP, editors. The Kelalis-King-Belman textbook of clinical pediatric urology. 6th ed. CRC Press; 2018.

Partin AW, Dmochowski RR, Kavoussi LR, Peters CA, Wein AJ. Campbell-Walsh-Wein urology. 12th ed. Elsevier; 2020.

71 Urinary Tract Infection in Children

Alpana Prasad and Subhasis Roy Choudhury

Urinary tract infection (UTI) is one of the most common infections in children. In young infants, the clinical picture is often nonspecific, and hence the diagnosis is often missed or delayed. In the first year of life, urinary infections are more common in boys, but thereafter, UTIs occur predominantly in girls. P-fimbriated *E. coli* are the most common and particularly potent pathogens by virtue of their adherence properties. Other common UTI-causing organisms are *Klebsiella*, *Proteus*, *Enterococcus,* and *Enterobacter* species. Less commonly, *Pseudomonas*, *group B Streptococcus,* and *Staphylococcus* aureus infections occur in the presence of genitourinary surgery, malformations of the urinary tract, foreign body (catheter), or after recent antibiotic treatment. The presence of foreskin may be a risk factor in boys with recurrent UTIs and similarly for those with congenital abnormalities of the kidney and urinary tract (CAKUT) or bladder bowel dysfunction (BBD). Preservation of kidney function and ensuring kidney growth is the main concern in the management of children with UTI.

A. Prasad (✉)
Department of Pediatric Surgery, Sir Gangaram Hospital, New Delhi, India

S. Roy Choudhury
Pediatric Surgery, Lady Hardinge Medical College and Associated Kalawati Saran Children's Hospital, New Delhi, Delhi, India

71.1 Clinical Features in Suspected UTI

In children with suspected UTI, clinical features may vary from life-threatening septicemia to asymptomatic bacteriuria (ABU). Infants younger than 3 months of age usually present with vague symptoms of fever, vomiting, lethargy, irritability, inadequate feeding, or failure to thrive. In older children, specific features like fever with dysuria, frequency, abdominal pain, loin tenderness, hematuria, cloudy urine, or foul-smelling urine may be present.

UTI can be classified according to site (cystitis / pyelonephritis), severity (mild / severe), episode (first / recurrent / breakthrough), symptoms (asymptomatic / symptomatic), and complicating factors (uncomplicated / complicated). This differentiation helps in making diagnostic and management decisions.

71.2 Symptoms of Lower Urinary Tract Infection

Children with only urinary symptoms without systemic signs and symptoms are considered to have lower urinary tract infection. Symptoms of lower urinary tract infection (UTI) include urinary frequency, urgency, hesitancy, dysuria, suprapubic pain, cloudy urine, daytime wetting, and new onset nocturnal enuresis.

© The Author(s), under exclusive license to Springer Nature Singapore Pte Ltd. 2025
S. Roy Choudhury (ed.), *Pediatric Surgery*, https://doi.org/10.1007/978-981-96-1257-4_71

71.3 Symptoms of Upper Urinary Tract Infection

Upper urinary tract infection is suspected if fever >38 °C is present with bacteriuria or in children with fever <38 °C and bacteriuria with additional findings of loin pain or tenderness.

Clinical diagnosis of UTI is based on confirmed growth of bacteria in urine in a symptomatic child. Urine sampling is required in the following scenario:

- Signs and symptoms of UTI.
- Unexplained fever >38 °C or higher for more than 24 h.
- Children with fever with an alternative site of infection who remain unwell despite adequate treatment.

71.4 Urine Sampling

A clean-catch mid-stream voided sample, after careful cleaning of external genitalia, is the preferred technique in toilet-trained children. For neonates, infants and children who are unable to void on command, urine is obtained by a plastic bag attached to the cleaned genitalia, clean-catch urine on spontaneous voiding with or without stimulation, urethral catheterization, and suprapubic aspiration (SPA). While performing SPA, the urine container should be ready, as this procedure may itself initiate voiding. Urine sampling from adhesive urine collecting bags or nappy pads should be avoided because of very high contamination rates.

Commonly used methods for urinalysis screening are:

1. Dipstick—leucocyte esterase and nitrite test
2. Microscopy—presence of WBCs and bacteria
3. Enhanced urinalysis by hemocytometer

Urine Biomarkers: Urine dipstick test is a widely available screening tool. The leucocyte esterase test detects the presence of leucocytes in the urine, whereas the nitrite test detects the presence or absence of coliform bacteria in urine. In UTIs with low bacterial count or those caused by non-E.coli bacteria, the leucocyte esterase test may be negative. Nitrite test is mostly negative in infants with UTI because of shorter bladder urine incubation time, infection caused by nonnitrite producing bacteria (Pseudomonas aeruginosa), or insufficient dietary nitrate intake. Combined positivity of both leucocyte esterase and nitrite tests is highly sensitive and specific for the diagnosis of UTI.

Other urinary biomarkers which may be useful in children to differentiate UTI from other febrile illnesses are neutrophil gelatinase-associated lipocalin (NGAL) and interleukin 8 (IL-8).

Urine Microscopy: Significant pyuria is defined as >10 WBC/mm^3 in an uncentrifuged specimen and is supposed to be more sensitive. Usually, centrifuged urine is tested and the presence of 5 WBC/ high-power field (equivalent to 25 WBC/mm^3) is considered significant. Pyuria is a hallmark of UTI and helps to distinguish UTI from ABU. The urine sample should be tested within 1 h if stored at room temperature or within 4 h if refrigerated.

Enhanced Urinalysis by Hemocytometer (≥10 WBC/μL in a counting chamber or any bacteria in 10 oil emersion fields) has greater sensitivity and specificity than standard urinalysis.

Urine Culture: It is considered the gold standard for the diagnosis of UTI. The criteria for the bacteriological diagnosis of urinary infection are growth of a single strain of bacteria $\geq 1 \times 10^5$ colony-forming units (CFUs) per ml. Growth of multiple strains of bacteria in most cases indicates contamination of the urine sample. The American Academy of Pediatrics (AAP) guidelines in 2011 have suggested modification of this criterion as bacteriuria $\geq 5 \times 10^4$ CFU/ml ± pyuria for diagnosis of UTI in children. Depending on the urine sampling technique, different cut-off levels for significant bacterial growth have been proposed. In specimens obtained by suprapubic aspiration, any growth of bacteria is significant in recent guidelines. Urine samples that cannot be cultured within 4 h should be refrigerated, or boric acid should be added to them.

Urine samples should be sent for culture in:

- Systemically unwell children of all ages
- All children under the age of 3 years
- Single positive result for nitrite or leukocyte esterase
- Recurrent UTI

Newer diagnostic techniques to replace urine culture are emerging which may help in early diagnosis of UTI within few hours of sample collection. These include polymerase chain reaction (PCR) for detecting 16S ribosomal RNA and new generation sequencing of urinary bacterial DNA, where not only the causative agent is identified but the genes for resistance and virulence factors can also be detected.

71.5 Imaging

Ultrasound: Renal and bladder ultrasound within 24 h is recommended after first-time UTI in all infants and after a febrile UTI in older children, and if the UTI is severe or atypical or recurrent. It helps to identify obstruction or dilatation of the upper or lower urinary tract and any major abnormalities in the size and location of the kidneys. In toilet-trained children with UTI, ultrasound assessment of postvoid residual urine is important. Ultrasound cannot reliably diagnose vesicoureteral reflux (VUR) or the degree of renal damage or renal scars, but it is readily available, noninvasive, and free of radiation.

Voiding Cystourethrography (VCUG): VCUG is the gold standard imaging modality for detection and grading of VUR as well as imaging the bladder and urethra and to diagnose posterior urethral valves in boys. It is recommended in children with abnormal ultrasound (hydronephrosis, renal scarring, findings suggestive of reflux or obstructive uropathy), infants below 6 months, severe, atypical, or recurrent UTI or those with urinary symptoms. Prophylactic antibiotic cover should be given prior to VCUG. Main drawbacks of VCUG are its invasiveness (need for catheterization which is distressing for both child and parent), risk of UTI due to catheterization, and radiation exposure.

Contrast-enhanced ultrasonography (CEUS) and indirect or direct radionuclide cystography (DRCG) are other modalities for diagnosis of VUR.

Radionuclide Scanning: Nuclear scintigraphy with dimercaptosuccinic acid (DMSA) is the gold standard for renal cortical imaging and helps in assessment of relative renal function. In the acute phase of febrile UTI (up to 6 weeks), perfusion defects on DMSA scan suggest pyelonephritis, whereas renal scars can be detected after 4–6 months. It is recommended in cases with atypical or recurrent infections. Disadvantages of acute DMSA scans are higher cost, radiation exposure, requirement of sedation in young children, need for intravenous access and special equipment.

Besides DMSA renal scan, acute pyelonephritis and late renal scars can be accurately diagnosed by diffusion-weighted MRI which avoids radiation exposure too but is expensive and not readily available.

There are two different strategies followed in diagnostic imaging for febrile UTI in children, which are *Bottom-Up Approach* and *Top-Down Approach*. In the "bottom-up" approach, renal ultrasound followed by VCUG is done first to assess bladder dysfunction, VUR, and other bladder abnormalities. In the "top-down" approach, renal ultrasound is followed by a DMSA renal scan first to detect kidney involvement. If the DMSA scan is positive, then only VCUG is done so that unnecessary VCUG examinations are avoided. Early identification and grading of VUR and its appropriate management is the aim of the bottom-up approach, whereas the focus in the top-down approach is early detection of kidney involvement and prevention of damage to renal function.

Definition of atypical UTI is the presence of:

- Septicemia, a seriously ill child
- Poor urine stream
- Deranged renal function test
- Failure to respond to treatment with antibiotics within 48 h.
- Infection with non-*E. coli* organisms
- Significant family history

71.6 Treatment

Oral antibiotics are preferred if tolerated. Children who are very sick and cannot take oral medication are given intravenous antibiotics till they are well enough for oral antibiotics. Delay in antibiotic treatment of febrile UTI increases the incidence of pyelonephritis leading to renal scarring. Children who do not respond to treatment within 24–48 h, should be suspected of having acute pyelonephritis for which antibiotics should be given for 7–14 days, whereas for lower urinary tract infection and afebrile cystitis, antibiotics are recommended for 3 days. In children with bladder bowel dysfunction and girls with dilating reflux, antibiotic prophylaxis decreases the risk of recurrent UTI. Correction of any anatomical abnormality of the urinary tract should follow. Dysfunctional voiding and constipation are frequent causes of UTI in young girls and should be treated with increasing intake of oral fluids, complete bladder emptying with voiding training, and avoidance of constipation. Children who have bilateral renal abnormalities, impaired kidney function, raised blood pressure, and/or proteinuria should receive monitoring and appropriate management by a specialist to slow the progression of chronic kidney disease.

Comparison of recent guidelines for UTI diagnosis and management

Guidelines	Method of urine sampling in nontoilet-trained	Significant bacteriuria (CFUs/ml)	Imaging Renal-bladder US RBUS	Imaging VCUG	Imaging DMSA
UK / NICE (2018)	MSU Pad Cath / SPA	Not defined	<6 mon.—all children >6 mon.—if atypical or recurrent UTI	<6 mon.: if atypical or recurrence 6–36 mon.: if associated risk factors	<3 yrs: if atypical or recurrent UTI >3 yrs: if recurrent UTI
USA / AAP (2016)	Cath / SPA MSU for screening	Cath/SPA— $\geq 5 \times 10^4$	All children	If abnormal RBUS or complicated or recurrent UTI	Not recommended
ESPU/ EAU (2021)	Cath/SPA/MSU Bag for screening	SPA: any growth Cath: $\geq 1 \times 10^3$ MSU: $\geq 1 \times 10^5$ ($\geq 10^4$ if sympt.)	All children with febrile UTI	<1 yr: all children >1 yr: atypical or recurrent febrile UTI	Alternative to VCUG in top-down approach, within 1–2 mon. from infection
Asian guidelines (2021)	Cath/SPA/MSU Bag for screening	SPA: any growth Cath: $\geq 5 \times 10^4$ MSU: $\geq 1 \times 10^5$	All children with febrile UTI	If abnormal RBUS or abnormal DMSA scan; if febrile recurrence	Severe acute pyelonephritis Hypodysplasia on RBUS If UTI, diagnosis is in doubt (acute scan)

Summary Box

- UTI in infants and children is a common condition which requires a high index of clinical suspicion followed by appropriate investigations for early diagnosis.
- Top-down approach which involves renal-bladder ultrasound followed by DMSA renal scan after the first febrile UTI in infants is recommended.
- Bottom-up approach involving an initial VCUG after a renal-bladder ultrasound is mandated in children with CAKUT and recurrent UTI.
- Delay in initiation of antibiotic therapy after missed diagnosis of UTI may result in renal scarring.
- Diagnosis and management of BBD are important for the treatment of UTI and VUR.
- Surgery is reserved for recurrent febrile UTI with high-grade VUR and CAKUT.

Suggested Reading

Brandström P, Hansson S. Urinary tract infection in children. Pediatr Clin N Am. 2022;69(6):1099–114. https://doi.org/10.1016/j.pcl.2022.07.003.

Cooper CS, Storm DW. Infection and inflammation of the pediatric genitourinary tract. Ch. 25. In: Campbell-Walsh-Wein urology. 12th ed. Philadelphia: Elsevier Saunders; 2021. p. 426–46.

Jerardi KE, Jackson EC. Urinary tract infections. Ch. 553. In: Nelson textbook of pediatrics. 21st ed. Philadelphia: Elsevier Saunders; 2020. p. 2789–95.

National Institute for Health and Care Excellence (NICE). Urinary tract infection in under 16s: diagnosis and management: NICE clinical guidelines, 2018. PMID: 31971701.

t'Hoen LA, Bogaert G, Radmayr C, et al. Update of the EAU/ESPU guidelines on urinary tract infections in children. J Pediatr Urol. 2021;17(2):200–7. https://doi.org/10.1016/j.jpurol.2021.01.037.

Wang HS, Cahill D, Panagides J, et al. Top-down versus bottom-up approach in children presenting with urinary tract infection: comparative effectiveness analysis using RIVUR and CUTIE data. J Urol. 2021;206(5):1284–90.

Yang SS, Tsai JD, Kanematsu A, et al. Asian guidelines for urinary tract infection in children. J Infect Chemother. 2021;27(11):1543–54.

Vesicoureteric Reflux

72

Priyank Yadav, Subhasis Roy Choudhury, and Sujit K Chowdhary

Vesicoureteric reflux (VUR) is retrograde flow of urine from the bladder into the upper urinary tract. If reflux extends into the renal papilla, then it is called intrarenal reflux (IRR). VUR is a significant concern in pediatric patients and can lead to complications such as urinary tract infections (UTIs), pyelonephritis, renal scarring, hypertension, and chronic renal insufficiency.

72.1 Incidence

Vesicoureteric reflux (VUR) is identified in 25% of cases of antenatally diagnosed hydronephrosis which brings its incidence to 1 in 2000–5000 live births. VUR is a heritable disorder with a high incidence in siblings of up to 50%. It is a common cause of pediatric UTI, and 30–50% of children with UTIs have VUR. Among infants diagnosed with VUR because of antenatal hydronephrosis, males predominate, while among older children who present with VUR due to an UTI, females predominate.

P. Yadav
Sanjay Gandhi Institute of Post Graduate Medical Education & Research, Lucknow, UP, India

S. Roy Choudhury
Pediatric Surgery, Lady Hardinge Medical College and Associated Kalawati Saran Children's Hospital, New Delhi, Delhi, India

S. K Chowdhary (✉)
Indraprastha Apollo Hospital, New Delhi, Delhi, India

72.2 Etiology

Mechanisms which prevent reflux across the ureterovesical junction (UVJ) are as follows:

1. Natural tone of the ureter muscle allows mild passive closure of the intramural ureter.
2. Ureteral peristalsis, characterized by rhythmic muscle contractions, promotes urine flow from the kidneys to the bladder, ensures unidirectional movement, and aids in the prevention of reflux.
3. Flap-Valve Mechanism: As the bladder distends, there is progressive obliquity of the intramural and submucosal ureter. Increase in intravesical pressure causes compression of this portion of the ureter against the detrusor muscle.
4. Trigone also contracts during micturition, anchoring the ureteric orifice and preventing its lateral displacement. This aids in the flap-valve mechanism.
5. The ratio of the length of submucosal ureteral tunnel to ureteric diameter is critical. This ratio is 5:1 in children without VUR (described first by Paquin) and is lesser in patients with VUR.

Disruptions of these mechanisms result in VUR.

© The Author(s), under exclusive license to Springer Nature Singapore Pte Ltd. 2025

S. Roy Choudhury (ed.), *Pediatric Surgery*, https://doi.org/10.1007/978-981-96-1257-4_72

72.3 Possible Embryological Reasons for VUR Are

- Abnormal distal origin of the ureteric bud from the mesonephric duct results in ureteric lateral ectopia and decreased length of submucosal ureter (Mackie and Stephens theory).
- Abnormal development of the trigone can also result in lateral ectopia and poor anchorage of the ureteric orifice.

Both the absolute and relative lengths of the submucosal tunnel tend to increase with age, thus accounting for the spontaneous resolution of VUR over time. The length of the intravesical ureter in neonates (0.5 cm) reaches the mature, adult length (1.3 cm) by 10–12 years of age.

72.4 Classification

72.4.1 Primary and Secondary VUR

Primary VUR is due to an anatomical abnormality of the vesicoureteric junction.

Secondary VUR is 7 and abnormal bladder function, commonly associated with neuropathic bladder and posterior urethral valve.

VUR is known to run in families. In females, it usually presents late (3–7 years), is of low grade (1–3), and is associated with dysfunctional voiding. In males, it presents early (0–2 years) and is usually of high grade (3–5), and anatomical factors are often associated.

72.4.2 Reflux Nephropathy

Acquired renal scarring is the consequence of symptomatic upper tract infection associated with VUR and intrarenal reflux (IRR). Congenital nephropathy and renal dysplasia may contribute a significant proportion of cases. Asymptomatic bacteriuria, a relatively common finding in older girls, does not give rise to renal scarring. To pose a risk of renal scarring, urinary infection must be sufficiently severe to give rise to symptomatic pyelonephritis. VUR per se does not cause renal damage but when associated with UTI, it results in acute pyelonephritis and subsequently renal damage.

Reflux nephropathy, also known as chronic pyelonephritis or chronic atrophic pyelonephritis, is a condition characterized by kidney damage caused by VUR. The "Big Bang Theory" of reflux nephropathy, put forth by Ransley and Risdon in 1978, suggests a sequence of events leading to kidney damage:

- Primary VUR: The theory starts with primary VUR, which is present from birth or develops early in life. The ureterovesical junction (UVJ) fails to function properly, allowing urine to flow back from the bladder into the ureters and kidneys during bladder contractions.
- UTIs: Primary VUR predisposes individuals to recurrent UTIs. Bacteria from the bladder can ascend the ureters and reach the kidneys more easily due to the refluxed urine. The UTIs contribute to renal damage over time.
- Acute Pyelonephritis: The recurrent UTIs can lead to episodes of acute pyelonephritis, an inflammation of the kidney tissue caused by bacterial infection. These episodes cause further damage to the renal tissue.
- Renal Scarring: The repeated insults of acute pyelonephritis result in renal scarring, also known as renal fibrosis. Scar tissue replaces healthy kidney tissue, leading to a loss of functional nephrons.
- Chronic Renal Damage: As renal scarring progresses, the kidneys lose their ability to function properly. Chronic kidney damage occurs, characterized by impaired filtration, decreased urine concentration, and reduced overall kidney function.

Renal scars typically form at the upper and lower poles, which are also the most common locations of pyelonephritis caused by VUR-related UTIs. This is because these locations have "fused" or "compound" calyces that have a concave papillary configuration that allows for the easy retrograde flow of fluid into the collecting system.

The incidence of UTI and resolution of VUR is affected by presence of voiding dysfunction which causes urinary stasis, incomplete emptying, and worsens reflux. Even in primary VUR, 18% of patients may have voiding dysfunction.

72.5 Presentation of VUR

72.5.1 Antenatal

In the antenatal period, VUR may only present with isolated hydronephrosis on prenatal scan. More commonly, there will be dilated ureter in addition to hydronephrosis. An enlarged bladder (megacystis) may also be seen sometimes on prenatal scan. VUR cannot be confirmed prenatally, therefore a suspicion of VUR antenatally merits postnatal follow-up and evaluation with ultrasound and VCUG.

72.5.2 Postnatal

Many children may not have any symptoms of VUR and may have incidental hydronephrosis or hydroureteronephrosis. The common postnatal symptoms of VUR include:

- Symptomatic UTIs with or without fever
- Urinary urgency, frequency, or incontinence
- Abdominal or flank pain
- Poor growth or failure to thrive
- High blood pressure
- Renal insufficiency

The evaluation of bladder and bowel dysfunction (BBD) in the context of vesicoureteral reflux (VUR) involves various clinical aspects and diagnostic procedures. Clinical aspects include assessing signs and symptoms such as increased or decreased urinary frequency, two or fewer defecations per week, daytime incontinence, urgency, nocturia, hesitancy, straining, weak or intermittent stream, holding maneuvers, sensation of incomplete voiding, and post-void dribbling.

72.5.3 Clinical Workup and Investigations

After detailed history and examination, a bladder diary helps to identify the child's voiding patterns, frequency, and any incontinence episodes, including their triggers. It is a 24-hour record of all fluid intake, urine output, and incontinence episodes, including fecal soiling. A 3-day diary is commonly used. A urinalysis and culture test checks for the presence of infection or abnormalities. Further investigations include:

Renal and bladder ultrasound (USG) assesses the size, shape, and structure of the kidneys and detects any abnormalities such as hydronephrosis and hydroureter, and identifies renal scars. USG may be normal in low-grade reflux, and up to one-fourth of high-grade refluxes may be missed on ultrasound.

Voiding/Micturating cystourethrogram (VCUG/MCUG) remains the gold standard investigation for the diagnosis and grading of VUR (Figs. 72.1 and 72.2). It is the principal method of assessing the lower urinary tract in children by visualizing the reflux, urethra, and bladder, and detecting other conditions predisposing to UTIs. Micturating cystourethrogram (MCUG) also helps in recognizing secondary VUR by detecting posterior urethral valve or neurogenic bladder. It requires catheterization and use of ionizing radiation, leading to concerns about nonphysiologic results and radiation exposure.

Radionuclide Studies:

Renal scanning with Tc99m-DMSA (dimercaptosuccinic acid) scan is excellent for visualization of the renal cortex. DMSA is very sensitive for the detection of scars associated with VUR and the determination of differential renal function. Direct radionuclide cystogram (DRCG) uses a catheter to inject a small quantity of a radioactive substance, typically Tc99m-DTPA, into the bladder, where it combines with urine, and a gamma camera captures the tracer's movement as the patient voids. DRCG offers continuous imaging and

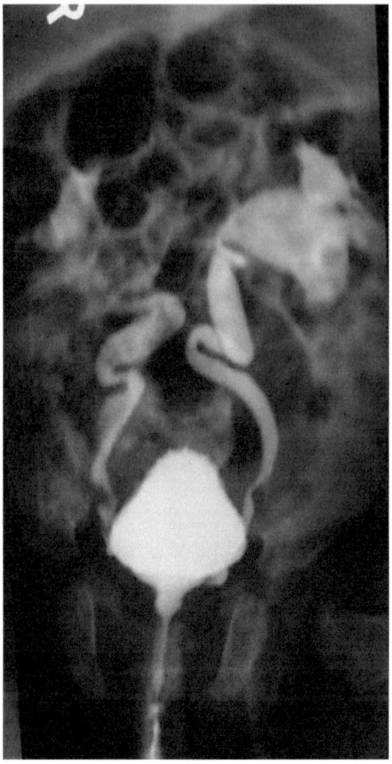

Fig. 72.1 MCU: bilateral VUR with trabeculated bladder

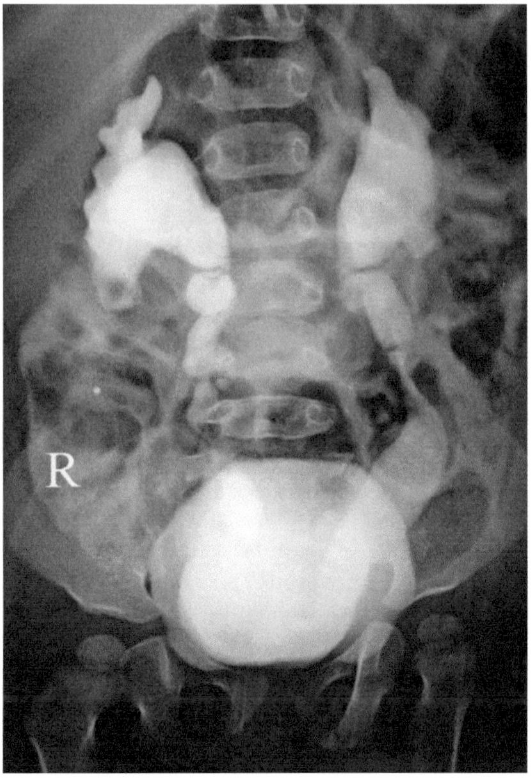

Fig. 72.2 MCU, bilateral grade V VUR

less radiation exposure than VCUG and is used for follow-up purposes. The disadvantages of DRCG are a lack of information about the grade of reflux and bladder and urethral anatomy.

Indirect cystography with intravenous MAG3 (mercaptoacetyltriglycine) may be used for follow-up investigation, particularly in older children.

Uroflowmetry and Postvoid Residual Volume (PVR)

Uroflowmetry is a noninvasive test that measures the rate and pattern of urine flow during voiding. It helps evaluate the bladder emptying function and can identify abnormalities such as weak flow, obstruction, or detrusor-sphincter dysfunction (when performed with electromyogram). Postvoid residual volume (PVR) measurement involves determining the amount of urine left in the bladder after voiding. A high PVR volume suggests incomplete emptying and may indicate bladder dysfunction, such as poor detrusor muscle contraction or obstruction. Persistent elevated PVR volumes in children with VUR may contribute to recurrent urinary tract infections and renal damage.

Urodynamic studies help identify abnormalities like detrusor overactivity and urethral obstruction that contribute to VUR, provide information on bladder pressure, capacity, and contractions during filling and emptying. Useful for children with voiding dysfunction and neurogenic bladder for diagnosis and monitoring of response to treatment. Results from urodynamic studies guide treatment decisions, such as medication (like anticholinergics), behavioral changes (like bladder training), or surgery (like intradetrusor botulinum toxin injection), for effective management of VUR.

72.6 Grades of VUR

International classification of vesicoureteral reflux (grades I to V): (Fig. 72.3).

Grade I—Ureter only.

Grade II—Ureter, pelvis, calices, no dilatation, normal caliceal fornices.

Grade III—Mild or moderate dilatation and/or tortuosity of the ureter, and mild or moderate dilatation of the pelvis, but no or slight blunting of the fornices.

Grade IV—Moderate dilatation and/or tortuosity of ureter and mild dilatation of renal pelvis and calices, complete obliteration of sharp angle of fornices but maintenance of papillary impressions in the majority of calices.

Grade V—Gross dilatation and tortuosity of ureter, gross dilatation of renal pelvis and calices, papillary impressions are no longer visible in majority of calices.

72.7 Top-Down Versus Bottom-Up Approach

The top-down and bottom-up approaches are two different methods for the initial imaging of children with UTI (Fig. 72.4).

- The top-down approach involves an initial DMSA scan, and only those with renal scarring undergo a VCUG.
- In contrast, the bottom-up approach involves an initial VCUG.
- Top-down approach is associated with slightly higher recurrent UTI compared to the bottom-up approach (24.4% vs. 18.0%)
- Top-down approach significantly reduced the need for VCUG (2.4% vs. 100%) and continuous antibiotic prophylaxis (0.4% vs. 25%).

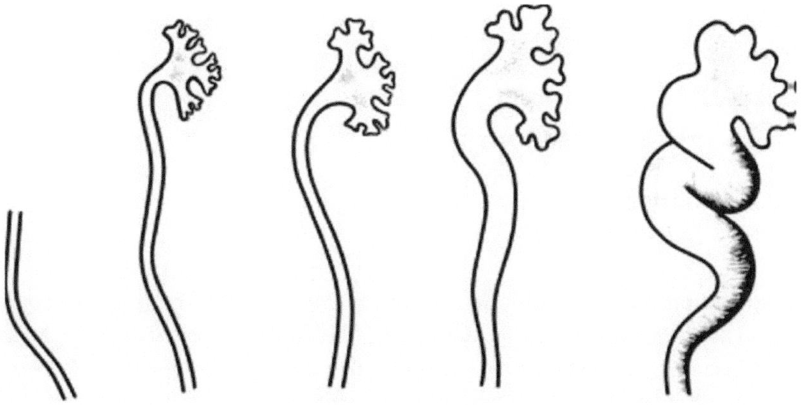

Fig. 72.3 Grades of vesicoureteric reflux

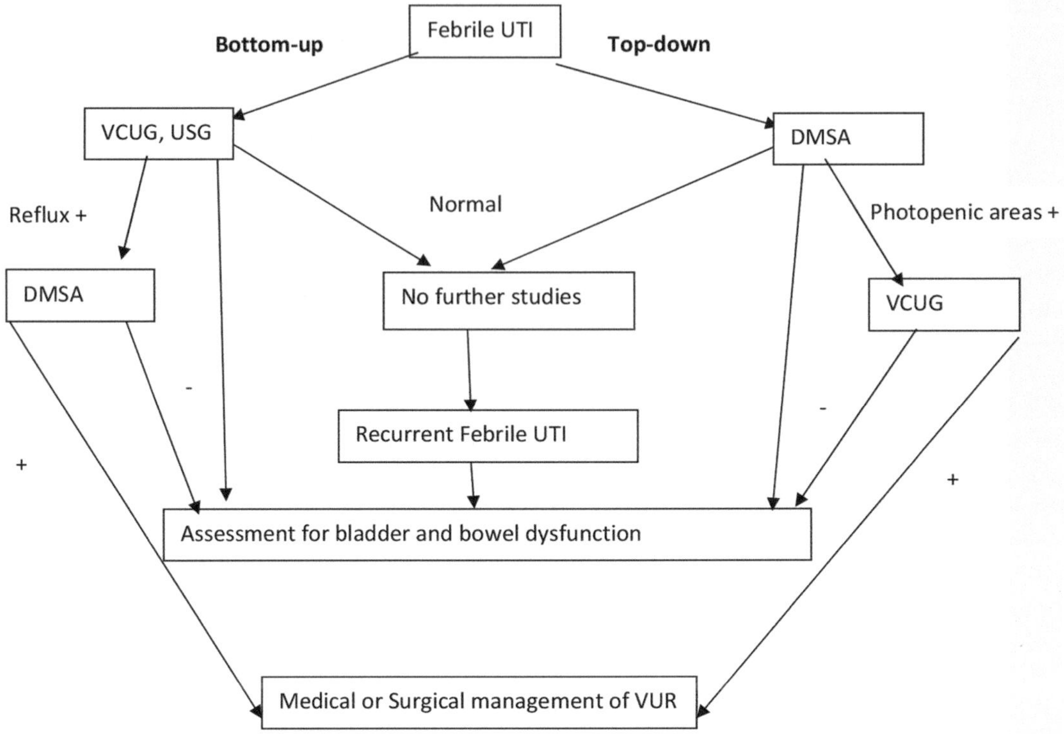

Fig. 72.4 Top-down versus bottom-up approach

72.8 Management of VUR

72.8.1 Conservative (Medical Management)

(a) Continuous antibiotic prophylaxis: Antibiotics are given at ¼ to ½ of the full dose, e.g., trimethoprim 1–2 mg/kg/day as a single nighttime dose. Nighttime dosing is preferred as there is residual urine for a prolonged bladder in the night.
(b) Regular urine examination (microscopy and culture sensitivity).
(c) Treatment of bladder dysfunction
   - *Urotherapy (bladder training)*—Regular voiding every 2–3 hours, double or triple voiding.
   - Anticholinergics like Oxybutynin, Tolterodine, Beta 3 agonist (Mirabegron) if bladder pressures are high or the bladder is overactive.
   - α-blocker therapy for functional bladder outlet obstruction.
   - Pelvic floor relaxation therapy and biofeedback therapy to help in the relaxation of the sphincter while voiding.
(d) Treatment of constipation if present.
   - Typically involves maintenance treatment with laxatives like polyethylene glycol powder or other osmotic, lubricant, or stimulant laxatives.

72.8.2 Follow-Up Management

General evaluation, including monitoring of blood pressure, height, and weight, is recommended annually. The follow-up interval is determined by the likelihood of resolution; for higher grades of VUR, resolution is less likely, and therefore, a longer interval of follow-up is appropriate. Generally, yearly USG, MCUG, and DMSA are recommended.

72.9 Indications for Surgical Intervention

72.9.1 Functional

Symptomatic breakthrough urinary tract infection despite medical management including antibiotic prophylaxis and treatment of constipation.

72.9.2 Anatomical

(a) VUR that occurs in conjunction with abnormalities such as paraureteric diverticulum or ureteric duplication has a lower tendency to resolve than uncomplicated primary reflux and needs surgical intervention.
(b) High-grade reflux (Grade IV or V) persisting after 12 months of age requires surgical intervention.
(c) If the child experiences poor renal growth or develops new renal scars, surgical treatment may be considered to prevent further kidney damage.
(d) Persistent dilating reflux in female patients who have attained full somatic potential needs surgical intervention to prevent acute pyelonephritis during future pregnancy.

72.9.3 Surgical Management (Fig. 72.5)

72.9.3.1 Endoscopic Injection Treatment

The endoscopic correction of VUR involves the placement of a bulking material near the ureterovesical junction (UVJ) to prevent the backflow of urine from the bladder to the kidneys. Different techniques are described:

- Subureteric Teflon Injection (STING): This technique, originally described by O'Donnell and Puri, involves injecting a bulking agent, such as polytetrafluoroethylene (PTFE) paste, submucosally at the ureterovesical junction. The injected material creates a bulge or mound that helps to prevent the backflow of urine into the ureter during bladder filling. Systemic migration of Teflon is an adverse effect.
- Hydrodistension Implantation Technique (HIT): This modified technique, introduced by Kirsch et al., involves hydrodistending the ureteral orifice to allow for injection of the material within the ureteral lumen, rather than injecting it subureterically. This technique aims to achieve greater coaptation of the ure-

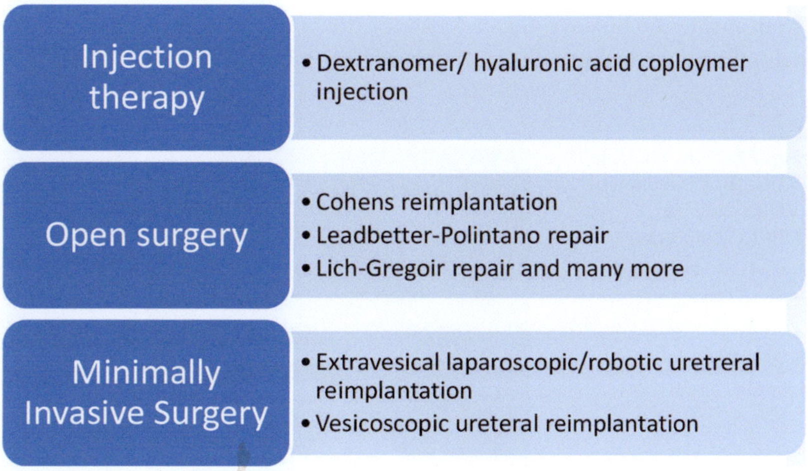

Fig. 72.5 Summary of interventional management of VUR

teral walls and has shown improved success rates compared to the standard STING technique.

- Double HIT: This technique, advocated by Cerwinka and Kirsch, involves performing two tandem intraluminal ureteric injections. The first injection is made at the mid-tunnel of the ureter, coaptating the tunnel, and the second injection is made at the distal aspect of the tunnel close to the ureteral orifice. This technique aims to enhance the coaptation of both the ureteral tunnel and the ureteral meatus.

Dextranomer–hyaluronic acid copolymer (Deflux, Dexell) is the most common material used for endoscopic correction of VUR. The success rate of endoscopic correction varies from 60 to 90% and is greater for low-grade reflux (grades I–III), but many patients with high-grade reflux respond well to injection with either complete resolution (Fig. 72.6a, b) or downgrading to a lower grade.

72.9.3.2 Open Ureteric Reimplantation for VUR

There are two types of techniques for ureteric reimplantation: intravesical and extravesical. In the former, reimplantation is carried out without opening the urinary bladder, while the latter involves opening the bladder to access the ureters from inside the bladder. Success rate of ureteric reimplantation exceeds 90%. If the ureters are dilated significantly, reimplantation may become difficult due to the bulk of the ureter within the submucosal tunnel. The ureter can be tapered via excision (Hendren) (Fig. 72.7a) or plicated without excision (Kalicinski and Starr) (Fig. 72.7b) in order to facilitate reimplantation.

72.9.3.3 Intravesical Techniques

1. Politano-Leadbetter Repair
   Following dissection of the ureter from the adjacent tissues, a right-angle clamp is passed through the original muscular hiatus in the bladder wall superiorly, marking the new muscular entrance for the ureter. The mucosa and muscle are incised on the clamp, and the ureter is transferred to the new hiatus. The ureter is relocated through a submucosal tunnel or mucosal flaps. The ureteral orifice is secured with sutures, and the original mucosal opening is closed (Fig. 72.8).
2. Cohen Cross-Trigonal Repair
   It is the most popular type of ureteric reimplantation. In this procedure, the submucosal tunnel is created along the posterior bladder wall without transferring the ureter to a new muscular hiatus, virtually eliminating kinking of the distal ureter that may happen with the Politano-Leadbetter repair. The ureter is transferred through the tunnel and brought out on the contralateral side above the other ureteric orifice and sutured to bladder mucosa (Fig. 72.9a, b).

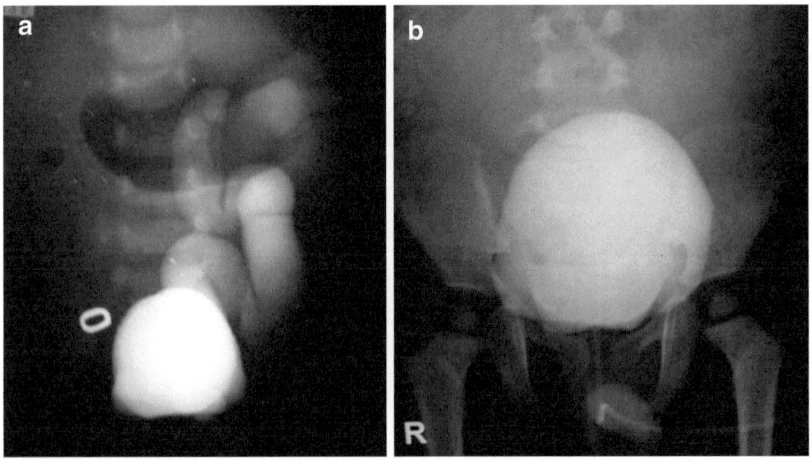

Fig. 72.6 (**a**) MCU: left VUR. (**b**) Resolution of VUR following DEFLUX injection

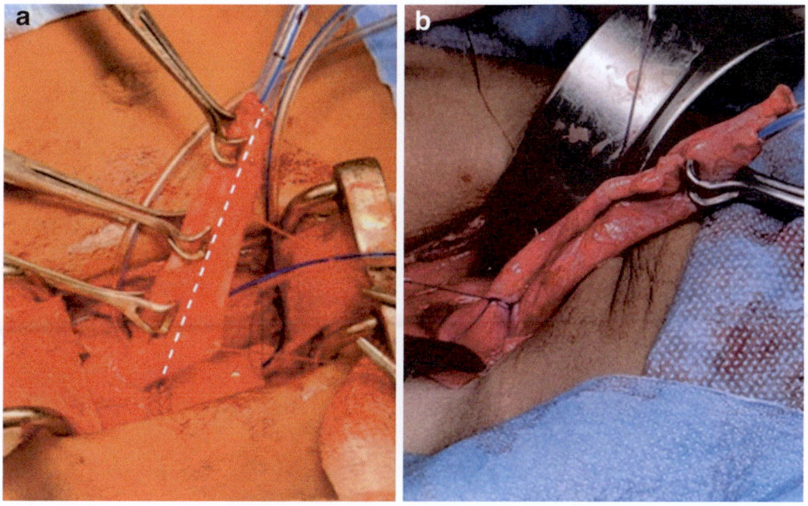

Fig. 72.7 (**a**) Hendren's excisional tapering (dashed line marks excision line), and (**b**) Kalicinski plication for refluxing megaureter

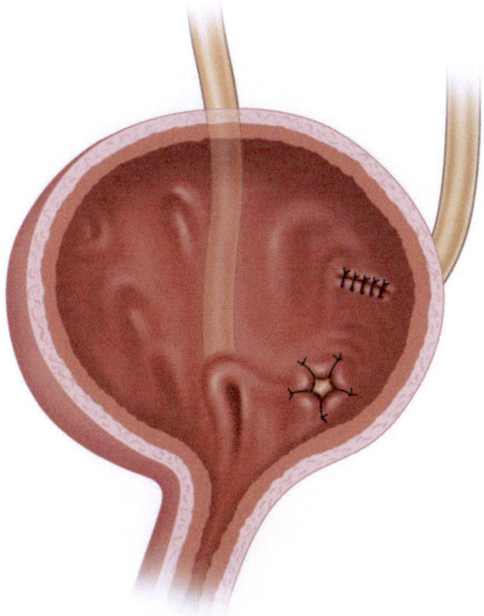

Fig. 72.8 Politano-Leadbetter technique of ureteric reimplantation

3. Glenn–Anderson's Advancement Technique
   Lateral and cephalad ureteral orifices are ideal for this technique. The ureters are advanced to an area superior to the bladder neck with an adequate submucosal tunnel (Fig. 72.10).
4. Gil-Vernet Trigonoplasty
   The principal is approximating the medial aspect of the ureteric orifices across the trigone by applying traction sutures (Fig. 72.11).

72.9.3.4 Extravesical Technique

Lich-Gregoir Technique

The bladder is rotated through a Pfannenstiel incision to expose the ureter extravesically. The detrusor muscle is incised, creating detrusor flaps to expose the surrounding bladder uroepithelium around the orifice. Synthetic absorbable sutures are used to invaginate the ureter into the bladder, forming a long subepithelial tunnel, and the hiatus is closed with absorbable sutures.

72.9.3.5 Laparoscopic and Robotic Approaches to Ureteric Reimplantation

Laparoscopic and robotic ureteric reimplantation offer advantages over open surgical approaches, including smaller incisions, reduced blood loss, shorter hospital stays, and quicker recovery while offering similar success rates. The principles of repair are the same as for open surgery. Extravesical approach is performed through the transperitoneal route, whereas intravesical approach is performed via vesicoscopic approach in which the ports are placed directly into the bladder and the bladder is distended with carbon dioxide (to create a pneumovesicum) (Fig. 72.12).

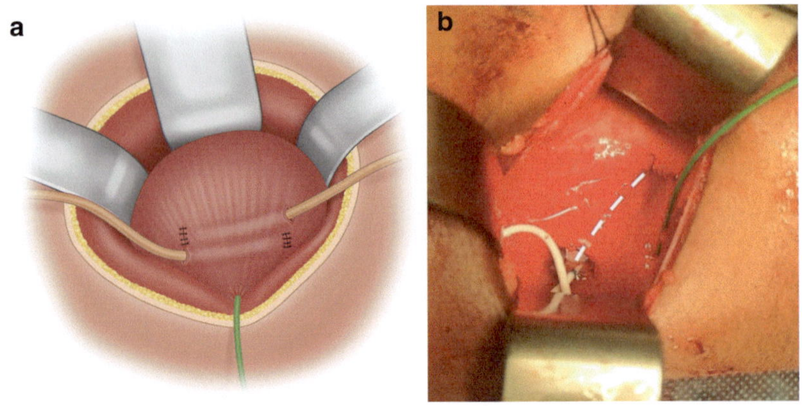

Fig. 72.9 (**a**) Cohen cross-trigonal repair, (**b**) dashed line indicating the tunnel

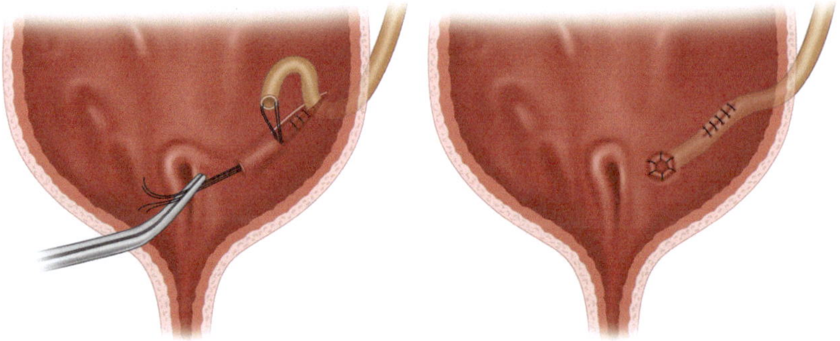

Fig. 72.10 Glenn–Anderson's advancement technique

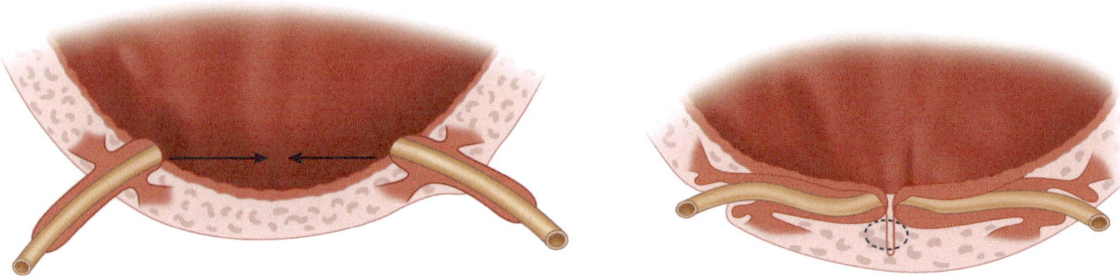

Fig. 72.11 Gil-Vernet trigonoplasty

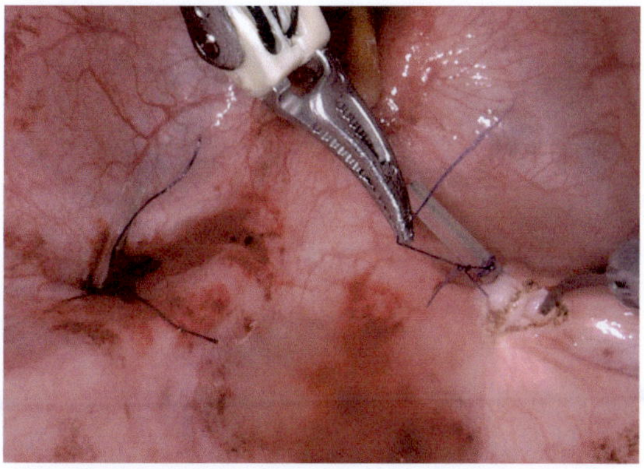

Fig. 72.12 Robotic intravesical ureteric reimplantation (dissection of the right ureter)

72.10 Summary

1. VUR can cause recurrent urinary tract infection leading to renal damage and scarring.
2. VCUG and DMSA scan help in planning management and follow-up of VUR patients.
3. Majority of VUR especially the lower grades resolve sopntaneously and can be managed with prophylactic antibiotic therapy and close follow-up.
4. Breakthrough infection, appearence of fresh scar with high grade VUR calls for intervention.
5. VUR associated with anatomical abnormality like paraureteric diverticulum also require surgical intervention.
6. Injection therapy and surgical ureteric reimplantation (open or minimally invasive) both offers effective treatment to stop VUR.
7. The end result often depend on the quality of the functional renal units in an individual patient.

Suggested Reading

Docimo SG, Canning D, Khoury A, Salle JLP, editors. The Kelalis-King-Belman textbook of clinical pediatric urology. 6th ed. CRC Press; 2018.

Partin AW, Dmochowski RR, Kavoussi LR, Peters CA, Wein AJ, editors. Campbell-Walsh-Wein urolosgy. 12th ed. Elsevier; 2020.

Neurogenic Bladder

73

Priyank Yadav, Subhasis Roy Choudhury, and Sujit K Chowdhary

Neurogenic or neuropathic bladder refers to a dysfunction of the urinary bladder caused by a neurological disorder or damage to the nerves that control bladder function. It can result in problems with bladder storage or emptying, leading to issues such as urinary incontinence, urinary retention, or abnormal bladder contractions. It can adversely affect the function of the kidneys with serious consequences.

73.1 Etiology of Childhood Neuropathic Bladder

- Neuropathic
  - Spinal cord
    Congenital
    - Neurospinal dysraphism
    - Other anatomic
    Acquired
    - Trauma
    - Tumor
    - Infection
    - Vascular (infarction)
    - Miscellaneous
  - Supraspinal cord
    Anatomic or congenital
    Trauma
    Tumor
    Infection
    Vascular
    Degenerative
    Miscellaneous
    Temporary
  - Peripheral
    Trauma
    Tumor
    Degenerative
    Guillain–Barré syndrome
- Nonneuropathic
  - Anatomic
  - Myopathic
  - Psychological
  - Endocrinologic
  - Toxic

Common Childhood causes are

1. Spina bifida and tethered cord, hydrocephalus
2. Spinal cord trauma, infarction, tumors
3. Transverse myelitis
4. Tumors, sacrococcygeal teratoma, and neuroblastoma

P. Yadav
Sanjay Gandhi Institute of Post Graduate Medical Education & Research, Lucknow, UP, India

S. Roy Choudhury
Pediatric Surgery, Lady Hardinge Medical College and Associated Kalawati Saran Children's Hospital, New Delhi, Delhi, India

S. K Chowdhary (✉)
Indraprastha Apollo Hospital, New Delhi, Delhi, India

© The Author(s), under exclusive license to Springer Nature Singapore Pte Ltd. 2025
S. Roy Choudhury (ed.), *Pediatric Surgery*, https://doi.org/10.1007/978-981-96-1257-4_73

73.2 Physiology of Bladder Function

Bladder function involves two main phases: storage and voiding.

- Storage Phase:
  - The bladder relaxes and expands to accommodate urine.
  - The detrusor muscle remains relaxed to allow the bladder to fill.
  - The bladder neck and the external urethral sphincter (EUS) remain closed to prevent urine from flowing out.
  - The urethra is also closed.
  - The pelvic floor muscles provide support to the bladder and help maintain continence.
  - The nervous system, including the brain and spinal cord, coordinates the storage phase by sending signals to inhibit bladder contraction and promote sphincter contraction.
  - Sensory nerves in the bladder walls detect bladder filling and transmit signals to the brain to convey the sensation of fullness or urgency.
- Voiding Phase:
  - When it is appropriate to empty the bladder, the detrusor muscle contracts.
  - The contraction of the detrusor muscle generates pressure, pushing urine out of the bladder.
  - The bladder neck and EUS relax, allowing the urine to flow through the urethra and out of the body.
  - The coordination between the detrusor muscle and the urethral sphincters ensures proper urine flow without leakage.
  - The nervous system coordinates the voiding phase by sending signals to promote bladder contraction and inhibit sphincter contraction.
  - The process of bladder emptying is under voluntary control, allowing individuals to initiate and control the voiding process.
  - After emptying, the bladder returns to the storage phase, and the cycle repeats as urine accumulates.

73.3 Types of Lesions

- *Suprasacral cord lesions* (contractile bladder) where the conus medullaris is intact, voiding occurs solely by detrusor contractions, almost always accompanied by detrusor–sphincter dyssynergia. These are upper motor neuron lesions.
- *Sacral cord lesions* (acontractile bladder) where the conus medullaris is destroyed, voiding occurs either by overflow or by raising intra-abdominal pressure. These are lower motor neuron lesions.
- *Intermediate bladder dysfunction is* characterized by a combination of detrusor hyperreflexia, typically generating low pressures, and some degree of sphincteric incompetence. Neuropathic bladder with meningomyelocele is mostly intermediate in nature.

73.4 Secondary Upper Renal Tract Complications

Secondary upper tract complications can occur in children with neurogenic bladder dysfunction, leading to potential damage and dysfunction of the kidneys and upper urinary tract. These complications may include:

- Hydronephrosis: Results from functional obstruction due to sphincter contraction or impaired urine flow into a persistently distended bladder.
- Vesicoureteral Reflux (VUR): Neurogenic bladder commonly causes secondary VUR which is a manifestation of backpressure changes due to high-pressure voiding.
- UTI: Frequent UTIs can occur due to incomplete bladder emptying, stasis of urine, or urinary catheter use.
- Pyelonephritis: Inflammation and infection of the kidneys which can cause severe illness and further renal damage if left untreated.
- Renal Insufficiency: Long-term, untreated upper tract complications can lead to impaired kidney function and eventual renal failure.

- Renal Calculi: Formation of kidney stones can result from concentrated urine, altered urinary pH, and chronic urinary stasis.

73.5 Types of Neurogenic Bladder

The types of neurogenic bladder can be classified as per Fig. 73.1.

Disorders of storage include increased detrusor tone, which limits the ability of the bladder to hold urine, and urine is stored under high pressures. This can be due to

- Nonelastic bladder
- Hyperreflexia or overactive bladder

Another reason for the bladder's inability to hold urine can be poor outflow resistance at rest. This can be due to

- Incompetent bladder neck
- Incompetent external sphincter

Disorders of evacuation include the inability of the bladder to contract effectively to empty. This can be due to

- Areflexic bladder (no contraction).
- Underactive bladder (unsustained contraction).
- Detrussor-sphincter dyssynergia, where the external sphincter fails to relax while the detrusor is contracting.

73.6 History

A detailed history of the following is taken

- Perinatal health
- Birth and development
- Bladder/ bowel habits
- Pattern of incontinence
  - Dry periods
  - Stream
  - Dribbling
- Urinary tract infections
- Bowel incontinence

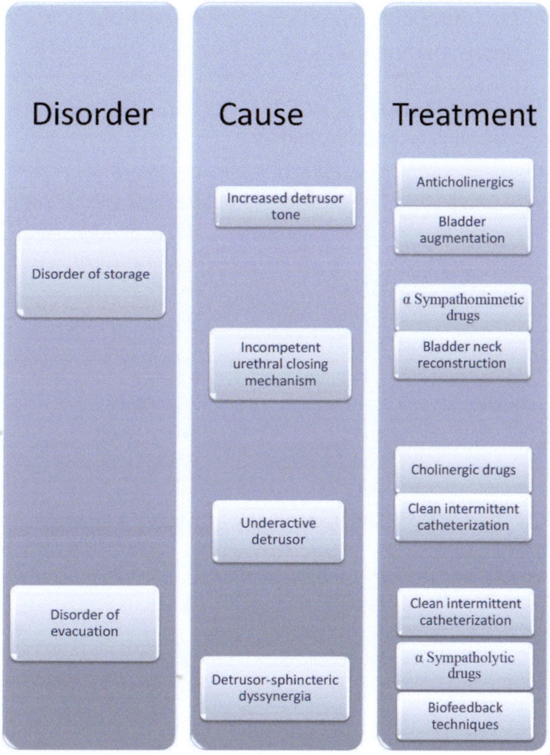

Fig. 73.1 Summary of pathophysiology and management of neurogenic bladder

73.7 Examination

- Anthropometry and blood pressure
- Spine examination
- Abdomen
  - Bladder palpable/ compressible
  - Palpable fecaloma
  - Renal lump
- Perineum
  - Ammoniacal dermatitis
  - Sensations
  - Anal tone
  - Bulbocavernous reflex
- Lower extremities
  - Deep tendon reflexes
  - Muscle mass and strength sensation
  - Gait
- Central nervous system (CNS)
  - Handedness
  - Fine and gross motor coordination

73.8 Assessment

- *Bladder expressibility* (expressing out urine by suprapubic pressure): An expressible bladder is pathognomonic of bladder neuropathy with some measure of sphincteric incompetence. A bladder that cannot be expressed, by contrast, implies either sphincteric competence or a bladder that is virtually empty due to gross sphincteric incompetence.
- *Conus Reflex* (anocutaneous, glansbulbar): Positive conus reflexes carry an excellent prognosis for continence. Most patients with positive reflexes become dry on clean intermittent catheterization (CIC) alone or in combination with an anticholinergic drug; few patients may need augmentation cystoplasty or other procedures.
- *Sacral Sensory sparing* (perineal sensation) is a favorable sign.

In a newborn, bladder expressibility, absence of conus reflex, and no sacral sensory sparing are signs of a neuropathic bladder.

73.9 Investigations (Table 73.1)

- Laboratory: Urine analysis and culture, urine-specific gravity, serum creatinine level
- Renal and Bladder Ultrasound: Presence of renal pelvic/ ureteral dilatation, cortical

Table 73.1 International Children's Continence Society recommendations for the diagnostic evaluation and follow-up of congenital neurogenic bladder

Age group	Type of investigation	Recommended frequency	Indication for investigation
Newborn to toddler	Ultrasonography	Every 6 months until 2 years of age	High risk for tethering with rapid growth
	UDS	Every 12 months	UTIs or lower extremity changes
	DMSA renal scan	When indicated	Consider if VUR on initial VCUG/RNC or febrile UTIs
Toddler to adolescent	Ultrasonography	Every 12 to 24 months	Low risk for tethering with slower growth
	UDS	When indicated	Change in ambulation or lower extremity function
	DMSA renal scan	When indicated	Febrile UTIs
Adolescent to adult	Ultrasonography	Every 12 months	Low risk for tethering with slower growth; may decrease to every 24 months once growth velocity has decreased
	UDS	When indicated	Development of hydronephrosis, more frequent CIC required for continence, new wetting, recurrent UTI
	VCUG/RNC	When indicated	Recurrent UTI
Adult	Ultrasonography	Every 36 months	Low risk for tethering without ongoing somatic growth
	UDS	When indicated	Development of hydronephrosis, more frequent CIC required for continence, new wetting, recurrent UTI

thickness and renal length, bladder wall thickness, postvoid residue—very important to determine

- DMSA scan for renal functional assessment and presence and location of scars
- Micturating cystourethrography (MCUG) (Fig. 73.2).
  - Bladder outline in a neurogenic bladder is usually elongated with sacculation giving a "Christmas tree" appearance (Fig. 73.2).
  - Vesicoureteric reflux (VUR) may be found.
  - Bladder neck incompetence—funnel-shaped bladder neck during filling phase.
  - Postvoid residue is frequently seen.
- MRI of Lumbosacral spine in children more than 3 months of age (Fig. 73.3). In children less than 3 months of age, spinal ultrasonography can provide necessary information.
- Urodynamics is used to identify the "unsafe" bladder, i.e., the bladder which can result in renal damage. "Unsafe" bladder has intravesical pressure of more than 40 cm H_2O during the filling phase

  Parameters recorded are:

(a) Bladder capacity
  - Expected bladder capacity in ounces is:
    - < 2 years age: Age (years) × 2 + 2
    - > 2 years of age: Age (years)÷2 + 6
  - Expected bladder capacity in ml is:
    - For 0–2 years, capacity = weight (kg) × 7
    - For 2–12 years, capacity = (age + 2) × 30

(b) Compliance can be assessed by pressure-specific volumes, i.e., bladder volume at bladder pressures of 10, 20, and 30 cm H_2O,

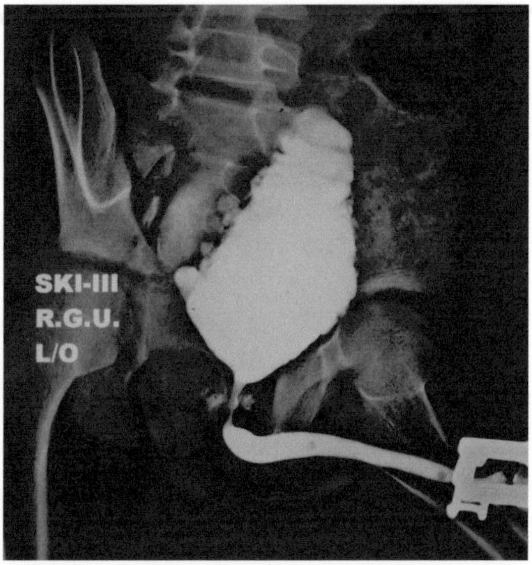

Fig. 73.2 MCU: neurogenic bladder (sacculation and christmas tree appearance) with VUR

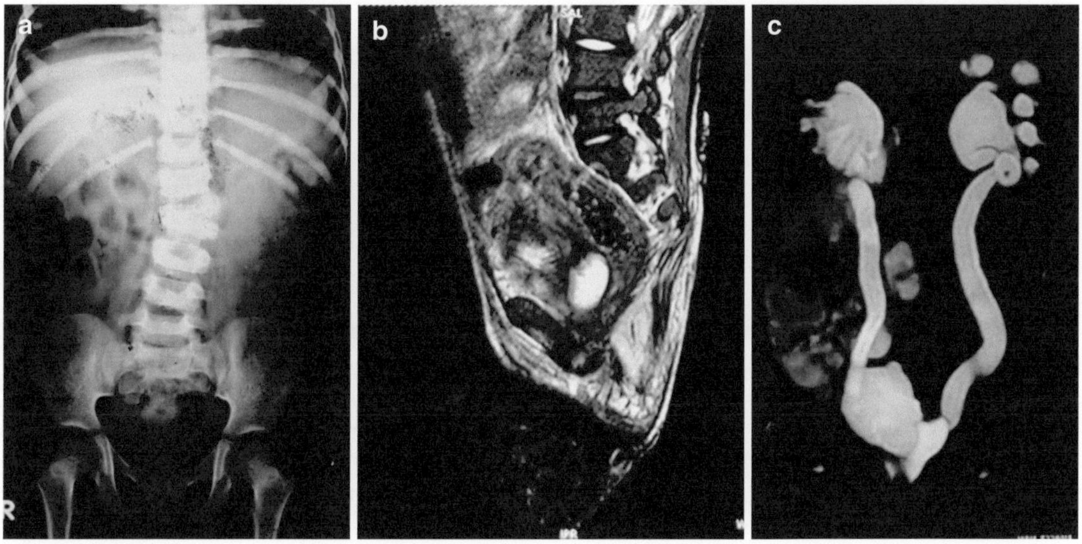

Fig. 73.3 (**a**, **b**) Neurogenic bladder due to (**a**) spinal deformity and (**b**) tethered cord, (**c**) Magnetic Resonance Urography (MRU) showing a small bladder with VUR

respectively. In normal children, more than 99% of bladder capacity can be stored at 30 cm H_2O pressure. Baseline pressures exceeding 20 cm H2O within the physiological range of capacity on conventional slow-fill urodynamics should be regarded as being "unsafe."

(c) Detrusor Leak Point Pressure (DLPP): It is the pressure at which urine starts leaking in the filling phase in the absence of bladder contraction. DLPP above 40 cm H_2O is dangerous for the upper tract.

(d) Detrusor Overactivity: Suprasacral and intermediate lesions typically cause detrusor overactivity. They are managed with anticholinergic treatment and sometimes even intravesical botulinum toxin injection.

(e) Detrusor Pressure During Voiding: Normal detrusor pressure during voiding typically remains under 40 cm H2O in children. Neurogenic bladder may frequently have low voiding pressure, suggesting detrusor underactivity. High-voiding pressure with increased sphincter activity on electromyogram is typical of detrusor-sphincter dyssynergia.

(f) Uroflowmetry and postvoid residue: Neurogenic bladder typically shows an interrupted flow curve with elevated postvoid residue (See Chapter on Urodynamics).

73.10 Management

73.10.1 Goals of Management

1. Preservation of the upper urinary tract by maintaining adequate bladder storage and emptying function, reducing high pressures within the bladder, and minimizing the risk of reflux.
2. Optimization of renal function by preventing or treating complications such as hydronephrosis, renal stones, or recurrent UTIs that can lead to renal damage.
3. Alleviation of bothersome symptoms associated with neurogenic bladder, such as urinary incontinence, urgency, frequency, nocturia, and difficulties with voiding initiation or completion.
4. Prevention of UTIs by ensuring adequate bladder emptying, sterile intermittent catheterization if necessary, and appropriate use of antimicrobial therapy when indicated.
5. Improvement of Quality of Life by minimizing bladder-related complications, improving social integration, reducing limitations in daily activities, and maximizing independence.

73.10.2 General Principles of Management

73.10.2.1 High Postvoid Residue

- Evaluate and identify the cause of the high postvoid residue, such as incomplete bladder emptying or impaired detrusor contraction.
- Children with borderline residues who can otherwise void with stream can be managed with double voiding (voiding in quick succession).
- Patients with detrusor-sphincter dyssynergia may require clean intermittent catheterization (CIC) or rarely an indwelling catheter.
- Children who find it difficult to catheterize their urethra due to neurological deficiency or a sensate urethra can be managed by creating an appendicovesicostomy (Mitrofanoff procedure). Appendix is used as a continent conduit between the bladder and skin (Fig. 73.4).
- Where the appendix cannot be used or is unavailable, a similar tube fashioned from the ileum (Monti tube) can be used.

73.10.2.2 Detrusor Overactivity

- Initial treatment options include conservative measures such as behavioral modifications (bladder training, fluid management).
- First-line pharmacological management may involve anticholinergic medications (Oxybutynin, Tolterodine) or beta-3 agonists (Mirabegron) to suppress involuntary bladder contractions.

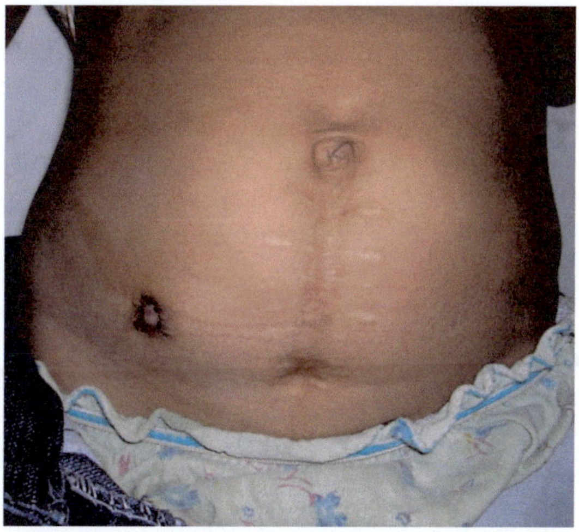

Fig. 73.4 Mitrofanoff stoma

- Consider second-line treatment like intravesical *botulinum toxin* injections if conservative measures and medications are ineffective.
- The effect of botulinum toxin wanes off in 6–9 months. It is safe to use repeated injections.
- Augmentation cystoplasty is the last resort for refractory detrusor overactivity.

73.10.2.3 Poor Bladder Outlet Resistance

- Identify the underlying cause of poor bladder outlet resistance, which may involve bladder neck dysfunction or urethral sphincter weakness.
- Sympathomimetics like pseudoephedrine or phenylpropanolamine can be used to increase bladder neck resistance, but the efficacy is limited.
- Surgical options include:
  - Bladder neck reconstruction/ tightening
  - Bladder neck suspension using fascial slings, especially in females
  - Artificial urethral sphincter
  - Bladder neck bulking agents (Deflux)
  - Bladder neck closure with Mitrofanoff stoma for CIC

73.10.2.4 Detrusor-Sphincter Dyssynergia

- Confirm the diagnosis of dyssynergia through urodynamic studies and electromyography (EMG) assessment.
- CIC is the only way to eliminate the effects of sphincter contractions during voiding.
- Implement strategies to improve coordination between the detrusor muscle and the urethral sphincter, such as biofeedback-assisted pelvic floor muscle training.
- Pharmacological management with alpha-blockers or anticholinergic medications may be considered to relax the sphincter or suppress detrusor overactivity, but the role is limited.
- In refractory cases, advanced interventions like or onabotulinumtoxinA injections into the sphincter can be considered. However, it can lead to incontinence due to total loss of outlet resistance (as the bladder neck is already open) and may only be suitable when incontinence is acceptable over renal deterioration.

73.10.2.5 Functional Voiding Disorders

- Not all children with a lesion in the brain or spinal cord will develop a neurogenic bladder. Some of these children may, however, develop symptoms like those of neurogenic bladder due to dysfunctional voiding or bowel bladder dysfunction.
- Conduct a comprehensive evaluation to identify any underlying factors contributing to the functional voiding disorder, such as anxiety, poor toileting habits, or inadequate fluid intake.
- Implement behavioral modifications, including regular toileting schedules, double or triple voiding, relaxation techniques, and adequate fluid intake.
- Pelvic floor muscle exercises and biofeedback-assisted training can help improve coordination and control during voiding.
- Anticholinergics may be required for overactive bladder symptoms.

- Treat constipation, which may be commonly found.
- Address any psychological or emotional factors contributing to the functional voiding disorder, such as anxiety or stress, through counseling or therapy.
- Regular monitoring and follow-up is necessary to assess progress and make any necessary adjustments to the management plan.

73.11 Clean Intermittent Catheterization (CIC) in Children

CIC is a valuable technique used in the management of various bladder dysfunctions in children. It involves the periodic insertion and removal of a catheter into the bladder to empty urine completely.

Indications:

- Neurogenic bladder
- Myogenic failure of the bladder, like that in some patients with PUV
- Following bladder augmentation
- Continent urinary diversion

Benefits of CIC in Children:

- Complete Bladder Emptying: CIC ensures thorough bladder emptying, reducing the risk of UTIs and bladder overdistention.
- Preservation of Renal Function: By maintaining adequate bladder emptying, CIC helps prevent kidney damage caused by backflow of urine into the kidneys.
- Continence Management: By eliminating residual volume, CIC decreases the chances of leakage due to bladder overdistension.
- Prevention of Complications: Regular CIC can prevent complications associated with urinary retention, such as urinary tract infections, bladder stones, and renal damage.
- Promotes Independence: CIC empowers children to take control of their own bladder management, leading to increased independence and self-esteem.

Technique

CIC should be demonstrated and taught to the patient/parent in the hospital or clinic, and followed at home. Proper hygiene should be maintained, including thorough hand washing and cleaning of the perineum/genitalia with soap and water. Size 6 to 10 Fr feeding tubes can be used for pediatric patients. A liberal amount of water-soluble jelly (2% lignocaine) is to be applied to the catheter insertion site. Allow urine to drain completely by pressing on the lower abdomen before removing the catheter. Clean the catheter by rinsing it with soap and water, then dry it in the sunlight. Store the catheter in a dry stainless steel container or boil it in water for 20 minutes before use. One catheter can be used for 1–2 weeks, but should be discarded if it gets dirty or damaged. CIC is generally recommended every 3–4 h interval to keep the patient dry and protect the upper urinary tract from any pressure effects. For patients at high risk of upper tract damage, a nighttime indwelling catheter is recommended.

73.12 Augmentation Cystoplasty

This procedure is required for high-pressure low compliant and small volume bladder which is considered unsafe for the upper renal tract (See Chap. 76).

73.13 Summary

1. Neurogenic bladder should be differentiated from functional voiding disorders by through histroty taking, physical examination, renal function tests and imaging studies.
2. The commonest cause of neurogenic bladder in children is spinal dysraphism.
3. Urodynamic study helps to categorize the different types of bladder dysfunction and helps to identify the “unsafe” bladder needing special attention.
4. CIC and pharmacotherapy are the cornerstone of management.

5. Botulinium toxin injection has a short term effect.
6. Bladder augmentation may be required in selected group of patients with high pressure, low compliant bladder to protect the function of the upper tracts.

Suggested Reading

Docimo SG, Canning D, Khoury A, Salle JLP, editors. The Kelalis-King-Belman textbook of clinical pediatric urology. 6th ed. CRC Press; 2018.

Franco I, Austin P, Bauer S, von Gontard A, Homsy Y. Pediatric incontinence: evaluation and clinical management. John Wiley & Sons; 2015.

Partin AW, Dmochowski RR, Kavoussi LR, Peters CA, Wein AJ, editors. Campbell-Walsh-Wein urology. 12th ed. Elsevier; 2020.

74 Posterior Urethral Valves

Prema Menon and Subhasis Roy Choudhury

74.1 Introduction

Posterior urethral valve (PUV) is the most common cause of urinary obstruction in males with an incidence of 1 in 5000–8000 male live births.

74.2 Embryology and Types

Hugh Hampton Young (1919) classified posterior urethral valves into three types:

Type I (95%) arises from the posterior lower end of the verumontanum and extends distally and anteriorly on either side, fusing in the midline and attaching to the anterior urethral wall and cause obstruction. As per one theory, an abnormal insertion of the mesonephric duct into the urogenital sinus affects its normal migration, with the valves being created by their anterior fusion.

Type II valves are folds which extend upwards from the verumontanum to the bladder neck. They should not be rightfully included in the classification as they are nonobstructive.

Type III (5–10%) is a circumferential ring in the membranous urethra distal to the verumontanum and is obstructive. They may be formed by the failure of complete canalization of the membranous urethra.

A common morphological diagnosis for all the types of PUV was proposed by Dewan in 1993 with the unique concept that all PUVs were in fact a congenital obstructing membrane with a hole, which he named as Congenital Obstructing Posterior Urethral Membrane (COPUM) (Dewan 1993). Following insertion of a catheter or an instrument, this would then appear as a type I valve.

74.3 Pathophysiology

The severity of changes in the upper tracts is related to congenital dysplasia, the gestational age at which the obstruction occurs and the degree of mechanical obstruction by the valve.

Early embryonic obstruction leads to smooth muscle hypertrophy and increased type III collagen extracellular matrix deposition in the bladder wall. Later, damage to the muscles and nerves of the bladder wall can occur from hypoxic injury. These changes lead to higher voiding pressure, reduction in compliance and capacity, followed by incomplete emptying of the bladder. Upper tract changes include injury to renal tubules, renal parenchymal fibrosis, and ureteral dilata-

P. Menon (✉)
Department of Pediatric Surgery, Level 3A, Advanced Pediatric Centre, Post Graduate Institute of Medical Education and Research, Chandigarh, India

S. Roy Choudhury
Pediatric Surgery, Lady Hardinge Medical College and Associated Kalawati Saran Children's Hospital, New Delhi, Delhi, India

© The Author(s), under exclusive license to Springer Nature Singapore Pte Ltd. 2025

S. Roy Choudhury (ed.), *Pediatric Surgery*, https://doi.org/10.1007/978-981-96-1257-4_74

tion. Obstruction in later gestation results in the typical sequelae of chronic bladder outflow obstruction and raised intravesical pressure, without renal dysplasia. The long-term prognosis in an individual with this disorder is determined by a combination of the degree of early abnormal development, involving the urethra, bladder, kidneys and the ureters, and the severity of late secondary effects of outflow obstruction on the bladder and the upper urinary tract.

74.4 Presentation

74.4.1 Antenatal Diagnosis

With improvement in fetal ultrasonography (USG), diagnosis can be established between 16 and 20 weeks of gestation. A distended hypertrophied bladder which does not empty completely, and a dilated posterior urethra give a "keyhole" sign. Other features include bilateral hydroureteronephrosis (HUN). The presence of oligohydramnios before 20 weeks of gestation is associated with renal dysplasia, i.e., cystic and echogenic kidneys, and carries a poor prognosis. When such pregnancies proceed to term, a severely affected infant often demonstrates features of Potter's syndrome at birth with characteristic facies and skeletal molding deformities. Early mortality is the norm due to pulmonary hypoplasia. In the absence of oligohydramnios, functional prognosis is linked to the severity of dilatation and other prognostic features on second-trimester USG.

When dilatation develops later in gestation, the prognosis is generally good. Fetal USG may also detect urinary ascites and perinephric urinomas. Other differential diagnoses should be kept in mind while interpreting fetal USG. The keyhole sign may be seen in prune belly syndrome, neurogenic bladder, and urethral atresia, and HUN may be seen with vesicoureteral reflux (VUR) per se or primary megaureter among other causes.

74.4.2 Postnatal Diagnosis

74.4.2.1 Neonates

The urinary stream is usually thin with associated dribbling. The baby strains while passing urine and may have dysuria due to a urinary tract infection (UTI). Listlessness, poor feeding, irritability, and failure to thrive are common. A thick-walled small bladder is usually palpable in the suprapubic region on careful examination. Due to hydronephrosis or pyonephrosis, one or both kidneys may be palpable. Perinephric urinoma can also cause a palpable swelling in the flanks. Abdominal distension may be secondary to uremia or urinary ascites. The latter occurs in 5–10% of cases and is usually secondary to renal fornix blowout, renal parenchymal rupture, or rarely bladder rupture. Although alarming, it is said to have a protective effect on the kidneys from the high-pressure bladder. In case of respiratory distress from the gross abdominal distension, bilateral bedside flank drains insertion gives good relief. In milder cases, a period of bladder catheter drainage reduces the ascites spontaneously. Due to absorption of urine from the peritoneum, the renal function tests (RFT) will be higher than their actual values. Abnormal RFTs are however common in neonatal PUV presentation, and the first RFT before catheterization should be noted.

Rarely, respiratory distress may be due to spontaneous pneumothorax or pleural effusion and should be managed by a chest drain.

74.4.2.2 Infants and Older Children

They present with poor stream and voiding dysfunction, in the form of dribbling, and enuresis. History of recurrent UTI is common. Renal failure will be associated with a lethargic child with pallor and poor physical growth. Older children may have a large palpable bladder due to decompensation and may also occasionally present with hematuria.

74.5 Investigations

1. Urine routine/microscopic examination, culture, and sensitivity.
2. Blood urea, serum creatinine, serum electrolytes, blood gas analysis.
3. Height and weight measurement.
4. Blood pressure recording.
5. USG Kidney, Ureter, Bladder, Urethra (KUBU): Features which should be looked for are bladder distension, bladder wall thickening, echogenic urine, postvoid residual urine, size of kidneys, anteroposterior diameter of renal pelvis, echogenic urine in pelvicalyceal system suggestive of pyonephrosis, renal parenchymal thickness, any cystic changes or echogenicity, corticomedullary differentiation, dilatation, and tortuosity if any of ureters with diameter, perirenal urinoma or urinary ascites, and dilatation of the posterior urethra (Fig. 74.1). The HUN may be due to VUR or nonrefluxing slow draining, or obstructed systems.
6. Micturating Cystourethrography (MCUG): This is the gold standard investigation for the definitive diagnosis. It should be performed under strict aseptic precautions after ensuring a sterile urine culture. It is done in the filling and voiding phase. While the former is done in the supine position, the latter should be done in an oblique fashion so that the posterior urethra shape can be correctly delineated. A dilated and elongated posterior urethra will be seen. Its diameter will be much more than that of the bulbar or anterior urethra. The ratio between them is a useful marker of the severity of the obstruction (Menon et al. 2010). A defect caused by the valve may be appreciated in the posterior urethra as a radiolucent area. A prominent bladder neck suggests bladder neck hypertrophy. The bladder is often small and trabeculated and may have sacculations and diverticulae (Fig. 74.2a). VUR is associated in nearly 50% of cases with two-thirds having unilateral reflux. Postvoid residual urine is usually significant. Sometimes the child does not pass urine on the table in the radiology suite, and the crucial anatomy of the posterior urethra does not get delineated. At other times, the MCUG is postponed by the radiologist because of recurrent UTIs. Abnormal RFTs may also cause a delay. If the treating surgeon is very convinced of the diagnosis, the child should be admitted, catheterized, treated adequately with appropriate intravenous antibiotics and intravenous fluids till dehydration, electrolyte imbalance, and RFTs are normalized. The investigation should then be carried out in the Radiology department or the operation theater under general anesthesia and antibiotic cover. In some cases, a suprapubic cystostomy or vesicostomy may have to be performed initially, and the study postponed to a later date (Fig. 74.3).

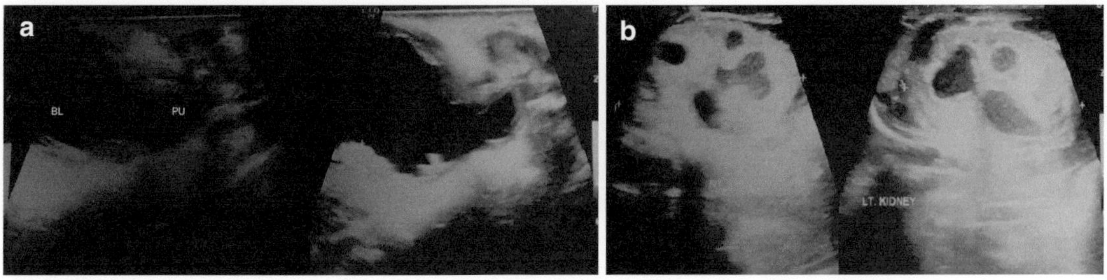

Fig. 74.1 Ultrasonography shows (**a**) distended, thick-walled bladder (BL) and dilated posterior urethra (PU); (**b**) dilated bilateral pelvicalyceal systems

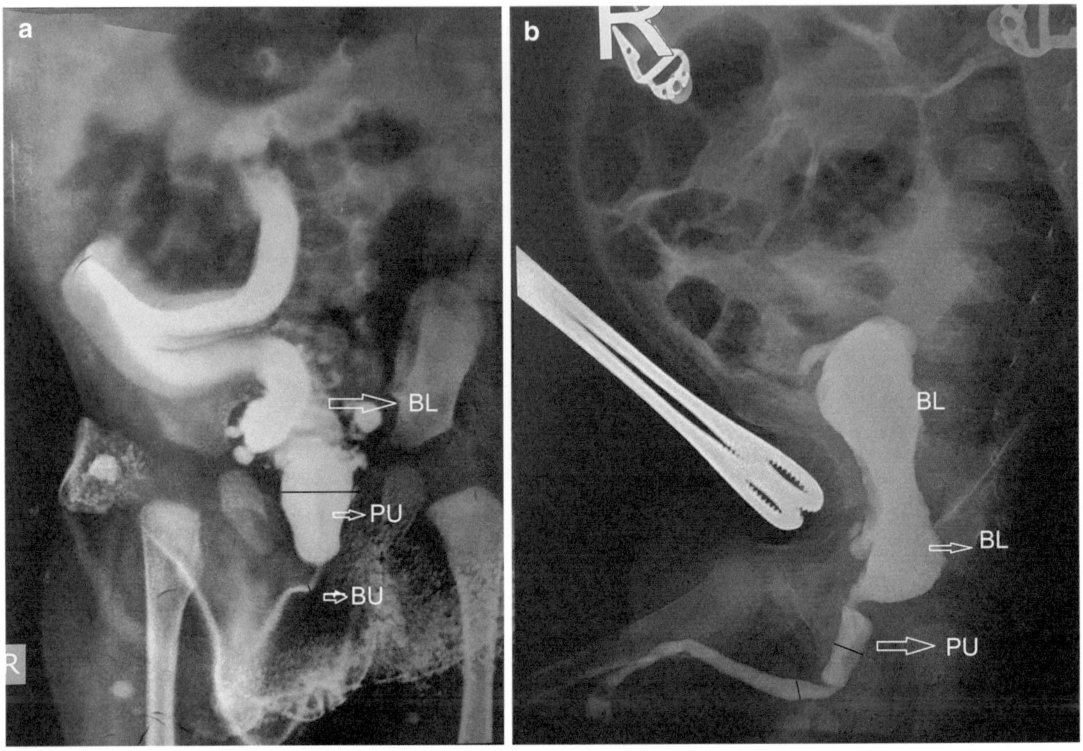

Fig. 74.2 Micturating cystourethrogram of a neonate with PUV. (**a**) Preoperative showing dilated posterior urethra (PU), small trabeculated bladder (BL) with multiple diverticulae, and grade V reflux on the right side. The ratio of the diameter of the PU to the bulbar urethra (BU) is 10:1. (**b**) Postoperative of the same patient 3 months after fulguration shows normalization of PU/BU ratio, grade I VUR on right side, and improvement in bladder characteristics

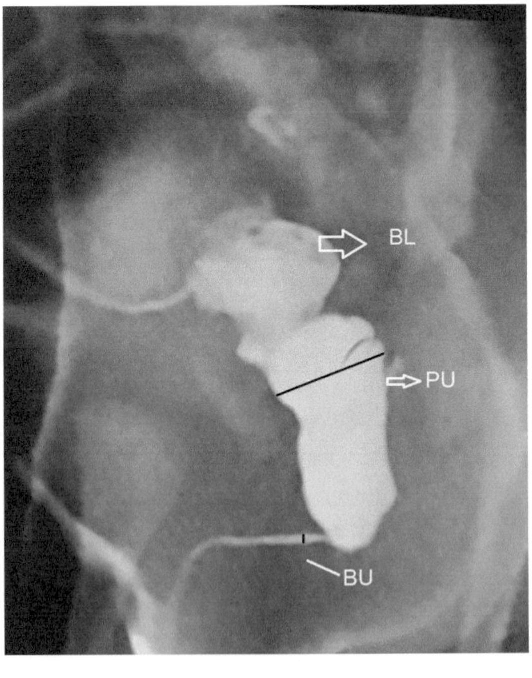

Fig. 74.3 Micturating cystourethrogram of a neonate with PUV performed through a suprapubic cystostomy showing dilated posterior urethra with a high PU/BU ratio

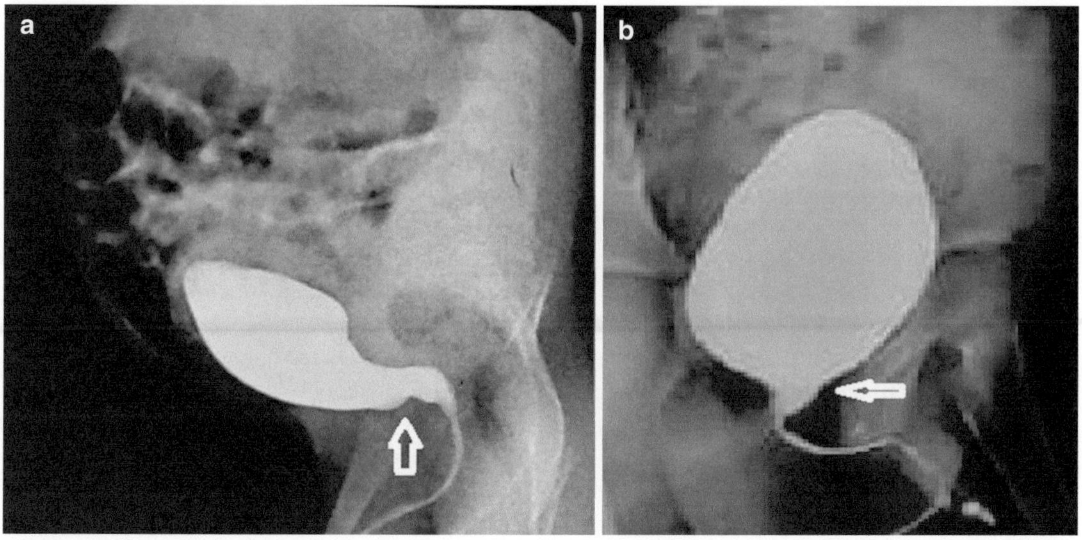

Fig. 74.4 (**a**) Appearance of bladder and posterior urethra in a child with (**a**) prune belly syndrome, (**b**) neurogenic bladder. Although the posterior urethra is dilated, the bladder neck (arrowhead) is open in both pictures

74.6 Differential Diagnosis

Dilatation of the posterior urethra can occur due to urethral obstruction below the prostatic urethra from various other causes like anterior urethral valve (which may be rarely associated with PUV), stricture due to trauma or prolonged catheterization, neurogenic bladder, prune belly syndrome, etc. (Fig. 74.4a and b). A good history, clinical examination, and interpretation of the MCUG and, if necessary, urethrocystoscopy will help to rule out these conditions.

74.7 Management

74.7.1 Fetal Management

The different options are as follows:

1. Early detection before 20 weeks of gestation associated with severe urinary tract dilatation, renal dysplasia as seen by echogenic kidneys or cystic changes in renal parenchyma, oligohydramnios, and the presence of malformations in other organs implies a poor outcome and the pregnancy should be terminated. Other poor prognostic factors are fetal urine analysis showing sodium >100 mmol/L, Cl >90 mmol/L, beta 2 microglobulin >4 mg/L, urine osmolality >210 mOsm, and urine output <2 ml/h.
2. If initial USGs were normal and performed by experienced radiologists, detection after 24 weeks with rapidly progressing late-onset urinary tract dilatation and decreasing amniotic fluid volume is an indication for preterm delivery at a tertiary care neonatal center. The pregnancy should be taken as close to term as possible, balancing the need for lung growth. However, if a certified medical board deems fit, termination can be carried out till 28 weeks under expert obstetric care.
3. An international randomized trial of percutaneous vesicoamniotic shunting versus conservative management for fetal lower urinary tract obstruction (PLUTO) was conducted, wherein 31 women with singleton male pregnancies with unknown causes of fetal lower urinary tract obstruction (i.e., PUV, urethral atresia, etc.) were recruited (Morris et al. 2013). The mean gestational age was around 20–21 weeks with most having oligohydramnios. About 15 were managed conservatively and 16 were allocated to the vesicoamniotic shunt group. There were 12

live births in each group. There were 12 neonatal deaths. Although the vesicoamniotic shunt group had better survival at 28 days (8/16) versus the conservative group (4/15), it did not affect renal parenchymal damage. Although the study had several flaws, it paved the way for a better understanding of fetal management of PUV.

4. Current Recommendations: If facilities are available, and there are upper tract features of obstruction, fetal intervention may be performed only if fetal urine analysis suggests good renal function. In such a scenario, the following procedures can be considered:
   (a) Vesicoamniotic Shunt: It helps in restoring amniotic fluid volume and lung development. The shunt under USG guidance is passed percutaneously and drains the bladder urine into the amniotic fluid cavity. It is associated with complications like dislodgement, occlusion, chorioamnionitis, and preterm labor.
   (b) Valve Ablation: Through an ultrasound-guided small incision in the lower abdominal wall of the fetus, the bladder is entered. The scope is negotiated through the bladder neck, valve visualized, and 1–2 small perforations are made in the valve membrane with a bugbee electrode. Inadequate opening, injury to the urethra and bladder, preterm labor, etc., are associated.
   (c) There is no data to show benefit in preventing end-stage renal disease (ESRD) following any of these interventions and we would still consider postnatal intervention to be safer in our current circumstances.

74.7.2 Postnatal Management

74.7.2.1 Medical Management

Any neonate suspected to have PUV antenatally should preferably be delivered in a tertiary care center so that assessment and treatment can start early. Parents should be asked to observe the urinary stream for 24 h and not put the baby in diapers, and an early USG KUB performed within 24–48 h of birth.

Initial management includes correction of dehydration, metabolic acidosis, and electrolyte imbalance, if any, with appropriate intravenous fluids (Table 74.1). Blood and urine samples should be sent for culture, and intravenous antibiotics should be started. Aminoglycosides should be avoided until renal function test reports are available. The bladder usually requires drainage in early presenters. A feeding tube is preferable over a balloon catheter but should be fixed properly. If a Foley catheter is being used, the balloon should not be overinflated. This is retained until optimization of renal function, correction of fluid and electrolyte imbalance, and infection. Sometimes it is difficult to insert a per urethral catheter as it may coil within the posterior urethra. While insertion of a finger in the rectum may be helpful in insertion, repeated attempts will cause trauma to the urethra, predisposing to stricture. Insertion of a suprapubic catheter is preferable. Full oral feeds should be allowed whenever possible. Following catheterization, diuresis is common. Urine output should be measured hourly and two-thirds of urine >4 ml/kg/hour should be replaced with half normal saline.

74.7.2.2 Surgical Management

(a) Valve Fulguration (ablation).

Once stabilized, under general anesthesia, transurethral fulguration of the valve at 12, 5, and 7 o'clock positions using a resectoscope and low intermittent cutting cautery is the method of choice (Fig. 74.5). Glycine [1.5%] should be used as the irrigating fluid. The insulation of the hook and instrument should be checked before use. The scope should be inserted into the bladder and then gradually withdrawn visualizing the bladder neck and then the verumontanum. The valves often fall as a white curtain just before the external sphincter as the scope is withdrawn. Occasionally, the valves can be thick and fleshy. A recent UTI can increase chances of bleeding and that situation should be avoided. The scope should be held carefully during fulguration so as not to injure the external sphincter, especially during fulguration

Table 74.1 Algorithm for management of PUV

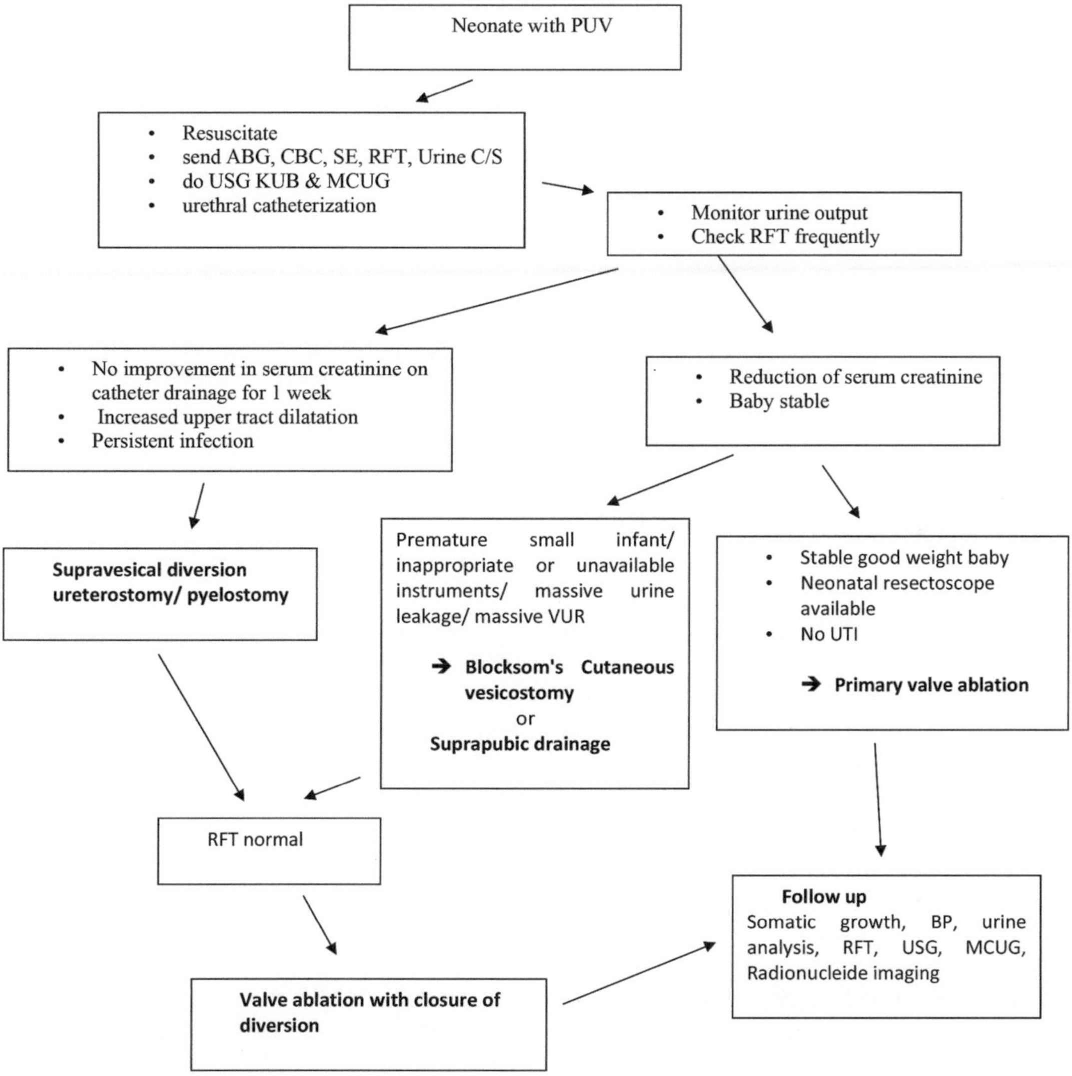

at 5 and 7 o'clock positions. Bladder neck incision should not be given. A bugbee electrode, cold knife, or NdYAg laser may also be used. Only an appropriate size scope (and not a larger size) should be used and the procedure should not be prolonged. In older children, the angulation between the anterior and posterior urethra may be more acute and needs skillful maneuvering of the scope. Overall, only an experienced surgeon should do the fulguration to avoid urethral injury. The stream of urine should be observed at the end of the procedure.

(b) Vesicostomy (Blocksom).

Indications include severe urosepsis, poor general condition, nonavailability of an appropriately sized resectoscope, low birth weight, or prematurity. It is useful where there is some improvement with a draining per urethral catheter, but the baby is not fit for fulguration. Severe VUR with abnormal RFT and urosepsis is also an indication. We have found vesicostomy to be lifesaving in babies with systemic/urosepsis unresponsive to broad-spectrum antibiotics and low

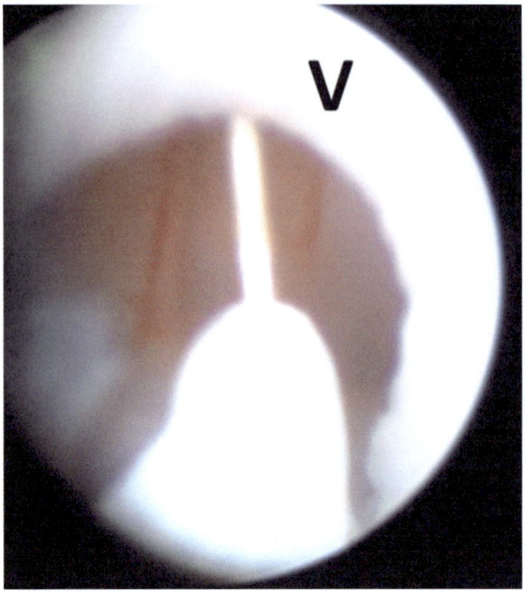

Fig. 74.5 Cystoscopic view of PUV (V) which usually appears as a white membrane with fulguration at 12 o'clock in progress. The veru is seen in the background

platelets not responding to even single donor platelet plasmapheresis who are not good candidates for fulguration.

(c) Supravesical Diversion (Ureterostomy, Pyelostomy).

If there is persistence of sepsis and metabolic acidosis, despite a period of catheterization or vesicostomy, and there is evidence of pyonephrosis on USG, a temporary percutaneous nephrostomy is very useful. This usually occurs in the presence of nonrefluxing obstructed systems due to the hypertrophied bladder musculature causing functional obstruction. Ureterostomy or pyelostomy can be considered in such patients with dilated and tortuous ureters. During ureterostomy, especially if purulent urine is found within, the ureters should be straightened by excising some part. While a Sobers ureterostomy allows bladder cycling, recurrent UTIs can still occur in the lower urinary tract if the baby has not yet been fulgurated. Often, there is an association with renal dysplasia in such cases, and the long-term outcome regarding renal failure does not change. The other concern is the lack of bladder cycling in divided ureterostomy because of which the bladder may not grow adequately. Refluxing ureterostomy (ureterostomy of the refluxing, poorly functioning side) maximizes drainage from the ipsilateral kidney and at the same time maintains bladder cycling.

74.8 Assessment of Renal Function

A baseline dimercaptosuccinic acid (DMSA) scan gives relative function of both kidneys and presence of pyelonephritis or scars. A di-ethylene triamine pentaacetic acid (DTPA) or ethylene dicysteine (EC) scan will provide information of relative function and drainage of both renal units.

74.9 Bladder Management

It is very important to check the adequacy of valve fulguration by a repeat MCUG around 3 months after the fulguration. A check scope may be performed if there is a doubt about the residual valve. A 3-month period allows adequate time in most cases for the posterior urethra size to normalize. The bladder will have smoother walls with an increase in its capacity. The VUR will also have reduced in severity (Figs. 74.2b and 74.6a and b) (Priti et al. 2004).

Bladder dysfunction occurs in 50–75% of patients with PUV. Urodynamic study (UDS) of the bladder helps to determine the bladder capacity and compliance of bladder. The urodynamic patterns are: (a) decreased compliance/small capacity bladder in infants, (b) detrusor hyperreflexia in older children, and (c) myogenic failure in postpubertal boys. Anticholinergics like oxybutynin relax the bladder muscle and reduce the frequency of micturition. Newer drugs like mirabegron, a beta 3 adrenergic agonist, also relax the detrusor muscle and improve bladder capacity. Alpha 1 blockers like tamsulosin and prazocin are useful in bladder neck hypertrophy and improve bladder emptying. Patients with dilated upper tracts and a history of urinary tract infection should be kept on prophylactic antibiotics. CIC (clean intermittent cauterization) is

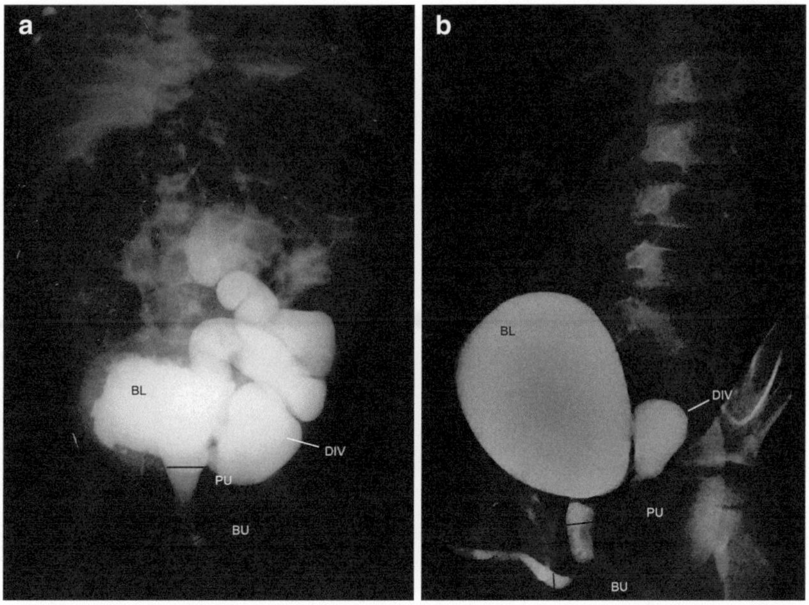

Fig. 74.6 MCUG films. (**a**) Preoperative shows dilated PU, trabeculated bladder with left large diverticulum (DIV) and left grade V VUR. (**b**) Postoperative of the same patient shows smooth bladder with increased capacity, normalization of PU/BU ratio, absence of VUR, and slightly smaller size of diverticulum

occasionally indicated. However, it is extremely important to first check the adequacy of fulguration and patency of the urethra before starting medication.

74.10 Valve Bladder

Some older patients with a noncompliant bladder and upper tract dilatation will manifest with incontinence. Renal tubular dysfunction due to prolonged back pressure causes acquired nephrogenic diabetes insipidus. The polyuria aggravates the upper tract dilatation and frequency of micturition and creates a vicious cycle. These patients may benefit from clean intermittent catheterization (CIC) during the day and overnight bladder drainage.

74.11 Vesicoureteric Reflux

Vesicoureteric reflux subsides in 30% of cases in 3 months and up to 70% in 9 months to 1 year after adequate fulguration (Priti et al. 2004). Around 30% of cases have persistent reflux. A poorly functioning kidney has more chance of persistent VUR. Kidneys with less than 10% function and VUR causing recurrent UTIs should undergo laparoscopic nephroureterectomy. This also helps to improve bladder cycling. If bladder dynamics have improved, and there is adequate renal function, dextranomer hyaluronic acid endoscopic subureteral injection may be given for persistent VUR. However, success rates are less as compared to primary VUR. Ureteric reimplantation is difficult if the bladder is still trabeculated and is not recommended.

74.12 Vesicoureteric Reflux Disease (VURD) Syndrome

This is an association of unilateral high-grade VUR with ipsilateral nearly nonfunctioning kidney/renal dysplasia. This unit takes the brunt of the high-pressure bladder before treatment protecting the contralateral kidney which may have normal function. Recurrent UTI is an indication for nephroureterectomy and is usually performed around 1–2 years of age. The tortuous ureter may be used for bladder augmentation where indicated.

74.13 Hydroureteronephrosis (HUN)

This is common in untreated patients with PUV. Glassberg has defined these dilated upper tracts as: type 1, where drainage is independent of bladder volume; type 2, which drains only when the bladder is empty; and type 3, which are obstructed irrespective of bladder volume. After adequate valve fulguration, nearly half will resolve, with one-fourth having persistent dilatation even in adulthood. One should differentiate HUN secondary to VUR from the ones due to partial obstruction from a thick-walled bladder. The diagnosis should be based on MCUG, and renal scans like DTPA/EC, and not USG alone. Slow drainage in a dilated system may persist for some time despite resolution of VUR on MCUG, and here USG and renal scans are useful.

74.14 Follow-Up Management

PUV patients should be under close long-term follow-up. Initially, they should be seen every 3 months in the first 1 year, then 6 months till 4–5 years, followed by yearly visits to the outpatient department. Patients with abnormal RFT, albuminuria, HN/HUN, single functioning kidney, and hypertension should be under regular pediatric nephrology clinic follow-up. Patients should always be seen in the peri-pubertal period associated with a growth spurt, which stretches renal reserves.

The following parameters should be closely monitored during each visit:

1. Height and weight.
2. Blood pressure.
3. USG KUB.
4. Urine routine, microscopy including protein, and culture at follow-up visit and during any unexplained febrile episode or urinary complaints.
5. Serum creatinine and electrolytes.
6. Calculation of glomerular filtration rate (GFR) based on modified Schwartz formula and CKD stage (Schwartz et al. 2009).
7. DMSA: at 6 months and 1 year as baseline, then once a year as indicated.
8. DTPA or EC scan in patients with nonrefluxing slow draining units at 6 months and 1 year as baseline, then once a year as indicated.

74.15 Prognosis and Outcome

After initial valve ablation, further management may include:

1. Continuous monitoring for UTI, hypertension, and proteinuria.
2. Surgical intervention:
   (a) If the urine stream has not normalized, repeat MCUG should be looked at carefully and the child planned for check cystoscopy, residual valve fulguration, or urethral dilatation for stricture.
   (b) Nephroureterectomy for nonfunctioning kidney: indications as mentioned earlier in the chapter.
   (c) Closure of diversions once the urethra/bladder are optimized.
   (d) Bladder Augmentation/Mitrofanoff: A small contractile bladder with severe upper tract dilatation despite adequate fulguration and medical treatment should be treated with bladder augmentation. It may be required before a renal transplant is performed. A Mitrofanoff channel should be created after making sure that patients will be compliant with CIC.
   (e) Endoscopic dextranomer injection for persistent VUR.
3. Valve Bladder Syndrome: Patients should be on CIC with overnight bladder drainage.
4. Dialysis Requirement and Renal Transplantation: End-stage renal failure is expected to occur in 25–30% of cases. Renal injury occurs not only due to dysplastic changes at birth but also from persistent obstruction and UTI. There is a reduction in GFR, proteinuria, stunting, and hypertension in children with renal insufficiency. Before okaying a patient for renal transplant, the pediatric surgeon should check the voiding stream, and do a MCUG, and urodynamic study. A persistent bladder dysfunction aggravates the renal insufficiency as well as reduces graft survival.

74.16 Indicators of Good Renal Function

1. Presentation in later childhood.
2. Protection of the upper tracts by a "pop-off"phenomenon like VURD syndrome and also urinary ascites, perinephric urinoma, and a large bladder diverticulum (Fig. 74.6a).

74.17 Predictors of Poor Outcome

74.17.1 Prenatal

(a) Maternal oligohydramnios, regardless of the gestational age.
(b) Early detection on prenatal ultrasound of "bright" echogenic kidneys and pelvicalyceal dilatation.

74.17.2 Postnatal

1. Neonatal or early infancy presentation.
2. Proteinuria: if present, is associated with poor outcome.
3. Nadir creatinine, i.e., the lowest creatinine during the first year after diagnosis if greater than 0.85 mg/dL (75 μmol/L) and the creatinine velocity, i.e., the rate of change of creatinine after initial bladder drainage of greater than 3 μmol/L/day (Coleman et al. 2015) are said to be associated with increased risk of chronic renal failure.
4. Angiotensin-converting enzyme (ACE) gene has been found to have a link with nephrogenesis as well as progression to end-stage renal disease (ESRD) in obstructive uropathies.

74.18 Conclusion

Management of PUV includes not only ablation of the valve but also long-term follow-up. This includes management of the bladder by appropriate drugs, improving voiding habits, removal of non-functioning kidneys, and appropriate lifelong management for hypertension, UTI, and renal function deterioration. It needs close coordination with the pediatric nephrology team during childhood, and later, as per renal status, the child should be handed over to the adult urologists and nephrologists.

74.19 Summary

1. Proper medical management of fluid and electrolyte imbalance, deranged RFT, and UTI, especially in neonatal presentation, is extremely important.
2. Adequate valve fulguration is the most important part of initial surgical management.
3. Further medical management should be closely coordinated right from the beginning with pediatric nephrology team.
4. Bladder should be managed with appropriate drugs and improved voiding habits.
5. Children with persistent problems should be handed over to adult urologists/nephrologists and renal transplant team as required at the appropriate time.

Suggested Reading

Coleman R, King T, Nicoara CD, Bader M, McCarthy L, Chandran H, et al. Combined creatinine velocity and nadir creatinine: a reliable predictor of renal outcome in neonatally diagnosed posterior urethral valves. J Pediatr Urol. 2015;11(214):e1–3.

Dewan PA. Congenital obstructing posterior urethral membrane (COPUM): further evidence of a common morphological diagnosis. Pediatr Surg Int. 1993;8:45–50.

Gearhart JP, Rink RC, PDE M. Posterior urethral valves in pediatric urology. Philadelphia, PA: 2nd, Elsevier Saunders; 2010. p. 437–45.

Menon P, Rao KLN, et al. Posterior urethral valves: morphological normalization of posterior urethra after fulguration is a significant factor in prognosis. J Indian Assoc Pediatr Surg. 2010;15:80–6.

Morris RK, Malin GL, Quinlan-Jones E, Middleton LJ, Hemming K, Burke D, et al. Percutaneous vesico amniotic shunting versus conservative management for fetal lower urinary tract obstruction (PLUTO): a randomised trial. Lancet. 2013;382:1496–506.

Priti K, Rao KL, Menon P, Singh N, Mittal BR, Bhattacharya A, Mitra SK. Posterior urethral valves: incidence and progress of vesicoureteric reflux after primary fulguration. Pediatr Surg Int. 2004;20:136–9.

Schwartz GJ, Munoz A, Schneider MF, Mak RH, Kaskel F, Warady BA, et al. New equations to estimate GFR in children with CKD. J Am Soc Nephrol. 2009;20:629–37.

Urinary Incontinence, Ectopic Ureter, Ureteral Duplications, and Ureterocele

75

Subhasis Roy Choudhury and Prema Menon

75.1 Urinary Incontinence in Children

Children are expected to have bladder control during the daytime by 2 years of age and at night by 3 years of age. A large majority achieve this by 5 years age.

As per the new International Children's Continence Society guidelines and terminology, enuresis is synonymous with nocturnal incontinence, or bed wetting, where there is involuntary voiding of urine while asleep in a child who is more than 5 years old. This is a functional type of incontinence. Diurnal (daytime) wetting is less common. If the child has never achieved control of urine, then it is termed primary enuresis. The term secondary enuresis, occurring in 25% of children, especially school-going children, includes those who had a preceding 3–6-month period of dryness and is usually due to voiding dysfunction. This is also known as dysfunctional elimination syndrome with features of infrequent voiding, dribbling, weak or intermittent stream, straining, urgency, frequency, and recurrent urinary tract infections (UTIs).

S. Roy Choudhury
Pediatric Surgery, Lady Hardinge Medical College and Associated Kalawati Saran Children's Hospital, New Delhi, Delhi, India

P. Menon (✉)
Department of Pediatric Surgery, Level 3A, Advanced Pediatric Centre, Post Graduate Institute of Medical Education and Research, Chandigarh, India

75.1.1 Causes of Urinary Incontinence

1. Constipation
2. Urinary tract infection
3. Medical causes leading to polyuria: renal failure, diabetes insipidus, drug intake, etc.
4. Abnormal bladder activity: meningomyelocele, detrusor instability
5. Central nervous system causes: developmental delay, cerebral palsy
6. Psychosocial issues: e.g., change in school, arrival of a new baby in the family, loss of a parent
7. Structural Causes:
   (a) Bladder outflow obstruction: posterior urethral valves, urethral stricture, etc.
   (b) Exstrophy/epispadias, Ectopic Ureter (girls), Congenital short urethra (girls), wide bladder neck seen with congenital pouch colon, Urogenital sinus anomaly (girls)

Structural causes usually lead to continuous incontinence, whereas in the others, the leak is intermittent. In girls, continuous incontinence with normal voiding strongly suggests the possibility of an ectopic ureter.

© The Author(s), under exclusive license to Springer Nature Singapore Pte Ltd. 2025

S. Roy Choudhury (ed.), *Pediatric Surgery*, https://doi.org/10.1007/978-981-96-1257-4_75

75.1.2 Diagnosis

A child with a history of incontinence should be taken to a separate room with his/her parents for a detailed history and examination, and not in busy outpatients where other patients are also present.

Lack of privacy often leads to the child not expressing his/her concerns, and it is also important that the family should not feel embarrassed in front of others. The leading questions to be asked are (a) whether the wetting is present since birth or occurred after a period of toilet training, (b) is it occurring only at night, only in the day or both, (c) is it continuous or intermittent, (d) association with dysuria, abdominal pain, (e) is the child aware of wetness, (f) does it occur only with stress, like coughing, sneezing, laughing, playing, etc., (g) bowel habits, (g) any posture used by the child to prevent leakage like squatting or crossing and bending legs (Vincent's curtsy), (h) toilet facilities at home and in school, (i) is the child facing bullying at school or in the playground, (j) is the child being reprimanded for scholastic ability or being compared with other siblings, etc.

In those with daytime variation, parents should be asked to maintain a voiding diary for the entire 24 hours for 3–7 days. It should mention the time of fluid intake and voiding, voided volume, and incontinence episodes. The sleep pattern and presence of snoring should be noted. Children with urinary tract infections will usually give a short period of complaints. A child smelling of urine, wetness of underwear, local excoriation, and use of diapers should be noted along with fecal soiling. If necessary, a rectal examination should be performed. A thorough physical examination, including weight, enlargement of adenoids and tonsils, abdominal examination for palpable bladder and fecaliths, genitourinary examination to rule out structural anomalies, change in posture/difficulty in walking, examination of the spine, and neurological examination, should be performed.

75.1.3 Investigations

1. Urine routine, microscopic examination, osmolality, culture, and sensitivity.
2. Blood urea, serum creatinine, electrolytes, sugar.
3. Ultrasound kidney, ureter, bladder: bladder distension, postvoid residual, bladder wall thickening, upper tract dilatation, stones, duplication anomalies (hydronephrosis, hydroureter, and dysplastic kidney).
4. Plain abdominal X-ray for fecal loading.
5. Psychological assessment in those between 6 and 18 years. Parents could be asked to fill a Child Behavior Checklist (CBCL) questionnaire.
6. MRI Spine in suspected neurogenic bladder dysfunction.
7. Micturating cystourethrogram.
8. Urodynamic study for suspected neurogenic bladder and dysfunctional voiding: noninvasive uroflowmetry and conventional urodynamics (cystometry, pressure flow study, video urodynamics, urethral pressure profiling) to see the coordination between the sphincter muscles and bladder.
9. Where structural anomalies are suspected, Intravenous urography (IVU) or Magnetic Resonance urography (MRU), renal scan, and Examination under anesthesia and cystourethroscopy can be performed.

75.1.4 Management

1. General Measures: Management of constipation by dietary changes. Based on the voiding diary, changes in pattern of fluid intake can be advised. Avoiding excess fluids late in the evening and before going to bed, inculcating regular voiding habits including double voiding especially before going to bed are useful.
2. Behavioral Treatment: Waking up at night to void, use of an alarm.

3. Medication: In older children with dysfunctional voiding, anticholinergics such as oxybutynin or tolterodine can be used. To decrease bed wetting, desmopressin orally or as a nasal spray can be used. Imipramine may also be used for a short period. Tamsulosin may be considered in children who have poor stream or difficulty in initiating voiding or prolonged duration of voiding. Urodynamic studies before and after initiating therapy for 3 months are useful.

75.2 Ureteral Duplication

This is a common abnormality, occurring in nearly 8% of children investigated for urinary tract infection. Ureteral duplication results when the ureteral bud divides after origin from the mesonephric duct (incomplete duplication) or two separate ureteric buds arise from the mesonephric duct (complete duplication). Most are asymptomatic and require no treatment. A duplex collecting system may open into a single ureter, or there may be partial ureteral duplication which joins distally (Fig. 75.1). Other rare anomalies have also been described. Duplications are termed complete when both the ureters open separately in the lower genitourinary tract. Usually, the upper moiety of the duplex system is associated with ectopic ureters and ureteroceles which often require surgical intervention. As per the Wiegert Meyer rule, the upper pole ureter will insert caudally and will have a more medial insertion in the bladder. The lower pole ureter usually has vesicoureteral reflux (VUR) as it opens more laterally and has a shorter intramural course. The lower part lies in a common sheath and knowledge of this will avoid injury to the normal system.

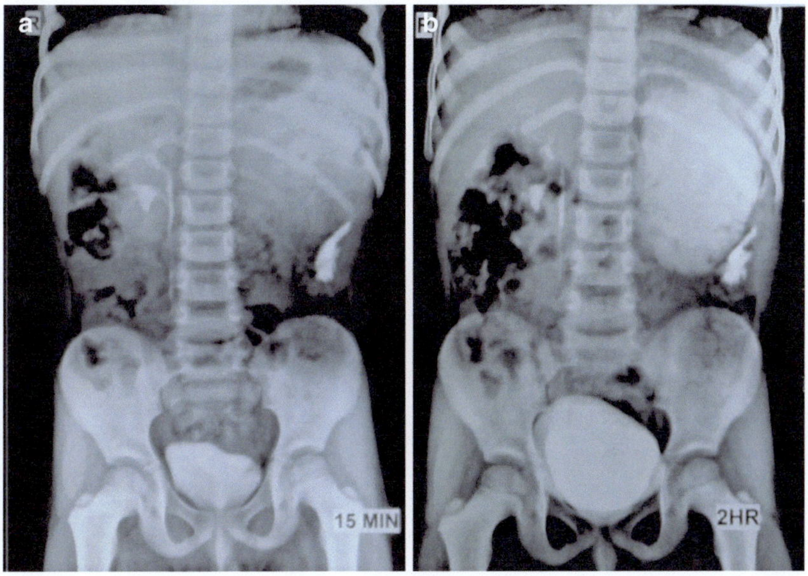

Fig. 75.1 IVU films (**a** early and **b** late) showing left-sided upper moiety pelviureteric junction obstruction in a partial duplex system. Function of the upper moiety is less as compared to the lower pole. This patient underwent pyeloureterostomy of the upper pole pelvis to the lower pole ureter

75.3 Ectopic Ureters

They are nearly six times more common in females, with the presentation being slightly different compared to males due to the difference in insertion of the ureteric orifice. It results when the ureteric bud arises more proximally than its usual location. In males, the mesonephric duct is incorporated in the proximal urethra and bladder trigone, resulting in the ectopic ureter opening proximal to the urethral sphincter. The child remains continent with the majority being associated with a single system. In females, the mesonephric remnants are in close relation with the anterolateral wall of the vagina. The majority are associated with a duplex system and can open below the sphincter as well as into the vagina or vestibule making the child incontinent. Bilateral single-system ectopic ureters are rare and associated with bladders with small capacity and poor musculature (Fig. 75.2).

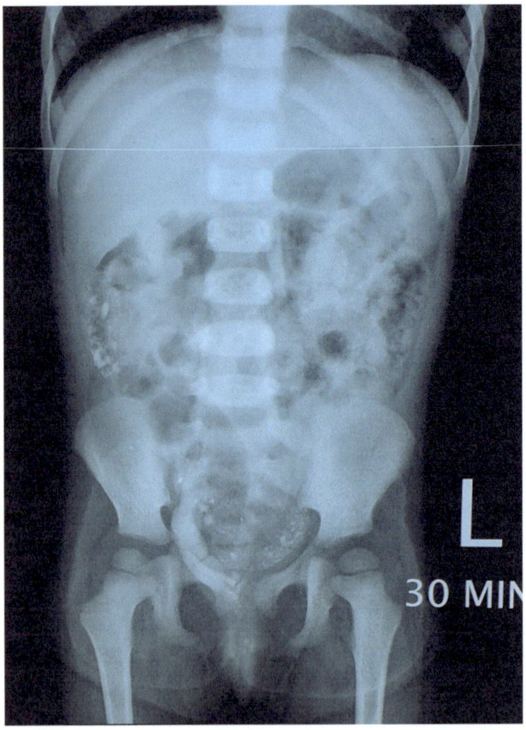

Fig. 75.2 Intravenous urography film at 30 minutes post-contrast in a child with continuous dribbling shows bilateral hydroureteronephrosis with no opacification of bladder and ureters appearing to open at or below the bladder neck suggestive of bilateral ectopic ureters

75.4 Ureterocele

Ureterocele is an abnormal dilatation of the terminal ureter which is usually stenotic. Like ectopic ureters, they are more common in females (4:1) in whom the majority are associated with duplex systems. In males, they are associated with a single system. They are classified as intravesical—confined within the bladder or ectopic, where some portion extends into the bladder neck or the urethra. Cecoureterocele is a variety of ectopic ureterocele which extends under the trigone into the urethra with its orifice into the bladder. Etiology remains unclear but abnormal muscular development of the terminal ureter has been implicated.

75.5 Presentation

Both these conditions may present with recurrent urinary tract infections (UTIs), failure to thrive, abdominal mass, and pain. Ectopic ureter in males can present as urgency, frequency, epididymo-orchitis, and pelvic pain. Females may present with continuous dribbling of urine with normal voiding pattern and vaginal discharge.

Ureterocele may present with bladder outlet obstruction in either sex or as an intralabial mass in females (ectopic or cecoureterocele) (Fig. 75.3).

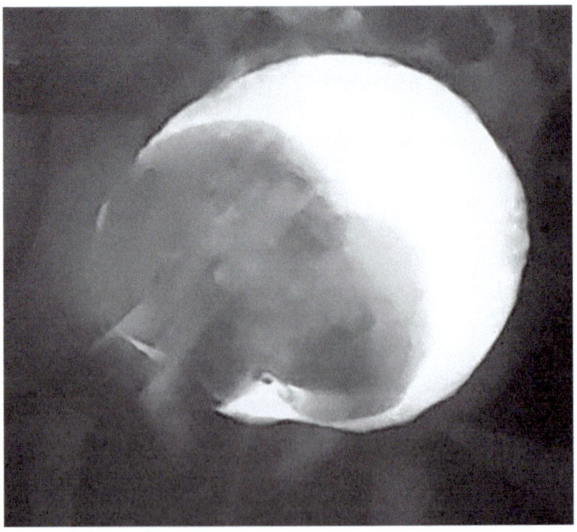

Fig. 75.3 MCUG in early filling phase in an infant with difficulty in voiding and palpable lower abdominal swelling shows a large space-occupying lesion in the bladder suggestive of right ureterocele. This was successfully treated with cystoscopic incision

75.6 Investigations

Duplex systems are unique in that multiple investigations are often required before the correct diagnosis is established. The surgeon should be able to interpret the results independently, regardless of the report given by the radiologist or nuclear medicine specialist. In the absence of Magnetic Resonance urography (MRU), often a combination of two superimposed films from investigations like IVU and MCUG clinches the anatomy and diagnosis.

75.6.1 Ultrasonography

Both ureterocele and ectopic ureter may present with hydroureteronephrosis. The duplex system may be identified especially in females. An ectopic ureter can often be traced very low in the pelvis. Ureterocele can be identified in a partially filled bladder as a thin-walled cystic protrusion in the posterolateral wall of the bladder which can be followed above into a dilated ureter.

75.6.2 Micturating Cystourethrogram

Ureterocele may be seen as a filling defect positioned in the area of the trigone (Fig. 75.3). If images are taken once the bladder has been filled significantly, then it may be effaced. In some cases, it may evert, giving the appearance of a diverticulum. The presence of ipsilateral reflux in the lower pole system is often seen because of associated lateral ectopia and distortion of the trigone. Ectopic ureters also often demonstrate VUR.

75.6.3 Retrograde Urography (RGU)

Under general anesthesia, with cystoscopic guidance, the ureteric orifices can be cannulated and a dye study performed to delineate the anatomy of the ureters (Fig. 75.4).

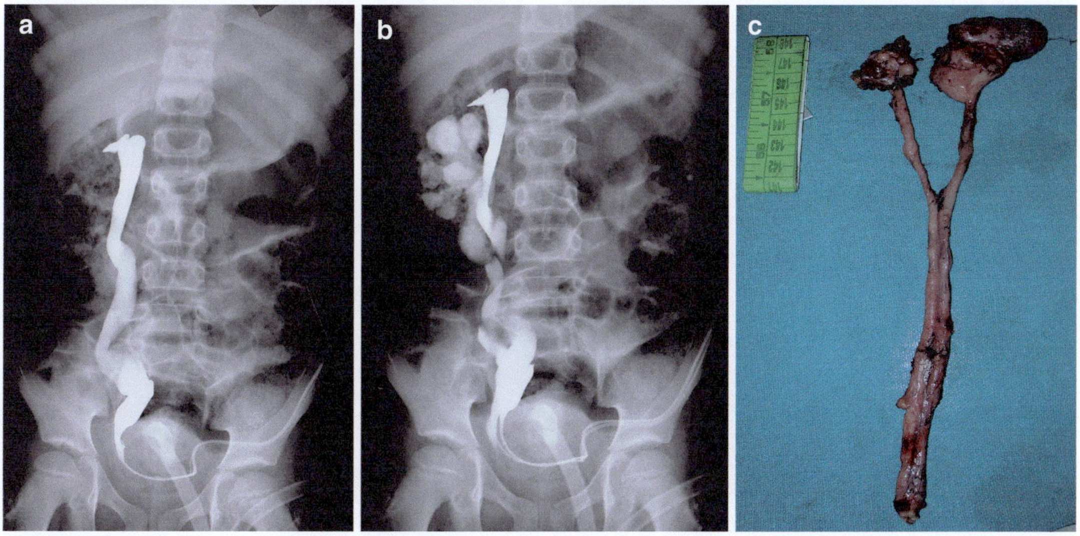

Fig. 75.4 Retrograde urography (RGU) (**a**) and (**b**) shows anatomical delineation of both moieties in a right-side complete duplex system; laparoscopic nephroureterectomy specimen (**c**) of another patient with both moieties nonfunctioning shows complete duplication and early start of common sheath

75.6.4 Examination Under Anesthesia, Cystoscopy/Cystovaginoscopy

This can be performed during the initial workup and helps to rule out bilateral ectopic ureters in bilateral duplex systems missed on previous imaging. It is useful just before the final surgical procedure of excision of a nonfunctioning moiety for RGU and inserting a DJ stent into the functioning moiety.

75.6.5 Renal Scintigraphy

It helps in determining if any functioning renal parenchyma is present and guides treatment planning. Split function of the upper and lower moieties helps in decision-making. For example, if the split function of the poorly functioning upper moiety is 20% and that of the lower 80% in a kidney whose differential function is 50%, then the actual function of this unit is only 10%. However, scans may not always detect a duplex kidney, especially if both moieties are functioning well or the capsule is not separate, or if one moiety is completely nonfunctioning. Presence of scars in only one pole may lead us to suspect a duplex system. Presence of reflux or a dysplastic dilated system may give falsely high function of the poorly functioning moiety. Other investigations and clinical judgment take precedence in such cases.

75.6.6 Intravenous Urography

It is a useful investigation, especially when the pathology is not defined by USG, MCUG, and renal scintigraphy. Ureterocele with functioning renal moiety may demonstrate contrast-filled "cobra head" at ureterovesical junction. If the associated moiety is nonfunctioning, then the ureterocele may appear as a filling defect when the bladder fills with contrast. Ectopic ureter with a functioning associated moiety may be seen to extend very low down in the pelvis and open in the proximal urethra in males or the genital tract in females (Fig. 75.2). Few findings may suggest presence of a nonfunctioning (occult) duplex with an ectopic ureter like "drooping lily sign" (inferior and lateral displacement of lower pole by the dilated upper pole system), lateral displacement of lower system ureter (i.e., away from the tip of the transverse processes of the lumbar vertebrae), and missing calyx (although in some cases, all major calyces in the functioning moiety may be seen) (Fig. 75.5).

75.6.7 CT Urography and MR Urography

They help in defining anatomy especially when the involved renal moiety is nonfunctioning (Figs. 75.5 and 75.6). MRU with contrast and 3D reconstruction is the best investigation to delineate all the components of the duplex system including functional status. Both T1 and T2 weighted and postcontrast images should be looked at carefully.

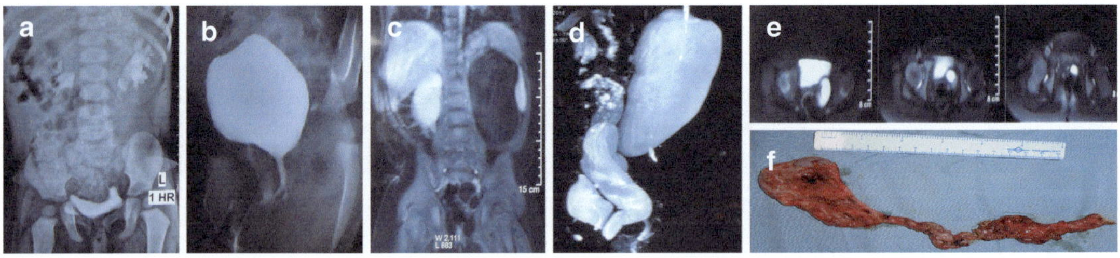

Fig. 75.5 IVU (**a**) shows the normally functioning left kidney which appears to be pushed downwards and laterally; MCUG (**b**) appears normal except for a faint shadow posterior to the urethra and bladder on the left side; MRU (**c**, **d**, **e**) shows functioning left lower moiety pushed laterally and a large nonfunctioning left upper moiety with ureter of the upper pole ending ectopically in the vagina; excised specimen (**f**) of left laparoscopic upper pole hemi-nephroureterectomy in this 18-month-old female infant

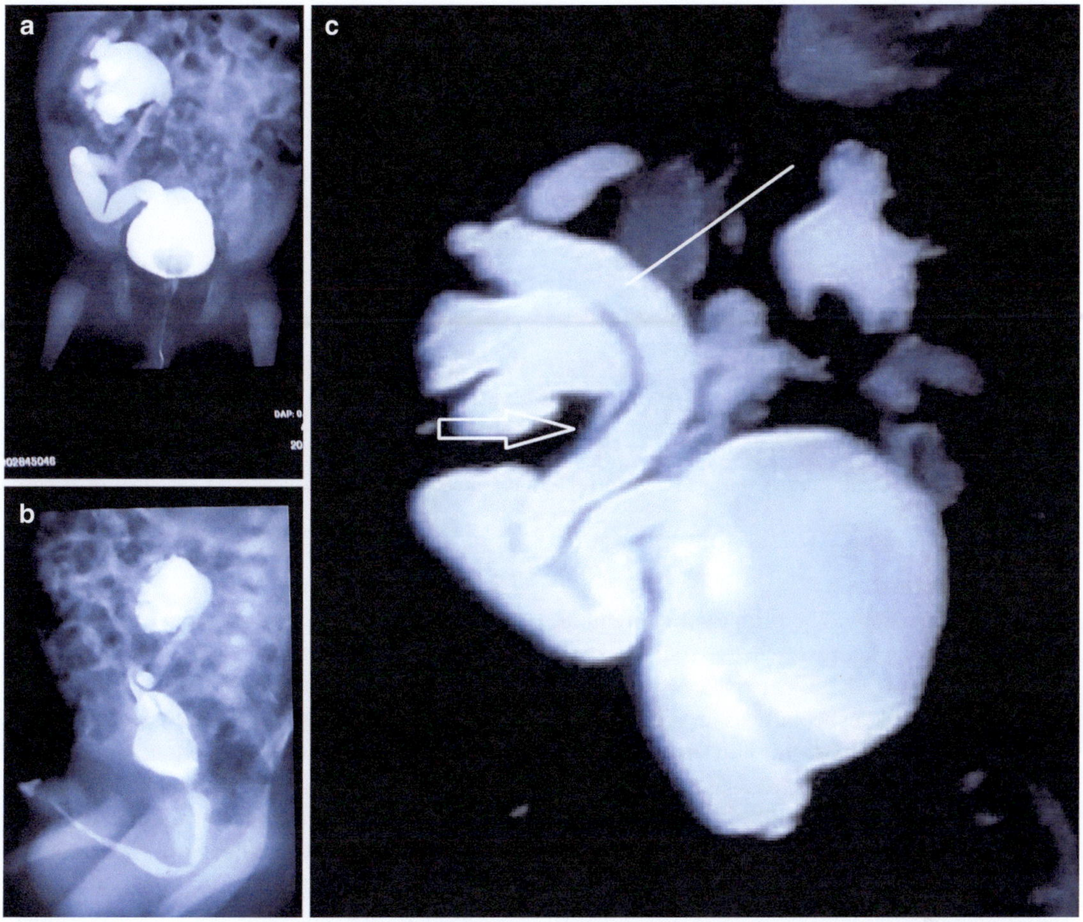

Fig. 75.6 MCUG (**a** and **b**) shows grade V vesicoureteric reflux right side with lateral and downward displacement of the kidney, with normal bladder and urethra. MRU (**c**) clarifies the anatomy and shows a dilated upper moiety ureter (straight line) with negligible renal parenchyma and a separate ureter of the lower moiety (arrow) which corresponds to the picture on the MCUG. This 10-month-old male infant underwent robotic right upper pole hemi-nephroureterectomy and lower pole extravesical ureteric reimplantation in the same sitting with good results

75.7 Treatment

75.7.1 Surgical

75.7.1.1 Ectopic Ureter

When associated with a dysplastic nonfunctioning kidney, nephroureterectomy (hemi or complete, depending on the anatomy) will be required (Figs. 75.4c and 75.5f). This can be easily performed laparoscopically. Care should be taken while excising the distal ureter. In duplex systems, it will share a common sheath with the functioning moiety. The ureter should not be traced in its entirety distally, as it will damage the sphincter area. Ectopic ureter in a functioning kidney merits renal preservation with either ureteric reimplantation or transureteroureterostomy (Fig. 75.7). The result of surgery is very gratifying in unilateral ectopic ureter as the chance to achieve complete dryness is very high. The same is not true for bilateral nonduplex cases due to absent or poorly formed trigone, small bladder, and insufficiency of the bladder neck. Ureteric reimplantation, bladder augmentation, and bladder neck repair or closure will be required.

Management of other causes of urinary incontinence is discussed in relevant chapters.

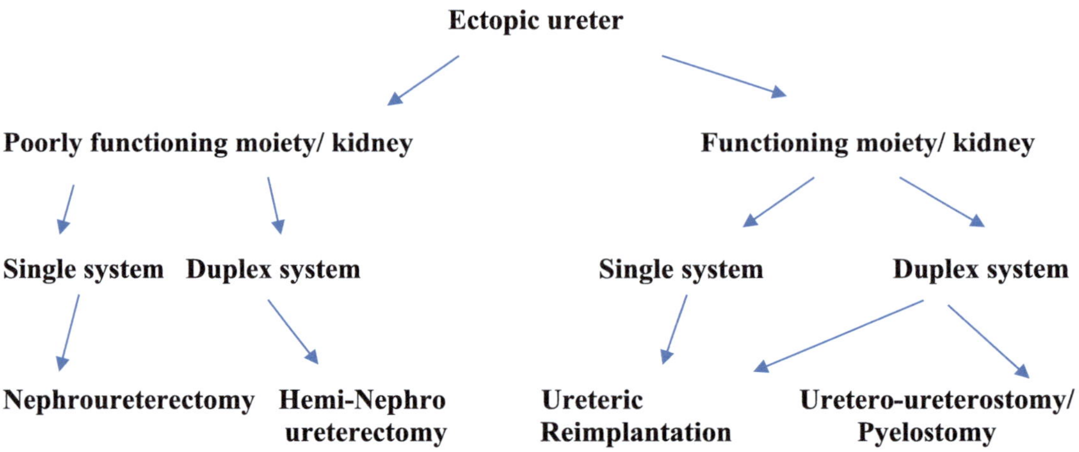

Fig. 75.7 Flow chart illustrating the management of ectopic ureter with arrows indicating the flow of decision making

75.7.1.2 Ureterocele

Endoscopic incision as a primary treatment is very useful. It can be done when associated with UTI, obstruction to the upper tract, or occlusion of the bladder neck, especially as an initial semi-elective procedure. These children should be kept on uroprophylaxis and an MCUG performed to rule out VUR after 3–6 months. Based on further investigations which reveal the function of this moiety, a decision should be taken regarding ureteric reimplantation with detrusor repair or excision of the moiety, or a wait-and-watch policy can be taken for lower grades of VUR. Results in ectopic ureteroceles are not as good as compared to single-system intravesical ureteroceles because of the more complex anatomy.

Heminephroureterectomy in duplex cases or nephrectomy in single systems for nonfunctioning units by open or laparoscopic techniques has good long-term results. The urine in a moiety with ureterocele, if this has not been drained earlier, can be sucked out during the procedure. In a duplex system with VUR in one, with both moieties functioning, a common sheath reimplantation is usually performed. A top-down approach is advocated by some, wherein ureteroureterostomy/pyeloureterostomy for diverting urine into the normal moiety in the duplex system is performed even with poorly functioning moieties. However, here there is a worry of injuring the normal system, recurrent UTI, and the requirement for removing this non-functioning moiety later.

75.8 Summary

1. Management of urinary incontinence in children requires a thorough histoty taking and physical examination.
2. Imaging studies with ultrasonography, nuclear scan, MRU, MCUG as nesessary.
3. Examination under anesthesia and cystourethroscopy and retrograde study if necessary.
4. Identification of the affected renal unit, restoration of the anatomy with preservation of functioning renal unit whereever possible.

Suggested Reading

Bauer SB, Nijman RJ, Drzewiecki BA, Sillen U, Hoebeke P. International children's continence society standardization report on urodynamic studies of the lower urinary tract in children. Neurourol Urodyn. 2015;34:640–7.

Choudhury SR, Chadha R, Bagga D, Puri A, Debnath PR. Spectrum of ectopic ureters in children. Pediatr Surg Int. 2008;24:819–23.

Nocturnal enuresis. In: Gearhart JP, Rink RC, Mouriquand PDE, editors. Pediatric urology, 2nd edn. Philadelphia: Elsevier Saunders; 2010a. p. 380–5

Pragmatic approach to the evaluation and management of non-neuropathic daytime voiding disorders. In: Gearhart JP, Rink RC, Mouriquand PDE, editors. Pediatric urology, 2nd edn. Philadelphia: Elsevier Saunders; 2010b. p. 366–79

76 Bladder Augmentation

Arvind Sinha

76.1 Introduction

Bladder augmentation is a reconstructive surgery of the lower urinary tract which is performed to add to the reservoir capacity of the bladder. Augmenting the bladder capacity increased the bladder's capacity, increasing compliance and reducing the bladder's pressure. The most common indications for the performance of the procedure are for a neurogenic bladder or an exstrophy bladder. Various bowel segments like the ileum, caecum, colon or stomach are commonly used. Ureter might be utilised in selected cases. Augmenting the bladder leads to long-term metabolic problems and a higher risk of malignancy, which requires a lifelong surveillance regimen.

76.2 Bladder Augmentation

Bladder augmentation, also known as augmentation cystoplasty, is a reconstructive surgery to increase the reservoir capacity of the bladder. The stated aims of augmenting the bladder capacity are mainly twofolds—i.e. to increase the reservoir capacity and to decrease the reservoir pressures.

76.3 Mechanism

Clinically augmenting the bladder capacity via augmentation is used to help in simplifying the following

1. Increase in the Bladder Capacity—A small capacity bladder may cause clinical problems, including increased frequency of micturition, enuresis, incontinence or upper tract damage. Optimal bladder capacity should allow a 4-h catheterisation or voiding interval during the day and an 8-h break at night without reaching excessive pressure or leading to urinary incontinence.
2. Prevention of Upper Tract Damage—High detrusor pressure either during storage or while voiding may be transmitted to the kidneys leading the upper tract dilatation/damage. The maintenance of storage pressures below 35–40 cm H_2O will optimise upper tract preservation.
3. Treatment of Incontinence—Many clinical scenarios exist where augmentation might be utilised to tackle urinary incontinence. The incontinence in these cases might be due to a combination of low bladder capacity, high pressures or a low pressure/damaged external urinary sphincter, and augmenting the bladder capacity contributes to better control of urinary continence. Aims in augmenting the bladder capacity in these cases may be to achieve social continence by measures that the patients

A. Sinha (✉)
Department of Pediatric Surgery, All India Institute of Medical Sciences (AIIMS), Jodhpur, Rajasthan, India

© The Author(s), under exclusive license to Springer Nature Singapore Pte Ltd. 2025
S. Roy Choudhury (ed.), *Pediatric Surgery*, https://doi.org/10.1007/978-981-96-1257-4_76

may practice independently eg. Clean intermittent catheterisation (CIC).

Augmenting the bladder is often combined with the creation of a continent catheterisable stoma using Mitrofanoff's Principle.

76.4 Indications

Augmentations of the bladder capacity may be done for the following indications:

- Neurogenic Bladder due to Spina bifida, Tethered cord syndrome, Transverse myelitis etc.—Neurogenic Bladder remains the most common indication for performing a bladder augmentation worldwide.
- Severe/Failed Congenital anomalies of the bladder, e.g. Cloacal Exstrophy, Bladder Exstrophy or Prune Belly Syndrome—One of the important indications for augmenting the bladder.
- Physical Loss of Bladder following surgery for tumour excision or following trauma. However, mutilating or extensive tumour surgery is being performed less frequently nowadays.
- Poorly Functional Bladder, e.g. Following Posterior Urethral Valves, Radiation injury to the bladder, bilateral single system ectopic ureters, interstitial cystitis, detrusor instability or chronic cystitis, e.g. Thimble bladder.

Augmenting the bladder for Neurogenic Bladder requires a thorough evaluation of the bladder dynamics via Urodynamic evaluation to identify the 'unsafe' bladder. Following parameters may be assessed:

1. Bladder Capacity—Normal bladder capacity in children
   (a) Less than 2 years, capacity = weight (kg) × 7 ml
   (b) For 2–12 years of age = (age + 2) × 30
2. Compliance—Normally, the whole bladder capacity of the child can be stored at 30 cm H_2O. Baseline pressures exceeding 20 cm H_2O within the physiological range of capacity should be regarded as 'unsafe'.
3. Bladder Pressures—Vesical Pressures greater than 40 cm H_2O either during storage or voiding are regarded as 'unsafe'.

The child should be considered for augmentation of bladder capacity only after all efforts towards managing the condition medically have been exhausted.

76.5 Pre-operative Assessment Before Bladder Augmentation

When contemplating urinary tract reconstruction, meticulous pre-operative evaluation is critical and to tailor the reconstruction according to the individual needs of the patient. The following factors need to be assessed:

1. Renal Function—Renal function may be assessed by measuring the serum creatinine and glomerular filtration rate. The kidneys can also be assessed by an ultrasonography to assess the anatomical integrity and status of the kidneys.
2. Vesicoureteric Reflux—Contrast Voiding cystourethrography along with an endoscopic evaluation should be performed to evaluate for reflux. Antireflux surgery may be combined with augmentation of the bladder.
3. Bladder and Sphincter Function—A thorough urodynamic evaluation of the bladder and the sphincter function should be performed to evaluate the competence of the bladder neck. Bladder neck procedures like bladder neck closure or bladder neck reconstruction may be combined with augmentation of the bladder depending on the clinical scenario.
4. Previous Urinary Diversion—The patients should always be evaluated for previous history of a previous urinary diversion because these patients might have a massively reduced bladder capacity and may benefit from an adequate regiment of bladder cycling without resorting to an augmentation cystoplasty.
5. Bowel Function—Using the bowel to augment the bladder capacity might affect the

post-operative bowel function. Patients with limited intestinal length might not be suitable candidates for an enterocystoplasty as they might not have adequate "reserve" of bowel to spare for use in augmenting the bladder.

6. Ability and Willingness to Catheterise—A thorough evaluation of the child and the caregivers need to be undertaken to assess the patients' intellect, dexterity and potential for self-care, including lifelong clean intermittent catheterisation. Patients and caregivers unwilling or unable to perform lifelong intermittent catheterisation are poor candidates for an augmentation of the bladder capacity.

76.5.1 Contraindications

- Unwilling or unable to perform lifelong intermittent catheterisation
- Patients with inflammatory bowel disease, short or irradiated bowel or bladder tumour
- Severe Renal Insufficiency
- Poor surgical candidates and patients with a short life expectancy

76.6 Physiological Considerations for the Reservoir

1. Management of the Native Bladder
   (a) An intact native bladder with the intact detrusor can continue to generate high pressures with its attendant risk to the kidneys.
   (b) This is avoided by an extended sagittal opening of the native bladder (clamshell bi-valving) (Fig. 76.1).
2. Management of the Donor Intestinal Segment
   (a) The donor intestinal segment with intact circular muscle can also continue to generate high pressures
   (b) This is avoided by the process of detubularisation of the intestinal segment which disrupts the intestinal segment abolishing the peristaltic wave. This entails opening the bowel along its antimesenteric border and closing it in a way which disrups the circular muscle of the intestine. This weakens the intensity of the muscular contractions of the augmented bladder.
   (c) Similarly, an adequate capacity of the reservoir is achieved by a process of reconfiguration of the bowel segment. The bowel segments are reconfigured in many configurations, e.g. U, S, W with each limb of the bowel segment adding extra capacity to the reservoir. Each extra limb in the reconfigured bladder approximately doubles the capacity.
   (d) Accommodation of the reservoir is also a phenomenon seen with the gradual enlargement of the reservoir with time.

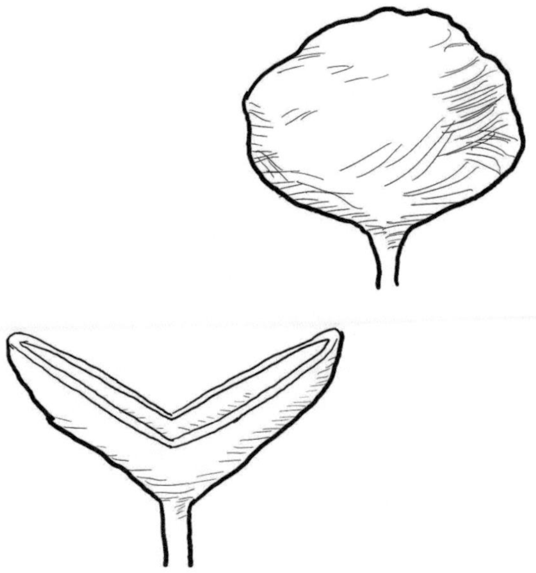

Fig. 76.1 Extended sagittal opening of the native bladder

Donor Tissues commonly utilised for augmentation

1. Ileum
2. Ileocaecal Region
3. Colon
4. Stomach
5. Ureter

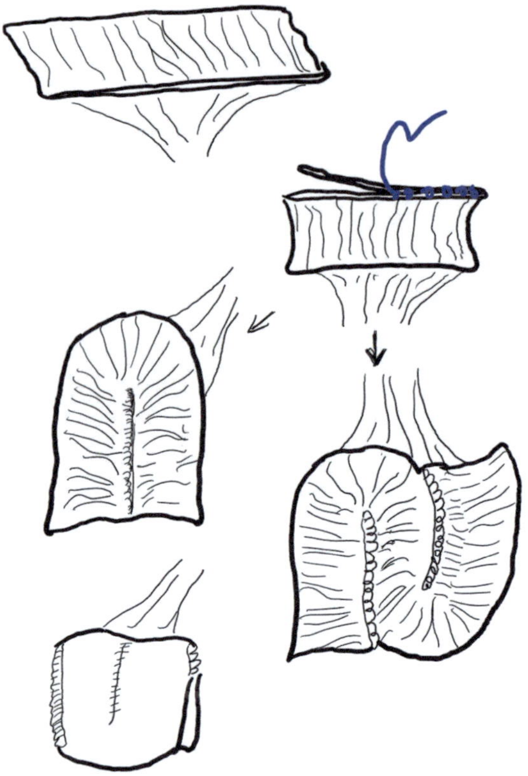

Fig. 76.2 Ileal segment detubularisation and reconfiguration

76.6.1 Small Bowel Procedures

Ileum or ileocystoplasty is the most commonly used augmentation technique.

About 20–40 cms segment of ileum which will easily reach the bladder is selected (Fig. 76.2)

76.6.1.1 Advantages

1. Most compliant and least contractile segment
2. Lower mucus production as compared to the colonic segment
3. Lower incidence of hyperchloremic acidosis

76.6.1.2 Disadvantages

1. Higher incidence of diarrhoea due to loss of absorptive surface (ileum)
2. Segment has poor muscular backing making implantation difficult, if not impossible.
3. Vitamin B12 deficiency - Terminal segment of ileum is the site for vitamin B12 absorption.
4. Cholelithiasis
5. Hyperchloremic Acidosis

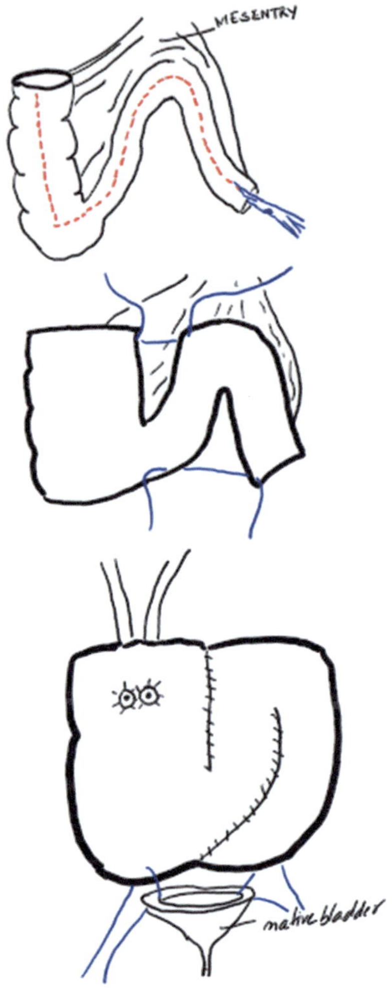

Fig. 76.3 Mainz pouch

76.6.2 Ileocaecal Segment Procedures

Caecum is capacious and provides a large volume reservoir. Ileocaecal valves have been utilised as antireflux mechanism with variable results. Indiana Pouch, Mainz Pouch, Penn Pouch and Florida pouch are some of the procedures performed.

Mainz Pouch (Mixed Augmentation with ileum and caecum)—One of the commonly used segments. Utilises the caecum along with a segment of terminal ileum (usually twice the length of the caecal segment). The intestine is opened along the antimesenteric border and is reconfigured in an S-shaped reconfiguration with the caecal segment being utilised for ureteric reimplantation. This segment is anastomosed to the native bladder (Fig. 76.3).

76.6.2.1 Advantages

1. Capacious Reservoir—Small segment provides a large reservoir
2. Allows reimplantation of the ureters
3. Attached Appendix or ileum may be used as a continent catheterisable stoma
4. Terminal ileum may also be utilised as a ureteral replacement

76.6.2.2 Disadvantages

1. Diarrhoea—Especially troublesome in neurologically impaired patients due to the loss of ileocaecal junction.
2. Significant B12 deficiency - Terminal segment of ileum is the site for vitamin B12 absorption.
3. Significant mucus production - All colonic segments produce large amounts of mucus.
4. Persistent high-pressure contractions - These high-pressure contractions are present even after adequate detubularisation of the colonic segments.

76.6.3 Colonic Segment Procedures

Sigmoid is a segment which is sometimes used for augmenting the bladder.

76.6.3.1 Advantages

1. Redundant sigmoid is available, especially in neurologically impaired patients (one of the common indications for doing an augment).
2. Excellent segment for tunneling ureters and catheterisable stoma.

76.6.3.2 Disadvantages

1. Very high mucus production
2. High-pressure coordinated contractions exceeding 40 cm H_2O - These high-pressure contractions are present even after adequate detubularisation of the colonic segments.
3. High incidence of Hyperchloremic Metabolic acidosis

76.6.4 Gastric Segment Procedure

Use of the stomach was popularised by Mitchell for its use in urinary tract reconstruction.

76.6.4.1 Advantages

1. Buffers the systemic acidosis and is the donor tissue of choice in the presence of renal failure.
2. Decreased mucus production and Stone formation.
3. Decreased incidence of urinary tract infection due to acid production. Acidic media being a poor medium for the growth of bacteria.
4. Segment has a good muscular backing and patients have the potential for spontaneous voiding.

76.6.4.2 Disadvantages

1. Haematuria—Dysuria syndrome especially with a sensate urethra. The passage of highly acidic urine leads to hematuria due to bladder mucosal ulceration and bleeding. The acidic urine also leads to features of dysuria while its passage through a sensate urethra.
2. Peptic Ulcer disease with risk of patch perforation
3. Hypochloremic Hypokalemic Metabolic Alkalosis
4. Less compliant and capacious reservoir than the intestinal or colonic segment reservoir
5. Higher incidence of malignancy

76.6.5 Uretrocystoplasty

It holds great promise in view of the use of native tissue for augmenting the bladder and avoids many of the problems with the use of intestinal segments.

Not every patient is suitable as it requires a non-functional renal unit with a dilated and tortuous ureter.

76.6.5.1 Advantages

1. Preserves native urothelium and avoids the attendant problems like acid-base disturbance and tumour formation with the use of intestinal segment. This is because the native urothelium is not designed for absorption of fluid or electrolytes.
2. No shrinkage with time.
3. Extraperitoneal procedure can be performed, allowing the use of the peritoneal cavity for peritoneal dialysis.
4. Higher incidence of spontaneous voiding.

76.6.5.2 Disadvantages

1. Not applicable to all, as a non-functional renal unit needs to be available.
2. Limited increase in reservoir capacity.

76.7 Choice of Segment and Approach

Enterocystoplasty improves bladder capacity and compliance in most cases after exhausting all options to manage these children medically. No single bowel segment is perfect and would fit the needs of all patients. All gastrointestinal segments continue to be used depending on the center and the expertise and the choice of the surgeon. In many cases, the personal preference and familiarity of the surgeon dictate the choice of the gastrointestinal segment. Ileum may be preferred if there is no obvious and overriding reason for choosing another segment. Children with renal failure with acidosis, short gut syndrome, or irradiated gut might be better served using the stomach. The sigmoid colon segment can be used without reservation but is especially useful if ureteric reimplantation is required and the bladder capacity is extremely small to preclude a bladder patch reimplantation of the ureter. Ureterocystoplasty is the procedure of choice in select patients with renal failure with a non-functional renal moiety with massive ureteric dilatation.

Choice of segment	Common indication
Ileum	Preferred choice, surgeons preference
Sigmoid	If ureteric reimplantation is required, preferred choice with surgeons preference
Stomach	In the setting of renal failure, where other segments might not be available
Ureter	In the setting of renal failure (in select cases), allows peritoneal dialysis

76.8 Bladder Dynamics After Augmentation

Adequate bladder capacity is usually achieved in all patients following an augmentation. The bowel segment utilised for the creation of the reservoir may continue to contract, leading to occasional problems with pressure after an augmentation cystoplasty. Rhythmic or sinusoidal contractions usually occur and are common, which may increase in amplitude near the capacity of the reservoir. These are usually of no clinical significance. Early high-pressure contractions may precipitate incontinence or upper tract damage. Significant contractions (above 40 cm H_2O) may be seen, particularly with colocystoplasty.

Post-operative problems with the use of intestinal segments for augmentations

1. Early Post-operative Management
   (a) Continuous drainage of the bladder should be achieved via the suprapubic catheter.
   (b) Suprapubic tube should be irrigated at least three times a day to prevent mucus buildup and to clear the collected mucus.
   (c) Cystogram should be done to document healing at the time of discharge.
   (d) A regimen of Clean Intermittent catheterisation (CIC) should be instituted every 2–3 h.
   (e) Suprapubic catheter is removed once the CIC regimen is instituted and the cystogram demonstrates no abnormality.
2. Hyperchloremic Metabolic Acidosis
   (a) These children with this metabolic derangement present with fatigue, weakness and polydipsia.
   (b) Patients with normal or near-normal renal function are usually able to handle the resorbed load of chloride and acid without obvious acidosis.
   (c) Ammonium in urine pretends to be sodium in the intraluminal Na/H Exchanger. With the entry of ammonium in the cells, bicarbonate moves out to maintain the ion balance in exchange for the entry of Chloride via with Chloride-Bicarbonate exchanger.
   (d) Prolonged storage of urine in the bladder contributes to this. It is mandatory to empty the bladder via CIC every 4–5 h, irrespective of the capacity of the neobladder created.

(e) Oral Alkalising agents like sodium citrate and citric acid solution intake are instituted to prevent hyperchloremic metabolic acidosis. Blockers of chloride transport like chlorpromazine and nicotinic acid inhibit c-AMP at the cell membrane level and are useful in preventing metabolic derangements.
(f) Oral Potassium replacements may also be required in cases with significant hypokalemia.

3. Impaired Bone Growth and Demineralisation: Prolonged acidosis leads to wasting of the bony calcium buffers, leading to bone demineralisation.
4. Decreased Growth Potential in Children: A delay in growth in height of the child is noted in approximately 20% of patients, even without major apparent metabolic derangement.
5. Bowel Dysfunction and Diarrhoea in 10–20% of Patients: Though the removal of a small segment of intestine rarely causes any bowel dysfunction, but inclusion of Ileocaecal valve may be a significant factor contributing towards bowel dysfunction and diarrhoea.
6. Vitamin B12 Deficiency: May require adequate supplementation. Terminal Ileum is the only site for Vit B12 absorption and the terminal 15–20 cms of ileum are not used for the construction of the reservoir. Up to a third of patients may develop subclinical or clinical features of B12 deficiency requiring surveillance and treatment as indicated.
7. Bladder Patch Perforation: Delayed perforation is noted in 5–10% of cases, especially with the use of colonic segment.
8. Mucus Production and Stone Formation: Requires a daily regimen of saline bladder wash to prevent this complication.
9. Infection: Bacteriuria is common after cystoplasty and is usually not clinically significant. Febrile urinary tract infections with haematuria need a more aggressive management.
10. Adenocarcinoma Bladder: Higher incidence of malignancy over decades.

76.9 Summary

1. Bladder augmentation increased the reservoir capacity of the bladder.
2. The technique aims to either make the bladder 'safe' for the upper tracts or to assist the child in attaining continence.
3. Ileum, caecum, colon, stomach or ureter are all utilised as a donor site to increase the bladder capacity.
4. Ileum is the most commonly utilised donor segment.
5. Hyperchloremic metabolic acidosis, infections, stone formations, high coordinated reservoir pressures and risk of malignancies are common problems.

Suggested Reading

Docimo SG. The Kelalis-King-Belman textbook of clinical pediatric urology. 6th ed. CRC Press; 2019.
Partin AW, Dmochowski RR, Kavoussi LR, Peters CA. Campbell-Walsh-Wein urology. 12th ed. Elsevier; 2020.
Snodgrass WT. Pediatric urology: evidence for optimal patient management. Springer; 2013.

Urinary Diversion

77

Arvind Sinha

77.1 Introduction

Urinary diversion is when the normal anatomical urinary tract structures are bypassed, and an opening/tube/stent is made/placed in the urinary system to bring the urine out via another way. It is used for a novel set of indications to address the unique surgical and technical challenges and diagnosis among the pediatric age group. A variety of techniques, including temporary and permanent diversion procedures, are utilized to divert the flow of urine safely.

Urinary diversion is a surgical procedure that reroutes/ bypass the normal flow of urine out of the body when urine flow is blocked/obstructed. Urinary diversion is indicated when the bladder is no longer able to safely function as a reservoir for urine storage in a socially safe/acceptable manner while keeping the kidneys safe.

The primary indications for diverting the flow of urine (urinary diversion) in children are as follows:

1. Renal function preservation: McGuire and colleagues demonstrated that elevated detrusor leak point pressures (higher than 40 cm H_2O) are associated with an higher and increasing risk of upper tract damage. These elevated passive bladder pressures lead to impaired ureteral drainage and/or reflux with secondary development of hydroureteronephrosis and renal damage.
2. Urinary incontinence: Lack of storage capacity of the bladder or a loss of sphincter function of the bladder may cause urinary incontinence. Diversion may be one of the approaches to manage Urinary incontinence.
3. Bypassing Obstructive lesions: Obstructive lesions like stricture urethra or posterior urethral valves may necessitate a temporizing urinary diversion before the definitive repair.
4. Egress for Infected Urine: Pyonephrosis in the setting of an obstruction may also require a temporizing urinary diversion to allow the infected urine to drain and for the infection to settle.

The choice of diversion depends on the diagnosis, body habitus, the attendant manual dexterity, psychological compliance for intermittent catherization and social circumstances. The majority of urinary diversions are performed for congenital anomalies of the spine and/or urinary tract and their consequences.

A. Sinha (✉)
Department of Pediatric Surgery, All India Institute of Medical Sciences (AIIMS), Jodhpur, Rajasthan, India

© The Author(s), under exclusive license to Springer Nature Singapore Pte Ltd. 2025
S. Roy Choudhury (ed.), *Pediatric Surgery*, https://doi.org/10.1007/978-981-96-1257-4_77

77.2 Indications for Urinary Diversion

1. Neurogenic Bladder
   (a) Spina Bifida, sacral deformities, spinal trauma, etc., are common indications leading to a need for urinary diversion.
   (b) The presence of hostile bladder dynamics, including high outlet resistance, detrusor sphincter dyssynergia, or a hypercontractile bladder, that are at risk for upper tract damage.
   (c) Medical management, including behavioral modifications, anticholinergic bladder relaxants, and clean intermittent catheterization are initial procedures of choice to manage these hostile bladder dynamics.
2. Exstrophy Bladder
   (a) An insufficient bladder plate of failed bladder reconstruction might push a child with exstrophy bladder towards a diversion procedure.
3. Posterior Urethral Valve
   (a) Usually, children with posterior urethral valves can be managed by neonatal cystoscopic fulguration of the valves.
   (b) However, a severely premature baby or a child with severe high-grade reflux with azotemia might require a diversion procedure as a stabilizing measure.
   (c) Later in life, children with deteriorating renal function due to "valve" bladder might be served by an augmentation with an urinary diversion.
4. Vesical/Perivesical Tumors and Trauma
   (a) Though the indications for performing extensive mutilating surgery is decreasing in the pediatric age group, cystectomy for tumor or trauma might necessitate a urinary diversion.
5. Other severe congenital anomalies: Cloacal exstrophy or common cloaca, urogenital sinus, etc., might require a diversion of the urinary stream.

Table 77.1 Common pediatric urinary diversion

Continent	Incontinent
Mitrofanoff	Cutaneous Vesicostomy
Monti Procedure	Ureterostomy
Continent catherizable Vesicostomy	Ileal/Urinary conduit
Continent Urinary Reservoir, e.g. Indiana Pouch, Kock Pouch, Gastroileal Pouch	
Augmentation Cystoplasty (Chap. 76)	
Ureterosigmoidstomy	

77.3 Urinary Diversion: Types

Urinary diversion has been variously classified as continent and incontinent. It has also been classified as temporary and permanent or even intubated and non-intubated.

Continent urinary diversion often tries to maintain the continence by utilizing a continent catherizable channel (Table 77.1).

77.4 Incontinent Urinary Diversion

77.4.1 Cutaneous Vesicostomy

Cutaneous vesicostomy was in vogue in the 1970s and 80 s. However, with the onset and increasing acceptability of clean intermittent catheterization and improvement in the size of neonatal endoscopes and its miniaturization, the indications for performing a cutaneous vesicostomy are steadily declining. Indications for performing a cutaneous vesicostomy include neonates with posterior urethral valve where cystoscopic ablation is not possible, children with myelodysplasia/neurogenic bladder with significant upper tract damage due to hostile bladder, and children with recurrent febrile urinary tract infections with worsening upper tract function. Other severe congenital anomalies like common cloaca with severe hydronephrosis might be best served by a cutaneous vesicostomy. It still remains the most common form of temporary incontinent urinary diversion.

77.4.2 Blocksom Technique for Vesicostomy Creation

A. A 2 cm midline transverse incision is made about 2 cms above the pubic symphysis. The rectus is separated and the bladder is exposed after adequate mobilization of the peritoneum in a cephalad direction. The top of the bladder is further mobilized and the posterior wall of the bladder is then exposed. The posterior bladder wall near the dome is then opened and the edges sutured to the skin.
B. Stenosis and mucosal prolapse are common complications.
C. It stabilizes the renal function in a majority of patients and the incidence of new urinary tract infections is reduced due to prevention of stasis and the presence of a low pressure reservoir.

77.4.3 Cutaneous Ureterostomy

Supravesical urinary diversion via a ureterostomy is rarely indicated or performed today. It has been utilized earlier for drainage of a massively dilated upper urinary tract, especially in the setting of urosepsis or to improve drainage of the renal units in settings of severe obstruction. High-grade vesicoureteric reflux and megaureter are usually managed surgically, especially with recurrent febrile urinary tract infections or with persistent or worsening urinary tract deterioration. However, cutaneous ureterostomy may be a temporizing measure in young children allowing the child to grow. A ureterostomy may be utilized in children with posterior urethral valves, especially when the renal function fails to improve after adequate bladder drainage.

To decompress massively dilated upper urinary tracts in children with urosepsis or severe obstruction, a low ureterostomy (performed near the bladder) or a high ureterostomy (near the pelvis of the kidney) might be performed depending upon the clinical situation.

Low diversion can be commonly performed either as a loop or an end cutaneous ureterostomy. However, the subsequent takedown often involves a ureteroneocystostomy because of a small residual ureteric stump. High diversion at the level of the kidney is done through a flank incision and can be accomplished as a loop ureterostomy, Sober's ureterostomy, or end ureterostomy (Figs. 77.1 and 77.2).

The Y-ureterostomy (Sober's Ureterostomy) and a loop ureterostomy allows antegrade urinary flow to the bladder, maintaining a semblance of bladder cycling. An end ureterstomy precludes any drainage of the urine from the renal unit to the bladder.

High ureterstomy are usually approached via a subcoastal or flank incision in an extraperitoneal fashion. The ureter is further mobilized and a wide patent anastomosis to the skin is created.

Ureterostomy creates a wide drainage to the renal unit. Stomal Stenosis and Pyelonephritis may be particularly troublesome complications.

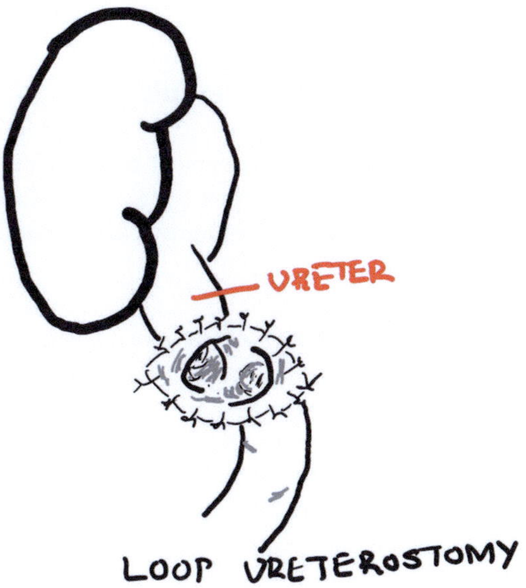

Fig. 77.1 Loop Ureterostomy

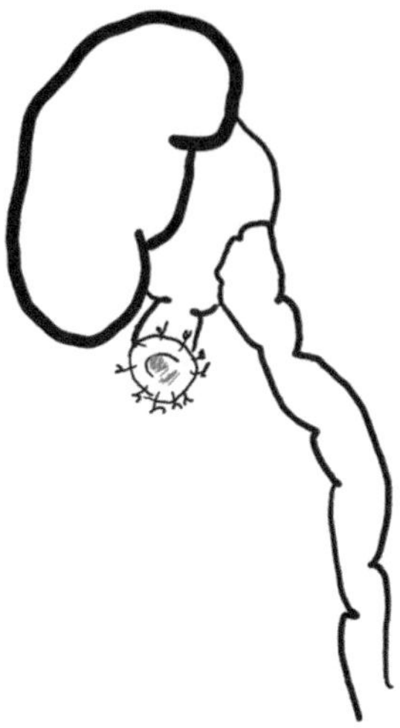

Fig. 77.2 Sober ureterostomy

77.4.4 Cutaneous Pyelostomy

Extremely rarely performed nowadays with the availability of interventional percutaneous procedures like a percutaneous nephrostomy. This procedure can only be performed easily in patients with a extrarenal pelvis which is dilated, which can reach the skin without tension and may be used as a diversion (temporary) in select cases of ureteropelvic junction obstruction and posterior urethral valve.

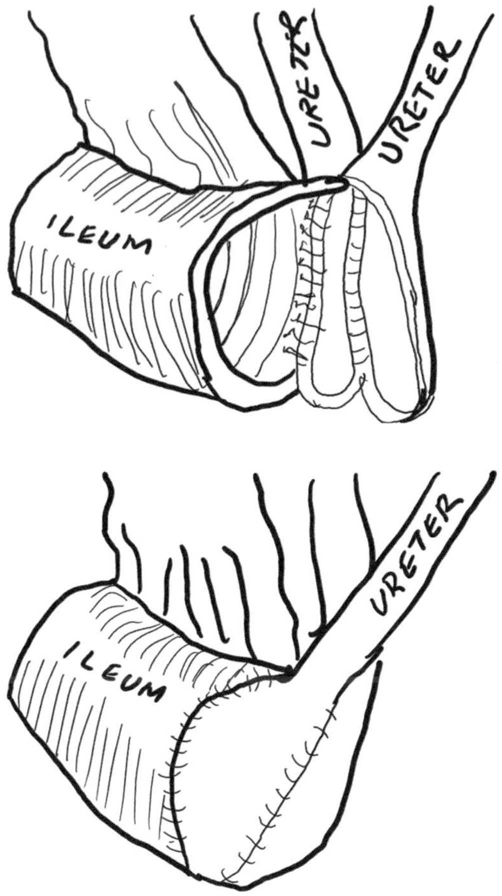

Fig. 77.3 Ureterointestinal anastomosis—refluxing

77.4.5 Urinary/Ileal Conduit

- A procedure where a segment of intestine is utilized to create a stoma for external diversion of urine. Less commonly used now after the advent of CIC.

Current indications for the use of a Urinary or Ileal conduit are

- Patients who lack the ability to care for themselves due to physical or mental disability.
- Children with malignancies after extensive pelvic/abdominal radiation.
- Deteriorating upper urinary tract with presence of limitation for continent diversion.

Ileum is used quite frequently. However, the use of colon as a conduit allows for the non-refluxing anastomosis of the ureters into the taenia. Use of Jejunal conduits have a high incidence of metabolic complications and are not used. However, the use of conduits for diversion of urinary stream is associated with high complication rate including a very high incidence of upper tract deterioration. Thus, ileal conduit is used very infrequently among children and is typically used in those children who have no other options for urinary diversion.

Types of ureterointestinal anastomosis that can be performed for creation of ileal/urinary conduit are simple refluxing type or a tunneled non-refluxing type of ureterointestinal anastomosis (Figs. 77.3 and 77.4).

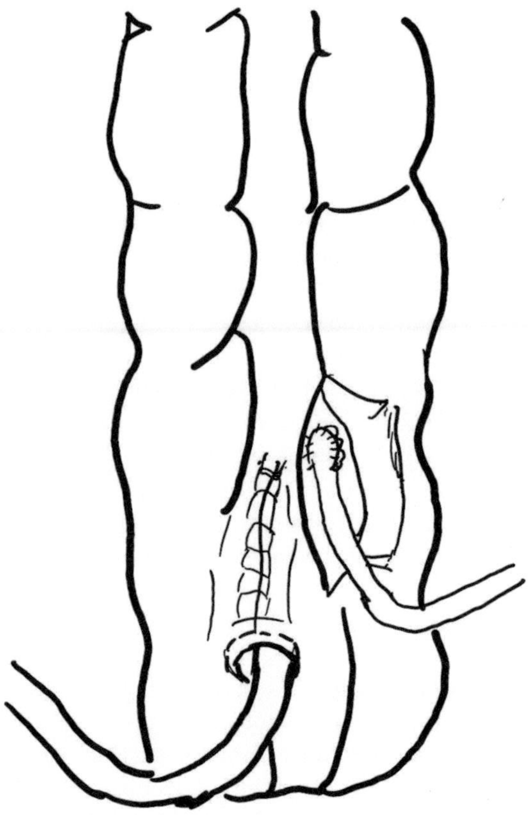

Fig. 77.4 Ureterointestinal anastomosis—non-refluxing

77.5 Continent Urinary Diversion

It involves the creation of a low-pressure reservoir with adequate volume which is continent via the means of intermittent catheterization of a non-refluxing channel without leakage or reflux. The creation of the low pressure, adequate volume reservoir is discussed in the chapter on bladder augmentation (Chap. 76). The creation of continent catherizable conduits will be discussed further.

77.6 Mitrofanoff Appendicovesicostomy

Described in 1980, Mitrofanoff created a continent-catherizable channel by utilizing the appendix which was submucosally implanted into the bladder. It is based on the principle that any supple tube, if implanted submucosally with sufficient muscle backing, acts as a flap valve, and results in a reliable continence mechanism (Mitrofanoff Principle).

Mitrofanoff appendicovesicostomy is a surgical procedure commonly performed in pediatric patients with bladder dysfunction or urinary incontinence. It involves using a section of the appendix to create a channel joining the bladder with the abdominal wall. This channel provides a pathway for urine to be drained from the bladder using a catheter, which can be accessed through a small opening in the abdomen.

The procedure is often used in children who have undergone extensive bladder surgery or have congenital anomalies affecting the urinary tract. Mitrofanoff appendicovesicostomy can improve bladder function, reduce the risk of urinary tract infections, and provide greater independence for children with urinary incontinence.

77.6.1 Advantages of Appendix

- Can be safely utilized safely without affecting the bowel function.
- A submucosal length of 2 cm is adequate for continence.
- It can be easily implanted into both the bladder or even the bowel segments.

77.6.2 Technique

A transverse abdominal incision or a low midline incision is utilized. The mobilization of the ascending colony along the line of Toldt is necessary to gain better access and to provide adequate length to the appendix and its mesentry. The appendix along with a small cuff of the cecum are amputated and the cecal cuff is closed. The appendix is further mobilized with mesoappendix to ensure an adequate blood supply. After adequate mobilization, the distal appendix is submucosally tunneled into the bladder and the tip is amputated to ensure continuity. The cecal end is fixed to the abdominal wall. Careful attention should be placed throughout the procedure to avoid kinking of the appendix and to ensure the ease of catheterization of the stoma.

Some of the possible complications of Mitrofanoff appendicovesicostomy in children include:

- Infection: There is a risk of infection at the site of the catheterization, which can lead to urinary tract infections and other complications.
- Blockage: The channel created by the Mitrofanoff procedure can become blocked, preventing urine from draining properly.
- Leakage: In some cases, urine may leak from the channel or around the catheter.
- Stenosis: Stenosis refers to the narrowing of the channel created by the Mitrofanoff procedure (seen in 6–10% of patients), which can make it difficult to catheterize.
- Fistula: In rare cases, a fistula (an abnormal connection between the bladder and another organ) can develop.

While the procedure is generally safe and effective, there are potential risks and complications, including infection, bleeding, and blockage of the channel, as detailed above. It is important for parents and caregivers, and health professionals to monitor children who have undergone the Mitrofanoff procedure for signs of complications and to seek medical attention if any issues arise.

77.7 Monti Procedure

During the Monti procedure, a segment of the patient's small intestine is used (instead of the appendix) to create a channel between the bladder and the skin of the abdomen. The segment of intestine is isolated, and the blood supply to it is carefully preserved. The intestine is then detubularized and folded and sewn to create a tube tunneled under the skin to the surface of the abdomen. This tube is then used as a channel for the patient to catheterize the bladder to empty urine. A 2–2.5 cm length of intestine is utilized. With the reconfiguration, the length of the donor intestine becomes the circumference of the tube and the circumference becomes the length of the tube. Thus, it is important to carefully measure a 2–2.5 cm segment of ileum for use as Monti's tube because a longer length would translate to a higher diameter channel requiring a longer length for a continent mechanism.

Monti and Yang technique: An isolated 2–2.5 cm of ileum is opened along its antimesenteric border. This patch of ileum is retubularized over a 12 French catheter which creates a channel which is then implanted into the bladder. The other end of the channel is attached to the abdominal wall, usually at the level of the umbilicus and an indwelling catheter is left in situ for 2–3 weeks to allow adequate healing and to keep the conduit patent.

Complications of the Monti procedure can include infection, bleeding, and obstruction of the channel. There is also a risk of bowel perforation during the procedure and long-term risks such as bladder stones, urinary tract infections, and reflux of urine from the bladder back into the kidneys. It has a higher incidence of stomal stenosis as compared to Mitrofanoff's procedure. In some cases, the valve mechanism may fail, leading to leakage of urine between catheterizations.

77.8 Casale's Modification

- Also known as the Spiral Monti
- The main advantage of "Spiral Monti" or Casale's Modification is that it provides a channel with twice the length without resorting to an end-to-end circular anastomosis, which is often quoted as a theoretical disadvantage of the classic double Monti tube.
- A 3.5 cm segment of ileum is divided partially.
- Both ends of the ideal segments are tubularized and reanastomosed, resulting in increased channel length.

77.9 Continent Urinary Reservoir

- Goal of a continent urinary reservoir is the creation of a reservoir of sufficient capacity and compliance with non-refluxing ureteric implantations and a continent cutaneous stoma.
- Colon and stomach are preferred more because of well-developed musculature of tenia coli of the colon and the muscle wall of the stomach allows for a more reliable non-refluxing ureteric and catheterizable channel anastomoses.
- The three most common types of continent reservoir in used in children are:
  1. Kock pouch
  2. Gastro-ileal pouch
  3. Indiana pouch

77.10 Kock Pouch

- A continent ileostomy described in 1971. It entails the construction of an efferent nipple for continence with an afferent limb for the prevention of urinary reflux.
- 60–70 cms of bowel segment is isolated approximately 50 cm from the ileocecal valve. It is positioned as the letter U with the ends directed toward the patient's head. The legs of the U are united at the antimesenteric border creating the reservoir. Intussusception of the afferent and efferent segments into the future reservoir is then done to prevent reflux or leakage and is secured with staples.

77.11 Gastro-Ileal Pouch

77.11.1 Advantages

- The theoretical and metabolic advantages of both gastric and ileal segments can be maximized.
- The metabolic derangements of both segments (gastric and ileal segment) complement each other with the acidic gastric secretion neutralizing the absorptive properties of colon or ileum.
- Useful in high-risk patients of short gut syndrome (Cloacal exstrophy) as it minimizes loss of absorptive tissue.

77.11.2 Demerits

- Complex reconstruction and requirement of a longer operating time.

77.12 Indiana Pouch

- Indiana pouch utilized the inherent continence or anti-reflux mechanism of the ileocecal valve. Gilchrist and Merritt's popularized the use of ileocecal valve as a continence mechanism in the 1950s. The Indiana group modified the pouch described by Gilchrist and Merricks and utilized an unique plication method.

77.12.1 Technique

- Detubularized cecum is used as a reservoir with ureters implanted in a non-refluxing manner into the taenia.
- A short segment of terminal ileum is used as efferent limb.
- This segment is deliberately kept as short and straight as possible to facilitate easy clean intermittent catherization.
- The ileum is then plicated to the ileo-cecal valve, which is re-enforced by lambert suture.

77.12.2 Advantages

- High continence rate: 95–99%.
- Simple technique with short learning curve.
- Very low complication rate (0.6%).

77.13 Ureterosigmoidostomy and Its Variants

- An effective form of continent urinary diversion in some patients. It allows for the spontaneous evacuation of urine with stool providing continence. However, it is not used anymore due to significant complications.
- Hyperchloremic acidosis—Significant and a major complication.
- Infection.
- Hydronephrosis.
- Colonic malignancy—Possibly the most significant complication which arguably precluded its further use.

77.14 Modifications of Ureterosigmoidostomy

- MAINZ II POUCH(Sigma Rectum)
  - The colon is incised along its antimesenteric border for approximately 6 cm proximal and distal to the rectosigmoid junction.
  - The ureters are implanted into an antirefluxing fashion into the colon.

Colon is then reconfigured and closed. The Mainz pouch II (sigma rectum) has been touted as a means of reconstructing a low-pressure ureterosigmoidostomy.

77.14.1 Advantage

- A recto-sigmoid reservoir of low pressure is created which protects the upper tracts.
- Continence is good.

77.14.2 Disadvantages

- Risk of Acidosis.
- Risk of adenocarcinoma is unaltered.
- Stricture at uretero-colonic anastomosis.

77.15 Summary

1. Urinary diversion in children is used to reroute urine flow in cases where the normal urinary system is damaged or not functioning properly.
2. The most common indication for urinary diversion in children is neurogenic bladder dysfunction, posterior urethral valves. or during the management of severe congenital anomalies.
3. There are several types of urinary diversion procedures, including continent and incontinent diversions. Continent diversions involve the creation of a reservoir to store urine, which can be emptied at regular intervals using a catheter. Incontinent diversions involve the creation of an opening on the abdominal wall, which allows urine to drain into a pouch or bag outside the body.
4. The choice of urinary diversion procedure in children depends on several factors, including the cause and severity of the underlying condition.

Suggested Reading

Docimo SG. The Kelalis-King-Belman textbook of clinical pediatric urology. 6th ed. CRC Press; 2019.

Partin AW, Dmochowski RR, Kavoussi LR, Peters CA. Campbell-Walsh-Wein urology. 12th ed. Elsevier; 2020.

Role of Urodynamics and Interpretation in Children

78

Priyank Yadav, Vikram Khanna, and Sujit K Chowdhary

78.1 Introduction

Pediatric urology encompasses a wide range of conditions affecting the urinary system in children, posing distinct challenges in terms of diagnosis and management. The specialized field of urodynamics plays a pivotal role in this domain by aiming to evaluate and comprehend the dynamic functionality of the urinary tract in a distinctive manner. Urodynamic analysis involves the examination of pressures and flow dynamics within the bladder and urethra, yielding valuable insights into the intricate interplay between storage and voiding functions.

Accurate diagnosis and prognosis of pediatric urological diseases hinge upon the assessment of urodynamic parameters in children. Over the past few decades, considerable progress has been made in the field of urodynamics, bolstered by improved instrumentation and software, thus facilitating a better understanding and more effective management of pediatric urological disorders.

P. Yadav
Sanjay Gandhi Post Graduate Institute of Medical Sciences, Lucknow, UP, India

V. Khanna
Pediatric Surgery, LHMC, New Delhi, India

S. K Chowdhary (✉)
Indraprastha Apollo Hospital, New Delhi, Delhi, India

This chapter provides a comprehensive overview of urodynamics in children, underscoring its significance in pediatric urology. It will cover the fundamental principles of urodynamic testing, the clinical applications of these studies across a spectrum of urological conditions and unique considerations and challenges associated with performing urodynamic studies on children.

78.2 Indications

Three situations may require urodynamic evaluation in children: Neurological disorders that affect vesicourethral function; Non-neurological disorders that affect vesicourethral function; and Lower urinary tract symptoms (LUTS) suggesting vesicourethral dysfunction but not known underlying cause. The common indications for performing urodynamic studies include:

- *Spinal dysraphism:* Urodynamics is essential for diagnosis and characterization of neurogenic bladder in patients with spinal dysraphism as well as identifying abnormal lower urinary tract (LUT) function and selection of appropriate therapies based on the risk of urinary tract deterioration.
- *Anorectal malformations:* Urodynamics contributes to the assessment of neurogenic bladder dysfunction resulting from spinal cord tethering or surgical injury to identify the type

© The Author(s), under exclusive license to Springer Nature Singapore Pte Ltd. 2025

S. Roy Choudhury (ed.), *Pediatric Surgery*, https://doi.org/10.1007/978-981-96-1257-4_78

of LUT dysfunction and guides the treatment process.

- *Dysfunctional voiding/ bladder and bowel dysfunction:* The combination of uroflowmetry with pelvic floor patch electromyography can enhance diagnostic accuracy. Urodynamics also helps assess the severity of voiding dysfunction as well as its relationship to vesicoureteral reflux (VUR).
- *Overactive bladder:* An overactive bladder can be diagnosed with urodynamics by confirming the overactivity of the detrusor during filling cystometry. However, treatment needs to be tailored to the patient's specific symptomatology rather than purely urodynamics findings.
- *Posterior urethral valves:* Urodynamics is indicated to assess bladder compliance, overactivity, contractility, and potential outlet obstruction.

78.3 Patient Preparation

It is imperative that both patients and their parents have a thorough understanding of the urodynamic test and its implications for treatment decisions. Before the test, it is particularly important to address any issues related to constipation, since this can affect the accuracy of pressure measurements.

A thorough medical history and physical examination should be done to guide the diagnostic process and determine appropriate treatment. Specific information about voiding habits, such as wet and dry diapers in infants or frequency of wetting and voiding characteristics in older children, is important in identifying potential issues. The history should also include details about bowel habits and symptoms associated with urinary tract infections (UTIs), as constipation and UTIs can impact urinary control. Medication use and the use of voiding diaries or home pad tests can provide additional insights. A 3-day voiding diary prior to the test helps understand the usual pattern of storage and voiding and also gives an idea about the functional capacity of the urinary bladder. The child should not have an active UTI, and the test is performed under an antibiotic cover. The child should arrive at the facility with preferably a full bladder so that a uroflowmetry can be performed at the beginning and the residual volume can be aspirated (and measured) after placement of the urodynamics catheter. Before the test, a sedative may be administered to a child experiencing high levels of anxiety or fear. However, anesthesia must be avoided as it may affect the bladder dynamics.

78.4 Procedure

A multichannel fluid-filled pressure recording is recommended by the International Children's Continence Society (ICCS) for the study of urodynamics in children.

- Conductive gel should be applied to the degreased surface of the skin before placing electrodes for EMG.
- Filling rates and temperatures will affect bladder function when retrogradely filling with saline.
- Estimated bladder capacity = (age [yrs] + 1 × 30); it is important to know it before starting the study as it will guide the filling volume and rate.
- More than one study may be required in children, especially those who are more anxious.
- Children should be seated or held by a caregiver during the study.

78.4.1 Catheter Insertion and EMG Electrode Placement

- Use a 6-fr double lumen transurethral catheter for bladder pressure measurement.
- Place the catheter per urethra using lubricating gel. Consider a suprapubic double lumen catheter for some cases (e.g., very high bladder neck).
- Record abdominal pressure with a fully fluid-filled open 8-fr feeding tube or a small air-free fluid-filled balloon catheter rectal catheter.

- Secure both catheters with tape and connect them to external transducers.
- Position surface EMG electrodes symmetrically near the external anal sphincter.

78.4.2 Pressure Positioning and Zeroing

- Preferably perform filling cystometry in a seated position.
- Zero the bladder pressure channel to atmospheric pressure (transducer at the level of symphysis).
- Test catheter and sensor function using gentle abdominal pressure or coughing.
- Regularly perform cough tests or Credé maneuvers during the study for quality control.

78.4.3 Filling Cystometry Procedure

- Fill the bladder at a rate of 5–10% of estimated capacity per minute using saline at body or room temperature.
- Record intravesical and abdominal pressures simultaneously.
- Mark specific filling states on the tracing: "first sensation of filling," followed by "normal desire," and "strong desire to void."
- Mark voiding or leakage as the end of filling.

78.4.4 Voiding Cystometry Procedure

- Record voiding pressures and uroflow measurements.
- Note is there is abdominal straining, look at the uroflow curve.
- If EMG is performed simultaneously, note whether the sphincter becomes silent during voiding.
- Measure the post void residual volume by aspirating through the catheter. If the catheter has been removed, the same can be measured using an ultrasound/bladder scanner.

78.4.5 Conclusion of the Test

- Remove all catheters and EMG electrodes.
- Instruct children to resume normal activities and drink extra water.
- Complete a clinical evaluation report immediately after the test.

78.5 Interpretation

A urodynamics study has two phases: the filling phase and the voiding phase. Both phases are important in order to understand the function of the bladder.

The following parameters are important during the filling phase:

- Bladder Capacity: Bladder capacity refers to the maximum volume of urine the bladder can hold during the filling phase. It is calculated by measuring the volume of infused fluid until the child expresses a desire to void or experiences leakage. Bladder capacity can be estimated based on age using the formula: Age (in years) + 1 × 30 = capacity (in mL). However, it is important to note that individual variations may exist.
- Bladder Compliance, $\Delta V/\Delta P$: Bladder compliance measures the ability of the bladder to stretch and accommodate increasing volumes of urine without a significant increase in pressure. It is calculated by dividing the change in bladder volume by the change in detrusor pressure during the filling phase. Normal bladder compliance ranges from 20–40 mL/cm H_2O. Higher values suggest increased elasticity and capacity, while lower values indicate reduced elasticity and stiffness.
- First Sensation of Filling: The "first sensation of filling" refers to the point at which the child first perceives the presence of urine in the bladder. It is an important landmark in assessing bladder sensation. This sensation is typically reported by the child during the urodynamic study and marked on the urodynamic tracing.

- Normal Desire to Void: The "normal desire to void" represents the sensation of a moderate urge to urinate. It occurs after the initial perception of bladder filling and indicates the child's awareness of a need to empty the bladder. Similar to the first sensation, the normal desire to void is marked on the urodynamic tracing.
- Strong Desire to Void: The "strong desire to void" signifies a strong urge to urinate and is a more intense sensation compared to the normal desire to void. It indicates a higher level of urgency and the child's increased need to empty the bladder. This sensation is also marked on the urodynamic tracing.

The voiding phase (pressure-flow study) consists of the following parameters:

- Detrusor Pressure: Detrusor pressure measures the pressure generated by the bladder muscle during voiding. It is calculated by subtracting the the abdominal pressure from the intravesical pressure. $P_{det} = P_{ves} - P_{abd}$. Normal detrusor pressure during voiding typically remains under 40 cm H_2O in children. An elevated detrusor pressure (>74 cm H_2O in boys and 63 cm H_2O in girls) along with a decreased urine flow is suggestive of static or dynamic obstruction. Failure of detrusor pressure to rise during the voiding phase is suggestive of underactive bladder (Fig. 78.1).
- Maximum Flow Rate: Maximum flow rate (Qmax) measures the peak rate of urine flow during voiding. Normal Qmax values vary based on age and gender, but typically range from 15 to 20 mL/s in children. Lower flow rates may suggest bladder outlet obstruction or impaired bladder contractility.
- Voided Volume: Voided volume refers to the total amount of urine expelled during voiding. It is measured directly during the urodynamic study and provides information about bladder emptying efficiency. Normal voided volumes vary depending on age and functional bladder capacity.

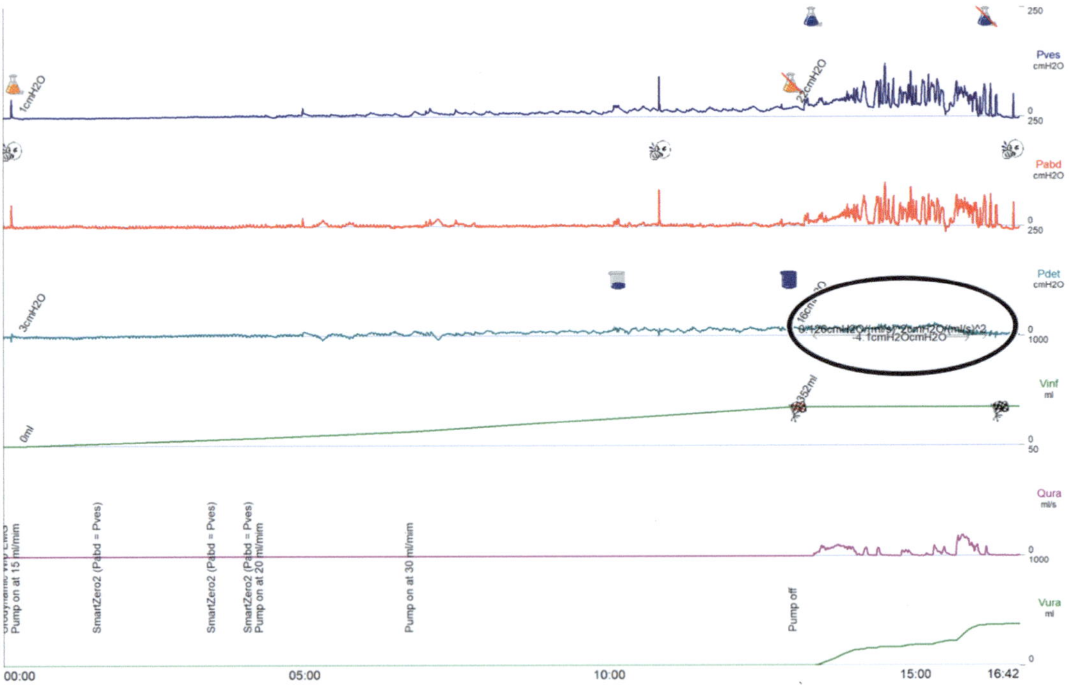

Fig. 78.1 Underactive bladder voiding by contracting abdominal muscles with no discernible detrusor contraction (circle) and interrupted uroflowmetry

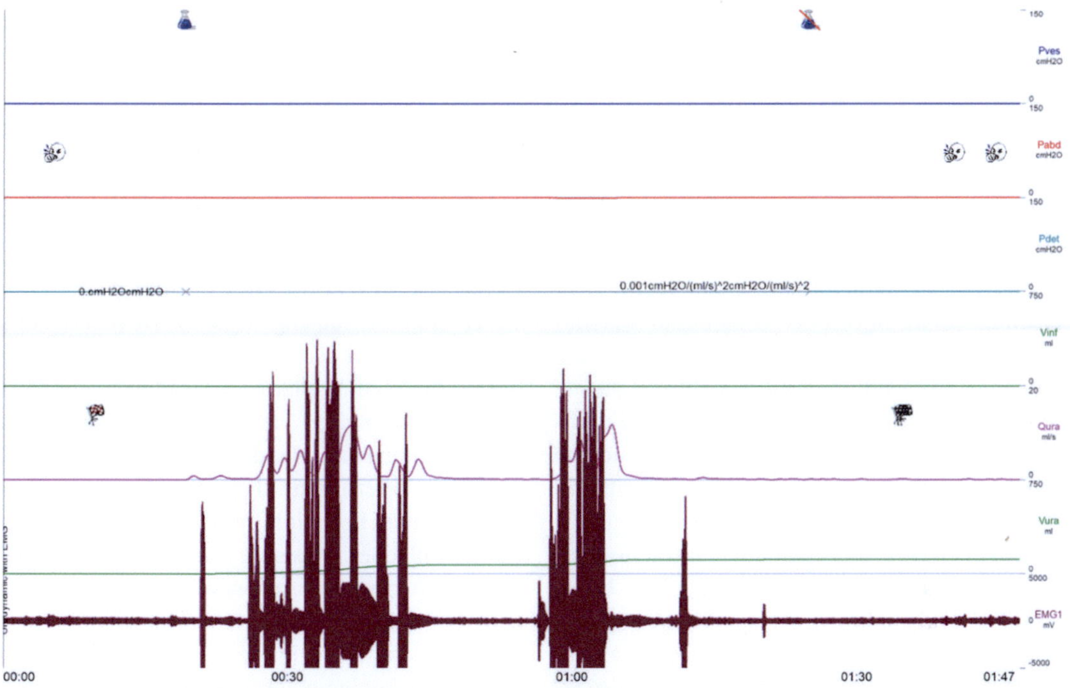

Fig. 78.2 Staccoto (sawtooth) pattern of Uroflow (Pink) with increased sphincter activity during voiding (EMG)

- Post-Void Residual (PVR) Volume: Post-void residual volume measures the amount of urine that remains in the bladder immediately after voiding. It is assessed using ultrasound or catheterization. Normal PVR volumes are typically less than 10% of the voided volume or less than 20–30 mL. Elevated PVR volumes indicate incomplete bladder emptying due to bladder outlet obstruction or impaired bladder contractility. Sometimes, children with VUR may have significant PVR that is essentially the refluxed fluid that drains back into the bladder.
- Flow Pattern: Flow pattern refers to the shape and characteristics of the urinary flow curve during voiding. It is assessed visually and can provide insights into the presence of voiding dysfunction. Normal flow patterns are typically smooth and continuous (bell shaped). Abnormal flow patterns, such as interrupted flow or a staccato pattern, may suggest bladder outlet obstruction or detrusor-sphincter dyssynergia.
- Detrusor-Sphincter Dyssynergia (DSD): DSD refers to the simultaneous contraction of the bladder muscle and the involuntary contraction of the urethral and/or periurethral striated muscles, often leading to obstructed or interrupted urinary flow (Fig. 78.2). DSD is suggested by high maximum detrusor pressure during voiding, or a staccato detrusor pressure curve synchronized with reductions in flow rate along with increased activity on EMG.

78.6 Specific Clinical Situations

78.6.1 Neurogenic Bladder

Urodynamic studies play a crucial role in the evaluation and management of neurogenic bladder, a condition commonly seen in patients with spinal cord injury, spina bifida, or other neurological disorders. These studies provide valuable information about bladder function and help guide treatment decisions. During the filling cystometry phase, urodynamic studies measure bladder compliance, capacity, and detrusor activity. These parameters are essential in understanding the storage function of the bladder in neurogenic patients. Reduced compliance and increased detrusor activity may indicate bladder overactivity, which can lead to symptoms such as urgency and urinary incontinence (Fig. 78.3). This information helps determine the appropriate management strategies, including the use of anticholinergic medications or botulinum toxin injections to modulate bladder contractions. Pressure-flow studies assess the bladder outlet and urethral resistance during voiding. In neurogenic patients, impaired coordination between the detrusor muscle and the external urethral sphincter can result in DSD. Pressure-flow studies can identify DSD by demonstrating simultaneous contractions of the detrusor and urethral sphincter. This information is crucial for selecting the appropriate treatment approach, such as the use of alpha-adrenergic blockers or intermittent catheterization to improve voiding efficiency and prevent complications like urinary retention or upper urinary tract deterioration.

78.6.2 Dysfunctional Voiding/Bowel and Bladder Dysfunction

Urodynamic studies provide essential information about bladder function, urethral dynamics, and pelvic floor muscle activity, allowing for a comprehensive evaluation of dysfunctional voiding. During the filling cystometry phase, urodynamic studies help identify bladder overactivity which may be causing urgency, frequency, and urinary incontinence, while bladder underactivity during the voiding phase can lead to incomplete bladder emptying and urinary retention. Understanding the bladder's storage function is crucial in determining the appropriate interventions, such as behavioral modifications, medications, or bladder retraining techniques. Abnormal EMG patterns, such as increased or decreased activity, can indicate incoordinated or poor sphincter control (Fig. 78.4). This information guides the implementation of pelvic floor exercises, biofeedback training, or other behavioral interventions to improve voiding patterns and enhance bladder control.

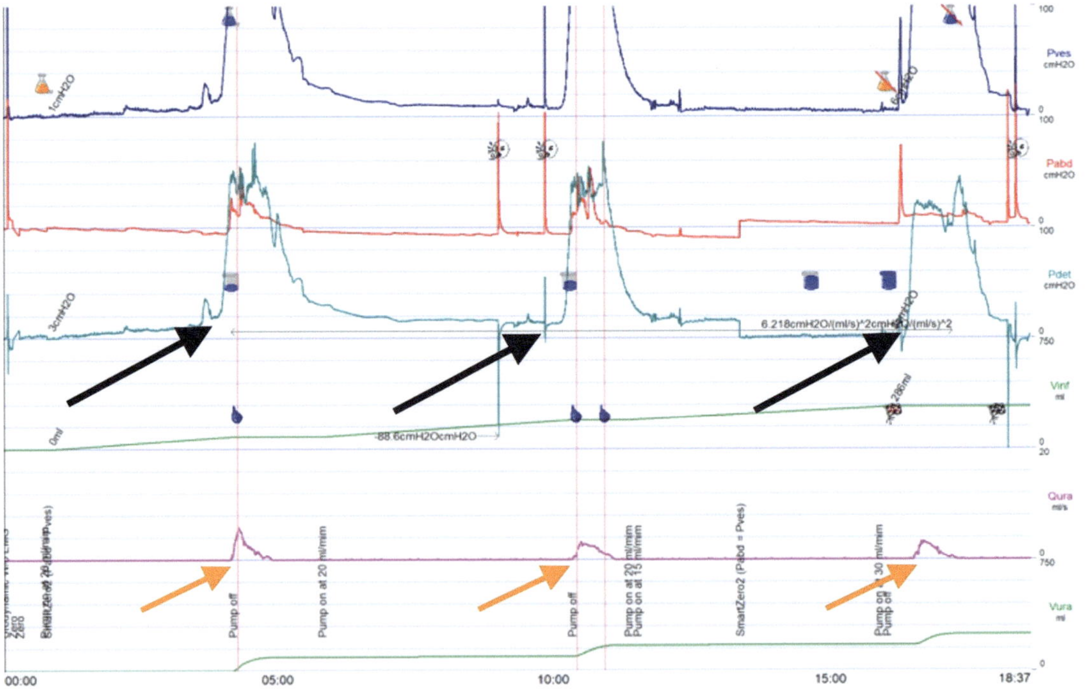

Fig. 78.3 Overactive bladder with phasic detrusor contractions (Black arrows) during the filling phase with some urine leak (Orange arrows)

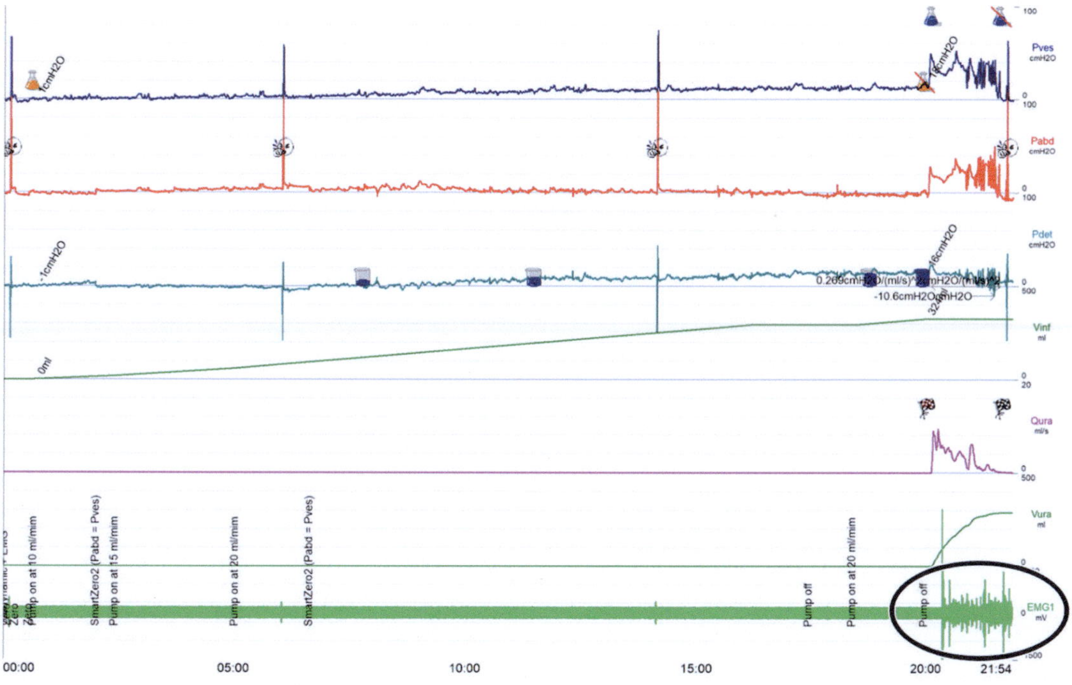

Fig. 78.4 Increased EMG activity (Black circle) during voiding giving the characteristic staccato uroflow pattern (pink)

78.6.3 Overactive Bladder (OAB)

Urodynamic studies are very important in the evaluation and management of OAB, a condition characterized by urinary urgency, frequency, and often urgency incontinence. Detrusor overactivity is identified by involuntary contractions of the bladder during the filling phase, which contribute to urgency and urinary frequency (Fig. 78.5). Evaluating detrusor activity assists in tailoring treatment options, such as antimuscarinic medications or beta-3 agonists, to suppress these involuntary contractions and alleviate OAB symptoms.

78.6.4 Nocturnal Enuresis

During the filling cystometry phase, urodynamic parameters help identify any abnormalities in bladder function that may contribute to nocturnal enuresis. For example, reduced bladder capacity or increased detrusor activity during the filling phase can lead to decreased nocturnal urine storage, resulting in bedwetting. During the voiding phase, detrusor underactivity may be detected which can lead to overflow incontinence. Identifying these abnormalities can guide interventions such as bladder training, timed voiding, double voiding, or pharmacotherapy to improve bladder control and reduce nighttime accidents.

78.6.5 Posterior Urethral Valves (PUV)

In PUV, bladder wall hypertrophy and trabeculation may develop due to increased resistance from the obstructed urethra. These changes can be detected during the filling phase leading to poor compliance with or without detrusor overactivity. During the voiding phase, the presence of high detrusor pressures during voiding after fulguration may indicate residual valves, high bladder neck, or even sphincter contraction due to coexisting dysfunctional voiding. The urodynamic findings help determine the severity of the obstruction, guide treatment decisions, and moni-

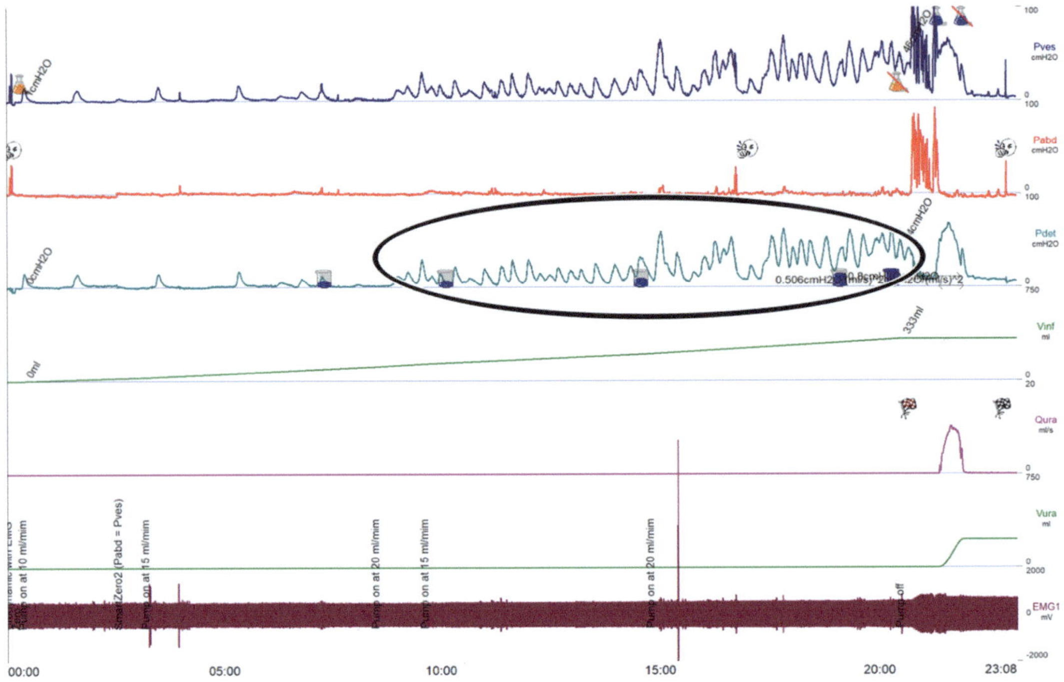

Fig. 78.5 Uninhibited detrusor contractions suggestive of detrusor overactivity (green) characterized by increase in Pdet >15 cm H_2O from baseline (black circle) during the filling phase associated with no leakage of urine

tor the response to interventions such as valve ablation, CIC, botulinum toxin injection, or even augmentation cystoplasty.

78.7 Summary

Overall, urodynamic studies provide valuable information that enhances the diagnosis, prognosis, and management of pediatric urological conditions. The comprehensive evaluation of bladder dynamics through urodynamics assists healthcare professionals in tailoring individualized treatment approaches and improving patient outcomes.

Suggested Reading

Ellison JS, Nicholls G, Woodward M. Urodynamics in children. In: Drake M, Hashim H, Gammie A, editors. Abrams' urodynamics. 4th ed. Wiley-Blackwell; 2021. p. 227–41.

Wen JG, Djurhuus JC, Rosier PF, Bauer SB. ICS educational module: cystometry in children. Neurourol Urodyn. 2018;37:2306–10.

Wen JG, Djurhuus JC, Rosier PF, Bauer SB. ICS educational module: pressure flow study in children. Neurourol Urodyn. 2018;37:2311–4.

79 Disorders of Sexual Differentiation

Sahaj Prajapati and Subhasis Roy Choudhury

79.1 Introduction

"Disorders of sexual development" (DSD) comprises a specific group of congenital conditions having abnormal development of external genitalia, gonads and chromosomal arrangement. Previously used terminologies like ambiguous genitalia, male or female hermaphroditism, intersex diseases, etc. have now been replaced with the term DSD.

79.2 Development of Gonads and Internal Genitalia (Table 79.1)

Urogenital ridge has three anatomical divisions as undifferentiated gonad (bipotential gonad), mesonephros, Wolffian ducts (mesonephric duct) and Mullerian duct (paramesonephric duct). It develops on the ventromedial aspect of intermediate mesoderm. Differentiation of the bipotential gonad to ovary or testis begins after the migration of primitive germ cells to this ridge during the third to fifth week of gestation. Steroidogenic Factor 1 (SF 1) is expressed in

Table 79.1 Normal development of gonads and genitalia

Structure	Male	Female
Gonad	Testis (needs presence of SRY gene present on Y chromosome)	Ovary was considered the default pathway in the absence of Y chromosome but recent evidence suggests the need for both X chromosomes for normal development
Internal genitalia	Mullerian ducts involute due to the secretion of MIS (Mullerian inhibiting substance) Wolffian ducts develop in the presence of testosterone Both MIS and testosterone secreted by testis (Sertoli cells)	Wolffian ducts involute in the absence of androgens, and Mullerian ducts develop in the absence of MIS
External genitalia	Develop in the presence of dihydrotestosterone (DHT)	Default pathway in the absence of androgens

S. Prajapati (✉)
Manjeet Children Hospital (DMICC), Jaipur, Rajasthan, India

S. Roy Choudhury
Pediatric Surgery, Lady Hardinge Medical College and Associated Kalawati Saran Children's Hospital, New Delhi, Delhi, India

© The Author(s), under exclusive license to Springer Nature Singapore Pte Ltd. 2025

S. Roy Choudhury (ed.), *Pediatric Surgery*, https://doi.org/10.1007/978-981-96-1257-4_79

bipotential gonad. In the presence of Y chromosome, SF 1 upregulates the function of SR Y gene which leads to the development of the testis from the bipotential gonad. This testis has Sertoli cells and Leydig cells which secrete Mullerian inhibiting substance (MIS) and testosterone, respectively. Another gene, SOX 9 also plays an important role in male sexual development. It stimulates FGF 9 to increase the activity of Sertoli cells, Leydig cells, their hormones and helps in the development of male reproductive structures. The SOX 9 gene suppresses the WNT 4 gene, which along with beta-catenin is responsible for the development of ovaries.

Development of internal genitalia depends on the ipsilateral gonad, and external genitalia development depends on the presence of testosterone and dihydrotestosterone (DHT). In the absence of testis, Mullerian structures lead to the development of uterus and fallopian tube, the bipotential gonads will develop into the ovary and the Wolffian ducts get involuted. External genitalia develops into female-like genitalia as the default pathway in the absence of androgens. If a testis is present, the internal genital duct (Wolffian duct) develops into male structures and an epididymis, vas deferens and seminal vesicle will be formed. Testes secrete anti-Mullerian hormone (AMH)/ Mullerian inhibiting substance (MIS) which leads to involution of Mullerian structures. Androgens released from the testes lead to the development of external genitalia into male phenotype. Children with DSD can also have two other varieties of abnormally developed gonads in the form of streak gonads or ovotestis. These gonads may lead to abnormal synthesis of testosterone and dihydrotestosterone (DHT) which in turn results in hypospadias due to defective urethral tubularization.

Few terminologies that need attention:

Gender Dysphoria—Dissatisfaction with one's assigned gender.

Gender Identity—A person's self-representation as male or female.

Gender Role—Psychological characteristics that are sexually dimorphic within the general population (toy preferences, clothing, play and playmate preferences and physical aggression).

Gender Orientation—Direction of erotic interest (behavior, fantasies and attractions)

The old and new nomenclatures of DSDs are

- 46 XX DSD (Female pseudohermaphroditism, Overvirilization of Female)
- 46XY DSD (Male pseudohermaphroditism, Undervirilization of male)
- Ovotesticular DSD (True hermaphroditism)
- Disorders of gonadal differentiation (includes syndromes of gonadal dysgenesis).

46 XX DSD (Female Pseudohermaphroditism)

It occurs because of excessive androgen exposure to the female fetus. The causes are:

- Congenital Adrenal Hyperplasia (most common) (Figs. 79.1 and 79.2)
- Maternal tumors of ovarian and adrenal origin.
- Placental aromatase deficiency
- Exogenous androgens received during pregnancy
- Tumors of the clitoris
- Idiopathic

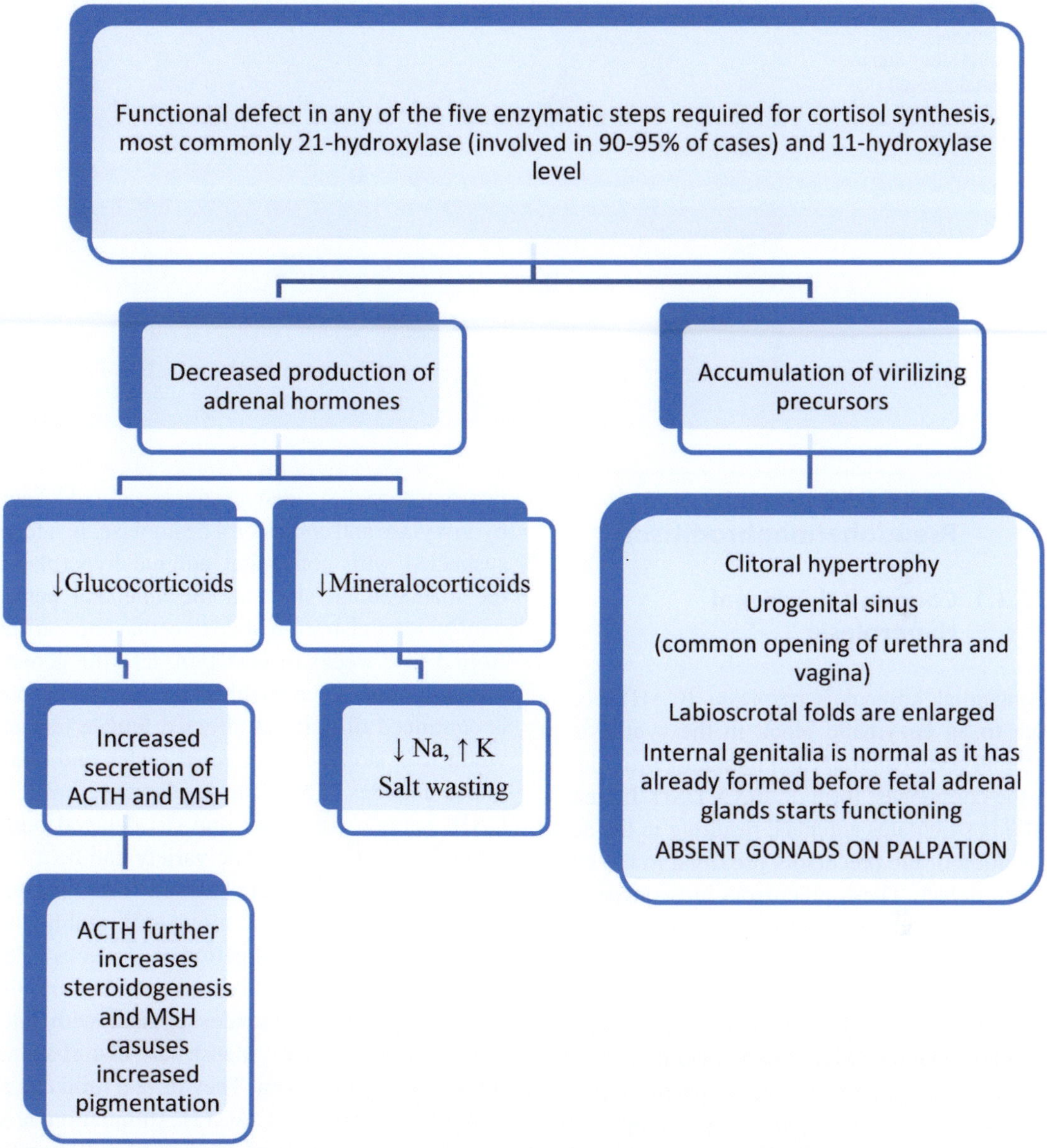

Fig. 79.1 Pathogenesis and clinical features of congenital adrenal hyperplasia. (ACTH—Adrenocorticotropic hormone, MSH—Melanocyte-stimulating hormone)

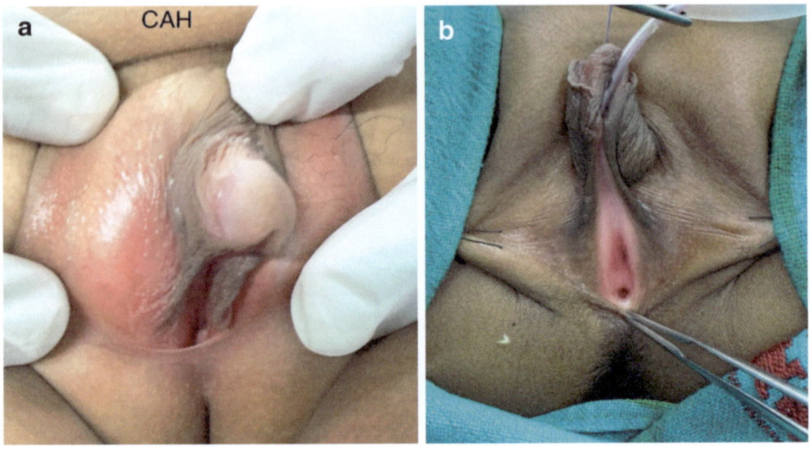

Fig. 79.2 (**a**) Clitoromegaly with urogenital sinus due to congenital adrenal hyperplasia. (**b**) Clitoromegaly (idiopathic)

79.3 46 XX DSD (Female Pseudohermaphroditism)

79.3.1 Congenital Adrenal Hyperplasia

Congenital adrenal hyperplasia (CAH) occurs due to an enzymatic block in the synthesis of adrenal corticosteroids and mineralocorticoids. It is the commonest form of 46XX DSD. Increased ACTH stimulates adrenals, resulting in the accumulation of the precursors proximal to the enzymatic defect. These precursors are converted to the potent androgens which lead to the typical virilization of the female child. The most common enzyme deficiency is 21-hydroxylase (90–95%) followed by 11-hydroxylase. This is an autosomal recessive genetic disorder.

The external genitalia has a spectrum of phenotypic appearance which can be a simple clitoral enlargement in mild form to the complete masculinization with urethral opening at the distal most end of the phallus in severe variety (Fig. 79.2a). Prenatal diagnosis is based on karyotype findings consistent with the presence of disease gene on the short arm of chromosome 6. The diagnosis can be confirmed by chorionic villous sampling. In 95% cases, there is a mutation in the CYP21 gene encoding the enzyme 21-hydroxylase (21-OHD). There are other enzyme deficiencies which can lead to CAH. These are 17 alpha-hydroxylase, 3-beta-hydroxysteroid dehydrogenase, 11-beta-hydroxylase and cholesterol desmolase. In a fetus suspected with congenital adrenal hyperplasia, the management starts in the antenatal period only by administration of dexamethasone starting from 5 to 6 weeks of gestation until the genetic testing results are available. The dexamethasone is continued till term in affected female fetuses, while it is stopped in affected males and unaffected females. There are two major forms of CAH, namely (i) classic and (ii) delayed onset (non-classic) CAH. Classic variety can be a salt loser or a non-salt loser. The salt losers present with vomiting and shock along with ambiguous genitalia in the neonatal period (1–4 weeks). The non-classic CAH usually presents late in the puberty age. These females present with late-onset clitoromegaly, menstrual disturbances, infertility and hirsutism. They have a mild elevation of 17-OHP after ACTH stimulation test. After birth, management consists of replacement steroid therapy. Glucocorticoids (hydrocortisone) and mineralocorticoids (fludrocortisone) are given along with oral salt supplementation to suppress the CRH-ACTH-adrenal axis. The differential diagnosis of clitoromegaly should exclude other idiopathic causes (Fig. 79.2b). The degree of musculinization of the female genitalia is classified into 5 stages as per Prader:

1. Clitoromegaly
2. Clitoromegaly with posterior labial fusion

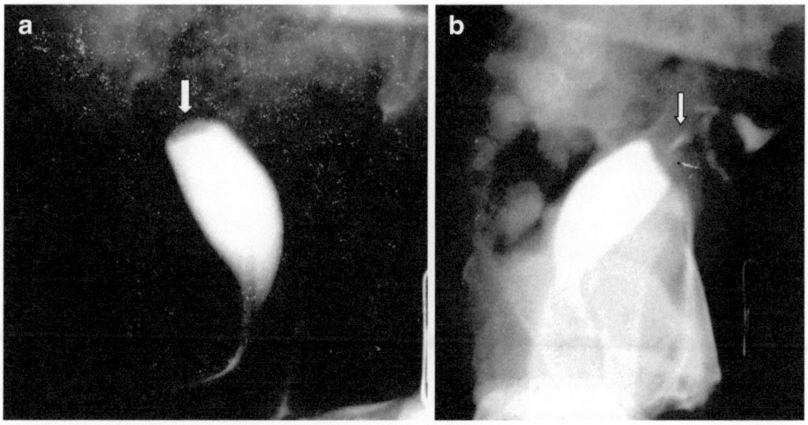

Fig. 79.3 Genitogram in a CAH patient. (**a**) Vagina with cervical impression (arrow). (**b**) Dye filling of cervical canal (arrow)

3. Clitoromegaly with complete labial fusion, UG sinus
4. Clitoris with a phallic appearance, chordee, fused labial folds
5. Penile transformation of the clitoris and urethra

A genitogram helps in identification of the vagina (Fig. 79.3a and b) and in determining the length of the common urogenital sinus which is confirmed on panendoscopy (cystourethroscopy and vaginoscopy). Along with the genitogram and panendoscopy, investigations like pelvis ultrasonography, karyotype, serum 17-OHP and testosterone, FSH, LH, serum electrolytes and gonadal biopsy are the other supportive investigations to help in diagnosis and decision making. Medical management with glucocorticoid and minerelocorticoid replacement can result in regression of mild to moderate masculinization. Genital reconstruction is required for persistent or severely masculinized genitalia. Cut-back or flap vaginoplasty with clitoral recession is recommended for low vaginal confluence. Children with high vaginal confluence proximal to the urethral external sphincter will require more extensive reconstruction by either total urogenital sinus mobilization (TUM) or bowel vaginoplasty. Such genital reconstruction should be delayed till puderty if possible and recommendation of a multidisciplinary team is mandatory. Long-term results of reconstructive surgery in female children show adequate sexual identification, reproduction, intellectual functioning and acceptable genitalia.

79.4 46XY DSD (Male Pseudohermaphroditism)

79.4.1 Androgen Insensitivity Syndrome (AIS), Male DSD (Testicular Feminization Syndrome)

Male DSD or AIS are genetic males with 46XY karyotype having female-like appearance of the external genitalia. They are inherited as X-linked recessive conditions and present mainly in two forms: complete and partial (Fig. 79.4). In the complete variety, the external genitalia look like normal female.

Partial androgen insensitivity is the result of partial resistance at the level of the androgen receptor. This leads to suboptimal response to androgens, subsequently affecting the development of external genitalia and also interferes with the descent of the testis. Patients with this disorder present with severe hypospadias often associated with undescended testis (Fig. 79.5a–c). A Quigley grade of severity from grade 1 to 6 (masculine to feminine appearance) can be applied.

Complete androgen insensitivity syndrome (CAIS) leads to complete feminization of the

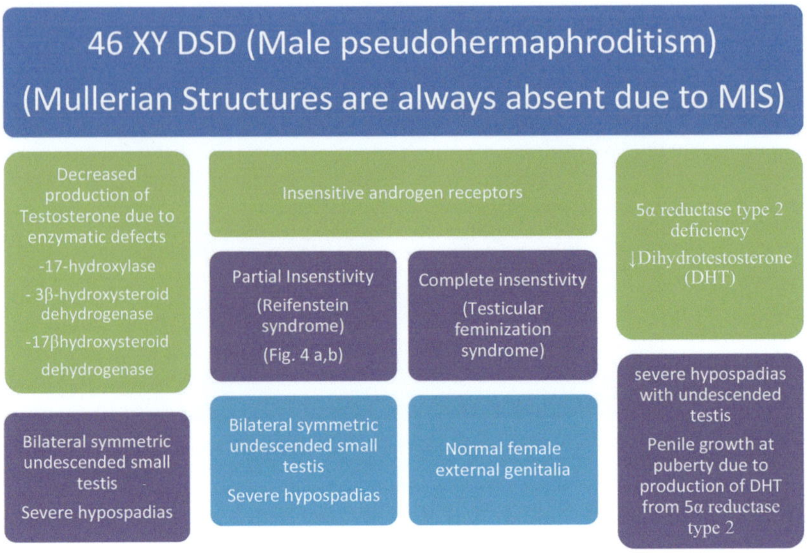

Fig. 79.4 Types and clinical features of various types of 46XY DSD. (MIS—Mullerian inhibiting substance)

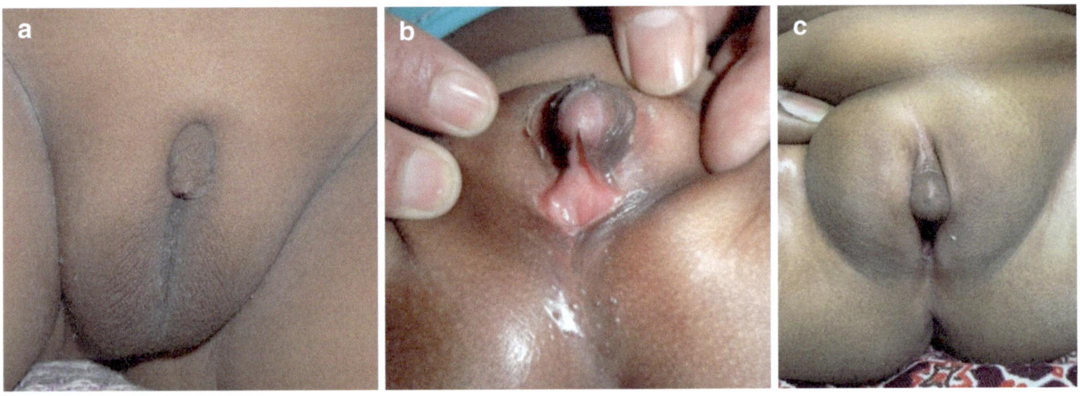

Fig. 79.5 46 XY DSD. (**a**) Micropenis. (**b**) Perineal hypospadias. (**c**) Both testis descended (AIS)

external genitalia into a normal female, and they present at the time of puberty with amenorrhea or a hernia containing testis in the hernia sac.

Evaluation should include karyotype, hormonal assays, pelvic ultrasound, urethrovaginogram and gonadal biopsy in some cases. The gene encoding androgen receptor protein is located on X chromosome (Xq11–12) and can be detected in gonadal/genital skin fibroblast biopsy. Due to the presence of MIS from the testis, these patients will never have menstruation or bear children as they do not have uterus or fallopian tube. These children have intra-abdominal testes; hence, malignant degeneration and chances of developing germ cell tumors of the gonads are increased (20–30%). Early gonadectomy is advised in these children to decrease the possible risk of malignancy and avoid the latter psychological trauma to the older child. However, survillence and delayed orchidectomy has its own advantage of pubertal breast development due to the production of estrogen from aromatization of high level of testosterone. They require hormonal replacement therapy (estrogen) and vaginal reconstruction later in life.

79.4.2 5α Reductase Deficiency:

A close differential diagnosis is 5α reductase type 2 (converts testosterone into dihydrotestosterone) deficiency (Fig. 79.4). The gene responsible for the deficient production of 5α reductase (SRD5A2) is located on chromosome 2p23 (ref1). However, as the Sertoli cells are intact and they produce MIS which prevents the formation of Mullerian structures. So phenotypically these babies have micropenis, bifid scrotum with testes as gonad, rudimentary vagina and can be reared as male with hormonal replacement therapy (androgens). Evaluation should include clinical genital ambiguity, karyotype, hormonal assays (increased testosterone-to-DHT ratio after HCG stimulation), pelvic ultrasound, urethrovaginogram and gonadal biopsy in some cases. Genetic evaluation includes molecular analysis of SRD5A2 gene to establish the diagnosis of 5-alpha reductase type 2 deficiency in children having abnormal hormonal assays.

Once diagnosed, these babies should be preferably reared as males as they virilize near puberty and will need genital reconstructive procedures along with testosterone supplementation. Those who are reared as girls will need feminizing genitoplasty, estrogen supplementation and rarely vaginoplasty.

46 XX male or De la Chapelle syndrome is a rare disorder with 90% being SRY positive. They usually present in adulthood with small testis, infertility, occasional gynaecomastia and hypergonadotropic hypogonadism. In vitro fertilization with a sperm donor is the fertility option for these patients.

79.5 Disorders of Gonadal Dysgenesis

79.5.1 Mixed Gonadal Dysgenesis

Mixed gonadal dysgenesis (MGD) is another form of DSD in which there is a streak gonad on one side and a palpable dysgenetic testis on the other side. The chromosomal abnormality is 45XO/46 XY mosaicism. These children have ambiguous genitalia comprising a small phallus with significant chordae. Vaginal and urethral openings may also be seen often, either separately or with wide meatus urogenital sinus. On one side, a testis may be palpable which is often dysgenetic, and the other side being a streak is never palpable (Fig. 79.6). Histologically, the dysgenetic testis might show pre-pubertal tubules lined by a few spermatogonia and immature Sertoli cells. Most of the time, female gender assignment is preferred, but in case of extreme virilization, male assignment is an alternative approach. Presence of a Y chromosome or a translocated fragment in the dysgenetic gonads poses a significant risk of developing malignant gonadoblastoma (though seminoma and dysgerminoma can occur). The risk is very high in children with pure gonadal dysgenesis, and hence, bilateral gonadectomy should be done at an early age. The child to be raised as a female will need clitoral recession and vaginoplasty in early infancy. If the child has to be raised as male, then various types of hypospadias repair can be done, gonads can be replaced with prostheses, the prepenile scrotum reconstructed and Müllerian structures removed. They should be screened for Wilms' tumor and has a high association with Denys-Drash syndrome.

Complete gonadal dysgenesis with 46 XY karyotype, also known as Swyer syndrome, is externally female with bilateral streak gonads. Treatment is early gonadectomy with hormonal replacement therapy.

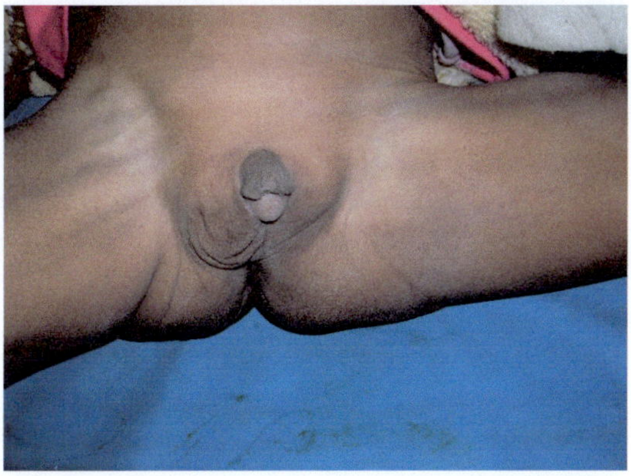

Fig. 79.6 Mixed gonadal dysgenesis (note asymmetric gonad)

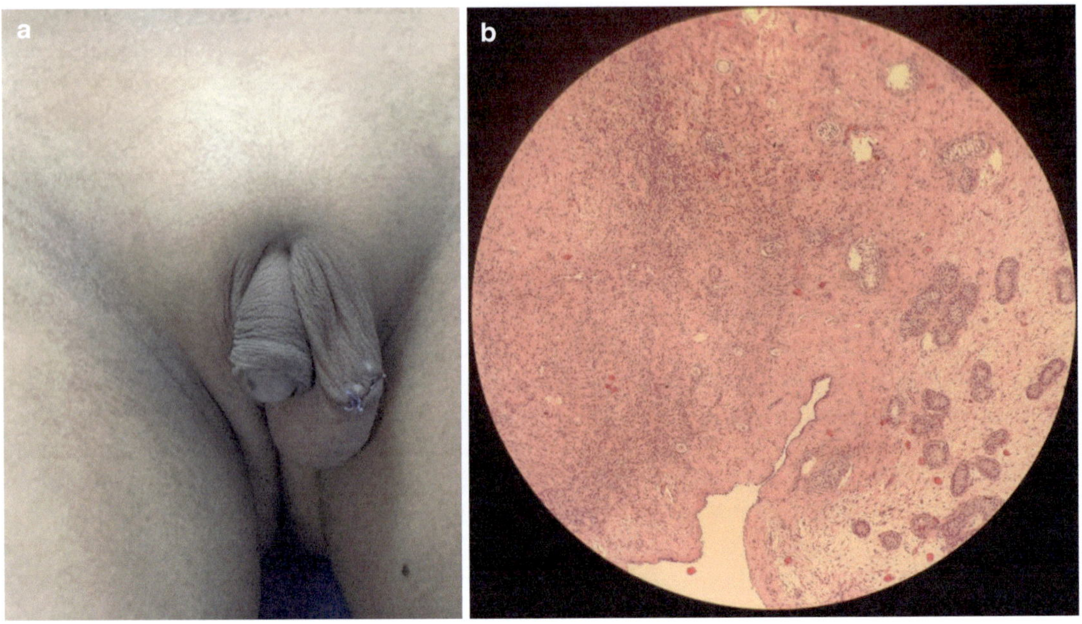

Fig. 79.7 (**a**) Ovotesticular DSD, gonadal biopsy taken. (**b**) Photomicrograph of ovotestis

79.6 Ovotesticular DSD (True Hermaphrodite)

These patients have both testicular and ovarian tissue. A few of the suggested etiologies are fusion of the two zygotes which were formed from two haploid ova early in the development, fertilization of an ovum by two sperm and SRY gene mutation. The most common configuration is of an ovary on one side and an ovotestis on the other side. The ovotestis is usually palpable, and the degree of descent is proportional to the testicular tissue in the gonad. Other gonadal combinations like bilateral ovotestis or ovotestis on one side and streak on other side are also possible. The mullerian structures ovary and fallopian tube on the side of the testicular tissue are regressed but are retained on the other side along with a midline uterus. A urogenital sinus defect is present along with a hypertrophied clitoris. The phenotype depends on the amount of testicular tissue and shifts more toward a male phenotype when the quantity of testicular tissue increases. The karyotype is usually 46,XX (74%), but 46,XX/XY (19%) and 46,XY (6%) are also seen. For the confirmation of the ovotesticular DSD, a laparoscopic visualization of internal genitalia and a gonadal biopsy is recommended. Biopsy of an ovotestis should be performed by opening the gonad widely and taking a deep biopsy as the testicular tissue is central and ovarian tissue is polar (Fig. 79.7). After biopsy report, corrective surgery including repair of hypospadias, orchidopexy and removal of ovarian tissue is done for true hermaphrodites raised as males. Hermaphrodites raised as females undergo clitoroplasty, vaginoplasty and removal of testicular tissue. Testicular tumors like seminomas, gonadoblastomas and dysgerminomas have been described but as the incidence is low (2.6–4.6%), and therefore, gonadectomy is rarely indicated.

79.7 Persistent Müllerian Duct Syndrome

This is an autosomal recessive disorder which is characterized by the presence of Mullerian structures (uterus, fallopian tubules, and upper 2/3 of vagina) in a phenotypic and genetic male. This disorder is caused by the absence of Mullerian inhibiting substance (MIS) or insensitivity of its

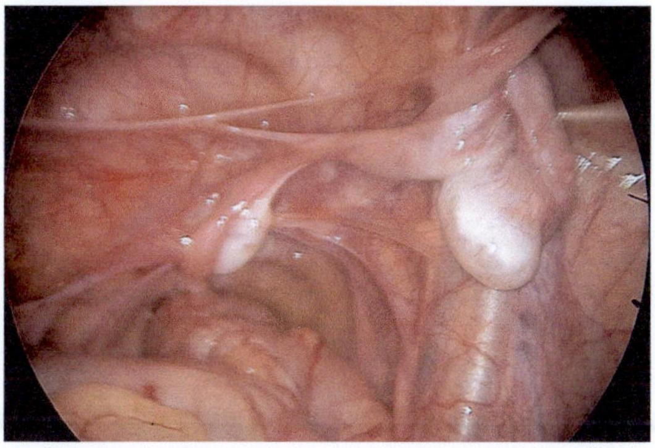

Fig. 79.8 Laparoscopic view of PMDS, note bilateral intra-abdominal testis with uterus, fallopian tubes and upper vagina

receptors. Mutations of the AMH gene (19p13) or AMHR2 (13q12) gene are the main causative factors for PMDS. The patients may present in the following three forms:

- Female form (10–20%): bilateral undescended gonads located in the pelvis on either side in the broad ligament
- Male form (80–90%):
  1. Hernia uteri inguinalis: One testis is located in the hernia sac along with fallopian tubules and/or uterus
  2. Transverse testicular ectopia: Both the testes along with Mullerian remnants are located in the hernial sac on one side.

These children often present with hernia or undescended testis, and the Mullerian structures are an intra-operative surprise. In the era of laparoscopy, these abnormalities are more often diagnosed with findings of bilateral intra-abdominal testis with uterus, fallopian tubes and upper vagina often ending at the prostatic urethra (Fig. 79.8). The current management recommendation is excision of Mullerian remnants with careful preservation of vas deferens and orchidopexy. The uterus may be split in the middle, and the removal of the endometrial by coring is done, avoiding dissection on the outer wall to prevent any injury to the vas deferens or testicular blood supply. Malignancies have been reported from the uterine segment. Often staged orchidopexy (2-stage Fowler-Stephens) is needed.

79.8 Principles of Diagnosis and Management of DSD

- A multidisciplinary approach with geneticists, neonatologists, pediatric and adult endocrinologists, gynecologists, pediatric surgeons/urologists, psychologists, ethicists and social workers.
- Goal of DSD treatment is the long-term physical, psychological and sexual well-being of the patient ("Patient-centered"). Late-onset gender dysphoria can be troublesome.
- When recognized in the neonatal period, the situation should be explained to the parents fully and kindly. Registering and naming the newborn should be delayed as long as necessary.
- As most of the parents don't accept the possibility of infertility, possible fertility preservation in conditions like CAH and ovotesticular DSD has to be explained to parents.
- Details of external appearance and sexual function should also be explained to the parents.

79.8.1 Various Components of Female Genitoplasty

As most of these children have clitoral hypertrophy, fusion of labia majora, absent labia minora and a common urogenital sinus, so they need either one or all of the following procedures for female genital reconstruction:

- **Panendoscopy**: Better visualization of the confluence and urethrovaginal anatomy.
- **Clitoroplasty** (Fig. 79.9a and b)—Clitoroplasty has evolved over the years through these phases:

  Clitorectomy—Leads to loss of sensation and orgasm on tactile stimulation

  ↓

  Clitoral recession—Maintains sensations but enlargement during orgasm causes pain.

Clitoral reduction—Most preferred technique involves resection of the corpora with preservation of neurovascular bundles.

Corpora preserving clitoroplasty (Pippi Salle)—This technique involves dissection of corpora from glans, division into two halves and fixation on either side of the labia and covered with clitoral prepuce to make labia minora.

- **Repair of Urogenital Sinus**

  Low confluence UG sinus—Only limited posterior vaginal wall mobilization is enough to restore the perineal anatomy (Fig. 79.10a–c).

  High confluence UG sinus—Total or partial urogenital sinus mobilization (TUM/PUM)

1. Total urogenital mobilization (Fig. 79.11a)—The urogenital sinus is mobilized circumferentially till the pubourethral ligament on the anterior aspect and posterior to the vaginal

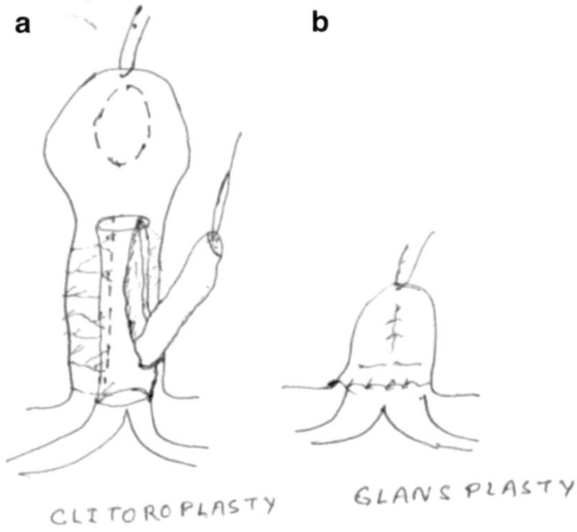

Fig. 79.9 (**a**) Excision of erectile tissue with the incision marking for the glansplasty. (**b**) Completed glansplasty and clitoroplasty

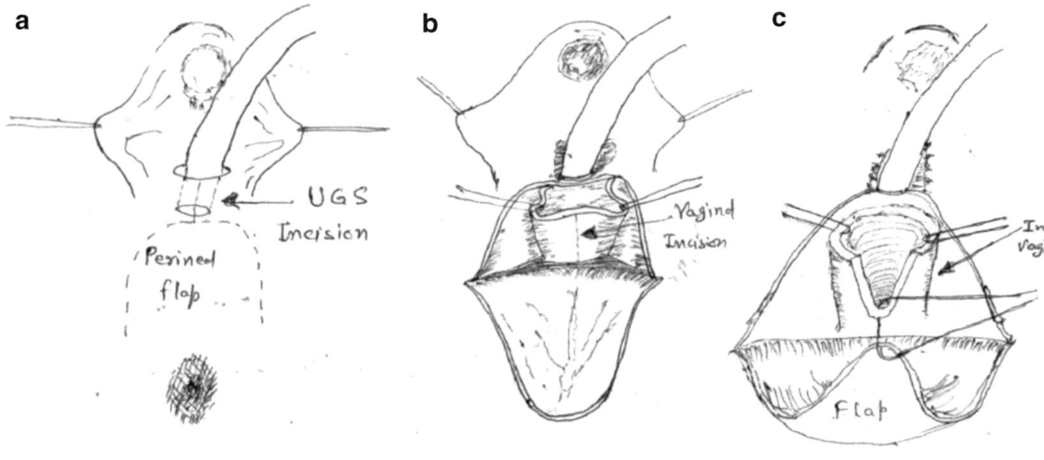

Fig. 79.10 Flap vaginoplasty. (**a**) Inverted perineal U-shaped flap based on the anus. (**b**) Vaginal dissection with outlining of back wall incision. (**c**) Inverted U-shaped flap sutured to the back wall of vagina

wall on the posterior aspect so that the entire unit moves outwards.

2. Partial urogenital mobilization (Fig. 79.11b)—The UG sinus is mobilized till the pubourethral ligament.
3. The excess UG sinus can be used to make mucosa-lined vestibule, or enhance the lower vaginal wall (Fig. 79.12a–d).

- *Labioplasty*

  The labioscrotal skin is used in the form of Y-V advancement flaps, and these flaps are placed on both the lateral side of UG sinus and sutured to the labia minora (made from clitoral hood) medially (Fig. 79.13a and b).

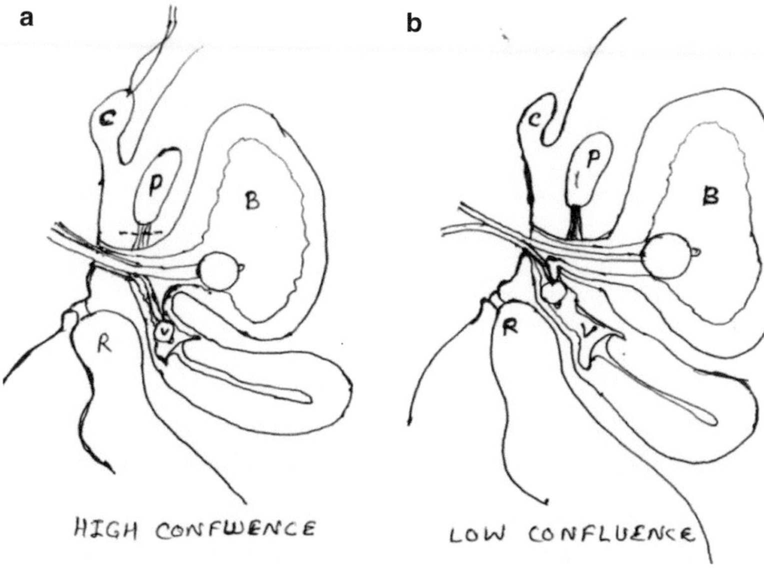

Fig. 79.11 (**a**) Total urogenital sinus mobilization; Mobilization of the UG sinus beyond the pubourethral ligament. (**b**) Partial urogenital sinus mobilization; circumferential mobilization of UG sinus stops at the pubourethral ligament. B—Bladder, V—Vagina, R—Rectum, C- —Clitoris, P—Pubic bone

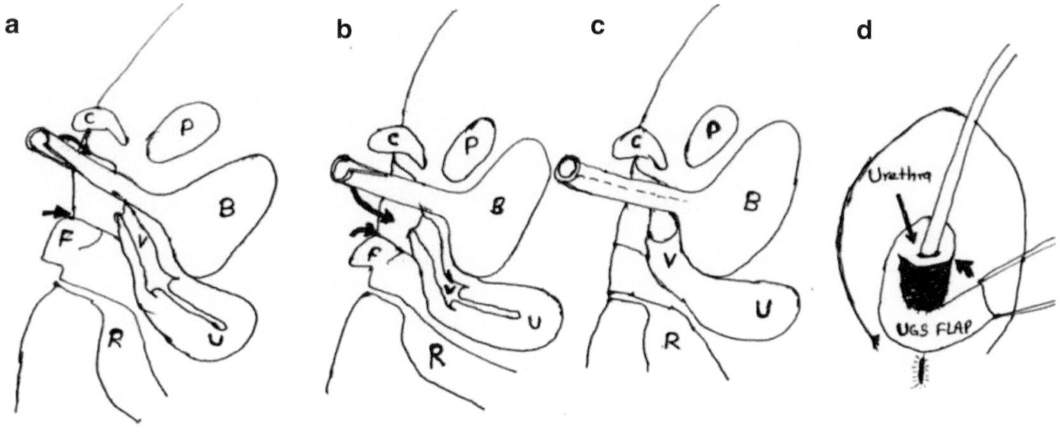

Fig. 79.12 Redundant UG sinus. (**a**) Split ventrally to make mucosa-lined vestibule. (**b**) Split dorsally to create a flap to enhance the anterior half of the vagina. (**c** and **d**) Split laterally to rotate and extend the vagina and completing the vaginoplasty

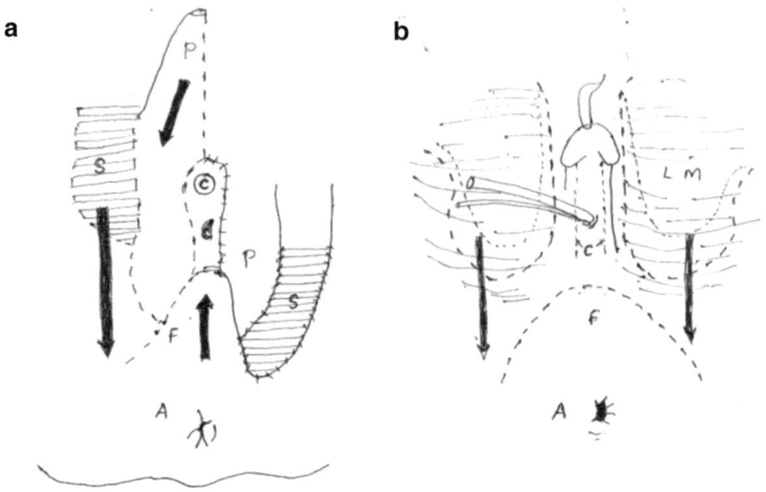

Fig. 79.13 (**a**) Clitoral prepuce split to create labia minora, labia majora Y-V plasty, flap vaginoplasty. (**b**) Bilateral Y-V plasty to create labia majora, flaps moved posteriorly to enhance vaginoplasty, medial aspects of skin flaps are sutured to the lateral aspect of preputial skin (now labia minora). C—Clitoris; P—Split prepuce; S—Labioscrotal fold; F—Flaps; LM—Labia Minora; A—Anus

- *Vaginal replacement is generally recommended after 10 years of age*
- *Removal of testicular tissue*

79.8.2 Various Components of Male Genitoplasty

- Orchidopexy
- Hypospadias repair
- Repair of penoscrotal transposition
- Removal of ovarian tissue
- Removal of Mullerian structures

Some patients may need hormonal (testosterone) replacement at puberty to help the development of secondary sexual characteristics.

79.9 Summary

79.9.1 Diagnosis of DSD

The following conditions merit work-up for DSD

- Genital ambiguity
- Female genitalia with palpable gonad/clitoromegaly or posterior fusion of labia minora
- Male genitalia with micropenis, severe hypospadias and hypospadias with undescended testis.
- Older patients with delayed/incomplete puberty, virilization in females, primary amenorrhea, gynaecomastia in males.

Common Principles in the Diagnosis of DSD

- CAH should be suspected in every case with ambiguous genitalia and non-palpable gonads. Plasma 17-hydroxy progesterone (17-OHP) is raised in CAH due to an enzymatic block. It is a useful marker for diagnosis and monitoring the response to treatment.

Position of the gonads should be observed carefully on clinical examination. Gonads are considered asymmetric if one gonad is above, and the other is below the superficial inguinal ring. If both gonads are present above or below the superficial inguinal ring, then they are called symmetric (Table 79.2).

Table 79.2 Rapid diagnosis of common DSD disorders

	Y chromosome present	Y chromosome absent
Symmetrical gonads	46XY DSD	46XX DSD
Asymmetrical gonads	Mixed gonadal dysgenesis (MGD)	True hermaphrodite (ovotesticular DSD)

79.9.2 Standard Investigations for the Diagnosis of DSD

- Pelvic ultrasonography—to look for gonads and Mullerian structures
- Karyotype
- Study for gene mutation for a specific type of DSD
- Genitogram—retrograde contrast study through the apparent urethral opening
- MRI pelvis—for Mullerian structures
- Diagnostic laparoscopy

In addition to the standard karyotyping, a rapid diagnosis can also be made by clinical examination along with determination of Y chromosome by PCR (polymerase chain reaction) or FISH (fluorescent in situ hybridization) test.

79.9.3 Summary of Treatment of DSD Due to CAH

Congenital adrenal hyperplasia (CAH) is managed well with oral hydrocortisone with or without fludrocortisone which may need to continue lifelong to counter the hormonal imbalance. Mild form of clitoromegaly reverses with medical management. Female gender assignment is the rule. In cases with severe masculinization, clitoroplasty and repair of the urogenital sinus are needed. Surgical reconstruction may be delayed until puberty to observe the response to medical treatment and a better gender identity.

79.10 Principles of Sex Assignment

Parental and patient preference should be carefully considered. It is preferable to delay the surgical genital reconstruction, if possible, till the patient can give valid consent. Early surgery should be restricted to emergency situations like relief of urinary obstruction. Both the patient and the gender assignment medical team should agree with the decision of surgical genital reconstruction. In mild to moderately virilized children, surgery should be avoided as they can be managed medically. Similarly, removal of gonads or genital mutilation should be avoided. Possibility of redo surgery should also be considered and explained to the parents.

Suggested Reading

Docimo SG, Canning D, Khoury A, Salle JLP, editors. The Kelalis-King-Belman textbook of clinical pediatric urology. 6th ed. CRC Press; 2018.

Kirtane J, Ravikumar VR. Disorders of sexual differentiation. In: Redkar R, Agarwal P, Raveenthiran V, Gosavi SJ, Bangar A, editors. IAPS textbook of pediatric surgery. 1st ed. Jaypee Brothers Medical Publishers; 2020.

Partin AW, Dmochowski RR, Kavoussi LR, Peters CA, Wein AJ, editors. Campbell-Walsh-Wein urology. 12th ed. Elsevier; 2020.

Ramsay M, Bernstein R, Zwane E, Page DC, Jenkins T. XX true hermaphroditism in Southern African blacks: an enigma of primary sexual differentiation. Am J Hum Genet. 1998;43(1):4–13.

Thigpen AE, Davis DL, Milatovich A, Mendonca BB, Imperato-McGinley J, Griffin JE, Francke U, Wilson JD, Russell DW. Molecular genetics of steroid 5 alpha-reductase 2 deficiency. J Clin Invest. 1992;90(3):799–809.

Van Niekerk WA, Retief AE. The gonads of human true hermaphrodites. Hum Genet. 1981;58(1):117–22.

Ovarian and Genital Disorders in Girls

80

Subhasis Roy Choudhury and Rajiv Chadha

80.1 Ovarian Cysts

Ovarian cysts are not uncommon in the neonatal period, and small (follicle) cysts are present in approximately 90% of newborn females. These cysts occur in response to maternal estrogens, and in 20–30% of cases, the cyst may be more than 1 cm in diameter. The cysts usually resolve gradually after birth as the gonadotrophin levels reach prepubertal levels by 2–3 years of age. Complex ovarian cysts are identified on ultrasonography (US) by a multi-septate appearance which is most commonly due to bleeding into the cyst or torsion.

80.2 Management of Ovarian Cysts

The management of ovarian cysts depends on the age at presentation, size of the cyst, and US findings including echogenicity of the cyst's contents. Most simple ovarian cysts in neonates can be managed expectantly with periodic observation and US scanning.

S. Roy Choudhury
Pediatric Surgery, Lady Hardinge Medical College and Associated Kalawati Saran Children's Hospital, New Delhi, Delhi, India

R. Chadha (✉)
Department of Pediatric Surgery, Lady Hardinge Medical College and Kalawati Saran Children's Hospital, New Delhi, Delhi, India

80.2.1 Simple Cysts

- Cysts less than 2 cm in diameter are not considered pathological.
- Cysts 2–5 cm in size can be managed by close follow-up with periodic US scanning.
- Cysts more than 5 cm should be considered for intervention due to the higher risk of torsion of the cyst and ovary. Although simple aspiration of the cyst is an option, fenestration of the cyst (either laparoscopically or open) is preferred to reduce the risk of recurrence.

Complex ovarian cysts carry the risk of bleeding, rupture of the cyst, and intestinal obstruction. Thus, these patients merit cystectomy, usually performed laparoscopically, with preservation of maximal ovarian tissue.

80.2.2 Ovarian Cyst in a Prepubertal Child

Ovarian cysts are very uncommon (2–3%) during the prepubertal period as gonadotrophin, and estradiol levels are very low. A single cyst of less than 1 cm can be considered non-pathological but a larger cyst needs evaluation. Presence of precocious puberty should be ruled out.

Cysts can be managed conservatively if (i) the cyst is clearly of ovarian origin, (ii) the cyst is not complex, (iii) serum ß-HCG and alpha-fetoprotein (AFP) levels are normal, and (iv) there are no sig-

© The Author(s), under exclusive license to Springer Nature Singapore Pte Ltd. 2025

S. Roy Choudhury (ed.), *Pediatric Surgery*, https://doi.org/10.1007/978-981-96-1257-4_80

nificant symptoms. The cyst usually undergoes significant spontaneous resolution over a 3–6 month time period. In the absence of spontaneous resolution, active intervention is warranted.

The goal of active intervention is to resolve the symptoms and risks of the cyst with maximal preservation of normal ovarian tissue. Simple ovarian cysts can usually be managed easily by cystectomy or fenestration. Complex cysts merit cystectomy or oophorectomy (as differentiation from mature teratoma is difficult). A laparoscopic approach is usually employed.

80.3 Ovarian Cysts in Adolescence

Ovarian cysts are very common in adolescent girls. The usual cause is 'dysfunctional ovulation' with persistence of the remaining follicle. Usually, these cysts are simple and filled with fluid. Another cause is a persistent corpus luteum. Complex cysts merit surgery as differentiation from teratomas is frequently difficult. The operative management is similar to that of an ovarian cyst in the prepubertal period.

80.3.1 Ovarian Torsion

Ovarian torsion is an uncommon condition resulting from partial or complete twisting of the ovarian pedicle on its axis causing congestion of the ovary, vascular compromise, and hemorrhagic infarction with necrosis (Fig. 80.1a). It is a known complication of ovarian cysts and is a surgical emergency as delay in diagnosis and management can lead to necrosis with loss of the ovary. Most girls present with a sudden onset of lower abdominal pain, nausea and vomiting, and low-grade fever. This presentation is quite similar to that of acute appendicitis. Although ovarian torsion can occur at any age, it is most frequently diagnosed in prepubertal girls. US with or without Doppler is the most feasible diagnostic modality, and the most consistent finding is of an echogenic solid mass with peripheral cysts in the pelvis along with non-visualization of the ipsilateral ovary. US also readily differentiates ovarian torsion from acute appendicitis. In neonates with ovarian torsion, US generally shows a cystic mass, confirmed at surgery (Fig. 80.1b), while a prepubertal child may have a complex mass on

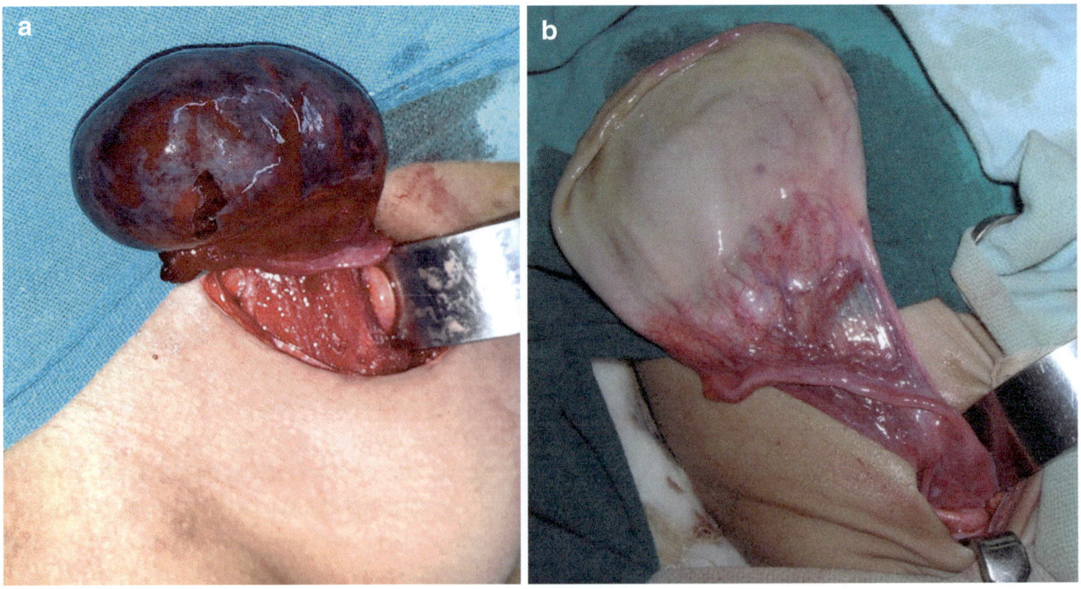

Fig. 80.1 (**a**) Ovarian torsion. (**b**) Twisted ovarian cyst in a neonate

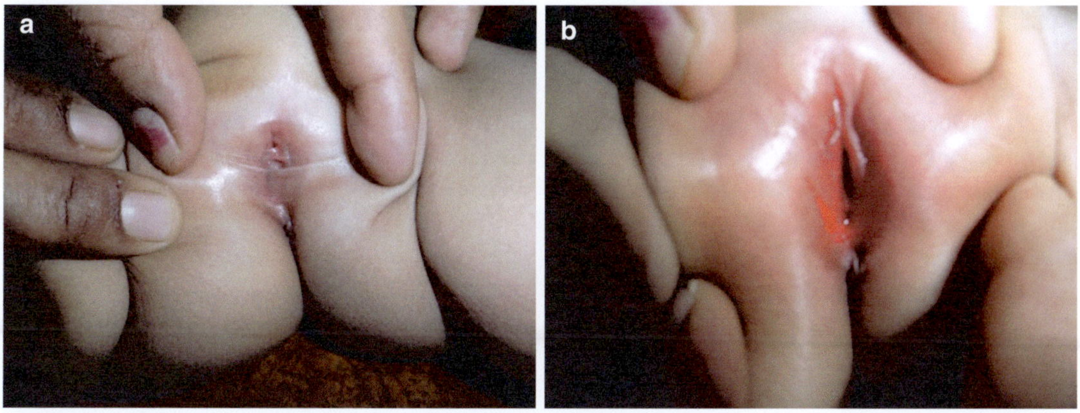

Fig. 80.2 (**a** and **b**) Labial adhesions, before and after separation

US. Color-Doppler US is useful to confirm the absence of ovarian blood flow in torsion, although the presence of vascular flow does not completely rule out ovarian torsion. In some cases, an emergency CT scan may be required to clarify the nature of the mass. Management is by either laparoscopic or open surgical exploration. The removal of a mass carrying a twisted ovary is recommended therapy, although a more conservative approach consisting of detorsion with or without cystectomy is an option as normal ovarian function has been reported after up to 72 h of torsion. Detorsion and observation in case of absence of a mass (normal ovaries) is an accepted mode of treatment. Contralateral oophoropexy in cases of torsion of normal adnexa is advisable.

80.3.2 Labial Adhesions in Infants

Labial adhesions or synechiae are a relatively common pediatric gynecologic problem seen most frequently in young girls, usually between 1 and 2 years of age. This condition can occasionally be confused with imperforate hymen or absence of the vagina and can cause a great degree of parental anxiety. Labial adhesions may relate to low estrogen levels and are rare in neonates who are likely protected by maternal estrogens. Local inflammation or irritation caused by diaper rash or other causes of vulvar dermatitis, trauma, and sexual abuse may also result in labial adhesions. A small opening near the clitoris allows urine to escape, and difficulty in micturition is infrequent. Other relatively rare symptoms include recurrent urinary tract infections (UTI) and wetting of the undergarments due to pooling of urine in the vestibule once the child gets up after voiding urine.

Asymptomatic patients may be managed by a 'wait and watch' approach. If treatment is required, daily local application of estrogen vaginal cream (0.1%) for 2 weeks is usually effective. Manual separation using an artery forceps or even the nozzle of an ointment tube is also a simple and effective minor out-patient department (OPD) procedure (Fig. 80.2a and b). In some cases, adhesions may recur, and treatment may need to be repeated. More aggressive management is not recommended unless the urethral meatus is covered. Prolonged use of estrogen cream can occasionally cause precocious sexual development and should be discouraged.

80.4 Vaginal Conditions

80.4.1 Mayer-Rokitansky-Küster-Hauser Syndrome (MRKH Syndrome)

The MRKH syndrome is characterized by an underdeveloped or absent vagina with a rudimentary uterus and normal ovaries, often associated with renal and skeletal abnormalities. The incidence of MRKH syndrome is 1 in 4000–5000 live female births.

80.4.2 Embryology and Pathology

This condition results from the failure of the Müllerian ducts to reach the urogenital sinus during embryonic development. The uterus is usually rudimentary, although rarely, a normal uterus and cervix may be present. The vagina is completely absent in most patients, while a small vaginal pouch may be present in about 20–25% cases. Associated renal abnormalities include renal agenesis or ectopia. Skeletal abnormalities most commonly involve the spinal vertebrae, although limb or rib defects have also been reported.

80.4.3 Presentation

- Primary amenorrhea noticed by age 16 years
- At puberty, lower abdominal pain may occur due to bleeding in the rudimentary uterus in response to hormones
- Absent vaginal opening noticed in the prepubertal period
- A rare presentation is rectovestibular fistula with vaginal agenesis

It is essential to differentiate this condition from complete androgen insensitivity syndrome (CAIS) which may have a similar presentation (Table 80.1).

Table 80.1 Differences between MRKH syndrome and CAIS

Features	MRKH syndrome	CAIS
Karyotype	46XX	46XY
Vaginal opening	Absent in most	Present in most
Uterus and ovary	Present	Both absent
Testis and testosterone	Absent	Present
Associated renal/skeletal defects	Present	Absent
Pubic hair at puberty	Present	Absent

80.4.4 Treatment

MRKH syndrome is best managed during the post-pubertal period when the presence and functional status of the uterus can be easily ascertained by imaging and other studies. A pull-through vaginoplasty can be considered in the presence of a uterus with cervix and proximal vagina. In other patients, hormones can suppress the rudimentary uterus, and a neo-vagina can be created with a bowel segment. In recent years, a uterine transplant has emerged as a possible treatment for infertility associated with the condition.

80.4.5 Imperforate Hymen

In newborn girls, the primary caretaker should inspect the external genitalia at birth to rule out an anatomical genital abnormality such as imperforate hymen [IH] (Fig. 80.3). In this uncommon condition, the hymen may completely obstruct the vaginal opening and result in retention of uterine and vaginal secretions. Several anatomical variations of IH exist, including microperforate, cribriform, or septate hymen (Fig. 80.4), and these variants often allow egress of secretions and blood. IH may occasionally present in newborns with a mass due to hydrocolpos or hydrometrocolpos (Fig. 80.5) due to obstruction of

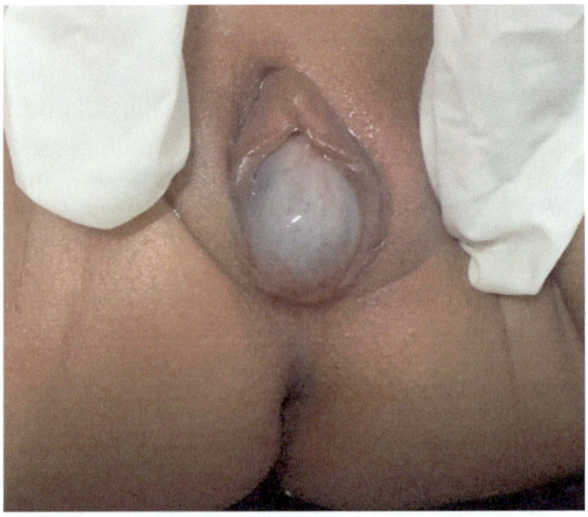

Fig. 80.3 Imperforate hymen in a new born

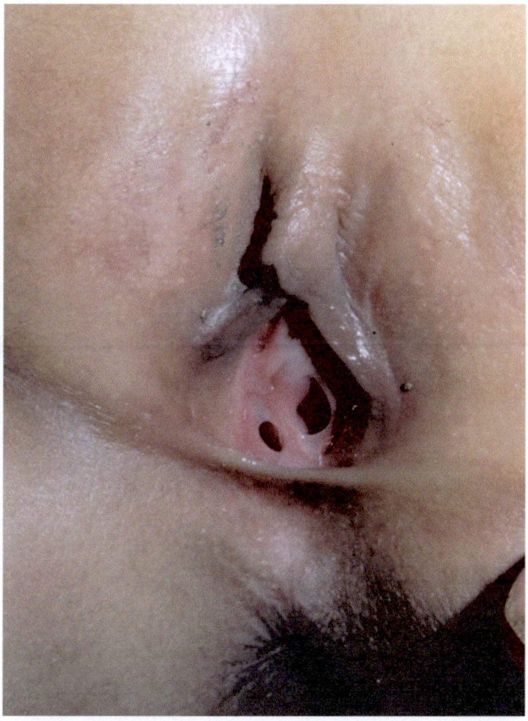

Fig. 80.4 Septate hymenal membrane

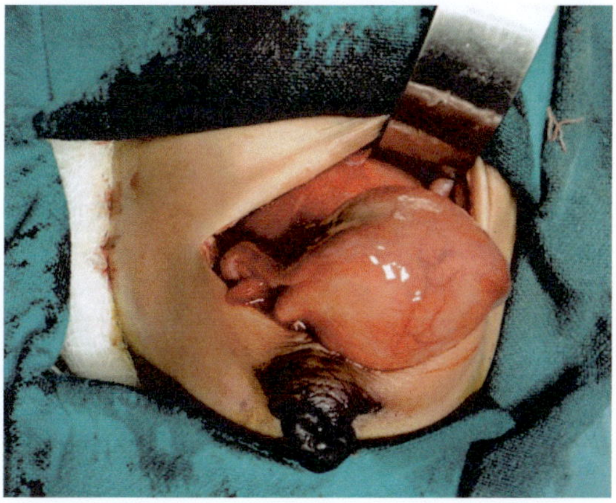

Fig. 80.5 Hydrocolpos due to persistent cloaca with vaginal obstruction

fetal secretions resulting from maternal estrogens. In these instances, it can often be picked up by antenatal or postnatal US. Infants and adolescent girls may present with recurrent UTI or an abdominal mass due to hydrometrocolpos. Most cases are diagnosed at puberty with amenorrhea, recurrent abdominal pain, or urinary retention. A careful genital examination with abdominopelvic US is diagnostic. Newborns with IH need immediate surgical intervention, but in older asymptomatic patients, surgical treatment should be deferred until puberty when the estrogen surge will help to minimize the risk of scarring and recurrence of obstruction that may occur with early surgical incision in a low estrogenic environment. A cruciate incision of the hymen has a high risk of recurrence, and removal of an elliptical piece of excess hymenal tissue is preferred.

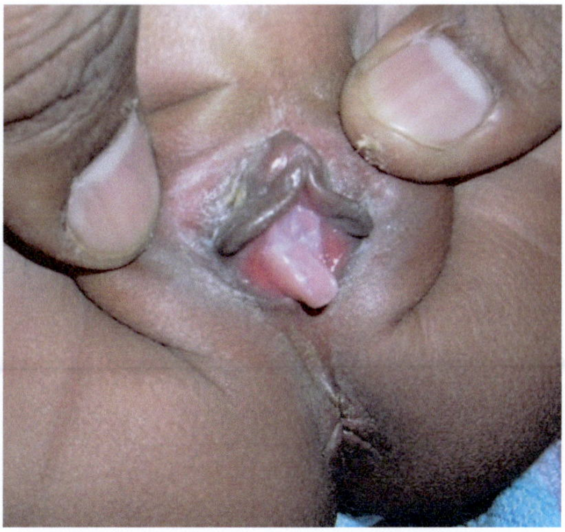

Fig. 80.6 Hymenal tag

Hymenal tag often presents as a protruding mass in newborn and infant girls (Fig. 80.6) and can cause significant parental anxiety. This is a simple, benign condition, and management requires observation with reassurance to the family.

80.5 Vaginal Septation

A *septate vagina* is a congenital abnormality where the vagina is divided, completely or partially, into two vaginal canals by a septum (Fig. 80.7). Vaginal septation by a longitudinal septum may be noticed only at adolescence when the patient starts to use tampons or engage in sexual activity. This type of septate vagina may be associated with other urogenital anomalies like persistent cloaca and is present in approximately 6% of girls with a rectovestibular fistula.

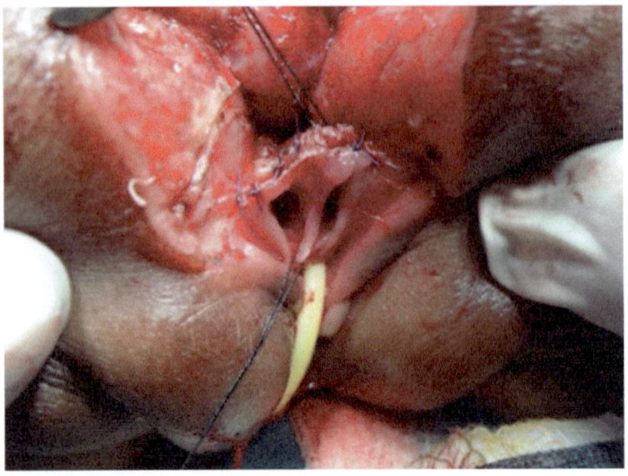

Fig. 80.7 Septate vagina

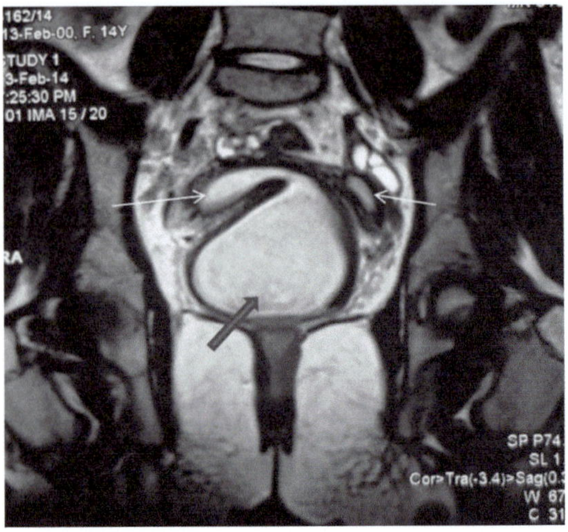

Fig. 80.8 OHVIRA syndrome. White arrows point to uteri and broad arrow, obstructed hemivagina

In congenital pouch colon (CPC), a septate/double vagina is always present along with a unicornuate uterus on each side in the pelvis. Physical examination including endoscopy is diagnostic. Most patients have 2 cervices. Surgical resection of the septum can be easily performed in the presence of complications such as dyspareunia or for the safe delivery of a baby.

Transverse vaginal septum is a congenital abnormality in which a horizontal 'wall' of tissue blocks the vagina. The septum blocks the passage of vaginal secretions causing primary amenorrhea and can produce hematocolpos and cyclic pelvic pain. Although the septum is most commonly located in the upper vagina, it can occur at many different levels in the vagina and can also vary in thickness. Physical examination along with pelvic US is diagnostic. Surgical resection of the septum, usually performed after menarche, is the recommended treatment. Postoperative dilation may be necessary to prevent re-stenosis and dyspareunia. Early diagnosis and surgical correction to drain accumulated blood from the vagina may restore fertility.

80.6 OHVIRA Syndrome

The OHVIRA syndrome consists of uterus didelphys, unilateral low vaginal obstruction due to a vaginal septum (Fig. 80.8), and ipsilateral renal agenesis or dysplastic kidney, all three components being secondary to mesonephric duct-induced Müllerian anomalies. Treatment invariably requires surgical intervention in the form of excision of vaginal septum to relieve obstruction and if present, removal of the dysplastic kidney with its ureter.

80.7 Vaginal Bleeding

Vaginal bleeding in the premenstrual female infant is a not uncommon and is distressing for patients and their families. Differential diagnosis of vaginal bleeding in this age group includes estrogen stimulation, vulvovaginitis or vulvar dermatosis, genital tract tumors, ovarian tumors, foreign bodies, and trauma. Transplacental estrogen stimulation (neonatal withdrawal bleeds) is the commonest cause of vaginal bleeding in newborns during the first 2 weeks after birth and is self-limiting. Poor vulvar hygiene practices can cause vulvovaginitis, the most common gynecological infection in children, due to ascending enteric bacteria and may need management with systemic antibiotics. Condylomas may cause painless vaginal bleeding. Tumors of the genital tract associated with vaginal bleeding include infantile hemangiomas of the vulva or cervix, uterine arteriovenous malformation, rhabdomyosarcoma botryoides (the most common malignant tumor of the lower genital tract in young females), endodermal sinus tumors, and endometrial carcinomas. Functional ovarian or adrenal tumors that produce estrogen such as juvenile granulosa cell tumors of the ovary can cause sexual precocity and vaginal bleeding. A vaginal foreign body is one of the most common causes of prepubertal vaginal bleeding and can produce local inflammation associated with a serosanguineous or foul-smelling discharge. Prolapse of redundant urethral mucosa through the urethral meatus may present as a friable polypoid lesion with bleeding. Childhood sexual abuse with trauma and genital injuries is also an important cause of vaginal bleeding.

80.8 Summary

Simple ovarian cysts in neonates can be managed expectantly. Simple ovarian cysts >5cm in diameter and complex cysts merits surgical intervention. Simple ovarian cysts can usually be managed easily by cystectomy or fenestration. Complex cysts merit cystectomy or oophorectomy. Torsion requires detorsion with or without cystectomy. Labial adhesion is generally managed with gentle separation and sometimes application of a week estrogen cream. MRKH syndrome requires complex surgical reconstruction with vaginal replacement. Vaginal bleeding in new born and infants can be physiological, however, a through examination should be done to exclude any pathological cause.

Suggested Reading

Chadha R, Khan NA, Shah S, Pant P, Gupta A, Roy Choudhury S, Debnath PR, Puri A. Congenital pouch colon in girls: genitourinary abnormalities and their management. J Indian Assoc Pediatr Surg. 2015;20:105–15.

Coran AG, Caldamone A, Scott Adzich N, Krummel TM, Laberge JM, editors. Pediatric surgery. 7th ed. Oxford: Elsevier; 2012.

Redkar R, Agarwal P, Raveenthiran V, Gosavi SJ, Bangar A, editors. IAPS textbook of pediatric surgery. 1st ed. Delhi: Jaypee Brothers Medical Publishers; 2020.

Part XI
Miscellaneous

Conjoined Twins

81

Mehak Sehgal and Prabudh Goel

81.1 Introduction

Conjoined twinning is an anomaly which features two identical twins sharing one or more organs. The condition is very rare, with most antenatally detected cases ending in stillbirths or miscarriages. An incidence of 1:50,000–2,50,000 is described in the literature, with a 3:1 female predominance. A higher incidence has been noted in African countries and Asia. The twins are always of the same sex, but differing personalities. These cases have elicited great fascination historically, and the literature over the years has described improving outcomes. The management has to be customized on a case-by-case basis and is preferably performed at a center with prior expertise. A thorough and planned undertaking by a multidisciplinary team of experts from all relevant fields leads to successful separation with reduced mortality.

81.1.1 Etiopathogenesis

The twinning in this anomaly results from a monoamniotic-monozygotic placentation.

The *'fission' theory* suggests that an incomplete cleavage of the embryonic axis results in conjoined embryogenesis. Kaufman suggested that this form of twinning occurs at the primitive streak stage around 13–14 days after fertilization in humans. Since the twins are symmetrical and often mirror images of each other, this theory very well explains these findings, except for parasitic twins.

The *'fusion' theory*, propagated by Rowena Spencer, proposes that there is a fusion of two separate embryonic disks resulting from a monoovular pregnancy at specific points after initial separation. The location of conjoinment is at vulnerable sites where the ectoderm is absent or disrupted during development. This fusion occurs at specific locations only, resulting in the predetermined types of conjoined twins.

According to the *'spherical'* theory, the embryonic disks are located either in the dorsal-ventral axis or rostro-caudal axis of each other, which explains the three-dimensional angles where the fusion can occur.

After the twinning event, adaptations in the form of division and diversion of the midline anatomical structures and aplasia of the sagittal and lateral structures occur, which leads to accommodation of this conjoinment. Associated anomalies often occur, predominantly in the structures which are joined.

M. Sehgal · P. Goel (✉)
Department of Paediatric Surgery, All India Institute of Medical Sciences, New Delhi, Delhi, India

© The Author(s), under exclusive license to Springer Nature Singapore Pte Ltd. 2025

S. Roy Choudhury (ed.), *Pediatric Surgery*, https://doi.org/10.1007/978-981-96-1257-4_81

81.1.2 Classification

Conjoined twins can be classified as symmetrical and parasitic. The common variety, symmetrical twins are further subclassified based on the site of attachment as described in Fig. 81.1. In dorsal union, each twin carries its own umbilicus and separate abdomen, while in ventral union twins share a single cord and peritoneal cavity. The description of each subtype is further elaborated in Table 81.1.

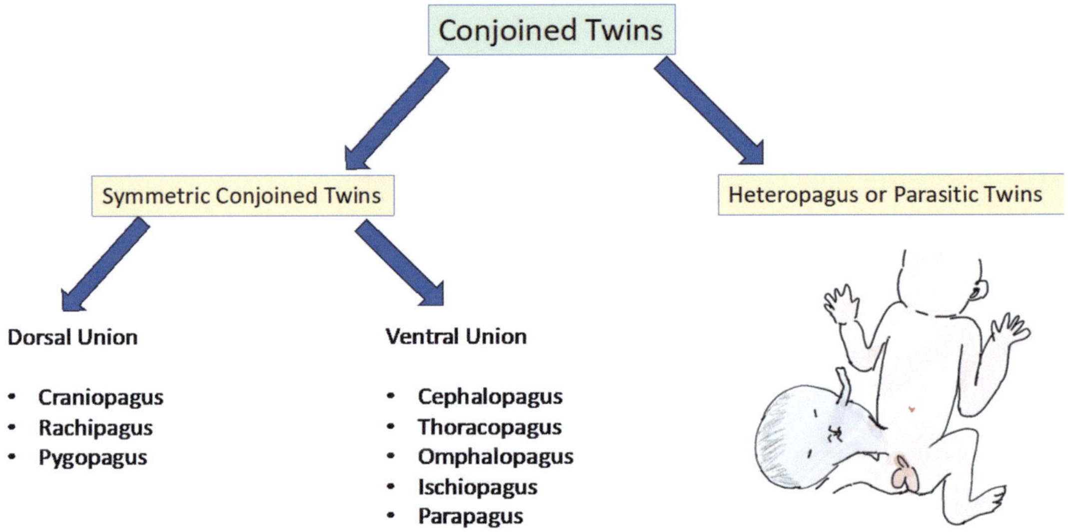

Fig. 81.1 Broad classification of conjoined twins

Table 81.1 Description of the types and charactertics of conjoined twins

Site of attachment (incidence)	Key Features	Figurative representation
1. Cephalopagus (11%)	Conjoined skull and head, fused thorax Common face or two separate faces Trachea, lung, heart separate May share the upper abdomen	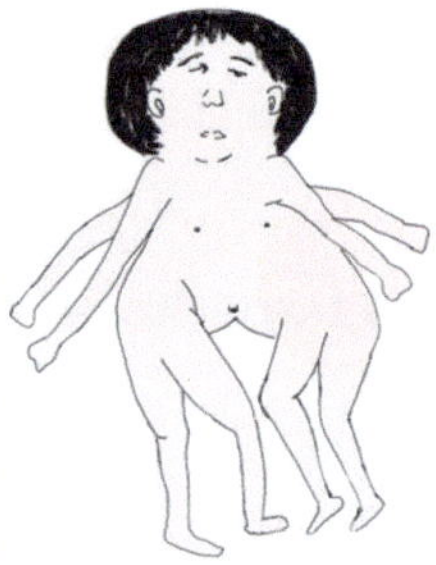
2. Thoracopagus (19%)	Ventral fusion from upper chest to upper abdomen, omphalocoele present Sternum, diaphragm, cardiovascular and liver shared Upper intestine shared in 50% Joined biliary tree in 25% Cardiac defects common	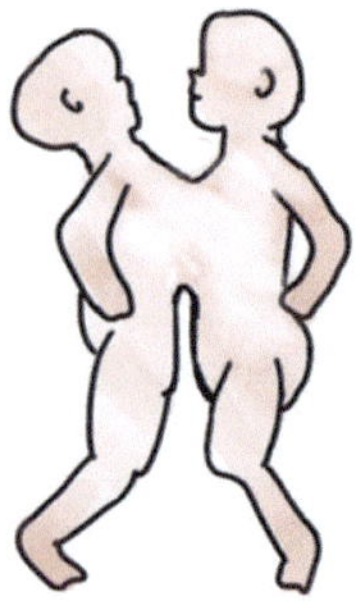

(continued)

Table 81.1 (continued)

Site of attachment (incidence)	Key Features	Figurative representation
3. Omphalopagus (18%)	Joined from lower thorax to groin May have a common pericardium, no sharing of cardia/vessels Omphalocoele present Liver and upper gastrointestinal organs shared Common terminal ileum and colon in 1/3rd	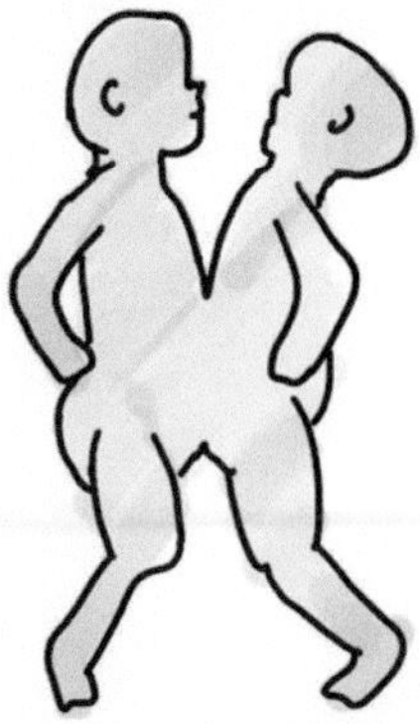
4. Ischiopagus (11%)	Joined primarily at the pelvic bones, cranially may be variably attached till the diaphragm Face to face or Back to back Genitourinary fusion and variable abnormalities Lower gastrointestinal fusion with anorectal malformation Based on number of legs—Bipus, tripus or tetrapus; altered orthopedic anatomy	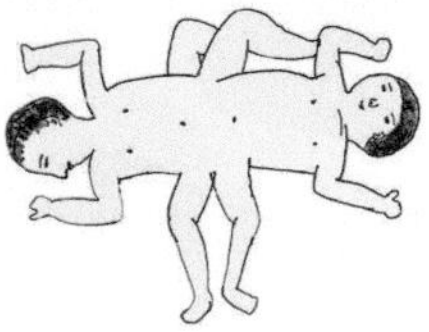
5. Parapagus (28%)	Extensive lateral fusion from diaphragm to pelvis Shared liver, diaphragm, intestine, genitourinary tract Anorectal anomalies common Subtypes based on extent of fusion: Diprosporus, dicephalus, Dithoracis	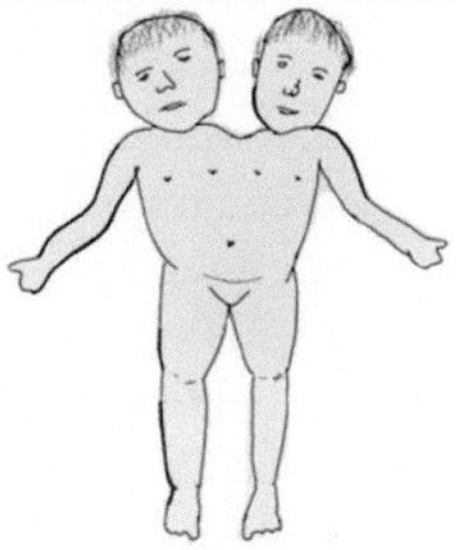
6. Craniopagus (5%)	Shared cranium, meninges, dura Degree of vascular sharing—Predominantly venous Variable cortical sharing Separate foramen magnum, skull base Types: Temporal, parietal or occipital	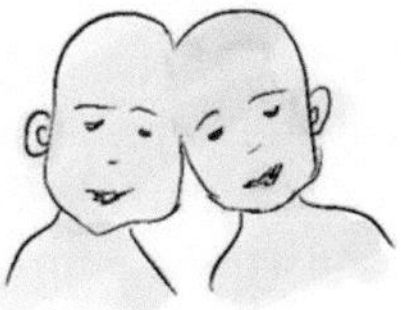

(continued)

Table 81.1 (continued)

Site of attachment (incidence)	Key Features	Figurative representation
7. Rachipagus (2%)	Dorsal fusion of vertebral canal Individual face, thorax, limbs, gastrointestinal organs and limbs Separation impossible	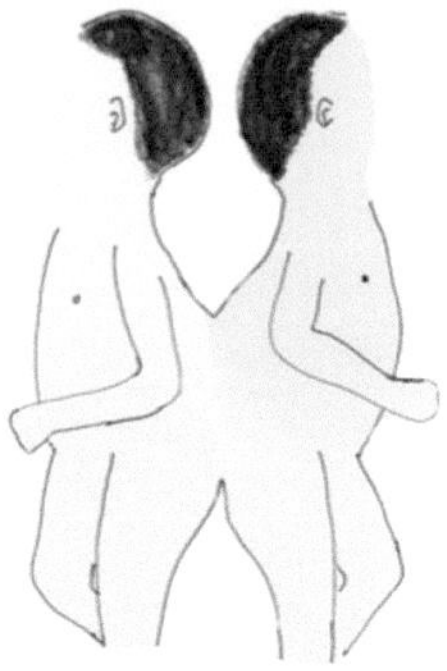
8. Pygopagus (6%)	Joined dorsally at sacrum and coccyx Conjoined spinal cords—Variable extent Single anal opening, common or separate rectum Genitourinary fusion in up to 15%	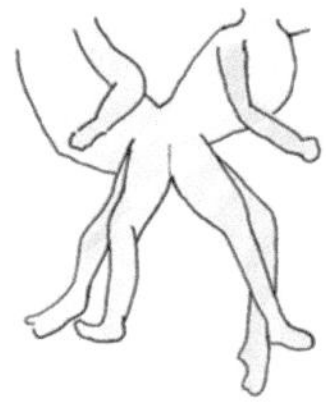

81.2 Prenatal Diagnosis

1. *Fetal Ultrasonography*: Most often, the diagnosis of conjoined twins is established on antenatal imaging. Using high-resolution ultrasonography and transvaginal sonography, visualization of a single yolk sac with a single placenta and no separating amniotic membranes between two apparently joined fetuses can provide evidence of conjoined twinning. There may be the presence of polyhydrominos as well. While suspicion can arise as early as 7–12 weeks, the diagnosis is usually confirmed by 20 weeks, when better anatomical delineation is possible. Newer modalities like three-dimensional ultrasonography can be utilized for better characterization. It is also important to identify other associated congenital anomalies, some of which may be incompatible with life.
2. *Fetal Echocardiography*: This is an important investigation utilized which is helpful in acertaining the prognosis of the fetuses. It may help us identify the presence of separate hearts, the degree of cardiac fusion and the presence of any structural anomalies.
3. *Magnetic Resonance Imaging (MRI):* MRI is a safe and more superior modality to help in the antenatal diagnosis, which helps in characterizing the anatomy and evaluating for associated anomalies, especially in the later part of pregnancy. This also helps in prognosticating the parents for the possible outcomes and obstetric planning. Ultrafast T2-weighted sequences have minimal image degradation and a good tissue contrast.

81.3 Obstetric Management

- *Termination of Pregnancy* can be considered and offered to those diagnosed antenatally with a poor prognosis, such as those with extensive cardiac anomalies, single heart, significant cortical sharing, and associated anomalies. It has been suggested occasionally that termination as an option should be offered to all parents with antenatally detected conjoined twins, owing to extensive morbidity in the surviving twins. Some studies have reported that more than half the parents would prefer to terminate their pregnancy if given the option.

Termination can be successfully performed up to 25 weeks of gestation.

- *Parental counseling* is important, especially with regards to the high risk of stillbirths and perinatal mortality.
- *Close follow-up* with serial scans to monitor the growth of the children and watch for any adverse signs of heart failure, oligo or polyhydramnios. There is an increased risk of preterm labor.
- *Elective delivery* by cesearean section is recommended at 35 weeks of gestation, after a dose of steroids to increase lung maturity in the fetus. Vaginal delivery can lead to trauma and has been done in very small fetuses or in those considered nonviable.
- *EXIT to separation* is known but rarely required or performed.
- The children are usually delivered in a tertiary care center with availability and presence of a pediatric surgeon. After delivery, they are admitted to the Neonatal Intensive Care Unit (NICU) for further stabilization and evaluation.

81.4 Postnatal Evaluation and Imaging

The aim of postnatal evaluation is to delineate the anatomy of the twins—the degree of conjoinment externally and internally. Imaging is required not only for the fused structures but also to look for any associated anatomical anomalies. This is achieved by a three-step approach:

1. *Basic Imaging* of the skeletal anatomy and baseline investigations: Chest and abdominal radiographs and ultrasonography aid in understanding the skeletal system and degree of fusion. The addition of ultrasonography adds to this information. Sonography of the cranium, spine and abdomen grossly defines the baseline anatomy we are dealing with. This can be further supplemented with Doppler imaging of the great vessels of the heart as well as complex abdominal vasculature, on a case-to-case basis. Limbs need screening for neuro-orthopedic deformities.

Echocardiography is performed for each twin due to a high incidence of congenital cardiac anomalies. It helps us answer three important questions: Are the hearts separate for each twin? Is there any great vessel abnormality or any anatomical cardiac defects? Would this child survive after cardiac separation? This is especially important in situations where a decision needs to be taken on the viability of the twins after separation. It also has a great bearing on anesthetic considerations. And it helps in prognosticating the parents on the outcome that can be expected.

2. *Advanced Imaging* by Computed Tomography (CT) and Magnetic Resonance Imaging (MRI) is performed next to further understand the anatomy.

Multidetector CT provides us with high-resolution imaging and is recommended while scanning conjoined twins. Contrast enhancement is routinely performed. Three-dimensional reconstruction of the images can then be performed to better understand the skeletal anatomy and degree of fusion. Electrocardiographic-gated cardiac CT is performed especially in thoracopagus twins.

Magnetic Resonance Imaging (MRI) has a better soft tissue resolution and is especially important for the spine and the brain. MR cholangiopancreatography is an important modality for biliary anatomy. Cardiac-gated MRI and Gadolinium-enhanced MRI can also be used for cardiovascular anatomy.

3. *Supplemental Imaging* is done by means of contrast studies, nuclear imaging and angiography. This can be done to understand the intestinal fusion. Barium meal, follow through and enema help detect the shared and independent bowel possessed of each twin. Selective angiography may be necessary to delineate any crossed vascular anatomy, especially in cases of craniopagus, thoracopagus and pyopagus twins. Nuclear medicine studies add to the information obtained by cross-sectional imaging. Renal scans can be used to estimate the baseline and split renal function and confirm the absence of any obstruction.

Hepatic scintigraphy is important in cases of shared liver, and however, most of this information is also obtained through MR cholangiography.

81.5 Pre-separation Considerations

- *Multidisciplinary Teams (MDTs):* Formation of multidisciplinary teams (MDTs) are essential and have been recommended even by centers where such surgeries are frequently conducted. MDTs should be constituted right at admission to plan for the evaluation and further management, keeping all aspects of care in view. Such teams usually include personnel from Pediatric Surgery and urology, Neurosurgery, Radiology, Vascular Surgery, Nuclear Medicine, Anesthesia, Plastic Surgery, Pediatrics, Intensivists, Nursing, etc. Since these surgeries are not routine, individual experience is often limited, and hence, the formation of such a team is of immense benefit. Each person involved in the care of these twins should have his or her role defined. A leader or coordinator should take charge of the organization of the team and be the source person.
- *Timing and Requirement of Surgery:* The twins after their detailed evaluation should be assessed with the involvement of the MDT with regard to their prognosis and feasibility for separation. Especially in cases with complex cardiac and cortical union, it may not be possible to separate the twins. In some instances where only a single twin remains viable due to a complex cardiac defect, a dead twin may need to be separated from the normal living twin in an emergency scenario to prevent mortality of the viable twin. However, in most cases the surgery is performed electively once the children are old enough to tolerate the morbidity of a prolonged anesthesia and stress. Staged procedures have also been advocated for the separation of certain types of craniopagus twins, and this must be predecided and planned accordingly.
- *Three-Dimensional (3D) Printing:* This is a novel technique used to understand the structural bony anatomy in a tangible method, which would help to plan the planes of division. The 3D reconstructed images of the skeletal anatomy obtained from CT scans can be utilized for printing and creating a replica of the skeletal anatomy.
- *Predefining Flaps and Skin Coverage Requirements:* During the process of separation, one major issue that needs to be addressed is the skin coverage. This can be done by plastic surgical involvement and predefining flaps along which the incisions are placed to maximize the available skin. Skin grafts can be obtained from the twins in a limited fashion or from cadavers. Cadaveric skin grafts hold in place, while epithelialization occurs on the underlying tissue. Alternatively, a mesh can also be placed for temporary coverage.
- *Tissue Expanders:* Tissue expanders have been described and used in the literature to increase the amount of local skin available to enable better coverage during the time of separation. Saline expanders are often used and can be sequentially expanded in volume over time prior to separation. However, while this would reduce reliance on alternative skin cover, they tend to get infected, and this leads to fibrosis and scarring around the areas of insertion.
- *Neuromonitoring:* This is an invaluable tool used especially in cases of conjoinment of neural structures, especially during spinal and cortical separation. It helps minimize functional damage and aids in separation along the correct plane. It can also be used to understand anal sphincter control and allocate to the twin with better control or divide accordingly.
- *Blood Products:* Adequate blood, blood products and colloids need to be kept on hand while planning the surgery due to extensive dissection and high probability of transfusion requirements.
- *Stoma:* In certain situations, especially when the anal canal is common, there could be a requirement for fashioning a stoma. This needs to be planned, and the site of the stoma

needs to be identified preoperatively. In some situations, the bowel can be hung out of the anal opening for 2–3 cm, to prevent contamination and subsequently trimmed after auto-anastomosis to the neo-anal opening.

- *Rehearsal:* The surgery should be divided into phases and each phase should be planned, prepared and discussed, often over months. It is advisable to have a rehearsal prior to the main surgery as it would help to understand areas which need deliberation, to avoid last-minute glitches. Some areas which need to be focused on include positioning and shifting of twins, table arrangements, anesthesia machine location, availability of another close-by theater to shift one of the twins after separation, etc.

81.6 Anesthetic Concerns

The assessment for anesthesia takes place soon after admission, and it is required for the separation procedure as well as various radiological investigations. This requires extensive planning, coordination and preparation as each twin is managed by a separate team. Each member of the team should be aware of their role and should restrain from monitoring the hemodynamics of their own twin. Additionally, separate equipment is required for each twin, while also ensuring no confusion ensues as a result. This is often obtained by color coding for individual twins' belongings and labeling all lines and tubings. Cardiovascular instability may be encountered as cardiac anomalies are often seen to be associated with these patients. While it is easier to prepare in cases of elective separation, emergency surgery in these patients is a challenge and is associated with a significantly higher mortality.

Induction is initiated simultaneously for both twins. An important point to consider is that there is a possibility of cross-circulation due to sharing of vasculature, and thus, the effect of the drugs given may be unpredictable. Due to the conjoint nature, intubation and securing the airway is challenging due to unusual positioning. The separation procedure is often prolonged and involves extensive fluid shifts and blood loss owing to exposed tissue and extensive dissection. Central venous access and arterial line blood pressure monitoring are often required and should be placed right after induction. Adequate blood and blood products need to be kept on hand. Hypothermia should be prevented, and temperature regulation should be optimal. Multiple position changes are also to be anticipated during the duration of the surgery, and thus, endotracheal tube stability needs to be ensured.

81.7 The Separation Procedure

- The procedure is individualized to the type and degree of conjoinment. Standard techniques are used for separation as described in the literature. The tissues are normal but the surgeon should be wary of the anatomical abnormalities that might be encountered.
- Each phase of the separation is planned while also keeping in mind the unexpected anatomy which may be encountered. Anomalies such as vascular crossovers and crossed ureters should be expected even if not detected in the imaging done prior. The allocation of the shared organs should be discussed and decided prior to ensure equitable distribution.
- Separation is often started after marking the incision in accordance with the flaps to be elevated which would aid in eventual skin coverage. Most surgeons prefer to start the procedure posteriorly first
- Availability of energy devices such as ultrasonographic dissector and vessel sealing devices is immensely beneficial, especially in thoraco-omphalopagus twins for division of the liver.
- Cysto-vaginoscopy is often very important prior to separation, especially in situations where pelvic organs are shared. Per-urethral catheter is placed to help identify the structures as well as monitor urine output. Pediatric urologists prefer that the more significant separation of the liver and intestines is performed prior to performing the pelvic component. The urological aspect is often dealt with first, prior to addressing the rectum and pelvis. This is performed anteriorly to maintain orientation.

If a urogenital sinus is encountered, it can be left for reconstruction at a later date.
- In cases of spinal separation, intra-operative neuromonitoring assists in a functional division rather than an anatomical division of the nerves. There may be a requirement for the placement of lumbo-peritoneal shunts to improve wound healing. Occasionally artificial dura material might also be required.
- Pelvic osteotomy has been decribed and is said to be required in cases of ischiopagus.
- After separation, one of the twins is shifted to another theater to complete the remaining reconstruction and skin cover.

81.8 Post-separation Care

- After the surgery, the twins are kept electively ventilated till the hemodynamic parameters, disturbed due to the stress of surgical separation, settle. The initial 1–2 weeks are very crucial as the twins adjust to the changes to their physiology. This is ideally done in an intensive care unit (ICU) setting, with an isolated space for the twins and separate nursing care.
- Routine investigations, including a coagulation profile, are sent immediate postoperatively once settled in the ICU. Central lines and arterial blood pressure monitoring are of immense benefit during this period.
- Since fluid loss during separation is quite extensive, meticulous calculation and replacement should be done to ensure good tissue perfusion. There may be a requirement for inotropes in the perioperative period. There may be losses from the wound site and drains, which need to be calculated and adequately replaced.
- Urine output should be carefully monitored. Renal function may be impaired secondary to nephrotoxic drugs, hypovolemia or systemic inflammatory response. Drug dosages and fluids should be modified accordingly.
- Analgesia and sedation must be adequately tailored to the requirement. Adequate pain relief is essential and enables early respiratory weaning and mobilisation.
- Nutrition should be started as early as possible to improve outcomes. Feeds may be initiated through nasogastric tubes if needed. Total parenteral nutrition may be required in some cases of extensive bowel dissection. Protein and albumin levels should be checked routinely, and twins must be weighed regularly.
- All strategies must be in place to avoid hospital-acquired infections and cross infections between twins. Dressings are done regularly and barriers placed between the anal opening and incision sites if possible. The invasive tubings and drains should be removed as early as possible.
- There may be a requirement for revision and additional surgeries in the post-separation phase. Split thickness skin grafting may be required for skin cover, or abdominal wall closure may be done in some cases.

81.9 Follow-Up

Conjoined twins are chronic patients, who apart from having a prolonged course in the hospital, require regular follow-up. Cardiac evaluation and follow-up are necessary in those with cardiac defects. Orthopedic follow-up is needed for further management of neuro-orthopedic deformities. Plastic surgery inputs may be needed for wound and scar management. Stoma care and bowel management programs are often a routine part of some of these twins. Follow-up investigations for neurogenic bladder and its management should be done, and twins should be initiated on clean intermittent catheterization. Furthermore, they often require a great deal of psychological support to deal with the complexities of their condition.

81.10 Heteropagus Twins

Asymmetric conjoined twins where tissues of a grossly defective fetus or its parts (parasite) are connected with a relatively normal twin (autosite) are called heteropagus twinning. The parasite is joined at the same sites as described for symmetric twins, omphalopagus being the most common. It is nonviable and is dependent upon the autosite. This condition technically is a clinical spectrum which includes not only the exoparasitic twins, but also endoparasitic twins (fetus-in-fetu), twin reverse arterial perfusion sequence and fetiform mature teratoms. The incidence ranges between 0.02 and 0.1 per 100,000, comprising 4.5–15% of all conjoined twins.

The theories for the embryogenesis of these twins include the fission theory and fusion theory. Another theory on the ischemic atrophy of one of the twins has also been described—vascular accident in the parasite causes it to be dependent on the autosite along with the development of the selective atrophy of the parasite's body.

These cases can be antenatally detected, and pregnancy is advised to be continued as the autosite generally has a good prognosis and outcome. The autosite has also been reported to have a high incidence of congenital cardiac anomalies, up to 25% in some cases. Fetal echocardiography and prenatal MRI is performed to confirm the viability of the autosite. Normal vaginal delivery can be advised in cases where the parasite is small but if a risk of obstructed labor is evident, elective cesarean section is preferred around 38 weeks of gestation.

Preoperative CT, MRI and echocardiography are advisable for diagnostic and anatomical clarity. Surgical excision of the parasite is usually straightforward and is performed in infancy. Early surgery is important not only for cosmetic and psychological reasons, as it enables bonding between the mother and the normal twin, but also because in some cases presence of a parasite may cause respiratory distress and hinder the growth of the autosite.

The incisions must be planned in a way to ensure adequate skin coverage of the autosite. Division of the vessels is done carefully and meticulously to divide the blood supply to the parasite. Sometimes parasite viscera may be located within the autosite, and it is important to thoroughly inspect the division site to ensure complete removal. Other anomalies if present are often repaired at the same time. The outcome is generally favorable in most cases.

Suggested Reading

Bajpai M, Sehgal M, Yadav D, Singh A, Goel P, Tomar S, et al. Multimodality management of two pairs of pyopagus twins. Natl Board Exam J Med Sci. 2023;1:18–26.

Mian A, Gabra NI, Sharma T, Topale N, Gielecki J, Shane Tubbs R, et al. Conjoined twins: from conception to separation, a review. Clin Anat. 2017;30:385–96. https://doi.org/10.1002/CA.22839.

O'Brien P, Nugent M, Khalil A. Prenatal diagnosis and obstetric management. Semin Pediatr Surg. 2015;24:203–6. https://doi.org/10.1053/j.sempedsurg.2015.06.002.

Pierro A, Kiely EM, Spitz L. Classification and clinical evaluation. Semin Pediatr Surg. 2015;24:207–11. https://doi.org/10.1053/j.sempedsurg.2015.06.003.

Sehgal M, Bajpai M, Jaryal A, Gupta U. Role of neuromonitoring in the spinal separation of pyopagus twins. Natl Board Exam J Med Sci. 2023;1:92–8.

Spitz L, Kiely EM, Pierro A. Conjoined twins. Pediatric Surg, 2-Volume Set: Expert Consult - Online and Print. 2012:1725–38. https://doi.org/10.1016/B978-0-323-07255-7.00137-9.

Breast Disorders in Children

82

Nitin Pant and Subhasis Roy Choudhury

82.1 Introduction

Paediatric breast problems can be categorized into three types. Firstly, they may present as congenital lesions. Also, they can present as part of normal breast development (developmental lesions) which can be subdivided into pre- or post-pubertal lesions. In addition, they can also develop secondary to a neoplastic process. Fortunately, most breast problems in children are benign, and many are self-limiting. Evaluation of breast problems in children starts with a thorough history and examination. Most congenital problems and those related to physiologic breast changes are clinically diagnosed and do not require any further investigation. For discretely palpable masses, ultrasound is the investigation of choice. Masses arising in adolescence, large masses with a rapid rate of progression, those with persistent pain, bloody nipple discharge, and any distortion in breast contour require in addition to an ultrasound, a biopsy to rule out malignancy.

N. Pant (✉)
King George's Medical University, Lucknow, Uttar Pradesh, India

S. Roy Choudhury
Pediatric Surgery, Lady Hardinge Medical College and Associated Kalawati Saran Children's Hospital, New Delhi, Delhi, India

82.1.1 Abnormalities of Embryogenesis

Amastia is a congenital or iatrogenic absence of breast tissue, nipples, and areola. The congenital form is seen in the case of Poland syndrome, first-trimester exposure to teratogens, whereas the iatrogenic form is associated with biopsy of the breast bud, trauma, or radiation to the breast tissue. Some cases have an absence of only the breast tissue, and the nipple and areola are present. This condition is known as *Amazia*. It is similar to amastia and can be congenital or iatrogenic, unilateral or bilateral. Treatment of both conditions includes psychological counselling and breast reconstruction.

Persistence of the remnants of the embryonic milk line (Hughes line) may lead to *Polythelia* "accessory nipples" (Fig. 82.1) and *Polymastia* "supernumerary breasts". Presentation of polymastia can vary from a breast without a nipple to a fully formed breast with axilla being the most common site of occurrence. It can sometimes be mistaken for a pigmented naevus. When associated with a nipple, milk production can occur in polymastia during pregnancy and lactation.

Rarely one encounters a *tuberous breast*, a congenital malformation of unknown aetiology, which occurs due to the underdevelopment of the nipple, areola, and base of the breast. Its aetiology is unknown and is a clinically benign condition. Treatment involves psychological counselling and breast reconstruction.

© The Author(s), under exclusive license to Springer Nature Singapore Pte Ltd. 2025

S. Roy Choudhury (ed.), *Pediatric Surgery*, https://doi.org/10.1007/978-981-96-1257-4_82

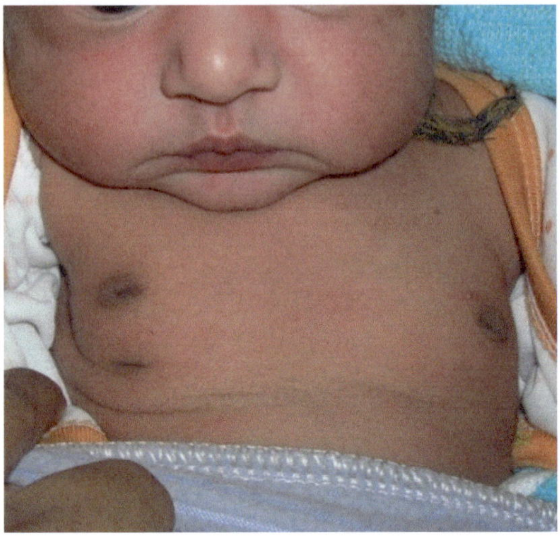

Fig. 82.1 Accessory nipple (polythelia)

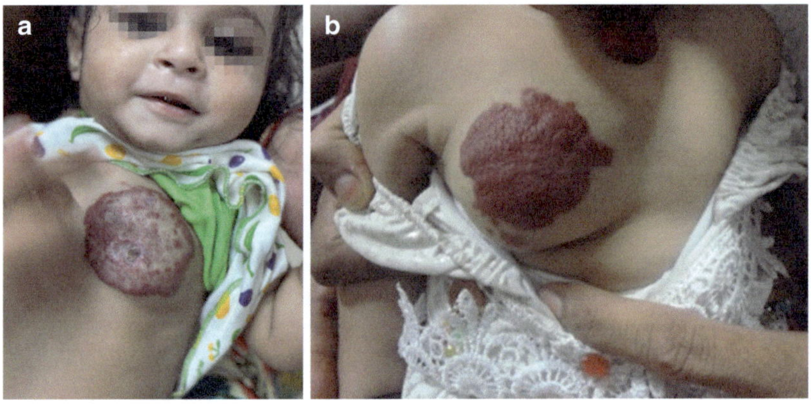

Fig. 82.2 (**a**) Hemangioma on the left breast. (**b**) Large hemangioma on the right breast leading to breast asymmetry

Sometimes *vascular lesions* like hemangiomas can also occur in the breast. Mostly they are superficial and small in size but occasionally can present as large masses causing breast asymmetry (Fig. 82.2a and b). Treatment varies from expectant waiting to oral propranolol and very rarely intralesional sclerosant injection.

82.1.2 Abnormalities in Breast Development in Pre-pubertal and Peri-pubertal Age

Early breast development can be asymmetric, with nearly a two-year difference in the growth pattern of the two breasts. *Breast asymmetry* is the most common problem seen in children less than 12 years. The typical presentation is a unilateral, subareolar breast mass secondary to asymmetrical breast development. One breast develops more rapidly than the other, leading to an asymmetry in shape, volume, and position of the breasts or nipple-areola complex (Fig. 82.3). Gradually, the asymmetry lessens in most cases, but if it is significant and persists even after full breast development, breast augmentation or reduction mammoplasty might be considered once the child reaches 18 years of age and has mature breasts. There are five Tanner stages of development from prepubertal till final adult form based on the pubic hair, female breast and male external genitalia.

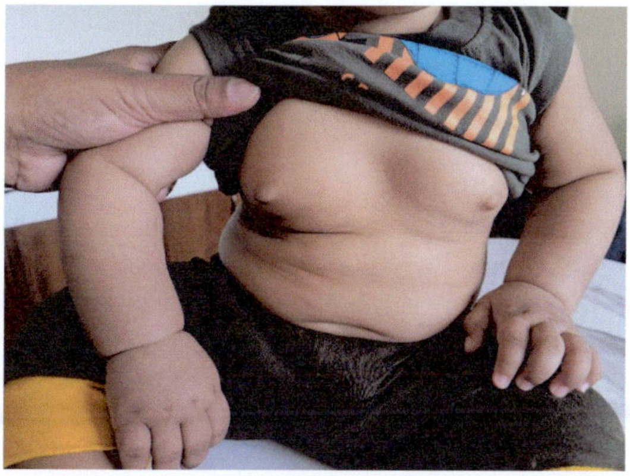

Fig. 82.3 Asymmetric breast enlargement

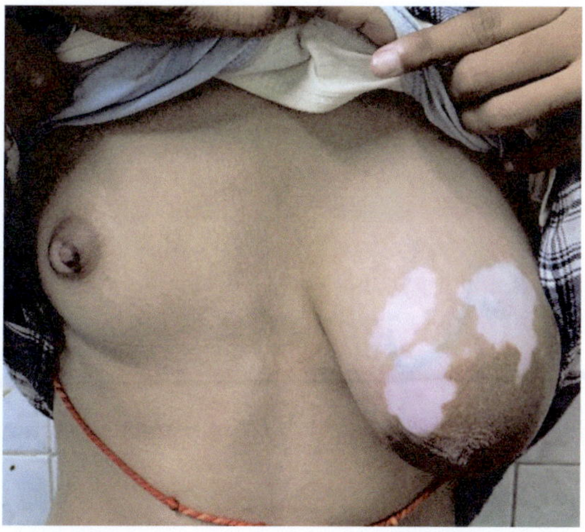

Fig. 82.4 Virginal hypertrophy of left breast

82.2 Premature Thelarche

This condition sometimes occurs in females of less than 7 years, usually at age 1–3 years, wherein breast development occurs without other signs of sexual maturity, i.e. the breast enlargement is unrelated to precocious puberty. An increase in oestrogen sensitivity or serum levels is supposed to play a role in its development. There is hypertrophy of only the breast buds without any change in the nipple or areola. Vaginal mucosa remains un-oestrogenized. Mostly presents as a palpable subareolar mass. In a bilateral presentation, the breast usually presents with Tanner stage III. However, in unilateral cases, they mostly present with Tanner stage II. The condition is mostly benign, and its clinical course can vary from completely regressive, to progressive or cyclical. Differential diagnosis includes precocious puberty, which is described as secondary sexual development occurring before the age of 7.5–8 years in the West. Patients should be closely monitored, every 3–6 months for signs of sexual development. Ultrasonography can be used to exclude an underlying breast mass and examine the pelvis to exclude early sexual development.

82.3 Virginal Breast Hypertrophy

Also known as "Juvenile Gigantomastia", it is a rare condition associated with rapid and excessive growth of the breast in pre-pubertal or peri-pubertal girls in the absence of any hormonal or physiological cause. By definition, the breast weight exceeds 3% of the total body weight or the breast tissue weight exceeds 1.5–1.8 kg. The presentation can be unilateral, bilateral, symmetrical, or asymmetric. The aetiology remains unknown. Clinical onset is typical with a history of sudden, spontaneous, rapid, and sustained increase in breast size in young women who have not experienced any previous breast development or hormonal changes. This massive and rapid breast growth leads to overstretching of breast skin, loss of areola morphology, ulcerations, and breast pain (Fig. 82.4). Further progression may result in physical discomfort and functional limitations, neck and back pain, and shoulder grooving from bra straps. Psychological problems of body image dissatisfaction, low self-esteem, and emotional distress also develop. One has to exclude other causes of breast enlargement before diagnosing this entity. Breast reduction surgery is the treatment of choice.

82.4 Gynecomastia

It is a condition due to the excessive development of breast tissue in males. Physiologic gynecomastia constitutes 65% of cases and can be observed in neonates, pubertal boys, or elderly men. *Neonatal breast enlargement* is a common transient condition seen in up to 90% of all newborns of both sexes. It is supposedly caused by transient elevations in oestrogen secondary to its transplacental passage. Clinically, the nipple is generally depressed, and colostrum milk (witch's milk) may be squeezed out from the nipple. The enlargement reduces gradually with the decrease of circulating maternal oestrogen in the baby. Parental reassurance is sufficient (Fig. 82.5).

Pubertal gynecomastia can be seen in boys aged 10–13 years, typically 6 months after the onset of secondary sexual characteristics (Fig. 82.6a and b). The aetiology is unknown, but few implicate the hormone Leptin present in the mammary epithelial cells which increases aromatase enzyme activity as well as activates oestrogen receptors in breast fatty tissue. Breast enlargement usually regresses within 2 years of onset in nearly 75% of cases but takes slightly longer in obese boys. About 50% of boys have a family history of gynecomastia.

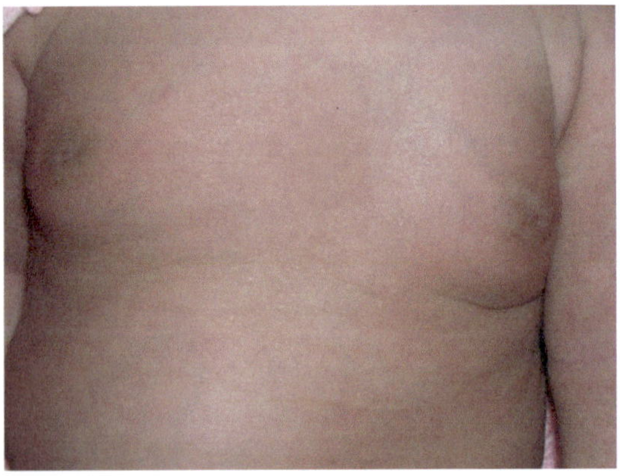

Fig. 82.5 Neonatal (physiological) gynecomastia

Pathologic gynecomastia can be secondary to an increase in oestrogen levels, a decrease in testosterone, medication, or drug use. Sometimes it may be idiopathic. The details of its aetiology and causes are provided in Table 82.1. A pathologic cause should be suspected when either puberty is early (tumours) or late (gonadal dysfunction), when there is rapid breast growth, or if there is associated nipple discharge. Surgery is reserved for cases where the breast size does not decrease over a year or if there is excessive fibrosis of the breast tissue. It is also indicated in those boys where there is a risk of malignant degeneration in the breast; e.g. Klinefelter's syndrome where a prophylactic mastectomy is indicated.

A good clinical examination suffices in most cases to confirm gynecomastia. An ultrasound is

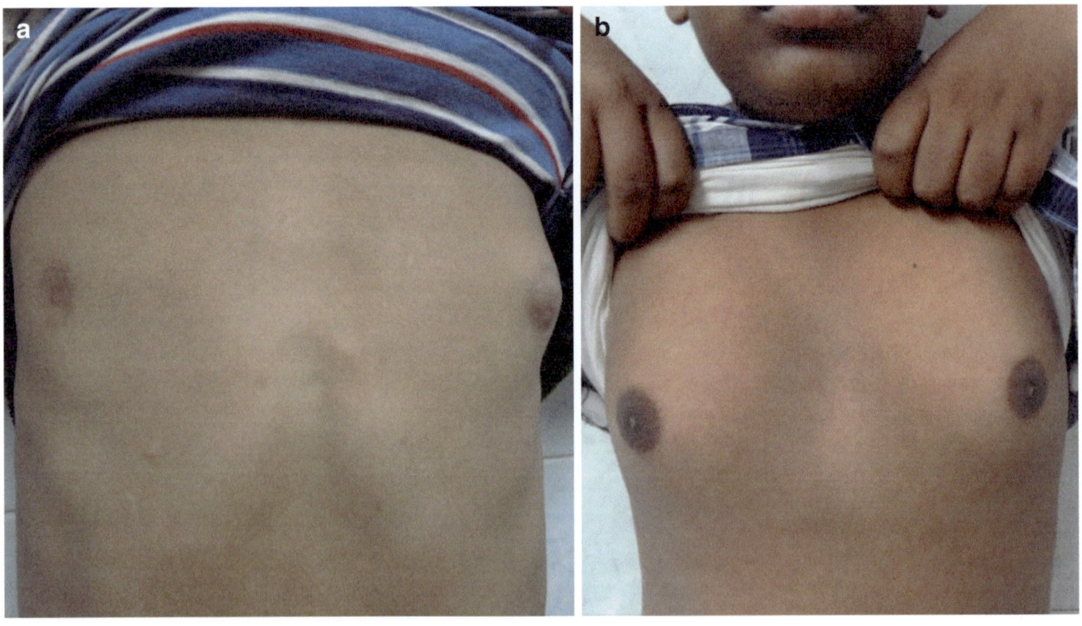

Fig. 82.6 (**a**) Unilateral gynecomastia. (**b**) Bilateral gynecomastia

Table 82.1 Aetiology of gynecomastia

Aetiology	Elevated serum oestrogen	Increased aromatization of the oestrogen precursors	Drugs displacing oestrogen from sex hormone-binding globulin	Decreased testosterone
1	Leydig cell tumour	Sertoli cell tumour	Ketoconazole	Congenital testicular aplasia/hypoplasia
2	Adrenocortical neoplasm	Sex cord testicular tumour	Spironolactone	Testicular torsion/ trauma
3		Testicular germ cell tumour	Cimetidine	Viral orchitis
4		Cirrhotic liver disease		Androgen insensitivity
5		Hyperthyroidism		Klinefelter syndrome
6		Klinefelter syndrome		

occasionally used if the physical examination is questionable. It allows verification of normal-appearing breast tissue and helps exclude an underlying mass. It also helps in revealing a paucity of breast tissue in patients with *pseudo-gynecomastia*, an entity where there is breast enlargement due to only fat deposition.

82.4.1 Abnormalities in Breast Development in Post-pubertal (Adolescence)

82.4.1.1 Fibroadenoma

These are the most common solid benign tumours of the breast, comprising nearly 90% of solid breast masses in adolescence and also the most frequently biopsied and/or excised breast masses in this age (Fig. 82.7). It occurs due to the overgrowth of the specialized connective tissue stroma of the breast lobule. The presentation can vary from unilateral to bilateral (10–15%), and single to multiple solid masses. The use of oral contraceptives before the age of 20 is associated with a higher incidence. The classic presentation is of an adolescent girl presenting with a self-palpated mass which has been present for many months. The mass is well-demarcated, mobile, smooth, and rubbery on palpation with no associated changes in the skin or nipple-areola complex. Ultrasonography is the investigation of choice. The typical sonographic appearance is of a well-circumscribed, homogeneous mass, without any acoustic shadowing. They may appear as round, oval, or macro-lobulated. Mammography is not preferred as it provides poor-quality images owing to the density of breast tissue at this age. Similarly, a biopsy should be selectively used as any iatrogenic injury to the developing breast can lead to permanent disfigurement. Complete regression occurs in 10–40% of cases.

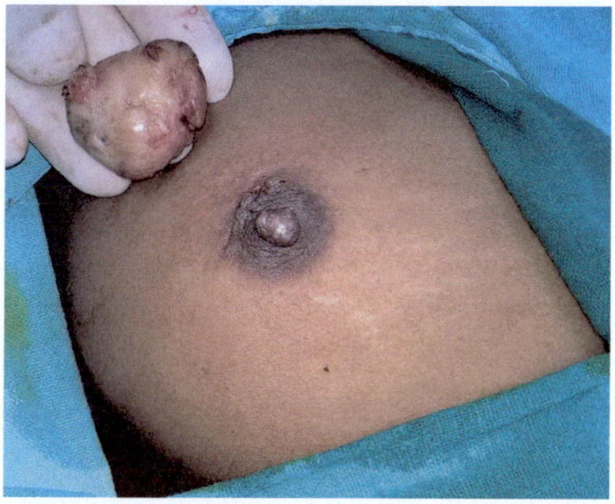

Fig. 82.7 Fibroadenoma breast (note the circumareolar cosmetic incision for its removal)

The treatment is a combined decision of the patient and the clinician. Small, <5 cm, lesions, not causing any morphological change to the breast or discomfort to the patient, can be safely followed both clinically and by ultrasound every 6 months for 2 years and then yearly. The indications for surgery are: gross morphological changes in the breast, multiple and/or bilateral lesions, symptomatic lesions, complex fibroadenoma or stromal hypercellularity at biopsy, rapid growth, size >5 cm, and cystic changes on ultrasound. The last three suggest a phyllodes tumour.

Phyllodes tumour comprises <1% of the adolescent breast masses. It arises from the periductal stromal cells. Clinically, it can attain a very big size (Fig. 82.8). The clinical course can vary from benign (85%) to malignant. Clinically, it is difficult to differentiate from fibroadenoma. As previously stated, rapid growth, size >5 cm, and cystic changes on ultrasound point towards its possibility. As ultrasound is not useful in differentiating between a benign and malignant phyllodes tumour. A tissue biopsy helps establish the diagnosis and its grade (Low/Intermediate/High). Surgical excision with a 2 cm margin is advised for all grades. The risk of recurrence and metastasis is present in all three grades.

82.4.1.2 Mastitis and Breast Abscess

In children, mastitis has a bimodal distribution. It is observed in babies (mostly girls) below the age of 2 months and in adolescence. The most frequent pathogen is Staphylococcus aureus (>75%). Neonatal mastitis is very uncommon. The aetiology involves the entry of pathogens through the skin or mucus membrane of the nipple and ducts. This is facilitated by a hormonally stimulated infant breast tissue. Adolescent mastitis is secondary to skin infections, instrumentation/piercings, or lactation. The usual presentation is an erythematous, warm, and tender breast with or without fever and leukocytosis (Fig. 82.9). In clinically equivocal cases, an ultrasound can differentiate it from an abscess (Fig. 82.10) and help in a needle-guided aspiration of pus for culture. For mastitis, antibiotic therapy for 7–10 days is the treatment of choice along with warm compresses and analgesics. An abscess requires formal drainage in addition.

82.4.2 Ductal Ectasia or Mammary Duct Ectasia

It is an inflammatory breast condition of the large duct (milk duct) of the breast. The inflammation causes ectasis, i.e. widening and thickening of the ducts. Further, the inflammation can extend to the nipple-areola complex or periductal region.

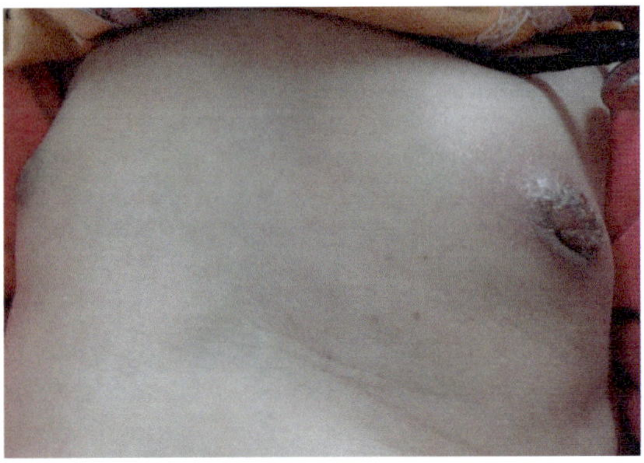

Fig. 82.9 Neonatal mastitis

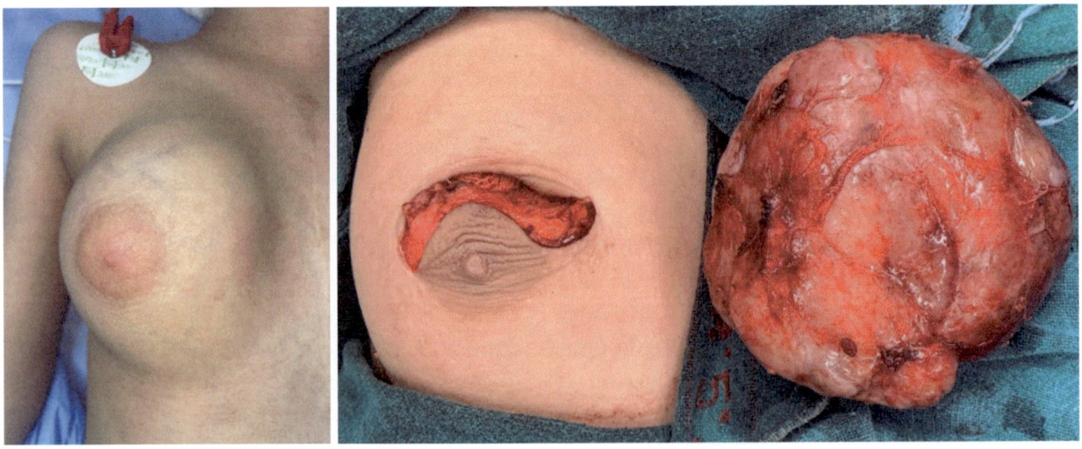

Fig. 82.8 Phyllodes tumour of the right breast: (**a**) clinical, (**b**) post excision

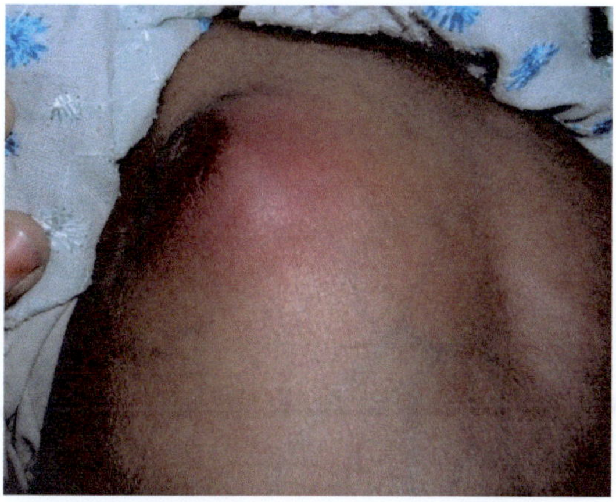

Fig. 82.10 Breast abscess

Subsequently, it causes periductal fibrosis. It has a non-proliferative and benign course. The patients frequently complain of pain at the site of the nipple and/or areola along with intermittent nipple discharge which can vary in colour, from white to green or grey. Nipple inversion or breast lump may be apparent in a few cases. This condition typically subsides on its own in 2–3 weeks, and therefore, a conservative and symptomatic treatment is recommended. Rarely a persistent nipple discharge requires a biopsy.

82.4.3 Malignancy of the Breast in Children

Primary malignancy of the breast is very rare in children with a reported incidence of <0.1 per 1000,000. Phyllodes tumour is the most common primary malignancy in children, and unlike adults, invasive ductal carcinoma is very rare. They are more likely to suffer from metastatic breast lesions, e.g. lymphoma than primary breast cancers. In clinically suspicious cases, one should also look for corroborative evidence of a strong family history of breast cancer, known extramammary malignancy, genetic mutation, or prior irradiation.

82.5 Summary

Most breast lesions can be diagnosed by a good history and clinical examination. Physiological breast changes can be clinically diagnosed and observed for spontaneous resolution.

Ultrasonography is the radiological investigation of choice in requisite cases.

Biopsy should be reserved for masses which arise suspicion of malignancy.

Suggested Reading

Adekeye A, Lung KC, Brill KL. Pediatric and adolescent breast conditions: a review. J Pediatr Adolesc Gynecol. 2023;36(1):5–13. https://doi.org/10.1016/j.jpag.2022.11.001.

Gao Y, Saksena MA, Brachtel EF, terMeulen DC, Rafferty EA. How to approach breast lesions in children and adolescents. Eur J Radiol. 2015;84(7):1350–64. https://doi.org/10.1016/j.ejrad.2015.04.011.

Kaneda HJ, Mack J, Kasales CJ, Schetter S. Pediatric and adolescent breast masses: a review of pathophysiology, imaging, diagnosis, and treatment. AJR Am J Roentgenol. 2013;200(2):204–12. https://doi.org/10.2214/AJR.12.9560.

Soliman SA, Algatheradi MA, Aljahwashi TA, Alhussan TH, Alqahtani RS, Ali NI. Virginal breast hypertrophy: a case report. Cureus. 2023;15(6):e40067. https://doi.org/10.7759/cureus.40067.

83 Short Cases in Pediatric Surgery

Praveen Jhanwar and Subhasis Roy Choudhury

83.1 Introduction

There are many pediatric surgical referrals for different conditions in children which are not organ-specific. They can be diagnosed by their clinical appearance in the outpatient clinic. In this chapter, an attempt has been made to present some of those conditions including their management.

83.2 Tongue-Tie

Ankyloglossia, commonly referred to as tongue-tie, is a prevalent congenital condition that affects the lingual frenulum. It is characterized by a limitation in the mobility of the tongue tip, which is unable to extend beyond the lower incisor teeth. It ranges in severity from a mild form to a severe variant in which the tongue is entirely anchored to the floor of the mouth. Assessment necessitates the use of a tongue depressor in young children or a request for tongue protrusion in older children to evaluate tethering and tongue mobility. A short and thick frenulum may limit tongue mobility (Fig. 83.1). A minor degree of ankyloglossia, characterized by the tongue's ability to easily protrude beyond the dental boundary, may be noted in relation to speech development. In older children, speech and articulation may be impacted; however, the association is inadequately documented, making it challenging to anticipate which patients would experience these difficulties. It frequently raises significant concerns for the family. The frenulum is thin and relatively avascular in neonates and young infants, and it can frequently be incised with sharp scissors as an outpa-

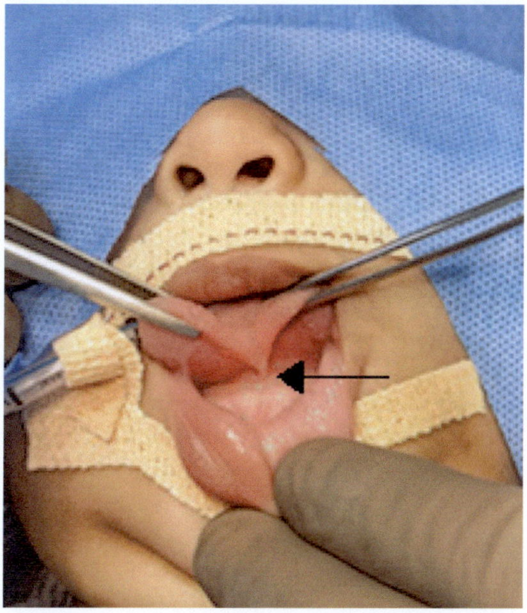

Fig. 83.1 Tongue-tie, severe grade, intra-operative picture

P. Jhanwar (✉)
Department of General surgery, Pediatric Surgeon, Pacific Medical College and Hospital, Udaipur, Rajasthan, India

S. Roy Choudhury
Pediatric Surgery, Lady Hardinge Medical College and Associated Kalawati Saran Children's Hospital, New Delhi, Delhi, India

© The Author(s), under exclusive license to Springer Nature Singapore Pte Ltd. 2025

S. Roy Choudhury (ed.), *Pediatric Surgery*, https://doi.org/10.1007/978-981-96-1257-4_83

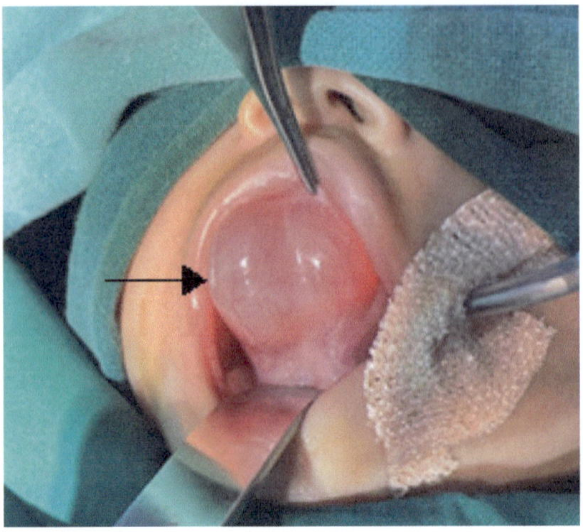

Fig. 83.2 Ranula, large lesion

tient surgery. Surgical intervention in older children may necessitate short general anesthesia for the procedure of frenulectomy.

83.3 Ranula

Ranula is a type of mucocele that can be found on the floor of the mouth. On clinical examination, it appears as a dome-shaped swelling that is blue, translucent, and fluctuating in the floor of the mouth (Fig. 83.2). The accumulation of salivary mucin from the salivary gland duct, which occurs as a consequence of minor trauma, is the most common cause of this condition. Small lesions that do not cause any symptoms can be seen. Surgery might be necessary for larger lesions. Both the excision of the sublingual gland and the marsupialization of the cyst wall to the floor of the mouth are potential treatments for this condition, the latter being more commonly practiced.

83.4 BCG Lymphadenitis

There is a 0.1–1% chance that recipients of the BCG vaccine would develop suppurative lymph adenitis (Fig. 83.3). In the majority of cases, they have a spontaneous resolution; nevertheless, chemotherapy may be required on occasion. The cold abscess might need to be aspirated in order to be treated. Excision of a suppurative draining node using surgical means is only occasionally prescribed.

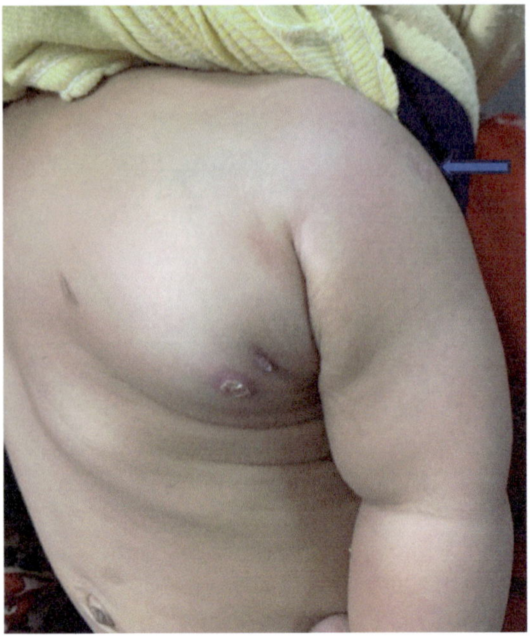

Fig. 83.3 BCG adenitis axilla, note the BCG injection site mark on the arm (arrow)

83.4.1 Tubercular Lymphadenitis

Lymph node tuberculosis typically manifests in the cervical, axillary, and inguinal regions. The staging of superficial tuberculous lymphadenitis by Jones and Campbell is as follows:

Stage I. Enlarged, firm, mobile discrete lymph nodes exhibiting non-reactive hyperplasia.
Stage II. Enlarged, rubbery nodes adhered to adjacent tissues as a result of periadenitis.
Stage III. Central softening resulting from abscess development.
Stage IV. Collar stud abscess.
Stage V. Rupture and sinus development (undermined edges with discolored margins)

Management involves antituberculous medicines (ATT) and surgical removal in a minority of instances.

Chemotherapy is almost invariably therapeutic in instances of superficial lymphadenitis prior to caseation and sinus development (Figs. 83.4a, b). Surgery is restricted to patients who do not exhibit improvement following a sufficient regimen of chemotherapy or who experience discomfort from swollen, tense, and fluctuating lymph nodes, as well as those with atypical mycobacterial infections frequently resistant to antitubercular therapy (ATT).

83.4.1.1 Caput Succedaneum

Caput succedaneum (Fig. 83.5a, b) occurs in certain instances of birth trauma, vacuum, and forceps delivery, resulting from the rupture of blood vessels within the dense connective tissue beneath the skin. The swelling extends across the suture lines due to subcutaneous fluid accumulation. Purpura and ecchymosis of the superficial skin are common. Hemorrhage is often minimal because of the tamponade action of dense connective tissue and generally resolves spontaneously within a few days.

A cephalhematoma (Fig. 83.5c) is a collection of blood located between the periosteum and the cranial bone. The sub-periosteal swelling is confined by the individual bone, in contrast to the caput, which is a subcutaneous extra periosteal fluid collection characterized by indistinct edges.

Both disorders are managed by vigilant observation and providing reassurance to the family. Administration of vitamin K is advised to rectify coagulation disorders in neonates.

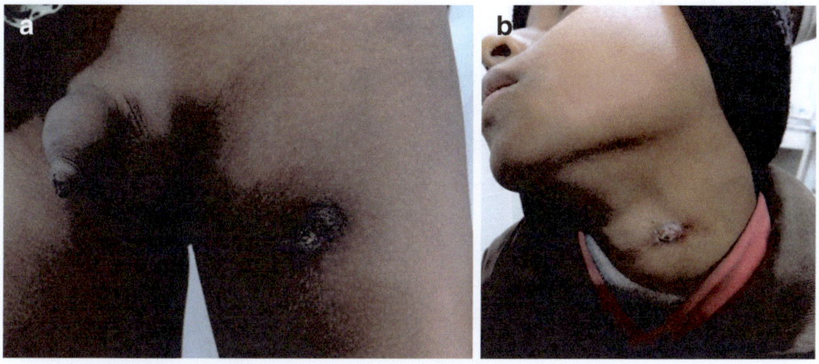

Fig. 83.4 (**a**) Tubercular sinus in the groin (**b**) Tubercular sinus in the neck

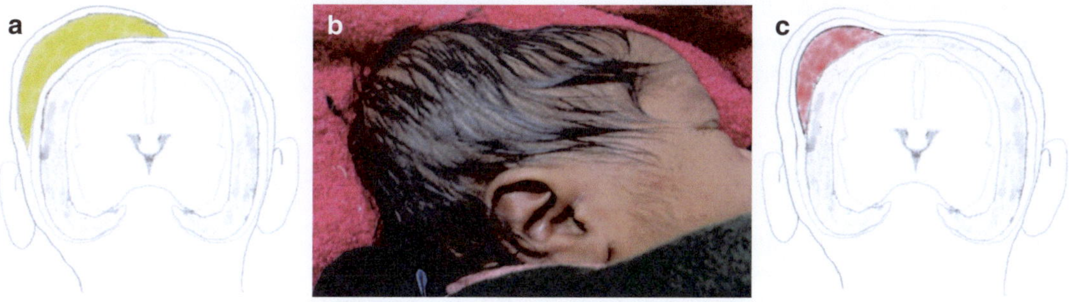

Fig. 83.5 (**a**) Caput succedaneum (line diagram) (**b**) Caput (**c**) Cephalhematoma (line diagram)

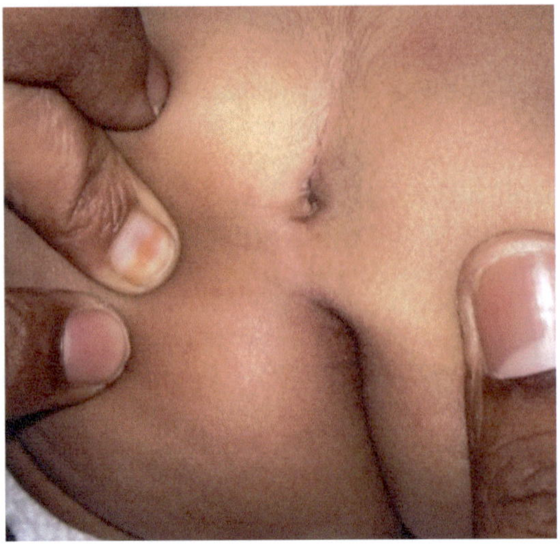

Fig. 83.6 Presacral cleft

83.5 Presacral Cleft

A presacral cleft (Fig. 83.6) is a minor, typically superficial indentation located in the lower back (lower end of the coccyx), just above or within the gluteal cleft. Sacral dimples are benign and require no intervention.

A sacral dimple often presents no complications and is not linked to any health hazards. The sole indication of a sacral dimple is a typically modest indentation located around the base of the tailbone and the upper region of the buttocks. In infrequent instances, a sacral dimple may signify an underlying spinal cord anomaly, such as spina bifida occulta or tethered cord syndrome.

83.6 Paraphimosis

Paraphimosis (Fig. 83.7) is an emergency characterized by the inability to reposition the retracted foreskin, resulting in restriction of the glans penis. This restriction may obstruct blood flow, potentially resulting in swelling and injury to the penis. Manual reduction with the help of warm compression is generally successful.

It is essential to differentiate from phimosis (Fig. 83.8), which is characterized by the inability to retract the foreskin over the glans, and paraphimosis, which occurs when the retracted foreskin cannot be repositioned to its original position.

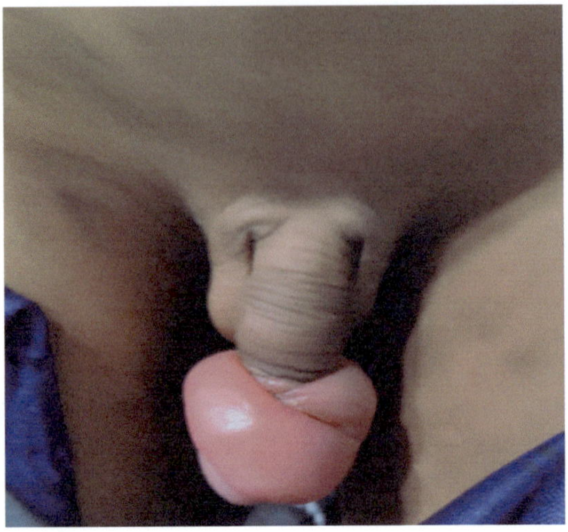

Fig. 83.7 Paraphimosis

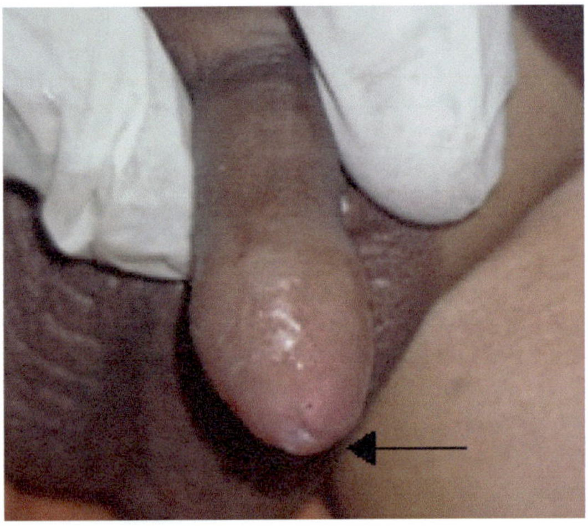

Fig. 83.8 Phimosis, note a pinpoint opening

83.7 Syndactyly

Syndactyly is a condition where two or more digits are fused together. It could affect either the hand (Fig. 83.9a) or the foot (Fig. 83.9b). Surgical release is only required in order to regain the ability to move the digits that are functional. Six to twelve months is the ideal time frame for surgical procedures.

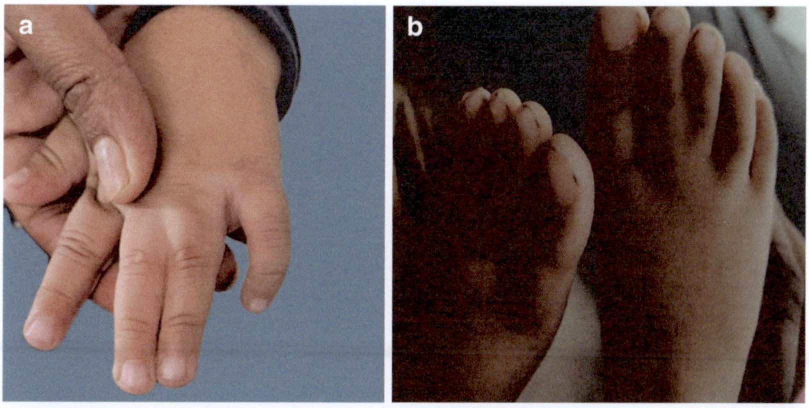

Fig. 83.9 Syndactyly of (**a**) hand, (**b**) foot

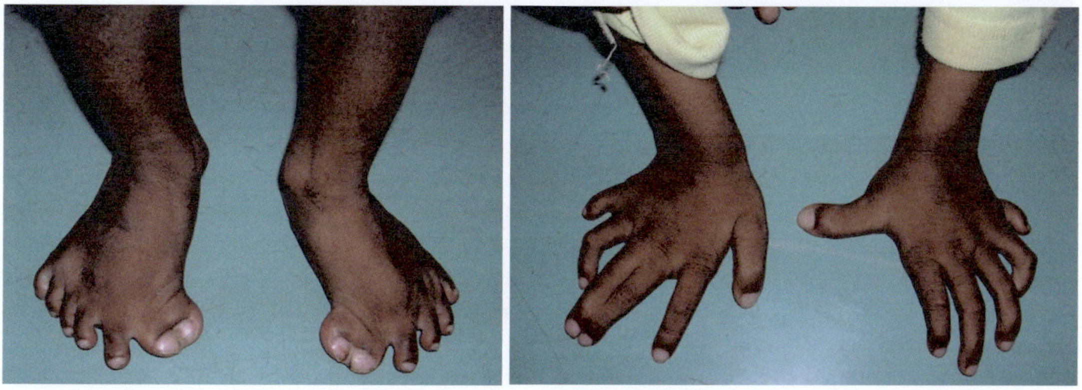

Fig. 83.10 Polydactyly (multiple digits) with syndactyly (28 fingers and toes in one patient)

83.7.1 Polydactyly

Polydactyly or multiple digits (Fig. 83.10). An accessory digit is an extra digit. A digit attached with a simple skin tag (accessory digit) can be easily removed (Fig. 83.11). Those with a bony attachment to the functioning digit require further evaluation with an X-ray and a planned surgery for separation.

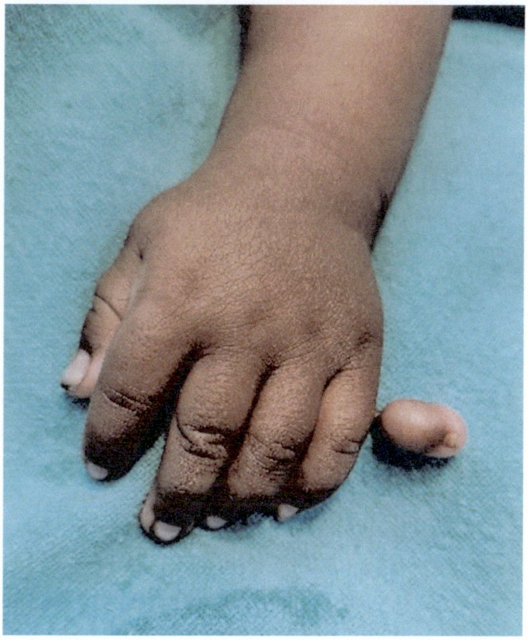

Fig. 83.11 Accessory digit

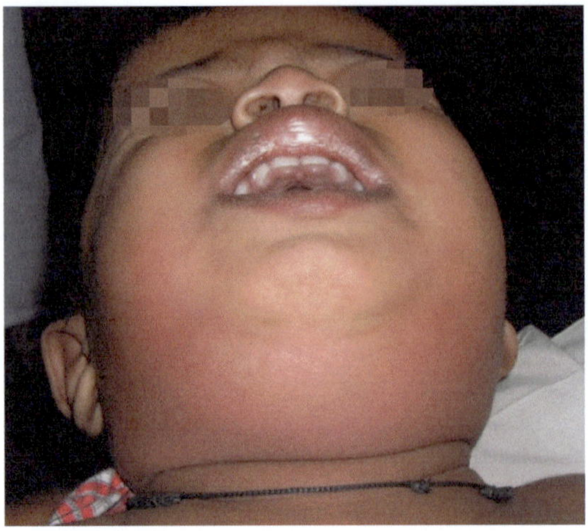

Fig. 83.12 Ludwig's angina

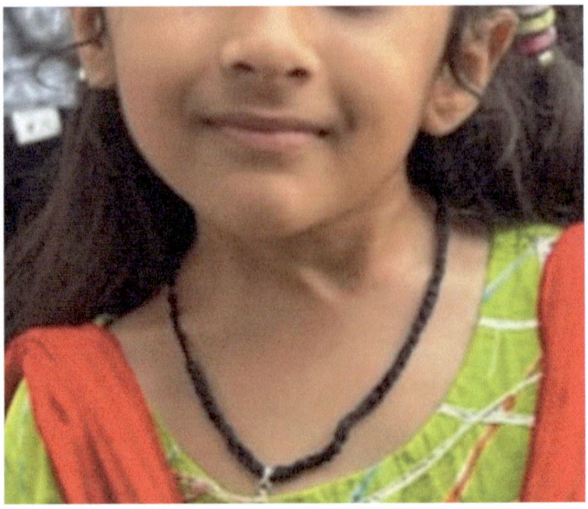

Fig. 83.13 Torticollis (left side affected short sternocleidomastoid muscle, patient forced to face toward right side, restricted movement of neck)

83.8 Ludwig's Angina

Ludwig's angina (Fig. 83.12) is an illness that affects the floor of the mouth, namely the submandibular, sublingual, and submental parts of the mouth that are affected. This infection is most frequently caused by a tooth that is already infected. It is a cellulitis that is aggressive and rapidly spreading, and it frequently does not have any noticeable lymphadenopathy. Additionally, it has the ability to restrict the airway. For the purpose of preventing hypoxia and aspiration pneumonia, aggressive treatment with hospitalization, intravenous antibiotics, and incision and drainage may be necessary. Airway obstruction may require a tracheostomy.

83.8.1 Torticollis (See Chap. 20)

When the muscles in the neck, particularly the sternocleidomastoid muscle, undergo tightening, it results in an abnormal tilt of the head, which becomes fixated in a static position, accompanied by a forward bending of the neck (Fig. 83.13). This condition is referred to as torticollis. Torticollis is not a standalone diagnosis; rather, it may serve as an indication of various other diseases and disorders that can either be present at birth (congenital) or develop subsequently. The congenital variant typically presents in isolation and within a few weeks following delivery. There exists a likelihood that the infant may exhibit squinting behavior when the head is oriented to one side. In most instances, the advised approach is to provide reassurance, as the condition generally resolves spontaneously by the age of 1 year. Alternative methodologies encompass the provision of physiotherapy, and in more advanced cases, surgical intervention may be required (see Chap. 20).

83.9 Amniotic Band

In addition to being referred to as Streeter bands, amniotic bands are strands of tissue that originate in the embryo and cross from one wall of the amniotic sac to the other. As a result, they have the ability to restrict any area of the developing fetus.

This has the potential to disrupt the regular development of that particular portion (Fig. 83.14). In some cases, they can lead to the amputation of body parts. If the bands are connected with neurocirculatory impairment, they can be loosened using Z-plasties that are performed once the child has reached the age of 2 years or as an emergency treatment.

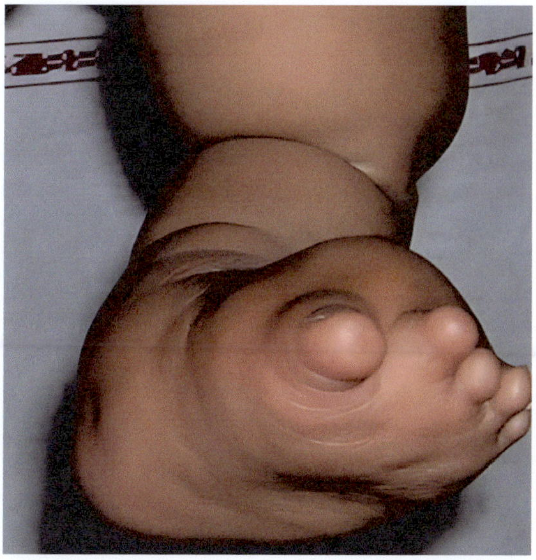

Fig. 83.14 Amniotic band

83.10 Mucous Cyst

Mucous cyst of the oral cavity is a common problem. A mucous cyst is a nonmalignant lesion located in the buccal mucosa, which arises from the rupture of a salivary gland duct, leading to the extravasation of mucin into the surrounding soft tissues. The lower inner lips are the most frequently affected site (Fig. 83.15a, b).

Management is generally by observation only. Rarely surgical marsupialization is required.

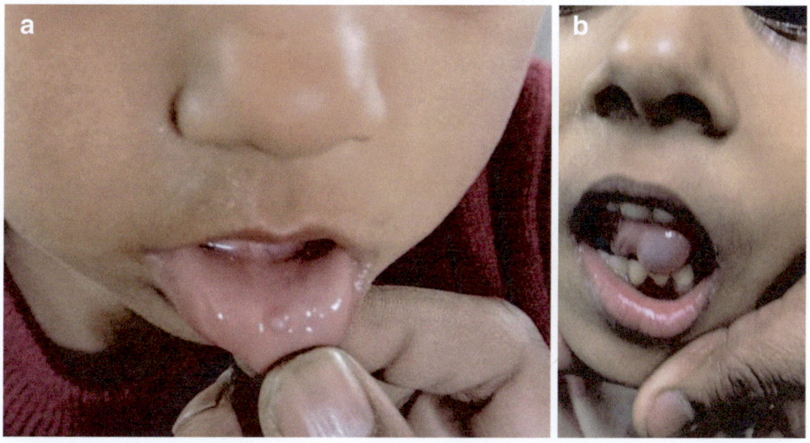

Fig. 83.15 (**a**) Mucous cyst, lower lip (**b**) Mucous cyst, tongue

83.11 Preauricular Tag

Preauricular tags are congenital abnormalities that are located anterior to the tragus and originate from the remnants of supernumerary brachial hillocks. These papules, also known as tags, are the outward manifestations of these lesions, which can be unilateral or bilateral, numerous or solitary. It is believed that they developed as a consequence of an imperfect merger of the first two branchial arches that occurred during embryonic growth.

Treatment of preauricular tag (Fig. 83.16) and preauricular sinus (Fig. 83.17): They are best left alone.

83.11.1 Ganglion Cyst

A ganglion cyst, also referred to as a synovial cyst, arises from the extravasation of synovial fluid from the joint into the adjacent tissue, typically within the tendon sheath. They present as firm swellings that are adherent to the underlying tendon sheath (Fig. 83.18). The initial approach to the management of a ganglion cyst involves observation and providing reassurance to the family concerning its benign characteristics. The likelihood of spontaneous resolution is exceedingly high. Historically, the Bible (heavy book) was used to rupture the cyst, facilitating the subsequent absorption of the fluid into the surrounding tissue. Symptomatic cases may be addressed through needle aspiration accompanied by the injection of a local steroid, like Kenacort, with or

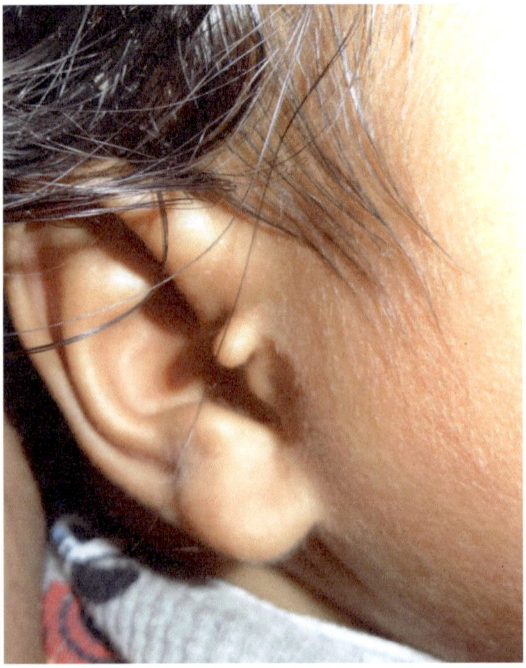

Fig. 83.16 Preauricular tag

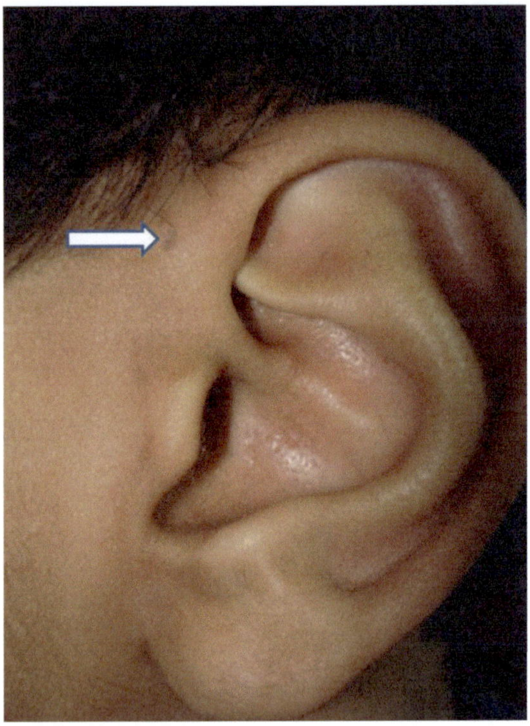

Fig. 83.17 Preauricular sinus

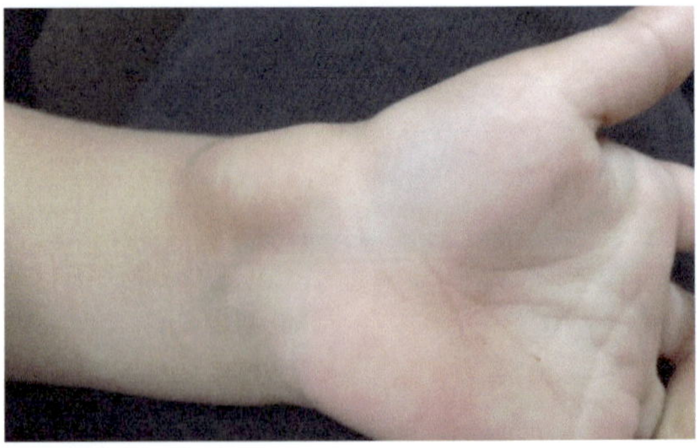

Fig. 83.18 Ganglion cyst

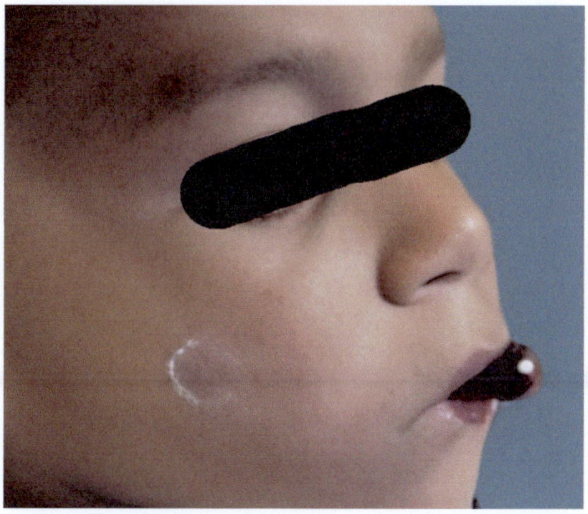

Fig. 83.19 Pyogenic granuloma

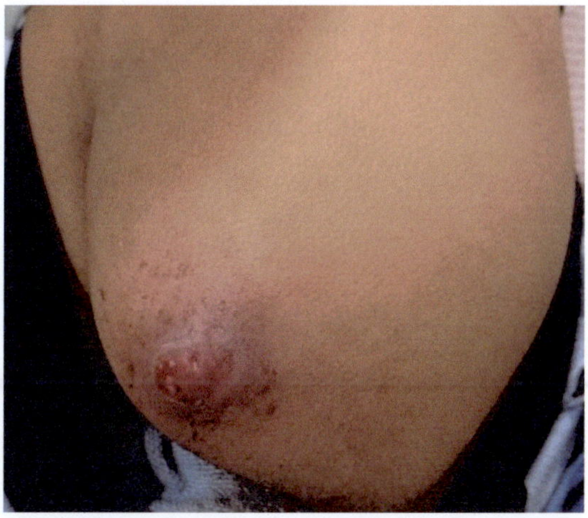

Fig. 83.20 Carbuncle on gluteal region

without the addition of hyaluronidase (Hyalase). However, it is important to note that there exists a significant likelihood of recurrence, then surgical excision may be required.

83.12 Pyogenic Granuloma

Pyogenic granulomas, as depicted in Fig. 83.19, are vascular lesions that manifest themselves as quickly expanding papules or nodules. As a result, they have the potential to bleed abundantly following minimal trauma. 'Pyogenic granuloma' is an incorrect title for this condition. In terms of their genesis, these lesions are vascular lesions and do not have an infectious cause. Surgical excision and skin suturing, electrocoagulation, or CO2 laser ablation are all equally effective treatments for the condition, although there is a possibility that it may recur in certain cases.

83.13 Carbuncle

An infection of the hair follicle that spreads into the neighboring dermal layers and the deeper subcutaneous tissue is referred to as a carbuncle (Fig. 83.20). This type of infection affects the hair follicles only. The most common manifestation of these conditions is a nodule that is erythematous, irritable, inflammatory, and fluctuating, and it is characterized by the presence of pustules or sinus tracts. Systemic symptoms are often noticeable, and there is a possibility that localized lymphadenopathy will appear. Treatment is usually conservative with antibiotics. Sometimes incision and drainage are required.

83.13.1 Ingrown Toenail

The condition known as ingrowing toenail (Fig. 83.21) is a painful ailment that occurs when the nail grows too far into one or both sides of the nail bed, which leads to inflammation and the creation of granulomas. Surgical excision of the nail, either in its entirety or in part, together with the germinal layer from the nail bed is the treatment for this condition.

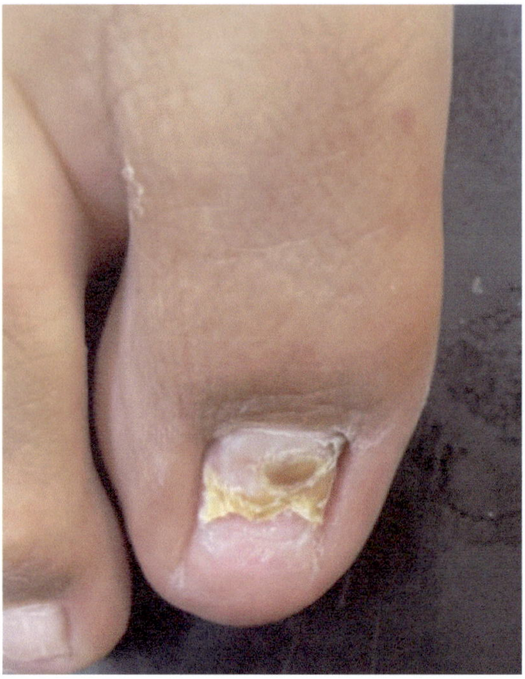

Fig. 83.21 Ingrown toenail

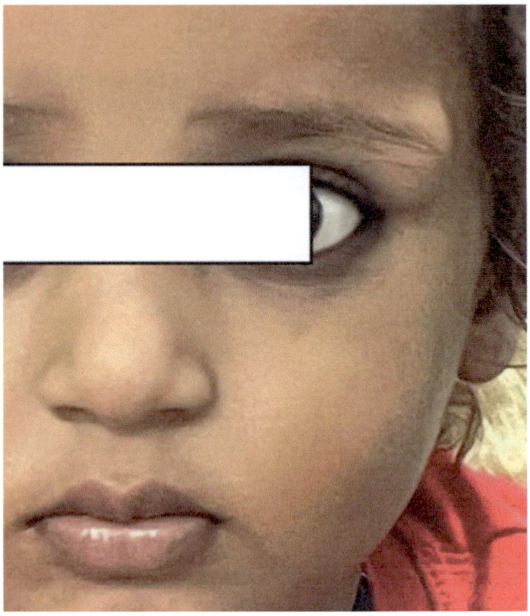

Fig. 83.22 Angular dermoid cyst

83.14 Dermoid Cyst

Dermoid cysts are seen either in the midline of the body or along the lines of embryonic fusion (Fig. 83.22). Treatment is by complete surgical excision.

83.15 Wound Granuloma

Treatment of wound granuloma (Fig. 83.23) is by chemical cauterization with copper sulfate or silver nitrate, or trichloroacetic acid.

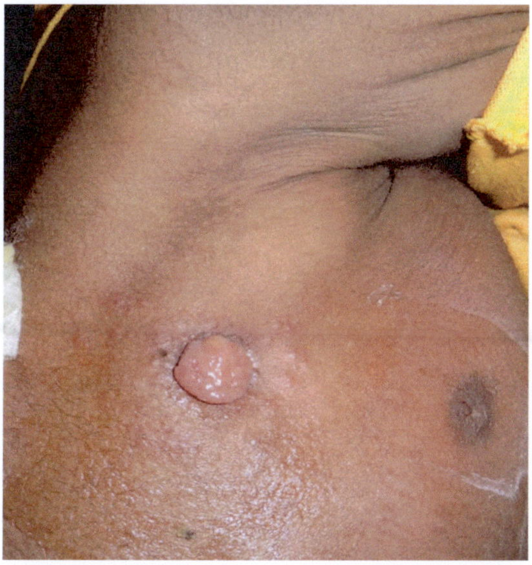

Fig. 83.23 Chest tube site wound granuloma

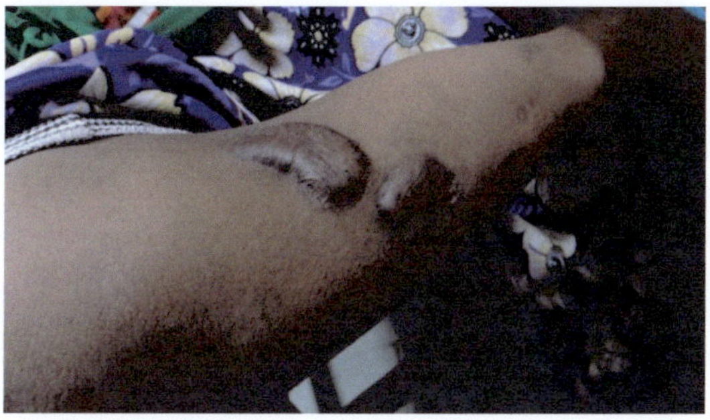

Fig. 83.24 Keloid over leg

83.15.1 Keloid

Management of keloid (Fig. 83.24) includes intralesional steroids (triamcinolone), surgical excision, cryosurgery, radiation therapy, interferon alpha, and pulse dye laser treatment.

83.15.1.1 Overgrowth of Limb

This benign overgrowth of the limb may be a type of congenital hamartomatous malformation (Fig. 83.25). Surgical correction requires the removal of the abnormal tissues and the reconstruction of the functional tissues.

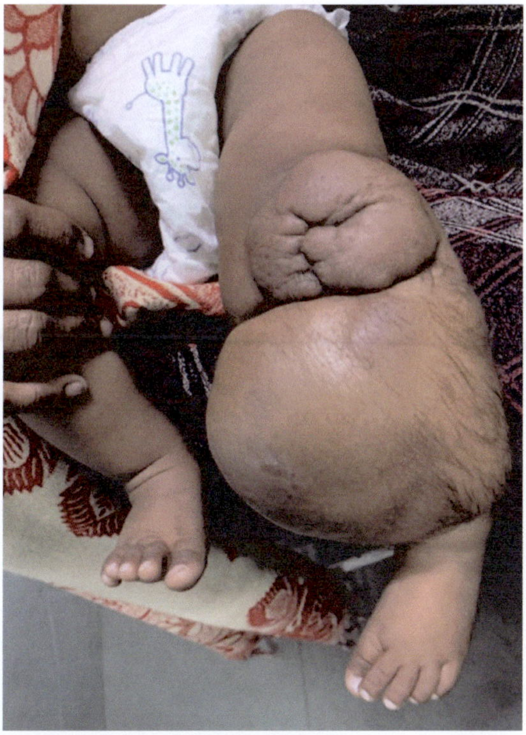

Fig. 83.25 Overgrowth of limb

83.15.1.2 Hair Thread Band Constriction

This is an iatrogenic insult which can lead to ischaemic damage to tissues often seen around the fingers, toes, or genitalia (Fig. 83.26). This condition once identified can be managed by removing the constricting band.

83.15.1.3 Accessory Limb

This is a type of heteropagus or parasitic twin (Fig. 83.27). Management is by surgical removal and local tissue reconstruction.

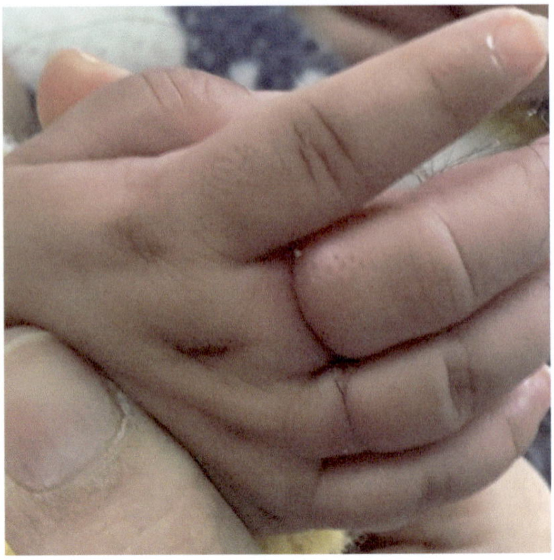

Fig. 83.26 Hair thread constriction of fingers

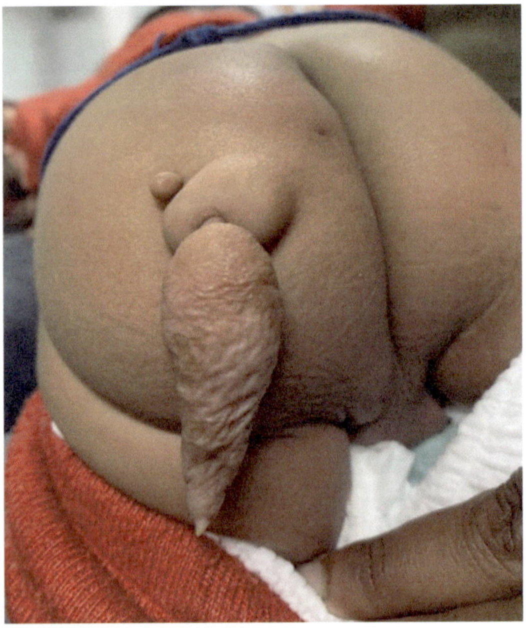

Fig. 83.27 Accessory limb

Suggested Reading

Hutson JM, O'Brien M, Woodward AA, Beasley SW. Jone's clinical pediatric surgery diagnosis and management. 6th ed. Oxford: Blackwell; 2008.

84 Minimal Access Surgery in Children

Ramesh Santhanakrishnan, Vinupriya Dasaratha, and Subhasis Roy Choudhury

Minimal access surgery (MAS) has now become an indispensable skill in the surgical armamentarium of all surgical branches. Pediatric surgery is no exception. Though a late entrant, it has advanced leaps and bounds that currently almost all the pediatric surgical procedures can be done using MAS techniques.

84.1 Advantages of MAS in Children

- A very important advantage of minimal access surgery (MAS) is minimal tissue damage caused by long access wounds. This results in reduced metabolic response of the body, reduced pain response, faster recovery and better cosmesis.
- The scars in children tend to grow with the child, and hence, it would be preferable to shorten the length of the scars in a child.
- Another major advantage of MAS is the magnified field of vision, and hence, the precision of the tissue handling is better.
- As the handling of the tissues is less, there are lesser chances of adhesions and a shorter duration of ileus.

R. Santhanakrishnan (✉) · V. Dasaratha
Pediatric Surgery, Indira Gandhi Institute of Child Health, Bangalore, Karnataka, India

S. Roy Choudhury
Pediatric Surgery, Lady Hardinge Medical College and Associated Kalawati Saran Children's Hospital, New Delhi, Delhi, India

84.2 Disadvantages of MAS in Children

- There is a need to procure additional equipment and familiarize the team with its functioning, acquire additional skills.
- The lack of tactile feedback and depth perception, which all surgeons are all too familiar is missing. Hence, an entirely new set of skills needs to be acquired, but this is not very difficult.
- The physiology of the child is quite fragile and poses significant challenges to the surgical and anesthetic team.
- Unlike in general surgery, the incidence of index cases like appendicectomy and cholecystectomy is lower in children. Hence, the bar in pediatric MAS is quite high.

84.3 Physiological Changes in MAS

There are a lot of physiologic changes in a child undergoing MAS, which the surgical and anesthetic team should be familiar with to ensure the safety of the child being operated. Pneumoperitoneum is a complex process and affects many systems

- Changes in the *acid-base metabolism* include increased $ETCO_2$, increased pCO_2 and decreased pH. Most of the changes are tran-

© The Author(s), under exclusive license to Springer Nature Singapore Pte Ltd. 2025

S. Roy Choudhury (ed.), *Pediatric Surgery*, https://doi.org/10.1007/978-981-96-1257-4_84

sient if the correct principles are followed. The $ETCO_2$ returns to baseline by 6–8 minutes. The other parameters also settle down with time.
- *Cardiovascular changes* in the form of direct arteriolar dilatation and myocardial depression are caused by high CO_2. It indirectly increases catecholamines, thereby increasing heart rate, blood pressure and cardiac output. High intra-abdominal pressure is associated with decreased venous return.
- *Renal effects* include reversible oliguria due to renal vein compression and direct parenchymal compression. However, there are no changes in serum creatinine level.
- *Neurological effects* like increased intracranial pressure can be due to hypercarbia.
- *Other effects* include.
  - Hypothermia.
  - Pneumothorax.
  - Pneumomediastinum.
  - Gas embolism.
  - Subcutaneous Emphysema.

It is always safe to start with lower CO_2 pressures and gradually increase the pressure allowing the child to adapt. The recommended CO_2 pressure and flow for children is 10 mm and 1 liter flow and 8 mm pressure and 0.8 liter flow. The pressure can be gradually increased once the baby is stable and tolerates the increased pressure. For thoracoscopy, the flow is generally 0.5 liters and the pressure is 5 mm. This is to ensure adequate working space without compromising the venous return.

It is highly recommended that the pressure setting is personally verified by the surgeon before connecting to the CO_2 insufflator to avoid sudden distention and its possible catastrophic consequences.

84.4 Ergonomics

It is very essential to maintain ergonomics during any form of MAS—be it laparoscopy or thoracoscopy or neuroendoscopy. The essential steps of ergonomics include:

- Positioning of the operating table, the Laparoscopy equipment including the monitor and the operating/anesthetic team is very crucial for the smooth conduct of the surgery (Fig. 84.1).
  - While the anesthetist is positioned at the head end of the table ensuring easy access to the child's airway and the other leads for patient monitoring.
  - The surgeon stands on the opposite side of the lesion or at the foot end between the two abducted limbs of the patient for surgeries in the upper abdomen (in this case, the anesthetic team moves to either side of the head end).
  - The monitor is placed in alignment to the surgeon's vision and the operative field. All three should be in the same straight line to reduce the stress on the surgeon.
  - The rest of the team—the assistants and the nursing staff are placed accordingly.
  - The child is placed as close to the side of the operation table toward the surgeon and in alignment with the monitor and the surgeon.
  - The child needs to be securely strapped to the OT table to ensure the safety of the child whenever the position of the patient is altered during the surgery.
  - The OT table can be tilted during surgery to ensure that the other viscera drop away from the operating field and can even be referred to as the "invisible port."
- *Port Placement.*
  It is essential to:
  Empty bladder—catheterize for infraumbilical procedure.
  Empty stomach—for supraumbilical procedure.
  - The telescopic port is generally placed at the umbilicus. However, in small children it may have to be shifted either below (for surgery in the epigastrium) or above (for pelvic surgery). It may also be placed in other locations in special circumstances. Open method of primary port placement (Hassen's technique) is preferred in children over Veeres' needle insertion.

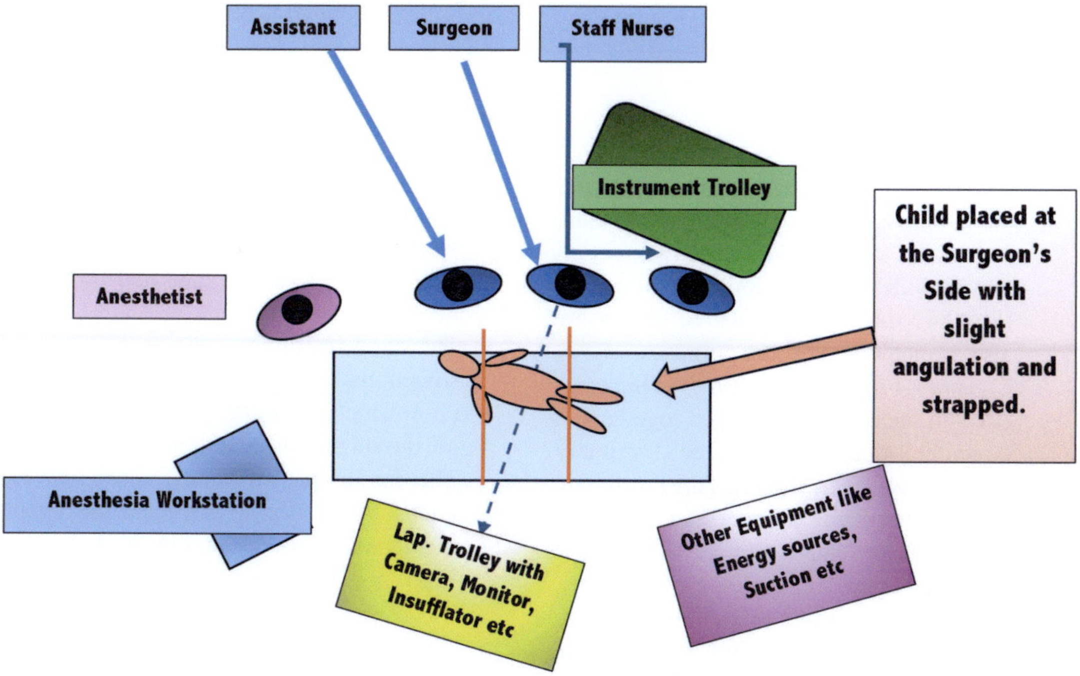

Fig. 84.1 Ergonomics of the OT Set-up

- The working ports are placed on either side by about 30 degrees from the primary trocar. This will ensure a comfortable working for the surgeon.
- Additional ports may be needed for retraction and can be placed based on the exigencies and requirements.
- The ports are fixed to the abdominal wall by using a sleeve on the trocar (either a rubber tube or a rubber band made of gloves). This is done to prevent the slippage of the trocar during the surgery.
- As there are too many types of equipment, tubing and wires in the OT, it is necessary to ensure that all the types of equipment are correctly placed and the tubing and cables do not clutter the area around the OT table.
- The surgeon has to comfortably positioned with the held straight looking at the monitor, the feet about a foot apart and the shoulders are relaxed, the elbow should be at an obtuse angle and the wrist should be slightly dorsiflexed (Fig. 84.2). The height and the tilt of the OT table can be adjusted accordingly.

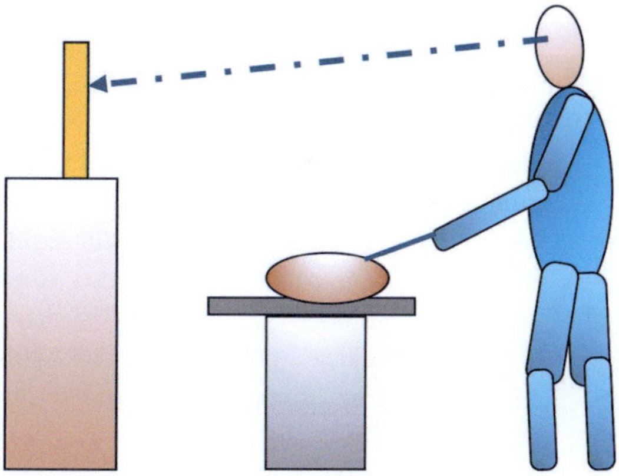

Fig. 84.2 Ergonomics for the Surgeon

- The importance of the correct position of the surgeon during surgery cannot be overemphasized to prevent joint problems in the operating surgeon in due course.

84.5 Laparoscopic and Thoracoscopic Instruments

- *Optics.*
  - *Telescopes*—Even though 0-degree scopes are easier to handle, 30-degree scopes are very useful to perform advanced surgery, as they provide a better visibility of the organs (Fig. 84.3). 45- and 70-degree scopes are also available for specific purposes.
  - *Camera*—From the era of single-chip cameras (all the colors transmitted together) to three-chip camera (where the 3 primary colors—red, green and blue, are separately sent to the camera and processed there for a better image), the optics in laparoscopy have advanced tremendously. Currently, both are outdated, and high-definition cameras and 4K cameras are the standard choice, and the image quality is outstanding. Three-dimensional cameras are also available at additional cost.
  - *Light Source and Cable*—The halogen light sources which used to provide light of lesser brightness with a yellow tinge were replaced by whiter and brighter Xenon light source. However, currently, LED light sources are most popular and effective in providing a good amount of bright light. The light source cables can be either fiber optic or gel-filled.
  - *Monitor*—Medical grade monitors with high resolution are essential if the tissue visibility has to be good.
- *CO_2 Insufflator*—It is quite important to have a good quality insufflator to ensure safety for all. The CO_2 that is used for insufflation should ideally be of medical grade, but not easily available.
- *Hand Instruments.*
  - Most of the working instruments are longer versions of the open surgical instruments. However, they are all modified for use in MAS.
  - The hand instruments are quite long and sometimes unwieldy. The port acts as a fulcrum which can either impede or exaggerate the surgeon's hand movements.
  - The tip of the instrument moves in the opposite direction of the hand movement (paradoxical movement, Fig. 84.4).
  - The range of movements is grossly reduced (to 6 ranges) in MAS as compared to open surgery. This has to be kept in mind and practiced for the safe performance of MAS.
  - Most of the laparoscopic instruments (those that have a connection for diathermy) have a sleeve of insulation. It is very crucial to ensure that this insulation is not damaged and that the insulation is visible in the field while using diathermy to prevent collateral diathermy injury.
  - There are a wide variety of graspers for handling the tissues—Maryland, toothed, non-toothed, Babcock, fenestrated, bowel holder, atraumatic, etc.
  - A variety of dissectors are also available—Hook, spatula, scissors, etc.
  - There are also a variety of retractors and other instruments available.

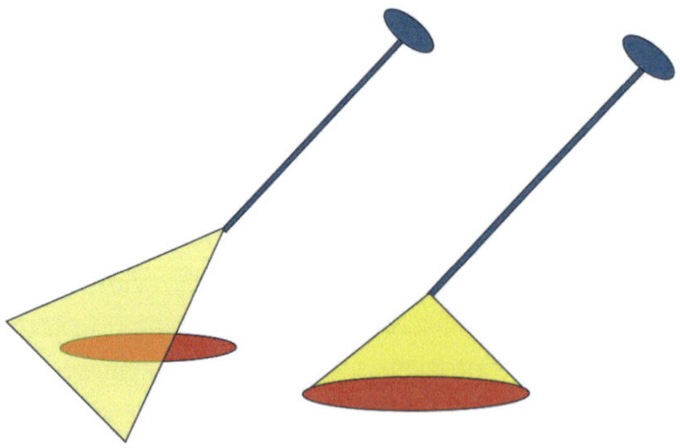

Fig. 84.3 Advantages of 30 degree telescope

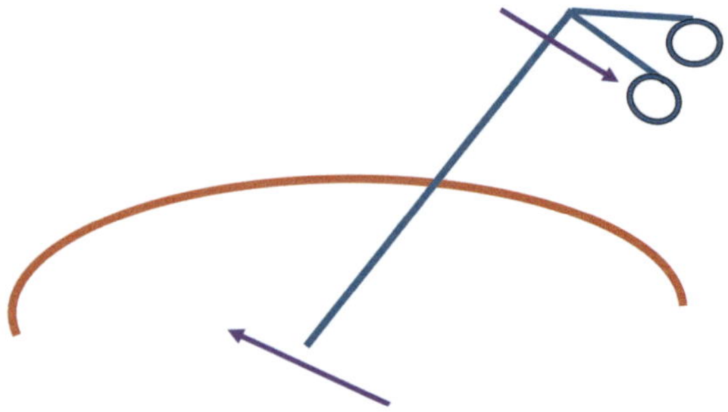

Fig. 84.4 Paradoxical Movement of Hand instruments

It is very essential that the operating surgeon should be familiar with the functioning of the instruments and to troubleshoot if there is a malfunction. It is also very safe to check these before the operation so as to avoid unnecessary issues during the surgery.

84.6 Energy Sources

Several energy sources are currently available.

- *Monopolar Diathermy* is the most frequently used energy source as it is easily available, economical and quite versatile. However, it is essential to keep in mind the possible damage that it can cause to the tissues if not used properly. Apart from charring the tissues, it can cause direct coupling damage to other organs if inadvertently touched and latent thermal damage. There have been many advances in the design of the instruments to render them safe by working on tissue impedance to avoid tissue damage.
- *Bipolar diathermy* is quite safe when compared to its monopolar counterpart as the travers of the electrical energy is limited between the blades of the tip. It would be useful to rotate the instruments to visualize the cautery process between the blades.
- *Ultracision—Harmonic Scalpel* ® works by rapid oscillation (up to 55,000 cycles per second) by the active limb of the tip. This denatures the tissues and helps in cutting the tissues as well. It can handle vessels up to 7 mm in diameter. It is quite crucial to keep in mind the high temperature of the tip after use and be cautious in handling the instrument after use.
- *Advanced Bipolar with Vessel Sealing—LigaSure ® and Thunderbeat ®* are very useful when handling vascular tissues and the vessel pedicles. It seals the vessels and hence very reliable when dealing with vessels.

84.7 Tissue Approximation

The real test for the MAS surgeon comes when performing reconstructive surgeries where a lot of suturing is required. The various types of tissue approximation include:

- *Extra-Corporeal Knotting*—This is the easiest method of knotting as the knot is tied outside and then slipped inside using a knot pusher or a Maryland grasper. There are several popular techniques for extra-corporeal knots including *Roeder's Knot*, *Meltzer's Knot* and *Tayside Knot*.
- *Intra-Corporeal (IC) Suturing*—The skills and the patience of an MIS surgeon will be put to the maximum test during intra-corporeal suturing (IC suturing). It needs a lot of practice on endo-trainers, good dexterity, plenty of patience and presence of mind to execute it smoothly.
  - *C-loop Technique* popularized by Sir Alfred Cuschieri and Zoltan forms the basis of most of the other techniques of suturing.
  - *Freehand Suturing*—While the C-loop technique is ideal and forms the basis of other suturing techniques, many surgeons find it rather unwieldy after the basics are mastered. Many of the senior surgeons resort to "freehand" suturing technique that we use in open surgery.
  - *Sliding Knot*—This is a fairly simple technique used where the tissues are far apart and need to be brought closer by the suture, or when the suture tends to get loose before the next knot.
- *Extra-corporeal suturing* is a handy technique particularly useful for situations which require secure but not necessarily finer suturing such as in diaphragmatic hernia repair. The bites are taken as in any surgery, but the needle is retrieved out where a conventional hand suture is made extra-corporeally and the knot is cinched in with the help of a knot pusher.

- The utility of *stay sutures* and *hitch sutures* cannot be overemphasized. Correct placement of a hitch suture will render the process of IC suturing efficient.
- *Endo-staplers* are very good for bowel anastomosis and are available in various sizes and thicknesses. The major limitations are cost and space constraints in small infants. Additionally, it is necessary to use a 12-mm trocar for introduction and deployment of endo-staplers.
- *Fibrin glue,* used as a tissue adhesive with minimal tissue handling, has been described to seal staple lines and vascular anastomoses. The outcomes have largely been unfavorable with respect to intestinal anastomoses, and its use is presently limited to skin approximation.
- *Laser tissue welding* is another experimental method using stay sutures and laser energy over a protein solder to weld the edges together. It has been attempted where a watertight seal is desirable such as in ureteral and bladder anastomoses. The challenges presently are precision in the procedure.

84.8 Common Indications for MAS in Pediatric Surgery

- There are several procedures in which MAS has become the gold standard and the procedure of choice:
  - Diagnostic laparoscopy for non-palpable testis, intersex conditions, intra-abdominal cysts, etc.
  - Simple laparoscopic procedures like appendicectomy, cholecystectomy, pyloromyotomy, etc.
  - Thoracoscopy for empyema thoracis, diaphragmatic hernia and eventration, biopsies, lung biopsies, sympathectomy, etc.
- Some procedures have become very popular and are being widely done by many pediatric surgeons.
  - Excisional surgeries like splenectomy, nephrectomy, ovarian cystectomy, adrenalectomy, etc.
  - Reconstructive surgery like pyeloplasty, fundoplication, pull-through for Hirschsprung's, anorectal malformation, choledochal cysts, etc.
- However, there are some advanced procedures which are practiced only by a select group of surgeons as the demand on the resources, skill and backup is tremendous.
  - Esophageal atresia + Tracheoesophageal fistula,
  - Duodenal atresia,
  - Pulmonary lobectomy,
  - Pericardiectomy,
  - Pancreatectomy, Puestow's procedure, etc.

Essentially, any surgical procedure which can be done by open technique can be done through MAS. However, it all depends on the skill and aptitude of the surgical team, the resource availability and the backup.

It is paramount to remember that the child has been brought to us for a problem and that needs to be fixed with no compromise on the essential surgical principles. Any new technology, including MAS, does not give any surgeon to violate the essential dictum of patient safety.

84.9 Training and Skill Development

Practicing on endo-trainers is an essential part of mastering the art of laparoscopic skills and endosuturing. Even practicing for about 30 minutes each day will go a long way in achieving mastery in MAS techniques. If sophisticated simulators are not available, local modifications of an endotrainer and improvisations of simple box trainers will be worthwhile (Fig. 84.5).

While the skills acquired by training on a simulator have been demonstrated to be transferable to actual surgical scenarios, the ultimate test awaits at the operating table.

Mastery in basic techniques of minimal invasive suturing and knotting with ex vivo practice sets up the platform for successful in vivo performance.

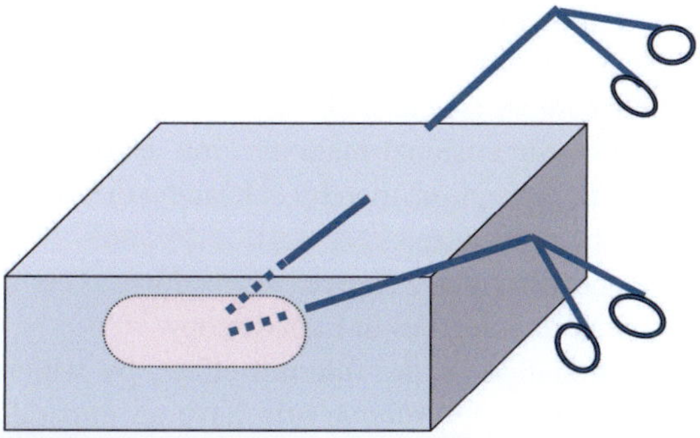

Fig. 84.5 Home made Endotrainer

84.9.1 Tips for the Beginner

Minimal access surgery (MAS) is here to stay and is the way forward. There is no way to miss the bus. Make a very earnest effort to start learning the right way and progress steadily.

- *MAS is no license to violate the basic surgical principles*—Always follow the basic surgical principles with no compromise on patient safety.
- *Primary aim is to "fix the problem"*—and unless that is achieved, your obligation is not complete. Treating the patient is the primary aim, and the means are secondary.
- *Conversion is never a failure, but a failure to convert is*. Do not hesitate to convert as that was the option if you had not chosen to do MAS.
- *MAS is a teamwork*—take the entire team along as a true captain.
- *It's never too late to learn*. Keep learning from everywhere at every opportunity.
- *Be ready to adapt to new technologies*. They can make your surgery easier and safer.
- *Start small and make steady progress. Don't be greedy.*
- *Read, discuss, see, rehearse the steps and alternatives with the entire team well before the surgery*, and do not hesitate to take suggestions from other team members during surgery.
- *Due diligence at all levels* is very essential for the safe performance of the procedure.
- *Utilize the available resources—Books/Journals/Internet.*
- *Discuss with colleagues and seniors* if you have any difficulties.
- *Record and review and be honest.*
- *Learn the trade... you will learn the tricks yourself!*

84.10 Robotic Surgery in Children

Robotic surgery is the latest entrant in the field of pediatric MAS. The modality is steadily gaining popularity over the last decade as it provides extraordinary precision in surgery and has very exciting potential.

Robot (the Czech word "robota" meaning slave) is defined as a machine capable of carrying out complex series of actions automatically as programmed by a computer.

84.10.1 Classification of Robot Based on Autonomy

- *Autonomous*—These robots carry out preoperative plan without any immediate control from the surgeon, and their applications are more in other branches like radiation oncology (Example: Robodoc, CyberKnife).
- *Surgical Assist Devices*—These are the next-generation robots in which the surgeon and robot share the control. These robots had limited applications as they just obeyed voice commands to retract tissues or hold the camera. (Example: AESOP.)
- *Teleoperators*—Whose every function is controlled by the surgeon with a "master-slave relationship." These robots are currently extremely popular as the machine augments the skills of the surgeon by precision movements and negates the drawbacks of the surgeon like tremors and violent movement. In addition, there are a lot of safety features installed in these robots making it truly safe for the child and the surgeon. (Example: Da Vinci system, SSI Mantra).

84.10.2 Components of a Robotic Surgery System (Fig. 84.6)

- *Surgeon's console* where the surgeon and the assistant sit and gain hand control of the instruments. There are many controls in the fingers and feet such that the surgeon operates in the console remote from the actual patient. There is also a provision for mentoring a trainee with a dual console with variable controls.
- *Patient side cart*, which is the actual set of instruments which perform the surgery. There is an array of bulky equipment, but with finer handles which do all the maneuvers as commanded by the surgeon. It is very essential to plan and place the equipment properly and "dock" the equipment before starting the surgery.
- *Vision cart* which is stack of the camera, light source and the monitors.

84.10.3 Advantages of Robotic Surgery

- Motion scaling, by which the movements of the surgeons' hands are smoothed without any jerky or rapid movement.
- Tremor reduction, by which the tremors of the surgeon's hands are eliminated completely.
- High-resolution stereo display ensures excellent magnification and hence the precision of the surgery is achieved-.
- Three-dimensional magnification enables the depth perception, thereby enhancing the safety of the procedure.
- Robot provides 7 degrees of freedom, as compared to 6 degrees in Laparoscopy.
- Elimination of the fulcrum effect, by which the tips of the robotic arm have an unparalleled range of dexterity and precise movements including reverse motion.
- Tele-surgery is possible, wherein a surgeon can sit in a remote place (even in a different country) and operate on the patient with the same amount of precision.

84.10.4 Disadvantages

- Absence of tactile feedback can actually be felt by senior surgeons, but is well compensated by the excellent vision and depth perception afforded by the surgical robot.
- The huge cost in procurement of the equipment (cost running into crores of Rupees) is a major hindrance in setting up in most of the hospitals.
- The high cost of the disposables for each case is a recurring cost, which again is a major deterrent in developing countries.

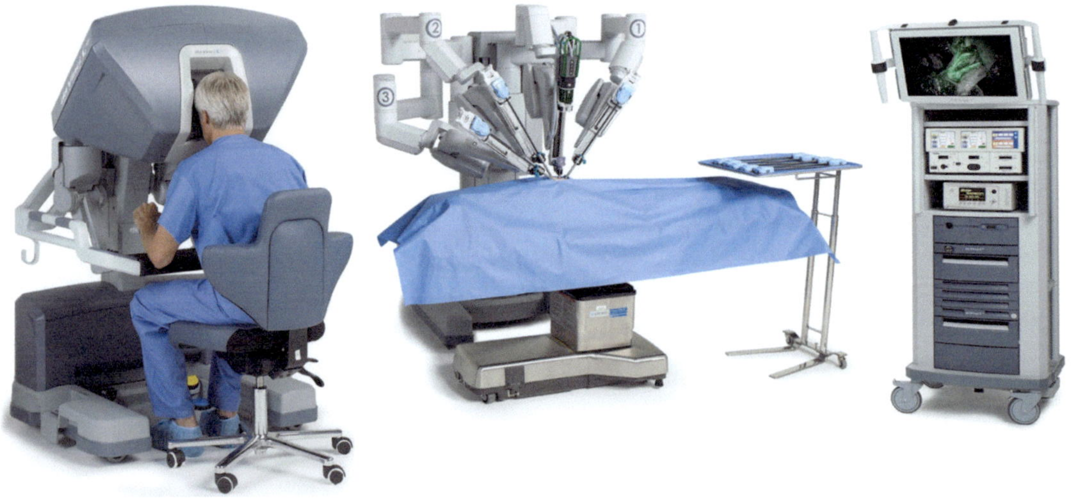

Fig. 84.6 Da Vinci surgical robot in action

- The equipment is very bulky and occupies a large portion of the operation theater. In addition, the hand instruments are still big and are 12 mm, 8 mm and 5 mm. This renders infants and small-sized children less suitable for robotic surgery.

84.10.5 Current Status of Robotics in Pediatric Surgery

Robotic surgery in children has grown significantly over the last decade even in developing countries. A wide variety of excisional and reconstructive surgery in all age groups have been reported from all over the world. Robotic pyeloplasty, choledochal cyst excision, ureteric re-implantation, bladder augmentation, fundoplication, etc. have all been successfully and routinely done across the world with good results.

The safety and effectiveness of robotic surgery are well established; however, the cost is still quite prohibitive in most centers. However, with further widespread use, the cost of the equipment and disposables is expected to come down. That is the time that the benefits of robotic surgery can be passed on to all the children who need surgical intervention.

Further Reading

Cave J, Clarke S. Paediatric robotic surgery. Ann R Coll Surg Engl. 2018;100(Suppl 7):18–21. https://doi.org/10.1308/rcsann.supp2.18. PMID: 30179047; PMCID: PMC6216751

Holcomb GW III, Murphy PJ, St Peter SD, editors. Holcomb and ashcraft's pediatric surgery. 7th ed. Philadelphia: Elsevier; 2020.

Mei H, Tang ST. Robotic-assisted surgery in the pediatric surgeons' world: current situation and future prospectives. Front Pediatr. 2023;11:1120831. https://doi.org/10.3389/fped.2023.1120831.

Shen LT, Tou J. Application and prospects of robotic surgery in children: a scoping review. World J Pediatr Surg. 2022;5:e000482. https://doi.org/10.1136/wjps-2022-000482.

Walsh DS, Ponsky TA, Burns NE. The Sages manual for pediatric minimally invasive surgery. Cham: Springer International; 2017.

Part XII

Recent Advances in Pediatric Surgery

Recent Advances in Pediatric Surgery

85

Narasimhan Kannan Laksmi, York Tien Lee, and Xuxin Lim

In the rapid pace of scientific development, the advancement of knowledge in pediatric surgery has been accelerating. Current medical knowledge is getting obsolete even faster and our need to upgrade frequently has become a necessity. We shall briefly delve into recent advances relevant to Pediatric Surgeons after the last edition of this book was published.

When the millennium began, one of the criticism against pediatric surgery was the lack of evidence-based practices in decision-making. We have changed our practice based on the available evidences in last few years because of intense pressure from peers in our pediatric specialties. In addition to technology, molecular biology, precision imaging, and novel instrumentation have changed our practices. The emergence of social media and ChatGPT in public platforms caused a paradigm shift in the way we give information to families and the way families are empowered to make decisions on their own surgical conditions. Emerging technologies are also helping poorer countries cope with Pediatric Surgical workload and improving their outcomes.

Global pediatric surgery research is focused on providing access to essential surgical procedures for children in a timely and affordable manner. The objective is to reduce pain, minimize length of hospital stay, and complications and increasing shift towards day surgery has been implemented in several countries.

The surgical community has looked at evidences to raise the standard of care. This is one the most significant developments in Pediatric Surgery.

N. K. Laksmi (✉)
Senior Consultant in Pediatric Surgery, Duke NUS School of Medicine, K Women's and Children's Hospital, Singapore, Singapore

Senior Consultant in Pediatric Surgery, KK Women's and Children's Hospital, Singapore, Singapore

Y. T. Lee
Senior Consultant in Pediatric Surgery, KK Women's and Children's Hospital, Singapore, Singapore

Pediatric Surgery, KK Women's and Children's Hospital, Singapore, Singapore

X. Lim
Senior Consultant in Pediatric Surgery, KK Women's and Children's Hospital, Singapore, Singapore

85.1 Evidence-Based Practices

Onventional opinions are constantly getting challenged and there are increasing numbers of well run trials/studies which is changing clinical practices in pediatric surgery over time. These include diagnostic modalities, indications and mode of surgery, and long-term follow-ups. Several treatment modalities have got refined, especially in the areas of anorectal malformations, Hirschsprung's disease, and pelvic-ureteric junction obstruction.

© The Author(s), under exclusive license to Springer Nature Singapore Pte Ltd. 2025

S. Roy Choudhury (ed.), *Pediatric Surgery*, https://doi.org/10.1007/978-981-96-1257-4_85

85.1.1 Appendicitis in Children

There is a paucity of high-quality evidence in the literature regarding timing of appendectomy for patients with acute appendicitis and its association with adverse events or resource utilization. Based on available evidence, appendectomy performed within the first 24 hour from presentation is not associated with an increased risk of perforation or adverse outcomes. Most patients randomized to antibiotic treatment for uncomplicated appendicitis did not require appendectomy during the 1-year follow-up period, and those who required appendectomy did not experience significant complications.

85.1.2 Timing of Neonatal Hernia Repair

Several studies have now established that neonatal hernias can be operated after a delay, safely in a larger sized baby. The risk of hernia incarceration and testicular atrophy did not increase with delayed elective hernia repair in neonates. Delayed hernia repair decreased the risk of perioperative and postoperative complications. Repair of inguinal hernia in premature infants before NICU discharge may increase the odds of recurrence, but not incarceration or surgical complications.

85.2 Technology

Minimally invasive surgery (MIS)is now increasingly prevalent in the field of pediatric surgery and has changed patient care radically. The novel types of approaches to surgery such as retro-peritoneal access vs transperitoneal access for kidney, ureter, bladder; better suturing and miniaturization and handheld robots have facilitated in decreasing the hospital stay, reduce pain and minimizing scars. These areas are fast evolving and biomedical scientists are constantly working on improving the devices used. The issue of costs of equipment in MIS is important and research to bring down costs is imperative to increase uptake of MIS approaches. Increase in the use of MIS in poorer countries is gradually happening because of better marketing by the instrument manufacturers. Instruments appropriate for the pediatric size have started appearing in the market and reuseable instruments and technology is also gaining traction.

Handheld robotic instruments that are lighter and allow better hand–eye co-ordination than plain laparoscopic instruments, but they are technologically simpler and seem to have a lot of scope in developing countries. They also bring down the cost of treatment to the patient. The use of Artificial Intelligence (AI) in handheld robots may also improve efficiency and precision of such instruments in clinical practice.

For minimally invasive surgery (MIS) to penetrate the developing world, certain adaptations are needed. An awareness that penetration to areas with unstable power and resources and with high population is necessary to ensure that these equipment are operable on battery power and reuseable. Scaling down the costs and improving ergonomics in laparoscopy will facilitate the use of laparoscopy all over the globe.

85.3 Artificial Intelligence (AI)

There are several areas where artificial intelligence is making its impact. Younger generations of surgeons are using ChatGPT for writing papers and research.

Jobs considered menial and boring are increasingly being replaced by robots.

Artificial Intelligence (AI) can facilitate learning tasks that are difficult or need steep learning skills. AI can do a lot in automation, image analysis, and give us a degree of freedom to improve clinical care.

The next few decades will see AI leading advancement along with medical device technology. AI may be able to integrate cross-sectional images, 3-dimensional visual impressions, and intra-operative ultrasound. This is likely to help refine our surgical techniques over time resulting in smaller scars and better surgical outcomes.

The other issue with medical devices is the enormous electronic waste it produces. Technology that is green and recyclable is needed. With governments going environmentally friendly, medical companies will hopefully shift towards sustainable technology.

85.4 Areas Where AI Can Help

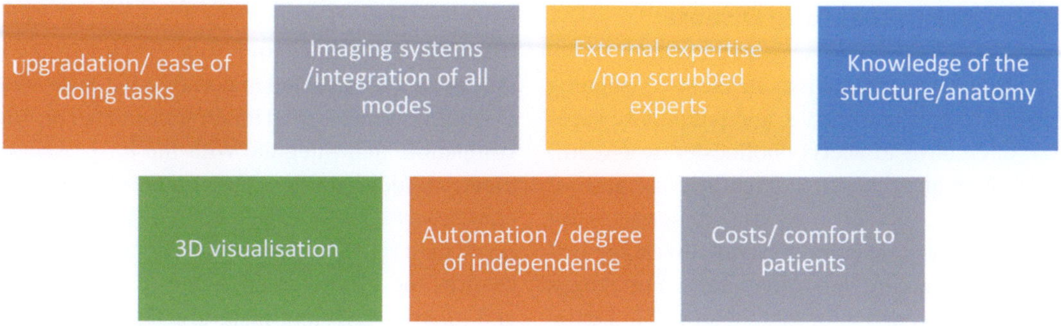

85.5 Training for Newer Technologies

Newer technologies come with a learning curve. Time and investment are needed to train manpower. Every 5 years, there is upgradation of technology and there is need for retraining. There is need to subspecialize so that one has adequate volume of cases and the necessary time to upgrade skills. In our life time, there were several technologies that got upgraded—such as intravenous lines and total parenteral nutrition, neonatal ventilation, diagnostic modalities, intervention radiology, chemoimmunotherapy, multidisciplinary team management, instrumentation technology, and use of information technology for all aspects of medical care. Phishing and data security breaches have also become more problematic with increasing use of paperless medical records. Medical litigation and the concept of "second victim" has become rampant. The medical practice has become increasingly complex.

Yet medical care needs to be standardized, easy to access, and accountable. The health care management systems are constantly impacting how we teach and coach our trainees. Most junior doctors are guideline-dependent and increasingly rely on radiologic investigation even for simple diagnosis, instead of developing their clinical acumen.

85.6 Access to Medical Care/ Remote Assistance

One of the common complaints in pediatric surgery is the difficulty of accessing affordable medical care in the United States, Canada, and the United Kingdom. Such developed countries have excellent access to medical care but the cost of medical is high. The COVID era saw a sudden boost in online consultations and Zoom consultations as never before. Indeed, the development of telemedicine was largely facilitated by COVID.

Better internet connectivity and AI will lead to better medical consultations over zoom or any other internet platform. Perhaps even overseas scrub assistants are a possibility wherein a technical expert from outside remotely scrubs and helps the surgeon and guides the surgery. With faster internet speeds, these are going to be available across the globe. Such platforms are being tested in developed world and will soon be released to the medical world.

85.7 Diagnostic Aids

85.7.1 Use of Calretinin Staining in Hirschsprung Disease

Calretinin immunohistochemical staining appears to be a reasonable, and potentially superior, alternative to acetyl-cholinesterase (AChE) staining as an adjunctive diagnostic method for evaluating suction rectal biopsies for Hirschsprung's disease. Several advantages of Calretinin staining are mentioned. For frozen section, identification of ganglion cells in hemotoxylin and eosin staining is the gold standard. The superiority of Calretinin staining over AChE staining is yet to be proven by prospective studies but may be a useful adjunct in diagnosis of Hirschprung's disease.

Newer non-invasive diagnostic models are being tried out for the diagnosis of Hirschsprung's disease including transrectal Raman spectroscopy and ultrasound. These devices are in the primitive stages and yet to be standardized but if there is a break through achieved, it will tremendously improve the care of the children with HD.

85.8 Tissue Engineering In Pediatric Surgery

Tissue engineering (TE) in pediatric surgery is a relatively new and growing field. Engineered tissue scaffolds can be used for various purposes such as wound healing and tissue regeneration in pediatric patients with congenital malformations or tissue defects after oncological resection. Tissue engineering involves interaction between three key components: cells, scaffolds, and growth factors. The interplay between these key components results in a dynamic biocompatible material which can integrate with the recipient site over time or accelerate the healing process. The benefit of using tissue engineered scaffolds is that it only requires a small amount of autologous cells which can be expanded and grown externally before transfer back to the host. Bioengineered scaffolds have been used to replace urethral tissue in hypospadias, epidermal and dermal layers in burns, as well as for tracheal reconstruction. However, the challenge of using tissue engineered materials in pediatric surgery is that these scaffolds and materials must grow with the child over time, and therefore needs to be biocompatible and integrate with the host environment. Additionally, the three-dimensional complexity of solid organs such as liver and kidney where there is an interplay of various factors such as the different cell types, growth factors, and microarchitecture make it a significant challenge to recapitulate such a construct artificially.

Tissue engineering combines the principles of engineering and biology and generally involves the use of some combination of the following: biomaterials, cells, and bioactive molecules. The appropriate contribution of each factor depends upon the application in question, the strategy for tissue replacement, and patient variables such as age, co-morbidities, and other factors. TE strategies can include both in vitro and in vivo approaches, and the optimal approach for each clinical situation is different.

The pediatric population has unique opportunities for application of the tissue engineering technology.

85.9 Tissue Engineering and Regenerative Medicine

Organ regeneration is one of the holy grails in pediatric surgery. It is particularly useful in babies with congenital defects where there is a deficiency in an organ or tissue which can be supplanted by tissue engineered materials and stem cells. It is an evolving field which holds a lot of potential. Induced pluripotent stem cells derived from differentiated cell lines and pluripotential stem cells present in placental amnion and chorion have been used as source of cells for regenerative purposes, particularly in wound healing and burns. Heart valves, tympanic membrane, tracheal cartilages and even bladder mucosa, have been constructed using tissue engineering. The challenges and opportunities in this area are still being explored.

85.10 Imaging

Several imaging modalities have been upgraded over the last decade as well. Magnetic resonance imaging (MRI) has advanced rapidly to replace computed tomography (CT) scans in many areas. The principal limitation in MRI in children was the inability of kids to hold their breath, causing artefacts and blurred images. The reduction of MRI time has been attempted and several new techniques of MRI are described. The replacement of intravenous urography (IVU) by magnetic resonance urography (MRU) in the recent years have resulting in better image quality with reduction in radiation. The use of MR spectroscopy is also increasingly explored but remains experimental at present.

Hybrid imaging techniques such as positron emission tomography combined with magnetic resonance imaging (PET-MRI) is a new combination that is being investigated. The field of paediatric oncology has benefitted the most in advance imaging techniques which helps detect minute cancerous foci in the body. FDG PET-CT has been available and is very useful in oncology in detecting tumors and monitoring cancer response to chemotherapy.

Indications for FDG PET/CT include, but are not limited to, the following:

- Differentiation of benign from malignant lesions.
- Searching for an unknown primary tumor when metastatic disease is discovered as the first manifestation of cancer or when the patient presents with a paraneoplastic syndrome.
- Staging patients with known malignancies.
- Monitoring the effect of therapy on known malignancies.
- Determining whether residual abnormalities detected on physical examination or on other imaging studies following treatment represent tumor or posttreatment fibrosis or necrosis.
- Detecting tumor recurrence, especially in the presence of elevated tumor markers.
- Selection of the region of tumor most likely to yield diagnostic information for biopsy.
- Guiding radiation therapy planning.

85.11 Can Robots Replace Human Surgeons?

AI algorithms and surgical robots may be able to achieve complication-free and faster surgery even in inaccessible areas as believed by data scientists. The following table compares the two skill sets.

Human abilities	Robotic abilities
Physical state and age , need to take coffee breaks etc	Insusceptibility to fatigue
Variation in skills and regional differences	Tremor resistance
Training and updating skills needed	Scalable movements
Minimum numbers to keep skill sets intact	Greater range of axial movement
	Reduced technical errors and reduced morbidities

The surgical robots at present are behaving as servants and are programmed to make our job simple. However, medical technology companies have yet to design better robots ro replace human surgeons which is well-nigh impossible. Even an automatic car or a plane on auto mode needs human supervision.

Nevertheless, one useful advantage of devices controlled by AI-based algorithms is that they may help with surgical skills training and upgrading.

For example, many Surgeons learn PSARP (posterior sagittal anorectoplasty) by watching live operative workshops and videos. Robots can machine learn the operation by going through all the PSARP videos done by Prof Alberto Pena and provide guidace to junior surgeons to improve technical success rates. This opens up the feasibility of trying to standardize surgical care across the globe and optimize the conditions to shorten the learning curve for surgical skills.

85.12 Technologies for the Future

85.12.1 Virtual Scrubbing Platforms

This seems an exciting proposition and some investigators have come out with novel ideas. It may be awhile before these technologies are freely available. In future, expertise may be available online for complex operations. One such platform is Proximie as shown below.

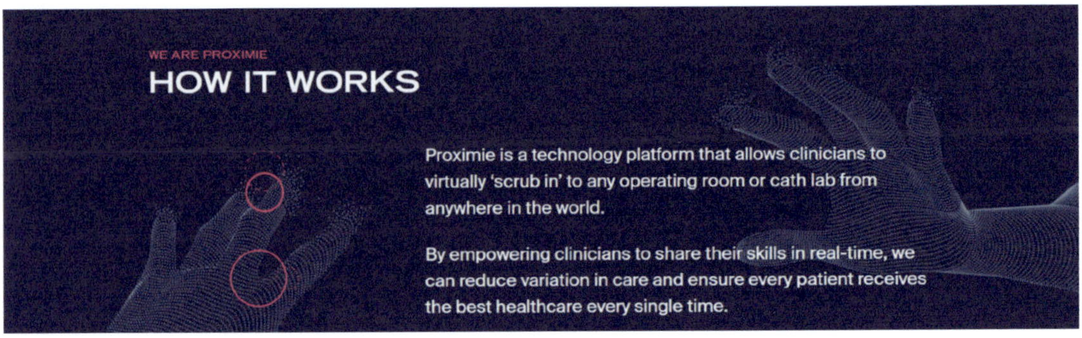

3D image-guided surgery is also a newer technology available for future. Several universities have developed their own 3D image-guided surgery or virtual reality surgical models. One of the examples given below is a model created by King's College London. Several other models are available and the 3D models can be generated from CT or MR images to help guide surgical planning.

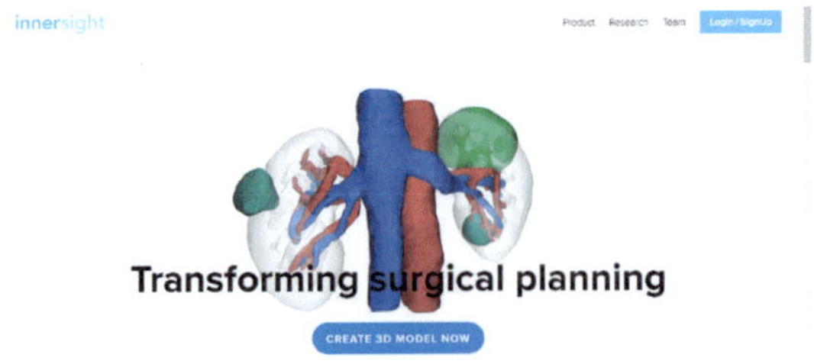

3D image-guided surgery—King's College London Tech Platform

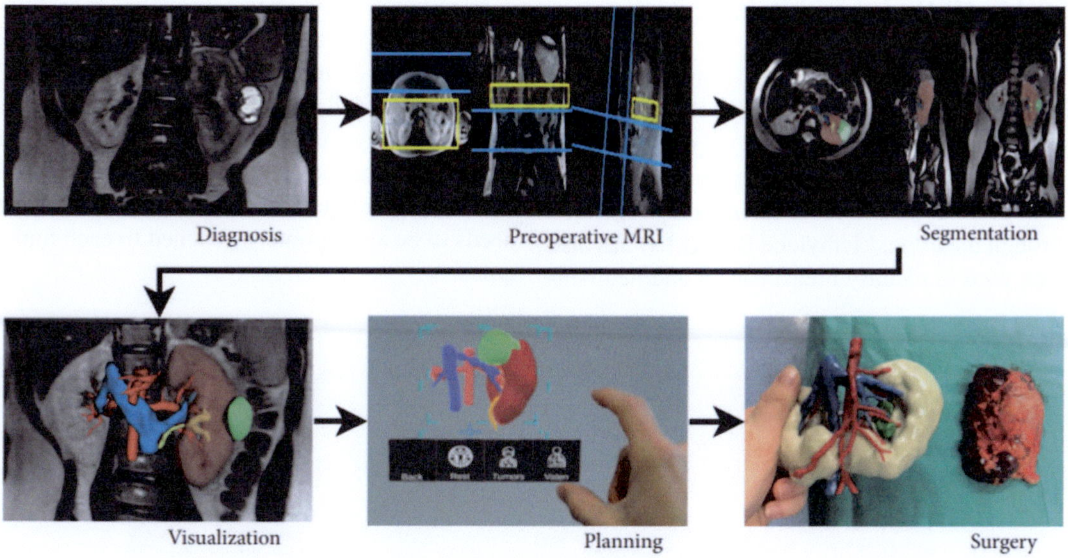

(Source: Matthijs Fitski. Journal of Healthcare Engineering Volume 2020)

Use of augmented reality and 3D technology has become a reality in Oncology. It may soon be used in complex ano-rectal and genito-urinary reconstructions as well.

85.13 Intra-operative Real-Time Imaging

85.13.1 Fluorescence-Guided Surgery (FGS): Non-Ionizing Optical Imaging

Intra-operative imaging with florescent dyes such as indocyanine green offers advantages and will be another tool in a surgeon's armamentarium to increase surgical precision. This has been in vogue for a long time but has picked up in momentum over the last 10 years. 20% of hepatobiliary minimally invasive surgery is done routinely using FGS.

These may become the standard of care for hepatobiliary surgery from laparoscopic Cholecystectomy to Kasai and Liver resection. They may be used for TEF surgery, chylothorax, and even confirming the vascular perfusion of organs. They are safe, provide high resolution and clarity and have been used in heminephrectomy and varicocelectomy as well. The fluorescent dyes used have an infrared wave length. Now, higher wave length (1000–2000 nm) are under investigation and when tagged with Anti-EGR and anti- VEGF monoclonal antibodies, they can even target specific cancers.

85.14 Indocyanine Green (ICG)

Indocyanine green (ICG) is a water-soluble, anionic FDA-approved compound. Its excitation peak is 780 nm and emission peak is at 820 nm, which places it outside the range of most tissue autofluorescence. ICG has maintained a high safety index. It also allows multiple repeated uses due to its short half-life of 150 to 180 s and is cleared exclusively by the liver. For instance, ICG fluorescence imaging can help identify primary hepatocellular carcinomas (HCCs) and in 40% of the cases also identified additional, small (3–6 mm) HCCs that would otherwise have gone undetected.

85.15 Methylene Blue (MB)

When sufficiently diluted, methylene blue acts as a near-infrared fluorescent dye that operates within the near infrared (NIR) optical window with an absorption peak at 670 nm and an emission peak at 690 nm. It is naturally excreted through the urine. Methylene Blue (MB) has also been used to identify breast cancer and neuroendocrine tumors, and is commonly used for sentinel lymph node (SLN) mapping, as well as the identification of urologic tumors and tumors in the parathyroid glands. Methylene blue is known to be relatively safe; Although MB accumulates in most tumors, the amount of accumulation varies with tumor type. Therefore, dye concentration needs to be appropriately matched to each tumor type.

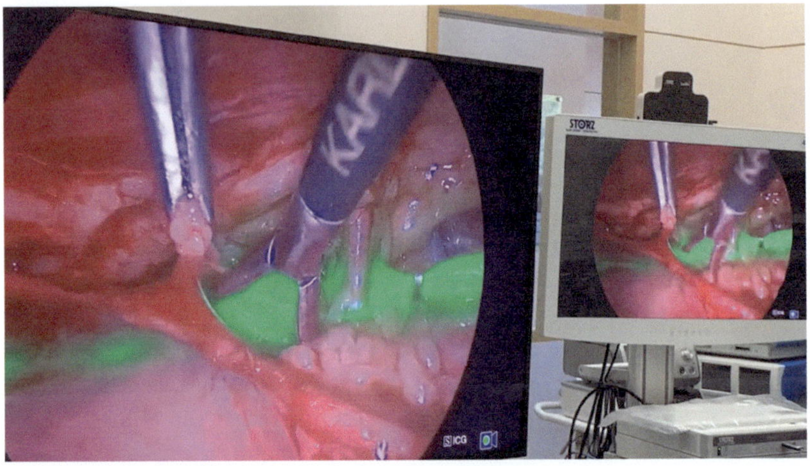

MIS thoracic duct ligation with Karl Storz Rubina in 4K ICG

85.16 Molecular Biology in Pediatric Malignancies

We would like to introduce a few terminologies before we proceed.

Chromosomal microarray Chromosomal microarray (CMA) is a high-resolution method for detecting copy number changes (gains or losses) across the entire genome in a single assay and is sometimes called a molecular karyotype.

FISH (fluorescence in situ hybridization) Fluorescence in situ hybridization (abbreviated FISH) is a laboratory technique used to detect and locate a specific DNA sequence on a chromosome.

Next-generation genome sequencing A new DNA sequencing technology which has replaced the old Sanger method (slow) to a rapid DNA sequencing and has a huge potential in future.

In the diagnosis of tumors, we use several markers to prognosticate the outcome.

Proteins—We use AFP, beta-HCG blood levels are used as tumour markers.

DNA—Wilms tumor- WT1,WT2, WAGR, Beckwith-Weidmann syndrome, 16q and 1p are markers for oncological prognosis.

RNA—DICER, DROSHA, etc., Subunit RNAs like mi-RNA, si-RNA can be used for gene silencing.

85.17 Precision Medicine

Precision medicine in oncology aims to identify an individualized treatment plan based on genomic aberrations in patient's tumor. The patients with cancer have biomarkers which can be selected to individualize the treatment plan of the patient.

Next generation sequencing (NGS) uses an approach to identify genetic alterations across hundreds of clinically relevant cancers biomarkers from biopsy samples of cancer tissue using a single assay. There is another terminology called homologous recombinant deficiency which refers to a cell that fails to repair double-stranded DNA by homologous repair system. Next generation sequencing has the technology to identify the causal genes and injuries. NGS can evaluate immunologic genomic signatures such as tumor mutation burden which can be used as a biomarker for immunotherapy in solid tumors.

85.18 Epigenetic Mechanisms

Epigenetics is the study of heritable and stable gene expression changes through chromosomal alterations rather than DNA material itself. Epigenetic mechanisms can regulate gene expression through chemical modification of DNA bases and change the chromosomal superstructure.

Histone proteins are an integral part of the packing of DNA. Alterations of histone proteins can induce the formation of an open euchromatin state, which allows gene expression by allowing transcription factors and enzymes to interact with DNA.

DNA methylation is another epigenetic mechanism associated with gene silencing. Epigenetic modifications can be affected by several mechanism like age, diet, smoking, stress, and disease state. Epigenetic mechanisms are reversible, but can pass through generations in human despite multiple cycles of cell replication.

Epigenetic mechanisms form a layer of control within a cell that regulates gene expression and silencing.

One of the applications of epigenetic mechanisms is its use in cancer. Drugs are formulated to block epigenetic regulators to treat various cancers. Two conditions with abnormalities in gene imprinting including Prader–Willi syndrome and Beckwith–Wiedemann syndrome. The study of epigenetic mechanisms can be useful in these conditions.

Epigenetic mechanisms, including DNA methylation, can influence gene activity without changing the DNA sequence. DNA methylation is a stable, heritable, covalent modification to DNA. Methylation is associated with normal developmental processes, as well as the changes that are observable during oncogenesis and other pathological processes, such as gene silencing of tumor suppressor or DNA repair genes. DNA methylation has been studied and used in several tumors.

The mutation rate in pediatric tumors is 14 times less than the mutation rate in adult tumors, implying that different mechanisms may be involved in pediatric-cancer development than in adult cancers. Of the mutations that have been identified in pediatric tumors, many are associated with epigenetic regulation. In many pediatric tumors, molecular profiling does not identify genomic abnormalities but does show abnormal DNA methylation patterns, suggesting that DNA methylation may play a critical role in tumorigenesis in these cases. This is definitely an area of looking for novel therapies.

85.18.1 Fetal Therapy and Surgeon (See Chap. 7)

There is a constant improvement in clarity of when to intervene in fetal abnormalities because of multicentric trials. The area of active research is congenital diaphragmatic area and neural tube defects. Recently, Scott Adzick from the Children's Hospital of Philadephia (CHOP) has developed a womb-like device that can be useful in extremely premature babies. The initial enthusiasm for every defect being amenable to fetal surgery has died down and there is a highly selected approach (see Chapter on Antenatal diagnosis and fetal surgery).

85.18.2 Nanotechnology and Surgery (See Chap. 87)

Nanomedicine's nanobots are so tiny that they can easily traverse the human body.

They can be made of carbon and be nonimmunogenic and they can be powered by body oxygen and glucose. The first useful applications of nanomachines, if such are ever built, might be in medical technology. They can be used for targeted drug delivery, cancer therapy, and as surgical tools for breaking down kidney stones.

Further Reading

Abbas TO, Mahdi E, Hasan A, AlAnsari A, Pennisi CP. Current status of tissue engineering in the management of severe hypospadias. Front Pediatr. 2018;5:283. https://doi.org/10.3389/fped.2017.00283. PubMed. 5 Raya-Rivera.

Behjati S, Tarpey PS. What is next generation sequencing? Arch Dis Child Educ Pract Ed. 2013;98:236–8.

Blog: Washington university in St Louis: how molecular biology is making medicine more precise. Tim Peterson, 31st Jan 2018.

Boulanger SC, Caty MG, Glick PL. Molecular biology for the pediatric surgeon. J Pediatr Surg. 1999;34(6):917–30.

Hamilton NJ, Kanani M, Roebuck DJ, Hewitt RJ, Cetto R, Culme-Seymour EJ, et al. Tissue-engineered tracheal replacement in a child: a 4-year follow-up study. Am J Transplant. 2015;15(10):2750–7. https://doi.org/10.1111/ajt.13318.

Hirsch T, Rothoeft T, Teig N, Bauer JW, Pellegrini G, De Rosa L, et al. Regeneration of the entire human epidermis using transgenic stem cells. Nature. 2017;551(7680):327–32. https://doi.org/10.1038/nature24487.

Paraboschi I, De Coppi P, Stoyanov D, Anderson J. Stepahno Giuliani: fluorescence imaging in pediatric surgery: Sate -of-art and future perspectives. J Pediatr Surg. 2021;56(4):655–62.

Uecker M, Kuebler JF, Ure BM, Schukfeh N. Minimally invasive pediatric surgery: the learning curve. Eur J Pediatr Surg. 2020;30(02):172–80.

Genetic and Genomic Advances in Pediatric Surgery

86

Ashutosh Halder

86.1 Introduction

The dissemination of genetic and genomic information is rapidly transforming the management of newborns and children with birth disabilities. Genetic and genomic research advances have enhanced our understanding of various disease causes at the gene level and beyond. Technological breakthroughs enable whole genome sequencing and provide individual genetic profiles in less than 24 h. Techniques like next-generation sequencing (NGS) and microarrays have significantly improved our comprehension of pediatric disorders.

Genetic disorders are prevalent in pediatric practice, with nearly every pediatric disability having a genetic component. The complexity of disease presentations in pediatrics, particularly with malformations, differences in sex development (DSD), and various cancers, necessitates updated diagnostic, prognostic, and treatment strategies. Effective management can be achieved by integrating clinical skills with genetic information.

Molecular genetic testing can yield essential insights for diagnosing and predicting outcomes and, in some cases, guide treatment. This is particularly important for conditions such as congenital malformations, DSD, and childhood tumors. DSD, in particular, has a profound impact on gender differentiation. An accurate genetic diagnosis is crucial for effective counseling and management.

In oncology, genetic analysis can reveal underlying etiological factors, inform targeted therapies, and facilitate predicting and preventing cases within families. Utilizing molecular genetic techniques will enhance the quality of care and lead to improved outcomes. This chapter will focus on pediatric surgical disorders with significant genetic underpinnings.

86.2 Congenital Disabilities

Congenital disabilities are structural or functional defects present at birth, arising during the embryonic or fetal period. These disabilities can affect various organs and have multiple underlying causes. They are often classified as multifactorial, where genetic and environmental factors play a role—for example, isolated neural tube defects (NTDs). They (syndromic NTDs) can also have a genetic origin, such as chromosomal abnormalities like trisomy 21, copy number variations (e.g., 22q11.2 microdeletion syndrome), or monogenic disorders like osteogenesis imperfecta (OI). On the other hand, some congenital disabilities are primarily due to environmental factors, such as teratogenic exposure—like congenital rubella syndrome.

Globally, the burden of significant congenital disabilities is approximately 7.9 million cases

A. Halder (✉)
Reproductive Biology, AIIMS,
New Delhi, Delhi, India

© The Author(s), under exclusive license to Springer Nature Singapore Pte Ltd. 2025

S. Roy Choudhury (ed.), *Pediatric Surgery*, https://doi.org/10.1007/978-981-96-1257-4_86

annually. The World Health Assembly has emphasized the need to address these disabilities and reduce their occurrence. This reduction can be achieved through primary preventive measures, such as periconceptional multivitamin or folic acid supplementation to prevent NTDs, rubella vaccination to avoid congenital rubella syndrome, careful medication management during early pregnancy to prevent teratogenic effects, and preimplantation genetic diagnosis to transfer unaffected embryos.

Secondary prevention strategies include prenatal diagnosis and considering termination of affected pregnancies. Non-invasive prenatal testing (NIPT) can detect chromosomal and copy number variations in early pregnancy. At the same time, second-trimester fetal ultrasonography (between 18 and 20 weeks) can identify fetal abnormalities, allowing for potential termination of pregnancy as a preventive measure. Although not all malformations can be detected, high-resolution ultrasound scans can identify most major fetal malformations. Additional imaging techniques such as fetal echocardiography, 3D ultrasonography, and ultrafast magnetic resonance imaging (MRI) are helpful in characterizing uncertain cases of fetal malformations, including cardiac defects, facial dysmorphisms, open fetal defects, central nervous system defects, skeletal abnormalities, and genitourinary defects. These investigations assist healthcare providers in planning the appropriate delivery setting for management and counseling.

Establishing an accurate etiological diagnosis is crucial for effective counseling and predicting the risk of future pregnancies. Unfortunately, the cause is unknown in the majority of cases. Therefore, gathering detailed clinical information and suitable biological materials for biorepositories is essential, followed by efforts to screen for genetic etiologies using high-throughput omics platforms.

Copy number variations (CNVs), which include microdeletion and microduplication syndromes, are commonly associated with multiple congenital anomalies. The common CNVs linked with malformation syndromes include 22q11.2 (DiGeorge/Velocardiofacial syndrome), 15q11–13 (Prader-Willi/Angelman syndrome), 7q11.23 (Williams syndrome), 17p11.2 (Smith-Magenis syndrome), 11p15 (Beckwith-Wiedemann syndrome), and 17p11.2 (Potocki-Lupski syndrome). SNP microarray technology effectively detects CNVs and unbalanced chromosomal abnormalities (including trisomy, triploidy, and partial aneuploidy), mosaicism, and uniparental disomy disorders. This testing has a high probability of providing a genetic diagnosis.

For reproductive counseling and future pregnancy planning, an etiological diagnosis is essential. Research involving families with multiple affected members is valuable, as these cases are more likely to reveal positive etiological associations. Studying early embryogenesis is crucial for understanding malformations. Maintaining a malformed fetal repository (including tissue, organ, and blood samples from the patient and family members, affected and unaffected) alongside detailed clinical history (at least three-generation pedigree) is the foundational step toward success in this field.

Pregnant women with fetal developmental disabilities should receive targeted assessments in specialized prenatal ultrasound facilities. It is vital to identify all associated anomalies and underlying causes. Every effort should be made for prenatal diagnosis, which may include invasive testing if necessary. Parents should also be encouraged to pursue fetal autopsy and establish biorepositories in the event of perinatal loss. Families with multiple affected members should be referred to a genetic center to investigate the underlying causes, ultimately contributing to advancements in this field.

Pediatric surgeons frequently manage congenital disabilities that include foregut anomalies such as esophageal atresia (EA), tracheoesophageal fistula (TEF), cystic adenomatoid malformations of the lung, and congenital diaphragmatic hernia (CDH) with lung hypoplasia; midgut abnormalities affecting the liver, pancreas, and small intestine; hindgut anomalies including anal atresia and cloacal deformities; dysmotility disorders like Hirschsprung disease; abdominal wall defects such as omphalocele, gastroschisis, and exstrophy of the bladder; urological and reproductive abnormalities, including differences in sex development (DSD); and various muscular, skeletal, and neurological anomalies. Pediatric surgeons should strive to uncover the molecular pathogenesis of these conditions and translate molecular knowledge into effective treatment strategies.

86.2.1 Neural Tube Defects (NTDs)

Neural tube defects (NTDs) are early embryonic congenital disabilities resulting from improper closure of the neural tube, leading to abnormalities in the cranium and spine. NTDs are the most common lethal developmental defect (Fig. 86.1), with a worldwide prevalence of approximately one per 1000 live births. They can be classified into two categories:

1. Open NTDs: These have no coverings over the exposed nerve tissue and include conditions such as anencephaly, open spina bifida (meningomyelocele), craniorachischisis, and anen-iniencephaly.
2. Closed NTDs: These are covered by skin and include spinal dysraphism and iniencephaly.

Other NTD malformations, such as encephalocele, are likely to arise from issues occurring after neurulation. Most NTDs occur in isolation (such as anencephaly or spina bifida, encephalocele, iniencephaly, craniorachischisis, etc.). They are rarely part of a syndrome (such as trisomy 18 or 13, monosomy X, sirenomelia, Meckel syndrome, or amniotic band syndrome).

A deficiency in the occipital region near the foramen magnum, spina bifida, and retroflexion of the spine characterizes iniencephaly. Associated malformations may include pulmonary hypoplasia, diaphragmatic hernia, and omphalocele, resulting from increased pressure in the thoracic and abdominal cavities due to retroflexion and crowding of ribs. Most cases of iniencephaly are sporadic and likely result from multifactorial inheritance, with chromosomal abnormalities being rare.

Craniospinal rachischisis presents with anencephaly and an open defect throughout the spine, leading to damage to the entire neural tissue, including both the brain and spinal cord.

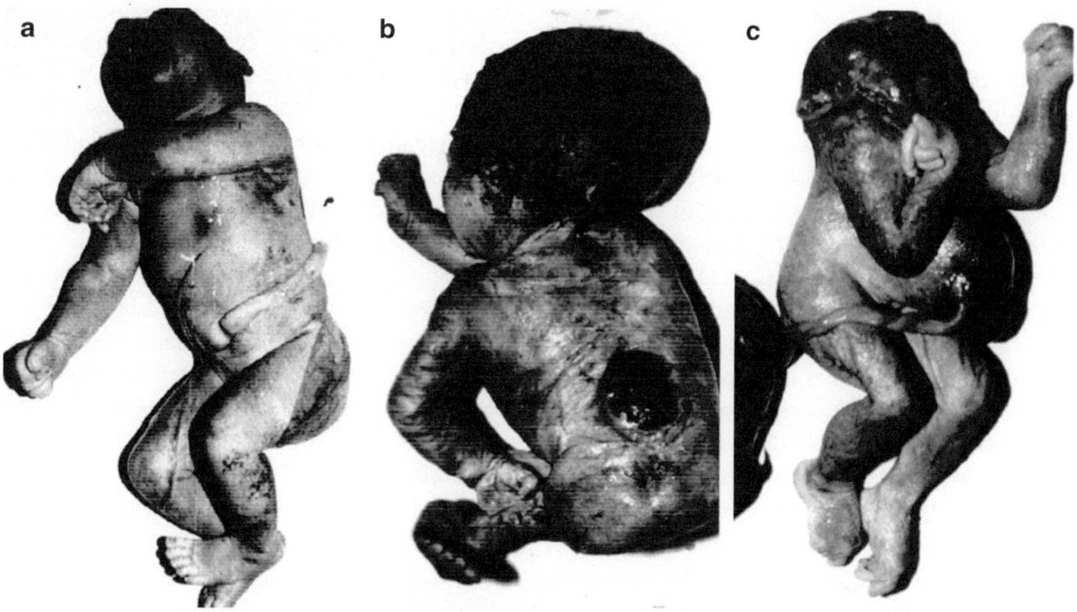

Fig. 86.1 Neural Tube Defect (NTD) showing Anencephaly (**a**) in a newborn, Spina Bifida Aperta (**b**) with ruptured meningocele after termination of pregnancy, and Iniencephaly (**c**) with hyperextension of neck, fusion of occiput with back and abdominal hernia in a newborn

The genetic mechanisms underpinning NTDs involve critical signaling pathways, such as the over-activation of the sonic hedgehog (SHH) signaling pathway or loss of function in the planar cell polarity (PCP) pathway. Specifically, loss of function in the PCP pathway, involving genes like *Celsr1* and V*angl2*, has been linked to craniorachischisis in mice. Moreover, double knockouts of the *Fzd3 or Fzd6 and Dvl* genes also display a craniorachischisis phenotype. Other significant pathways include retinoid and inositol signaling. Mutations in the *Fkbp8* gene are associated with isolated spina bifida.

Genes linked to human NTDs, such as spina bifida and craniorachischisis, include *VANGL1, FZD6, FKBP8, and MED12*. Rarely, conditions like spina bifida may be associated with other malformations (such as omphalocele, cardiac abnormalities, and choroid plexus cysts) with chromosomal abnormalities like trisomy 18.

Meckel-Gruber syndrome (MKS) is an autosomal recessive disorder characterized by central nervous system developmental defects, including occipital encephalocele. It is recognized as the most common syndromic form of neural tube defect, with key contributing genes *MKS1, MKS2/TMEM216, MKS3/TMEM67, RPGRIP1L, and CC2D2A*.

The recurrence risk for isolated NTDs after having one affected child is approximately 3–5%, which is ten times higher than in the general population. This risk increases to around 10% after two affected children and 25% after three, resembling an autosomal recessive pattern. After the birth of a child with an NTD, couples should be informed about prevention strategies for subsequent pregnancies. These include periconceptional folic acid supplementation (primary prevention) and antenatal maternal serum alpha-fetoprotein (MSAFP) screening, followed by an ultrasound examination and potential selective termination of affected pregnancies (secondary prevention). However, syndromic NTDs present different recurrence risks, ranging from sporadic occurrences to 25% in cases like Meckel syndrome. Therefore, an accurate etiological diagnosis is essential for effective counseling.

86.2.2 Amniotic Band Syndrome (ABS)

Amniotic band syndrome (ABS) and limb body wall complex (LBWC) arise from the rupture of the amnion during early embryogenesis, which leads to secondary effects on morphogenesis, resulting in deformations and disruptions (Fig. 86.2). The prevalence of ABS is estimated to be between 1 in 1300 and 1 in 2000 births. This syndrome is often underdiagnosed, and its presentation can vary significantly. Various mechanisms have been proposed in the literature, including those related to the germ disc, genetics, vascular issues, and amniotic disruptions.

The amniotic band theory proposed by Torpin in 1965 suggests that these defects are exogenous and result from the rupture of the amniotic sac. When the amnion ruptures, the fetus is positioned outside the amniotic cavity. Mesodermal bands develop from the chorionic side of the amnion, entrap different parts of the fetus, and disrupt normal fetal movement and development. An early rupture often leads to severe malformations, while a late rupture tends to result in milder phenotypes. Oligohydramnios, commonly associated with ABS, can further exacerbate deformities due to compression.

Another proposed mechanism, the vascular disruption theory, suggests that abnormal blood supply during embryogenesis interrupts normal morphogenesis or disrupts previously established structures. The embryonic dysplasia theory indicate that fetal disruptions may occur due to imperfect histogenesis.

Amniotic band syndrome (ABS) is a constellation of malformations that lacks a precise pathway and a satisfactory pathogenetic explanation. Various literature has documented familial cases of amniotic band syndrome. In some families, the defect appears to be an autosomal dominant trait. Genes implicated in ABS include *COL3A1*, which is associated with vascular Ehlers-Danlos Syndrome and an increased risk of ABS; *COL7A1*, related to dystrophic epidermolysis bullosa and a higher risk of ABS; and *IQCK*, which is linked to an increased risk of LBWC. Additionally, temporal and geographic

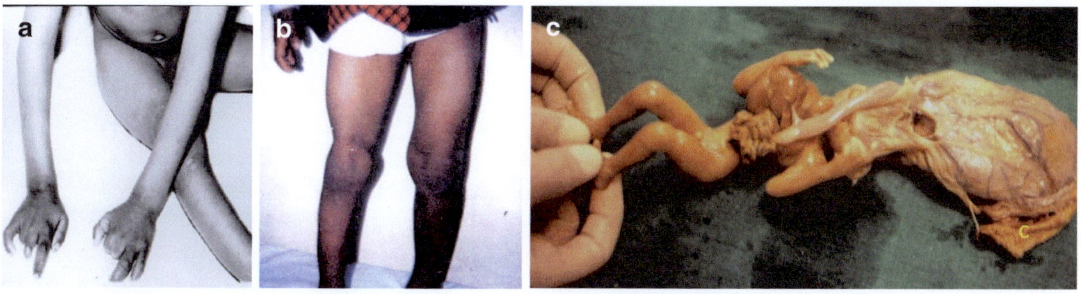

Fig. 86.2 Amniotic Band Syndrome/Limb Body Wall Complex (LBWC) showing amputation of fingers, syndactyly (**a**), constriction above knee joint (**b**), and complete disruptions of abdomen, thorax, and head with constriction bands at lower thigh along with attachment of placenta with disrupted vault (**c**)

clustering of cases suggests environmental teratogens may be a causative factor.

86.2.3 Skeletal Dysplasia

Skeletal dysplasias commonly encountered in pregnancy include thanatophoric dysplasia, osteogenesis imperfecta, achondrogenesis, short rib polydactyly syndrome, Roberts syndrome, hypophosphatasia, campomelic dysplasia, chondrodysplasia punctata (rhizomelic type), and atelosteogenesis, among others. Thanatophoric dysplasia and osteogenesis imperfecta are common and notably severe forms that can lead to fetal lethality (Fig. 86.3).

Severe shortening of the limbs, a large head, frontal bossing, a depressed nasal bridge, a narrow thoracic cage, short ribs, platyspondyly, hypoplastic iliac bones, and significant shortening of long bones, including bowed femora, characterize thanatophoric dysplasia. A mutation causes the condition, typically de novo, in the fibroblast growth factor receptor 3 (*FGFR3*) gene. Early prenatal diagnosis is often possible.

Osteogenesis imperfecta (OI) is a connective tissue and skeletal disorder resulting from a mutation in the *COL1A2* gene. Genetic tests and prenatal ultrasonography can be used for prenatal diagnosis. Osteogenesis imperfecta type II is the most severe form of this condition. In postnatal life, the presence of blue sclera, along with bone fractures, supports the diagnosis. Prenatal mesenchymal stem cell therapy shows promise as a treatment for severe OI.

Achondrogenesis is an autosomal recessive lethal skeletal dysplasia presenting with intrauterine growth failure, micromelia, defects in ossification of the skull and spine, short beaded ribs, and deformed and short long bones. Achondrogenesis Type 1A is caused by mutations in the *TRIP11* (thyroid hormone receptor interactor 11) gene, leading to a deficiency of the golgi microtubule-associated protein 210. In contrast, achondrogenesis Type 2 results from mutations in the *COL2A1* (collagen type II) gene, also associated with Kniest dysplasia and spondyloepiphyseal dysplasia congenital.

Short rib polydactyly syndrome features short limbs, polydactyly, thoracic hypoplasia, heart defects, and renal dysplasia. There are four types of this syndrome: type I (Saldino-Noonan), type II (Majewski), type III (Verma-Naumoff), and type IV (Beemar-Langer).

Roberts syndrome is a rare autosomal recessive disorder characterized by symmetrical limb defects (tetra-amelia or hypomelia), craniofacial abnormalities (including microcephaly, cleft lip and palate, down-slanted palpebral fissures, widely spaced eyes, shallow orbits, underdeveloped nasal alae, and ear malformations), growth retardation, oligodactyly, thumbs that are aplastic or hypoplastic, syndactyly, clinodactyly, and flexion contractures. It is caused by a mutation in the *ESCO2* (cohesion one homolog 2) gene.

Camptomelic dysplasia is a heterogeneous and lethal skeletal dysplasia linked to abnormal bone and cartilage development. It is an autosomal dominant disorder caused by a mutation in

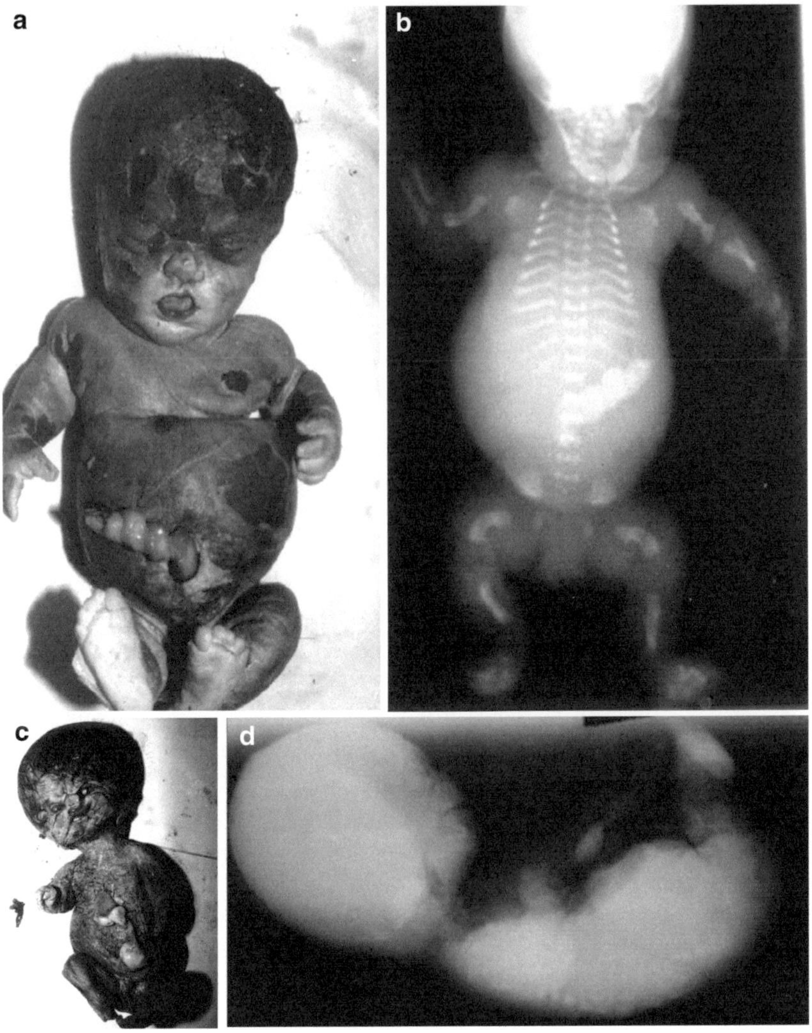

Fig. 86.3 Skeletal Dysplasia showing terminated fetus with extremely short limbs, large head (**a**), and marked shortening of long bones including bowing of femora, short ribs, platyspondyly, hypoplastic iliac bones, etc. (**b**) in a case of Thanatophoric Dysplasia. Terminated fetus with deformed limbs (**c**), multiple fractures in ribs & long bones (**d**) in a case of Osteogenesis imperfecta type II

the *SOX9* gene. The clinical features associated with the Pierre Robin sequence include cleft palate, shortening and bowing of the long bones, and sex reversal. Other findings may include laryngotracheomalacia, which can lead to respiratory compromise.

Atelosteogenesis types I and III are also autosomal dominant skeletal dysplasias characterized by vertebral abnormalities, hypoplastic long bones, and joint dislocations. These conditions are caused by mutations in the *FLNB* gene (filamin B).

Hypophosphatasia is an autosomal recessive/dominant disorder resulting from decreased alkaline phosphatase activity, leading to defective bone mineralization. Molecular diagnosis can be achieved through mutational analysis of the *TNSALP* gene.

Achondroplasia, which falls under the category of growth plate dysplasia, is characterized by impaired cartilage formation due to a mutation in the *FGFR3* gene. This condition is also autosomal dominant with 100% penetrance, and more than 80% of cases arise de novo. Advanced paternal age is recognized as a risk factor.

FAM111A-related skeletal dysplasias include Kenny-Caffey syndrome and osteocraniostenosis. Kenny-Caffey syndrome presents with proportionate short stature, relative macrocephaly, a large anterior fontanel with delayed closure, cortical thickening of long bones with stenosis of the medullary cavity, along-with eye and dental abnormalities. Osteocraniostenosis is characterized by growth retardation, microcephaly, decreased skull ossification, cortical thickening of long bones, stenosis of the medullary cavity, and thin ribs. This condition can also be associated with thoracic and pulmonary hypoplasia and is inherited in an autosomal dominant fashion. Primary hypoparathyroidism with hypocalcemia and hyperphosphatemia can be associated with this condition.

Craniosynostosis is characterized by premature fusion of skull sutures and caused by mutations in genes such as *FGFR1* (Pfeiffer syndrome), *FGFR2* (Apert syndrome, Pfeiffer syndrome, Crouzon syndrome), *FGFR3* (Crouzon syndrome, Muenke syndrome), *EFNA4* (Craniofrontonasal dysplasia), *EFNB1* (Craniofrontonasal dysplasia), *TWIST* (Saethre-Chotzen syndrome), *RAB23* (Carpenter syndrome), etc.

Osteopetrosis is characterized by abnormal bone growth and remodeling, resulting in generalized osteosclerosis, fractures, pancytopenia, hepatosplenomegaly, and often cranial neuropathies. This disorder is primarily due to osteoclast dysfunction and is associated with mutations in *CLCN7, TCIRG1, OSTM1, PLEKHM1, SNX10, TNFSF11, and TNFRSF11A* genes.

Next-generation sequencing (NGS) tests, including whole exome, whole genome, or skeletal dysplasia gene panels, are now commonly employed to screen for genes associated with skeletal dysplasias quickly. Prenatal diagnosis can be achieved through invasive techniques (for all types of inheritance) or non-invasive methods such as non-invasive prenatal diagnosis (NIPD) from maternal blood for autosomal dominant disorders like achondroplasia and thanatophoric dysplasia, either inherited paternally or arising from de novo mutations. Non-invasive prenatal testing (NIPT) using methods such as gene SAFE (Italy) or the NATERA platform can also screen for single-gene disorders like osteogenesis imperfecta.

86.2.4 Hirschsprung Disease

Hirschsprung disease, also known as congenital intestinal aganglionosis, is a developmental disorder characterized by the absence of parasympathetic intrinsic ganglion cells in the submucosal and myenteric plexuses of the hindgut. This condition arises from the failure of enteric neural crest cells to migrate, proliferate, and differentiate adequately in the bowel wall during embryonic development. As a result, areas of the gastrointestinal tract become aganglionic. The disease can be classified into three types based on the extent of aganglionosis: short-segmental (where the aganglionic segment is limited to the rectosigmoid colon), long-segmental (where it extends into the sigmoid colon), and total (where the entire small and large intestines are affected). In the absence of parasympathetic ganglia, the intestines lose their propulsive motility, leading to symptoms such as chronic constipation, abdominal distension, and bilious vomiting. Complications can include bowel perforation and enterocolitis. The prevalence of Hirschsprung disease is approximately 1 in 5000 live births, with variations among different ethnic groups; it is particularly more common in Asians and males.

The genetics of Hirschsprung disease is complex. Syndromic forms, such as Mowat-Wilson syndrome and Waardenburg syndrome type 4, follow a Mendelian mode of inheritance. In contrast, isolated Hirschsprung disease shows non-Mendelian inheritance patterns, often associated with copy number variations (microdeletions). In severe cases, the inheritance may appear dominant with incomplete penetrance, while milder cases may exhibit multifactorial or recessive inheritance with low penetrance.

Numerous genes have been implicated in causing the disease, including *ABCC9, BACE2, CCT2, COMT, ECE1, EDN3, EDNRB, ERBB2/3/4, GDNF, GFRA1, GLI1, 2, 3, HOXB5, KIAA1279, KIFBP, L1CAM, LRBA, NKX2.1, NRG1, NRG3, NRTN, NTRK3, PHOX2B, RET, RORA, SEMA3A/C/D, SLC6A20, SOX10, SSPO, STIM2, TCF4, TELO2, VRK2, ZEB2, ZFXH1B,* etc., among others. Hirschsprung disease is associated with genetic heterogeneity, variable penetrance and expressivity, and gene interactions.

Molecular testing, such as DNA microarray analysis, should be the first-tier approach for exploring the etiology of Hirschsprung disease. Next-generation sequencing (NGS) is recommended to detect other potential genetic causes if the results are negative. The ultimate goals of genetic studies on Hirschsprung disease are to translate genetic information into predictions of risk and clinical outcomes and, in severe cases, to enable prevention through prenatal diagnosis.

86.2.5 Infantile Hypertrophic Pyloric Stenosis (IHPS)

Infantile hypertrophic pyloric stenosis (IHPS) is the most common reason for performing laparotomy in the first year of life, with a prevalence of approximately 1 in 500 live births. This condition can be isolated or associated with several genetic syndromes, including Apert, Denys-Drash, Kallmann, and Marden-Walker.

There is a genetic component to IHPS, as evidenced by the frequent occurrence of the condition within families; however, it does not follow a Mendelian inheritance pattern. Research has shown an association between IHPS and nitric oxide, which plays a role in relaxing smooth muscle cells. Additionally, mutations in the neuronal nitric oxide synthase (*NOS1 or nNOS*) genes are linked to IHPS. Other genes associated with this condition are *SOS1, BARX1, and EML4-MTA3*.

86.2.6 Esophageal Atresia/Tracheoesophageal Fistula (EA/TEF)

Esophageal atresia (EA) is a congenital abnormality that results from incomplete embryonic compartmentalization of the foregut. It is commonly associated with a tracheoesophageal fistula (TEF). EA may be linked to syndromic conditions such as VACTERL association, CHARGE syndrome, and various chromosomal abnormalities or arise from specific signaling pathways or monogenic defects. Molecular methods like DNA microarray and next-generation sequencing (NGS) are essential to explore the genetic etiology of EA.

Approximately 6–10% of patients with EA/TEF have chromosomal aberrations. The most frequently associated abnormalities include trisomy 13, 18, and 21 and the 13q-, 17q-, and 22q11-deletion syndromes. Over 50 genetic syndromes have been identified in association with EA/TEF. Specific genes linked to these syndromes include *MYCN* in Feingold syndrome type 1, *GLI2* in Pallister-Hall syndrome, *CHD7* in CHARGE syndrome, *GDF3* in Klippel–Feil syndrome, *SOX4* in Coffin-Siris syndrome, among others.

In cases of isolated EA/TEF, the associated genes include *APC2, AMER3, CTNNA3, EFTUD2, FANCA/B/C, FGFR3, FOXF1, FOXC2, FOXL1, GTF3C1, HNF1B, ITSN1, MYCN, NRXN1, PCDH1, POLR2B, RAB3GAP2, SOX2, and TCF4*. Therefore, a microarray test is recommended as the first line of genetic testing to identify chromosomal abnormalities and microdeletion syndromes. If the microarray test is negative, next-generation sequencing should be conducted.

Understanding the genetic information related to EA is crucial for establishing the etiology, preventing family recurrence, and predicting long-term outcomes.

86.2.7 Congenital Diaphragmatic Hernia (CDH)

Congenital diaphragmatic hernia (CDH) occurs in approximately 1 in every 2500 live births or 1 in every 1000 early pregnancies. Genetics plays a significant role in the development of CDH. Genetic associations include various chromosomal abnormalities (such as those on 15q, 8p, and 12p), copy number variations (located at 1q41–42.12, 15q26, and 22q11), and gene mutations involving *COUP-TFII, DISP1, FOG2, FOXF1, GATA4, GATA5, GATA6, GLI1, GLI2, LRP2, ROBO1, SLIT3, STRA-6, WT1*, and others.

86.2.8 Omphalocele, Gastroschisis, Exstrophy, etc.

Omphalocele, gastroschisis, and exstrophy are congenital malformations of the anterior abdominal wall.

In the case of omphalocele, a membranous sac covers the herniated organs, which protrude through a relatively large abdominal wall defect at the umbilicus. The intestines and liver remain morphologically and functionally normal, but omphalocele is often associated with other malformations.

Conversely, in gastroschisis, the bowel is exposed as it does not have a protective covering and is damaged. The abdominal wall defect in gastroschisis does not include the umbilicus. While chromosomal anomalies are commonly associated with omphalocele, they are rare in cases of gastroschisis.

Bladder and cloacal exstrophy occur due to a failure to close the anterior abdominal wall at the ventral end of the cloacal membrane. Bladder exstrophy is frequently associated with other genitourinary anomalies. In contrast, cloacal exstrophy may be accompanied by omphalocele, imperforate anus, diastasis of the pubis, and absent genitalia. Prenatal ultrasonography can diagnose bladder exstrophy by identifying the absence of the urinary bladder.

The OEIS complex represents a combination of severe congenital anomalies, including the oculo-auriculo-vertebral sequence (cranial defects) and caudal anomalies resembling those found in omphalocele and exstrophy of the bladder, imperforate anus, and spine defects. The caudal anomalies may also resemble the caudal deficiency sequence or the OEIS complex itself or indicate a defect in blastogenesis. This malformation can be caused by a generalized alteration in mesodermal cell migration during the primitive streak period.

86.2.9 Lymphatic Malformations (LM)/Lymphangioma (With/Without Overgrowth Syndromes)

Lymphatic malformations (LM) are congenital conditions caused by developmental abnormalities in the lymphatic vessels (Fig. 86.4). Examples of LM include primary lymphedema, hereditary lymphedema, lymphedema-distichiasis, hypotrichosis-lymphedema-telangiectasia, primary lymphedema associated with myelodysplasia, and lymphedema-choanal atresia, among others. LM is often linked to various syndromes, such as Klippel-Trenaunay syndrome, Parkes-Weber syndrome, Sturge-Weber syndrome, Megalencephaly with capillary malformations, microcephaly with capillary malformations, CLOVES syndrome, Proteus syndrome, and Cowden syndrome.

LM and other overgrowth syndromes' genetic basis typically involve germline and somatic

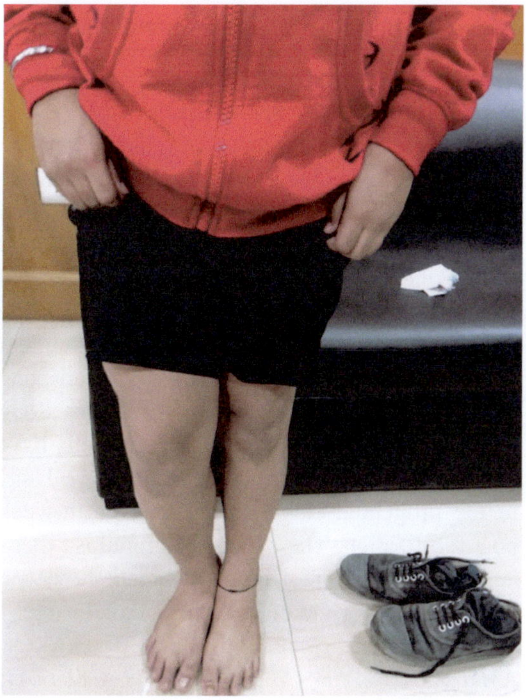

Fig. 86.4 Lymphatic malformation (LM)/localized overgrowth syndrome in a girl shows overgrowth of the right thigh and leg (mainly adipose tissue) and lengthening of the right lower limb (overgrowth of femur and tibia)

mutations. Germline mutations are present in every body cell, regardless of whether the tissue is affected or normal, and can be passed on to future generations. In contrast, somatic mutations occur post-zygotically, meaning they arise after fertilization and typically affect only the cells or tissues involved.

Common gene mutations associated with LM include *AKT1, CX47, EPHB4, FOXC2, GATA2, GJC2, GNAQ, mTOR, PIK3CA, PTEN, PTEN14, RAS, RASA1, SOX18, STAMBP, and VEGFC.* Among these, somatic mutations of the PIK3CA gene significantly contribute to developing LM and related overgrowth syndromes.

Several signaling pathways play a role in the development and progression of LM. Specific inhibitors targeting these pathways, such as PI3K/AKT/mTOR inhibitors like rapamycin (sirolimus), are being researched for clinical applications. Additionally, molecular diagnostics can assist families in reproductive counseling, potentially helping to prevent future births of children affected by these conditions.

86.3 Differences of Sex Development (DSD)

Differences in Sex Development (DSD) are characterized by abnormalities in the determination and differentiation of chromosomal, gonadal, and phenotypic sex. Chromosomal sex is assigned at fertilization and initiates the differentiation of the gonads, ultimately determining the development of internal and external genitalia. Gonads and genitalia originate from the same structures along the urogenital ridge. Primordial germ cells have an epiblast origin and migrate from the yolk sac to the urogenital ridge during the fourth-week post-fertilization. The origins of granulosa-theca and Sertoli-Leydig cells are debated; however, they generally originate in the urogenital ridge.

Several genes (including *AKR1C2, AKR1C4, AMH, AMHR2, AR, CBX2, CYP11A1, CYP17A1, DHH, DMRT1, DMRT2, ESR1, FOXL2, GATA4, LHCGR, MAP3K1, NR0B1, NR5A1, RSPO1, SOX3, SOX9, SRY, STAR, WT1, WNT4, ZFPM2,* etc.) are required for gonadal development, and abnormalities in these genes can lead to atypical sex development. The indifferent gonads differentiate into testes through genes such as *AMH, CYP17A1, GLI1, SF1, SOX9, SRY, WT1,* etc., and into ovaries through ETV5, FOXL2, LIN28, RSPO1, WNT2B, and WNT4.

Around 6 weeks post-fertilization, the Müllerian ducts appear adjacent to the Wolffian ducts. Anti-Müllerian Hormone (AMH), secreted from Sertoli cells of the testes, induces the regression of Müllerian ducts. In contrast, testosterone, secreted from Leydig cells of the testes, initiates the differentiation of the Wolffian ducts. Various genes, such as *AMH, AMHR2, AR, EMX2, EGF, FGF, HOXA10, HOXA11, HOXA13, IGF, LHX1, LIM1, PAX2, PAX8, RAR, TCF2, WNT4, WNT1,* etc., are involved in the development of the Müllerian and Wolffian ducts. Dihydrotestosterone (DHT), derived from testosterone by the enzyme 5-alpha-reductase, promotes the masculinization of external genitalia. Fetal androgen levels and their receptors are crucial in determining the extent of masculinization. Elevated testosterone levels during fetal development influence the brain's maturation toward male sexual orientation later in life.

Any defects in this developmental pathway can lead to genital ambiguity. This may manifest as under-virilization in XY individuals, virilization in XX individuals, or, more rarely, complications with gonadal differentiation or gender dysphoria (Fig. 86.5). AMH is essential for the regression of the Müllerian duct in males, and incomplete regression may arise from inappropriate synthesis or action of AMH. Cases of 46, XY DSD and 46, XY gonadal dysgenesis are frequently associated with Müllerian duct remnants.

Androgen Insensitivity Syndrome (AIS) results from defects in the androgen receptor, causing insufficient masculinization in 46, XY individuals. The causes of 46, XX DSD include early antenatal androgen exposure from fetal adrenal sources, maternal androgen-producing tumors, maternal exogenous androgen exposure, fetal aromatase deficiency, or *WNT4* mutations. The most common cause of 46, XX DSD is virilizing congenital adrenal hyperplasia (CAH) due

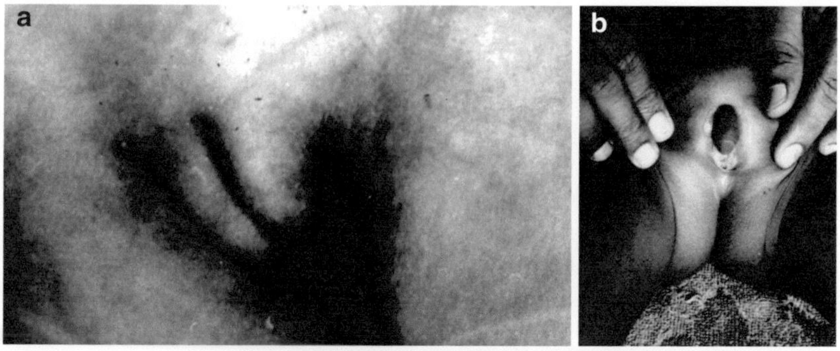

Fig. 86.5 Differences of Sex Development (DSD) showing genital ambiguity. No virilization of external genitalia (despite gonadal/testis prominence in right labia majora) of an XY individual, i.e., androgen insensitivity syndrome (AIS) (**a**) and virilization (proximal labial fusion and extreme clitoromegaly) of an XX individual (**b**) with normal vaginal opening and female urethra

to 21-hydroxylase deficiency (*CYP21A2*). Other causes are 11-hydroxylase (*CYP11A1, CYP11B1, CYP11B2,* etc.), 3-beta-hydroxysteroid dehydrogenase (*3β-HSD*), P450-oxidoreductase (*POR*), etc., deficiencies. In these cases, females may be born with varying degrees of external genital ambiguity, including occasional complete masculinization of external genitalia while retaining feminine internal genitalia. Aromatase deficiency (*CYP19A1*) can also lead to partial virilization of 46, XX fetuses due to an altered testosterone/estrogen ratio.

Patients with ovotesticular DSD exhibit well-developed ovarian and testicular tissues (histologically confirmed). The chromosomal makeup in ovotesticular DSD can be 46, XX/46, XY or just 46, XX, and rarely 46, XY. Cases of gonadal dysgenesis typically show a female phenotype, normal to tall stature, dysgenetic gonads, sexual infantilism, and a 46, XY karyotype. In these cases, the internal genital structures are female, often consisting of bilateral fallopian tubes, a uterus, and an infantile vagina. Some 46, XY gonadal dysgenesis cases may have gene mutations such as *MAP3K1, NR5A1, SOX9, or SRY.* SRY mutations are found in about 10–20% of these cases. Mixed gonadal dysgenesis refers to a condition where one gonad shows some development, such as an immature ovary or testis, while the other is streak gonad. Patients with this condition often possess testicular tissue on one side and a streak gonad on the other side. Some of these cases have *NR5A1* gene mutations.

Genetic diagnosis is critical for managing DSD cases effectively, as well as for counseling regarding prognosis, recurrence, prevention (prenatal or preimplantation diagnosis), and screening for family members. Commonly implicated genes in DSD include *AMH, AMHR2, AR, CYP11A1, CYP11B1, CYP11B2, CYP17A1, CYP19A1, CYP21A2, GATA4, HSD3B2, HSD17B3, MAMLD1, MAP3K1, NR5A1, RSPO1SF1, SF1, SOX9, SRD5A2, SRY, and WT1.* Due to low clinical and biochemical diagnostic yield, genetic etiology is particularly important in 46, XY DSD. Genomic screening of sex reversal DSD cases suggests an oligogenic nature in many instances, complicating the counseling process. Oligogenic inheritance represents an intermediate genetic model involving multiple genes contributing to the condition. Many of these cases are monogenic, meaning they involve a single gene, but genetic modifiers can influence the expression of the phenotype. The mutation of the *MAP3K1* gene is associated with complete gonadal dysgenesis. This mutation may disrupt interaction with the RHOA gene, contributing to complete gonadal dysgenesis. Additionally, interpreting genetic tests necessitates a comprehensive understanding of genetics, such as monogenic, oligogenic, polygenic, copy number variations (CNVs), and other disorders.

86.4 Pediatric Cancer

Cancer is a genomic disorder characterized by genetic changes in cancer cells, which can either be inherited (as in neonatal cancers) or arise from somatic mutations (as seen in older patients). Researchers can create neoplastic cells in the laboratory by genetically manipulating normal cells. Specifically, the ectopic expression of three genes, such as hTERT, simian virus 40 large-T oncoprotein, and H-RAS, can transform normal cells into cancer cells. This finding suggests that only a few genetic changes are required to distinguish early cancer cells from normal cells. Initially, tumor development is a finite process that necessitates only a handful (3–4) of genes. However, genetic changes in cancer cells during the advanced stages can become chaotic (Fig. 86.6).

The initiation of neoplastic transformation can occur through genetic abnormalities that arise during normal cell division or are inherited from parents. This initial event creates a foundation for additional genetic changes. Once the appropriate combination of genetic alterations accumulates, the cell becomes neoplastic. Neoplastic cells exhibit numerous genetic abnormalities, including chromosomal changes (such as aneuploidy and polyploidy), sub-chromosomal alterations (like deletions, duplications, and amplifications), gene mutations, and epigenomic changes (such as hypermethylation and deacetylation). These genomic changes result from multi-step processes linked to failures in cell cycle checkpoint regulations.

Key hallmarks of cancer cells include genetic instability, continued proliferation, evading growth suppressors, resisting cell death, enabling replicative immortality, inducing angiogenesis, activating invasion and metastasis, and achieving prolonged survival. Cancer cells are genetically distinct in advanced stages and exhibit various genetic changes (markers) that can assist in diagnosis, prognosis, and treatment selection. Ideally, these genetic changes should diminish with treatment, and this information is crucial for evaluating remission and potential relapse.

Despite extensive knowledge of cancer genomics, advancements in cancer survival rates remain limited, primarily due to late diagnosis when effective control becomes challenging. Global genomic approaches, such as next-generation sequencing and DNA microarrays, have provided vast insights into genomic altera-

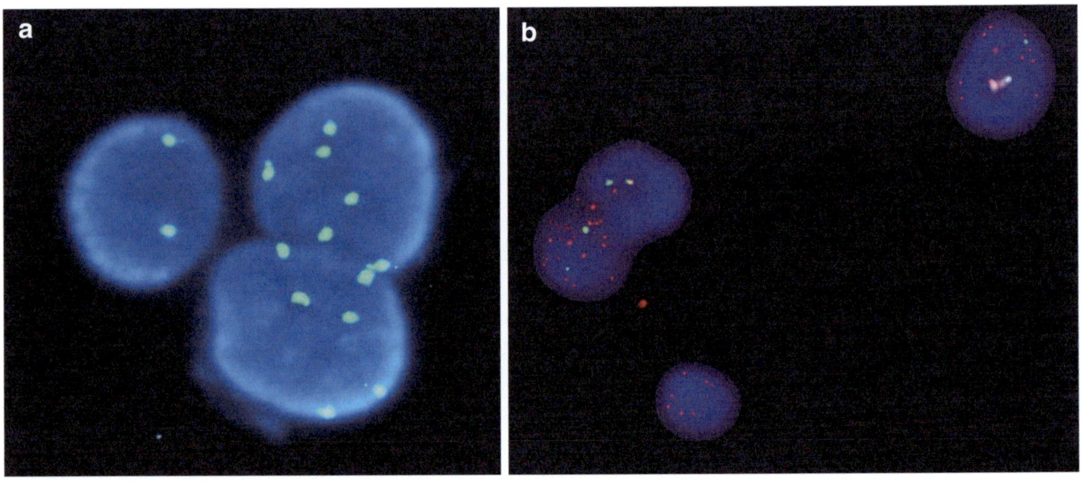

Fig. 86.6 Fluorescent in situ hybridization (FISH) image on cancer cells showing chromosomal changes (single chromosome)/aneuploidy (**a**). Note cell-to-cell heterogeneity. The number of copies varies from 2 to 6 (usually should be two copies) and gene amplification/N-MYC (**b**). Note cell-to-cell heterogeneity, few copies to 100 s of copies (green fluorescent signals are centromere of chromosome 2, and red fluorescent signals are 2p24.3/N-MYC gene)

tions (including mutations, copy number variations, aneuploidy, and loss of heterozygosity) in cancer cells. Advanced-stage cancer cells often harbor hundreds of copy number variations (CNVs), thousands of mutations, and epigenetic changes. The DNA sequences for many cancers are publicly accessible, offering a comprehensive view of cancer-related genetic modifications.

Understanding cancer biology through cancer genetics has advanced significantly. However, the dynamic nature of cancer cells and the challenge of distinguishing driver mutations (which provide growth advantages and contribute to metastasis) from passenger mutations (which do not confer growth advantages) remain major hurdles. Successfully targeting driver mutations can inhibit tumor growth, while focusing on passenger mutations may not be beneficial. Hence, differentiating driver mutations from passenger mutations is essential for identifying relevant treatment targets while avoiding unnecessary, costly, and potentially harmful interventions. It is also important to note that some passenger mutations may be detrimental to cancer cells, making any targeted approach potentially harmful. Additionally, mutations in non-coding genomic regions—often left untested—also play a role in cancer development and progression, adding complexity to the issue.

Extensive information regarding most cancers at genomic, epigenomic, and proteomic levels is available in public databases. Integrating these data into systems biology will require substantial effort in the coming years. Cancer genomics can potentially guide detection, management, predictions, and prevention. Pharmacogenomics is aimed at reducing drug toxicity-related deaths from cancer chemotherapy or radiotherapy as part of personalized medicine. Furthermore, prevention strategies can be implemented through preimplantation genetic diagnosis in cases of inherited cancers.

Common cancers in the pediatric age group include Burkitt's lymphoma, glioma, osteosarcoma, Ewing's sarcoma, rhabdomyosarcoma, adrenocortical carcinoma, medulloblastoma, neuroblastoma, T-cell acute lymphoblastic leukemia, B-cell acute lymphoblastic leukemia, acute myeloid leukemia, Wilms tumor, retinoblastoma, and hepatoblastoma. Pediatric cancer genomics requires special attention, as many of these cancers are often inherited. Germline mutations are responsible for most familial pediatric cancers, including retinoblastoma, nephroblastoma, and hepatoblastoma. Hereditary predisposition is most commonly observed in cases of bilateral early-onset retinoblastoma (100%), adrenocortical carcinomas (50%), high-grade gliomas, atypical teratoid/rhabdoid tumors (ATRTs), sonic hedgehog (SHH) pathway cancers, medulloblastomas, and unilateral retinoblastomas (15–25% each). Most germline gene variants are associated with tumor suppressor genes (such as *RB1, p53, and BRCA1*) and DNA repair genes (like *MSH2, MSH6, PMS2, TP53, BRCA2, and CHEK2*). Individuals carrying *TP53* germline mutations are at a higher risk of developing adrenocortical carcinomas, B-cell acute lymphoblastic leukemia, medulloblastomas, and high-grade gliomas. Inherited mutations in the RB1 gene are known to cause retinoblastoma.

In today's era of genome sequencing, cancer diagnosis is undergoing significant transformation. These molecular advancements are creating opportunities for more precise and earlier detection of tumors. The possibility of predicting, preventing, and providing early precision treatment for cancer is now a reality.

86.5 Organoids and Organ Transplantation

Organoids are three-dimensional structures that resemble miniature versions of parent organs in structure and function. Often referred to as "organs-in-a-dish," they are derived from stem cells or progenitor cells through a process known as self-organization. Organoids can be created from adult stem cells (sourced from tissues like the intestine, breast, prostate, etc.), intact tissue fragments (which contain both parenchymal and stromal elements), pluripotent stem cells (PSCs), and induced pluripotent stem cells (iPSCs). In 2017, the organoid research method, 3D culture, was awarded Method of the Year by Nature Methods.

The key characteristics of organoids include:
1. They are 3D multicellular tissue constructs grown in vitro.
2. They contain multiple cell types specific to the corresponding parent organ.
3. They mimic the key components of the parent organ, including its architecture, cell populations, and functions.
4. They possess the ability for self-renewal and function.

Organoids derived from adult stem cells are limited to epithelial organoids, whereas those created from tissue fragments incorporate both parenchymal and stromal elements, better reflecting the complex in vivo microenvironment. Epithelial organoids lack the mesodermal components typically found in native tissues. PSC-derived organoids are valuable for studying developmental processes, physiological functions, and disease models in vitro. They are also utilized in drug development and screening.

Research is ongoing into the feasibility of using organoids to replace or treat conditions such as esophageal and tracheal replacement, correction of short bowel syndrome (as seen in Hirschsprung's disease), biliary atresia correction, and liver organoid transplantation for chronic end-stage liver failure. However, using organoids for therapeutic or replacement purposes will take time due to challenges such as the mass expansion of organoids and overcoming immune rejection. Despite their promise, technical challenges remain in creating vascularized multilineage organ systems.

86.6 Concluding Remarks

The rapid advancement of new technologies has greatly enhanced medical care, particularly in diagnosis and targeted therapies. These innovations have improved our understanding of diseases, leading to more personalized medicine. Such developments have significantly benefitted pediatric surgery practices. Understanding the genetic basis of diseases can help predict and prevent disorders within families. A specific molecular diagnosis can also assist families in comprehending why their child is different and provide accurate counseling for future pregnancies. Applying molecular genetic techniques for diagnosis and therapy will undoubtedly result in better care and higher success rates in pediatric surgery.

Suggested Reading

Ahmed SF, Alimusina M, Batista RL, Domenice S, Lisboa Gomes N, McGowan R, et al. The use of genetics for reaching a diagnosis in XY DSD. Sex Dev. 2022;16(2–3):207–24.

Copp AJ, Greene ND. Genetics and development of neural tube defects. J Pathol. 2010;220(2):217–30.

Gröbner SN, Worst BC, Weischenfeldt J, Buchhalter I, Kleinheinz K, Rudneva VA, et al. The landscape of genomic alterations across childhood cancers. Nature. 2018;555(7696):321–7.

Grody WW, Thompson BH, Hudgins L. Whole-exome/genome sequencing and genomics. Pediatrics. 2013;132:S211–5.

Halder A. Amniotic band syndrome and/or limb body wall complex: split or lump. Appl Clin Genet. 2010;3:7–15.

Halder A. Lethal developmental defects: an overview. Open J Obstet Gynecol. 2014;4:1006–36.

Heuckeroth RO. Hirschsprung disease—integrating basic science and clinical medicine to improve outcomes. Nat Rev Gastroenterol Hepatol. 2018;15:152–67.

Nature Methods Editorial Board. Method of the year 2017: organoids. Nat Methods. 2018;15:1.

Padia R, Zenner K, Bly R, Bennett J, Bull C, Perkins J. Clinical application of molecular genetics in lymphatic malformations. Laryngoscope Investig Otolaryngol. 2019;4(1):170–3.

Tang CS, Karim A, Zhong Y, Chung PH, Tam PK. Genetics of Hirschsprung's disease. Pediatr Surg Int. 2023;39(1):104.

Application of Nanotechnology in Medicine

87

Amit K. Dinda

87.1 Introduction

Nanotechnology is a discipline of science and engineering pertaining to fabricating structures, devices, and systems by manipulating atoms and molecules at nanoscale. In 1959, noble laureate physicist Richard Feynman first introduced the concept of nanotechnology in an invited talk at the annual meeting of American Physical Society at California Institute of Technology, USA. Reduction of a material from macro to nano form/nano size results in changes in its physical, chemical, and other properties. These unique properties of nanomaterials can be utilized for diverse applications like industrial processing, energy sector, metallurgy, agriculture, packaging, textile, cosmetics, medicine, and so on. The area of medical application of nanotechnology is also termed as "Nanomedicine." Now it has become one of the most promising technologies of the twenty-first century along with digital technology like artificial intelligence. The nanoparticles are made from different organic and inorganic materials. Examples of organic material are lipid, protein, carbohydrate, biopolymer, etc. Large number of inorganic materials are also used like metal, metal oxide, ceramics, silica, carbon, etc.

A. K. Dinda (✉)
Emeritus Scientist (ICMR), Department of Pathology, Centre for Medical Innovation & Entrepreneurship, All India Institute of Medical Sciences, New Delhi, Delhi, India

87.2 Applications

There are innumerable applications of nanotechnology in medicine and health care. They can be broadly categorized as therapeutic and diagnostic.

The important examples of therapeutic use of nanotechnology are:

- Targeted drug delivery system
- Photothermal therapy
- Regenerative Medicine, tissue engineering, and implants

Targeted drug delivery system The drug or therapeutic biomolecules may be loaded in suitable nanoparticles which can be targeted at the disease site. Targeted nanodrug delivery has become a reality in cancer treatment. Abraxane (Nab-paclitaxel loaded albumin nanoparticle), Doxil (Doxorubicin-loaded liposome) are examples of nanoformulation widely used for different types of cancer treatment. The nanosized particles are accumulated in the cancer tissue due to enhanced permeability of cancer vasculature and retained in the cancer tissue, which enhances therapeutic effect of the drug and reduces systemic as well as off-target toxicity. Such mechanism of targeted drug delivery for cancer is called EPR (Enhanced Permeability & Retention) effect. The drug targeting may be done by attaching a ligand on the surface of the drug loaded nanoparticle for a specific receptor of the targeted cell. For example,

© The Author(s), under exclusive license to Springer Nature Singapore Pte Ltd. 2025

S. Roy Choudhury (ed.), *Pediatric Surgery*, https://doi.org/10.1007/978-981-96-1257-4_87

highly expressed folate receptors on cancer cells can be targeted with conjugating folate on the nanoparticle. The nanodrug delivery system can be used to cross different physiological barriers which cannot be achieved by conventional drug molecules. This enables drug-loaded nanoparticles to easily cross blood-brain barrier for treatment of central nervous system diseases like malignancy, infection, and others. Similarly, several drugs cannot cross gastrointestinal barrier and can be administered only through parenteral routes. Nano drug delivery system can help them to cross gastrointestinal barrier. Thus, it is possible to make oral nanoformulation of injectable drugs or vaccine. With the help of nanotechnology, it is possible to target subcellular systems like mitochondria and delivery of genetic material into the nucleus. Non-viral systems are being fabricated for safer gene therapy. Stimuli responsive drug delivery at the site of action (cancer area) is also a reality where ultrasound induced or magnetic stimulation induced drug release can be done in the cancer tissue as and when needed. There are large number of functional nanosystem, which can be fabricated for pH dependent or temperature sensing drug release. Thus, targeted nanodrug delivery system is enhancing efficacy with lower requirement of drug molecules as well as reduces toxicity. Lipid nanoparticles are used for development of mRNA vaccine for COVID. In wound care, silver nanoparticle-based dressings are highly effective preventing biofilm formation and development of antimicrobial resistance. Such formulations are being used in wound care in burn and plastic surgery. Similarly, nanomaterial impregnated catheters are becoming important to prevent infection. There are several such nanopharmaceuticals will be available in the market at near future for treatment of cancer and other diseases.

Photothermal therapy Several metal nanoparticles like gold and silver when exposed to specific wavelength of light produces heat due to the phenomenon of surface plasma resonance (SPR). This property can be utilized for thermal ablation of cancer tissue, which can be substituted for radiotherapy with much less side effect. Near infrared light which can pass long distance from the surface can be used for thermal ablation of cancer in different viscera.

Regenerative Medicine, Tissue engineering, and implants Exosome/extracellular vesicles (EVs) are heterogeneous cell-derived vesicles mostly in nanoscale size (endogenous nanoparticles) generated by almost all cells in the body through diverse mechanisms that undertake cell-to-cell communication by transferring divergent biological molecule based signals like non-coding RNAs, coding RNAs, DNA strands, proteins, lipids to counterpart cells. They are found in almost all body fluids like blood, urine, saliva, sweat, tears, breast milk, ascites, plural fluid, cerebrospinal fluid, etc. Due to unique properties of exosome, its stable and biocompatible structure and capability of modulation of cellular functions, it is emerging as an important mode of diagnostic and therapeutic interventions specially in regenerative medicine. In the area of tissue engineering, nanofibers (thickness in nanoscale) from different materials can be made for making scaffold to repair and replace damaged tissue with controlled release of growth factors. Implants with nanostructured surface as well as surface functionalization have shown better compatibility in orthopedic and dental practices.

Diagnostics There is a diverse application of nanotechnology in diagnostics which can be broadly discussed under the following categories:

Imaging and Theragnosis
Nano-Biosensor, biological microelectromechanical systems (BioMEMS)/biological nanoelectromechanical systems (BioNEMS)
Point of Care Diagnosis, Lab on a Chip

Imaging & Theragnosis Fast and accurate imaging of tissue microstructures and characterization of lesion/abnormalities are current challenges, which could be achieved by use of nanoparticles acting as nontoxic contrast agents with a longer circulation time. Nanoparticle-based contrast agents can be used for many common biomedical imaging currently being practiced in imaging like CT, MRI, PET, SPECT, and Ultrasound. In addition, in vivo florescence imaging with receptor-based targeting of cancer cells using nanoparticles with diverse functionalization can help to detect early micro-metastasis. Therapeutic molecule/drug can be loaded in these nanoparticles, which can kill the cancer cells under imaging surveillance. Such combined procedure of imaging diagnosis and therapy is termed as *"Theragnosis."*

Nano-Biosensor, BioMEMS/BioNEMS The area of Nano-Biosensor is expanding rapidly. Technically sensor can detect specifically gases, chemicals, biological agents, light, electric fields, heat, pressure, and may other parameters. Nanotechnology can create a large reactive surface area with a very small mass of material increasing the sensitivity of detection. There are large number of diagnostic, prognostic biomarkers present in body fluids, exhaled air, cellular, and tissue extracts which can be detected by nanosytems working as molecular sensors. These nano sensors can be used as chemical sensor for specific protein, enzyme, nucleic acid, and other biomolecules. BioMEMS (biological microelectromechanical systems) has been developed earlier where the micro component has been replaced by nano structures leading to generation of BioNEMS (biological nanoelectromechanical systems). The electrochemical techniques commonly used in diverse types of sensors which include potentiometric, chronometry, voltammetry, impedance measurement, field effect transistor (FET), etc. Exploiting the advantage of nanotechnology, new generation of nano-sensors have a high sensitivity. These are used in large number of wire able devices, implanted systems used in operation theatre, ICU, and portable systems monitoring ambulant patients. Integration of multiple nanosensors with Artificial Intelligence (AI)-based data analytics and remote monitoring through Bluetooth and other web-based technologies is revolutionizing clinical management in different specialties.

Utilizing the technology of BioNEMS microfluidic devices are being made. Few microliter of serum or other body fluid can be put on these devices, which flows to reaction site with nanosensors that can detect reaction between antigen and antibody, enzyme and substrate, hybridization of complementary nuclei acid strand, and so on. The sensing can generate various signals like optical, mechanical, electrical, etc., which can be detected and analyzed with generation of data (result). Such microfluidic nanotechnology-based devices are low cost, portable, and can be used peripheral rural areas at the point care (bedside practice). These technologies use less energy, consumables, and instrumentation facility and easy to use. This has given rise to designing small portable point-of-care "Lab on a Chip" devices, which can do larger number of serum chemistry as well as PCR and replace current practice of laboratory medicine, which requires large laboratory set ups and human resources.

There is rapid advancement of nanotechnology applications in all specialties of medicine with a lot of products in the clinical trials as well as being commercialized. The quality safety and efficacy of these emerging therapeutics should be regulated with greater stringency considering the health and environmental impacts. The use of nanomaterials in agriculture and food has also shown many benefits. Thus, this enabling technology is going to enter all spheres of human life. In the coming era of precision medicine, all medical students and practitioners should know about this emerging technology, which is going to revolutionize health care practices in near future.

Suggested Reading

Haleem A, Javaid M, Singh RP, Sc R, Suman R. Applications of nanotechnology in medical field: a brief review. Glob Health J. 2023;7(2):70–7.

Han X, Xu K, Taratula O, Farsad K. Applications of nanoparticles in biomedical imaging. Nanoscale. 2019;11(3):799–819.

Huang X, Zhu Y, Kianfar E. Nano biosensors: properties, applications and electrochemical techniques. J Mater Res Technol. 2021;12:1649–72.

Loizidou M, Seifalian AM. Nanotechnology and its applications in surgery. Br J Surg. 2010;97(4):463–5.

Zhenga X, Zhanga P, Fub Z, Mengb S, Dai L. Applications of nanomaterials in tissue engineering. RSC Adv. 2021;11:19041–58.

88 Recent Advances in Pediatric Radiology and Imaging

Shayeri Roy Choudhury

In the recent years, pediatric radiology has progressed immensely due to technological and scientific advancements that have improved image quality while reducing scan times, welcomed new possibilities of imaging techniques and provided deeper insights into well known as well as rarer pathologies. Children are vastly different from adults and the "one size fits all" principle cannot be applied to them. Therefore, pediatric radiology has a different set of requirements and challenges which all surgeons should be keenly aware of.

Due to the sheer volume of scientific developments, it is not always possible to keep up with all the advances; therefore, in this chapter we will discuss the key trending developments in the field of pediatric radiology in the last few years. Readers are encouraged to peruse through recent journals and articles on a regular basis to keep abreast of the new and upcoming advancements in radiology.

88.1 Advances in Ultrasound (US)

Ultrasound is a safe, highly cost-effective and useful tool in pediatric imaging. It is easily accessible, portable, and can be used in point-of-care settings. It is one of the most preferred investigations in many cases due to absence of harm from non-ionizing radiation. Due to improvements in the equipment as well as invention of new techniques beyond the conventional grayscale imaging, the utility of ultrasound in diagnostic and interventional imaging has grown.

88.1.1 Contrast-Enhanced Ultrasound (CEUS)

The use of tiny microbubbles which are coated in a stabilizing phospholipid-shell is the backbone of CEUS. These small particles, once injected, circulate through the vessels and reach the small vasculature (i.e., the capillaries). The US beam causes the microbubbles to oscillate within the vessels. Using a low mechanical index ($MI < 0.2$), the microbubbles are compressible, and behave in a linear pattern. Their distribution within the vessels can be analyzed and hence they behave as "blood pool agents." Increasing the mechanical index, causes the micro-bubbles to expand due to increased acoustic power of the beam, and eventually they burst. These contrast agents are excreted primarily by lungs and liver, and therefore are safe to use even in renal insufficiency.

The older generations CEUS contrast agents were relatively unstable, and afforded only very transient imaging. The newer (second) generation agents are more stable, for example, sulfur hexafluoride microbubbles coated in a lyophilized

S. R. Choudhury (✉)
Department of Radiodiagnosis, PGIMER, Chandigarh, India

© The Author(s), under exclusive license to Springer Nature Singapore Pte Ltd. 2025
S. Roy Choudhury (ed.), *Pediatric Surgery*, https://doi.org/10.1007/978-981-96-1257-4_88

powder. The utility in pediatric radiology is currently off-label and under research.

Applications in pediatric imaging include

1. Imaging of various parenchymal lesions like liver, renal, and pancreatic lesions for assessing vascularity and determining the nature of lesions
2. Assessment of organ perfusion in trauma and transplantation
3. Transcranial imaging for intra-cranial vascular malformations
4. Acute abdominal pathologies like acute appendicitis, intussusception and Meckel diverticulitis
5. Intra-cavitary uses such as contrast enhanced voiding uro-sonography in vesicoureteral reflux or posterior urethral valves, and for evaluation of ano-genitourinary malformations.

88.1.2 Ultrasound Elastography

Elastography is a sonographic technique for evaluating the stiffness of tissues using the US beam and measuring variations in its speed in different tissues. Two main techniques are currently present—the semi-quantitative strain elastography, and the quantitative shear wave elastography. The strain elastography technique employs manual compression of the tissues to cause linear deformation, which is visualized in color-coded maps to evaluate relative stiffness. Shear wave elastography employ the use of high-intensity US pulses which propagate through tissues and the resultant tissue deformation leads to lateral propagation of the pulses, which is transmitted back to the transducer and is recorded for absolute quantification of tissue stiffness. When a broadband pulse is applied onto the tissues of interest, there is formation of two different waves. The primary wave is the compression wave which is along the direction of the pulse and has high velocity. The secondary wave is perpendicular to the direction of the US pulse, and has relatively low velocity. This is called shear wave, and the velocity increases with increasing tissue stiffness.

Shear wave elastography is commonly used for estimation of liver fibrosis and liver parenchymal disease. Similarly, it can be utilized for evaluation of splenic stiffness in patients with chronic liver parenchymal disease for the prediction of formation of esophago-gastric varices. Further research is warranted in the utility of elastography in many areas, but it is showing promise in diagnosis of biliary atresia, bowel inflammation vs fibrosis in inflammatory bowel disease, thyroid disorders, chronic kidney disease, and muscle stiffness in congenital muscle dystrophies.

88.1.3 3D and 4D Ultrasound

Three-dimensional US has many applications in diagnostic radiology, particularly in the field of obstetric imaging. It is based on combining a series of two-dimensional images along with positional and planar data, which are reconstructed to make a 3D dataset. Thereafter, many post-processing tools can be applied based on the software availability. Multiplanar reconstructions and 3D surface and volume rendering are few of the commonest available tools. Due to faster computer processors, higher frame rates are now achievable, and we have 4D US, which is real-time visualization of 3D dataset.

The application of 3D US in pediatric neurosonography afford production of a 3D dataset, which is comparable to CT or MRI. It can be used to diagnose and evaluate developmental disorders, vascular malformations and ventricular volumes. It also has utility in uro-sonography to assess the bladder volumes in irregular shaped neurogenic bladder, depiction of renal tissue in grossly hydronephrotic kidneys, evaluation of small bladder diverticulae or urethral valves, polyps etc. Trans-perineal 3D US can be used for urogenital anomalies in the pediatric female and help in evaluating any uterine anomalies.

It is important to note, that obtaining 3D datasets requires the stillness and cooperation of patients, which may be difficult in infants and pediatrics especially in abdominal and genitourinary US; therefore, operator expertise is necessary and timing the data acquisition with the respiratory cycle, or when the child is sedated or sleeping are few of the practiced techniques.

88.2 Advances in Computed Tomography

88.2.1 CT Dose Reduction

The most debated topic in pediatric radiology is undeniably the reduction in CT dose for children. This is based on the age-old adage that "children are not small adults." Modern CT scanners are now equipped with software to minimize the dose according to the size and weight of the patient, without significant compromise on the image quality. Use of pediatric specific CT protocols with limited area of interest and limiting to single phase acquisition wherever possible is encouraged. Automatic tube current modulation is used in most studies to reduce dose. Miliampere second (mAs) has a linear relationship with radiation dose but reducing it significantly may lead to loss of spatial resolution and increase in image noise. Similarly, kilovoltage peak (kVp) has a nonlinear relationship with radiation dose, and reducing kVp also leads to dose reduction. Use of iterative reconstruction allows for dose reduction while optimizing image noise to acceptable levels.

88.2.2 Dual Energy CT

Dual energy CT (DECT) uses separate X-ray beam spectra at the same time and allows interrogations of different tissues having different attenuation values at different spectra. Both low and high (80 and 120 kVp, respectively) energy acquisition can be done simultaneously on the latest generation DECT scanners with no discernible increase in radiation exposure. The low kVp acquisition allows us to visualize subtle enhancement and therefore detect small hypo- or hyper-enhancing lesions, and quantitative analysis of the degree of enhancement can be done by making iodine maps using information from both low and high energy acquisition. Virtual non-enhanced sequences can also be obtained by using post-processing technology, which reduces the need to acquire non-contrast sequences and therefore, reduces the dose.

DECT has the ability to improve characterization of masses and lesions, by allowing quantitative iodine estimation to predict the degree of enhancement and virtual non enhanced images providing information on calcification versus enhancement. Its utility in adult onco-radiology is well established and applications in pediatric oncology like mediastinal tumors, lymphomas, and gastrointestinal tumors are also under active development. It can also be used for assessing disease extent and response to treatment. In non-oncological applications, it can be used for characterizing renal calculus composition, for small pulmonary embolus detection in CT pulmonary angiograms, and for vascular lesions like arteriovenous malformations, hemangiomas, etc.

88.3 Advances in Magnetic Resonance Imaging (MRI)

Innovations in MRI are currently dominating in the field of radiology. It has vast utility in pediatric imaging, with applications in almost every body organ. The major challenge to overcome in pediatric MRI is to reduce the scan duration for children to provide images that are free from respiratory and motion artifacts. Sedation, scanning in infants after feeding, use of pediatric-size body coils, respiratory, and cardiac motion triggered imaging are some of the commonly practiced techniques during MRI.

88.3.1 Pediatric Magnetic Resonance Urography (MRU)

MRU combines both anatomical and functional dataset in a single imaging modality, and therefore presents an irreplaceable tool in pediatric uro-radiology. Both static and dynamic imaging can be performed. The heavily T2 weighted images provide an anatomical depiction of the kidney and the collecting system including the ureters and the bladder. Volume rendering and maximum intensity projection images from the 3D data set are useful in situations with complex anatomical structures. T2 weighted sequences are also important for assessing renal parenchymal thickness and morphology as well as in bladder to look for ureteroceles, ectopic ureteric insertion, ureteric valves, etc. There is established role of pre-procedure hydration and diuretic (typically furosemide at 0.5–1.0 mg/kg) injection to allow for distension of the collection system, and therefore, better evaluation. Intra-venous Gadolinium contrast administration in patients is considered safe in those with total estimated GFR of more than 60 mL/min, and can even be used (with some caution) in patients with levels between 30 and 60 mL/min. For post contrast dynamic imaging, the contrast is administered with a constant infusion rate using a power injector (between 0.1 and 0.2 mL/s). Sequential post contrast imaging over the first 5 min after contrast injection allows for evaluation of the renal nephrograms. Between 5 and 10 min, few interval sequences are acquired. The dynamic datasets help in assessing contrast accumulation, concentration, and excretion in the kidneys. Using post-processing techniques and algorithms, the split-renal function or differential renal function can also be calculated. This makes MRU a very attractive tool for evaluation of pediatric hydronephrosis and obstructive uropathy. It has better contrast resolution that CT urography with the advantage of lack of ionizing radiation. However, the long scan times and the requirement of a perfectly still patient during the sequences means that small children need to be sedated for the duration of the study, otherwise respiratory and motion artifacts will degrade the image quality and lead to suboptimal evaluation.

88.3.2 Whole Body MRI (WB-MRI)

There are many multi-focal and systemic diseases that occur commonly in the pediatric population. Evaluating the extent of these diseases becomes difficult with multimodality imaging, and therefore WB-MRI is an excellent tool in such cases. It can help in diagnosis and in treatment response of many pathologies. The recent developments allow for fast acquisition of multiple sequences from head to toe. Use of dedicated multi-channel surface coils of length 95–125 cm is usually sufficient for pediatric patients. These coils allow for a high signal-to-noise ratio and spatial resolution. Multiple parts of the body can be sequentially acquired in the same sitting. Later, post-processing stitching can be done to obtain seamless images of the entire body in coronal planes. The sequences that are most in use are Short-tau inversion recovery (STIR), T2-wieghted, and T1 weighted sequences. STIR imaging allows for a homogeneous and uniform fat suppression and helps in detecting pathological bone lesions, even in small children who have hyper-cellular bone marrow. T2-weighted sequences are also complementary, although fat saturated T2 weighted sequences may have relatively inhomogeneous fat suppression. To overcome this, the newer T2-weighted Dixon sequence is used, which has a high signal-to-noise ratio and shorter scan duration. It also accurately depicts small anatomic details. T1 weighted sequences is exceptionally good for detecting bone marrow lesions in hypo-cellular marrow, and therefore, has better utility in adolescents and adults. It is useful for post-radiation and post-treatment fatty marrow change and changes in chronic inflammatory arthritis with fatty marrow metaplasia. The T1- Dixon technique generates four images (fat, water, in-phase, and opposed-phase sequences) from a single acquisition. This allows better evaluation of marrow-replacement lesions and marrow-infiltration pathologies; and can be combined with post-contrast sequences to further improve lesion detection. Diffusion weighted imaging (DWI) along with apparent diffusion coefficient (ADC) map is an indicator of tumor cellularity. In viable tumors, there is reduced diffusion, i.e., diffusion restriction, with corresponding low signal intensity values on ADC maps. WB-DWI is useful for evaluating pediatric lymphoma and other multifocal malignancies. It can be used to monitor therapy, and an increase in ADC values after treatment reflect a favorable response.

In pediatric oncology, it has role in tumor staging, with capability of detecting bone as well as soft tissue lesions throughout the body. In post-treatment imaging, the addition of diffusion weighted imaging (DWI) can help differentiate viable tumor from post-treatment changes. It is useful for early detection of tumors in cancer-predisposition and various neurocutaneous syndromes like Neurofibromatosis I and II, Li-Fraumeni syndrome, Von Hippel Lindau syndrome, Multiple endocrine neoplasia (MEN) syndromes, etc. The extent of various lymphovascular and vascular malformations like Klippel Trenaunay syndrome, Parks-Weber syndrome can be evaluated with WB-MRI. In patients with widespread lymphangiomatosis, WB-MRI can predict clinical outcome and prognosis of patients by detected poor prognostic indicators such as chylous pleural effusion, extensive mediastinal, and laryngeal involvement. It also has a role in pediatric rheumatology, in diseases like dermatomyositis and rheumatoid arthritis. It can help to detect and characterize neuromuscular involvement patterns as well as evaluated disease activity and joint damage in rheumatoid arthritis, as evidenced by synovitis and bone erosions.

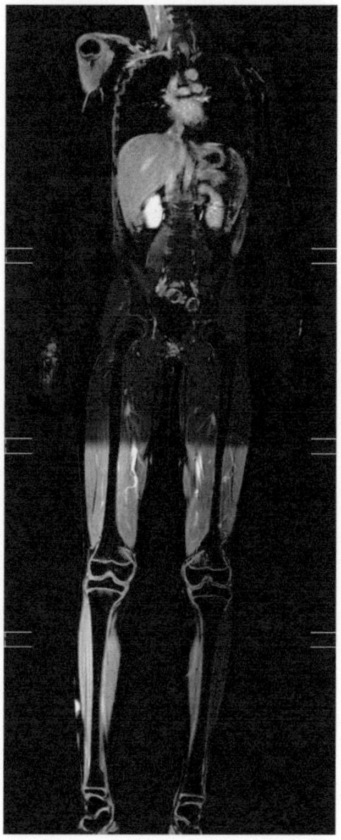

88.4 Nuclear Medicine in Pediatric Radiology

Nuclear medicine has a role in molecular imaging due to its ability to evaluate tissue viability by use of radio-isotopes, which undergo cellular uptake and metabolism. In the field of pediatric uro-radiology, nuclear medicine has great utility, in the context of antenatal hydronephrosis or non-functional kidney, recurrent urinary tract infections (UTIs), obstructive uropathy, etc.

The radiopharmaceuticals used in uro-radiology are Tc 99m dimercaptosuccinic acid (DMSA) and Tc-99m-mercapto-acetyl-triglycine (MAG3). Static scintigraphy using DMSA is the gold standard for assessing the renal parenchyma and total renal parenchymal function. Dynamic scintigraphy using MAG3 provides information on renal perfusion, function, and excretion. Use of these studies in recurrent UTIs, congenital hydronephrosis, megaureter, and other congenital anatomic renal anomalies is established and widely practiced.

Nuclear medicine is also being used for pediatric oncology, for disease detection and staging, assessing response to chemo or radiotherapy and for recurrence. For positron emission tomography (PET) scan, the metabolite used is 18 fluoro-dexoy-glucose (18-FDG). A PET and a CT are both acquired for accurate anatomical localization of small lesions. This adds to the radiation dosage. It is used commonly for staging of pediatric lymphoma. Other uses of PET-CT include infection and inflammatory disorders, autoimmune diseases, and musculoskeletal conditions like chronic recurrent multifocal osteomyelitis (CRMO). Meta-iodo-benzyl-guanidine (mIBG) labelled iodine (I-123 or I-131) is used for scintigraphy scanning for neuroblastoma staging and distant metastases detection. Hepatobiliary scintigraphy has its place in neonatal imaging for diagnosis of biliary atresia. The radiopharmaceutical used is Tc-99m labelled mebrofenin.

88.5 Artificial Intelligence in Pediatric Radiology

Artificial intelligence (AI) is rapidly emerging as a transformative tool in pediatric radiology, particularly in supporting surgical care. Its integration into preoperative, intraoperative, and postoperative phases of pediatric surgery is enhancing diagnostic precision, improving surgical planning, and enabling safer interventions. In the preoperative setting, AI algorithms assist in the segmentation and 3D reconstruction of complex anatomical anomalies, such as congenital heart defects, anorectal malformations, and tracheoesophageal fistulas. These reconstructions support virtual surgical simulation, personalized planning, and 3D printing of anatomical models for surgeon rehearsal and patient-family education. AI-enhanced volumetry also aids in surgical decision-making for hepatic resections, nephrectomies, or tumor debulking procedures by providing accurate organ and lesion measurements. Intraoperatively, AI applications include augmented reality overlays and image fusion, which guide surgeons during minimally invasive procedures. Real-time ultrasound enhanced by AI improves vascular access, regional anesthesia, and identification of vital structures, particularly in neonates and infants where precision is critical. Postoperatively, AI algorithms are increasingly used to monitor for complications such as anastomotic leaks, abscess formation, or vascular compromise, especially following transplant or gastrointestinal surgeries. AI-enabled comparison of follow-up studies helps assess healing, detect early recurrence, or evaluate graft viability. In pediatric trauma and emergency surgical settings, AI aids in rapid triage and prioritization by identifying critical findings on radiographs or CT, including internal bleeding, organ lacerations, or pneumoperitoneum. Despite its promise, challenges remain, such as the limited availability of pediatric-specific imaging datasets, the need for age-appropriate algorithm training, and ongoing ethical and regulatory considerations. Nonetheless, AI represents a major advancement in pediatric surgical radiology, offering enhanced accuracy, speed, and individualized care for complex pediatric surgical cases

Suggested Reading

Gottumukkala RV, Kalra MK, Tabari A, Otrakji A, Gee MS. Advanced CT techniques for decreasing radiation dose, reducing sedation requirements, and optimizing image quality in children. Radiographics. 2019;39(3):709–26.

Guimarães MD, Noschang J, Teixeira SR, Santos MK, Lederman HM, Tostes V, Kundra V, Oliveira AD, Hochhegger B, Marchiori E. Whole-body MRI in pediatric patients with cancer. Cancer Imaging. 2017;17:1–2.

Hwang M, Piskunowicz M, Darge K. Advanced ultrasound techniques for pediatric imaging. Pediatrics. 2019;143(3):e20182609. https://doi.org/10.1542/peds.2018-2609.

Lee EY, Liszewski MC, Gee MS, Daltro P, Restrepo R, editors. Pediatric body MRI: a comprehensive, multidisciplinary guide. Springer Nature; 2020.

89 Biomarkers in Pediatric Surgery

Sukrit Singh Shah

Biomarkers are biologically measured substances that are expressed by malignant/injured tissues, circulating tumor components, or generated by the host in response to the injury/insult and constitutively serve as essential tools to aid clinicians in making diagnosis, staging, and risk assessments.

89.1 Types

1. Based on disease state
   prediction, detection, diagnostic, and prognostic marker
2. Based on biomolecule
   DNA, RNA, proteins, and carbohydrates
3. Miscellaneous
   imaging markers and radiological markers

Where do biomarkers come from?

Tests (OMICS, ELISA), imaging (CT, PET, etc.), cytological (FNAC), IHC, electrophysiological (EEG, ECG)

Characteristics of an Ideal Biomarker?

A. Have great sensitivity specificity and positive predictive value
B. Safe and easy to perform
C. Cost efficient to follow up
D. Consistent across gender and ethnic groups

S. S. Shah (✉)
Lady Hardinge Medical College,
New Delhi, Delhi, India

Uses of Biomarkers

Clinical trials-drug development
Screening of diseases
Risk assessment
Diagnosis
Monitor therapy

Biomarker Identification Technologies

A. Genomics
B. Transcriptomics
C. Proteonomics
D. Metabolomics
E. Imaging
F. Other techniques like nuclear magnetic resonance (NMR), fluorescence in situ hybirdization (FISH), nanotechnology

89.2 Applications in Pediatric Surgery

89.2.1 Pediatric Urology

A. Pelviureteric Junction Obstruction (PUJO)—for antenatal detection—amniotic fluid indices (Na < 100 mg/dl. Chloride <110 osmolarity <210 mosm/l and beta 2 microglobulin <6 indicate good prognosis
B. Vesico-Ureteric Reflux (VUR)—laminin, TGF beta1, VCAM—all indicate renal scarring in children with VUR
C. Urinary Tract Infection (UTI)—MMP-9, tissue inhibitor of proteinases, chemokine IL8,

© The Author(s), under exclusive license to Springer Nature Singapore Pte Ltd. 2025
S. Roy Choudhury (ed.), *Pediatric Surgery*, https://doi.org/10.1007/978-981-96-1257-4_89

and urinary alpha 1 macroglobulin indicate urinary tract infection

D. Acute Kidney Injury (AKI)—kidney injury molecule 1, neutrophil gelatinase-associated lipoprotein, IL 18, cystatin c, chemokine interferon-inducible protein −10
E. Progressive renal damage—TFF1, TFF3, NGAL, Microalbumin
F. Bladder Malignancy—NMP22, BTA stat/TRAK, Immunocyt/ucyt+

89.3 Biomarkers in Pediatric Gastro Surgery

89.3.1 Necrotizing Enterocolitis (NEC)

A. Epidermal growth factor, intestinal fatty acid-binding protein, and fecal calprotectin have all been identified as potential biomarkers of NEC in human infants.
B. Several interleukins (ILs) and other inflammatory factors are either up-regulated (IL 1, 6, 8, and 12, tumor necrosis factor-alpha, interferon, and platelet-activating factor), down-regulated in infants with NEC despite promising results, no single biomarker has proven useful as a stand-alone diagnostic test in clinical practice.

89.4 Newer Biomarkers in NEC

A. Alpha-2macroglobulin (which shares homology with A2ML1) and Fibrininogen A are components of the coagulation cascade, (coagulation necrosis is a common pathologic finding in NEC resection specimens).
B. VASN is an inhibitor of transforming growth factor-beta and is down-regulated after vascular injury (lower urine levels in the surgical NEC cohort).
C. The pattern recognition receptor CD14 is a regulator of the innate immune system—plays a role in response to bacterial lipopolysaccharide (LPS) (elevated in surgical NEC)
D. Although these associations are intriguing, further investigation is needed.

89.5 Application in Pediatric Oncology

Survival rates for children with primarily leukemias and lymphomas have improved partly owing to their early detection, 5-year survival rates for pediatric solid tumors have not changed over the past 2 decades.

Difficulty in discriminating and diagnosing solid masses by using standard techniques has hindered progress in this area.

The role of biomarkers here is to not only accurately determine the type of masses but also detect tumor recurrences at the earliest.

For solid tumors, there has been increasing interest in several adult cancers where EV-based (extracellular vesicle) biomarkers are correlated with both disease stage and outcome. Due to significant differences in the development of adult and pediatric cancers, the results of studies cannot simply be extrapolated. For example, cancer development and progression are often driven by multiple genetic aberrations. In contrast, tumors in children have distinct genomic landscapes typically characterized by a paucity of recurrent mutations and structural variations.

The examples of current status of EV-based biomarkers are mentioned along with the specific malignancy in which they are being used.

89.5.1 Neuroblastoma

The most validated prognostic markers are age, stage, and amplification of the MYCN oncogene.

NB is designated as a neuroendocrine-related tumor—secretion of various regulatory peptides e.g., secretory granule proteins chromogranin A (CgA) and synaptophysin & the cytosolic enzyme neuron-specific enolase (NSE) is used for diagnosing the tumor.

Other NB secretory proteins include neural-specific protein gene product 9.5, neuropeptide Y (NPY), vasoactive intestinal peptide (VIP), gastrin-releasing peptide (GRP), galanin, somatostatin, peptide histidine isoleucine, pituitary adenylate cyclase–activating peptide, atrial natriuretic factor, etc.

The spectrum of released NB-related proteins is diverse and underscores the biological complexity involved in the regulation and modulation.

The plasma catecholamines dopamine (DA) and norepinephrine and their metabolites in urine, such as homovanillic acid (HVA) and vanillylmandelic acid (VMA), are diagnostic and have been used in clinical diagnosis and screening programs.

Both CgA and NSE are well-established intracellular neuronal markers used to monitor NB disease activity and treatment response.

Research on EV-based markers showed that expression of miR-199a-3p was significantly higher in patients especially high-risk groups compared to healthy age- and gender-matched controls.

Specifically, it was found that a combination of three miRNAs (miR-29c, miR-342-3p, and let-7b) can discriminate between patients with a poor clinical response and patients with a good clinical response. This combination of three miRNAs has tumor-suppressor functions, and further analysis has shown that they play a role in tumor progression, survival, and development of chemoresistance.

89.5.2 Wilms' Tumor (WT)

Angiogenetic regulation plays an important role in the formation of new blood vessels involved in the growth and metastatic spread of solid tumors, but the clinical significance remains to be understood.

The theory supports that angiogenesis regulators such as basic fibroblast growth factor (bFGF), vascular endothelial growth factor (VEGF), and hepatocyte growth factor (HGF) may be of clinical value in Wilms' tumor.

Currently the role of circulating tumor DNA (ct- DNA) and liquid biopsy in diagnosing and prognosticating Wilm's tumor is not significant but research is being done regarding "Driver Mutations" that can detect Wilms' tumor (WT) at an earlier stage.

There are around 40–50 proven or suspected WT drivers, which may reflect the histological heterogeneity and differences in founder cell types. Mutations of WT1, CTNNB1, and WTX, as well as loss of imprinting (LOI) of IGF2/H19 to name a few.

The Wnt/β-catenin signaling pathway is an attractive target for WT patients because CTNNB1 mutations are relatively common. The ongoing COG phase 1/2 study of tegavivint, inhibitor of Wnt/β-catenin signaling (NCT04851119) is of interest for patients with recurrent WT.

89.5.3 Hepatoblastoma

- Most patients with HB have extremely high serum levels of AFP [up to 100,000 ± 1,000,000 times the normal value] (<10 ng/Ml)
- Measurement of serum AFP—valuable diagnostic test, owing to the correlation between AFP level and disease activity.
- Serial determinations of AFP determine the effectiveness of therapy.
- Can also be associated with—inappropriate secretion of peptide hormones and other associated proteins.
- Marked thrombocytosis secondary to the release of tumor-derived factors with thrombopoietin-like activity.
- Current research on EV have shown that levels of miR-21 are increased in hepatoblastoma.
- Also, studies have found that levels of miR-34a, miR-34b, and miR-34c are lower in patients of hepatoblastoma as compared to controls.

89.5.4 Pediatric Germ Cell Tumors

- Predicting the biological behavior in GCTs can be confusing owing to other factors such as patient age, histologic subtype, anatomic site, and clinical stage.
- Serum levels of alpha-fetoprotein (AFP), beta-human chorionic gonadotropin (β-hCG), and lactate dehydrogenase (LDH) are well validated in their utility as non-invasive diagnostic as well as prognostic indicators of GCTs and also detect recurrences.
- In infants, significant elevation of serum AFP or β-hCG rules out pure mature teratoma or seminoma and indicates "secreting" components of YST or choriocarcinoma, respectively.

89.5.4.1 Pediatric Soft Tissue Sarcomas

- Includes rhabdomyosarcoma (RMS) (common in children <14 yrs) or non-RMS soft tissue sarcomas (NRSTS- more predominant in adolescents and young adults)
- A growing number of molecular genetic changes have been described in sarcomas, resulting in accurate categorization into either subgroup.
- Histologically RMS is divided into embryonal (further divided into polypoidal and spindle cell types) and alveolar types with the latter having a poor prognosis.
- Circulating clinical markers reported include NSE polysialylated neural cell adhesion molecule (PS-NCAM) creatine kinase MB and CA125-
- However, no routine serum biomarker has had efficient clinical application to date.
- In vitro studies on EV-based biomarkers have shown that two miRNAs—miR-1246 and miR-1268—are abundant in patients of RMS.
- Rhabdomyosarcoma-derived EVs were also shown to increase the proliferation of recipient fibroblasts and rhabdomyosarcoma cells. Moreover, these EVs also induced the migration and invasion of normal fibroblasts. They have a role in the promotion of angiogenesis that leads to early metastasis.

Suggested Reading

Eleveld TF, Oldridge DA, Bernard V, Koster J, Colmet Daage L, Diskin SJ, et al. Relapsed neuroblastomas show frequent RAS-MAPK pathway mutations. Nat Genet. 2015;47(8):864–71.

Gunasekara TDKSC, et al. Te utility of novel renal biomarkers in assessment of chronic kidney disease of unknown etiology (CKDu): a review. Int J Environ Res Public Health. 2020;17:9522.

Samuel G, Crow J, Klein JB, Merchant ML, Nissen E, Koestler DC, et al. Ewing sarcoma family of tumors-derived small extracellular vesicle proteomics identify potential clinical biomarkers. Oncotarget. 2020;11(31):2995–3012.

Spreafico F, Fernandez CV, Brok J, et al. Wilms tumor. Nat Rev Dis Primers. 2021;7(1):75.

Walz AL, Ooms A, Gadd S, et al. Recurrent DGCR8, DROSHA, and SIX homeodomain mutations in favorable histology Wilms tumors. Cancer Cell. 2015;27(2):286–97.

Wegert J, Ishaque N, Vardapour R, et al. Mutations in the SIX1/2 pathway and the DROSHA/DGCR8 miRNA microprocessor complex underlie high-risk blastemal type Wilms tumors. Cancer Cell. 2015;27(2):298–311.

WHO. CureAll framework: WHO global initiative for childhood cancer: increasing access, advancing quality, saving lives. Geneva: WHO; 2021.

Key Features of This Book

- Covers an up-to-date approach to diagnosis and management of general and specialized areas of Pediatric Surgery.
- Provides easy-to-follow text along with photographs, diagrams and algorithms.
- Information compiled in a concise form from commonly available resources.
- Updated information on application of recent advances in technology.

The new edition comprises 89 chapters divided into 12 Parts. In addition to revised and updated chapters, the new areas included are organ transplantation, pediatric airway management, pediatric anesthesia, tropical pediatric surgery and recent advances like robotic surgery and artificial intelligence. Several histopathological photomicrographs are added.

This book covers all the common surgical diseases affecting children, reflecting the latest available information. In addition, it discusses recent advances in pediatric surgery, including fetal diagnosis and management, organ transplantation and robotic surgery.

The text is presented in a concise and reader-friendly style and complemented by numerous photographs and illustrations to aid in comprehension. Each chapter is structured in a systematic uniform pattern, examining the embryology, incidence, and approach to diagnosis and management, along with flow charts and algorithms where appropriate.

The book is primarily intended for fellows-in-training and surgeons in pediatric surgery and pediatric specialties. In addition to familiarizing readers with common pediatric surgical conditions and helping them plan simple approaches to their management, it also offers an essential on-the-go guide to clinicians.

This book is suitable for medical students, residents preparing for postgraduate entrance and exit examinations, and nursing and medical professionals in the field of clinical practice.

© The Editor(s) (if applicable) and The Author(s), under exclusive license to Springer Nature Singapore Pte Ltd. 2025

S. Roy Choudhury (ed.), *Pediatric Surgery*, https://doi.org/10.1007/978-981-96-1257-4

MIX
Papier aus verantwortungsvollen Quellen
Paper from responsible sources
FSC® C105338

If you have any concerns about our products,
you can contact us on
ProductSafety@springernature.com

In case Publisher is established outside the EU,
the EU authorized representative is:
Springer Nature Customer Service Center GmbH
Europaplatz 3, 69115 Heidelberg, Germany

Printed by Libri Plureos GmbH
in Hamburg, Germany